Cardiovascular Genetics and Genomics

Dhavendra Kumar • Perry Elliott
Editors

Cardiovascular Genetics and Genomics

Principles and Clinical Practice

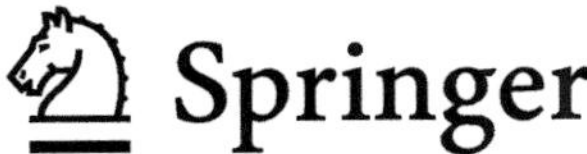

Editors
Dhavendra Kumar
Institute of Cancer & Genetics
University Hospital of Wales
Cardiff
United Kingdom

Perry Elliott
Barts Heart Centre
St Bartholomew's Hospital
London
United Kingdom

ISBN 978-3-319-66112-4 ISBN 978-3-319-66114-8 (eBook)
https://doi.org/10.1007/978-3-319-66114-8

Library of Congress Control Number: 2017964381

Printed on acid-free paper

This Springer imprint is published by Springer Nature
The registered company is Springer International Publishing AG
The registered company address is: Gewerbestrasse 11, 6330 Cham, Switzerland

Dedicated to Sir William Harvey (1578–1657)
Discovered circulation of the blood through arteries, veins and the heart

Foreword

The pace of advance in genetics and genomics in the last decade, underpinned by increasingly powerful technologies to interrogate the genome, has been such that it has moved from just being a field of elegant discovery science explaining disease mechanisms to one of progressively greater clinical utility and applicability. It is no longer beyond the realm of possibility, as is currently being explored in the UK 100,000 Genome Project, that all of us may one day have our genomes sequenced as a matter of course to aid with clinical diagnosis and management. All these new developments are laying the foundation for genomic and precision medicine, a concept that is being increasingly promoted globally as one way to tackle the increasing costs of healthcare.

In this context it is no longer possible for clinicians to ignore the potential and value of genetics and genomics to their practice as well as understand the limitations. Genetics affects many aspects of cardiovascular diseases—from causing Mendelian disorders such as hypertrophic cardiomyopathy and Marfan syndrome to contributing to the development of common and multifactorial disorders such as coronary artery disease and hypertension.

Building on their first edition published in 2010, in this revised and practically re-written new textbook on "Cardiovascular Genetics and Genomics-Principles and Clinical Practice", Dhavendra Kumar and Perry Elliott have assembled an outstanding group of contributors to cover the full spectrum of cardiovascular disorders where genetics makes a contribution. The book not only updates the state of the art with respect to conventional cardiovascular genetic disorders but also explores less traditional aspects such as the contribution of genetic analysis to the investigation of sudden cardiac death syndrome. Throughout the focus is on providing factual and easy to follow information that can help to inform clinical practice. The first section provides helpful background information about the nomenclature and approaches in genetics and genomics while other chapters deal with important issues such as principles and practice of genetic counselling and the value of the multi-disciplinary team approach.

With almost daily reporting of new associations of genetic variants with diseases, a book of this type cannot serve as a comprehensive compendium of such associations. What it does provide is a framework for clinicians to understand the genetic basis of cardiovascular diseases and when and how to incorporate genetic information into their clinical practice. It is also an excellent primer for those in training and those allied health professionals interested in genetic/genomic medicine.

I am confident that you will find the book of great value as you dip in and out of it!

Nilesh J. Samani
BHF Professor of Cardiology, University of Leicester,
The Medical Director, British Heart Foundation
London, UK

Preface

Where is the Life we have lost in living? Where is the wisdom we have lost in knowledge? Where is the knowledge we have lost in information?—T. S. Eliot

In 2010, we compiled, authored, and edited the first textbook on clinical cardiovascular genetics—"*Principles and Practice of Clinical Cardiovascular Genetics*" (ISBN-10:0195368959 & ISBN-13:978-0195368956, Oxford University Press, NY, USA). It was an ambitious project given many unproven hypotheses, incomplete evidence, loose fragmented scientific concepts, and controversial clinical applications. Nevertheless, the project was completed with the help of several experts from clinical cardiology, cardiovascular surgery, clinical genetics, genetic counseling, basic genetics and genomics, laboratory genetics, and many other health professionals. Fortunately, we were encouraged to receive largely welcome and positive feedback from medical, scientific, and allied health professionals.

Following the launch of the book, we were humbled to receive instructions and commission from Oxford University Press to produce a user-friendly specialist handbook for ready use and quick reference on factual clinically relevant information on inherited cardiovascular conditions. This Oxford specialist handbook further strengthened the new field of clinical cardiovascular genetics within the large field of clinical cardiovascular medicine. Subsequent years examined the purpose and applications of this new specialist field within the broad landscape of clinical medicine and clinical genetics.

The next five years witnessed exponential growth and enhanced genetic and genomic scientific applications and translations in many medical and health fields. The practice of cardiovascular medicine and surgery incorporates genetics and genomics that led to significant changes to the training curriculum and aspects of continued professional development necessary for enhancing the scientific basis of the clinical cardiology practice. This development is in line with other medical specialist fields, such as clinical oncology, medical ophthalmology, clinical rheumatology, clinical neurology, and many more. Genomic medicine is now a reality, not just a hypothetical scenario. This is now the agreed basis for personalized, precision and preventive medicine.

With the rapidly increasing quantitative and qualitative growth in the genetic and genomic knowledge base and evidence in cardiovascular medicine, the peer demands and expectations grew and persuaded us to revise and produce a new textbook. We debated and consulted many colleagues, trainees, and students on the likely format and title of the new book. It became clear that despite controversies surrounding the use of genetics and genomics, the new title would need to reflect these two intricately connected scientific fields. Further, we agreed to give the book much needed clinical focus moving away from the conventional scientific introduction. We are convinced that the title and the format of the new textbook on inherited and genetic aspects of cardiovascular medicine and surgery clearly reflect the genetic and genomic basis of the clinical practice.

The book includes 31 chapters written and contributed by leading experts in specific scientific fields and recognizable inherited cardiovascular conditions. The first five chapters cover the basic aspects including one chapter on cardiovascular pharmacogenomics and pharmacogenetics. The format is largely clinically focused with examples reflecting patient and family stories managed by evidence-based clinical and genetics input. Wherever possible and applicable, the key practice points are highlighted in the box style. Concluding 3 chapters focus on interventional cardiology, the multidisciplinary care and public/population health. Readers will have the benefit of the detailed and carefully compiled glossary with most commonly used terms and phrases in the emerging new field of clinical cardiovascular genetics and genomics. Each section of the book is thoroughly indexed in the end to assist the reader fast and efficient access to any term or description to the respective page and paragraph.

Finally, this book could not have been written and presented in the current format without sincere and painstaking efforts of all contributors and the publishing team. We remain greatly indebted for their kindness and generosity. We humbly submit this book to all students, trainees, and practitioners in clinical cardiovascular medicine and surgery, clinical genetics, genetic counseling, cardiac specialist nursing, public health practitioners and professionals, and other health professionals. The feedback and reflections on the book would be welcome in whatever quantitative or qualitative manner. We remain aware of possible errors and omissions and collectively take full responsibility.

Cardiff, UK
London, UK
September 2017

Dhavendra Kumar
Perry Elliott

Contents

Contributors

Anna Abou-Raya Department of Internal Medicine, University of Alexandria Hospital, Alexandria, Egypt

Suzan Abou-Raya Department of Internal Medicine, University of Alexandria Hospital, Alexandria, Egypt

Mohammed Majid Akhtar Barts Heart Centre, Department of Inherited Cardiovascular Diseases, St Bartholomew's Hospital, London, UK

Eloisa Arbustini IRCCS Foundation Policlinico San Matteo, Center for Inherited Cardiovascular Diseases, Pavia, Italy

Julie de Backer Department of Cardiology and Medical Genetics, Ghent University Hospital, Ghent, Belgium

Ilaria Bartolomei Department of Neuroscience, Bellaria Hospital, Bologna, Italy

Cristina Basso Department of Cardiac, Thoracic and Vascular Sciences, Pathological Anatomy-Cardiovascular Pathology, University of Padua Medical School, Padua, Italy

Cardio-Thoracic and Vascular Sciences, Policlinico Universitario di Padova, Padova, Italy

Barbara Bauce Department of Cardiac, Thoracic and Vascular Sciences, Pathological Anatomy-Cardiovascular Pathology, University of Padua Medical School, Padua, Italy

Cardio-Thoracic and Vascular Sciences, Policlinico Universitario di Padova, Padova, Italy

Elijah R. Behr Reader in Cardiovascular Medicine, Cardiovascular and Cell Sciences Research Institute, Tooting, London, UK

Paul Brennan Northern Genetic Service, Institute of Genetic Medicine, International Centre of Life, Newcastle Hospitals NHS Foundation Trust, Newcastle upon Tyne, England, UK

Gerry Carr-White Guys and St Thomas' NHS Foundation Trust, South East Thames Regional Genetics Centre, Guys Hospital, London, UK

Mark J. Caulfield Department of Clinical Pharmacology, Barts and the London, William Harvey Research Institute, Queen Mary University of London, London, UK

Patrick F. Chinnery Department of Clinical Neurosciences, Addenbrooke's Hospital, University of Cambridge, Cambridge Biomedical Campus, Cambridge, UK

Angus Clarke University Hospital of Wales, Cardiff, Wales, UK

Cardiff University School of Medicine, Institute of Medical Genetics, Cardiff, Wales, UK

John C.S. Dean North of Scotland Regional Genetics Service, Aberdeen Royal Infirmary, Aberdeen, Scotland

Nimesh D. Desai Division of Cardiovascular Surgery, Hospital of the University of Pennsylvania, Philadelphia, PA, USA

Mark Drury-Smith Department of Cardiology, University Hospital of Wales, Cardiff, UK

Girish Dwivedi Wesfarmers Chair in Cardiology, Harry Perkins Institute of Medical Research, Nedlands, WA, Australia

Perry Elliott, MBBS, MD, FRCP, FESC, FACC Barts Heart Centre, Department of Inherited Cardiovascular Diseases, St Bartholomew's Hospital, London, UK

Cardiovascular Medicine, University College London, London, UK

Clinical Research, UCL Institute of Cardiovascular Science, London, UK

Valentina Favalli IRCCS Foundation Policlinico San Matteo, Center for Inherited Cardiovascular Diseases, Pavia, Italy

Siv Fokstuen Department of Genetic Medicine and Laboratories, University Hospitals of Geneva, Geneva, Switzerland

Michael Frenneaux University of East Anglia, Norwich Medical School, Norwich Research Park, Norwich, Norfolk, UK

Christian Gagliardi Department of Experimental, Diagnostic and Specialty Medicine, Alma Mater Studiorum University of Bologna, Bologna, Italy

Lorenzo Giuliani IRCCS Foundation Policlinico San Matteo, Center for Inherited Cardiovascular Diseases, Pavia, Italy

Michael Hanna Department of Clinical Neurology, UCLH National Hospital for Neurology and Neurosurgery, London, UK

Sophie Herbert Department of Congenital Heart Disease, Bristol Heart Institute, Bristol, UK

Michael Ibrahim Division of Cardiovascular Surgery, Hospital of the University of Pennsylvania, Philadelphia, PA, USA

Syeda N.S. Jahangir Department of Clinical Pharmacology, Barts and the London, William Harvey Research Institute, Queen Mary University of London, London, UK

Sharon Jenkins Inherited Heart Diseases Unit, UCL/St Barts Partnership, London, UK

Department of Medical Genetics, King's College, London, UK

Human Molecular Genetics with Counselling, Imperial College, London, UK

Juan Pablo Kaski Paediatric Inherited Cardiovascular Diseases, Centre for Inherited Cardiovascular Diseases, Great Ormond Street Hospital, London, UK

Michael J. Keogh Department of Clinical Neuroscience, Cambridge Biomedical Campus, Cambridge, Cambridgeshire, UK

Caroline Kirwan Institute of Medical Genetics, University Hospital of Wales, Cardiff, Wales, UK

Dhavendra Kumar, MD, DSc, FRCP, FRCPCH, FACMG Institute of Medical Genetics, University Hospital of Wales, Cardiff, UK

Pier Lambiase Department of Cardiology, Barts Heart Centre, Institute of Cardiovascular Science, UCL, London, UK

Robert Leema Guys and St Thomas' NHS Foundation Trust, South East Thames Regional Genetics Centre, Guys Hospital, London, UK

Krystien V.V. Lieve Academic Medical Centre, Department of Clinical and Experimental Cardiology, New Amsterdam, The Netherlands

Bart Loeys Department of Clinical Genetics, Center for Medical Genetics, Antwerp University Hospital, Antwerp, Belgium

Pradeep P.A. Mammen Internal Medicine and Integrative Biology, University of Texas Southwestern Medical Center, Dallas, TX, USA

James Marangou Department of Cardiology, Fiona Stanley Hospital, Perth, WA, Australia

Hugh S. Markus Stroke Research Group, Department of Clinical Neurosciences, Cambridge Biomedical Campus, Cambridge, UK

Claire Martin Department of Cardiology, UCL, Barts Heart Centre, London, UK

Andrea Mazzanti Istituti Clinici Scientifici Maugeri SpA SB, Pavia, Italy

Agnese Milandri Department of Experimental, Diagnostic and Specialty Medicine, Alma Mater Studiorum University of Bologna, Bologna, Italy

Lorenzo Monserrat Health-in-Code, Le Coruna, Spain

Patricia B. Munroe Department of Clinical Pharmacology Barts and the London, William Harvey Research Institute, Queen Mary University of London, London, UK

Elaine Murphy Charles Dent Metabolic Unit, National Hospital for Neurology and Neurosurgery, London, UK

Anne de Paepe Department of Cardiology and Medical Genetics, Ghent University Hospital, Ghent, Belgium

Efstathios Papatheodorou Cardiovascular and Cell Sciences Research Institute, St George's University Hospital, Tooting, London, UK

Kalliopi Pilichou Department of Cardiac, Thoracic and Vascular Sciences, Pathological Anatomy-Cardiovascular Pathology, University of Padua Medical School, Padua, Italy

Cardio-Thoracic and Vascular Sciences, Policlinico Universitario di Padova, Padova, Italy

Sir Munir Pirmohamed The Wolfson Centre for Personalised Medicine, Institute of Translational Medicine, University of Liverpool, Liverpool, Merceyside, UK

Pieter G. Postema Academic Medical Centre, Department of Clinical and Experimental Cardiology, New Amsterdam, The Netherlands

Silvia G. Priori Department of Cardiology, University of Pavia, Pavia, Italy

Salvatore Maugeri Foundation IRCCS, Pavia, Italy

Fondazione Salvatore Maugeri, University of Pavia, Pavia, Italy

Candida Cristina Quarta Department of Experimental, Diagnostic and Specialty Medicine, Alma Mater Studiorum University of Bologna, Bologna, Italy

Claudio Rapezzi Department of Experimental, Diagnostic and Specialty Medicine, Alma Mater Studiorum University of Bologna, Bologna, Italy

Fabrizio Salvi Department of Neuroscience, Bellaria Hospital, Bologna, Italy

Mary N. Sheppard CRY Cardiovascular Pathology Unit, Institute of Cardiovascular and Cell Sciences, St. George's University Hospital, Tooting, London, UK

Hannah E. Steele Neurology Department, The Newcastle Upon Tyne Hospitals NHS Trust, Institute of Genetic Medicine, Newcastle University, Newcastle Upon Tyne, Tyne and Wear, UK

Douglas A. Stoller Division of Cardiovascular Medicine, University of Nebraska Medical Center, Omaha, NE, USA

Rhea Y.Y. Tan Stroke Research Group, Department of Clinical Neurosciences, Cambridge Biomedical Campus, Cambridge, UK

Gaetano Thiene Department of Cardiac, Thoracic and Vascular Sciences, Pathological Anatomy-Cardiovascular Pathology, University of Padua Medical School, Padua, Italy

Cardio-Thoracic and Vascular Sciences, Policlinico Universitario di Padova, Padova, Italy

J. Peter van Tintelen Department of Clinical Genetics, Academic Medical Center, Amsterdam, The Netherlands

Alessandro Di Toro IRCCS Foundation Policlinico San Matteo, Center for Inherited Cardiovascular Diseases, Pavia, Italy

Robert M.R. Tulloh Department of Congenital Heart Disease, Bristol Heart Institute, Bristol, UK

Chris Turner Centre for Neuromuscular Diseases, National Hospital for Neurology and Neurosurgery, London, UK

Richard Myles Turner The Wolfson Centre for Personalised Medicine, Institute of Translational Medicine, University of Liverpool, Liverpool, Merceyside, UK

Umesh Vivekananda MRC Centre for Neuromuscular Disease, National Hospital for Neurology and Neurosurgery, London, UK

Oliver Watkinson Department of Inherited Cardiovascular Disease, St Bartholomew's Hospital, London, UK

Arthur A.M. Wilde Academic Medical Centre, Department of Clinical and Experimental Cardiology, New Amsterdam, The Netherlands

Dirk G. Wilson Children's Heart Unit for Wales and Adult Congenital Heart Disease Unit, University Hospital of Wales, Cardiff and Vale NHS Trust, Cardiff, UK

Princess Al-Jawhara Al-Brahim Centre of Excellence in Research of Hereditary Disorders, Jeddah, Kingdom of Saudi Arabia

Yoshiji Yamada Department of Human Functional Genomics, Advanced Science Research Promotion Center, Mie University, Tsu, Mie, Japan

Department of Medical Genomics and Proteomics, Institute of Basic Sciences, Mie University Graduate School of Medicine, Tsu, Mie, Japan

Research Center for Genomic Medicine, Mie University, Tsu, Mie, Japan

Yoshiki Yasukochi Department of Human Functional Genomics, Advanced Science Research Promotion Center, Mie University, Tsu, Mie, Japan

Zaheer Yousef Department of Cardiology, University Hospital of Wales, Cardiff, UK

Paul A. van der Zwaag Department of Genetics, University Medical Center Groningen, Groningen, The Netherlands

Introduction to Genes, Genome and Inheritance

1

Dhavendra Kumar

Abstract

The introductory chapter introduces genes, genome, genetics and genomics in simplified manner that, irrespective of any specialty, any clinician or healthcare professional should know. In addition to core basic information on nucleic acids, structure of the gene and organisation of the whole genome, the text includes clinical examples relevant to cardiovascular medicine and surgery. Selected examples might be of interest to medical and healthcare professionals predominantly engaged with cardiovascular conditions. Emphasis is given on developing reasonable grasp of genetic or genomic factors, heritable, incidental or somatic, that is either etiologically relevant or capable of influencing the natural course of any cardiovascular disease, acting alone or in combination with environmental (infection and toxins etc.) or life style factors (nutrition and occupation etc.). The text is supported with generous illustrations, tables and boxes with key learning points.

Keywords

Nucleic acids • DNA • RNA • Gene • Genome • Genomic variation • Single nucleotide polymorphism • Copy number variation • Mendelian inheritance Complex disease • Genomic medicine

D. Kumar, MD, DSc, FRCP, FRCPCH, FACMG
Institute of Medical Genetics, University Hospital of Wales, Cardiff, UK
e-mail: kumard1@cf.ac.uk

D. Kumar, P. Elliott (eds.), *Cardiovascular Genetics and Genomics*,
https://doi.org/10.1007/978-3-319-66114-8_1

1.1 Introduction

Most medical practitioners and specialist physicians are oblivious of basic biological facts that govern the whole body and organ specific structure and function. In this context, understanding genes, genome, genetics and other intricately related facts are most fundamental to structure and function of any form of life. Higher mammals, including humans, have evolved over several thousands of years through repetitive cycles of transmission of genetic traits under enormous environmental pressures. Thus it is not surprising to find many unexplained and complex elements with the human genetic make up or genome. The human biology is perhaps one of the most complex and intriguing life sciences. Major organs and arbitrarily set out body systems have specifically assigned parts of the genome as the common denominator of structure and life long functioning. Nevertheless, system wide approach is relevant to medicine. In this context, understanding the role of genes and related elements of the human genome are pertinent to any medical practitioner, whether general or system specialist, such as the cardiovascular physician.

The present chapter introduces genes, genome, genetics and genomics in simplified manner that any clinician or healthcare professional should know. The broad spectrum of genetics and genomics includes many aspects of the genome (Fig. 1.1). Cardiovascular genetics and genomics are broadly similar to any other body system. Selected examples might be of interest to medical and healthcare professionals predominantly engaged with cardiovascular conditions. Emphasis is given on developing reasonable grasp of genetic or genomic factors, heritable, incidental or somatic, that is either etiologically relevant or capable of influencing the natural course of

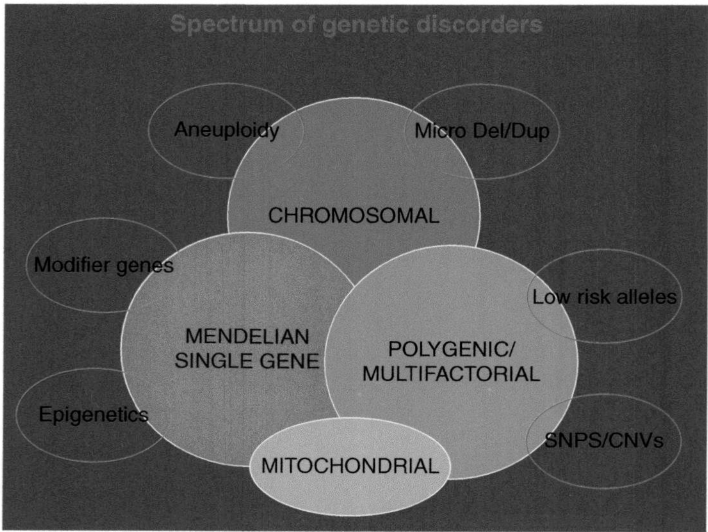

Fig. 1.1 Spectrum of genetic and genomic disorders; a genetic or inherited cardiovascular condition may be caused by one of these mechanisms

any cardiovascular disease, acting alone or in combination with environmental (infection and toxins etc.) or life style factors (nutrition and occupation etc.). The text is supported with generous illustrations, tables and boxes with key learning points. An interested reader or student might like to choose any book or resource listed under 'Further reading'.

1.2 Basic Facts: Cell Biology, Nucleic Acids, Gene, Genome

1.2.1 Human Genome: Structure and Functional Organization

Living organisms have two types of cells- nucleated, called *eukaryotes* and non-nucleated, called *prokaryotes*. Bacteria are essentially prokaryotes and all other multi-cellular organisms are basically eukaryotes. The total genetic constitution in either cell is called genome. In eukaryotes, it is contained within the nucleus and hence referred to as *nuclear genome*. However, the cytoplasm of a eukaryote cell also contains another genome within the energy rich intracellular organelle, mitochondria, referred to as the *mitochondrial genome*. Morbid changes in both genomes are associated with a number of human disorders. The cardiovascular system, by virtue of its diversity, complexity and high energy turnover, has many disorders caused by pathogenic changes in either the nuclear DNA (nDNA) or the mitochondrial DNA (mtDNA).

Genetic information is transferred from one generation to the next by small sections of the nucleic acid, deoxyribonucleic acid (DNA), which is tightly packaged into subcellular structures called *chromosomes*. Prokaryotes usually have a single circular chromosome, while most eukaryotes have more than two, and in some cases up to several hundred. In humans, there are 46 chromosomes arranged in 23 pairs, with one of each pair inherited from each parent (Fig. 1.2a, b). Twenty-two pairs are called *autosomes,* and one pair is called *sex chromosomes*, designated as X and Y; females have two X chromosomes (46, XX) and males have an X and a Y (46, XY).

A chromosome consists of a tightly coiled length of DNA and the proteins (e.g., chromatins) that help define its structure and level of activity. DNA consists of two long strands of nucleotide bases wrapped round each other along a central spine made up of phosphate and sugar (Fig. 1.3). There are four bases: adenine (A), guanine (G) cytosine (C), and thymine (T). Pairing of these bases follows strict rules: **A** always pairs with **T**, and **C** with **G**. Two strands are, therefore, complementary to each other.

Genes are made up of specific lengths of DNA that encode the information to make a protein, or ribonucleic acid (RNA) product. RNA differs from DNA in that the base thymine (T) is replaced by uracil (U), and the sugar is ribose. It acts as a template to take the coded information across to ribosomes, a major intracellular organelle, for final assembly of amino acids into the protein peptide chain (Fig. 1.3). The bases are arranged in sets of three, referred to as *codons*. Each codon "codes" for a specific amino acid; hence the term *genetic code*. Codons are located in *exons*, which contain the coding sequences. A gene may consist of several such coding DNA segments. Exons are separated from each other by non-coding sequences of

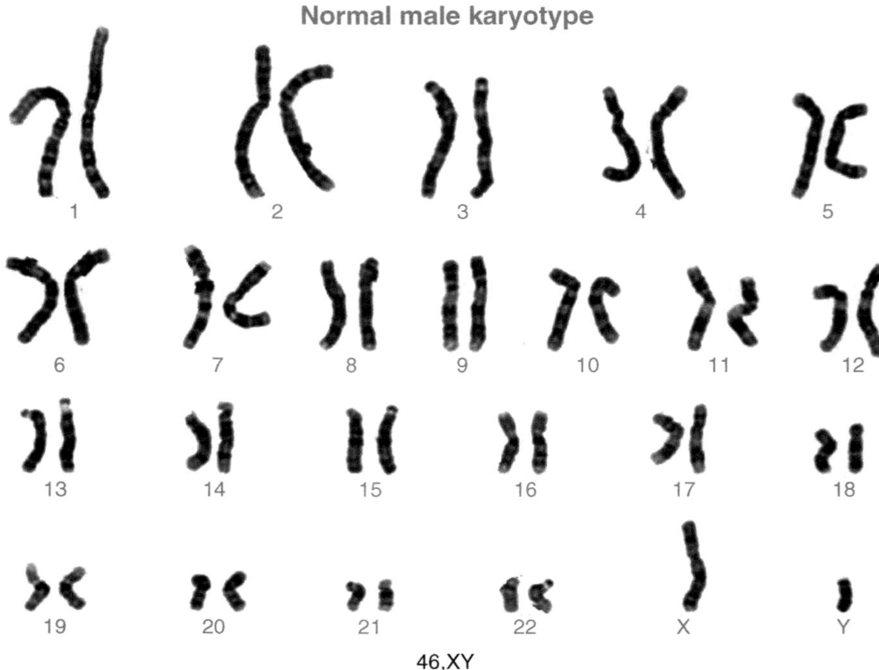

Fig. 1.2 A normal male karyotype- note small Y chromosome in the last chromosome pair

DNA, called *introns*. Although they are not yet known to be associated with any specific function, it is likely that some of these introns might be of evolutionary significance, or associated with other fundamental biological functions. During the transcription of DNA, the introns are spliced out, and the exons then attach to messenger RNA (mRNA) to start the process of protein synthesis (Fig. 1.4).

Proteins are one of the major constituents of the body's chemistry. These are remarkably variable in their structure, ranging from tough collagen that forms connective tissue and bone, through the fluid hemoglobin that transports oxygen, to thousands of enzymes, hormones, and other biological effectors and their receptors that are essential for the structures and functions of the body. Each protein is made up of one or more peptide chains consisting of series of amino acids, only of which 20 occur in living organisms. The different structures and functions of proteins depend on the order of amino acids as determined by the genetic code (Table 1.1: List of amino acids and Table 1.2: The Genetic code).

DNA has the remarkable property of self-replication. The two strands of a DNA molecule separate as chromosomes divide during cell division. There are two types of cell division; *mitosis* in all body cells, and *meiosis,* which is specifically confined to the gonads in making sperm and eggs. During mitosis, no reduction of the number of chromosomes takes place (*diploid*, or 2n), while meiosis results in half the number of chromosomes (*haploid*, or 1n). The new pairs of DNA are identical to those from which they were synthesized. However, sometimes mistakes or mutations occur. These usually result from substitution of a different base, or are due to extensive structural changes to genes. In other words, any "spelling mistake" in the letters A-T or C-G could result in either complete absence of the coded information (*nonsense mutation*) or a different or alternative message (*missense mutation*). However, not all mutations or spelling mistakes have an adverse effect (*neutral mutations*). Conversely, some changes in the genes might result in a favorable property; for example, resistance to disease or other environmental hazard. This is the basis for the gradual changes in species over millions of years of evolution. On the other hand, mutations may result in defective gene functions, leading to a disease, or susceptibility to a disease, due to qualitative or quantitative changes in the gene product, the peptide chain. However, these changes may also result from epigenetic mechanisms, abnormal RNA molecules, and post-translational modifications (see Glossary).

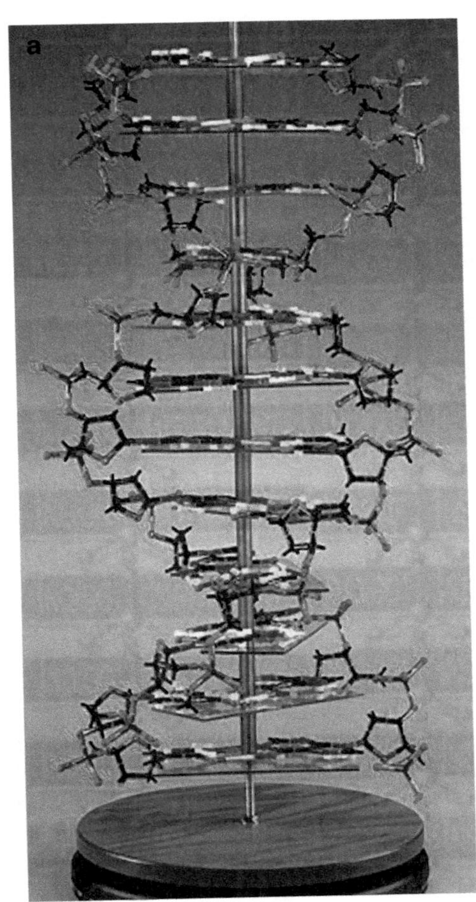

Fig. 1.3 The Watson-Crick double helix model of the nucleic acid (DNA) molecule. (**a**) Replica of the original model. (**b**) Graphic display of position of 4 bases (nucleotides), deoxyribose sugar, phosphate molecule back bone and the hydrogen bonds

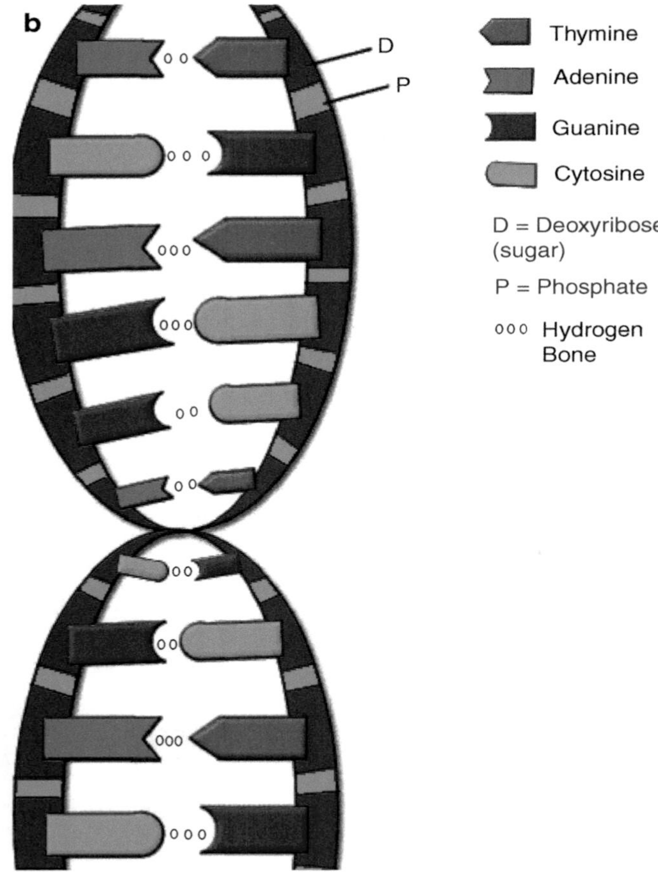

(continued)

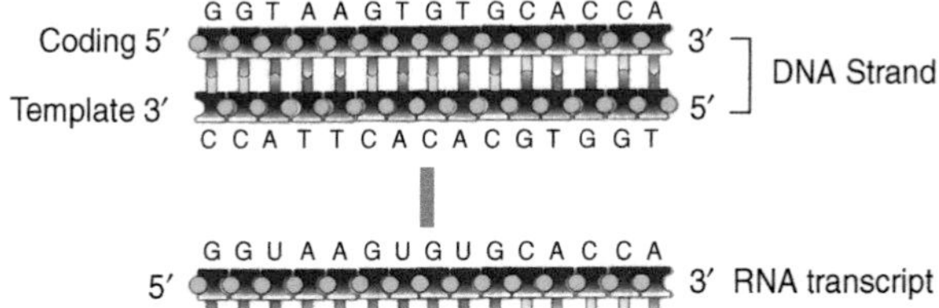

Fig. 1.4 Relationship of the double stranded DNA molecule (coding strand and the template) and the single stranded RNA molecule showing the transcript for translation

In brief, the human genome includes all coding and non-coding sections of DNA, interspersed sections of DNA of possible evolutionary or epigenomic significance, variable length of repetitive DNA sequences (polymorphisms), sections of RNA involved in transcription and translation, other RNA sequences involved in supporting biological functions, the compact mitochondrial genome (see next section) and ribosomal RNA. Apart from reproduction, genes, gene-sequence variation, genomic variation, and epigenetic factors are important in growth, development, aging, and

Table 1.1 List of amino acids with abbreviations

Alanine	A	Ala
Arginine	R	Arg
Asparagine	N	Asn
Aspartic acid	D	Asp
Cysteine	C	Cys
Glutamine	Q	GLN
Glutamic acid	E	Glu
Glycine	G	Gly
Histidine	J	His
Isoleucine	I	Ile
Leucine	L	Leu
Lysine	K	Lys
Methionine	M	Met
Phenylalanine	F	Phe
Proline	P	Pro
Selenocysteine	U	Sec
Serine	S	Ser
Threonine	T	Thr
Tryptophan	W	Trp
Tyrosine	Y	Tyr
Valine	V	Val

Table 1.2 The genetic code

BASE 1	BASE 2	BASE 3
U	Phe Ser Tyr Cys	U
U	Phe Ser Tyr Cys	C
U	Leu Ser STOP STOP[a]	A
U	Leu Ser STOP Trp	G
C	Leu Pro His Arg	U
C	Leu Pro His Arg	C
C	Leu Pro Gln Arg	A
C	Leu Pro Gln Arg	G
A	Ile Thr Asn Ser	U
A	Ile Thr Asn Ser	C
A	Ile Thr Lys Arg	A
A	Met Thr Lys Arg	G
G	Val Ala Asp Gly	U
G	Val Ala Asp Gly	C
G	Val Ala Glu Gly	A
G	Val Ala Glu Gly	G

[a]Codon UGA can also code for selenocysteine (Sec) under specific circumstances

senescence. Some of these may be evolutionarily conserved across species, but relevant to human health. Mutations and alterations in several of these genomic elements are linked to a broad range of medical conditions. A detailed description of the human genome is beyond the scope and remit of this chapter (see Further Reading resources).

1.3 The Mitochondrial Genome: Structure and Function

The mitochondrial genome is very different from the nuclear genome (Fig. 1.5). In many respects, it has more in common with bacterial genomes than the eukaryotic nuclear genome. Apart from the mitochondrial genome, a number of nuclear genes encode the great majority of mitochondrial proteins. Although the mitochondrial genome is very small compared to its nuclear counterpart, because there are many copies, mtDNA often makes up 1% or so of total cellular DNA.

As in bacteria, the mitochondrial genome is circular and closely packed with genes. There are no introns and little inter-genic non-coding DNA. Mitochondrial genes overlap on the same strand, using the same template but read in different reading frames. Twenty-four of the 37 genes specify functional RNAs (two ribosomal

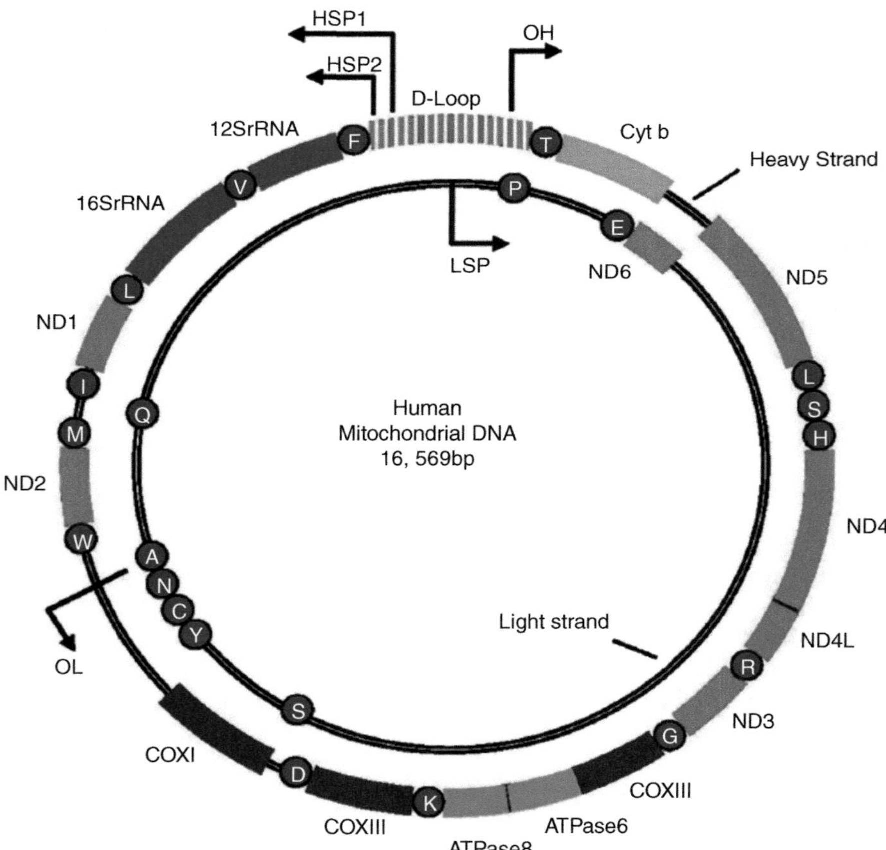

Fig. 1.5 The mitochondrial genome- note no introns; all circular compact mtDNA molecule is compact with coding stands; bulk of the mtDNA codes for the synthesis of transfer RNA (tRNA), ribosomal RNA (rRNA), ATPase and respiratory enzymes

RNAs and 22 tRNAs); the other 13 genes encode components of the electron transport pathway.

A short segment of the mitochondrial genome is triple-stranded of which the D-loop (displacement loop) is non-coding produced by replication forks overlapping as they travel in opposite directions around the circular DNA. The D-loop contains the only significant amount of non-coding DNA in the mitochondrial genome. Perhaps because of this, it is the location of many of the DNA polymorphisms that are such useful tools for anthropologists researching the origins of human populations. Because there is no recombination among mtDNAs, complete haplotypes of polymorphisms are transmitted through the generations, modified only by recurrent mutation. This makes mtDNA a highly informative marker of ancestry, at least along the maternal line.

Mutations in mtDNA are important causes of disease, and perhaps also of aging. Most energy dependent organs, such as heart and skeletal muscle, are predominantly affected (Table 1.3). Clinical picture is often described as dilated cardiomyopathy or myopathy (see Chap. 10). Phenotypes caused by variation in mtDNA are

Table 1.3 Diseases caused by mutations or pathogenic polymorphisms in the mtDNA molecule

Chronic progressive external ophthalmoplegia [CPEO]	External ophthalmoplegia, bilateral ptosis, mild proximal myopathy	tRNA	A3243G, T8356C Rearrangement (deletion/ duplication)
Kearns-Sayre syndrome [KSS]	PEO onset <20 years, pigmentary retinopathy, cerebellar ataxia, heart block, CSF protein >1 g/L		Rearrangement (deletion/ duplication)
Pearson syndrome	Sideroblastic anemia of childhood, pancytopenia, renal tubular defects, exocrine pancreatic deficiency		Rearrangement (deletion/ duplication)
Diabetes and Deafness	Diabetes mellitus, sensori-neural hearing loss	tRNA	A3243G, C12258A Rearrangement (deletion/ duplication)
Leber's hereditary optic neuropathy [LHON]	Subacute painless bilateral visual loss, age of onset 24 years, males>females (~4:1), dystonia, cardiac pre-excitation syndromes	Protein encoding	G11778A, T14484C, G3460A
Neurogenic ataxia with retinitis pigmentosa [NARP]	Late-childhood or adult onset peripheral neuropathy, ataxia, pigmentary retinopathy	Protein encoding	T8993G/C
Leigh syndrome [LS]	Subacute relapsing encephalopathy, cerebellar and brainstem signs, infantile onset	Protein encoding	T8993G/C
Exercise intolerance and myoglobulinuria	Exercise induced myoglobulinuria	Protein encoding	Cyt B mutations

(continued)

Table 1.3 (continued)

Mitochondrial encephalomyopathy with lactic acidosis and stroke-like episodes [MELAS]	Stroke-like episodes before 40 years, seizures and/or dementia, ragged-red fibers and/or lactic acidosis, diabetes mellitus, cardiomyopathy (HCM/DCM), deafness, cerebellar ataxia	tRNA	A32343G, T3271C, A3251G
Myoclonic epilepsy with ragged-red fibers [MERRF]	Myoclonus, seizures, cerebellar ataxia, myopathy, dementia, optic atrophy, bilateral deafness, peripheral neuropathy, spasticity, multiple lipomata	tRNA	A8344G, T8356C
Cardiomyopathy	Hypertrophic cardiomyopathy [HCM] progressing to dilated cardiomyopathy [DCM]	tRNA	A3243G, A4269G
Infantile myopathy/ encephalopathy	Early onset progressive muscle weakness with developmental delay	tRNA	T14709C, A12320G, G1606A, T10010C
Nonsyndromic sensorineural deafness	Early onset progressive bilateral moderate to severe sensorineural hearing loss	rRNA	A7445G
Aminoglycoside-induced nonsyndromic deafness	Early-onset nonprogressive sensorineural deafness secondary to aminoglycoside administration	rRNA	A1555G

transmitted exclusively down the maternal line (matrilineal inheritance), but most genetic diseases where there is mitochondrial dysfunction are caused by mutations in nuclear-encoded genes, and so follow normal Mendelian patterns. As cells contain many copies of the mitochondrial genome, they can be heteroplasmic, containing a mix of different sequences (Fig. 1.6). Unlike mosaicism for nuclear variants, mtDNA heteroplasmy can be transmitted by a mother to her children).

1.4 The Morbid Genome

1.4.1 Genetic Variation or Genetic Differences

The most direct way to measure genetic differences, or genetic variation, is to estimate how often two individuals differ at a specific site in their DNA sequences—that is, whether they have a different nucleotide base pair at a specific location in their DNA. First, DNA sequences are obtained from a sample of individuals. The sequences of all possible pairs of individuals are then compared to see how often each nucleotide differs. When this is done for a sample of humans, the result is that individuals differ, on average, at only about one in 1300 DNA base pairs. In other words, any two humans are about 99.9% identical in terms of their DNA sequences.

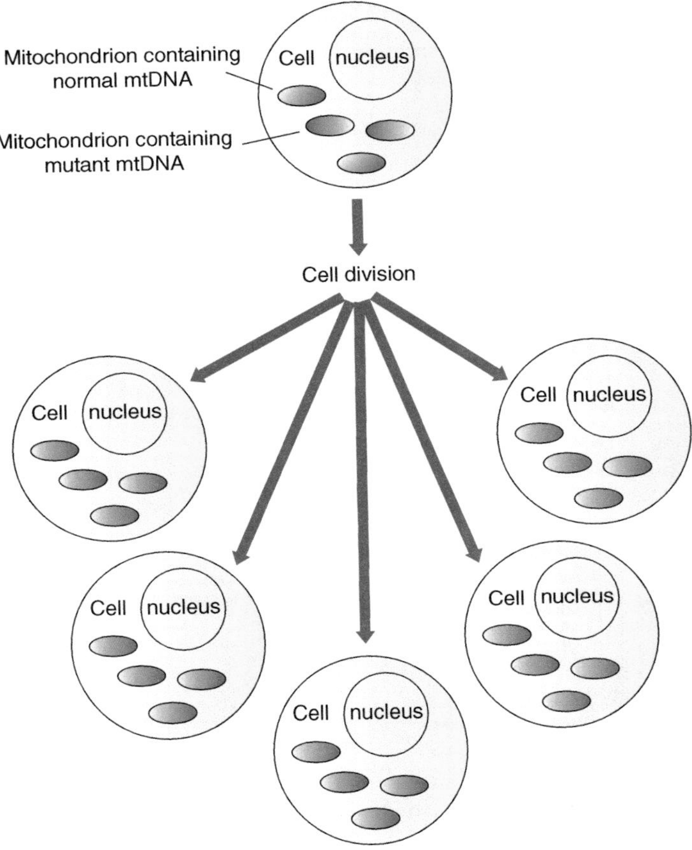

Fig. 1.6 Heteroplasmy in mitochondrial DNA mutation distribution- note from 100% to 0% distribution of mtDNA mutations compared to wild alleles

During the past several years, a new type of genetic variation has been studied extensively in humans: *copy-number variants* (CNVs) - DNA sequences of 1000 base pairs or larger are fairly distributed across the genome. In some instances, CNVs could be deleted, duplicated, or inverted in some individuals with mild phenotypic effects. Several thousand CNVs have been discovered in humans, indicating that at least 4 million nucleotides of the human genome (and perhaps several times more) vary in copy-number among individuals. CNVs thus are another important class of genetic variation and contribute to at least an additional 0.1% difference, on average, between individuals [1]. Despite significant progress, the medical and health implications of CNVs are not entirely clear.

Apart from CNVs, genomic variation at the single base pair level, the single nucleotide polymorphism (SNP) has attracted a lot of attention. The position of SNPs in the context of the gene could have impact on functionality of the gene.

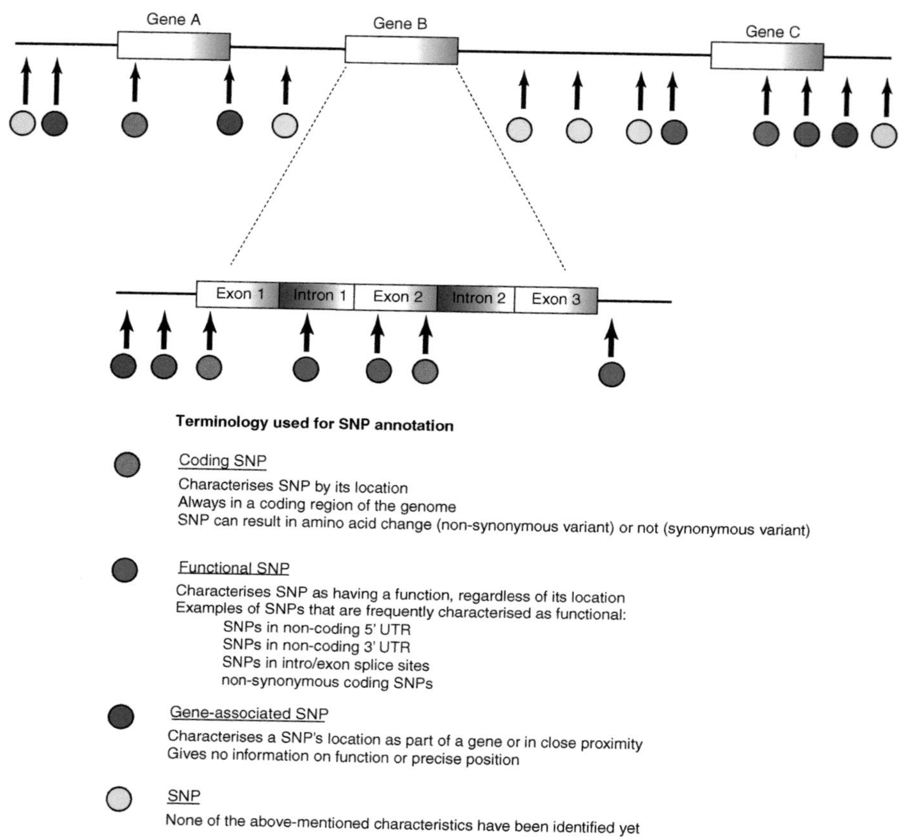

Fig. 1.7 Functional impact of the coding and non-coding single nucleotide polymorphisms (SNPs)

These could be located in the coding region where an amino acid change may occur (non-synonymous variant) or may not occur (synonymous variant) [2]. The position of the non-coding SNP is also important, for example occurring in 5′ UTR or in the intron/exon splice site region (Fig. 1.7).

An important approach is to use SNPs in planning and carrying out the genome-wide association studies (GWAS) in many complicated and multi-factorial conditions, such as essential hypertension [3] and coronary artery disease [4]. This approach and necessary laboratory and computational bioinformatics tools are now accepted as the 'must have' components to plan and carry out GWAS or limited genetic association studies [5]. Despite many limitations and disappointing lack of the clinical utility, GWAS using either SNPs or CNVs remain a very useful method in analyzing the genetic or genomic elements in the etiology and pathogenesis of complex traits. The classic display of GWAS based loci associated with a complex trait or phenotype, such as essential hypertension, is shown by chromosome specific peaks, commonly referred to as the Manhattan chart (Fig. 1.8). This approach has

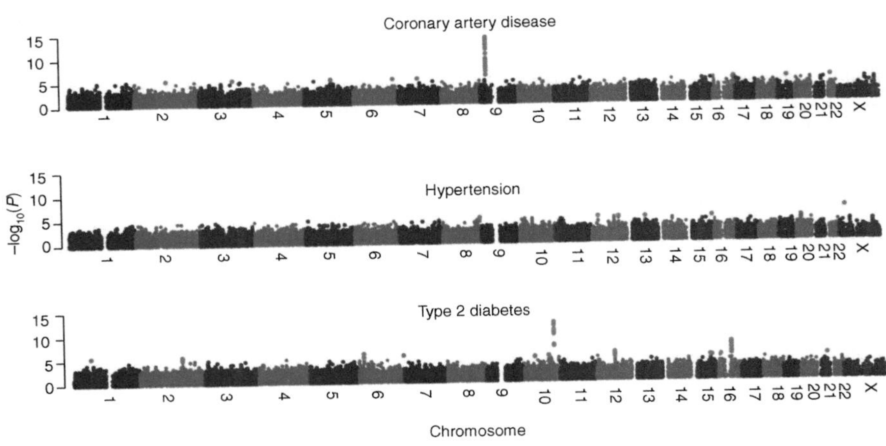

Fig. 1.8 Manhattan plots for genome wide association scan data from the Wellcome Trust Case Control Consortium contrasting results for the common cardiovascular disorders of coronary disease, type 2 diabetes with hypertension- The Wellcome Trust Case Control Consortium. Adapted from The Wellcome Trust Case Control Consortium [6]. The Manchattan chart of the coronary artery disease (CAD) genome wide association study (GWAS)- note high peak for 9p polymorphisms. From Lusis [7]; with permission

allowed estimate the heritability (see Glossary) at much higher levels that was missed (missing heritability) by conventional twin, family and population level studies [8].

1.4.2 Coding and Non-Coding Genome

Conventionally, functionality of the genome is divided into two parts- the coding and non-coding. Undoubtedly, the coding genome, only a small fraction (2–3%) of the whole genome remains the main focus in understanding the genetic or molecular basis of many normal and morbid phenotypic traits. The coding genome comprises of all exons, separated from the non-coding regions as introns by the splice site junctions. Some facts about the coding genome remain undisputed- the 3 nucleotides bases set of the codon as set out in the genetic code assigned to a particular amino acid that is selected for the peptide molecule assembly in the ribosome and transfer of the coded instruction (transcription) to the messenger RNA (mRNA) template for transport to the ribosome.

The ribosome, through highly complex system of ribosomal RNA (rRNA), receives the transcribed information on mRNA assisted by the transfer RNA (tRNA) for initiating the peptide molecule assembly. Many such peptide molecules take part in the triple helical structure of the protein molecule. In addition to the key RNA molecules required for transcription, transport, transfer and eventual translation of the coded instructions, many other forms of the RNA indirectly influence or interfere in the whole process, collectively called RNA interference (RNAi). Within this highly complex molecular make up of the RNAi, many different forms exist, for example nucelolar RNA, small nucleolar RNA, micro RNA etc. The precise role of the RNAi remains unclear in shaping the protein molecule and eventually the phenotype of interest. It is generally agreed that to some extent protein structural and functional variations are probably due to post-translational interference or influence of the RNAi [9].

In summing up, the exons in the genome constitute the major part of the coding genomes. The non-coding genome makes the bulk of the genome comprising of genome wide polymorphic variations, epigenome (see next section), 5′ and 3′ untranscribed region (UTR), splice sites between exons and introns and all introns. The non-coding genome plays a crucial role in the functionality of the coding genome [10].

1.4.3 Epigenome

The concept of epigenetics and later on epigenomics originated from earlier biological observations of genetic imprinting [11]. Animal studies and later observations in humans indicated specific 'parent of origin' effect on the outcome of certain phenotypic traits. This led to the debate on the existence of possible genetic imprinted information assigned to either paternal or maternal homologue. This phenomenon was conclusively demonstrated by the presence of interstitial micro-deletion or micro- duplication and uniparental disomy (UPD) unmasking the 'parent of origin' effect. The classic example is that of 15q deletion resulting in Prader-Willi syndrome due to the loss of paternal effect shown by the deletion in the paternal homologue or conversely by the maternal uniparental disomy (Fig. 1.9). Conversley, the phenotype of Angelman syndrome is known to exist due to maternal micro deletion of the same 15q region or the paternal UPD [12].

The central theme of the genetic imprinting lies with the fact that the phenotypic variation results from without any change within the specific coding regions of the gene or many genes in specific genomic locations. There are many such critical loci that control the imprinting process assigned the universally agreed term of the *imprinting control center* (ICC) [13]. Since most ICCs or loci are located outside and proximal to the 5′ UTR of the gene, the term *epigenetics* was coined and almost instantaneously accepted. Apart from the quantitative genome architectural disruptions (microdeletion or uniparental disomy) involving the critical parental homologue, other mechanisms involved include methylation of the CPG islands, histone modifications and point mutations in the ICC. Many examples of *epigenetics* are now increasingly discussed under the broad generic term of *epigenomics* that in addition to specific imprinted genes, compasses many critical loci that collectively exert imprinting effect on the penetrance, phenotype variation, and perhaps more importantly on the pharmacological responses including adverse drug reactions. Such evidence exists in relation to cancer pharmacotherapy [14].

Recent advances in neuro-developmental and neuro-muscular disorders provide good evidence for clinical applications of epigenetics and epigenomics. Autism spectrum disorder is highly complex and heterogeneous condition that carries devastating consequences. There are many clinically recognizable phenotypes including Rett syndrome, which is caused by mutations in the methyl-DNA binding protein MECP2, mapped to the X chromosome. The mammalian dosage compensation pathway involved

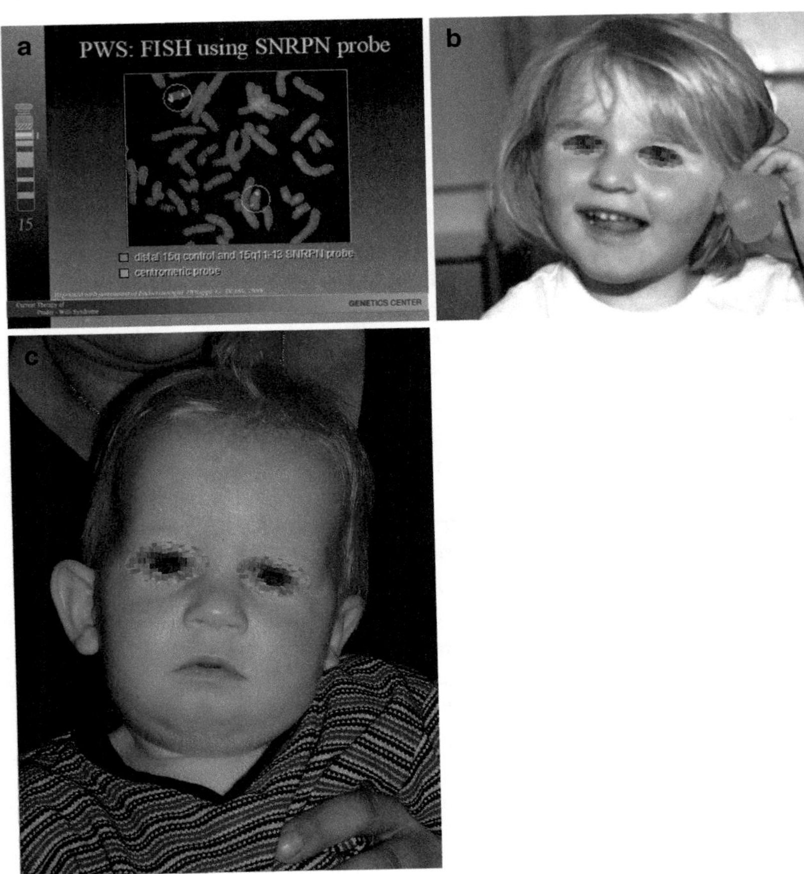

Fig. 1.9 (**a**) The 15q 11.2 microdeletion (FISH: green-centromere; red- 15q paint): Deleted maternal homologue or Paternal UPD- the Angelman syndrome (**b**); Deleted paternal homologue or maternal UPD- the Prader-Willi syndrome phenotype (**c**). (**b**) Maternal 15q Del Angelman Syndrome. (**c**) Paternal 15q Del Prader-Willi syndrome

in the X-inactivation or Lyonization regulates the *MECP2* gene function [15]. Another disease of importance might be the progressive dominantly inherited clinically variable neuro-muscular degenerative disease facio-scapulo-humeral muscular dystrophy (FSHD), a complex disease that is impacted by many epigenetic influences [16].

The medical importance of *epigenomics* in cardiovascular medicine is not yet fully understood. There is limited evidence for this to be of major importance in high risk Mendelian disorders. However, it is likely to be of greater significance in complex and multi-factorial conditions, particularly the adult and late onset disorders like coronary artery disease, chronic heart failure and essential hypertension. Recent reports on the role of epigenomics phenomenon on the transgenerational grandparental transmission of cardiovascular risks and related phenotypes have highlighted the significance of genetic and genomic imprinting in cardiovascular medicine [17].

1.5 Traditional Inheritance

1.5.1 Chromosomal

Understanding the chromosomal basis of inheritance is a very fundamental approach to grasp the concept of inheritance. This is essentially the holistic nuclear genomic inheritance that one could envisage. The diploid genome is spread across the 23 pairs of human chromosomes including the sex chromosome pair designated as XX in a female and XY in the male. Each haploid chromosome has defined genomic content that includes coding and non-coding nuclear DNA (nDNA) sequences. Thus any variation in number (aneuploidy) will result in either loss (monosomy) or gain (trisomy) of the respective chromosome. Mechanisms that underpin origin of trisomy 21 are complex and broadly include non-disjunction (error in chromatid polar movement during meiosis 1 or meiosis 2) or malsegregation of chromosome 21 in case of balanced parental chromosome rearrangement between chromosome 21 and another acrocentric chromosome (13–22), commonly referred to as Robertsonian translocation. The net chromosome numbers in the parental Robertsonian translocation carrier is 45 since two chromsomes, for example 14; 21, are attached and look one large chromosome (see *Further Reading* resources).

In the case of Down syndrome, additional copy of chromosome 21 (trisomy 21) results in copy number gains of several gene sequences, polymorphic sequences and many other elements of genome that are yet not fully understood. The outcome of additional genomic content belonging to chromosome 21 is universally recognized in the distinct Down syndrome phenotype with multi-system involvement (Fig. 1.10). The diverse cardiovascular manifestations in Down syndrome point to critical genomic elements involved in cardiovascular development and function.

Another category of chromosomal inheritance refers to structural changes where the apparent diploid number ($2 \times 23 = 46$) is maintained but the actual genomic content or organization could be disrupted either due to loss (deletion), gain (duplication), reversal of copy sequences (inversion), joining of chromosome ends following two breaks (ring chromosome) and two identical copies of a chromosome homologue (isochromosome).

There are a number of possible explanations for structural chromosome abnormalities. In most cases, a microdeletion or microduplication probably results from non-homologous allelic recombination (NHAR) of the chromosome region flanked with copy number variation on either side of the deleted or duplicated chromosomal segment involved (Fig. 1.11; [18]).

All these chromosomal structural variations account for genomic dysfunction manifesting with diverse physical features and molecular abnormalities. This is also referred to as disorder of genome architecture. Since each chromosome segment involved is likely to contain series of genes involved, the term *contiguous gene syndrome* is often used. By far the best example is the 22q deletion syndrome with a number of major anatomic cardiac out flow tract abnormalities (Fig. 1.12).

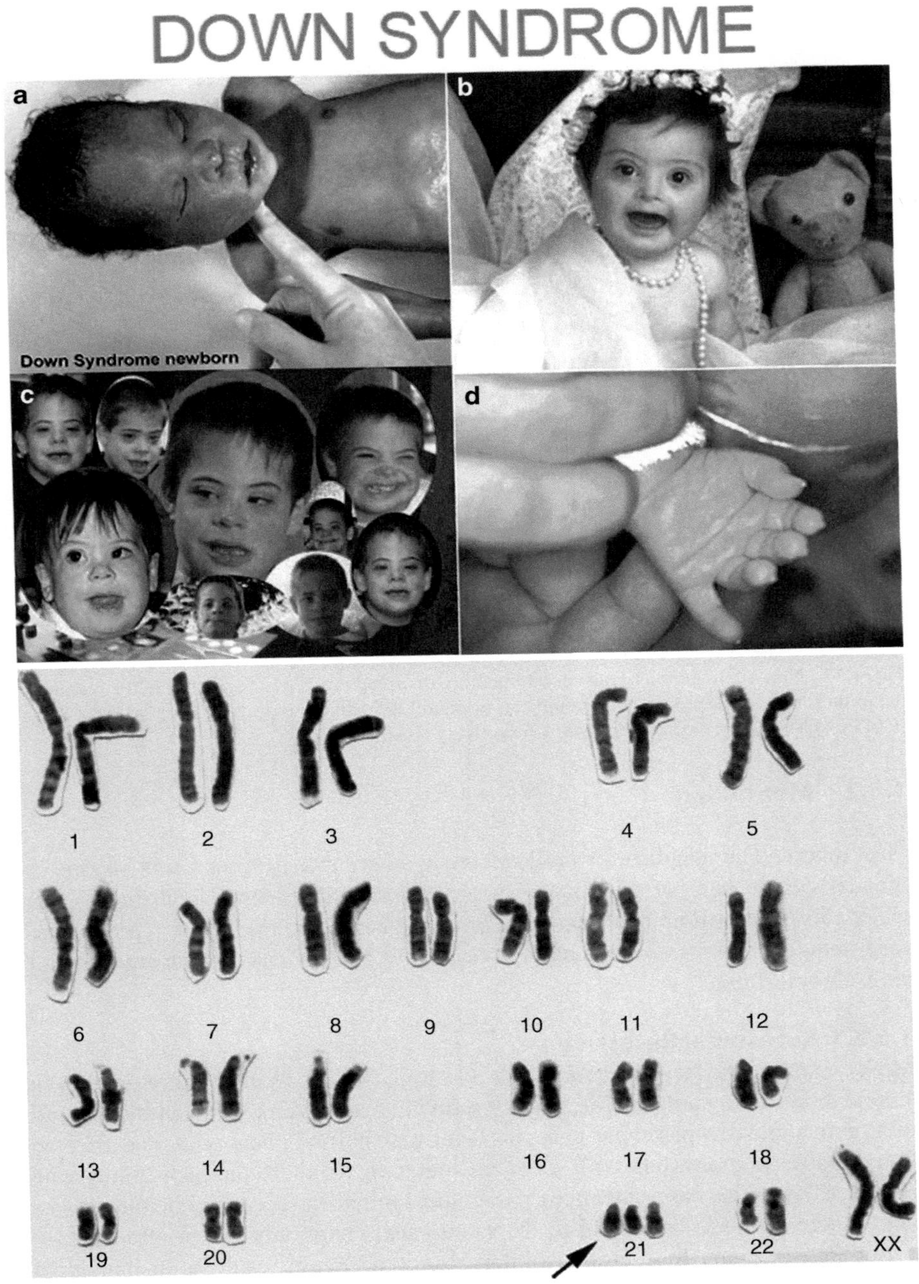

DOWN SYNDROME

a

Down Syndrome newborn

b

c

d

1 2 3 4 5

6 7 8 9 10 11 12

13 14 15 16 17 18

19 20 21 22 XX

Fig. 1.10 Down syndrome (Trisomy 21; 47 + 21)- note characteristic facial appearance (**a–c**) and single palmer (Simian) crease (**d**)

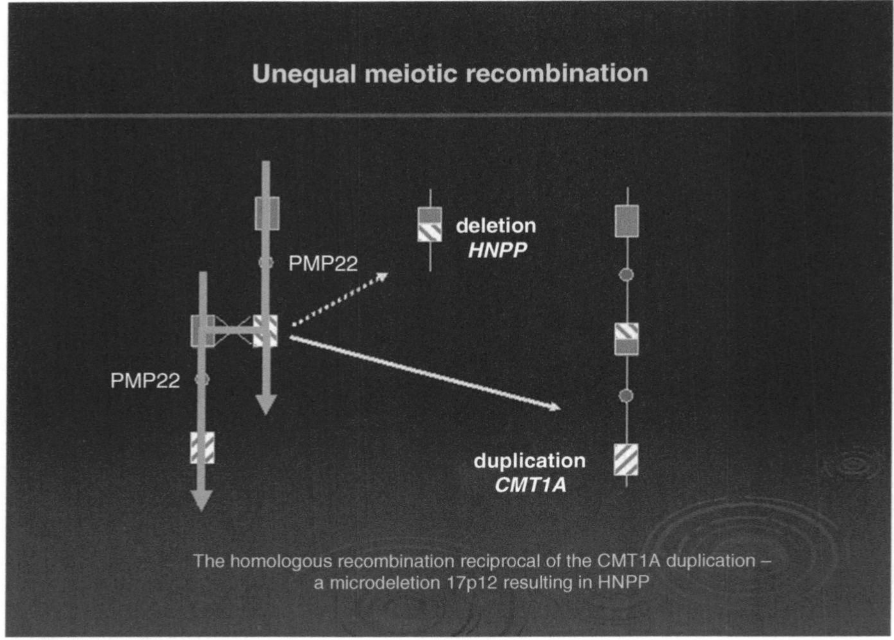

Fig. 1.11 Non-allelic homologous recombination involving the 17p12 region- deletion results in hereditary nerve pressure palsy and duplication manifests with the type 1A Charcot-Marie-Tooth (CMT1A) hereditary motor and sensory neuropathy (HMSN) [29]

1.5.2 Mendelian

Most inherited human disorders follow classic inheritance patterns based on Gregor Mendel's basic laws of inheritance- genes assort independently and manifest in either recessive or dominant manner. For convenience, morbid phenotypes or disease states are classified on the basis of respective genes located on an autosome or an X chromosome.

1.5.2.1 Autosomal Recessive

Most common inherited diseases follow autosomal recessive inheritance pattern. In simple terms, both parents of an affected individual are heterozygote with the mutation or an allele of a particular gene, however with normal phenotype. The affected individual is homozygous with identical mutation or allele on each homologue (Fig. 1.13). In some cases, an affected individual might carry a different mutation or allele (heterozygote) belonging to the same gene, commonly referred to as *compound heterozygote*. In contrast, similar phenotype might result in an individual heterozygous for two different genes, but functionally related. Such an individual is described as a *double heterozygote*.

Typically at each fertilization event, the probability of having a homozygous offspring is 1 in 4 (25%). In the remaining three situations, two offspring would be heterozygote (50%) and one (25%) would have normal genotype. In other words, an

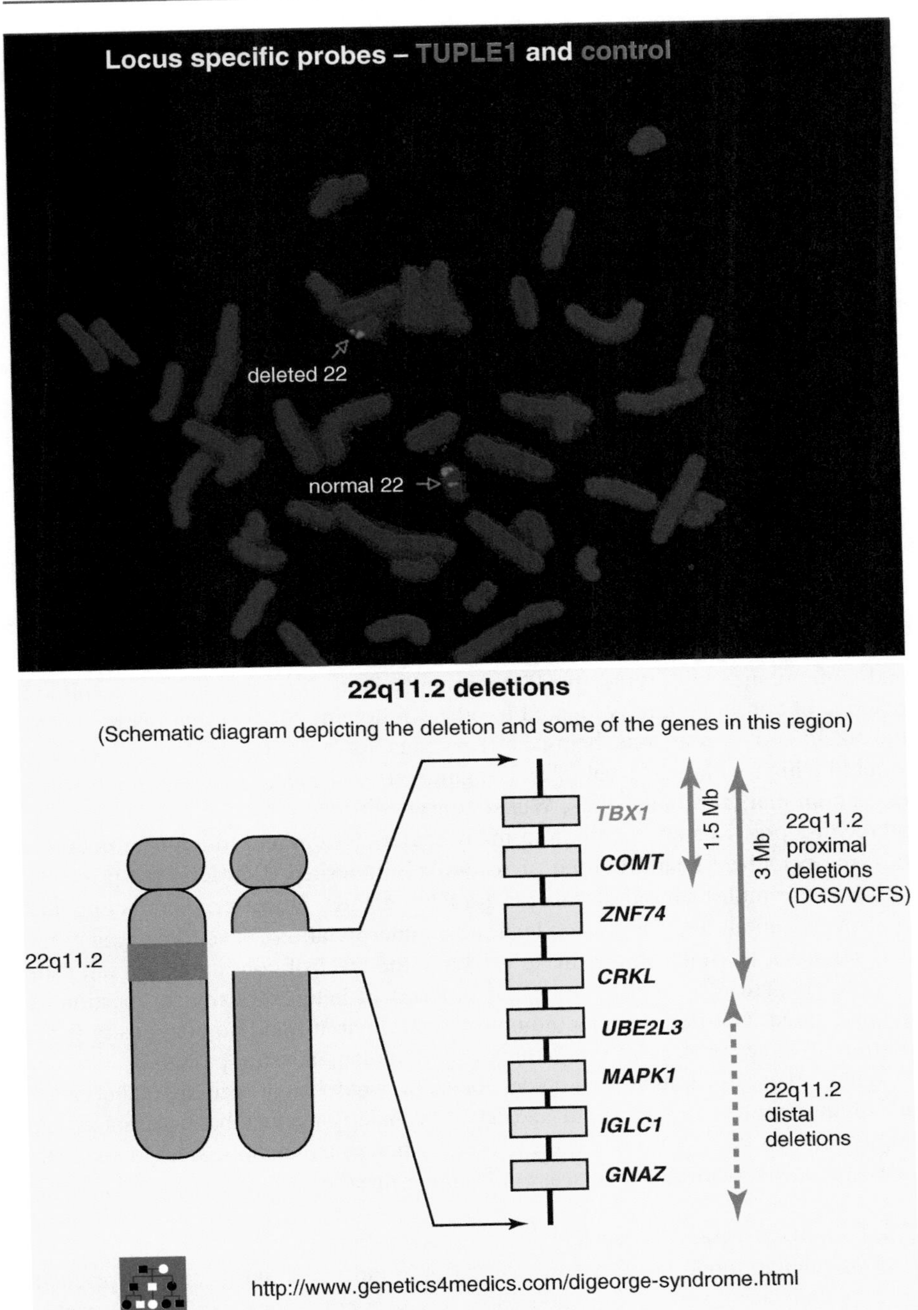

Fig. 1.12 The 22q deletion syndrome- (**a**) FISH showing normal and deleted 22q region (**b**) 22q deleted segment- different sizes deletion result in variable phenotypes; an example of contiguous gene syndrome

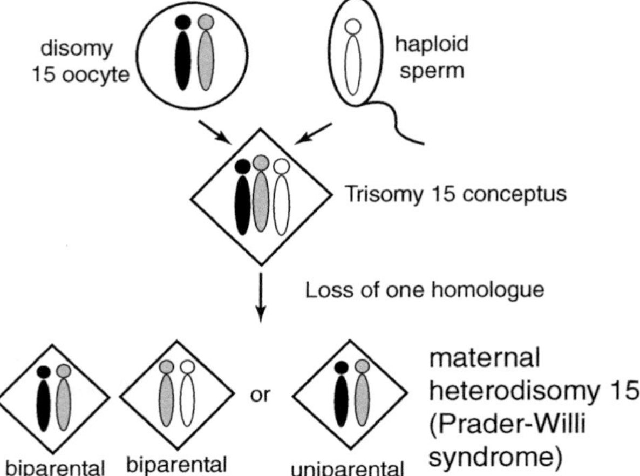

Fig. 1.13 Typical pedigree showing autosomal recessive inheritance- note each parent heterozygote with the mutated allele and the affected offspring homozygous for both alleles. Multiple affected members spread over more than one generation might falsely be interpreted as a dominant trait, also referred to pseudo-dominant

apparently clinically normal offspring of an affected sibling would carry a 2 in 3 probability for being heterozygote or carrier.

In the population context, for common autosomal recessive disorders, for example cystic fibrosis in European people and beta thalassemia in the Mediterranean, heterozygotes enjoy some advantages. This is probably more important for people and communities with wide spread community inbreeding and the socio-cultural practice of consanguinity compared to others following the assorted mating. Thus the likelihood of someone being heterozygous for an autosomal recessive trait would be high with high level of consanguineous marriages compared to selective or random marital relationships. Whilst consanguineous marriages and communal inbreeding practices are common in many social-cultural and religious communities, the perceived health burden of recessively inherited disorders and probably polygenic or multifactorial diseases is arguably greater. However, there is ongoing controversy about bias for data collection and interpretation. Nevertheless, in clinical practice it is vitally important to establish the level of consanguinity and estimate the degree of genetic relationship in terms of heterozygosity (proportion of alleles shared inherited from a common ancestral parent) and homozygosity (proportion of alleles inherited from parents with common ancestral parents).

Inherited cardiovascular phenotypes that follow autosomal recessive inheritance are often complex, multi system and have an underlying metabolic pathology. A large heart in a sick new born requires consideration of a metabolic storage disorder, for example glycogen storage disease or Pompe's disease (see elsewhere in this text).

1.5.2.2 Autosomal Dominant

This Mendelian mode of inheritance is probably most relevant in clinical practice dealing with a number of inherited cardiovascular conditions. Notable examples include hypertrophic cardiomyopathy, arrhythmogenic right ventricular cardiomyopathy, dilated cardiomyopathy with conduction defect, long QT syndrome, Brugada syndrome, familial cardiac conduction disease and many more (see specific chapters for these disorders). There are several genes spread across the human genome that are associated with a number of ICCs inherited in the autosomal dominant manner.

Typically the affected person, one of the parents, would be the heterozygous with a pathogenic mutation in a specific gene at a specific location (exon or exon-intron splice site) or a polymorphic variant located either upstream or downstream of the splice site junction or even within the exon or intron capable of interfering in the transcription and thus eventually either loss or abnormal gene product. In a true autosomal dominant situation, the correlation with the genotype and the phenotype should be consistent in all cases. However, in clinical practice, this is uncommon. The transmission from the affected parent would essentially be 50% or 1 in 2 (Fig. 1.14). This is the basic distinction of autosomal dominant inheritance from any other Mendelian inheritance (see X-linked dominant in later section). Another important observation is the major clinical distinction between the heterozygous and the homozygous persons with the same autosomal dominant disease. For example, parents heterozygous with an LDLR mutation affected with familial hypercholesterolemia (FH), would be at 25% risk for an affected child who could have extremely high plasma cholesterol levels, so called homozygous FH. It is likely similar examples occur in clinical practice that are probably not recognized due to either lethality or death at a very young age. This might be applicable to ICCs with relatively high prevalence rate, for example sarcomere related hypertrophic cardiomyopathy with a general population incidence of around 1 in 500.

Many mutations and polymorphic variants located in critical positions within the gene, could disrupt the coding sequences and thus might result in either a qualitative (abnormally functioning gene product) or quantitative (absent or insufficient gene product) alteration in the gene function. In simple words, heterogeneity at different genetic and molecular levels is highly likely and is often encountered.

In addition to the genetic heterogeneity, clinical variation or clinical heterogeneity is a likely to be associated. There are number of factors underlying the clinical variation including gender variation, age related penetrance, personal, life-style and environmental pressures. Thus it is mandatory to carry out detailed analysis on all background factors and carefully interpret the family history. The interpretation might well be misleading due to some family members manifesting with unrelated phenocopies.

1.5.2.3 X-Linked Recessive

Among all human chromosomes, the X chromosome is probably most relevant to many biological functions. The proportion of human genome shared by the X chromosome pair is relatively high with many genes encoding several proteins involved in complex metabolic pathways and multi-system physiological roles [19]. There are many X-linked Mendelian disorders listed in OMIM, of which a significant proportion involves the cardiovascular system.

Most mutations in genes mapped to the X chromosome behave in recessive manner. However, the transmission pattern is different from autosomal recessive since the male carrier, often clinically affected, would be *hemizygous* compared to the female carrier, often unaffected, would be *heterozygous* for the mutation (Fig. 1.15). Interpretation of the family history related to the X-linked recessive disorder

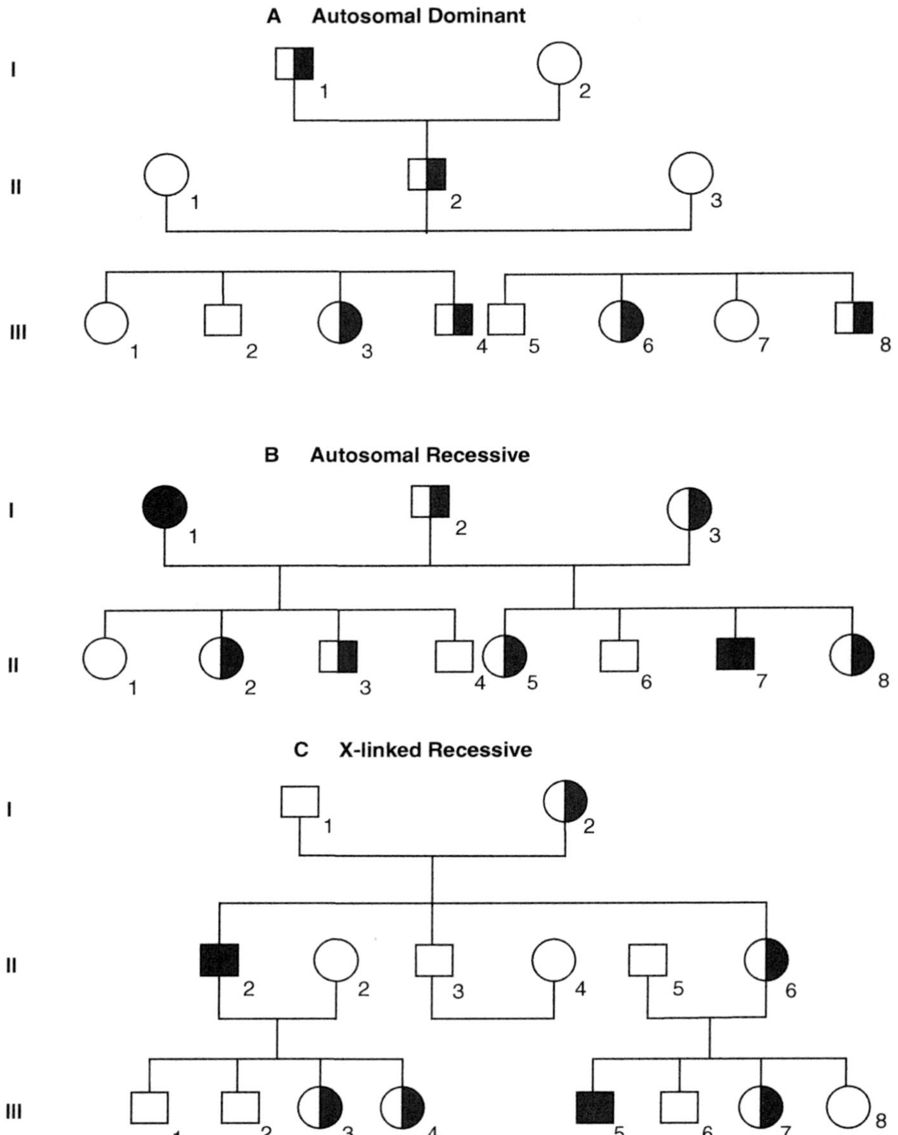

Fig. 1.14 Pedigree showing autosomal dominant inheritance- note affected father and son; male-male transmission of the heterozygous trait is confirmatory for the autosomal dominant inheritance. When both parents are heterozygotes then 25% risk for severely affected homozygous offspring, for example homozygous familial hypercholesterolemia with massively elevated plasma cholesterol requiring emergency plasmapheresis

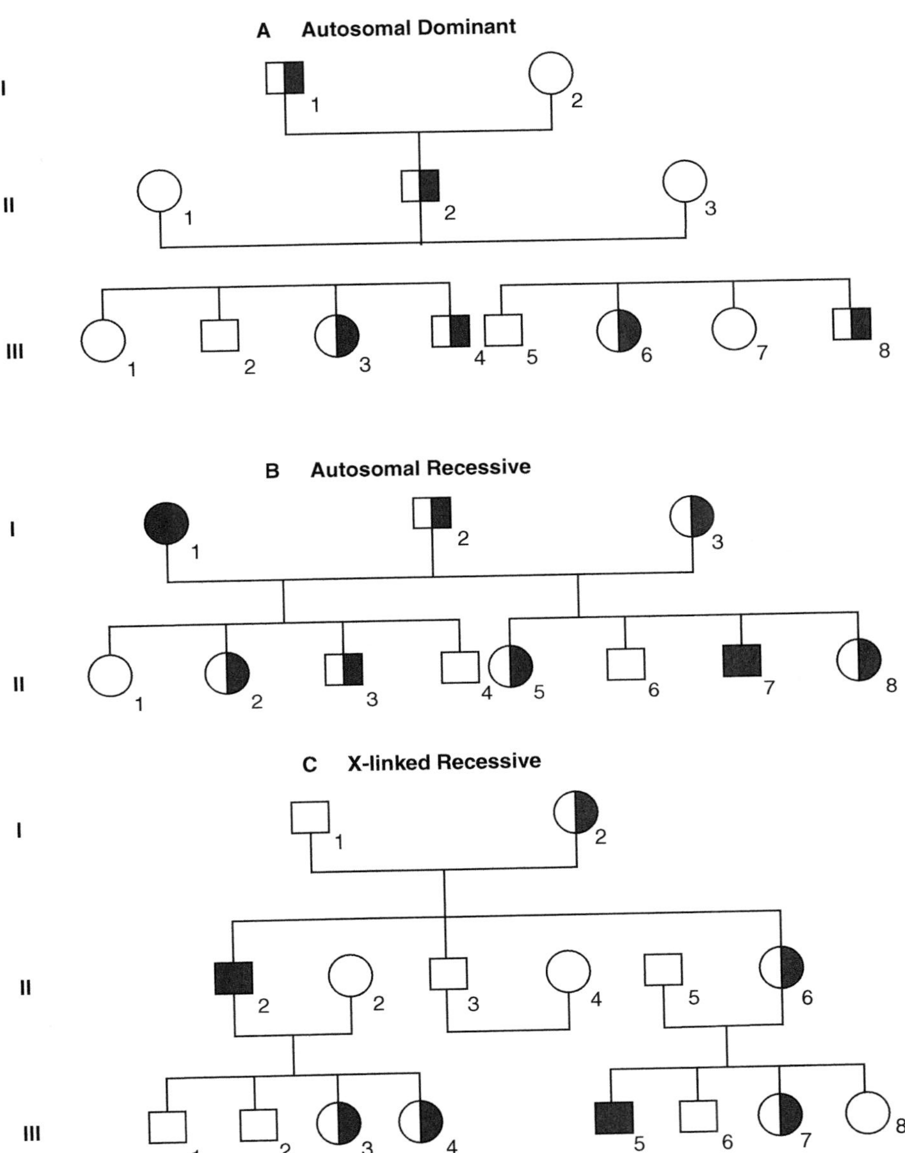

Fig. 1.15 Typical pedigree for X-linked inheritance; note hemizygous male (affected) and heterozygous female (normal phenotype) born to an obligate carrier mother

typically reveals affected males spread over 2 or more generations with evident maternal lineages. Most intervening female relatives (sister, mother, maternal aunt and maternal female cousin) are clinically asymptomatic and are deduced to carry the same pathogenic mutation or polymorphic variant shown in the affected male. In some situations, the female carrier could become symptomatic, for example progressive heart failure in a female carrier of Duchene or Becker muscular dystrophy or lysosomal storage metabolic Fabry's disease. This could be erroneously interpreted as a dominantly inherited disorder.

In simple segregation terms, in the X-linked recessive inheritance, typically the female carrier carries the probability of 50% (1 in 2) for passing on the mutation to both female and male offspring. This would be shared with other 1st degree female relatives (sister and mother) with a 50% or 1 in 2 probability. In contrast, the affected male carrier would carry 100% risk to pass the mutation to all female offspring and none to his sons. This is based on the simple biological fact that the conception of the male requires a Y chromosome bearing sperm compared to the X chromosome bearing sperm involved in the female offspring conception.

1.5.2.4 X-Linked Dominant

This mode of Mendelian inheritance in man is probably least understood or appreciated. As the name implies, the putative mutation in a gene located on one of the X chromosomes in a female (heterozygous) and in the only X chromosome in the male (hemizygous) should manifest with clinical symptoms, physical signs or any other recognizable clinical, electrophysiological, biochemical, molecular, pathological or imaging phenotype. However, in clinical practice, a proper recognition might not always be possible due to high level of lethality in the hemizygous male and extreme clinical variation in the heterozygous female. The mode of transmission would also follow simple rule of segregation- 100% chance to all female offspring from the hemizygous male and none to male offspring. In contrast, a heterozygous female would carry a 50% chance for passing on the mutation equally to male or female offspring. However, in reality, the clinical severity might be more intense in the male child.

In clinical cardiovascular medicine practice, it is rare to come across an inherited cardiovascular condition apparently inherited in the X-linked dominant manner. There is no doubt that clinically some of these disorders are often under diagnosed due to apparent unclear family history and disparity in the gender specific clinical phenotypes. It is possible that some of the X-linked recessive disorders, for example Fabry's disease, might behave in an apparent X-linked dominant manner given the fact that a significant proportion of heterozygous females might manifest with cardiac dysfunction [20]. Similarly, in the case of Fragile-X syndrome (FRAXA), the mode of transmission does not always follow the classic X-linked recessive inheritance and is often described as X-linked semi-dominant, a term that needs to be avoided as it has not clear scientific explanation. In other words, there could be paradoxical relationship between the gender specific clinical phenotypes and segregation in the family. This was first observed in FRAXA and is referred to as the Sherman paradox [21].

1.5.3 Mitochondrial

The mitochondrial genome was introduced in the earlier part of this chapter. There are many uncommon disorders that are directly or indirectly related to mitochondrial DNA (mtDNA) gene mutations or polymorphic variants. However, there are probably more rare Mendelian genetic diseases that result from mutations or polymorphic variants interfering with the function of certain nuclear DNA (nDNA) genes. These are Mendelian disorders with the phenotype of mitochondrial dysfunction, for example Freidreich's ataxia with dilated cardiomyopathy [22].

Most mtDNA diseases commonly present with variable complex phenotypes predominantly involving the energy rich organs and body systems, for example cerebral cortex, endocrine glands, choroid and retina, cochlea, skeletal muscles, myocardium and many others. In the cardiovascular medicine practice it is not uncommon to encounter these conditions that are often missed or under diagnosed (see elsewhere in this text). Typically, the pedigree analysis with a mitochondrial disease reveals negligible transmission from an affected male. In contrast, the pattern of transmission from an affected female, for example mother, might be variable from 100% to less than half.

Apart from the quantitative variation, the distribution of clinical manifestations in a given family with the same mtDNA mutation commonly indicates wide diversity. This is largely due to heteroplasmy, a term commonly used in the mitochondrial genetics. It implies that the proportion of wild and mutated mtDNA is inadvertently inconsistent in different tissues and organs, for example heteroplasmy of the mtDNA mutation in sensori-neural deafness associated with type 2 diabetes mellitus and dilated cardiomyopathy might result in a combination of affected family members with only one condition or a combination of the main manifestations [23].

1.6 Polygenic/Multi-Factorial

In clinical genetics, most apparently inherited diseases do not comply with either chromosomal or Mendelian inheritance. In such a case, the consideration would be either for multifactorial/ polygenic inheritance or one of the uncommon non-traditional inheritance patterns (see next section). The multi-factorial or polygenic inheritance is included within the traditional inheritance category. As the term implies, several genes with small additive effect are involved that are spread across the whole genome (Fig. 1.16). Collectively morbid mutations or biologically important polymorphic variants modify the threshold of tolerance to a host of environmental factors. A lower threshold could result in structural or functional phenotypes interpreted as a complex disorder, for example systemic hypertension, coronary artery disease, a congenital developmental heart anomaly and diabetes mellitus (both type 1 and 2).

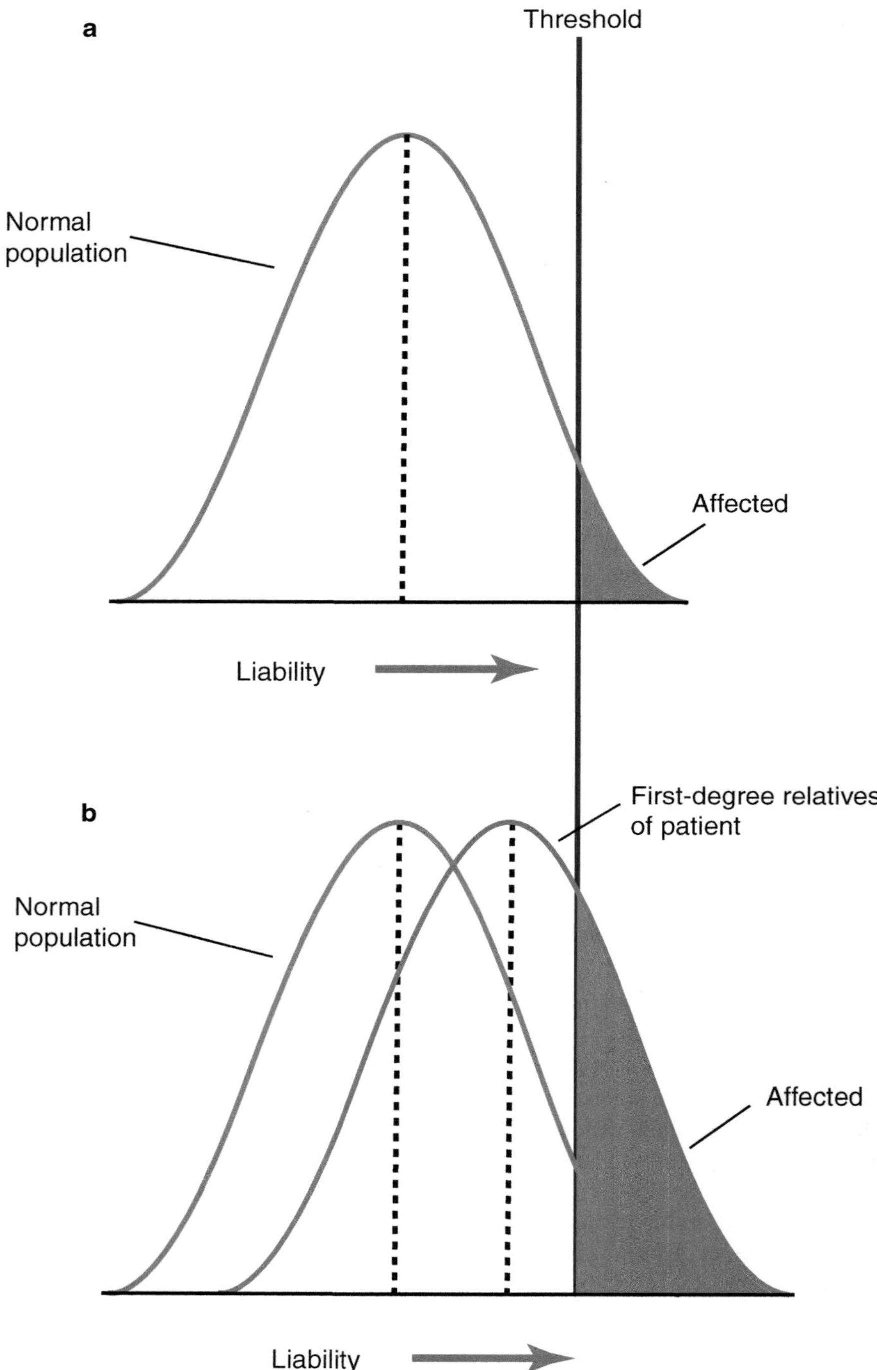

Fig. 1.16 Polygenic/ Multifactorial inheritance- note (top) the liability curve showing normal threshold for a trait or phenotype (**a**) and another curve (lower) showing a 'shift to the right' with increased liability (**b**)

Interpretation of the family history for a multi-factorial/ polygenic inheritance typically reveals one or more of the following observations:

1. Most affected family members are randomly distributed.
2. Both maternal or paternal lineages are likely
3. Affected persons may not have a set age related pattern but often in adults
4. Transmission of a phenotypic trait does not follow either a Mendelian or mitochondrial inheritance pattern
5. Variation in the pattern and/or severity of the phenotype is possible

Genetic counseling for a polygenic/multifactorial disease requires few important principles to follow-

1. Most are common but without any clear detectable mutations or pathogenic variants
2. Risk of recurrence if often small, less than 5% in most cases
3. Affected *parent-child* or *sibling-sibling* pairs might indicate higher recurrence risk
4. Affected cousins or distant relatives might not have significant impact on recurrence risk
5. Recurrence risk could be high if the affected person happens to be of the low prevalence gender; for example pyloric stenosis in a female would carry higher recurrence risk since incidence is much lower in the female (The Carter effect)
6. Recurrence risk could be approximately equal to the square root of the birth incidence; for example recurrence risks for ventricular septal defect (VSD) with a birth incidence of approximately 1 in 100 [$\sqrt{1/100} = 0.31$] could be just under 3% (Ref.)
7. Heritability estimates, based on dizygotic vs. monozygotic twin studies, provide a reasonable guide for recurrence risks in 1st degree relatives. The higher concordance probably reflects greater level of heritability in a given phenotype.
8. Data from complicated large genome wide association (GWAS) studies is often unhelpful in recurrence risk calculation. Typically GWAS provides genetic susceptibility data for a given complex medical disease. Most such studies require several hundreds and thousands of affected people with perceived similar clinical phenotypes. It is likely that GWAS data might also help in revising the heritability estimates by adding the previously unknown genetic component, commonly referred to as the *missing heritability* [24, 25, 26]. Whilst the outcomes of GWAS might look very attractive and encouraging, in clinical practice most of these observations have extremely limited applications [27].
9. In some cases and for certain complex medical diseases, the genetic counseling might help in good case selection for high profile and technically complicated and expensive surveillance in asymptomatic family members; for example an echocardiogram or CT coronary angiography

10. The final outcome might be specific prophylactic measures, such as a drug, for example the role of biguanide oral anti-diabetic (metformin) in obese and overweight individuals. The risk for type 2 diabetes mellitus (T2DM) is considerably high in obesity and overweight persons that are evidently complex medical conditions and perfect examples for multi-factorial/ polygenic inheritance.

1.7 Nontraditional Inheritance

1.7.1 Epigenetics/Genetic Imprinting/Uniparental Disomy

In the previous section, the concept of epigenetics and epigenomics was introduced. This has swept into the clinical arena relatively faster compared to other new genetic and genomic mechanisms.

In clinical practice, the genetic imprinting and different directions through which this might manifest are commonly taken into consideration. This is particularly important in terms of the inheritance pattern, segregation of the clinical phenotype, clinical variation and recurrence risks. The genetic imprinting is predominantly focused on the *parent of origin* phenomenon. It is now widely accepted that inactivating mutations of the imprinting control centre (ICC) genes and methylation of the CpG islands located proximal to the 5′ end of the untranscribed region (UTR) probably account for the loss of the *parent of orgin* effect. However, uniparental disomy, practically nil contribution of the critical parental set of genes or the whole chromosomal homologue, also account for a significant proportion of clinical outcomes of genetic imprinting. In addition, post-translational histone modifications also account for a small proportion of epigenetic changes.

Most genetically imprinted disorders clinically manifest with isolated or multiple developmental malformations or neuro-developmental delay. In addition, genetic imprinting is probably relevant in cancer, particularly in developing novel tumour markers for diagnosis, prognosis and therapy. However, it is as yet of limited practical use in the clinical cancer genetics dealing with inherited cancers and the cancer family syndromes.

In cardiovascular medicine, particularly dealing with inherited cardiovascular conditions, the evidence for genetic imprinting is gradually building up. In most cases, it is restricted to multiple malformation dysmorphic syndromes with structural cardiovascular manifestations and possibly in some rare inherited metabolic diseases. However, it is likely that environmental influences during mammalian development lead to stable changes in the epigenome that alter the individual's susceptibility to chronic metabolic and cardiovascular disease, and discuss the clinical implications [28].

1.7.2 Trinucleotide (Triplet) Repeats

Apart from a small fraction of the coding genome, the large part is full of apparently non-coding DNA and RNA sequences including evolutionary conserved sequences, biologically important sequences that regulate essential functions, such as gene organization and function, mitotic and meiotic cell divisions, cellular repair and ageing (apoptosis) processes. Within the non-coding genome, there are many variable length repeat sequences that are tandemly distributed, commonly referred to satellite DNA. Within the broad group of variable number tandem repeats (VNTRs), microsatellite repeats (more than 50 to few hundreds base pairs) and minisatellite repeats (up to 50 base pairs) are included. Microsatellites and minisatellites occur at thousands of locations in the human genome and are notable for their high mutation rate and diversity in the population. The name "satellite" refers to the early observation that centrifugation of genomic DNA in a test tube separates a prominent layer of bulk DNA from accompanying "satellite" layers of repetitive DNA. Microsatellites are often referred to as *short tandem repeats (STRs)* by forensic geneticists, or as *simple sequence repeats (SSRs)* by plant geneticists. They are widely used for DNA profiling in kinship analysis and in forensic identification. They are also used in genetic linkage analysis/marker assisted selection to locate a gene or a mutation responsible for a given trait or disease.

Apart from VNTRs and STRs, there are is another class of DNA sequence repeats that occur in the vicinity of coding regions of the genome. These are commonly in the form of triplets, however longer sequence repeats involving 4 or more also occur. The precise functional role of the DNA triplet repeats is not clearly understood. However, it is agreed that these take important part if gene regulation and expression. Normally the trinucleotide repeats occur up to certain numbers that provide a stable threshold for a specific gene. These are a subset of unstable microsatellite repeats that occur throughout all genomic sequences. If the repeat is present in a healthy gene, a dynamic mutation may increase the repeat count and result in a defective gene. The trinucleotide or triplet repeats are sometimes classified as insertion mutations and referred to as a separate class of mutations within the broad group of non-traditional inheritance. There are now many recognizable *Trinucleotide repeat disorders*, also known as trinucleotide repeat expansion disorders, triplet repeat expansion disorders or codon reiteration disorders) (Table 1.4). Most of the triplet repeats disorders include progressive inherited neurodegenerative diseases, for example fragile X syndrome, spinocerebellar ataxia, Huntington's disease and dystrophia myotonica. In most cases, the abnormal number of triplet repeats occur proximal to the 5′ end of the gene, except for myotonic dystrophy in which abnormal expansion is located at the 3′ end. Exceptionally, in Friedreich's ataxia, the triplet repeats expansion is located at the intronic 1 splice site (Ref.). There are not many examples of triplet repeats disorders within the group of inherited cardiovascular conditions. It is likely, however, that most of the triplet repeats disorders happen to be heterogeneous and pleiotropic, thus highly likely to impact up on cardiovascular system.

1.7.3 Nonallelic Homologous Recombination

Conventional and molecular cytogenetic techniques are the cornerstone for investigating a number of genetic conditions and syndromes. The basic classification of chromosome disorders rests on numerical and structural categorization. Both groups indicate gross and minimal genome disorganization. Within the structural

Table 1.4 The triplet (trinucleotide) repeat disorders

Disorder	Triplet	Location	Normal#	Mutation#
Fragile X syndrome	CGG	5'UTR	10–50	200–2000
Friedreich's ataxia	GAA	Intronic	17–22	200–900
Kennedy disease [SBMA]	CAG	Coding	17–24	40–55
Spinocerebellar ataxia 1[SCA1]	CAG	Coding	19–36	43–81
Huntington disease	CAG	Coding	9–35	37–100
Dentatorubral-Pallidoluysian Atrophy (DRPLA)	CAG	Coding	7–23	49>75
Machado-Joseph disease[SCA3]	CAG	Coding	12–36	67>79
Spinocerebellar ataxia 2[SCA2]	CAG	Coding	15–24	35–39
Spinocerebellar ataxia 6[SCA6]	CAG	Coding	4–16	21–27
Spinocerbellar ataxia 7[SCA7]	CAG	Coding	7–35	37–200
Spinocerebellar ataxia 8[SCA8]	TG	UTR	16–37	100>500
Myotonic dystrophy	CTG	3'UTR	5–35	50–4000
Fragile site E [FRAXE]	CCG	Promoter	6–25	>200
Fragile site F [FRAXF]	GCC	?	6–29	>500
Fragile site 16 A [FRA16A]	CCG	?	16–49	1000–2000

UTR-untranslated region

chromosome abnormalities, deletions and duplications involving variable chromosomal segments are clinically recognizable with salient phenotypes and recorded accordingly, for example 4p deletion (Wolf- Hirschhorn syndrome), 5p deletion (Cri-du-Chat syndrome), 7q deletion (Williams syndrome), 11 q deletion (Jacobson syndrome), 15 q deletion (Prader-Willi (Pat) and Angelman (Mat) syndromes based on the parent of origin), 17 p deletion (Hereditary nerve pressure palsy), 17p duplication (Charcot-Marie-Tooth disease type 1A), 20 q deletion syndrome (Alagile syndrome) and 22 q deletion (di George syndrome). These are good examples of disorders of the genome architecture [29].

With the completion of the human genome sequencing and emergence of many next generation genome sequencing (NGS) technologies, it is now possible to carry out in depth genome analysis in any case with multiple malformations or complex clinical phenotypes. Techniques like array comparative genome hybridization (aCGH), whole exome sequencing (WES) and whole genome sequencing (WGS) are now in routine clinical use. These are extremely powerful for deciphering copy number variations (CNVs) and single nucleotide polymorphisms (SNPs), the hall mark for documenting genome level disorganization involving loss, gain or reversal of the genome content in a specific chromosomal location.

There are recurrent regions in the human genome that are frequently encountered in multiple malformations, developmental delay, intellectual difficulties and behavior problems like autistic spectrum disorder. Why are these prone to deletions or duplications? This has been debated and discussed in a number of reports and reviews [30]. One of the arguments includes non-allelic homologous recombination, NAHR. Essentially, each recurrent specific genomic region is flanked with variable repeat sequences at proximal and distal ends. The presence of repeat sequences might interfere in meiotic recombination during the reduction phase in meiosis, thus resulting in another homologue with either loss or addition of the critical region. Since it is unrelated to any specific allelic groups or combinations and involves the two homologues, it is appropriately named the non-allelic homologous recombination (NAHR) [30].

The concept of NAHR is probably correct and offers understanding of the complex genome level mechanisms in the pathogenesis of a number of rare and common conditions. It is likely that a number of rare genetic conditions encountered in clinical cardiovascular medicine are due to genome level disorganization that is best explained by NAHR.

1.8 Digenic, Oligogenic and Multigenic Inheritance

In the previous section, an introduction to the polygenic/ multi-factorial inheritance is given. Conceptually, a genetic disorder, resembling a single gene Mendelian disorder, could also result from mutations in few different genes that share physiological roles, either belonging to the same *gene-molecule* pathway or biologically related functions. Terms like oligogenic (2–3 genes) or multigenic (10–20 genes) are used in some what arbitrary manner. It is argued that there is usually a single gene that behaves in dominant manner and other genes act like modifier genes [31]. However, it is also likely that altered gene function of few genes (less than 5) collectively manifest with the recognizable clinical phenotype.

It is now increasingly apparent that modifier genes have a considerable role to play in phenotypic variations of single-gene disorders. Intra familial variations, altered penetrance, and altered severity are now common features of single gene disorders because of the involvement of several genes in the expression of the disease phenotype. It is now certain that cancer occurs due to the action of the environment acting in combination with several genes. Although modifier genes make it impossible to predict phenotype from the genotype and cause considerable difficulties in genetic counseling, they have their uses [32].

The clinical presentation and the pattern of transmission in oligogenic disorders might follow one of the Mendelian patterns. Most of these diseases have a major central phenotype, for example progressive visual impairment, deafness, progressive muscle disease, joint hypermobility, chronic heart failure and many others. There are now several groups of genetic disorders that are discussed in the context of oligogenic or multigenic diseases. Examples include cortical heterotopia, retinitis pigmentosa, macular degeneration, congenital cataract, sensori-neural deafness, congenital myopathy, demyelinating neuropathy, joint hypermobility, Hirschprung's disease and many others. In cardiovascular medicine practice, inherited cardiovascular conditions like hypertrophic cardiomyopathy, dilated cardiomyopathy, ventricular non-compaction, atypical long QT syndrome, Brugada syndrome, cardiac conduction disease and probably familial atrial fibrillation could also be regarded as oligo/multi- genic diseases. This conceptual approach has led to studies looking into prospects of potential therapeutic applications [33].

1.9 Mosaicism: Somatic and Gonadal

In biological terms, the mosaicism implies a combination of differential cellular and molecular phenotypes arising from a single cell line. In comparison, a chimaera indicates a combination of different cells and molecules related to two different cellular lineages.

The mosaicism could be limited to somatic distribution, established at very early embryonic mitotic cell divisions leading to germinal layer differentiation. In such a case, the ultimate phenotype would be dependent up on the destined tissue or organ. In most cases, clinically this might manifest as a localized unusual growth or developmental anomaly. Examples might include asymmetric congenital heart anomaly and possibly atypical septal hypertrophy, mimicking variable expression of a Mendelian cardiovascular condition. Most of these are probably phenocopies rather than the true phenotype. Genetic analysis of the unusual tissue compared to the apparently normal tissue might indicate a detectable abnormality. For example, in certain pigmentary disorders, the cultured skin fibrobalsts might reveal confined chromosome abnormality compared to the normal looking adjoining region. In any such case, risk of recurrence is consistently low and the parents are convincingly reassured.

The mosaicism involving the germ cell lines and limited in the gonadal cellular lineages often create clinical dilemmas. The gonadal mosaicism evidently arose from the meiotic cell division, most likely in meiosis II, and might result in a combination of germ cell lines- wild and with a mutation or chromosomal rearrangement. In any such situation, the parental analysis should be normal. Apart from the theoretical possibility of clarification in a testicular biopsy, it would be practically impossible to offer any conclusive evidence. The evidence is mostly in the form of recurrence of a phenotype or disorder in the absence of a family history and with entirely normal parents. However, there are exceptions that might confuse the clinical picture. In Mendelian genetics, examples include recurrence in another sibling with similar detectable mutation but without any parental link [34]. Risk of recurrence (for example, recurrent hypertrophic cardiomyopathy or long QT syndrome) could be small but would need to be considered in genetic counseling, particularly in situation like prenatal diagnosis [35].

Conclusions

The practice of clinical cardiovascular genomic medicine and the clinical management of inherited cardiovascular conditions requires the clinician, specialist trainee, nurse and allied healthcare practitioner and the student understand and apply the following facts about basic genetics and genomics:

- Nucleic acids- nucleotides and the double helix structure
- The concept of gene and its organization, specifically exons, introns and splice sites
- The position of genes or the coding part of the genome in relation to rest of the genome

- Broad structural and functional organization of the genome
- Importance of the non-coding genome
- Importance of the RNA interference (RNAi)
- Clinical importance of genome variation including variable sequence repeats, copy number variation and single nucleotide polymorphisms
- Clinical utility of genetic heterogeneity and pleiotropism
- Mutational heterogeneity- understand and interpreting different mutations
- Traditional inheritance patterns
- Core concepts of the Mendelian inheritance
- Understanding concepts and different forms of the non-traditional inheritance
- Clinical importance of genome disorganization- deletion, duplication, insertions etc.
- Clinical importance of digenic, oligogenic or multigenic basis of inherited cardiovascular phenotypes
- Clinical relevance of epigenetics and genetic imprinting
- Understanding somatic and gonadal mosaicism with clinical applications

References

1. Conrad DF, Pinto D, Redon R, Feuk L, Gokcumen O, Zhang Y. Origins and functional impact of copy number variation in the human genome. Nature. 2010;464(7289):704–12.
2. Chen R, Davydov EV, Sirota M, Butte AJ. Non-synonymous and synonymous coding SNPs show similar likelihood and effect size of human disease association. PLoS One. 2010;5(10):e13574. https://doi.org/10.1371/journal.pone.0013574.
3. Eheret GB. Genome-wide association studies: contribution of genomics to understanding blood pressure and essential hypertension. Curr Hypertens Rep. 2010;12:17–25.
4. Schunkert H, König IR, Kathiresan S, Reilly MP, Assimes TL, Holm H, et al. Large-scale association analysis identifies 13 new susceptibility loci for coronary artery disease. Nat Genet. 2011;43:333–8.
5. Welter D, MacArthur J, Morales J, Burdett T, Hall P, Junkins H, et al. The NHGRI GWAS catalog, a curated resource of SNP-trait associations. Nucleic Acids Res. 2014;42:D1001–6.
6. Wellcome Trust Case Control Consortium. Genome-wide association study of 14,000 cases of seven common diseases and 3,000 shared controls. Nature. 2007;447(7145):661–78.
7. Lusis AJ. Genetics of atherosclerosis. Trends Genet. 2012;28(6):267–75. https://doi.org/10.1016/j.tig.2012.03.001
8. Eichler EE, Flint J, Gibson G, Kong A, Leal SM, Moore JH, Nadeau JH. Missing heritability and strategies for finding the underlying causes of complex disease. Nat Rev. Genet. 2010;11:446–50.
9. Mercer TR, Dinger ME, Mattick JS. Long non-coding RNAs: insights into functions. Nat Rev. Genet. 2009;10:155–9.
10. Esteller M. Non-coding RNAs in human disease. Nat Rev. Genet. 2011;12:861–74.
11. Reik W, Dean W, Walter J. Epigenetic reprogramming in mammalian development. Science. 2001;293(5532):1089–93.
12. Chamberlain SJ, Lalande M. Angelman syndrome, a genomic imprinting disorder of the brain. J Neurosci. 2010;30:9958–63.
13. Reik W, Walter J. Genomic imprinting: parental influence on the genome. Nat Rev. Genet. 2001;2(1):21–32.

14. Dawson MA, Kouzarides T. Cancer epigenetics: from mechanism to therapy. Cell. 2012;150:12–27.
15. Hoffbuhr K, Devaney JM, LaFleur B, Sirianni N, Scacheri C, Giron J, et al. MeCP2 mutations in children with and without the phenotype of Rett syndrome. Neurology. 2001;56(11):1486–95.
16. Cabianca DS, Casa V, Bodega B, Xynos A, Ginelli E, Tanaka Y, Gabellini D. A long ncRNA links copy number variation to a polycomb/trithoraxeEpigenetic switch in FSHD muscular dystrophy. Cell. 2012;149:819–31.
17. Ordovás JM, Smith CE. Epigenetics and cardiovascular disease. Nat Rev. Cardiol. 2010;7(9):510–9.
18. Slavotnek AM. Novel microdeletion syndromes detected by chromosome microarrays. Hum Genet. 2008;124:1–17.
19. Yang X, Deignan JL, Qi H, Zhu J, Qian S, Zhong J, et al. Validation of candidate causal genes for obesity that affect shared metabolic pathways and networks. Nat Genet. 2009;41:415–23.
20. Whybra C, Kampmann C, Willers I, Davies J, Winchester B, Kriegsmann J, et al. Anderson–Fabry disease: clinical manifestations of disease in female heterozygotes. J Inherit Metab Dis. 2001;24:715–24.
21. Crawford DC, Acuña JM, Sherman SL. FMR1 and the fragile X syndrome: human genome epidemiology review. Genet Med. 2001;3:359–71.
22. Chinnery PF. Searching for nuclear-mitochondrial genes. Cell. 2003;19:60–2.
23. Goldstein AC, Bhatia P, Vento JM. Mitochondrial disease in childhood: nuclear encoded. Neurotherapeutics. 2013;10:212–26.
24. Maher B. Personal genomes: the case of the missing heritability. Nature. 2008;456(7218):18–21.
25. Clarke AJ, Cooper DN. GWAS: heritability missing in action? Eur J Hum Genet. 2010;18(8):859–61.
26. Clarke AJ, Cooper DN. GWAS: heritability missing in action? Eur J Hum Genet. 2010;18:859–61.
27. Sun X, Yu W, Hu C. Genetics of type 2 diabetes: insights into the pathogenesis and its clinical application. Biomed Res Int. 2014;2014:926713.
28. Gluckman PD, Hanson MA, Buklijas T, Low FM, Beedle AS. Epigenetic mechanisms that underpin metabolic and cardiovascular diseases. Nat Rev. Endocrinol. 2009;5:401–8.
29. Kumar D. Disorders of the genome architecture: a review. Genome Med. 2008;2:69–76.
30. Stankiewicz P, Lupski JR. Genome architecture, rearrangements and genomic disorders. Cell. 2002;18:74–82.
31. Katsanis N. The oligogenic properties of Bardet–Biedl syndrome. Hum Mol Genet. 2004;13(suppl 1):R65–71.
32. Badano JL, Katsanis N. Beyond Mendel: an evolving view of human genetic disease transmission. Nat Rev. Genet. 2002;3:779–89.
33. Pinsonneault J, Sadée W. Pharmacogenomics of multigenic diseases: sex-specific differences in disease and treatment outcome. AAPS Pharm Sci. 2003;5:49–61.
34. Mettler G, Fraser FC. Recurrence risk for sibs of children with "sporadic" achondroplasia. Am J Med Genet. 2000;90:250–1.
35. Clemens PR, Fenwick JS, Chamberlain RA, Gibbs M, de Andrade M, Chakraborty R, Caskey CT. Carrier detection and prenatal diagnosis in Duchenne and Becker muscular dystrophy families, using dinucleotide repeat polymorphisms. Am J Hum Genet. 1991;49:951–60.

Suggested Reading

Brendan M. The case of the missing heritability. Nature. 2008;456(7218):18–21.

Ellard S, Turnpenny P. Emery's elements of medical genetics. 15th ed. New York: Churchill Livingstone; 2015.

Kumar D, Antonarakis S, editors. Medical and health genomics. Philadelphia: Academic Press/Elsevier; 2016.

Read A, Donnai D. New clinical genetics. 3rd ed. Scion: Oxford; 2015.

Spectrum and Classification of Inherited Cardiovascular Disease

2

Paul Brennan

Abstract

Since early times, clinicians and researchers have sought to explain the world around them using classification systems. Some of these are simply catalogues and others attempt to capture complexity in simple form. So it is with inherited cardiac conditions (ICCs). Early classification systems—which remain useful—were based on anatomical/pathological description. As the genetic mechanisms and genes responsible for ICCs were identified, initial attempts at molecular classification looked promising. But as knowledge increases, so often does complexity, and over the past 20 years the underlying heterogeneity that characterises so much human disease has been reported in every ICC. While this has lead to some fascinating insights into biology and therapy, this heterogeneity remains challenging to classify and, ultimately, a combined approach is necessary. As genomic medicine progresses and we enter an era of personalised medicine, our ability to develop an organic classification system able to deal with complexity will be key.

Keywords

Spectrum • Classification • Aortopathy • Cardiomyopathy • Online Inheritance in Man (OMIM) • Ion channelopathy • Phenotype • Genotype • Heterogeneity

P. Brennan
Northern Genetic Service, Institute of Genetic Medicine, International Centre of Life, Newcastle Hospitals NHS Foundation Trust, Newcastle upon Tyne, England, UK
e-mail: paul.brennan@nuth.nhs.uk

D. Kumar, P. Elliott (eds.), *Cardiovascular Genetics and Genomics*,
https://doi.org/10.1007/978-3-319-66114-8_2

2.1 Introduction: Why Classification is Challenging

For centuries, scientists and clinicians have sought to describe and classify the world around them. Once a simple cataloguing exercise, disease classification systems are now being elegantly refined by increasing knowledge about the molecular causes of disease and the advent of targeted therapies.

In order to understand how we can classify and categorise inherited cardiovascular conditions (ICC), we need to think about the heart not as a single organ but as a multi-dimensional complex of tissues and processes: so complex, in fact that we are only beginning to understand it. Classification—as we will see—is a major challenge at present. Why bother? We need a framework to work within, not only to identify common disease mechanisms and common opportunities for therapeutic intervention but also to understand the clinical and pathophysiological differences between sub-types of disease. Ideally, such a framework should also enable us to predict the phenotypic impact of a gene mutation. Early classification systems introduced bias, whereas more modern, precise classifications may seem unduly complex. Ultimately, however, biology is complex, and the challenge is to reduce that complexity to a clinically useful tool.

In this chapter we will consider ways in which we can group ICCs together into common themes; in doing so we will frequently discover that this often doesn't work. To some extent this reflects underlying heterogeneity: both phenotypic (or 'variable expression'; different effects of a single aetiology; or different genetics aetiologies giving rise to the same phenotype. In the following pages, the word 'phenotype' is used as a substitute for 'clinical or pathological presentation'. This chapter does not attempt to classify all inherited cardiovascular disease but instead considers specific disease groups to illustrate some of the inherent difficulties in classification and suggest future improvements.

2.1.1 Are You a 'Lumper' or a 'Splitter'?

These terms, first used by Charles Darwin, were introduced into medicine by Victor McKusick, one of the early founders of medical genetics [1]. 'Lumpers' tend to spot similarities between diseases and create phenotypic relationships; early classification systems were often based on lumping, which has proven extremely successful in gene discovery. 'Splitters', on the other hand, focus on the differences between diseases and tend to sub-categorise. The increasing ability of science to identify genetic mutations encourages such reductionism but this creates a problem too: diseases affecting a complex organ such as the heart cannot necessarily be reduced to the level of a single gene mutation. Increasingly—as we will see later—we need to adopt a more (w)holistic approach which explains a phenotype in terms of its major genetic predisposition (for example, a single gene mutation), its modifying genotype and its environmental modifiers. Such an approach has been termed 'organicism' [2].

2.1.2 The Central Paradigm: A Simple Disease Model

First, consider the most straightforward paradigm for an inherited disease. In very simple terms, a disease phenotype occurs as a result of a genetic predisposition in the context of an environment. For inherited cardiovascular diseases, the most conceptually straightforward genetic predisposition is a single gene mutation that significantly impacts on the function of a gene or its product (e.g. a protein); and for many such diseases that predisposing mutation is so significant that it is highly likely to lead to the development of that disease—that is, it is *highly penetrant*. Much of our current knowledge is based on highly penetrant single gene disease; and many of the genes we have come to know and understand were originally identified in large families with multiple cases of disease.

Penetrance may be increased by the presence of a significant environmental modifiers (e.g. diet in someone with familial hypercholesterolaemia) or co-inheritance of a mutation in a different gene (or more than one gene). These 'modifiers' may also give rise to differing expressions of the main predisposing gene mutation ('variable expression') within the same family or between different families, depending on the genetic background of the individuals concerned (a little like the range of interpretations of a symphony using different combinations of conductor and orchestra). It is also becoming clear that some modifiers may *reduce* the penetrance of a disease. As genomic medicine develops over the coming decade, many such modifiers will be identified. Inevitably, without all of this fine detail, classification of inherited disease, and the clinic use of such tools, will be limited.

2.2 Current Classification Systems

In the following sections we will consider three classification systems: classification based on structure, molecular pathway and genetic mechanism. These are frequently difficult to disentangle, however.

2.2.1 Classification Based on Pathology/Anatomy/Physiology

Anatomical classification systems have emerged as the standard starting point, and the attempt to incorporate further reductionist elements (see below) has become challenging.

2.2.1.1 ICD10

The World Health Authority's International Statistical Classification of Diseases and Related Health Problems version 10 (ICD10; WHO 2016 [3])) attempts to classify heart diseases according to anatomy/pathology but this currently lacks the fine detail required for hereditary disease (see Box 2.1). ICD10 is not designed to be a rare disease classification system, however: its use is mainly as a clinical coding system in health care organisations. Future revisions of this system may improve matters, although a separate rare disease classification system is required.

2.2.1.2 Online Inheritance in Man (OMIM)

OMIM started life in the 1960s as a paper-based catalogue of human inherited disease phenotypes and genes (Mendelian Inheritance in Man, MIM) compiled by Dr. Victor McKusick [1, 4]. After 12 subsequent revisions the catalogue was so large that a web-based format was required. OMIM is a carefully curated catalogue of phenotypes and genotypes.

At the time of writing, OMIM has detailed information concerning almost 5000 inherited phenotypes where the genetic cause is known; approximately 1600 phenotypes with unknown cause (including those in which the genetic locus has been localised to a specific chromosomal region but the gene itself has not been identified); 1800 phenotypes thought to have an inherited basis and, in addition, information about more than 15,000 genes.

In general, OMIM catalogue numbers are assigned in sequence based on the date on which the phenotype or gene is described in the literature. So, for example, the entry for hypertrophic cardiomyopathy type 4, 115,197, was created in May 1993, 2 years before the causative gene had been published, at which point the gene was added to OMIM and the two entries linked. Information is added in temporal sequence, with revision if necessary. Each entry is given a code number; those starting with 1 are autosomal dominant, 2 = autosomal recessive; 3 = X-linked. Since May 1994 all entries start with 6.

In a sense, OMIM provides one way of classifying inherited disease, although in reality it is simply a comprehensive catalogue. It records genetic (or, locus) heterogeneity (see Box 2.2a, using the example of hypertrophic cardiomyopathy) and captures all published genetic sub-types of a particular inherited disease. This might suggest a clear relationship between phenotype and gene: in reality, however, the phenotype of, for example, hypertrophic cardiomyopathy is not directly predictable from the genotype in anything other than a general sense.

OMIM also demonstrates that, for mutations in any given gene, a range of phenotypes may present (phenotypic heterogeneity, see Box 2.2b). Some of this variability is caused by genetic and non-genetic modifiers. However, these are generally ill-defined and therefore not catalogued by OMIM. Again, this serves to reinforce the difficulty in using genotype to predict phenotype.

OMIM, while useful as a catalogue, cannot resolve the fundamental challenge in classifying inherited disease by both phenotype and genotype.

2.2.1.3 Sequential Anatomical Classification

The most traditional way of classifying congenital heart malformation (CHM) is in a sequential fashion, starting with the pulmonary veins and ending at the Great Vessels. This commonly used system is well described elsewhere and is entirely based on anatomical description (e.g. IPCCC 2016 [5]). In a sense this represents the work of 'splitters', who sub-classify according to anatomical variation without needing to infer underlying pathophysiology. From a clinical viewpoint, being able to describe, categorise and classify structural defects in great detail is useful because specific anatomical variants may correlate with specific treatments and different surgical outcomes [6].

A relatively small but significant proportion of CHM arises as the result of an underlying single genetic mutation. In some cases this mutation is inherited from an affected parent and in others the mutation appears to arise *de novo*. CHM may therefore present as familial or sporadic 'single gene' disease. Most sporadic CHM, however, appears to be the result of a more complex multigenic mechanism which remains poorly understood. This chapter focuses on single gene disease.

Further, CHM can present as a single malformation in an otherwise normal individual or may be part of a more complex set of problems affecting other elements of the heart and/or other organ systems. It has become standard practice, therefore, to describe CHMs as either 'isolated' or 'syndromic'.

Familial CHM is a challenge to classify accurately at present. In some families the phenotype breeds true so that affected relatives who share the same pathogenic gene mutation develop the same CHM. However, this is not always the case: in some families, relatives with the same gene mutation develop apparently different CHMs (phenotypic heterogeneity). This is likely to reflect the presence of modifying factors or chance. The complexity of genetic and phenotypic heterogeneity is illustrated in Boxes 2.3a, 2.3b, 2.3c, and 2.3d.

Sequential anatomical classification can be extended to all ICCs (Table 2.1) although, as we will see, not all ICCs have an anatomical phenotype. Classification based on anatomy alone is therefore limited.

2.2.2 Classification Based on Genetic Mechanism

CHM provides a relatively straightforward example of the way in which diseases can be classified according to the underlying genetic mechanism (Box 2.4). Hereditary CHMs—whether isolated or present as part of a wider malformation syndrome—can be cause by a range of different mutational mechanisms but there is rarely a useful correlation between the precise mechanism and the phenotype; the most obvious exception is 'contiguous gene deletion' (also known as microdeletion), in which a block of genes is deleted from a chromosome and where the overall phenotype is related to the size of the deletion and therefore the specific genes deleted.

The same spectrum of genetic mechanisms can be associated with any ICC. Some mechanisms are more common in particular settings: for example, although contiguous gene deletion in relatively common in syndromic CHM, it is rare in autosomal dominant hypertrophic cardiomyopathy where single nucleotide mutation is the norm.

In isolation, the mutational mechanism is not a helpful way to classify ICDs, although, as we will see later, it does form part of a broader classification system.

Table 2.1 Sequential anatomical classification of inherited cardiovascular conditions

Site	Congenital malformation	Electrical disease	Heart muscle disease	Aneurysm/dissection
Atria	Atrial isomerism	Familial atrial standstill	–	–
	Atrial septal defect (primum/ secundum)	Sick sinus syndrome		
		Familial atrial fibrillation		
Atrioventricular junction	Atrioventricular septal defect	Congenital heart block	–	–
	Mitral valve prolapse	Familial progressive heart block		
	Hypoplastic left heart spectrum			
	Tricuspid atresia			
Ventricle	Ventricular septal defect	Short QT syndrome	Hypertrophic cardiomyopathy	–
	Hypoplastic left heart spectrum	Long QT syndrome	Dilated cardiomyopathy	
	Epstein anomaly	Catecholaminergic polymorphic VT	Arrhythmogenic cardiomyopathy	
		Brugada syndrome		
	Tetralogy of Fallot	Familial ventricular fibrillation	Restrictive cardiomyopathy	
			Left ventricular non-compaction cardiomyopathy	

Ventriculoarterial junction	Bicuspid aortic valve/aortic stenosis	–	–	–
	Supravalvar aortic stenosis			
	Hypoplastic left heart spectrum			
	Pulmonary stenosis			
Great Arteries	Transposition of the Great Arteries	–	–	Familial thoracic aortic aneurysm/dissection
	Patent ductus arteriosus			Marfan syndrome
				Beal syndrome
	Coarctation of the aorta			Ehlers Danlos syndrome
				Loeys Dietz syndrome

This list is not intended to be exhaustive. Many other congenital malformations are reported as apparently sporadic events. This table focuses on key reported *familial* phenotypes

2.2.3 Classification Based on Molecular Pathway

Such a system provides broad classification based on current understanding of common underlying pathophysiology.

2.2.3.1 Ion Channelopathy

One class of ICCs that generally appears to fit a simple classification system, at least superficially, is 'ion channelopathy'. Most of the founder members of this classification system were originally identified through electrophysiological experiments that revealed specific perturbations in transmembrane ion currents that had been known about for years before the advent of molecular genetics.

Thus, the commonest forms of Long QT syndrome (LQTS), now termed types 1 and 2, associated with abnormalities in the outward I_{Ks} and I_{Kr} currents respectively, were explained by mutations in major subunits of the cardiac *potassium* ion channel (*KCNQ1* [previously named *KVLQT1*] and *KCNH2* [*HERG*]). Additional cardiac potassium ion channelopathies were subsequently identified, each corresponding to a known electrophysiological abnormality and encoding a component of the potassium ion channel (Box 2.5a).

More recently, a number of rarer phenotypes have also been linked to mutations in the same potassium ion channel genes. Short QT syndrome and familial atrial fibrillation, for example, are both associated with *activating* mutations in *KCNQ1* and *KCNH2*, whereas Long QT syndrome is associated with *inactivating* mutations. This broadens the concept of a cardiac potassium ion channelopathy to the point where the phenotypes are so different that simple classification based on ion channel alone becomes limited.

A similar situation exists for type 3 long QT syndrome (LQTS3), which can be classified as a cardiac *sodium* channelopathy, caused by mutations in the *SCN5A* gene; a phenotypically distinct disorder, Brugada syndrome, is also associated—in about 20% of cases—with mutations in the same gene. Both disorders are therefore 'alleleic' (caused by mutations in the same gene) but their phenotypic difference is explained in the majority of cases by the fact that LQTS3 is associated with activating mutations in *SCN5A* whereas Brugada syndrome is associated with inactivating mutations. In some rare families, this dichotomous classification doesn't work, however, and both phenotypes can manifest in different members of the same family. Further molecular causes of Brugada syndrome have now been described (Box 2.5b).

While long QT syndrome might once have been considered a sodium and potassium ion channelopathy, and Brugada syndrome a sodium channelopathy, these simple classifications can no longer be used now that the full extent of genetic heterogeneity is being revealed by modern research. Likewise, catecholaminergic polymorphic ventricular tachycardia (CPVT) initially appeared to fall neatly into a class of cardiac *calcium* channelopathies. A more appropriate class might now be termed 'excitation-contraction coupling defect', although even this is not an exclusive category. Mutations in some, but not all, of the genes encoding components of the cardiac L-type calcium channel have been associated with inherited arrhythmia syndromes quite separate from CPVT (Box 2.5c).

Overall, ion channelopathies present us with a challenge: resolving down to the level of the specific ion channel gene mutation is acceptable as a general cataloguing system—this is one example of a system that initially made a great deal of sense as the initial molecular genetic data emerged in the 1990s—however, for such a system to be useful in clinical practice it is perhaps more helpful to consider both the underlying genetic mechanism (which may tell us something about therapy) *and* the phenotype (which tells us about arrhythmia risk).

2.2.3.2 Familial Cardiomyopathy

No-where is the need for a combined pathway/phenotype classification more essential than in the huge range of phenotypes collectively known as cardiomyopathy. Anatomical division into hypertrophic, dilated, restrictive, arrhythmogenic (etc.,) is possible. Mapping such an anatomical/pathological classification onto the underlying genetic mechanism reveals the enormous complexity of this group of diseases, however.

Familial Hypertrophic Cardiomyopathy (fHCM)

This is perhaps the archetypal inherited heart muscle disease. In the early molecular era, fHCM was considered to be a set of inherited diseases of the cardiac *sarcomere*: initial linkage and candidate gene studies of large, well-characterised families revealed mutations in the genes encoding the major protein components of the cardiac sarcomeric complex (*MYH7*, *TNNT2*, *MYBPC3*). Over the past 20 years, many more families have been described with autosomal dominant mutations in other genes encoding sarcomeric protein components. Furthermore, as with almost every other genetic disorder, more recent studies have also identified mutations in genes encoding *non-sarcomeric* proteins in families affected with fHCM.

Mimics may also give rise to a cardiac hypertrophy phenotype ('phenocopies'). For example, cardiac hypertrophy is common in lysosomal storage diseases such as Anderson-Fabry disease and Danon disease; infiltrative disorders such as cardiac amyloidosis, often familial; and defects in the RAS/MAP kinase signalling pathway (e.g. Noonan syndrome). However, in reality, it is often possible to distinguish between these on clinical grounds, based on imaging findings, biochemical testing and/or clinical history, without the need to resort to genetic testing.

The different genetic sub-types of fHCM are catalogued by OMIM as 'CMHX'; it is also clear, however, that considerable phenotypic heterogeneity exists for mutation in any given sarcomeric protein gene (Boxes 2.2a, and 2.2b). So, not all fHCM is sarcomeric disease and not all sarcomeric disease is fHCM.

Heterogeneity in Dilated Cardiomyopathy: Multiple Molecular Mechanisms

The challenge we have seen with arrhythmia syndromes and fHCM is compounded in familial *dilated* cardiomyopathy (fDCM) . Box 2.6a illustrates the considerable genetic heterogeneity of fDCM. For many of the genes so far found to be implicated there are robust data linking definite pathogenic mutation to familial disease. For some, data are less strong but two key principles emerge from our current state of knowledge: (1) that defects in a wide range of different molecular systems can result in fDCM and (2) that fDCM is not the only phenotypic consequence of mutation in a single gene. In fact, for some genes (e.g. *PSN1&2*) the consequences can be very different). In a sense this is no different to other examples presented in this chapter, but in the case of fDCM, is perhaps more marked. Contractile failure of heart muscle is a non-specific end-point for many diseases that have no discriminating features.

Although natural history data are limited across all sub-types (some of the sub-types in Box 2.6a are restricted to a single family or a very small number of families), this tends to be an adult onset disorder with variable outcome. Classifying fDCM by mechanism is on the whole meaningless at present from a clinical viewpoint, except for those with other potential cardiac or non-cardiac complications. In such cases there may be discriminating clinical features which may highlight a specific diagnosis, for example:

Laminopathy

The lamin protein is a large protein located just inside the nuclear membrane and part of a complex network of interacting proteins. It has many different functions, both structural and non-structural. Many mutations have been described along the entire length of the *LMNA* gene; these result in a wide range of very different phenotypes (see Box 2.6b; see also [7]). The exact phenotype depends very much on the location of the mutation and the impact this has on not only the structure of lamin but also its specific and multiple interactions with other proteins. Dilated cardiomyopathy is generally associated with missense mutations in exons 1–3 which affected the head and early rod domains, although the precise effects on protein function remain poorly understood.

LMNA-related fDCM is also associated with cardiac arrhythmias and conduction defects, the presence of which in someone with DCM (or an affected relative) should suggest the diagnosis; this is one sub-type of familial DCM with additional therapeutic implications beyond the management of heart failure.

In Emery-Dreifuss muscular dystrophy (type 2 and 3), similar cardiac problems occur in addition to a slowly progressive skeletal muscle disorder characterised by contractures and muscle weakness. Mutations in most parts of *LMNA* have been reported in these patients: in EDMD type 2 these appear to result in partial or complete loss of function. The practical implication of this is that individuals with *LMNA*-related fDCM should be assessed for skeletal muscle problems.

So, in keeping with observations elsewhere in this chapter, *LMNA* mutations do not all result in fDCM and only a fraction of all cases of fDCM is the result of *LMNA* mutation. Stating that someone has a *LMNA* mutation must be qualified by a description of the phenotype, which cannot always be predicted from the underlying genotype.

Titinopathy

Titin is a large protein expressed in cardiac and skeletal muscle that spans from Z line to M line with a critical role in sarcomere structure and function. It therefore comes as no great surprise that mutations in the *TTN* gene cause a number of different phenotypes (Box 2.6c), but unlike laminopathies, titinopathies appear to only cause diseases of skeletal and cardiac muscle.

Limb Girdle Muscular Dystrophies (LGMD)

DCM can occur in association with progressive muscle weakness involving limb girdle muscles; there are many different genetic subtypes of LGMD, often with specific discriminating clinical or imaging features. From a mechanistic/classification viewpoint these disorders are usually (but not always) the result of mutations in gene encoding components of the dystrophin/glycoprotein complex or sarcomere. Again, classification by molecular pathway/mechanism is not straight-forward and is beyond the scope of this chapter. Two key principles have emerged over the past 20 years of research, however:

(1) Mutations in some genes that cause LGMD may also cause DCM without features of LGMD (e.g. *SGD* [OMIM 601411; LGMD type 2F and DCM type 1 L] and *FKTN* (OMIM 697440; LGMD type 2 M and DCM type 1X]) and
(2) DCM (and cardiac arrhythmia) may occur in a number of different sub-types of LGMD. The clinical consequences are discussed elsewhere and summarised well by Norwood et al. [8].

Metabolic Disorders

A number of DCM-associated mutations are found in genes whose role is primarily metabolic. From a mechanistic viewpoint it is not difficult to imagine that failure of energy production can result in failure of an energy-dependent organ. As with LGMD, the two key principles are:

(1) Mutations in some genes that cause a metabolic phenotype may also rarely cause DCM in isolation (e.g. a homozygous *SDHA* mutation reported in a single Bedouin tribe in which 15 individuals had developed childhood-onset DCM [OMIM 600857.0004) and
(2) DCM may occur in a number of different inherited metabolic diseases characterised by impaired cellular energy production (e.g. Barth syndrome) and mitochondrial DNA disorders [e.g. the common point mutation m.8344A > G; see Bates et al. 2012 [9]].

Right Ventricular Cardiomyopathy and Desmosomal Diseases

The archetypal ICC under this category is known as arrhythmogenic right ventricular cardiomyopathy (ARVC), also known as dysplasia (ARVD). Both terms are still used in the literature. Debate exists about the precise terminology, however: cardiomyopathy is a simple pathological description whereas dysplasia (defined as an abnormal development of cells, tissues or organs) makes an assumption about the underlying mechanism that should be avoided until proven.

In addition, the correlation between phenotype and the underlying highly penetrant predisposing genotype is not always predictable: involvement of the left ventricle is commonly seen, even in the same family in which right-dominant disease is more typical, giving rise to biventricular or even left-dominant cardiomyopathy [10, 11]. These clearly cannot be classified as ARVC; the modifying factors have yet to be identified. For the moment, a broader classification term such as 'arrhythmogenic cardiomyopathy' is probably better to use.

Many cases of arryhthmogenic cardiomyopathy appear to be caused by germline mutations in genes encoding components of the cardiac desmosome, a multi-protein cell adhesion complex. This has given rise to the term 'desmosomal disease', which has been considered almost synonymous with 'ARVC'. Classification of arrhythmogenic cardiomyopathy as a purely desmosomal disease is not appropriate, however, since families have been described—albeit uncommonly—with germ line mutations in other genes. At least 4 different families have been described in which ARVC has been associated with mutations in specific conserved regions of the *RYR2* gene [12]; several families have been reported with mutations affecting the *TMEM43* gene [13]. This encodes a nuclear envelope protein; there are some data to suggest that—for at least one of the reported mutations, expression of plakoglobin appears to be reduced in such patients, suggesting that although *TMEM43* is not a desmosomal protein it may be involved in desmosomal biology in some way. In addition, mutations affecting the regulatory elements of the *TGFB3* gene (and apparently up-regulating TGFβ3 signalling activity) have been reported in two families with ARVC [14].

Interestingly, since many of the cardiac desmosomal proteins involved in arrhythmogenic cardiomyopathy are also expressed in the skin and hair, mutations in desmosomal protein genes are also known to cause hereditary primary skin disorders (e.g. palmoplantar keratoderma, PPK) and overlap syndromes with cardiomyopathy, skin and hair phenotypes (e.g. Naxos disease ['ARVC plus' and Carvajal disease ['dilated cardiomyopathy-plus']). This complexity is summarised in Box 2.7b.

So, not all arrhythmogenic cardiomyopathy is ARVC; not all ARVC is caused by desmosomal gene mutations and not all desmosomal gene mutations cause a pure cardiac phenotype. This current complexity is a challenge to resolve: ultimately, as we have seen elsewhere, an individual patient is best classified by both genotype and phenotype.

Familial Thoracic Aneurysm/Dissection

Until comparatively recently, familial clustering of thoracic aortic aneurysm and/or dissection (TAAD) remained unexplained. Marfan syndrome had been described in the late 1800s and was considered to be the major cause of 'genetic' thoracic aortic *aneurysm* until the 2000s; by contrast, vascular Ehlers Danlos syndrome (vEDS) was considered to be the major cause of 'genetic' aortic *dissection*. It proved difficult to reconcile the fact that both of these 'exemplar' conditions are associated with a range of extra-cardiovascular phenotypic features, against the observation that many families affected by TAAD display no additional features.

In time, a number of clearly autosomal dominant gene mutations associated with 'non-syndromic' TAAD were identified. In some families the genes involved would, in other families, cause syndromic disease. This degree of variable expression is so far unexplained but not entirely unexpected. One common theme is, however, emerging: in most of the familial forms of TAAD there appears to be dysregulation of the transforming growth factor-beta (TGFβ) signalling pathway, initially described in animal models of Marfan syndrome [15] and now reported more widely [16]. Disordered TGFβ signalling is associated with ultrastructural changes in the aortic media, leading to tissue failure and the characteristic histological feature known as 'cystic medial degeneration' (not restricted to Marfan syndrome).

It is therefore possible to classify familial TAAD according to the specific molecular defect in the canonical TGFβ signalling pathway (Box 2.8a) This is potentially helpful from a therapeutic point of view, since pharmacological manipulation of TGFβ signalling using angiotensin receptor blockers appears to correct or stabilise the underlying ultrastructural changes in the aortic media and reduce the risk of aortic aneurysm in at least one form of familial TAAD, raising the possibility that this intervention may be successful in other members of the same class of disease [17].

Classification is, however, problematic. For example, OMIM has catalogued a number of FTAAD sub-types (known as AAT sub-types): some are caused by genes currently known to be involved in TGFβ signalling, whereas others are caused by genes whose role is currently less certain. Furthermore, the OMIM 'AAT' classification does not overlap completely with the Loeys Dietz syndromes, which themselves are caused by mutations in genes known to be involved in TGFβ signalling. In addition to these two classifications, it is worth noting the large number of other inherited conditions known to be associated with TAAD, not least of which are in fact Marfan syndrome and vascular Ehlers Danlos syndrome. For many of the additional diseases, the underlying molecular defect is known but the association with dysregulated TGFβ signalling is not clear.

At present, no single classification system appears to work well, although in time it may be possible to resolve familial TAAD into a set of closely related 'TGFβ signallopathies' once the molecular defect is known. However, the range of phenotypes associated with mutations in individual genes in the same pathway—both syndromic and non-syndromic—is likely to confound a simple classification system.

2.3 The Future: Combining Classification Systems

In reality, all of the above classification systems have limitations, depending on the context in which they are being used. For example, in the early days of gene discovery it was acceptable to classify disease by the most likely underlying genetic mechanism: for example, fHCM as sarcomeric protein disease. From the point of view of identifying novel therapies, classification based on molecular pathway is important, as is increasingly the case with FTAAD.

In clinical practice, each individual member of an ICC family often requires a combination of systems to allow for the fact that, at any given time, different members of the same family may be manifesting in different ways. Indeed, with the advent of cascade genetic testing we commonly identify people who carry a single highly penetrant gene mutation without apparent phenotypic effect. It might be possible to give an overall 'ball-park' diagnosis, qualified by additional information that describes the individuals person's specific phenotype and modifiers. This will become increasingly important in years to come. Figure 2.1 illustrates this with examples of fHCM, long QT syndrome and FTAAD.

Fig. 2.1 Combined classification of inherited cardiovascular conditions in clinical practice. *The following pedigree is an imaginary family in which a 25 year-old male (II:2) is found to have an ICC. The challenge is now to classify his relatives' phenotypes to allow for variable penetrance and expression. In this figure, precise gene mutations are entirely fictitious and designed to illustrate principles. Example 1: familial hypertrophic cardiomyopathy. II:2 presents with an out-of-hospital cardiac arrest from which he is successfully resuscitated and is found to have classical HCM. He has a paternally-derived pathogenic mutation in the MYBPC3 gene and a maternally-derived genetic modifier in the ACE gene. II:2 might best be described as: ICC diagnosis familial hypertrophic cardiomyopathy. Phenotype (1) severe asymmetric septal hypertrophy with LVOT obstruction. (2) systolic anterior motion of mitral valve. (3) non-sustained VT. (4) previous VF cardiac arrest. Inheritance (autosomal dominant). Major genotype. c. 2364A > G MYBPC3 pathogenic mutation (pat). Modifiers (1) rs4746279 ACE polymorphism (mat). (2) essential hypertension. His father (I:2) has a milder phenotype: ICC diagnosis (familial hypertrophic cardiomyopathy).*

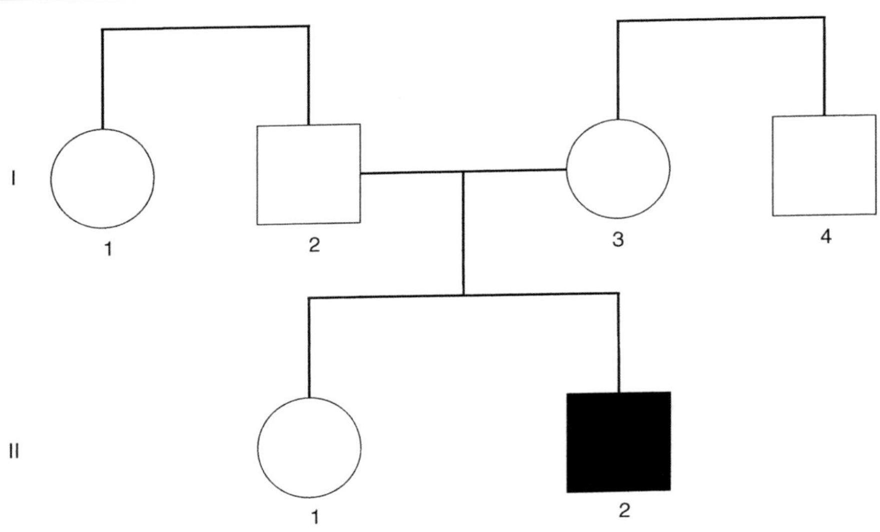

Phenotype (mild asymmetric septal hypertrophy (IVSd 18 mm)). Inheritance (autosomal dominant). Major genotype (c. 2364A > G MYBPC3 pathogenic mutation (origin unknown)). Modifiers (none). Example 2: long QT syndrome. II:2 presents with an out-of-hospital cardiac arrest while swimming from which he is successfully resuscitated and is subsequently found to have long QT syndrome. He has a maternally-derived pathogenic mutation in the KCNQ1 gene and a paternally-derived genetic modifier in the QTMOD gene. II:1 might best be described as: ICC diagnosis (long QT syndrome). Phenotype (1) out of hospital cardiac arrest. (2) recurrent Torsades de Pointes. (3) QTc > 580 ms. Inheritance (autosomal dominant). Major genotype (c. 1234delCC KCNQ1 pathogenic mutation (mat)). Modifiers (1) rs4746279 QTMOD polymorphism (pat). (2) corrected hypokalaemia. (3) nadolol. (4) implantable cardiac defibrillator. As is commonly found, I:3 has a normal ECG at rest: ICC diagnosis (long QT syndrome). Phenotype (normal QTc). Inheritance (autosomal dominant). Major genotype (c. 1234delCC KCNQ1 pathogenic mutation (origin unknown)). Modifiers (amitryptiline stopped). Example 3: familial thoracic aortic aneurysm. II:2 collapses after a rugby match and at hospital is found to have a thoracic aortic dissection arising in an aneurysmal sinus of Valsalva. As a child he had a cleft lip and palate repair. He has a paternally-derived pathogenic mutation in the TGFBR2 gene. II:2 might best be described as: ICC diagnosis (Loeys-Dietz syndrome type 2). Phenotype (1) thoracic aortic aneurysm/dissection. (2) cleft lip and palate (repaired). Inheritance (autosomal dominant). Major genotype (c. 321 delCCinsTTGG TGFBR2 pathogenic mutation (pat)). Modifiers (1) corrected hypertension (irbesartan). (2) valve-sparing aortic root replacement. On screening with echocardiography and magnetic resonance angiography, I:2 is classified as: ICC diagnosis (Loeys Dietz syndrome type 2). Phenotype (1) dilated aortic root (Z score + 4.5, sinuses of Valsalva). (2) splenic artery aneurysm (Z score + 4.0). Inheritance (autosomal dominant). Major genotype (c. 321 delCCinsTTGG TGFBR2 pathogenic mutation (origin unknown)). Modifiers (irbesartan). On similar screening, II:1 has a normal aorta: ICC diagnosis Loeys Dietz syndrome type 2. Phenotype (normal arterial system on whole body MRA). Inheritance (autosomal dominant). Major genotype (c. 321 delCCinsTTGG TGFBR2 pathogenic mutation (pat)). Modifiers (none)

2.4 Summary

There are many ways of classifiying ICCs, depending to some extent on your viewpoint as either a researcher or a clinician. Genetic and phenotypic heterogeneity remain challenging to classify and, as the genetic basis of each of the ICCs expands to include new genes and genetic modifiers, current classification models will fail to capture the evolving complexity. Ultimately, however, a clinician's starting point is always to describe the phenotype—after all, this usually predicts the patient's prognosis more accurately than genetics at present for most ICCs. Having done that, each individual patient can be classified using additional information, some of which will be clinical and some genetic. Such a combined approach (the organism of Gilbert & Sarkar [2]) will become essential as we move into an new era of personalised, genomic medicine.

Box 2.1 ICD10 version 2016 classification of cardiomyopathy

Section	Phenotype
I42.0	Dilated cardiomyopathy
I42.1	Obstructive hypertrophic cardiomyopathy
I42.2	Non-obstructive hypertrophic cardiomyopathy
I42.3	Endomyocardial (eosinophilic) disease
I42.4	Endocardial fibroelastosis
I42.5	Other restrictive cardiomyopathy
I42.6	Alcoholic cardiomyopathy
I42.7	Cardiomyopathy due to drugs and other external agents
I42.8	Other cardiomyopathy
I42.9	Cardiomyopathy, unspecified
I43.1	Cardiomyopathy in metabolic disease
	Cardiac amyloidosis
E85.2	Heredofamilial amyloidosis, unspecified
E75.2	Other sphingolipidosis
	Includes Fabry disease

Section	Phenotype
Q87.1	Congential malformation syndromes predominantly associated with short stature
	Includes Noonan syndrome

ICD10 is not designed as a stand-alone classification system for hereditary disease; as a result, it does not enable fine sub-classification. Indeed, many rare diseases are excluded from ICD10 (in this case, Danon disease, a rare X-linked lysosomal storage disease associated with cardiac hypertrophy). Rarer causes of hypertrophic cardiomyopathy such as Fabry disease or Noonan syndrome, are not classified in section I42. Furthermore, sub-classification of hypertrophic cardiomyopathy into obstructive and non-obstructive implies that they are different disease, whereas in reality they lie on the same spectrum

Source: http://apps.who.int/classifications/icd10/browse/2010/en#/I42 accessed 27.04.2017

Box 2.2a Genetic heterogeneity in hypertrophic cardiomyopathy: online inheritance in man classification

OMIM phenotype	OMIM number	Gene	Protein	Protein function
CMH1	192,600	*MYH7*	β myosin heavy chain 7	Sarcomeric contractile protein
CMH2	115,195	*TNNT2*	Troponin T2	Sarcomeric thin filament component
CMH3	115,196	*TPM1*	Tropomyosin	Actin-binding myofibrillar protein
CMH4	115,197	*MYBPC3*	Myosin binding protein C3	Sarcomeric protein
CMH5	*No longer used*[a]			
CMH6	600,858	*PRKAG2*	Protein kinase, AMP-activated, noncatalytic, gamma-2	AMP-activated protein kinase
CMH7	613,690	*TNNI3*	Troponin I3	Actin-binding myofibrillar protein
CMH8	608,751	*MYL3*	Ventricular myosin light chain 3	Sarcomeric contractile protein
CMH9	188,840	*TTN*	Titin	Structural and tensile sarcomeric protein
CMH10	160,781	*MYL2*	Cardiac myosin light chain 2	Sarcomeric contractile protein

OMIM phenotype	OMIM number	Gene	Protein	Protein function
CMH11	612,098	*ACTC1*	Cardiac α-actin	Sarcomeric contractile protein
CMH12	612,124	*CSRP3*	Cysteine- and glycine-rich protein 3	Cardiomyocyte stretch sensor protein
CMH13	613,243	*TNNC1*	Troponin C	Actin-binding myofibrillar protein
CMH14	613,251	*MYH6*	α myosin heavy chain 6	Sarcomeric protein
CMH15	613,255	*VCL*	Vinculin	Cell junction protein
CMH16	613,838	*MYOZ2*	Myozenin-2	Regulator of calcineurin
CMH17	613,873	*JPH2*	Junctophilin-2	Plasma membrane: endoplasmic reticulum junction protein
CMH18	613,874	*PLN*	Phospholamban	Regulator of intracellular calcium
CMH19	613,875	*CALR3*	Calreticulin 3	Calcium-binding chaperone
CMH20	613,876	*NEXN*	Nexilin F-actin-binding protein 3	Filamentous actin
CMH21	614,676	7p21.2-q21	–	
CMH22	615,248[d]	*MYPN*	Myopalladin	Structural sarcomeric protein
CMH23	612,158	*ACTN2*	Actinin α-2	Actin-binding structural sarcomeric protein
CMH24	601,493	*LDB3*	LIM domain-binding protein 3	Structural sarcomeric protein
CMH25	607,487	*TCAP*	Titin-cap	Structural sarcomeric protein
CMH26	617,047	*FLNC*	Filamin C	Actin-binding structural sarcomeric protein
Fabry disease[b]	301,500	*GLA*	α-galactosidase	Lysosomal enzyme
Danon disease[b]	300,257	*LAMP2*	Lysosome-associated membrane protein 2	Lyosomal membrane glycopotein
Noonan syndrome[b]	163,950	Multiple	See OMIM entry	RAS/MAP kinase signalling proteins

OMIM phenotype	OMIM number	Gene	Protein	Protein function
CMH1, digenic	192,600	*MYLK2*	Myosin light chain kinase 2	Regulator of myosin light chain
CMH, unclassified	192,600	*CAV3*	Caveolin 3	Component of dystrophin-glycoprotein complex
Cardiomyopathy, hypertrophic	590,035[c]	*MTTG*	Mitochondrial glycine transfer RNA	Transfer RNA
Cardiomyopathy with or without skeletal myopathy	590,050[c]	*MTTI*	Mitochondrial isoleucine transfer RNA	Transfer RNA

OMIM refers to this as Cardiomyopathy, Familial Hypertrophic (CMH)

Notes

[a]CMH 5 is no longer used. The original family on which this annotation was based was found to have both MYH7 and MYBPC3 mutations, once genetic analysis was possible

[b]Fabry disease, Danon disease and Noonan syndrome are not primarily classified as cardiomyopathy syndromes; rather, they all feature HCM as a phenotypic manifestation in some individuals

[c]590,035 and 590,050 are not phenotypic codes but gene codes, denoting mitochondrial tRNA genes. Phenotypes associated with mutations in these genes are broad and varied; cardiomyopathy is the presenting feature in some families

[d]615,248 represents a single large published Northern American family in which genetic linkage analysis localised the gene to chromosome 7; the identity of the gene itself has not yet been reported

Box 2.2b Phenotypic heterogeneity: consequence of sarcomeric protein gene mutations using OMIM classification

Gene	Phenotype	OMIM number
MYH7	Hypertrophic cardiomyopathy 1	192,600
	Dilated cardiomyopathy type 1S	613,426
	Left ventricular non-compaction type 5	613,426
	Laing distal myopathy	160,500
	Myosin storage myopathy, autosomal dominant	608,358
	Myosin storage myopathy, autosomal recessive	255,160
	Scapuloperoneal syndrome, myopathic type	181,430
TNNT2	Hypertrophic cardiomyopathy 2	115,195
	Dilated cardiomyopathy type 1D	601,494
	Left ventricular non-compaction type 6	601,494
	Restrictive cardiomyopathy type 3	612,422

Gene	Phenotype	OMIM number
TPM1	Hypertrophic cardiomyopathy 3	611,878
	Dilated cardiomyopathy type 1Y	115,196
	Left ventricular non-compaction type 9	611,878
MYBPC3	Hypertrophic cardiomyopathy 4	115,197
	Dilated cardiomyopathy type 1MM	615,396
	Left ventricular non-compaction type 10	615,396
PRKAG2	Hypertrophic cardiomyopathy 6	600,858
	Wolf Parkinson White syndrome	194,200
	Congenital lethal cardiac glycogen storage disease	261,740
TNNI3	Hypertrophic cardiomyopathy type 7	613,690
	Dilated cardiomyopathy type 1FF	613,286
	Restrictive cardiomyopathy type 1	115,210
MYL3	Hypertrophic cardiomyopathy type 8	608,751
TTN	Hypertrophic cardiomyopathy type 9	613,765
	Dilated cardiomyopathy type 1G	604,145
	Limb girdle muscular dystrophy 2J	608,807
	Tibial muscular dystrophy	600,334
	Early onset myopathy with cardiomyopathy	611,705
	Proximal myopathy with early respiratory involvement	603,689
MYL2	Hypertrophic cardiomyopathy type 10	608,758

Reported cardiac and non-cardiac phenotypes associated with mutations in genes which encode sarcomeric proteins. This table presents data corresponding to the genes responsible for the first 9 catalogued OMIM hypertrophic cardiomyopathy sub-types

Note: hypertrophic cardiomyopathy type 5 is a redundant term (see note 1 Box 2.2a)

Source: Online Mendelian Inheritance in Man, OMIM®. McKusick-Nathans Institute of Genetic Medicine, Johns Hopkins University (Baltimore, MD), {accessed 27.04.2017}. World Wide Web URL: https://omim.org/

Box 2.3a Heterogeneity in non-syndromic *secundum*-type atrial septal defect

OMIM type	OMIM number	Gene/ locus	Protein	Protein function
ASD1	108,800	5p	–	–
ASD2	607,941	*GATA4*	GATA-binding protein 4	Transcription factor
ASD3	614,089	*MYH6*	α-myosin heavy chain	Sarcomeric contractile protein
ASD4	611,363	*TBX20*	T-box 20	Transcription factor
ASD5	612,794	*ACTC1*	α-cardiac actin	Sarcomeric contractile protein
ASD6[a]	613,087	*TLL1*	Tolloid-like 1	Metalloprotease
ASD7	108,900	*NKX2.5*	NK2 homeobox 2	Transcription factor

OMIM type	OMIM number	Gene/ locus	Protein	Protein function
ASD8	614,433	*CITED2*	CBP-interacting transactivator 2	Transcription factor
ASD9	614,475	*GATA6*	GATA-binding protein 6	Transcription factor

As we have seen in Box 2.2a in the context of cardiomyopathy, atrial septal defects caused by highly penetrant single gene mutations are also characterised by genetic heterogeneity; as in Box 2.2b, mutations in ASD genes can present with a range of different phenotypes Note that many—but not all—of the genes implicated in ASD encode transcription factors that regulate expression of other genes

[a]Missense mutations reported in isolated cases

Other phenotypes associated with mutations in selected genes

Gene	OMIM phenotype	OMIM number
GATA4	Atrioventricular septal defect type 4	614,430
	Ventricular septal defect type 1	614,429
	Tetralogy of Fallot	187,500
NKX2.5	Ventricular septal defect type 3	614,432
	Tetralogy of Fallot	187,500
	Hypoplastic left heart syndrome type 2	614,435
	Conotruncal malformations	217,095
	Congenital hypothyroidism type 5	225,250
GATA6	Atrioventricular septal defect type 9	614,474
	Tetraology of Fallot	187,500
	Persistent truncus arteriosus	217,095
	Pancreatic agenesis with CHM	600,001

Box 2.3b Heterogeneity in non-syndromic *primum*-type atrial septal defect/ atrioventricular septal defect

OMIM type	OMIM number	Gene/ locus	Protein	Protein function
AVSD1	606,215	1p31-p21	–	–
AVSD 2	606,217	*CRELD1*	Cysteine-rich protein with EGF-like domains	Cell adhesion?
AVSD 3	600,309	*GJA1*	Gap junction protein 1 (connexin 43)	Cell adhesion
AVSD 4	600,576	*GATA4*	GATA-binding protein 4	Transcription factor
AVSD 5	614,474	*GATA6*	GATA-binding protein 6	Transcription factor

OMIM type	OMIM number	Gene/ locus	Protein	Protein function
AVSD 6	601,656	18q11	–	–

Other phenotypes associated with *GJA1* mutations (see Box 2.3a for *GATA4* & *GATA6*)

OMIM phenotype	OMIM number
Hypoplastic left heart syndrome type 1	241,550
Oculodentodigital dysplasia (dominant)	164,200
Oculodentodigital dysplasia (recessive)	257,850
Syndactyly type 3	186,100
Craniometaphyseal dysplasia (recessive)	218,400
Palmoplantar keratoderma with alopecia	104,100
Erythrokeratoderma variabilis et progressiva	133,200

Box 2.3c Heterogeneity in familial ventricular septal defect

OMIM type[a]	OMIM number	Gene/ locus[b]	Protein	Protein function
VSD1	614,429	*GATA4*	GATA-binding protein 4	Transcription factor
VSD2	614,431	*CITED2*	CBP-interacting transactivator 2	Transcription factor
VSD3	614,432	*NKX2.5*	NK2 homeobox 2	Transcription factor

[a]There are fewer reported familial sub-types of VSD. Familial clustering of a common heart defect may simply represent chance rather than Mendelian disease

[b]Note also that none of these genes are exclusively associated with VSD—all have differing phenotypic manifestations

Box 2.3d Heterogeneity in tetralogy of fallot

OMIM type	OMIM number	Gene/ locus	Protein	Protein function
Tetralogy of Fallot	187,500	*GATA4*	GATA-binding protein 4	Transcription factor
Tetralogy of Fallot	187,500	*GATA6*	GATA-binding protein 6	Transcription factor
Tetralogy of Fallot	187,500	*NKX2.5*	NK2 homeobox 2	Transcription factor
Tetralogy of Fallot	187,500	*ZFPM2*	Zinc finger protein, multi-type 2	Modulator of GATA4
Tetralogy of Fallot	187,500	*GDF1*	Growth/differentiation factor 1	Transcription factor

OMIM type	OMIM number	Gene/ locus	Protein	Protein function
Tetralogy of Fallot	187,500	*JAG1*	JAGGED 1	Ligand of NOTCH receptor
Tetralogy of Fallot	187,500	*TBX1*	T-box 1	Transcription factor

Source: Online Mendelian Inheritance in Man, OMIM®. McKusick-Nathans Institute of Genetic Medicine, Johns Hopkins University (Baltimore, MD), {accessed 27.04.2017}. World Wide Web URL: https://omim.org/

[a]OMIM does not sub-classify this entry

[b]*GDF1* appears to play a role in left-right differentiation; mutations in this gene are also associated with double outlet right ventricle, right atrial isomerism and transposition of the Great Arteries

Box 2.4 Classification of Congenital Heart Malformation by underlying genetic mechanism

Anatomical sub-classification	Genetic mechanism[a]	Complexity	Example	OMIM reference
	Simple	Isolated	Familial atrioventricular septal defect	606,215
		Syndromic	Down syndrome	–
Primum	Complex	Isolated	Sporadic primum ASD	–
		Syndromic	–	–
Secundum	Simple	Isolated	Familial ASD	108,800
		Syndromic	Holt Oram syndrome	142,900
	Complex	Isolated	Sporadic ASD	–
		Syndromic	Fetal alcohol syndrome	

[a]Mechanisms:

Example: ASD atrial septal defect

Simple: highly penetrant mutations such as single gene mutation, intragenic deletion/duplication, contiguous gene deletion, chromosomal aneuploidy (e.g. trisomy)

Complex: low penetrance multigenic susceptibility, environmental exposures

Box 2.5a Molecular classification of long QT syndrome

OMIM type	OMIM number	Gene/locus	Protein	Protein function
LQT1	192,500	*KCNQ1*	KQT-like voltage- gated potassium channel-1	Potassium Ion channel subunit
LQT2	613,688	*KCNH2*	Potassium channel, voltage-gated, subfamily H, member 2	Potassium Ion channel subunit

OMIM type	OMIM number	Gene/locus	Protein	Protein function
LQT3	603,830	*SCN5A*	Sodium channel, voltage-gated, type V, alpha subunit	Sodium ion channel subunit
LQT4	106,410	*ANK2*	Ankyrin2	Ion channel anchoring protein
LQT5	176,261	*KCNE1*	Potassium channel, voltage-gated, Isk-related subfamily, member 1	Potassium ion channel subunit
LQT6	613,693	*KCNE2*	Potassium channel, voltage-gated, Isk-related subfamily, member 2	Potassium ion channel subunit
LQT7[a]	170,390	*KCNJ2*	Potassium channel, inwardly rectifying, subfamily J, member 2	Potassium ion channel subunit
LQT8[b]	601,005	*CACNA1C*	Calcium channel, voltage-dependent, L-type, alpha-1C subunit	Calcium channel subunit
LQT9	611,818	*CAV3*	Caveolin-3	T-tubule component
LQT10	611,819	*SCN4B*	Sodium channel, voltage-gated, type IV, beta subunit	Sodium channel subunit
LQT11	611,820	*AKAP9*	A-kinase anchor protein 9	Scaffolding protein
LQT12	612,955	*SNTA1*	Syntrophin alpha-1	Regulator of SCN5A
LQT13	613,485	*KCNJ5*	Potassium channel, inwardly rectifying, subfamily J, member 2	Potassium ion channel subunit
LQT14	616,247	*CALM1*	Calmodulin-1	Regulator of L-type calcium channels
LQT15	616,249	*CALM2*	Calmodulin-2	Regulator of L-type calcium channels

Although initial gene cloning studies implicated mutations in genes encoding potassium and ion channels as causes of long QT syndrome, subsequent studies have revealed the typical heterogeneity seen in most other ICCs

[a]Also known as Anderson-Tawil syndrome or Anderson cardiodysrhythmic syndrome

[b]Also known as Timothy syndrome

Box 2.5b Molecular classification of Brugada syndrome

OMIM type	OMIM number	Gene/locus	Protein	Protein function
BRGDA1	601,144	*SCN5A*	Sodium channel, voltage-gated, type V, alpha subunit	Sodium ion channel subunit
BRGDA2	611,777	*GPD1L*	Glycerol phosphate dehydrogenase-like 1	Regulates SCN5A
BRGDA3	611,875	*CACNA1C*	Calcium channel, voltage-dependent, L-type, alpha-1C subunit	Calcium channel subunit
BRGDA4	611,876	*CACNB2*	Calcium channel, voltage-dependent, beta-2 subunit	Calcium channel subunit
BRGDA5	612,838	*SCN1B*	Sodium channel, voltage-gated, type I, subunit B	Sodium ion channel subunit
BRGDA6	613,119	*KCNE3*	Potassium channel, voltage-gated, Isk-related subfamily member 3	Potassium ion channel subunit
BRGDA7	613,120	*SCN3B*	Sodium channel, voltage-gated, type III, beta subunit	Sodium ion channel subunit
BRGDA8	613,123	*HCN4*	Hyperpolarisation-activated cyclic nucleotide-gated potassium channel 4	Potassium ion channel subunit
BRGDA9	616,399	*KCND3*	Potassium channel, voltage-gated, SHAL-related subfamily member 3	Potassium ion channel subunit

As with long QT syndrome, studies have also revealed that Brugada syndrome can no longer be consider a sodium channelopathy but a common phenotype arising from disruption of a number of different ion currents

SCN5A: sequential classification of extreme phenotypic heterogeneity

SCN5A **is unusual because mutations have been reported in the gene in many different ICCs:**

OMIM phenotype	OMIM number
Sick sinus syndrome type 1	608,567
Familial atrial fibrillation type 10	614,022
Non-progressive heart block	113,900
Progressive heart block type 1A	113,900
Brugada syndrome type 1	601,144
Familial ventricular fibrillation type 1	603,829
Long QT syndrome type 3	603,830
Familial dilated cardiomyopathy type 1E	601,154

Box 2.5c Molecular classification of catecholaminergic polymorphic ventricular tachycardia

OMIM type	OMIM number	Gene/ locus	Protein	Protein function
CPVT1	604,772	*RYR2*	Ryanodine receptor protein2	Ryanodine-sensitive calcium channel
CPVT2	611,938	*CASQ2*	Calsequestrin-2	Calcium reservoir regulator
CPVT3	614,021	*7p22-p14*	–	–
CPVT4	614,916	*CALM1*	Calmodulin-1	Regulator of L-type calcium channels
CPVT5	615,441	*TRDN*	Triadin	Mediator of excitation-contraction coupling

Other cardiac calcium channel diseases:

Gene	OMIM phenotype	OMIM number
CACNA1C	Brugada syndrome type 3	611,875
	Timothy syndrome/long QT syndrome type 8	601,005
CACNB2	Brugada syndrome type 4	611,876

Source: Online Mendelian Inheritance in Man, OMIM®. McKusick-Nathans Institute of Genetic Medicine, Johns Hopkins University (Baltimore, MD), {accessed 27.04.2017}. World Wide Web URL: https://omim.org/

Box 2.6a Genetic heterogeneity of familial dilated cardiomyopathy

OMIM sub-type	OMIM number	Gene/locus	Protein	Function	Additional reported phenotypes
1A	115,200	*LMNA*	Lamin A/C	Intermediate filament, nuclear lamina component	See Box 2.8
1B	600,884	9q13	–	–	–
1C	601,493	*LDB3*	LIM domain-binding protein 3	Z-disk integrity	LVNCC, HCM. MM
1D	601,494	*TNNT2*	Troponin T2	Sarcomeric thin filament component	LVNCC, HCM, RCM
1E	601,154	*SCN5A*	SCN5A	Sodium ion channel subunit	See Box 2.5
1F[a]	–	*DES*	Desmin	Desmosomal protein	See Box 2.7

OMIM sub-type	OMIM number	Gene/locus	Protein	Function	Additional reported phenotypes
1G	188,840	*TTN*	Titin	Structural and tensile sarcomeric protein	See Box 2.2
1H	604,288	2q14-q22	–	–	
1I	604,765	*DES*	Desmin	Desmosomal protein	Myofibrillar myopathy
1J	605,362	*EYA4*	Eyes absent 4	Developmental regulator	ADSNHL
1K	605,582	*6q12-16*	–	–	
1L	606,685	*SGD*	δ-sarcoglygan	Dystrophin/ glycoprotein complex comonent	LGMD
1M	607,482	*CSRP3*	Cysteine- and glycine- rich protein 3	Z disc protein	HCM
1N[a]					
1O	608,569	*ABCC9*	ATP-binding cassette C9	ATP-sensitive potassium ion channel	FAF
1P	609,909	*PLN*	Phospholamban	Endoplasmic reticulum calcium regulator	HCM
1Q	–	7q22.3-q31.1	–	–	
1R	613,424	*ACTC1*	Cardiac α-actin	Sarcomeric contractile protein	HCM LVNCC ASD
1S	613,426	*MYH7*	β myosin heavy chain 7	Sarcomeric contractile protein	See Box 2.2
1T	613,740	*TPMO*	Thymopoeitin (lamina-associated protein 2)	Nuclear architecture, interacts with lamin A/C	
1U	613,694	*PSEN1*	Presenilin 1	γ-secretase Endoplasmic reticulum calcium regulator	Familial dementias
1V	613,697	*PSEN2*	Presenilin 2	γ-secretase Endoplasmic reticulum calcium regulator	Familial dementias

OMIM sub-type	OMIM number	Gene/locus	Protein	Function	Additional reported phenotypes
1W	611,407	*VCL*	Metavinculin	Cytoskeletal protein	HCM
1X	611,615	*FKTN*	Fukutin	α-dystroglycan glycosylation	LGMD
					Dystroglycanopathy
1Y	611,878	*TPM1*	Tropomyosin 1	Actin-binding myofibrillar protein	LVNCC
					HCM
1Z	611,879	*TNNC1*	Troponin C	Actin-binding myofibrillar protein	HCM
1AA	612,158	*ACTN2*	α-2 actinin	Actin-binding proetin	HCM
1BB	612,877	*DSG2*	Desmoglein 2	Desmosomal protein	ARVC
1CC	613,122	*NEXN*	nexilin	Actin-binding protein	HCM
1DD	613,172	*RBM20*	RNA-binding motif protein 20	Spliceosomal protein	
1EE	613,252	*MYH6*	α myosin heavy chain 6	Sarcomeric protein	ASD
					HCM
					SSS
1FF	613,286	*TNNI3*	Troponin I3	Actin-binding myofibrillar protein	HCM
					RCM
1GG	613,642	*SDHA*	Succinate dehydrogenase subunit A	Mitochondrial flavoprotein	fPGL
					Leigh syndrome
					Mitochondrial complex II deficiency
1HH	613,881	*BAG3*	BCL-associated athanogene 3	Hsp70 (molecular chaperone) regulator	MM
1II	615,184	*CRYAB*	α-B crystallin	Heat shock protein	Cataract
					MM
1JJ	615,235	*LAMA4*	α-4 laminin	Basement membrane glycoprotein	
1KK	615,248	*MYPN*	myopalladin	Sarcomeric protein	RCM
					HCM
1LL	615,373	*PRDM16*	PR domain-containing protein 16	Zinc finger transcription factor	LVNCC
1MM	615,396	*MYBPC3*	Myosin binding protein C3	Sarcomeric protein	See Box 2.2

OMIM sub-type	OMIM number	Gene/locus	Protein	Function	Additional reported phenotypes
2A	613,286	*TNNI3*	Troponin I3	Actin-binding myofibrillar protein	HCM RCM
2B	614,672	*GATAD1*	GATA zinc finger domain-containing protein 1	Zinc finger transcription factor	
3A[a]	302,060	*TAZ*	Tafazzin	Mitochondrial transacylase	Barth syndrome
3B	302,045	*DMD*	Dystrophin	Dystrophin/glycoprotein complex component	Duchenne muscular dystrophy Becker muscular dystrophy

Genetic and mechanistic sub-types of familial dilated cardiomyopathy. Those starting with '1' are autosomal dominant, '2' autosomal recessive and '3' X-linked. Note the huge range of different molecular mechanism which give rise to a simple common phenotype: left ventricular systolic dysfunction/heart failure

LVNCC left ventricular non-compaction cardiomyopathy, *HCM* hypertrophic cardiomyopathy, *MM* myofibrillar myopathy, *RCM* restrictive cardiomyopathy, *ADSNHL* autosomal dominant sensorineural hearing loss, *LGMD* limb girdle muscular dystrophy, *FAF* familial atrial fibrillation, *ASD* familial atrial septal defect, *LGMD* limb girdle muscular dystrophy, *SSS* sick sinus syndrome, *fPGL* familial paragangliomatosis

[a]No longer used

Box 2.6b Diverse phenotypes associated with *LMNA* mutations

OMIM phenotype	OMIM number	Inheritance
Familial dilated cardiomyopathy type 1A	115,200	AD
Emery-Dreifuss muscular dystrophy type 2	181,350	AD
Emery-Dreifuss muscular dystrophy type 3	616,516	AR
Charcot-Marie Tooth disease type 2B1	605,588	AR
Congenital muscular dystrophy	613,205	AD
Limb girdle muscular dystrophy type 1B	159,001	AD
Heart-hand syndrome	610,140	AD
Hutchinson-Gilford progeria	176,670	AD
Familial partial lipodystrophy type 2	151,660	AD
Malouf syndrome	212,112	AD
Mandibuloacral dysplasia	248,370	AR
Restrictive dermopathy, lethal	275,210	AR

See text for further explanation

Box 2.6c Diverse phenotypes associated with *TTN* mutations

OMIM phenotype	OMIM number	Inheritance
Familial dilated cardiomyopathy type 1G	604,145	AD
Familial hypertrophic cardiomyopathy type 9	181,350	AD
Limb girdle muscular dystrophy type 2J	608,807	AR
Early onset myopathy with fatal cardiomyopathy	611,705	AR
Proximal myopathy with early respiratory involvement	603,689	AD
Tardive tibial muscular dystrophy	600,334	AD

See text for further explanation

Source: Online Mendelian Inheritance in Man, OMIM®. McKusick-Nathans Institute of Genetic Medicine, Johns Hopkins University (Baltimore, MD), {accessed 27.04.2017}. World Wide Web URL: https://omim.org/

Box 2.7a Arrhythmogenic cardiomyopathy

OMIM Sub-type	OMIM number	Gene/locus	Protein	Protein function
ARVD1[a]	107,970	*TGFB3*	Transforming growth factor beta 3	Growth factor
ARVD2	600,996	*RYR2*	Ryanodine receptor 2	Ryanodine-sensitive calcium channel
ARVD3	602,086	14q12-q22	–	–
ARVD4	602,087	2q32.1-q32.3	–	–
ARVD5	604,400	*TMEM43*	Transmembrane protein 43	Nuclear envelope protein
ARVD6	604,401	10p14-p12	–	–
ARVD7[b]	601,419	*DES*	Desmin	Desmosomal protein subunit
ARVD8	607,450	*DSP*	Desmoplakin	Desmosomal protein subunit
ARVD9	609,040	*PKP2*	Plakophilin 2	Desmosomal protein subunit

OMIM Sub-type	OMIM number	Gene/locus	Protein	Protein function
ARVD10	610,193	*DSG2*	Desmoglein 2	Desmosomal protein subunit
ARVD11	610,476	*DSC2*	Desmocollin 2	Desmosomal protein subunit
ARVD12	611,528	*JUP*	Junction plakoglobin	Desmosomal protein subunit
ARVD13	615,616	*CTNNA3*	Alpha-3 catenin	Cell junction protein

[a]Published data are difficult to interpret (Beffagna et al. 2005): one of these mutations was present in 3 *unaffected* individuals in the same family; one mutation was only reported in a single individual; and 2 families previously linked to the same genomic region did not have detectable mutations in the *TGFB3* gene. By contrast, neither reported mutation was found in normal controls. Mutations within the coding sequence of *TGFB3* are associated with Loeys Dietz syndrome (see main text). It remains possible that up-regulated TGFβ3 activity may represent a further non-desmosomal mechanism leading to ARVC

[b]Reclassified as myofibrillar myopathy

Box 2.7b ARVC + hair/skin phenotypes

Disease name	OMIM number	Gene
Naxos disease	601,214	*JUP*
Carvajal disease	605,676	*DSP*
ARVC with mild PKK and wooly hair	610,476	*DSC2*

Box 2.8a Familial thoracic aortic aneurysm/dissection

OMIM phenotype	OMIM number	Gene/locus	Protein	Protein function	Alternative nomenclature	OMIM number
AAT1	607,086	11q23.3-q24				
AAT2	607,087	5q13-q14				
AAT3	–	*TGFBR2*	Transforming growth factor beta receptor subunit 2	TGF-beta signal transduction	Loeys-Dietz 2	610,168
AAT4	132,900	*MYH11*	Myosin heavy chain 11 (smooth muscle)	Smooth muscle myosin		
AAT5	–	*TGFBR1*	Transforming growth factor beta receptor subunit 2	TGF-beta signal transduction	Loeys-Dietz 1	609,192
AAT6	611,788	*ACTA2*	Actin, alpha-2, smooth muscle	Smooth muscle myosin		
AAT7	613,780	*MYLK*	Myosin light chain kinase	Myosin light chain phosphorylation		
AAT8	615,436	*PRKG1*	Protein kinase, cGMP-dependent, regulatory type 1	Vascular smooth muscle contraction		
AAT9	616,166	*MFAP5*	Microfibril-associated protein 5	Component of fibrillin-containing microfibrils		
–	–	*SMAD3*	Homolog of Drosphila Mothers Against Decapentaplegic, 3	Mediator of TGF-beta ligand-receptor interaction	Loeys-Dietz 3/ Osteoarthritis-aneurysms syndrome	613,795
–	–	*TGFB2*	Transforming growth factor beta-2	TGF-beta signalling	Loeys-Dietz 4	614,816
–	–	*TGFB3*	Transforming growth factor beta-2	TGF-beta signalling	Loeys-Dietz 5	615,582
–		*FBN1*	Fibrillin 1	Microfibrillar protein	Marfan syndrome	154,700

OMIM phenotype	OMIM number	Gene/locus	Protein	Protein function	Alternative nomenclature	OMIM number
–		*FBN2*	Fibrillin 2	Microfibrillar protein	Beal syndrome[a]	121,050
–	–	*COL3A1*	Collagen type III, alpha-1	Extracellular matrix protein	Vascular Ehlers Danlos syndrome	130,050
–	–	*COL1A1*	Collagen type I, alpha-1	Extracellular matric protein	Ehlers-Danlos syndrome with a propensity to arterial rupture	130,000
–	–	*ELN*	Elastin	Elastic fibre component	Cutis laxa 1 (AD)	123,700
–		*FBLN5*	Fibulin 5	Extracellular matrix protein	Cutis laxa 1A	219,100
–	–	*EFEMP2*	EGF-containing fibulin-like extracellular matrix protein	Extracellular matrix protein	Curus laxa 1B (AR)	624,437
–		*SLC2A10*	Solute carrier family 2, member 10	Glucose transporter	Arterial tortuosity syndrome	208,050
–	–	*SKI*	V-SKI avian sarcoma viral oncogene homolog	Regulator of TGF-beta signalling	Shprintzen-Goldeberg syndrome	182,212
–	–	*FLNA*	Filamin A	Cytoskeletal protein	Perinodular heterotopia, 'ehlers danlos type'	300017.17-19
–	–	*MED12*	Mediator complex subunit 12	Transcriptional regulator	Lujan-Fryns syndrome	309,520

A note on nomenclature

A variety of terms exists in the literature which needs to be resolved in time including: *AAA* familial abdominal aortic aneurysm (OMIM), *AAT* familial thoracic aortic aneurysm (OMIM), *FAA* familial aortic aneurysm, *FTAA* familial thoracic aortic aneurysm, *FTAAD* familial aortic aneurysm/dissection

In addition, 'cystic medial necrosis' is a non-specific histological term which was often felt to be synonymous with the medial changes observed in thoracic aortic aneurysms from patients with Marfan syndrome

The Loeys-Dietz syndromes overlap with other classification systems and generally describe syndromic forms of thoracic aortic aneurysms

[a]Prevalence of thoracic aortic aneurysm is not well-documented; phenotypic features overlap with Marfan syndrome

Box 2.8b Molecular classification of familial abdominal aortic aneurysm

OMIM phenotype	OMIM number	Locus
AAA1	100,070	19q13
AAA2	609,782	4q31
AAA3	611,891	9p21
AAA4	614,375	12q13

None of the following genes have been identified or characterised. All have been localised through linkage studies in families with significant clustering of abdominal aortic aneurysms

References

1. McKusick V. On lumpers and splitters, or the nosology of genetic disease. Birth Defects. 1969;5:23–32.
2. Gilbert SF, Sarkar S. Embracing complexity: organicism for the twenty-first century. Dev Dyn. 2000;219:1–9.
3. World Health Authority. International statistical classification of diseases and related health problems. 10th revision. 5th ed; 2016. Accessed online 12 Oct 2016
4. Online Mendelian Inheritance in Man, OMIM®. McKusick-Nathans Institute of Genetic Medicine, Johns Hopkins University (Baltimore, MD); 2016. Accessed 27 Apr 2017. http://omim.org/ber.
5. IPCC-EATS-STS-Diagnostic-Shortlist-v3.3-January-1-2016(1).xls. Available at http://ipccc.net/ipccc-download-form/. Accessed 04 Jan 2017.
6. Sithamparanathan S, Padley SPG, Rubens MB, Gatzoulis MA, Ho SY, Nicol ED. Great vessel and coronary artery anatomy in transposition and other coronary anomalies. A universal descriptive and alphanumerical sequential classification. J Am Coll Cardiol. 2013;6:624–30.
7. Capell BC, Collins FS. Human laminopathies: nuclei gone genetically awry. Nat Rev Genet. 2006;7:940–52.
8. Norwood F, de Visser M, Eymard B, Lochmuller H, Bushby K, Members of EFNS Guideline Task Force. EFNS guideline on diagnosis and management of limb girdle muscular dystrophies. Eur J Neurol. 2007;14:1305–12.
9. Bates MDG, Bourke JP, Giordano C, d'Amati G, Turnbull GM, Taylor RW. Cardiac involvement in mitochondrial DNA disease: clinical spectrum, diagnosis, and management. Eur Heart J Adv. 2012;33(24):3023–33. https://doi.org/10.1093/eurheartj/ehs275.
10. Sen-Chowdhry S, Syrris P, Ward D, Asimaki A, Sevdalis E, McKenna WJ. Clinical and genetic characterization of families with arrhythmogenic right ventricular dysplasia/cardiomyopathy provides novel insights into patterns of disease expression. Circulation. 2007;115:1710–20.
11. Sen-Chowdhry S, Syrris P, Prasad SK, Hughes SE, Merrifield R, Ward D, Pennell DJ, McKenna WJ. Left-dominant arrhythmogenic cardiomyopathy: an under-recognized clinical entity. J Am Coll Cardiol. 2008;52:2175–87.
12. Tiso N, Stephan DA, Nava A, Bagattin A, Devaney JM, Stanchi F, Larderet G, Brahmbhatt B, Brown K, Bauce B, Muriago M, Basso C, Thiene G, Danieli GA, Rampazzo A. Identification of mutations in the cardiac ryanodine receptor gene in families affected with arrhythmogenic right ventricular cardiomyopathy type 2 (ARVD2). Hum Mol Genet. 2001;10:189–94.
13. Christensen AH, Andersen CB, Tybjaerg-Hansen A, Haunso S, Svendsen JH. Mutation analysis and evaluation of the cardiac localization of TMEM43 in arrhythmogenic right ventricular cardiomyopathy. Clin Genet. 2011;80:256–64.

14. Beffagna G, Occhi G, Nava A, Vitiello L, Ditadi A, Basso C, Bauce B, Carraro G, Thiene G, Towbin JA, Danieli GA, Rampazzo A. Regulatory mutations in transforming growth factor-beta-3 gene cause arrhythmogenic right ventricular cardiomyopathy type 1. Cardiovasc Res. 2005;65:366–73.
15. Neptune ER, Frischmeyer PA, Arking DE, Myers L, Bunton TE, Gayraud B, Ramirez F, Sakai LY, Dietz HC. Dysregulation of TGF-beta activation contributes to pathogenesis in Marfan syndrome. Nat Genet. 2003;33:407–11.
16. Renard M, Callewaert B, Baetens M, Campens L, MacDermot K, Fryns J-P, Bonduell M, Dietz HC, IM GR, Cavaco D, Stattin E-L, Schrander-Stumpel C, Coucke P, Loeys B, De Paepe A, De Backer J. Novel MYH11 and ACTA2 mutations reveal a new role for enhancing TGF β signaling in FTAAD. Int J Cardiol. 2013;165:314–21.
17. Habashi JP, Judge DP, Holm TM, Cohn RD, Loeys BL, Cooper TK, Myers L, Klein EC, Liu G, Calvi C, Podowski M, Neptune ER, Halushka MK, Bedja D, Gabrielson K, Rifkin DB, Carta L, Ramirez F, Huso DL, Dietz HC. Losartan, an AT1 antagonist, prevents aortic aneurysm in a mouse model of Marfan syndrome. Science. 2006;312:117–21.

3 Principles and Practice of Genetic Counselling for Inherited Cardiac Conditions

Sharon Jenkins and Caroline Kirwan

Abstract

The definition of Genetic Counselling is a "…communication process which aims to help individuals, couples and families understand and adapt to the medical, psychological, familial and reproductive implications of the genetic contribution to specific health conditions". Genetic counselling can be applied within different medical settings and can therefore be tailored to provide specific information relevant to the particular condition present within the family. This chapter outlines the essentials and gives guidance to those providing genetic counselling for individuals and families with Inherited Cardiac Conditions (ICCs).

Keywords

Genetics • Inheritance • Counselling • Cardiac • Genetic testing • Consent Reproductive genetic testing

S. Jenkins (✉)
Inherited Heart Diseases Unit, UCL/St Barts Partnership, London, UK

Department of Medical Genetics, King's College, London, UK

Human Molecular Genetics with Counselling, Imperial College, London, UK
e-mail: sharon.jenkins@bartshealth.nhs.uk

C. Kirwan
Institute of Medical Genetics, University Hospital of Wales, Cardiff, Wales, UK
e-mail: caroline.kirwan2@wales.nhs.uk

D. Kumar, P. Elliott (eds.), *Cardiovascular Genetics and Genomics*,
https://doi.org/10.1007/978-3-319-66114-8_3

3.1 Introduction

Inherited cardiac conditions (ICCs) present many challenges for genetic counsellors and clinicians. Sadly for a few families, the first sign that an ICC is present is a sudden death or cardiac event. It is important that these patients are seen by genetic counsellors who will be able to work directly with the patient and their family to provide information on the condition and support them in making the appropriate decisions for themselves and their family. Genetic counsellors help educate and support individuals and families with regards to their particular condition. This enables them to disseminate accurate information to other at-risk family members, ensuring they are able to access appropriate screening and testing.

There have been huge advances in our understanding of ICCs and it is essential that those working with families with ICCs keep abreast of current guidelines allowing them to identify families at risk and accurately interpret information about the disorder to fully support families. Genetics and cardiology need to continue to work closely to strive to develop the services provided to families with ICCs.

This chapter outlines the essentials of the genetic counselling process when working with families with ICCs. It cannot attempt to cover all the details but hopes to overview the key elements of genetic counselling for ICCs.

3.2 Family History

Taking a detailed family tree is an important and complex task that is an essential role of the genetic counsellor. A detailed family tree helps to define the type of inheritance, identify who else may also be at risk within the family and therefore require screening, and, in some cases, aid in directing genetic testing. The type of inheritance can only be fully confirmed when the specific pathogenic variant can be identified. It is only then that family members who are at risk can seek predictive genetic testing at the appropriate age for the condition.

It is important when taking the family history to obtain details of age and severity of diagnosis, gender and diagnoses of other family members. The focus should not just be on cardiac history but include strokes, renal history, muscle weakness, deafness and diabetes. In addition, the nature, age and circumstances surrounding all deaths within the family must be documented- i.e. progressive, sudden, cot death, drowning, road traffic accident (RTA) etc.

When taking a family tree, it is important to note that there are a few things which may complicate the interpretation of the family history. Skewed X inactivation, other non-cardiac conditions running within the family (which may or may not run in tandem with the cardiomyopathy), de novo pathogenic variants, consanguinity and more than one pathogenic variant running within the family may all complicate the interpretation of the family tree.

3.2.1 Information Gathering

ICCs are complicated in the fact that a negative family history resulting from unexamined, asymptomatic family members does not necessarily rule out a family history of the condition. This is due to reduced penetrance and variable expressivity that is present with most of the ICCs [1–3]. Therefore it is not possible to fully confirm or refute familial disease without examining family members or accessing current or past clinical data. It is important that consent is obtained to access family members medical records, post mortems or death certificates are obtained to help clarify information obtained so as to guide as accurately as possible.

Specific attention with regards to relevant questioning must be used when interviewing the individual. Past medical history including; shortness of breath, chest pain, palpitations, black outs or light-headedness, blood pressure, previous drug use and treatment.

3.2.2 Inheritance Patterns

For the vast majority of ICCs, the type of inheritance is autosomal dominant (AD), although X-linked (XL), mitochondrial and, more rarely, autosomal recessive (AR) are seen [4–6]. The latter is more often seen with ICCs associated with a syndrome [7, 8]. There is often great variation in the clinical presentation of ICC's even within the same family which can complicate the interpretation of a family tree.

3.2.3 Red Flags

As well as factors that may complicate the interpretation of a family tree and possibly the diagnosis within the family, there are red flags to be aware of which are often warning signs for a particular condition. It is extremely important to be alert to these when interpreting the family history of an ICC and knowledge of these will help in defining the specific condition within the family as well as the possible genetic cause. Some red flags are varied (sometimes age-related) severity within a family, males > females, additional non-cardiac conditions, and conduction disease.

3.2.4 Conduction Disease

Conduction disease is a red flag for ICCs, particularly in the young, and can be associated with certain ICCs as well as other non-inherited types of cardiac disease. Dilated cardiomyopathy with conduction disease coupled with a family history of sudden cardiac death with or without pacemakers is a strong indicator for LMNA associated DCM [9]. This is an important diagnosis to pick up as it often necessitates the implantation of an ICD due to the high likelihood of dangerous arrhythmias, although the clinical indication may initially only be for a pacemaker. The knowledge that LMNA is the gene responsible for the phenotype in the family would provide useful information for counselling other family members as well as valuable clinical information that would assist in the management of the patient.

Cardiomyopathies due to the PRKAG2 gene can also present with conduction disease (Wolff-Parkinson-White [WPW] syndrome. The course of the disease mimics other glycogen-storage and metabolic cardiomyopathies but is dissimilar from HCM caused by sarcomeric gene mutations. This is due to the fact that the cardiac hypertrophy in PRKAG2 mutations is due to increased intracellular glycogen deposition, rather than myocyte disarray and fibrosis. It is important to exclude this gene as a cause as risk-assessment for an individual or family with non-sarcomeric disease may be different as opposed to HCM that due to conventional sarcomeric disease [10].

3.2.5 Alternative Inheritance and Other Non-Cardiac Features

Although the majority of ICCs are inherited in an AD manner, there are other types of inheritance that are possible. X-linked inheritance is the second most common type of inheritance in ICCs and it is important to identity this as a possibility of the inheritance as the diagnosis within the family may be dependent on this. A more severe and early onset presentation in males versus females is a red flag for an X-linked pedigree. The identification of an X-linked inherited ICC will be informative for which individuals within the family require screening and/or genetic testing. In a few cases, there may be available treatment for the condition.

Anderson Fabry disease (AFD) is an X-linked lysosomal storage disease for which treatment exists (see also Chap. 7). The classical form presents in males in the first decade of life and signs include episodes of pain, burning sensation in the extremities, and angiokeratomas. Patients develop progressive renal damage and cardiomyopathy. Milder forms of AFD have now been recognised with cardiac and renal variants of AFD. The cardiac variant is the result of a specific gene change and presents after the 4th decade with cardiac hypertrophy and proteinuria. The renal variant presents around the 2nd decade of life and results in cardiac hypertrophy and can lead to end stage renal failure. There It is thought to be a rare condition affecting 1 in 50,000 males, although evidence from new-born screening indicates that there may be rare, later onset and milder variants that are present at a much more common frequency (1 in 3000) [11, 12].

If AFD is diagnosed early enough it can be treated by enzyme replacement therapy. Recombinant a-galactosidase A was originally trialled in patients with AFD to determine its safety and efficacy in 2001 [13, 14]. There is evidence that ERT decreases cardiac mass, improves LV function, decreases frequency of pain crises, improves pulmonary and GI symptoms, increases sweating, improves hearing and sensation and slows down renal deterioration. There is also more benefit when ERT is started at milder degrees of LVH and before the development of severe renal impairment [12, 15].

The diagnosis of AFD is more difficult in females as the presentation can be much more varied and can exhibit mild-to-moderate symptoms due to random X-inactivation. In addition, standard diagnostic enzyme testing for plasma alpha

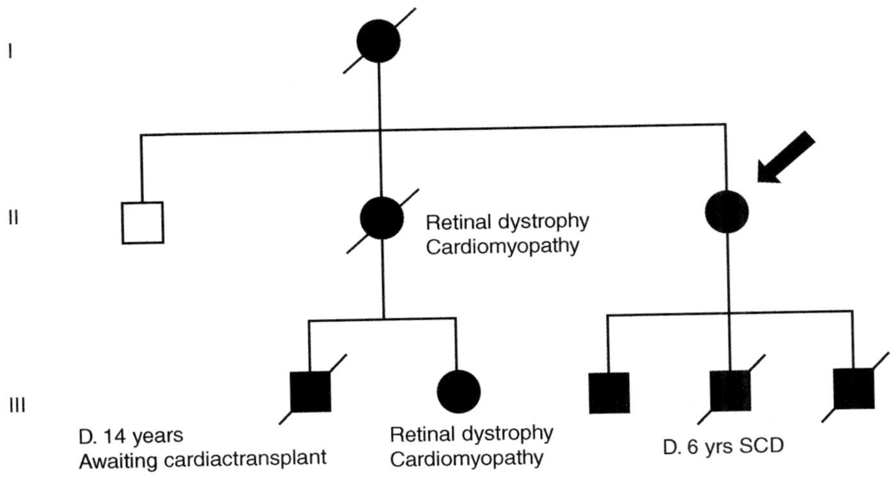

Fig. 3.1 Pedigree showing mitochondrial cardiomyopathy. *In this pedigree, the proband, indicated by an arrow, had extensive investigations for a potential mitochondrial cardiomyopathy given the retinal dystrophy and cardiomyopathy present within the family. A biopsy was inconclusive. The family history was significant for severe early onset Hypertrophic cardiomyopathy in males necessitating cardiac transplant. In addition, there was a high incidence of sudden cardiac death. Further questioning revealed that the proband's sister had retinal dystrophy in one eye only. Variable, and even unilateral, expression of retinal dystrophy is often a feature of X-linked retinal dystrophy female carriers. Consequently, X-linked inheritance was considered and genetic testing was performed for the LAMP-2 gene, which is the cause of Danon disease. A pathogenic mutation was identified confirming the diagnosis within the family*

galactosidase activity is not accurate for identifying an affected female, so DNA testing, rather than enzyme testing, must be performed if AFD is suspected. The presentation of other non-cardiac features should be a red flag as well as possible X-linked inheritance and should guide the appropriate diagnostic testing in order to make the diagnosis of AFD and enable time-sensitive treatment.

Danon disease is an X-linked glycogen storage disease with variable disease presentation and severity (see also Chap. 7). In addition, there is marked variability amongst female carriers. Like AFD, the presentation of Danon disease can vary and the severity of disease in females can complicate the interpretation of family history. Similarly, investigations performed on females can be inconclusive in carriers and it is important to consider this when investigating a family for Danon disease [16]. See pedigree below (Fig. 3.1).

3.3 Genetic Testing

A key task of genetic counselling for ICCs is to offer genetic testing, where possible, to the appropriate individual within the family. It is important that the individual understands the utility of genetic testing, as well as the possible outcomes, and that appropriate consent is obtained.

There are two main types of genetic testing for ICC's; diagnostic testing and predictive testing. Reproductive genetic testing can be performed, in certain circumstances, to provide a couple with the possibility of having a child who does not carry the familial pathogenic variant.

Genetic testing for inherited cardiac conditions is available both on the NHS and in the private sector; however, genetic counselling prior to going ahead with genetic testing should always be obtained due to the psychologically challenging nature of the impact of obtaining a result [17]. Even if a pathogenic variant is found, there is still uncertainty as to when or if the condition will present, as well as how severely it may present. This uncertainty can create more concerns and worries about the future and can often replace the worry of 'not knowing'.

3.3.1 Diagnostic Genetic Testing

Diagnostic genetic testing is usually performed on an affected individual to try and identify a specific pathogenic variant that is causative for their condition. Diagnostic testing for ICCs is complicated in that there is not one pathogenic variant or specific gene that is universally responsible for causing the condition. As is the case with other genetic conditions, there is usually one private pathogenic variant unique to that individual or family that is the cause of the ICC. However, there are several examples for ICCs in which more than one pathogenic variant has been responsible for the condition within the family [18]. In addition, depending on the particular ICC, the yield for genetic testing is considerably below 100% with a range of around 30-70% [19], implicating both the possibility of other yet un-associated causative genes. The yield improves significantly; however, with an established family history of the disease [3, 18, 20].

The considerable clinical variability displayed by individuals who are gene carriers further complicates the interpretation of genetic findings, with complete non-expression being observed for some ICCs [19, 21]. Given this, it is important that diagnostic testing be performed on an affected individual within the family, as a negative result from a genetic test on an unaffected family member would not be as informative. However, there are circumstances in which extensive genetic testing could be performed on someone who is at high risk but unaffected when there are no living relatives or sample available for testing. These are unusual examples and the genetic findings would need to be interpreted carefully along with the clinical results in order to be informative and meaningful to the individual or individuals being tested.

3.3.2 When to Offer a Diagnostic Test?

Genetic testing for ICCs should ideally be performed when the yield from the test and the benefits to the family are likely to be high. Two factors that determine a high yield are positive family history of the condition and a well-defined phenotype. In addition, it may be important to test for certain ICCs where affected status within a family can be difficult to assign due to diverse clinical variability. In extreme cases, there can be multiple sudden cardiac deaths within a family in presumably unaffected individuals having clinical screening. TNNT2 is a gene whereby pathogenic variants have been known to cause classically defined HCM as well as SCD in undiagnosed individuals without any obvious left ventricular thickening [22], although this is not always the case. The identification of a pathogenic variant in such families would allow for more directed clinical screening and possibly earlier clinical treatment. Genetic testing will also confirm the type of inheritance within a family and can direct clinical screening for family members.

From the clinician's point of view, genetic testing is warranted when there are potentially clinically actionable pathogenic variants in genes. For example, a pathogenic variant in the LMNA gene would identify the potential for fatal arrhythmias where the detectable clinical indication may only be that of conduction disease [23]. Therefore, in this instance, the implantation of an ICD would be merited, rather than a pacemaker.

From the individual perspective, genetic testing may be sought for reproductive purposes, career choices, or to reduce anxiety and eliminate long-term clinical screening. Entry into the Armed Forces often requires an extensive medical examination followed by a thorough family history questionnaire. It is possible that acceptance into such a career may be denied for a family history of an ICC, even if the individual is presently unaffected. In the past, genetic testing within the family has provided the only opportunity for a family member to gain entrance following a negative result.

3.3.3 Who Should Have a Diagnostic Test?

When considering diagnostic testing, it is important to consider who to offer a diagnostic test to. Ideally this would be the most informative individual within the family and for many of the ICCs this would be the most severely affected individual within the family. This is due to the fact that a percentage of families with ICCs have more than one pathogenic variant as a cause of the condition [18]. This can sometimes be indicated due to an observed discrepancy in phenotypic severity within a family; however this is not always a reliable indicator. Given this, it is advisable to confirm the identified pathogenic variant within a family in all affected members before proceeding to predictive testing. See pedigree (Fig. 3.2).

The concern over a second pathogenic variant within a family is becoming less important as panel testing is now becoming more commonplace, although selection of the most appropriate individual for pathogenic variant detection still needs to occur. Panel testing involves testing several genes at once and often includes a spectrum of genes associated with the particular ICC which includes both common genes and genes more rarely associated with the ICC in question. Due to the technology involved, it is more cost effective and quicker to test more genes than fewer

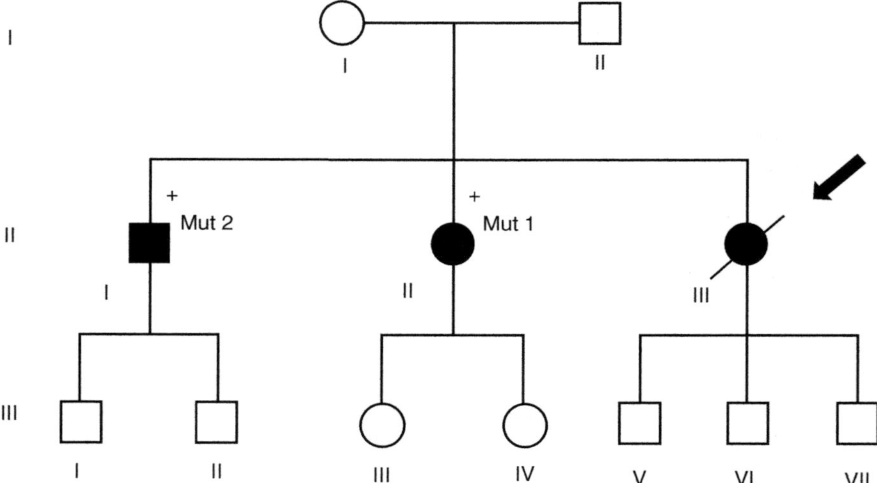

Fig. 3.2 In this example, the proband indicated by the arrow was diagnosed with severe Hypertrophic Cardiomyopathy at a young age and died before she could undergo genetic testing. Testing was therefore performed on an affected relative (II.II), who was more mildly affected, and a pathogenic sarcomeric mutation was identified. There was clinical suspicion of a second mutation within the family due to the phenotypic variability and confirmatory testing in another affected relative (II.I) was sought before predictive testing was offered to the proband's children. This affected relative did not carry the original mutation and so further testing was commenced and a second pathogenic mutation was identified. The assumption was that the proband carried two pathogenic mutations as a cause of her severe HCM. This could not be proven, but in this instance, predictive testing could then be offered to the proband's children

genes and so panel testing is now becoming the standard. However, due to the fact that more genes are being tested, it is becoming increasingly important to be able to interpret the genetic results in the context of the clinical phenotype. This is due to the inevitable expansion of our knowledge of genotype/phenotype association with the increased use of panel testing.

3.3.4 What Type of Sample to Test?

Genetic testing on blood, saliva or fresh tissue is usually preferred given the quality and quantity of DNA that is obtained from these samples. Occasionally it is possible to perform genetic testing on other types of sample; particularly paraffin embedded tissue obtained following a post-mortem. However, this type of sample is notoriously difficult to analyse given the amount of DNA that is usually available as well as the quality of the sample. It is often best to reserve paraffin-embedded tissue for clarification of carrier status within the family once a pathogenic variant has been identified in another living family member, thus also preserving the precious sample.

Genetic testing prior to pathogenic variant detection should include a discussion about the possible diagnostic outcomes, as well as any clinical, familial, psychological and insurance implications.

3.3.5 Possible Outcomes of Diagnostic Testing in an Affected Family Member

- A definite disease-causing pathogenic variant is identified. This could be in a gene directly linked to the condition being tested for or in a gene unrelated to the condition being tested for if panel testing is used. If it is in a gene directly related to the condition, predictive testing can be offered to at risk relatives. It is important that the phenotype and genotypes match so if a disease-causing pathogenic variant is identified in an unrelated gene it would be advisable to discuss this further with cardiology and genetics to clarify this. It is important to be cautious as there may be another causative pathogenic variant that is responsible for the condition. At this stage, it would be advisable (although not necessary) to offer a diagnostic test to all other affected family members, called segregation, to confirm that this is the only pathogenic variant within the family.
- A variant of unknown significance (VUS) is identified. These are variations within the gene in which there is insufficient evidence to clearly categorise the variant as disease-causing. In this instance, segregation testing should be performed within the family to prove or disprove the association of the VUS with the disease. This can be challenging if many of the affected family members have died. Until further evidence is obtained, it is not possible to offer predictive testing for a VUS.
- No disease-causing pathogenic variant is identified. In this instance, clinical screening should continue for at-risk family members. It is important to note that the absence of an identifiable disease-causing pathogenic variant does not mean that the ICC is not genetic. For instance, with Brugada syndrome, there is only an identifiable pathogenic variant in approximately 30% of cases [24]. Genetic testing should be revisited in the future when there may be additional testing available.

Classification of whether an identified variant is potentially disease-causing is based on whether the majority of the following criteria can be met as below (derived from [25]).

1. The identified sequence variation is absent from a large group of ethnically matched control populations.
2. The sequence variant co-segregates with disease within the family. This may not always be possible due to small family size, unavailable family members, or those that are unwilling to be tested.
3. The nature of the amino acid change is significant and it is predicted to cause a significant disruption in protein function and/or structure.

4. The sequence variation has been reported previously as disease-causing.
5. The sequence variant is in important functional domain of the gene and is widely conserved amongst different species.

This information is determined by the laboratory which are performing the testing and the relevant evidence for or against the variant being disease-causing is detailed on the report.

3.3.6 Predictive Genetic Testing

The predictive genetic testing is offered to relevant unaffected family members. This is done to determine whether someone is at high risk of developing the condition within the family. Those found not to have the familial pathogenic variant can then stop long term clinical screening.

Predictive genetic testing can only be offered if a definite disease-causing pathogenic variant has already been identified within the family. It is important that individuals receive genetic counselling prior to having a predictive genetic test. This is so that they understand the implications of a predictive test in relation to the specific ICC that they are being tested for. This includes the outcomes of both a positive and negative result, implications for insurance, any financial implications, and the psychological impact on the individual as well as implications for the extended family.

3.3.6.1 Possible Outcomes of Predictive Testing

1. The pathogenic variant previously identified in the family is present. This does not necessarily mean that the individual is affected with the condition, or that they will definitely develop the ICC; however they are at increased risk of doing so and would need regular clinical screening. This is almost always necessary even in the absence of symptoms as many of the ICCs present with little or no symptoms.
2. The pathogenic variant previously identified in the family is not present. This means that the individual is no longer at increased risk for developing the ICC that is present in the family and do not require additional screening. However, they are still at risk of heart disease and should get advice from their GP if they have concerns in the future. They will also not pass on the pathogenic variant to their children.

3.3.7 Genetic Testing in Children

When considering genetic testing in children there are a number of different ethical, moral and legal issues that need to be taken into account. The topic of genetic testing in children has been extensively deliberated [26–28] and whilst this chapter cannot cover in detail all the different aspects of genetic testing in children, it aims to highlight some pertinent considerations, particularly those related to ICCs.

First and foremost, one needs to consider if there is a clear advantage to the child and whether this is the right time to test. Is the condition being tested for a childhood onset condition, or an adult onset condition? There are a number of different tests that can be offered, ranging from single gene tests, gene panels, through to genome sequencing. When a gene panel, whole exome or whole genome sequencing is used it is important to consider that the result may come back indicating a pathogenic variant for a condition that would not affect the child during childhood. The genetic counsellor also needs to consider whether the child would receive screening and treatment if they were found to have a pathogenic variant and when this screening and treatment would start.

The challenges of genetic testing in children has been recognised for a number of years but it has always been agreed that “timely medical benefit to the child should be the primary justification for genetic testing in children and adolescents” ([29], p. 1233). This has been further supported throughout the literature [26, 30]. Thus it is essential to balance the potential benefits and harms of testing when considering genetic testing in children.

Predictive testing in children involves testing an unaffected child for a known familial genetic condition. It is usually agreed that testing should be offered when the onset of such a condition occurs in childhood [26, 31]. However, it is recommended that caution is taken and the timing of the test considered and discussed with the parents and child, if appropriate.

There are many questions to consider when offering predictive testing in children, which can help to determine the best time to carry out the genetic test:

- Is screening/treatment available immediately or would the child have to wait a number of years?
- Is the condition likely to present at any time?
- Is the child asking for the genetic test themselves?

It may be that a child attends the genetics clinic with an older sibling and has a number of questions of their own. Therefore it is important for the counsellor to make time for the child, to speak at their level and to also take into account what is going on in the child’s life at that point in time. For example, receiving a bad news result could have a huge impact on the child if they have just suffered the sudden loss of a close relative. In this instance it may be more suitable to delay testing and perhaps to consider if screening is more appropriate for the immediate future and review the situation at an agreed time.

It is important to always consider if the test is in the best interest of the child. This can be particularly challenging with ICC’s due to:

- Variability and penetrance within families
- Continued uncertainty
- Age of onset
- Loss of confidentiality

Variability refers to the diversity of signs and symptoms that present in different people with the same genetic condition. In ICC's the features can vary widely with some family members having only mild symptoms, while others may have life-threatening complications or sudden death [32]. Penetrance refers to the number of individuals with a pathogenic variant having signs and symptoms of the condition. As ICC's can show reduced penetrance these can greatly add to the challenges when offering genetic testing in children [19].

This uncertainty can increase anxiety within families, which in itself may cause more harm than good. It is therefore important to discuss the reasons for requesting a genetic test at a particular time, this may allow the genetic counsellor to allay particular fears and clarify any misconceptions supporting the child and family to make the right decision for them. Ormonroyd et al. [33] carried out a study looking at 22 families with ICC's who had undergone predictive testing. This study highlighted some of the parents' concerns when considering genetic testing of children. These included:

- Children's activity levels
- Whether or not to restrict these
- Lack of information

Although these are areas that can be explored with the parents and children this is not an exclusive list. It is important that each family is seen as individual and given time for their own fears and concerns to be raised and explored fully. This work is backed up by Mangset and Hofmann [34] who carried out qualitative interviews of 13 parents of children with Long QT syndrome (LQTS) and also found these were key points raised by parents when considering genetic testing for their children.

Another consideration is whether the child is mature enough and has sufficient understanding to make their own decision. In cases where an ICC is not likely to present within the near future, it is important to consider the child's own capacity to make an autonomous decision as an adult. In the UK the rights of the child to make their own autonomous decision, separate to that of the requests of the parents, are recognised in law by Gillick v West Norfolk and Wisbeck Area Health Authority [35]. This ruled that health professionals must balance the best interest and welfare of the child, while also hearing their views and opinions, and it may not be that the parents' views and requests are the overriding factor. It is important to be mindful not to alienate a parent or guardian in clinic but to try to draw all parties into discussions for predictive genetic testing. This is supported by the report from the British Society of Human Genetics [26] on the genetic testing of children.

When offering predictive testing in children the possible loss of confidentiality of their information needs to be considered. When undergoing genetic testing as an adult, one can choose to whom they disclose their information. However, as a child the parent or guardian may disclose the information to others whilst looking for their own support, as such the child is not able to control or determine who can and cannot know their result.

When carrying out genetic testing in a child, whether it is diagnostic or predictive testing, it is important to consider what and how to tell the child. This will be dictated by the age of the child and their level of understanding. The condition that is being tested for also needs to be considered and the depth of the information needs to be tailored to the individual child. It is important to strike the right balance between possibly frightening a child due to providing information they do not understand, against not providing sufficient information. One should consider whether information is best given piecemeal or all at once. Mangset and Hofmann's [34] study demonstrated that parents believed that information for children should be open and honest and children were best supported by allowing them to find out information over time.

Thus, as highlighted, it is important to discuss through the pros and cons of going ahead with genetic testing with the family (and child if appropriate), ensuring they are aware of all the options that are available. These then need to be balanced with the individual family and child.

3.3.8 Consent for Genetic Testing

There is numerous legislation and guidelines for health professionals to adhere to when obtaining consent including: Human Tissue Act [36], Code of Practice 1: Consent [37], Reference guides for consent [38] and Consent: Patients and doctors making decisions together [39]. The government has also set out the requirements for consent within the Human Tissue Act [36]. However, although these provide the fundamental basis of informed consent and the requirements to be adhered to, they do not focus on consent with regards to genetic testing directly and it is often added in as an adjunct to previous regulations. The Joint Committee on Genomics in Medicine (JCGM) (formerly Joint Committee of Medical Genetics) originally reviewed the literature in a document focusing on "Consent and Confidentiality in Genetic Practice" [40]. They have updated their guidance in line with the ever changing field of genetic testing to ensure it is current and appropriate to acknowledge the way we are now able to offer genetic testing [41]. All of these documents [36, 37, 39–41] need to be taken into account when obtaining informed consent from patients to maintain best practice.

Government regulations regarding consent stipulate that a number of requirements must be met in order for consent to be valid. These requirements include; identifying who should give consent, whether or not the individual has got sufficient information regarding the issue for which consent is being obtained, how the consent will be recorded, and whether or not a record of consent will remain with the sample [37].

3.3.8.1 Is Consent Required?

When considering genetic testing it is important to be aware that the Human Tissue Act [36] states:

> "A person commits an offence if –(a)He has any bodily material intending –(i)that any human DNA in the material be analysed without qualifying consent"(HTA [36], Part 1, section 45;(1)(a))

If tissue such as blood or saliva is being taken for DNA analysis consent must be obtained from the appropriate person before testing can be carried out. It is the responsibility of the health professional requesting the test to ensure that adequate consent has been obtained.

3.3.8.2 Who Should Give Consent?

Living competent adult: Where an adult has capacity to consent to genetic testing they should give their consent.

Living adult who lacks capacity: If an adult lacks capacity, then the best interests of that individual needs to be considered before going ahead with genetic testing. The Mental Capacity Act [42] details the requirements for making a judgement in the case of best interest. However, the [41], p. 14) argue that this could include "indirect benefit: the well-being of relatives could be a valid justification...if this had a positive effect on the care of the adult".

Deceased adult: If DNA needs to be extracted from a deceased adult in order to be tested, and the deceased individual made their wishes regarding genetic testing clear prior to their death their wishes should be followed. However, if they did not make a decision in relation DNA testing, consent needs to be obtained from their appointed representative. The decision by this representative will not be able to be overridden by those in a qualifying relationship (see below). If there is no appointed representative, then anyone in a qualifying relationship can give consent for DNA testing [36].

3.3.8.3 Qualifying Relationships

1. Spouse or partner
2. Parent or child
3. Brother or sister
4. Grandparent or grandchild
5. Niece or nephew
6. Stepfather or stepmother
7. Half-brother or half-sister
8. Friend of long standing.

One area that is not covered by the Human Tissue Act [36] is if DNA is already extracted and stored prior to the individual's death. In this situation it would be advisable to discuss testing with the deceased family before going ahead [41].

3.3.9 Living Child

When considering genetic testing in children it is important to be aware that a child is defined as being under 18 years old in England and Wales and under 16 years old in Scotland [36, 43]. Children can consent to genetic testing if they are competent to do so. This is defined by Gillick competency in which Lord Scarman stated a child could consent if they were found to have sufficient comprehension to fully understand the proposed procedure [35].

Genetic testing should be discussed with the child, if the person obtaining consent feels that they fully understand what is proposed they can consent to the test.

However, the Human Tissue Authority [37] recommend that those with parental responsibility are also consulted. It is important that the child is not influenced significantly by others and that the person taking consent is confident that this is in the best interest of the child. If a child is not competent to consent to genetic testing or they choose not to make a decision, then the person who has parental responsibility can give consent [37].

3.3.9.1 Deceased Child

Similar principles apply to deceased children as to deceased adults. If the child was competent at the time of their death and gave consent to genetic testing prior to their death, their consent will still be valid and their wishes should be upheld. The Human Tissue Authority [37] advises that it should be discussed with those with parental responsibility whether or not the child was competent to consent at the time.

If the child was not competent at the time of their death, or did not make a decision, then those with parental responsibility should give consent. Only if there isn't anyone with parental responsibility should consent be obtained from someone in a qualifying relationship [37].

3.3.10 Have They Sufficient Information to Understand?

Sufficient information regarding the test and its implications should be given. The patient should be aware if the test is diagnostic or predictive. If it is predictive a full discussion of the condition they are being tested for should be given as well as making them aware of their risk of being affected. They should also have a chance to discuss the implications of genetic testing not just for themselves but for other family members.

Practical aspects of the test itself should be discussed, from what the test involves, when a result will be obtained, the different types of results that maybe obtained including incidental findings. The Joint Committee for Genomic Medicine has set out clear guidance as to what should be discussed with patients when obtaining consent for genetic testing ([41], p. 5).

3.3.11 How Will the Consent Be Recorded?

Although written consent for genetic testing is not a legal requirement, both the General Medical Council (GMC) and JCGM consider it best practice to document clearly the discussion and agreement in the clinical notes [39, 41].

3.3.12 Scope of Consent

Obtaining consent can be more difficult when gene panels, whole exome or whole genome sequencing is being carried out. These tests can produce a broad range of results which may not be directly related to the condition diagnosed in the proband. In this situation it is not possible to discuss all the conditions which could be identified. However, if general consent to undergo genetic testing is obtained, with an explanation that unexpected results could arise, then this is considered to be sufficient [41].

3.3.13 Consent to Share Information

Genetic test results are not only relevant to the individual tested but also to the extended family. Thus during the consent process the implications and release of genetic information to other family members should be discussed. This can be invaluable in identifying those who wish to withhold consent to release information and there reasons for withholding this information. In such situations the genetic counsellor may be able to provide support and explore this further, allowing the genetic counsellor to put support in place if needed. It is also important to consider that it may be distressing for these individuals to have someone they have not met contact them at a later stage if consent about releasing their genetic result is not discussed at the time of testing.

3.3.14 Withdrawal of Consent

It is important when obtaining consent that patients are aware they are able to withdraw their consent at any time [37, 39]. However, in relation to genetic testing, once a result is given the information cannot then be withdrawn. A patient may withdraw their consent in relation to the test or if a family rift occurs a patient may withdraw their consent to share the information with other family members.

The requirement for obtaining consent has been around for many years, yet the specifics of consent continually change. It is important that genetic counsellors and health professionals keep abreast of these changes and local policies that are in place for the area they work in.

3.4 Reproductive Genetic Testing

Reproductive genetic testing gives couples an opportunity to avoid passing on the pathogenic variant to their children. There are two different types of testing; prenatal and pre-implantation genetic diagnosis (PGD).

Prenatal testing involves testing the pregnancy. A chorionic villus sample (CVS) is carried out at around 11–14 weeks gestation and involves placing a needle through the abdomen guided by ultrasound and sampling a small amount of the chorionic villus. This carries around a 1–2% risk of miscarriage [44]. An amniocentesis can be offered from around 15 weeks of pregnancy. This involves removing amniotic fluid from around the baby again via a needle inserted into the womb guided by ultrasound. This carries around a 0.5–1% risk of miscarriage [45]. The results for ICC testing take around 5–7 working days. However, it is important to discuss with patients that these will not be the only results and the results will be staged. Patients should be given the option of how they wish to receive the results and also the difficulties of the procedures such as low lying placenta and maternal cell contamination should be discussed.

Prenatal testing is not agreeable for every couple as it involves a risk of miscarriage and the possibility of a termination of pregnancy if the fetus is found to carry the pathogenic variant. PGD on the other hand involves checking for the pathogenic variant of an embryo that has been specifically created through assisted reproductive technology (ART) and implanting only those embryos that do not carry the pathogenic variant. However, in order to undergo PGD, the specific condition, gene, and pathogenic variant particular to the family must be licensed by the Human Fertilisation and Embryo Authority (HFEA). Presently, over 250 conditions are licensed, including HCM, ARVC, DCM, CPVT and LQT. Other syndromic conditions that have a cardiomyopathy as part of the phenotypic spectrum are also licensed [46]. If a condition is not presently licensed, it is often a couple interested in having PGD that starts the process towards being licensed. However, the HFEA must agree that a particular genetic condition is sufficiently serious before clinics are permitted to test for that condition using PGD. Provided the condition is licensed, PGD is available on the NHS for couples who fulfil certain criteria. These include having a healthy BMI, being a non-smoking couple, female age under 39 years, and no previous healthy child. If the couple do not qualify for PGD on the NHS, they can pay for it privately. However it should not be underestimated how emotionally challenging PGD can be.

3.5 Insurance and Genetic Testing

The Concordat and Moratorium on Genetics and Insurance in the UK has now been extended until 1st November 2019 [47]. This was drawn up with collaboration between Her Majesty's Government and the Association of British Insurers. In essence this is an agreement by which the insurance companies agree to be transparent and fair in the use of genetic information, in order not to deter individuals from going ahead with genetic testing due to financial considerations.

The Concordat and Moratorium only covers predictive genetic tests. There are three financial products currently affected by the concordat and moratorium. These include: life insurance, critical illness insurance and income protection. Life insurance pays out a lump sum if you die and is often a requirement for obtaining a mortgage; critical illness insurance covers an individual if they are diagnosed with or requiring treatment for certain conditions and payment protection insurance provides cover when someone is incapacitated and unable to work.

Insurance companies are able to ask details of diagnostic genetic tests which include those of family members [47]. Disclosure of a predictive genetic test result is only requested when three specified criteria are met. This is due to be reviewed in 2016. The implications of genetic testing on insurance should be discussed with patients undergoing genetic testing. It is important that genetic counsellors are aware of the current guidance and are able to advise and signpost their patients accurately. The Genetic Alliance UK publication [48] is a patient friendly review of the information, patients can also be directed to the actual Concordat and Moratorium (2014).

3.6 Psychological Implications of Inherited Cardiac Conditions

The impact of living with inherited cardiac conditions cannot be underestimated. The sudden and unexpected loss of a child, sibling, parent or close relative is a devastating and highly emotional event. Discovering this could be hereditary, and that other close family members may have an increased risk of sudden death, only exacerbates an already tragic situation. It is therefore essential that health professionals are able to communicate information in a clear and concise manner.

There are a range of emotions which those affected and their family members can go through; including fear, guilt, anger, denial, grief and despair. It is important for clinicians and genetic counsellors to be aware of these so they are able to fully support the patient and families as effectively as possible to adjust to the diagnosis. There are also many different reactions that families can have in response to having a relative experience a cardiac event or sudden death. This chapter will not attempt to cover all of these; however some of the more common reactions are highlighted here.

3.6.1 Information

It is essential that patients and families receive clear and accurate information so that they can process the many issues they may have to deal with, such as trying to explain to children why a parent or sibling has suddenly died, while at the same time being terrified of losing another relative to sudden death. Merlevede et al. [49] interviewed 74 relatives of individuals who had died suddenly. The interviews were carried out at three different time periods following their loss to look at their perceptions and needs. Although they were not looking specifically at relatives of sudden cardiac death, they demonstrated that relatives of those who died suddenly and unexpectedly have a need for information. In addition, they found they were often unable to ask questions in the immediate aftermath.

Families with inherited cardiac conditions are likely to attend the initial genetic counselling consultation with many questions. Thus it is important for the clinician and genetic counsellors to have access to up to date knowledge in order to give these families accurate information in a timely manner to help them process all of the information and the situation they find themselves in.

3.6.2 Uncertainty

Genetic testing for inherited cardiac conditions is available on the NHS and in the private sector. However, prior to going ahead with genetic testing, genetic counselling should always be obtained because of the psychologically challenging nature of the impact of obtaining a result [17]. Even if a pathogenic variant is found there is still uncertainty as to when the condition will present and how severely, due to the variability of these conditions even within families.

The European Society of Cardiology et al. [50] recommend screening of first-degree relatives when a possible inherited cardiac condition is found. It is estimated that around one third of families, in which no cause of sudden death is identified, are found to have inherited cardiac conditions [51]. However, for many families a pathogenic variant will not be detected and these families will continue to have uncertainty regarding risk and the hereditary nature of the condition. It is therefore essential that all of the possible outcomes are discussed prior to any testing, so that families are fully informed when considering genetic testing.

In a qualitative study by Hidayatallah et al. [52] they found that families often do not know or understand why their apparently healthy relative has died, this was found to be the case particularly with cardiac channelopathies. The study looked at 50 participants from 32 families, who were personally affected by a cardiac event, or had a relative who had a cardiac event or sudden death. This study found that genetic testing is not commonly requested following autopsy and as such "Families are frequently left with the ambiguous conclusion that a loved one died from 'unknown' causes" creating further anxiety ([52], p. 3). They also comment that since these deaths often occur during sleep there is very little information surrounding the death. This lack of information only further compounds the uncertainty.

3.6.3 Bereavement and Grief

Bereavement and grief is multifaceted and individuals will experience grief in different ways and at different times. There are five recognised stages of grief as identified in the seminal work of Elizabeth Kübler-Ross [53]. These include; denial, anger, bargaining, depression and acceptance.

3.6.3.1 Five Stages of Grief

Denial is a common reaction in the early stages of the grief process. Many people will think 'it didn't happen, it must be a mistake'. Whereas some may be numb and appear to others as if they are not grieving. This numbness may act as a form of defence to prevent being overwhelmed by the situation [54]. Patients may be aware they are in denial and not ready to let go of their loved one, others however, may not even realise they are in denial. It may be they are not able to cope, so by only accepting parts of the reality they prevent themselves from being overwhelmed. This reaction is more common in those who experience sudden deaths. Worden [54] suggests those who experience sudden and unexpected deaths are also more likely to take longer to accept the loss.

Anger is a common response in the grieving process but can be confusing to those experiencing this. It is hard for them to feel anger at their loved one for dying and leaving them, as a result this can get directed at others when looking for a sense of blame to try to reason with the loss [53]. By acknowledging and exploring their anger, but remaining detached and non-judgemental, it can allow the patient to voice the reality they are facing.

Bargaining sometimes happens with patients who have experienced a sudden loss or cardiac event. This is a time when they say "if I do this then...", this is not meant in reality but it is a form of adjustment. It may be reflected in wanting to ensure genetic testing and screening of all family members occurs immediately. This can make it more challenging when discussing the pros and cons of testing and the timing of testing with patients.

Depression is considered by Elisabeth Kübler-Ross foundation [53] to be the full reality of grief. Those experiencing it may withdraw from others, suffer from sleep disturbance or refuse to eat. They may consider 'what is the point'. This can be difficult and frustrating for relatives who may still be in the bargaining phase and want to be proactive but are unable to bargain with those in the depressive phase of grief.

Acceptance is a part of the grief process in which genetic counselling can play an important role. There are different aspects to acceptance that need to be considered. The relatives need to accept their loss on a practical level whilst adjusting to the impact on their everyday life. This may be financial and/or bringing up children alone. Relatives of the deceased will also need to come to terms with how the death affects their own sense of self. For many families the bereavement can also impact on their beliefs and values [54]. It is therefore important for genetic counsellors to be aware if someone appears to be suffering from complicated grief and ensure that further support is available and offered if required.

Anxiety: Due to the sudden and unexpected loss or near death experience of a family member, families can sometimes be left extremely anxious. Worden [54] states that anxiety in the bereaved can range from a lack of confidence in one's ability to cope to having a strong panic attack. Guidelines and strategies for extended family care were reviewed by Vincent [55] and these describe how families are left wondering who will die next. Patients often describe the fear of letting a family member out of their sight in case they don't come back.

Merlevede et al. [49] highlighted how patients can sometimes feel they are left with unanswered questions following the sudden death of relatives, which only adds to their anxiety. They may have been informed it is a hereditary condition but given little further information other than to see their GP. Even when they have further information in relation to the condition, patients still worry about how they are going to tell their relatives or when and how they are going to tell their children.

Guilt: Relatives may feel guilt and self-reproach in relation to the loss of a loved one. These may be irrational thoughts but it is common for people to feel they should have seen them more or been there more for them. In addition relatives can struggle with the guilt of having passed on a pathogenic variant to their child/children. This is highlighted in a study by Mangset and Hofmann [34], a small study of 13 parents of children with Long QT syndrome (LQTS). They demonstrated parents need to know the genetic status of their children and they looked specifically at the challenging issues that arise for parents of children at risk and affected by LQTS. The study highlighted the high levels of anxiety of having an affected child, as well as the parents struggle with guilt.

3.7 Family Communication

In order to ensure as many relatives as possible are screened or tested to prevent an adverse event occurring, genetic counsellors need to discuss with each family how they are going to disseminate the information to other family members. Some may wish to have a letter they can pass on to relatives to help them accurately convey the information.

It is important to make clear what information will and won't be released to other family members to ensure misconceptions and misunderstandings do not arise within the family, as this may prevent access to screening and testing. Mangset and Hofmann [34] support the importance of genetic counsellors assisting the family to convey the information to other family members. This may not be just after an initial consultation when informing a family member, it may be sometime later when a child is older and requiring more detailed information about the condition. Patients and families should be made aware that they can re-contact the genetics department if they wish to be seen again. Genetic counsellors and clinicians can help to support family communication in difficult times, for example when children get older and become more questioning.

3.7.1 Impact on Family Relationships

Family relationships can be deeply affected when a genetic condition is identified in the family. The ways in which different family members respond to the information may create tensions within the families. Parents can often feel guilty about having passed on a risk of early sudden death to their children. Siblings found not to be affected may suffer 'survivors' guilt' and question why it was not them or have many questions surrounding the death to try to come to terms with this sudden loss [56]. Affected children may be treated differently by parents who become over protective of them or distance themselves as a form of self-protection. This can then create issues between affected and non-affected siblings.

At risk individuals whose work may be impacted by such information may resent others for raising this information with them when they may have chosen not to know.

3.7.2 Support

In order to help reduce patients anxiety when going through genetic testing it is recommended, in other genetic conditions, that they bring a relative or friend to support them through the testing process [57]. It is important that the genetic counsellor who is taking the patient through diagnostic or predictive testing explores the patient's support network and who they will look to outside of the clinical setting to support them through the process. This will help to ensure they have support when they leave the clinic. Literature has shown that those with a good support network may have reduced anxiety compared to those without [58, 59].

3.7.3 Multiple Bereavements

Some families may have experienced multiple sudden deaths within the close family. Genetic counsellors need to be aware that bereavement due to multiple losses can have additional characteristics. In these families individuals can often suffer from increased personal vulnerability, depression and suicidal thoughts [54].

3.7.4 Adjustment: Living with Risk

In time most patients and their families will adjust and adapt to the new diagnosis within the family. Genetic counsellors need to have an understanding of how individuals and families process the information and adapt so they are better able to support these families and intervene with those who struggle to adapt.

Conclusion

It is important for clinicians and genetic counsellors to ensure patients undergoing genetic testing (diagnostic or predictive) are given as much information as they need, are fully supported and have time to consider the implications of the genetic test prior to going ahead. Genetic testing requires an understanding of the testing being offered, the limitations of the test, and all possible results that may arise. With their specific training, genetic counsellors are well placed to be able to provide the individual with all of this information and enable them to make an informed choice about testing. It is encouraging that the literature indicates that the majority of those going ahead with genetic testing for ICC's found that it promoted a sense of control and provided reassurance for the patient [60].

References

1. Goldenberg I, Zareba W, Moss AJ. Long QT syndrome. Curr Probl Cardiol. 2008;33(11):629–94.
2. Jensen MK, Havndrup O, Christiansen M, Andersen PS, Diness B, Axelsson A, Skovby F, Kober L, Bundgaard H. Penetrance of hypertrophic cardiomyopathy in children and adolescents: a 12-year follow-up study of clinical screening and predictive genetic testing. Circulation. 2013;127(1):48–54.
3. Van Driest SL, Ackerman MJ, Ommen SR, Shakur R, Will ML, Nishimura RA, Tajik AJ, Gersh BJ. Prevalence and severity of "benign" mutations in the beta-myosin heavy chain, cardiac troponin T, and alpha-tropomyosin genes in hypertrophic cardiomyopathy. Circulation. 2002;106(24):3085–90.
4. Arad M, Monserrat L, Haron-Khun S, Seidman JG, Seidman C, Arbustini E, Glikson M, Freimark D. Merits and pitfalls of genetic testing in a hypertrophic cardiomyopathy clinic. Isr Med Assoc J. 2014;16:707–13.
5. Ellaway C. Paediatric fabry disease. Translat Paediatr. 2016;5(1):37–42.
6. Gourraud J-B, Barc J, Thollet A, Le Scouarnec S, Le Marec H, Schott J-J, Redon R, Probst V. The Brugada syndrome: a rare arrhythmia disorder with complex inheritance. Front Cardiovasc Med. 2016;3:9.
7. El-Hattab AW, Scaglia F. Mitochondrial cardiomyopathies. Front Cardiovasc Med. 2016;3:25. https://doi.org/10.3389/fcvm.2016.00025.

8. Koeppn AH, Becker AB, Feustel PJ, Gelman BB, Mazurkiewicz JE. The significance of intercalated discs in the pathogenesis of Friedreich cardiomyopathy. J Neurol Sci. 2016;367:171–6.
9. Sen-Chowdhry S, McKenna WJ. Sudden death from genetic and acquired cardiomyopathies. Circulation. 2012;125(12):1563–76.
10. Wolf C, Michael A, Ferhaan A, Atsushi S, Scott B, Okan T, Tetsuo K, Gregory M, Jeffrey R, Seidman JG, Christine S, Charles B. Reversibility of PRKAG2 glycogen-storage cardiomyopathy and electrophysiological manifestations. Circulation. 2008;117(1):144–54.
11. Spada M, Pagliardini S, Yasuda M, Tukel T, Thiagarajan G, Sakuraba H, Ponzone A, Desnick RJ. High incidence of later-onset fabry disease revealed by newborn screening. Am J Hum Genet. 2006;79(1):31–40.
12. Zarate YA, Hopkin RJ. Fabry's disease. Lancet. 2008;372(9647):1427–35.
13. Eng CM, Guffon N, Wilcox WR, German DP, Lee P, Waldex S, Caplan L, Linthorst GE, Desnick RJ. Safety and efficacy of recombinant human α-Galactosidase a replacement therapy in Fabry's disease. N Engl J Med. 2001;345(1):9–16.
14. Mehta A, Beck M, Eyskens F, Feliciani C, Kantola I, Ramaswami U, Rolfs A, Rivera A, Waldek S, Germain DP. Fabry disease: a review of current management strategies. Q J Med. 2010;103(9):641–59.
15. Schiffmann R, Kopp JB, Austin HA III, Sabnis S, Moore DF, Weibel T, Balow JE, Brady RO. Enzyme replacement therapy in Fabry disease: a randomized controlled trial. J Am Med Assoc. 2001;285(21):2743–9.
16. Nishino I, Jin F, Kurenzai T, Takeshi Y, Sadatomo S, Tateo K, Marina M, Riggs JE, Oh SJ, Yasutoshi K, Sue CM, Ayaka Y, Nobuyuki M, Sara S, Edward B, Eduardo B, Ikuya N, Salvatore DM, Michio H. Primary Lamp-2 deficiency causes X-linked vacuolar cardiomyopathy and myopathy (Danon disease). Nature. 2000;406:906–10.
17. Ingles J, Semsarian C. Sudden cardiac death in the young: a clinical genetic approach. Intern Med J. 2007;37(1):32–37.
18. Richard P, Charron P, Carrier L, Ledeuil C, Cheav T, Pichereau C, Benaiche A, Isnard R, Dubourg O, Burban M, Gueffet JP, Millaire A, Desnos M, Schwartz K, Hainque B, Komajda M. Hypertrophic cardiomyopathy: distribution of disease genes, spectrum of mutations, and implications for a molecular diagnosis strategy. Circulation. 2003;107(17):2227–32.
19. Jacoby D, McKenna WJ. Genetics of inherited cardiomyopathy. Eur Heart J. 2012;33:296–304.
20. Ackerman MJ. Genetic testing for risk stratification in hypertrophic cardiomyopathy and long QT syndrome: fact or fiction? Curr Opin Cardiol. 2005;20:175–81.
21. Priori SG, Barhanin J, Hauer RN, Haverkamp W, Jongsma HJ, Kleber AG, McKenna WJ, Roden DM, Rudy Y, Schwartz K, Schwartz PJ, Towbin JA, Wilde A. Genetic and molecular basis of cardiac arrhythmias; impact on clinical management. Study group on molecular basis of arrhythmias of the working group on arrhythmias of the european society of cardiology. Eur Heart J. 1999;20(3):174–95.
22. Keren A, Syrris P, McKenna WJ. Hypertrophic cardiomyopathy: the genetic determinants of clinical disease expression. Nat Clin Practice Cardiovasc Med. 2008;5(3):158–68.
23. Van Rijsingen I, Arbustini E, Elliott PM, Mogensen J, Hermans-van JF, van der Kooi AJ, van Tintelen P, van den Berg MP, Pilotto A, Pasotti M, Jenkins S, Rowland C, Aslam U, Wilde AAM, Perrot A, Pankuweit S, Zwinderman AH, Charron P, Pinto YM. Risk factors for malignant ventricular arrhythmias in Lamin a/C mutation carriers. J Am Coll Cardiol. 2012;59(5):493–500.
24. Antzelevitch C, Brugada P, Borggrefe M, Brugada J, Brugada R, Corrado D, Gussak I, Le Marec H, Nademanee K, Ricardo A, Riera P, Shimizu W, Schulze-Bahr E, Tan H, Wilde A. Brugada syndrome report of the second consensus conference. Circulation. 2005;111:659–70.
25. Cotton RG, Scriver CR. Proof of disease casuing2 mutations. Hum Mutat. 1998;12:1–3.
26. British Society of Human Genetics. Report on the genetic testing of children. 2010. www.bsgm.org.uk/media/678741/gtoc_booklet_final_new.pdf. Accessed Apr 2016.
27. Clarke A. The genetic testing of children. J Med Genet. 1995;32(6):492.
28. McConkie-Rosell A, Spiridigliozzi GA. "Family matters": a conceptual framework for genetic testing in children. J Genet Couns. 2004;13:9–29.

29. American Society of Human Genetics Board of Directors, American College of Medical Genetics Board of Directors. Points to consider: ethical, legal, and psychosocial implications of genetic testing in children and adolescents. Am J Hum Genet. 1995;57(5):1233–41.
30. Heart Rhythm UK Familial Sudden Death Syndromes Statement Development. Clinical indications for genetic testing in familial sudden cardiac death syndromes: and HRUK position statement. Heart. 2008;94:502–7.
31. Clarke A. The genetic testing of children. Working Party of the Clinical Genetics Society (UK). J Med Genet. 1994;31(10):785–97.
32. Bos MJ, Towbin JA, Ackerman MJ. Diagnostic, prognostic and therapeutic implications of genetic testing for hypertrophic cardiomyopathy. J Am Coll Cardiol. 2009;54(3):201–11.
33. Ormonroyd E, Oates S, Parker M, Blair E, Watkins H. Pre-symptomatic genetic testing for inherited cardiac conditions: a qualitative exploration of psychosocial and ethical implications. Eur J Hum Genet. 2014;22(1):88–93.
34. Mangset M, Hofmann B. LQTS parents' reflections about genetic risk knowledge and their need to know or not to know their children's carrier status. J Genet Couns. 2014;23(6):1022–33.
35. Gillick v West Norfolk & Wisbeck Area Health Authority. AC 112 House of Lords. 1986.
36. Human Tissue Act. Chapter 30. Crown copyright. 2004.
37. Human Tissue Authority. Code of practice 1: consent. Crown Copyright. 2014. https://www.hta.gov.uk/guidance-professionals/codes-practice/code-practice-1-consent. Accessed 25 Apr 2016.
38. Department of Health. Reference guide to consent for examination or treatment. Crown Copyright. 2009. https://www.gov.uk/government/uploads/system/uploads/attachment_data/file/138296/dh_103653__1_.pdf. Accessed 25 Apr 2016.
39. General Medical Council. Consent: patients and doctors making decisions together. 2008. http://www.gmc-uk.org/static/documents/content/Consent_-_English_1015.pdf. Accessed 25 Apr 2016.
40. Joint Committee on Medical Genetics. Consent and confidentiality in genetic practice: guidance on genetic testing and sharing genetic information. Report of the Joint Committee on Medical Genetics. Copyright © 2006 Royal College of Physicians. 2006.
41. Joint Committee on Medical Genetics. Consent and confidentiality in genetic practice: guidance on genetic testing and sharing genetic information. 2011. http://www.bsgm.org.uk/media/678746/consent_and_confidentiality_2011.pdf. Accessed 25 Apr 2016.
42. Mental Capacity Act. Chapter 9. Crown copyright. 2005.
43. Human Tissue (Scotland) Act. (asp 4). Crown copyright. 2006.
44. Brambati B, Lucia T. Chorionic villus sampling and amniocentesis. Curr Opin Obstet Gynaecol. 2005;17(2):197–201.
45. Wilson DR. Amniocentesis and chorionic villus sampling. Curr Opin Obstetr Cardiol. 2000;12(2): 81–6.
46. Human Fertilisation and Embryology Association. 2016. Available at: www.hfea.gov.uk. Accessed May 2016.
47. Her Majesty's Government and Association of British Insurers. Concordat and moratorium on genetics and insurance. 2014. https://www.gov.uk/government/publications/agreement-extended-on-predictive-genetic-tests-and-insurance. Accessed 06 May 2016.
48. Genetic Alliance UK. Genetic conditions and insurance: what you need to know and what you need to tell. 2012. www.geneticalliance.org.uk/docs/genetics-and-insurance.pdf. Accessed 06 May 2016.
49. Merlevede E, Spooren D, Henderick H, Portzky G, Buylaert W, Jannes C, Calle P, Van Staey M, De Rock C, Smeesters L, Michem N, van Heeringen K. Perceptions, needs and mourning reactions of bereaved relatives confronted with a sudden unexpected death. Resuscitation. 2004;61:341–8.
50. European Society of Cardiology, Priori SG, Blomström-Lundqvist C, Mazzanti A, Blom N, Borggrefe M, Camm J, Elliott PM, Fitzsimons D, Hatala R, Hindricks G, Kirchhof P, Kjeldsen K, Kuck KH, Hernandez-Madrid A, Nikolaou N, Norekvål TM, Spaulding C, Van Velhuisen DJ. European Society of Cardiology Guidelines for the management of patients with ventricular arrhythmias and the prevention of sudden cardiac death. Eur Heart J. 2015;36:2793–867.

51. Van der Werf C, Hofman N, Tan HL, van Dessel PF, Alders M, van der Wal AC, van Langen IM, Wilde AA. Diagnostic yield in sudden unexplained death and aborted cardiac arrest in the young: the experience of a tertiary referral centre in the Netherlands. Heart Rhythm. 2010;7(10):1383–9.
52. Hidayatallah N, Silverstein LB, Stolerman M, McDonald T, Walsh CA, Plajevic E, Cohen LL, Marion RW, Wasserman D, Hreyo S, Dolan SM. Psychological stress associated with cardiogenetic conditions. Pers Med. 2014;11(7):631–40.
53. Elisabeth Kübler-Ross foundation. 2016. Available at: http://www.ekrfoundation.org/. Accessed 11 May 2016.
54. Worden W. Grief counselling and grief therapy: a handbook for the mental health practitioner. 4th ed. London: Routledge; 2009. p. 978–0415559.
55. Vincent GM. Sudden cardiac arrest in the young due to inherited arrhythmias: the importance of family care. Pacing Clin Electrophysiol. 2009;32:S19–22.
56. Clements PT, Garzon L, Milliken TF. 'Survivors' guilt following sudden traumatic loss: promoting early intervention in the critical care setting'. Crit Care Nurs Clin North Am. 2006;18(3):359–69.
57. MacLeod R, Tibben A, Frontali M, Evers-Kiebooms G, Jones A, Martinez-Descales A, Roos R. Recommendations for the predictive genetic test in Huntington's disease. Clin Genet. 2013;83(3):221–31.
58. Mikulincer M, Shaver PR. The attachment behavioral system in adulthood: activation, psychodynamics, and interpersonal processes. In: Zanna MP, editor. Advances in experimental social psychology. San Diego: Elsevier Academic Press; 2003. p. 53–152.
59. Pietromonaco P, Feldman Barrett L, Powers SI. Adult attachment theory and affective reactivity and regulation. In: Snyder DK, Simpson JA, Hughes JN, editors. Emotion regulation in couples and families: pathways to dysfunction and health, vol. 1. Washington: American Psychological Association; 2006. p. 57–74.
60. Christiaans I, van Langen IM, Birnie E, Bonsel GJ, Wilde AA, Smets EM. Genetic counselling and cardiac care in predictively tested hypertrophic cardiomyopathy pathogenic variant carriers: the patients' perspective. Am J Med Genet. 2009;149A:1444–51.
61. Resta R, et al. A new definition of genetic counelling: NSGC task force report. J Genet Couns. 2006;15(2):77–83.

Genetic and Genomic Technologies: Next Generation Sequencing for Inherited Cardiovascular Conditions

4

Lorenzo Monserrat

Abstract

What is NGS? Basically, we give this name to a group of technologies that allow the sequencing of thousands or millions of DNA or RNA fragments in parallel, while with the Sanger methods we were amplifying and evaluating those fragments one by one. The result is an enormous increase in the sequencing capacity and speed, and a huge decrease in the cost per sequence. As an example, one of the currently available NGS machines is able to perform the same work as 100,000 Sanger sequencers. In the "Sanger Sequencing era" we had to focus our analysis in a limited number of fragments or genes, and the cost of the studies was a major determinant in the decision to perform genetic studies in patients affected by inherited diseases. Now, we can use the huge capacity of the NGS technologies to perform not only more comprehensive studies, but also cheaper ones. NGS is very useful for the evaluation of many genes, or even a whole genome, in individual patients. It is also very appropriate for the evaluation of lower numbers of genes in multiple patients at the same time, which is very important to increase the accessibility to the genetic tests.

Keywords

Next generation sequencing • NGS • Bioinformatics • Inherited cardiovascular conditions

L. Monserrat
Health-in-Code, Le Coruna, Spain
e-mail: lmonserrat@healthincode.com

D. Kumar, P. Elliott (eds.), *Cardiovascular Genetics and Genomics*,
https://doi.org/10.1007/978-3-319-66114-8_4

4.1 Introduction: What Is "Next Generation Sequencing" and Why We Need It in Inherited Cardiovascular Conditions

Since the discovery of the DNA structure by Watson and Crick in 1953 there has been a continuous, but relatively slow, progress in our capacity to read and interpret DNA and RNA sequences. Sanger and Gilbert published their sequencing method in 1977, but the first automated sequencer was not commercially available until 1987. This technological advance was essential for the beginning of a new era of scientific and medical advances, with the discovery of the genetic basis of thousands of different diseases. For example, the first mutation associated with the development of hypertrophic cardiomyopathy was published in 1989. The Human Genome Project, which began in 1992 and resulted in the first sequence of the human genome in 2007, should be considered the culmination of what we could call "the Sanger Sequencing era". Hundreds of scientists and machines all over the world had to work together during 15 years to get that sequence, which now we can get in one day in a single machine for approximately 1000 euros. This extraordinary achievement is the consequence of the irruption of what we call "Next Generation Sequencing" or NGS [1].

What is NGS? Basically, we give this name to a group of technologies that allow the sequencing of thousands or millions of DNA or RNA fragments in parallel, while with the Sanger methods we were amplifying and evaluating those fragments one by one. The result is an enormous increase in the sequencing capacity and speed, and a huge decrease in the cost per sequence. As an example, one of the currently available NGS machines is able to perform the same work as 100,000 Sanger sequencers. In the "Sanger Sequencing era" we had to focus our analysis in a limited number of fragments or genes, and the cost of the studies was a major determinant in the decision to perform genetic studies in patients affected by inherited diseases. Now, we can use the huge capacity of the NGS technologies to perform not only more comprehensive studies, but also cheaper ones. NGS is very useful for the evaluation of many genes, or even a whole genome, in individual patients. It is also very appropriate for the evaluation of lower numbers of genes in multiple patients at the same time, which is very important to increase the accessibility to the genetic tests.

The inherited cardiovascular conditions, including cardiomyopathies, channelopathies, familial aortic and vascular diseases and inherited dyslipidaemias constitute one of the most appropriate scenarios for the application of NGS technologies for several reasons:

1. They are usually monogenic (or oligo-genic) diseases with a familial presentation: genetic testing has the highest impact in the management of those diseases that are due, and explained, by the presence of a single or a small number of mutations.
2. They show a high degree of genetic heterogeneity: Each one of these groups includes a number of diseases of genetic origin, and each one of those diseases may be caused by hundreds of different mutations affecting a number of different genes. This genetic heterogeneity found in inherited cardiovascular diseases explains a great part of their clinical heterogeneity. The understanding of the

genetic basis of each condition allows the clinicians to establish a more precise and individualized prognosis, through a better knowledge on the clinical characteristics associated with each gene and each particular mutation. NGS is the best tool for the evaluation of multiple candidate genes.

3. Overlapping or intermediate phenotypes are quite frequent: It is not rare that the same patient shows clinical characteristics that point to different diagnoses (for example, dilated, hypertrophic and arrhythmogenic cardiomyopathies may appear as overlapping phenotypes). In those cases, the genetic testing is especially useful to define the disease and the genetic screening has to include genes that have been associated with the different "suspected" phenotypes.
4. There are many cases with mild or incomplete clinical expression: genetic testing is very useful for an early and correct diagnosis in those cases that will allow a better programming of the follow up and risk stratification. The selection of the candidate genes is more difficult in cases with subtle or incomplete expression, and the possibility of including many genes in the screening is especially interesting in that situations.
5. They are associated with sudden death risk: In fact, inherited cardiovascular diseases are the main causes of sudden death in young individuals, and are also associated with sudden death risk in older patients. Sudden death may be the first manifestation of the disease, and for that reason it is essential to obtain an early diagnosis in affected individuals and in their relatives. Genetic testing offers a unique opportunity for early diagnosis, confirmation of clinically suspected (but not confirmed) conditions, and for the familial screening.

The impact of NGS in the evaluation of inherited cardiovascular conditions is clearly explained by the following example. In 2011, the HRS/EHRA expert consensus statement on the estate of genetic testing for the channelopathies and cardiomyopathies [2] said about genetic testing in dilated cardiomyopathy that "none of the >25 known disease-associated genes has been shown to account for ≥5% of this disease", and for that reason, it did not recommend to perform genetic testing in dilated cardiomyopathy except in cases with cardiac conduction defects or multiple sudden deaths (looking for mutations in the LMNA gene). Nowadays it has been shown that with the current NGS panels that allow the evaluation of all the candidate genes in parallel, including "giant" genes as TTN (encoding titin), we are able to find mutations responsible for the development of idiopathic dilated cardiomyopathy in more than 50% of the cases, and up to 70% in some circumstances [3].

4.2 Next Generation Sequencing Technologies

4.2.1 General Overview of the Process

The main differential characteristic of NGS versus the previously available sequencing technologies is its capacity to perform the evaluation in parallel of multiple DNA fragments (up to the level of millions) at the same time. This may be obtained through the application of different technologies at several steps in a complex process. We will briefly review this process, from the perspective of a clinician, in the following sections.

In summary, we can divide the process in four steps: sample preparations, sequencing, bioinformatics analysis and interpretation of the results. All those steps may vary depending on the selected technologies and objectives of the study. Figure 4.1 provides a general overview of the whole process.

4.2.2 Sample Preparations

We call "sample preparations" to all the processes that are required before the samples are introduced in the sequencer, including the DNA or RNA extraction and the enrichment or direct amplification technologies that will finish with the preparation of the fragments that will later enter in the sequencer.

4.2.2.1 DNA, RNA Extraction

The first step in the process is to extract DNA or RNA from the available sources. Genomic DNA may be obtained from any sample containing nucleated cells. Most often, DNA is extracted from either blood, saliva or tissue samples. It is of the maximum relevance for the quality of the NGS result to start with a sufficient quantity of good quality DNA. Both manual and automated DNA extraction methods are able to provide excellent quality DNA when we use fresh or refrigerated blood, extracted in the previous 48–72 h. When it is not possible to extract the DNA in that period, blood may be kept frozen (at least −20 °C) even for prolonged periods. However, frozen blood samples that are kept for a long time may be of suboptimal quality. Once the DNA has been extracted, it may be kept at −80 °C for very long periods without a relevant effect in its quality. Saliva samples are currently a good alternative for blood as DNA source for NGS. Several commercial kits are available that allow an easy collection and transport of the saliva samples. The yield and quality of the obtained DNA are good when the collection is adequately performed, even when the kits are maintained for several days at room temperature. Mouth swaps are an alternative for a non-invasive samples collection that is especially interesting in infants and small children who are not able to collaborate for saliva collection. In these cases it may be required to get more than one swap to warrant the obtaining of a sufficient DNA quantity. Fresh or frozen tissue samples from or autopsy or biopsies of organs with high cellularity are usually a good DNA and RNA source. DNA may also be obtained from paraffin embedded tissues, but this source should only be considered when there are not other samples available. The preservation process undergone by the samples before the paraffin inclusion is associated with DNA damage and degradation. Even thought it is possible to obtain DNA suitable for NGS sequencing from these samples, it is usually of lower quality and in a proportion of cases it will not be possible to obtain analysable sequences.

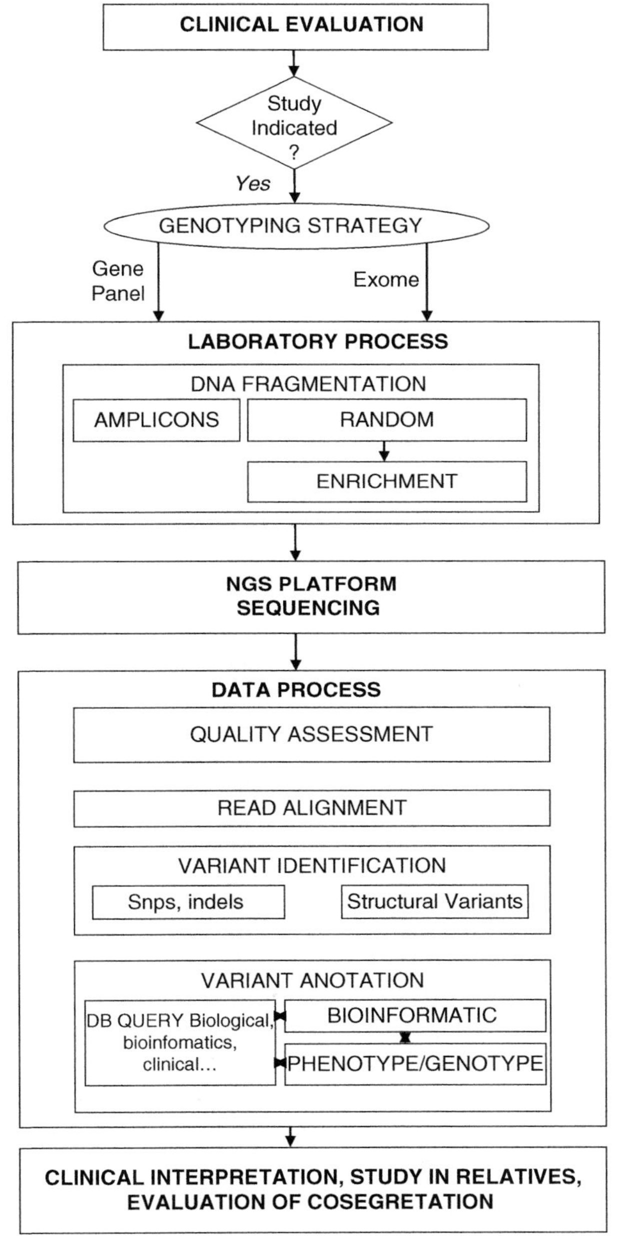

Fig. 4.1 Overview of the Next Generation Sequencing genetic testing process for the evaluation of patients with inherited conditions

A special situation is when we are interested in the evaluation of mitochondrial DNA. There are mitochondria in both nucleated and non-nucleated cells. When we extract whole DNA from any one of the previously described samples, we obtain both nuclear and mitochondrial DNA, and there are usually many copies of the mitochondrial DNA per each nuclear DNA copy. Nuclear DNA includes multiples sequences that are homologous to sequences found in the mitochondrial DNA. If we want to obtain pure mitochondrial DNA, we have to separate the mitochondria before doing the DNA extraction. However, in many cases the sequencing of the mitochondrial DNA is performed from extractions done from the whole samples, assuming that most of the copies of the sequences of interest will come from the mitochondrial DNA and not from the homologous sequences present in the nuclear DNA.

While genomic DNA is the same in all our diploid cells, RNAs (and cDNAs) are different in different cells and even in the same cells in different moments. For that reason, when we want to sequence RNA we have to obtain the sample from the specific cells or tissues we want to evaluate. Something similar occurs in a special situation for DNA analysis: when we suspect the presence of a somatic mosaicism.

4.2.2.2 DNA/RNA Fragmentation

Our objective is to evaluate multiple fragments of either DNA or RNA in parallel, so that, we need to obtain those fragments. The size of the fragments is critical for the NGS process. The sequencers can be programmed to make reads of different lengths, usually ranging between 50 and 200 pair bases from each side of the fragments. If the fragments are too small we will have too much overlap in the readings from each side, generating duplications in the reads and loosing sequencing capacity. The subsequent alignment of the reads versus the reference sequence is also more difficult or even impossible if the fragments are too small. On the other side, if the fragments are too big they will not be appropriately captured.

We can do the fragmentation either by mechanical or enzymatic processes.

Mechanical fragmentation is performed using ultrasounds. The currently available machines are able to process up to 96 samples at the same time and may be programmed to generate fragments of variable size. The objective is to obtain overlapping fragments and one of the main advantages of mechanical fragmentation is that it is more random than the enzymatic processes. However, it is not completely random and biases dependent on sequence characteristics are one of the potential bases for variations in coverage between different regions [4]. Enzymatic fragmentation is a faster and cheaper process than mechanical one. It is performed with restriction enzymes that are designed to break the DNA/RNA in multiple points trying also to get a random fragmentation.

4.2.2.3 Enrichment Technologies

When we perform NGS we can either evaluate the whole genome or to concentrate the analysis in those genomic regions we consider most relevant (we will comment on the advantages and disadvantages of both options in a subsequent section). Currently, most of the clinical studies use the second strategy and concentrate the sequencing in specific genomic regions. In those cases, we apply enrichment technologies in order to increase the proportion of fragments of interest in the studied sample. These processes increase the efficiency of the sequencing. As a comparison, if we want to make copies of the first and third chapters of one book, it is more efficient to extract those two chapters and copy them than to make copies of all the book and then select the two chapters of interest; especially if we have a limited amount of paper.

In order to select the fragments of interest, we have to generate a library of probes complementary to those regions. Commercial companies provide software that helps in the design process. Those probes are attached to molecules, such as biotin, that will be able to bind to a substrate, such as streptavidin, attached to magnetic beads. After the hybridization of the denaturalized DNA with the probes, the streptavidin coated magnetic beads are added, and the fragments of interest are captured with a magnet.

The fragments of interest will then undergo a process of amplification to obtain multiple copies of them. With some technologies, the DNA is introduced in a flow cell where the fragments are attached to the surface of a plate where they are replicated to generate clones. Other systems do the amplification in solution.

Usually we will pool multiple samples in the amplification step, so that previous to the amplification, the fragments are hybridised with short tags of bases, which will allow the identification of the origin of each one of the fragments and their separation during the bioinformatics analysis.

4.2.2.4 Direct Amplification Technologies

Instead of capturing the fragments of interest, we can make a direct amplification of them. We have to design specific primers for the sequences of interest and perform polymerase chain reactions (PCRs) that result in the generation of the corresponding "amplicons". Once we get those amplicons we continue with the ligation of the tag SNPs (for the identification of the origin of the samples prior to their mixing with amplicons from other cases) and the sequencing. These techniques of direct amplification may be very cost-efficient when we want to sequence a relatively small number of fragments, but they are not usually the best option if we need to sequence multiple genes, because it may be very difficult to amplify many fragments in a joint reaction. Direct amplification techniques are also not appropriate when we want to analyse copy number variations through some of the available bioinformatics methods.

4.2.3 Sequencing Process and Equipment

After samples preparation has finished the individual or pooled samples have to be sequenced. As for today, there are two main commercial alternatives for next generation sequencing, Illumina technologies and Ion Torrent (Life Technologies) that use very different methods.

Ion Torrent uses a method called ion semiconductor sequencing. The DNA to be sequenced is deployed in a chip with multiple microwells, in a way that each microwell will contain multiple copies of a single DNA fragment. Then, the four nucleotides are sequentially added to the chip in the presence of DNA polymerase. When the added nucleotide is complementary to the first base of the template sequence, it will be incorporated and it will generate the release of a single hydrogen ion. This ion produces a modification in the pH that is detected by the chip sensitive layer located beneath the microwells. The electronic signal is then transmitted to the computer that annotates that in that fragment it has been recorded the presence of the added nucleotide. If there are consecutive repetitions of the same nucleotide in the sequence, the corresponding number of hydrogen molecules will be released and the detected signal should be proportional to the number of nucleotides. One of the main limitations of Ion Torrent technology is the lack of precision in the identification of the number of consecutive nucleotides when there are long homopolymers (repetitions of the same nucleotide) in the sequences. This gives place to the generation of a large number of false positive genetic variants (usually frameshift deletions or insertions) and a limited capacity for the detection of real variants in regions with homopolymers. The system has also a lower throughput as compared with Illumina technologies [5].

Illumina sequencers use a very different approach. Once the samples are prepared and multiplexed, the first step of the sequencing is the cluster generation. First, DNA fragments are fixed to a flow cell where individual molecules are amplified to generate tens of millions of clusters of up to 1000 copies of each one of the fragments. The sequencing process involves the "visualization" of the nucleotides that are sequentially incorporated to each fragment, and in order to obtain the required signal is necessary to perform this amplification. Sequencing is performed with the successive addition of one of the four nucleotides in each cycle. Those nucleotides are fluorescently labelled and the label serves as terminator of the polymerization. The incorporation of the added nucleotide generates a signal that is captured by the imaging system of the equipment only in those clusters where the available position in the sequence is complementary to that nucleotide. Then an enzyme cleaves the fluorescent label and another cycle can start. This system allows a very precise sequencing, including homopolymers, with a high throughput [6].

There are different Illumina machines with different capacities and precision. The smallest is MiniSeq, with a amaximum output of up to 7.5 Gb. One of the most popular machines is the MiSeq (output up to 15 Gb). The NextSeq may generate up to 120 Gb of data. The HiSeq 2500 may generate up to 1 Tb, and the NovaSeq up to 3 Tb. There is an inverse relation between the size of the panels multiplied by the number of samples we study and the coverage we get, and it is important to use a machine with the adequate capacity in order to maximize the cost-efficiency of the tests.

4.2.4 Bioinformatics Analysis

Here we refer to the specific bioinformatics processes that allow the conversion of the data generated by the sequencers into the list of genetic variants present in the evaluated samples. We can differentiate the following steps:

4.2.4.1 Base Calling

Different algorithms are used to infer the nucleotide sequence of each one of the read fragments. The algorithms also provide a quality score for the calls. The result of this process is the generation of the "raw sequencing data": a great number of small sequences associated with their qualities and other parameters.

4.2.4.2 Demultiplexing

It is performed when multiple samples have been pooled in the same run. Reading the tags that had been attached to the fragments the computer separates the sequences corresponding to each sample.

4.2.4.3 Alignment

Different software tools may be used to align the raw data against a known reference sequence. We will usually have problems that may require specific solutions with sequences for which it will not be possible to establish a univocal alignment, for example in repetitive sequences, regions that are homologous to other regions in the genome, or presence of structural variants that complicate the analysis.

4.2.4.4 Identification and Annotation of the Variants Present in the Sample

The identification consists in the determination of the variants present in the sample through the SNPs/Indel calling and the genotype calling. The SNP/Indel calling, localizes the genomic positions where there are differences versus the reference sequence. The genotype calling is the process that using probabilistic models assigns a genotype to each variant with a quality score indicating the confidence of this assignment. A high quality score means that the probability that the detected variant is not really present is very low, while low values suggest that it could be a false positive result.

One of the most relevant parameters in the variants identification is the coverage, which is the number of times that a position in the sequence has been read. A good coverage provides higher quality and confidence on the variants calling and identification.

4.2.4.5 Copy Number Variation Analysis

Different strategies can be used to identify copy number variations that may correspond to big insertion or deletions: read-pair, split-read, de novo assembly and read depth and loss of heterozygosity.

4.2.4.6 Variants Annotation

It is the first step of the interpretation. Variants are classified according to the chromosome, gene, genomic region, type of variant (exonic, intronic, splicing, UTR, missense, non-sense, insertion/deletion, frameshift/non-frameshift), frequency in different populations, presence in public or private databases, and bioinformatics predictors. Once the variants have undergone this "automatic" annotation, we need to interpret their biological and clinical relevance, something that can also be considered as part of the bioinformatics processes.

4.3 The Interpretation of Next Generation Sequencing Results in Inherited Cardiovascular Conditions

NGS technologies have the capacity to analyse from individual mutations to hundreds of genes or even the whole genome, generating a huge amount of genomic data. The progression of these technologies makes the generation of those data (genetic variants) easier and cheaper. While the cost of the sequencing becomes lower, the cost and effort required for the management and interpretation of these data becomes higher. As an example, in our studies of inherited cardiovascular diseases, covering approximately 250 genes, we usually find more than 1000 different genetic variants per patient. We have to classify and give an accurate interpretation for each one of them. This interpretation is complex and requires a real multidisciplinary approach. We need good bioinformatics, molecular biologists and clinicians with expert knowledge of the genes and diseases we are evaluating, and we need tools that will help those experts to reach their conclusions in a reproducible and efficient way. In the next sections we will review the different aspects that should be covered in a good interpretation of the genetic results obtained from NGS studies.

4.3.1 Quality of the Results and Validation

NGS results are generated after a complex process of sample preparation, sequencing and bioinformatics. None of them is free of potential errors and limitations that depend on multiple parameters, including the quality of the sample, of the employed reactives, human errors, variability in the chemical reactions, number of samples that are multiplexed in the analysis (one of the main determinants of the coverage), quality and maintenance of the equipment (pipettes, sonicator, termociclers, PCR machines, sequencers…), variations in environmental conditions (temperature, humidity), and many other. One of the main sources of erroneous results arises from the probabilistic approaches that are used for variants´ annotation by bioinformatics software. It is usual that using the same raw data, different bioinformatics tools annotate different genetic variants. For all that reasons, one of the essential parameters that have to be considered in the annotation and interpretation of a genetic variant is its quality.

Variant callers always provide an individual estimation of the quality of the results.

We also have to consider other levels of "quality". Some of the most relevant are related to the sensitivity, specificity, positive and negative predictive values of the test. These depend on the technical aspects of the sample's preparation and sequencing, the quality of the design of the study, the quality of the bioinformatics process and the quality of the interpretation and reporting.

4.3.2 Pathogenicity of the Identified Variants

Once we have correctly identified the genetic variants present in a given individual we need to establish the pathogenicity of each one of them. This is not an easy task and in many cases we will not reach a definitive conclusion.

We could define the "pathogenicity" of a genetic variant as the causal or predisposing relation between the presence of a given variant with the development of a particular disease. It is important to remember that the classification of a variant as pathogenic or likely pathogenic does not mean that all the carriers of that variant will invariable develop the related disease. We define as "penetrance" the proportion of carriers of a genetic variant that express the related disease at a given age. It is very easy to identify as pathogenic genetic variants with a high penetrance at a young age: most of the carriers show the disease and there are very few healthy carriers; but it may be extremely difficult to establish the pathogenicity of disease associated variants with a low penetrance and incomplete clinical expression: we may find healthy carriers not only in affected families, but also in control populations.

Another aspect we need to consider is that disease expression may follow different inheritance patterns. While in autosomal dominant conditions a pathogenic variant may be sufficient for disease expression, in autosomal recessive, or recessive X-linked diseases the problem will only appear when both alleles of the gene are mutated. So that, a recessive variant could be considered pathogenic in homozygous carriers but it would not behave as pathogenic in heterozygous ones.

Many genetic variants are not sufficient cause for disease development even in homozygous carriers, but may be predisposing or susceptibility factors that contribute in a significant way to disease expression. We usually do not label those variants as "pathogenic", but as "risk factors" or "modifiers". There are also many variants that instead of "pathogenic" are "protective" factors.

Taking into account the previous considerations lets comment the processes employed for the definition of the pathogenicity of the genetic variants.

We have to consider and integrate three different aspects: epidemiology, molecular biology and clinical information.

4.3.3 Epidemiological Information

The frequency of a pathogenic genetic variant should be higher in patients than in controls. If the penetrance of the variant is very high, the variant should not appear in healthy individuals. Variants that appear frequently in the general population (in more than 0.5–1% of the population, depending on the definitions) are traditionally called "polymorphisms". Most polymorphisms are not pathogenic, and especially we would not expect that a polymorphism would explain the development of a very rare disease. However, polymorphisms may be predisposing factors for disease development, and some recessive pathogenic variants associated with the development of relatively rare diseases are not so rare in the general population (i.e. genetic variants associated with hemochromatosis or cystic fibrosis). Inherited cardiovascular diseases, such as hypertrophic cardiomyopathy or long QT syndrome are usually considered monogenic conditions caused by variants that are very rare in the general population (classically called "mutations" in opposition to the "polymorphisms"). However, in approximately 40% of the patients with hypertrophic cardiomyopathy and 20% of those with long QT we are currently not able to find a disease causing mutation, even studying hundreds or thousands of genes. In that cases it is possible that the mutation is located in deep intronic or regulatory regions that are usually not studied, but an alternative possibility is that in some of those patients the disease is secondary to the combination of several genetic variants that are present in the general population and are not sufficient to cause the disease in isolation. In conclusion, the presence of a genetic variant in control individuals does not completely exclude its pathogenicity: it may have incomplete penetrance, or it may be a contributing factor for disease development. Only properly developed case control studies will be able to help us to solve this difficult situation.

To establish the frequency of a given variant in the general population we need to study a sufficient number of controls. In genetic studies published before the widespread use of NGS technologies the study of a number between 100 and 400 controls were usually considered sufficient to discard the presence of the variant in controls. NGS has been fundamental to increase the number of controls that we generate and now it has become evident that those old numbers of controls were extremely low. A genetic variant that appears with a frequency of 1/1000 in the general population is not likely the cause of a disease like hypertrophic cardiomyopathy, which has a prevalence of 1/500 and may be caused by thousands of different mutations. However, if that genetic variant shows incomplete penetrance, we cannot completely discard its contribution to the disease development. Currently there are public access databases that provide information about the frequency of genetic variants in different populations that facilitate the interpretation of the genetic testing, such as the Exome Aggregated Consortium Database [7].

4.3.4 Information Related to Molecular Biology

The study of the characteristics of a mutation from the molecular biology point of view is essential in the evaluation of its pathogenicity. We will consider aspects like the type of mutation, functional consequence of the mutation in terms of gain or loss of function, relevance of the regions and isoforms affected by the mutation, in-silico bioinformatics predictions of the effect of the mutation, functional studies and evidence coming for the expression of the mutations in animal models [8].

4.3.4.1 Types of Mutations

We may define several types of mutations with different consequences. Firstly, we can distinguish between point mutations (change of a single nucleotide for other), small insertions or deletions (a few nucleotides are inserted or deleted from the sequence), big insertions or deletions (usually called "copy number variations), and structural abnormalities, including inversions, translocations, chromosomal rearrangements, monosomies or trisomies. NGS sequencing is especially focused in the analysis of point mutations, small insertions or deletions and copy number variation analysis, and not in the evaluation of chromosomal abnormalities.

We may also distinguish between mutations affecting intronic or exonic regions. Exonic regions include the nucleotides that constitute the codons that generate the messenger RNA and finally the protein sequence. Introns are non-coding regions that are not translated into messenger RNA. However, mutations affecting introns may be deleterious, especially when they affect intronic regions involved in the splicing process that "cut and paste" the exons and remove the introns in the DNA transcription process. Those mutations that affect coding regions (exons) are more likely relevant than mutations affecting then non-coding/non-splicing intronic regions. However, even point mutations affecting non-splicing intronic regions may be pathogenic (for example creating alternative splice sites, or affecting regulatory regions, like the promoters) [9]. The splicing process is not only dependent on the intronic consensus sequences that are close to the exons, but also exonic nucleotides (usually the first and last ones of the exons) participate in the splicing processes.

So that, we may classify point mutations and small insertion/deletions in: intronic, intronic-splicing, exonic and exonic-splicing categories.

Amongst the exonic mutations we may have the following types:

- Silent mutations: In these mutations there is a change in a nucleotide that does not cause a change in the corresponding amino acid. These mutations are usually non-pathogenic, but there are exceptions in cases where the mutation affects regions implicated in the DNA splicing process.
- Nonsense mutations: Point mutations that cause the introduction of a stop codon that may result in a truncated RNA. This truncated RNA may generate a truncated protein, or may be degraded, producing a decrease in the amount of available protein, which may produce what we call haploinsufficiency.
- Missense mutations: The change in one nucleotide results in a change in the resulting amino acid.
- Frame-shift mutations are caused by nucleotide insertions and or deletions that alter the reading frame of the sequence and may result in truncated (or abnormally elongated) transcripts.

Intronic variants may consist on changes of one nucleotide, insertions or deletions. When they occur in regions involved in the splicing process they may result in the generation of abnormal transcripts, with either loss of one or more exons, or the generation of a truncated RNA. Similar effects may happen due to intronic mutations affecting regions that are far from the "consensus splicing regions" in several circumstances. For example, when they create a new alternative splicing acceptor or donor. RNA splicing is a complex process that implies not only the sequences of the splicing region, but also other regulatory sequences and the participation of different enzymes. It is also a "probabilistic" process, and depending on the efficiency of the signals, the splicing may generate different transcripts even under the same circumstances. Alternative splicing is the mechanism that allows the generation of different protein isoforms from the same DNA sequence. Bioinformatics algorithms are used to try to predict the consequences of either intronic or exonic variants in the splicing process, but it is important to know that those predictions may be not accurate, and the demonstration of the real effect of splicing site mutations may require complex experiments.

4.3.4.2 Functional Consequences of the Mutations in Terms of Gain or Loss of Function

Loss of function mutations are those that produce a decrease in the function of the protein either because of a decrease in the amount of functional protein (usual mechanism of nonsense, frameshift and many splicing site mutations) or a decrease in the intrinsic activity of the protein, for example, a mutation that compromises the active site of a enzyme causing a diminution of its activity, or a mutation in a sarcomeric gene, such as MYH7, that causes a decrease in the contractile force generation. On the contrary, examples of "gain of function" mutations are those that increase the activity of a transcription factor, or mutations that increase the permeability and current generated through a cardiac channel. Loss of function mutations in the SCN5A gene are associated with a decrease in sodium currents and may cause Brugada syndrome, while gain of function mutations in the same gene delay its closure, causing prolonged sodium currents and are responsible for the development of long QT syndrome type 3. The terms "gain" and "loss" of function may be a bit confusing, because both types of mutations provoke a loss of the "normal" function of the protein. To increase the complexity of the interpretation of these terms, the same mutation may produce both effects: for example there are SCN5A mutations that produce a decreased early opening of the channel ("loss of function" and Brugada pattern) and a delayed closure of the same channel ("gain of function" and long QT) [10]. In any case, depending on the particular function of the protein, one type of mutation may be either pathogenic or protective. For example, loss of function mutations in the LDLR gene, encoding the LDL receptor, are pathogenic and associated with familial hypercholesterolemia, because they decrease the LDL uptake and increase the circulating cholesterol levels; however, loss of function mutations in the PCSK9 gene are protective, because the function of the protein is to down-regulate the expression of the LDL receptors, so that, when we decrease the levels of PCSK9, we have more LDL receptors available and a protective effect due to the decrease in circulating LDL cholesterol.

4.3.4.3 Relevance of the Regions and Isoforms Affected by the Mutation

The effect of the mutations depends on the functional relevance of the affected region of the protein and mutations in critical points are more likely pathogenic than mutations in regions with less critical functions [11]. As we have commented, one single gene may generate different versions of the encoded protein, called isoforms. Some isoforms may be preferentially expressed in certain tissues or organs. A deleterious mutation may not have any effect in an organ where the predominantly expressed isoforms of the protein are not affected by that genetic variant. A pathogenic effect is more likely when a mutation affects an amino acid that is highly conserved in homologous regions of different species and between different isoforms of the same protein, something we can evaluate comparing the sequences of different species.

4.3.4.4 Bioinformatics Studies

Bioinformatics programs that incorporate diverse algorithms provide calculations on the potential effects of the mutations in protein structure and function. Those programs evaluate multiple parameters, including the physicochemical differences in mass, charge, hydrophobicity and polarity between the original and the newly encoded amino acid. These parameters are combined with the characteristics of the affected protein regions. For example, change of charge is extremely important for mutations affecting amino acids involved in hydrogen bonds. Information about previous mutations described and structural data about the protein are also considered in those programs. There are also programs that estimate the likelihood that a mutation alters the splicing process. In any case, all the predictive software gives only indicative information and should not be considered sufficient to either confirm or discard the pathogenicity of a given variant.

4.3.4.5 Functional Studies and Animal Models

In vitro studies may provide very relevant information about the functional consequences of a mutation. The mutations may be expressed in cellular models to evaluate their consequences at cellular level. For example, we may study ion currents generated by the expression of mutated ion channels in cells. The study may also be done at a molecular level, for example through the evaluation of the velocities of contraction and relaxation in mutated myocardial filaments. The abnormalities generated by mutations in the splicing process may be studied by the expression of those mutations in mini-genes or in cellular models. Functional studies not only are used to evaluate the deleterious effects of mutations, but also the potential effect of different therapies.

The generation of transgenic animals with a given mutation may provide strong evidence about its pathogenicity. However, this approach is limited by the cost and difficulties to obtain those models and also because animals and humans have different genes, proteins and physiology, so that the consequences of a mutation in the animal and the human may be different.

4.4 Clinical Information

Clinical information is the essential part for the interpretation of the pathogenicity of genetic variants. A correct interpretation requires a good knowledge about the clinical manifestations, diagnostic criteria, differential diagnosis and heritability and pattern of inheritance associated with both the involved gene and the disease. We need information about the prevalence of the genetic variant in the general population, and in the particular sub-populations which the individual patient belongs to. We need also to know about the individual and environmental factors that may be key determinants for the expression of the disease in carriers of pathogenic variants. In general, the evaluation of the genotype-phenotype correlations, and co-segregation of genetic variants with disease expression is not a simple and one-way process, but it has to take into consideration multiple aspects. For that reason, specialized knowledge on the disease and genes we are evaluation are key for a correct interpretation.

If the mutation is related to disease development, its frequency in patients should be higher than in control populations. When the penetrance of the mutation, and its severity are high, we should not find that variant in controls. However, for mutations with milder effects and/or incomplete penetrance, or late clinical expression, we may find asymptomatic carriers amongst the control population, and in the patients´ families. The study of the cosegregation of the mutation with the disease expression within the family is one essential step in the interpretation of its pathogenicity and consequences. We always should remember that the presence of a genetic variant in two, three, four or even more affected members of the same family is not a definitive proof of its pathogenicity. Relatives from the same family may share many genetic factors, and just by chance they may share both the disease and a particular variant. However, when the number of affected carriers and unaffected non-carriers increases, the probability of a spurious association decreases, especially when more distant relatives are included. This is correct for mutations with an autosomal dominant pattern of inheritance, but not for recessive conditions, where heterozygous carriers are usually not clinically affected. Different patterns of inheritance have to be considered when we evaluate the cosegregation of a variant with a particular condition.

Previous descriptions of the same or similar genetic variants should be registered and compared with the phenotype of our patients. When a variant appears in multiple, and completely different phenotypes it may not be really associated with any of them. It is true that there are genetic variants that may show variable clinical expression, and generate overlapping phenotypes. The knowledge of the potential variations in the expression of pathogenic mutations in a given gene is very important in the evaluation of the cosegregation of variants with disease development, and to avoid false positive incidental associations.

4.4.1 Pre-Test and Post-Test Probabilities

The definition of the pathogenicity of a variant requires a probabilistic approach. As a consequence of the application of the Bayes theorem, the post-test probability of a genetic testing finding to be really associated with the disease we are studying or with other conditions (incidental findings) would depend on several pre-test probabilities:

1. The pre-test probability of the patient to be affected by the condition: the probability of finding a disease causing mutation is higher when the patient is defini-

tively affected by the disease we are looking for, and much lower if the patient is not clinically affected. Variants identified in healthy individuals have a lower probability of being pathogenic.

2. The pre-test probability of an association between the genes we are testing and the patient's disease: mutations in genes that have not been previously associated with the disease are less likely pathogenic. Genetic variants are more likely associated with the corresponding disease when they are found in genes that have been convincingly linked to the condition. Genetic variants identified in genes previously associated with the disease we are testing have a higher probability of being pathogenic than variants in "novel" genes.

4.4.2 The Yield of the Tests

The probability of identifying one or more disease causing genetic variants that explain a particular inherited cardiovascular disease is highly variable and we could say that it never reaches 100%. For that reason, it is important to remember that a negative genetic testing does not exclude the presence of a genetic disease. Genetic testing laboratories are usually asked about the yield of their tests, and in our opinion, the correct answer is "it depends…" It depends on the technical characteristics of the test, on the quality of bioinformatics analysis, on the interpretation of what is a "positive result", and especially on the criteria for the selection of the tested individuals (their pre-test probability of having a genetic condition caused by the studied genes).

4.4.2.1 Relation Between Yield of the Test and Experiment Design: Panel, Exome or Whole Genome Sequencing?

The same inherited cardiovascular disease may be caused by mutations in different genes, and the most relevant advantage of next generation sequencing technologies versus the classical Sanger sequencing is its capacity to test many genes at the same time. The question is how many genes and which genes have to be tested in each patient. To get the maximum cost-benefit relation, we usually design libraries that allow the study of a panel of genes that includes at least the most frequent genes that have been unequivocally associated with the disease of interest. What we may call "basic panels". The main advantages of basic panels including a limited number of genes are that the pre-test probability of a mutation in those genes to be associated with the disease is high, that usually most of the pathogenic mutations that we may find are included in those "major" genes, and that as the size of those panels is relatively small, we can obtain a good coverage of the genes of interest even when we put in the same assay samples from multiple patients, which decreases the cost of the studies. This strategy of "basic" panels is of special interest when we use sequencers with the lowest capacity (for example if we use Illumina MiSeq instead of HiSeq), and it may be the only feasible strategy when we are doing the studies preparing the samples through direct amplification (amplicons), as it may be difficult to combine in the same design many genes.

However, when we use "basic panels" it is not rare to get a negative result. In those cases we usually would like to have evaluated all those candidate genes or genes that are associated with the disease in a minority of the cases that are not included in a "basic" study. For example, in hypertrophic cardiomyopathy a typical basic panel includes between 3 and 25 genes, and there are extended panels that cover more than 100 genes. Many of the genes included in the extended panels have been related with the evaluated condition with low levels of evidence, but may be relevant for individual patients; and in some cases those genes turn out to be a relevant cause for the disease in terms of frequency. As an example of this, the FLNC gene was included in by our group in the extended panels for hypertrophic, dilated, restrictive and arrhythmogenic cardiomyopathies, and in a "cardiomyopathy panel" after the description of a limited number of cases with an unspecified cardiomyopathy in two families where FLNC mutations were associated with a skeletal myopathy. After sequencing more than 2700 samples with different phenotypes, we discovered that truncating mutations in this gene are responsible for approximately 4% of cases of idiopathic dilated cardiomyopathy, 3% of restrictive cardiomyopathies, almost 4% of cases of arrhythmogenic cardiomyopathy, and a higher proportion when we specifically evaluate patients with a diagnosis of arrhythmogenic left ventricular cardiomyopathy [12]. Now this gene is included in basic panels for those diseases. The difference between the cost of sequencing a basic and an extended panel is not very relevant, but there is a significant difference in the complexity and cost of the interpretation of the results. Incidental findings and variants of unknown significance are much more frequent with big panels, and it is very important to make a correct interpretation and avoid false positive diagnoses.

But even with the extended panels a relevant number of cases with a positive clinical diagnosis of an inherited (or potentially inherited) cardiovascular disease will have a negative result, considering as negative the absence of variants that explain the disease, including variants of uncertain significance with low probability of being pathogenic. For that reason many experts and laboratories consider performing Exome sequencing instead or after sequencing a gene's panel. Exome sequencing consists in the evaluation of the exonic and flanking intronic regions of all the genes (this would be a whole Exome sequencing) or of all the genes that are considered clinically relevant (for example what is called a clinical Exome). The advantage is clear: all the genes are evaluated. The disadvantages are very relevant for clinical application: lower coverage that usually results in the absence of full coverage of relevant regions in the main genes, and higher cost, both of sequencing and of interpretation. Currently, in our opinion, the advantage of covering genes of unknown relation with a particular condition using Exome sequencing does not provide any relevant advantage over the sequencing of a well designed panel, while it increases the probability of false negative results related to insufficient coverage of the main genes, and problems for the evaluation of copy number variations [1, 8]. However, Exome sequencing offers the possibility of identifying novel gene-disease association in the context of familial studies, through the evaluation of several affected and unaffected members of the same family. Finally, the evolution of Next Generation Sequencing technologies has made feasible to consider whole genome sequencing as a real alternative in clinical practice. In this case, we would not only evaluate exons and flanking intronic regions, but also deep intronic regions (which in any case is not always possible) and genomic regions of still unknown significance. We think that due to the complexity and cost of the interpretation, and the cost of sequencing, the role of genome sequencing is still limited to a research context.

4.4.2.2 Relation Between Yield of the Test and Clinical Pre-Test Probability of Finding a Disease Causing Mutation

It is something obvious, but usually not well understood, that the probability of identifying a disease causing mutation depends on the real presence of the condition we are evaluating. For example, if we are evaluating the presence of hypertrophic cardiomyopathy genes in young patients with a classical phenotype, the probability of finding a disease causing mutation is high, while if we are evaluating elderly hypertensive patients with a borderline diagnosis of HCM, the pretest probability of finding a pathogenic mutation in a sarcomeric gene is very low. At the same time, for any given mutation of uncertain significance we may find, it is more likely that the mutation is pathogenic when it is found in the first case (typical presentation and certain clinical diagnosis) than in the second (low pre-test probability). The indication for genetic testing is stronger in cases with high pre-test probability, where the identification of the disease causing mutation is more likely and the test will likely provide relevant information for the management of the patient and his/her relatives. However, the test is usually also useful in patients with intermediate or lower pre-test probability, where the identification of a pathogenic mutation may allow a diagnosis that is not clear in the clinical evaluation. In Fig. 4.2 we propose an algorithm for the indication of genetic testing in patients with inherited cardiovascular diseases that is based in the previous considerations.

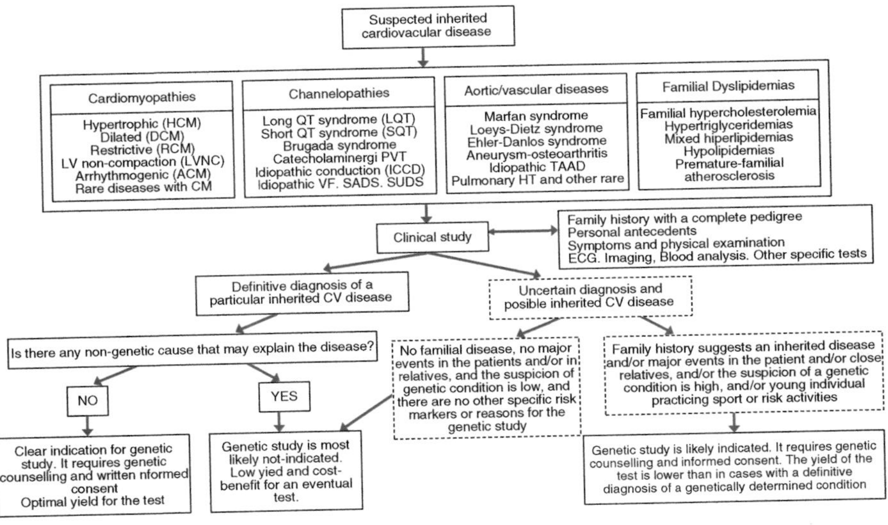

Fig. 4.2 Algorithm for the indication of genetic testing in patients with inherited cardiovascular diseases

4.4.3 From Diagnosis to Prognosis

The objective of genetic testing in clinical practice is not to find one or several pathogenic genetic variants, but to provide information useful for the clinical management of the patient and the affected families. For that reason, it is not sufficient with the classification of the identified variants according to their pathogenicity. Whenever we find a variant that is considered relevant we should try to answer several additional questions:

1. Do the identified variants explain the patient's phenotype?
2. Do they explain the phenotypes identified in the family?
3. What are the expected clinical manifestations of the disease and its prognosis?

The first two questions are related to the value of genetic testing for disease early diagnosis and confirmation of a previous clinical diagnosis. There is general consensus with respect to the value of genetic testing in this aspect. On the contrary, many experts consider that currently, the identification of a genetic mutation does not have prognostic implications, except for some particular genes (for example LMNA in dilated cardiomyopathy patients) or mutations. This opinion is based in the concept that the expression of the mutations is highly variable between families and even within members of the same family, and in the lack of reproducibility of previously established genotype-prognosis correlations. In our opinion, the relation between mutations and prognosis could be consider equivalent to the well established relation between individual viruses or bacteria and the prognosis of the related diseases. No one expects that through the description of a very small number of patients affected by a particular virus we can establish the exact clinical course and prognosis of an individual patient, but any clinician or biologist understand that through the evaluation of a sufficient number of patients we may be able to understand the natural history of the disease and its prognosis, to better identify individual clinical predictors of risk, and to guide the clinical follow up and management of the affected patients. It is interesting to remember that viral diseases are also "genetically determined" conditions. The viral genome suffers mutations that results in variations of the virus pathogenicity that we are used to evaluate and consider in the prognostic evaluation of our patients.

The major limitation for the use of genetic testing results in the prognostic evaluation of patients with inherited cardiovascular diseases is the lack of clinical details about the affected patients and families. In many instances, in the more prestigious publications, information about functional studies or animal models is considered more relevant than the publication of the clinical details of the identified patients. And the lack of clinical data on the identified patients is the major limitation of most of the available databases. However, even with these limitations in many of the available information sources, our group and others have shown that the systematic collection of data from reported patients and families allow identifying relevant genotype-phenotype-prognosis correlations [1, 8, 12, 13]. The collaboration of clinicians, molecular biologists and bioinformatics supported by knowledge management systems is the key for the development of an efficient personalized medicine in this new era of genetics powered by Next Generation Sequencing technologies.

References

1. Monserrat L, Ortiz-Genga M, Lesende I, Garcia-Giustiniani D, Barriales-Villa R, de Una-Iglesias D, et al. Genetics of cardiomyopathies: novel perspectives with next generation sequencing. Curr Pharm Des. 2015;21(4):418–30.
2. Ackerman MJ, Priori SG, Willems S, Berul C, Brugada R, Calkins H, et al. HRS/EHRA expert consensus statement on the state of genetic testing for the channelopathies and cardiomyopathies: this document was developed as a partnership between the Heart Rhythm Society (HRS) and the European heart rhythm association (EHRA). Europace. 2011;13(8):1077–109.
3. Cuenca S, Ruiz-Cano MJ, Gimeno-Blanes JR, Jurado A, Salas C, Gomez-Diaz I, et al. Genetic basis of familial dilated cardiomyopathy patients undergoing heart transplantation. J Heart Lung Transplant. 2016;35(5):625–35.
4. Poptsova MS, Il'icheva IA, Nechipurenko DY, Panchenko LA, Khodikov MV, Oparina NY, et al. Non-random DNA fragmentation in next-generation sequencing. Sci Rep. 2014;4:4532.
5. Ion Semiconductor Sequencing. In Wikipedia, the free encyclopedia. 2017. Retrieved 02 July 2017, from https://en.wikipedia.org/w/index.php?title=Ion_semiconductor_sequencing&oldid=780682285.
6. Illumina Dye Sequencing. In Wikipedia, The Free Encyclopedia. 2017. Retrieved 02 July 2017, from https://en.wikipedia.org/w/index.php?title=Illumina_dye_sequencing&oldid=776525060.
7. Lek M, Karczewski KJ, Minikel EV, Samocha KE, Banks E, Fennell T, et al. Analysis of protein-coding genetic variation in 60,706 humans. Nature. 2016;536(7616):285–91.
8. Monserrat L, Mazzanti A, Ortiz-Genga M, Barriales-Villa R, Garcia D, Gimeno-Blanes JR. The interpretation of genetic tests in inherited cardiovascular diseases. Cardiogenetics. 2011;1:e8.
9. Li H, Chen D, Zhang J. Analysis of intron sequence features associated with transcriptional regulation in human genes. PLoS One. 2012;7(10):e46784.
10. Makita N, Behr E, Shimizu W, Horie M, Sunami A, Crotti L, et al. The E1784K mutation in SCN5A is associated with mixed clinical phenotype of type 3 long QT syndrome. J Clin Invest. 2008;118(6):2219–29.
11. Herman DS, Lam L, Taylor MR, Wang L, Teekakirikul P, Christodoulou D, et al. Truncations of titin causing dilated cardiomyopathy. N Engl J Med. 2012;366:619–28.
12. Ortiz-Genga MF, Cuenca S, Dal Ferro M, Zorio E, Salgado-Aranda R, et al. Truncating FLNC mutations are associated with high-risk dilated and arrhythmogenic cardiomyopathies. J Am Coll Cardiol. 2016;68(22):2440–51.
13. García-Giustiniani D, Arad M, Ortíz-Genga M, Barriales-Villa R, Fernández X, Rodríguez-García I, et al. Phenotype and prognostic correlations of the converter region mutations affecting the β myosin heavy chain. Heart. 2015;101(13):1047–53.

5 Pharmacogenetics and Pharmacogenomics in Cardiovascular Medicine and Surgery

Richard Myles Turner and Sir Munir Pirmohamed

Abstract

Cardiovascular disease is a principal cause of global morbidity and mortality. Multiple drugs are used clinically to improve the population-level prognosis of cardiovascular conditions. However, there is a noticeable difference in the response of individual patients to a given drug, observed in both intermediate phenotypes (e.g. platelet function tests) and clinical outcomes. The aetiology underlying this drug response interindividual variation is multifactorial, incompletely understood, but is comprised from demographic, clinical, environmental and genetic factors. Pharmacogenomics aims to understand the genomic determinants of drug response, and to translate findings into clinical practice to reduce adverse drug reactions and/or improve drug effectiveness through genotype-informed dose and/or drug selection. Pharmacogenomic associations have been implemented for a few drugs after they have been licensed (e.g. abacavir in HIV disease), and there is a growing array of newly developed therapeutics that require a genomic companion diagnostic test, particularly in oncology. However, pharmacogenomics is yet to be adopted into widespread cardiovascular clinical practice. Several obstacles, including evidential, logistical, financial, and knowledge-based, have been identified. Nevertheless, substantive progress has been made, and early adopter sites are pioneering cardiovascular pharmacogenomics in practice. There is an undeniable large genomic influence affecting warfarin response, and strong evidence of pharmacogenomic associations with simvastatin myopathy, and stent thrombosis on clopidogrel. Variants that modulate responses to beta blockers, antiarrhythmics and angiotensin-converting enzyme inhibitors are also being identified. The integration of genomics into systems pharmacology approaches may further resolve interindividual drug response variability; the prospects are good, but the challenges are prodigious.

R.M. Turner • S.M. Pirmohamed (✉)
The Wolfson Centre for Personalised Medicine, Institute of Translational Medicine, University of Liverpool, Liverpool, Merceyside, UK
e-mail: Richard.Turner@liverpool.ac.uk; munirp@liverpool.ac.uk

D. Kumar, P. Elliott (eds.), *Cardiovascular Genetics and Genomics*,
https://doi.org/10.1007/978-3-319-66114-8_5

Keywords
Cardiovascular • Pharmacogenomics • Precision medicine • Translation Warfarin • Clopidogrel • Statin • Beta blocker • Antiarrhythmic

5.1 Introduction

Cardiovascular disease (CVD) is the leading cause of death, responsible for 30% of all deaths worldwide [1]; CVD currently accounts for ~17.5 million deaths per annum [1], and this is projected to extend to >23.6 million by 2030 [2]. Disability-adjusted life years (DALYs) measure overall disease burden by integrating mortality and morbidity measures into a single metric, and CVD underlies ~10–18% of all DALYs lost [2]. By 2020, global medicine use and spending will likely reach 4.5 trillion doses and $1.4 trillion, respectively [3]; CVD drugs account for ~13% of this global pharmaceutical spending [4, 5].

Underlying this huge spend on drugs for disease is a notable interindividual heterogeneity in drug response; just 50–75% of patients respond beneficially to the first drug offered in the treatment of a broad range of diseases [6], 6.5% of hospital admissions are related to an adverse drug reaction (ADR) [7], and 14.7% of inpatients experience an ADR [8]. The World Health Organisation definition of an ADR is: "a response to a drug which is noxious and unintended, and which occurs at doses normally used in man for the prophylaxis, diagnosis, or therapy of disease, or for the modification of physiological function" [9]. Understanding and overcoming this heterogeneity in drug response would improve clinical outcomes and lead to major savings for all healthcare systems.

The reasons for the interindividual variability are manifold, incompletely understood and vary between drugs. However, sources of this variability include demographic (e.g. age, sex), clinical (e.g. liver and renal impairment, adherence, heterogeneity in underlying disease mechanisms), environmental (e.g. smoking, alcohol) and genetic factors. Pharmacogenomics is the study of the genetic determinants of drug response. Pharmacogenomics aims to improve drug effectiveness and reduce ADRs through incorporating genotype information into dose and/or drug selection prescribing decisions, and is integral therefore in the drive for Precision Medicine. Technological and statistical advances have fuelled a rapid development in the conduct of pharmacogenomic investigations, which have evolved from candidate gene studies, to non-hypothesis driven genome-wide association studies (GWAS'), through to the emergence of next-generation sequencing (NGS) high-throughput platforms for whole exome and increasingly whole genome sequencing (Fig. 5.1). As a result of this intensive research, the US Food and Drug Administration (FDA)-approved drug labels for over 160 drugs now contain pharmacogenomic information [10].

It has been broadly anticipated that pharmacogenomics will be one of the first translational successes of the 'post-genomics' era, but notwithstanding a few notable exceptions, pharmacogenomics research has yet to be translated into widespread

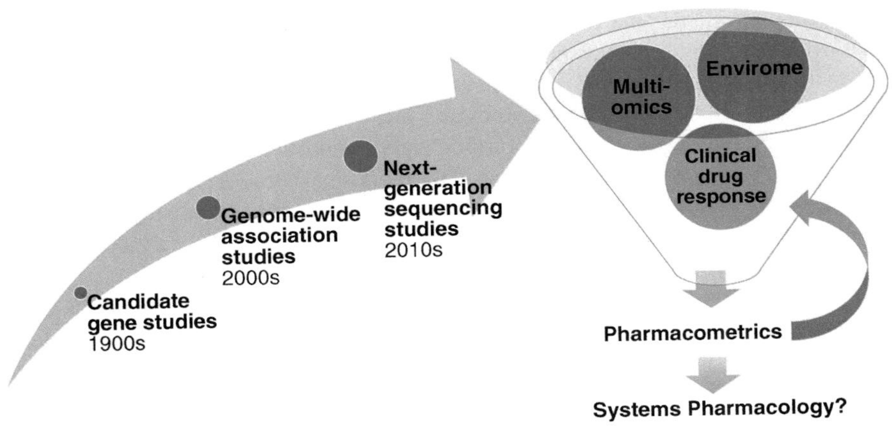

Fig. 5.1 The evolution of pharmacogenomic investigations. With continued technological and bioanalytical developments, systems pharmacology studies may increasingly occur. Systems pharmacology encompasses both systems biology and quantitative pharmacometrics approaches. The systems biology studies will integrate genomic data with data from other biological levels (e.g. the epigenome, transcriptome, proteome, metabolome, tissue and organ systems) and environmental factors to identify novel factors associated with drug response. These factors will be combined into pharmacometrics models; subsequent simulation predictions will inform further empirical investigations, leading to iterative model development. It is hoped that systems pharmacology approaches will produce sufficiently detailed, but not unduly burdensome, models to adequately parse interindividual variability in drug response for clinical application.

clinical care. These exceptions include: companion testing for the human leukocyte antigen (*HLA*)-*B*57:01* with the antiretroviral, abacavir, to avoid abacavir hypersensitivity syndrome [11]; and prescribing ivacaftor in patients with the cystic fibrosis transmembrane conductance regulator (*CFTR*) G551D mutation and the ivacaftor/lumacaftor combination in those with the common *CFTR* F508del variant. Furthermore, an increasing number of targeted anticancer drugs with therapeutic activity restricted to patients harbouring specific tumour gene variants are being licensed. These include crizotinib in non-small cell lung cancers carrying oncogenic anaplastic lymphoma kinase (*ALK*) gene rearrangements, and both vemurafenib and the dabrafenib/trametinib combination in V600E and V600E/K proto-oncogene B-Raf (*BRAF*)-positive advanced melanoma patients, respectively.

Several barriers obstructing widespread implementation of pharmacogenomics exist, including evidential, logistical, financial and the contemporary pharmacogenomics knowledge base of healthcare professionals [12]. Importantly, challenges to developing a sufficient research evidence base have included small underpowered studies leading to conflicting results, insufficient regard for the impact of ethnicity on pharmacogenomics, and the multifactorial nature of interindividual drug response variability. However, progress in these areas is being made. Notably, systems pharmacology is emerging as a potential approach, which combines systems biology and pharmacometrics [13]. Systems pharmacology recognises the necessity but insufficiency of pharmacogenomics alone to account for the observed variability of many drugs. Systems pharmacology has the potential to integrate clinical outcomes data with multi-omics patient-derived data at genomic, epigenomic, transcriptomic, proteomic, metabolomic and/or organ system levels, to identify novel drug response factors. These factors will be incorporated into pharmacometrics models; subsequent model predictions will shape further experimental studies and lead to iterative model development to further parse interindividual drug response variability (Fig. 5.1). However, whilst systems pharmacology is highly promising, it remains nascent. Therefore, this chapter focuses on pharmacogenomics, although some exemplars of non-genomic biomarkers are also included.

A second challenge facing pharmacogenomics implementation is 'genetic exceptionalism [14],' whereby the evidence threshold for clinical uptake required for a drug-genotype association appears to be higher than for clinically accepted factors that perturb drug activity, such as renal impairment, even if the magnitudes of effect (e.g. on systemic drug exposure) are equivalent. This barrier appears particularly pronounced in cardiology, where practice-changing results are expected to come from randomized controlled trials (RCTs) and meta-analyses of RCTs, which represent the highest tiers of the evidence hierarchy. Whilst striving for evidence from RCTs is highly commendable in general, treating all interventions the same irrespective of their benefit: risk profiles appears suboptimal. It is clear that a consensus pharmacogenomics evidence threshold is required, because conducting an RCT for every drug-gene associations is unfeasible. However intuitively, the evidence base for a dose-modifying pharmacogenomic variant should not need to be the same as a genetic test associated with life changing surgery (e.g. known deleterious *BRCA* variants and prophylactic mastectomy/salpingo-oophorectomy).

Finally, it should also be noted that the rate of recent cardiovascular drug development has been slow compared to oncology. Therefore, the majority of cardiovascular drug pharmacogenomic studies have focussed on licensed drugs, and changing entrenched clinical practices represents an additional hurdle to cardiovascular pharmacogenomics implementation.

Nevertheless, over the last decade meaningful advances in cardiovascular pharmacogenomics have been made. Therefore, this chapter provides an overview of contemporary cardiovascular pharmacogenomics in relation to warfarin, statins, antiplatelet drugs, beta blockers (βBs), antiarrhythmics and angiotensin-converting enzyme (ACE) inhibitors (ACEIs). Points for consideration include:

- The impact of pharmacogenomics on the effectiveness and/or safety of cardiovascular drugs;
- The impact of specific variants on drug pharmacokinetics (PK) or pharmacodynamics (PD), and an appreciation that the function of several associated variants remain uncertain;
- The current variable evidence base underlying specific drug-genotype associations.

Simple clinical cases are provided to illustrate some of the healthcare contexts that could benefit from cardiovascular pharmacogenomics.

5.2 Warfarin

5.2.1 Case Study

A 66-year old lean Caucasian woman visits her general practitioner (GP) with a two-month history of intermittent palpitations. She has a background of hypercholesterolemia and controlled hypertension, and takes atorvastatin 20 mg daily and amlodipine 10 mg daily. She drinks 20 units of alcohol per week. Electrocardiography (ECG) confirms atrial fibrillation (AF). Routine electrolyte and thyroid tests are normal, and an outpatient echocardiogram is arranged. She is commenced on rate control with bisoprolol 5 mg daily, and her GP initiates warfarin (CHA_2DS_2-VASc score of three, HAS-BLED score of two) with a loading dose regimen (10 mg, 10 mg and 5 mg on days one, two and three). On day four, her international normalized ratio (INR) is 7.4. She complains of purpura on her forearms, one episode of epistaxis, and is concerned and disheartened by these side effects.

5.2.2 Overview

Warfarin was initially developed as a rodenticide, but was approved for anticoagulant use in 1954. Warfarin is a coumarin-derived drug administered orally as a racemate; S-warfarin is 2–5× more potent than the R-warfarin enantiomer [15]. Warfarin inhibits the hepatic vitamin K cycle, which impairs post-translational γ-carboxylation leading to hypofunctional clotting factors II, VII, IX, X and proteins C and S (Fig. 5.2). The

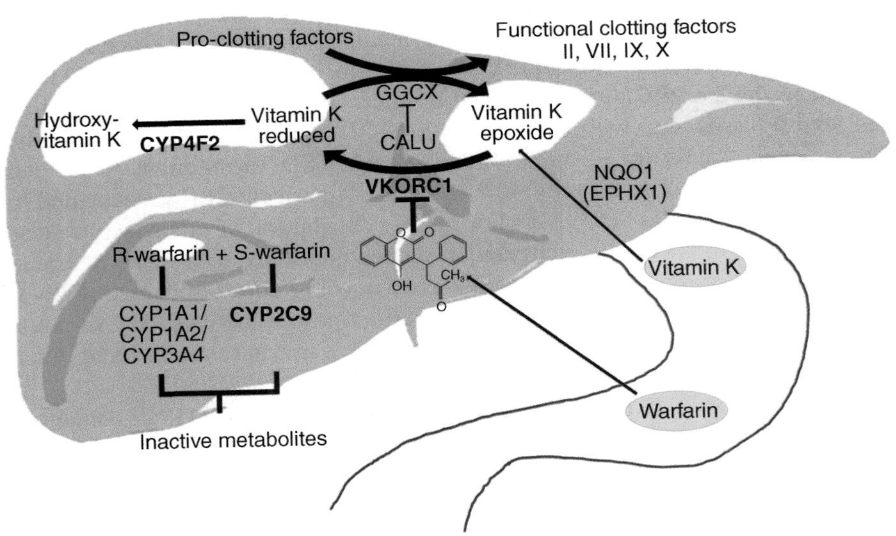

Fig. 5.2 An overview of the mechanism of action and metabolism of warfarin. Adapted from Wadelius et al. [58]. *CALU* calumenin, *CYP* cytochrome P450, *EPHX1* epoxide hydrolase 1, *GGCX* gamma-glutamyl carboxylase, *NQO1* NAD(P)H dehydrogenase (quinone) 1, *VKORC1* vitamin K epoxide reductase

degree of anticoagulation is reported as the INR, which is derived from the prothrombin time (PT) assay of the extrinsic pathway of anticoagulation. Warfarin is indicated in the prophylaxis and treatment of thromboembolism; most conditions (e.g. AF, venous thromboembolism (VTE)) require a target INR of 2.0–3.0, but a higher range is indicated following a mechanical mitral valve implantation (e.g. 2.5–3.5). For the 2.0–3.0 INR range, there is a ~40-fold interindividual variation in warfarin stable dose (WSD) requirements, ranging from 0.6 to 15.5 mg/day [16]. Clinical factors that affect response to the first warfarin dose include, age, sex, ethnicity, body mass index (BMI), smoking, co-mediations and warfarin adherence [15, 17–19]. Patients typically spend just ~45–63% of the time within the therapeutic range (TTR) [20, 21]; elevated INRs increase the risk of warfarin-associated bleeding (as in the clinical case) [22] and a 10% increase in time outside the TTR is associated with increased thromboembolic events and mortality [23]. Therefore, given its widespread use, narrow therapeutic range, the multifactorial aetiology of its varying activity, and serious type A bleeding/thrombosis ADRs, warfarin is the leading cause of preventable ADRs, and a priority for precision medicine. Multiple validated and candidate warfarin pharmacogenomics variants have been identified (Table 5.1).

5.2.2.1 VKORC1

VKORC1 encodes vitamin K epoxide reductase (VKORC1), the rate limiting enzyme in the vitamin K cycle and the on-target for warfarin inhibition (Fig. 5.2). A common *VKORC1* single nucleotide polymorphism (SNP) is rs9923231 (-1639G>A; G3673A). The -1639A allele frequency is ~13% and ~40% in Africa-American and Caucasian populations, respectively. However, it is ~90% in Asian populations, indicating minor allele reversal. Carrying -1639A has been associated with reduced WSD requirements to maintain a therapeutic INR [24] and over-anticoagulation [25], but not with bleeding [25]. rs9923231 is located in the *VKORC1* promoter region, alters a transcription factor binding site, and is associated with decreased *VKORC1* expression [26]. Importantly, rs9923231 accounts for ~20–25% of observed WSD variation in Asian and Caucasian populations, but only ~6% in Africa-Americans [14] perhaps due to the lower frequency of -1639A and/or larger contribution of other factors (discussed below). Interestingly, a targeted re-sequencing study in African-American patients demonstrated that the minor allele of a novel *VKORC1* SNP, rs61162043, is associated with increased WSD [27]. Furthermore, rare *VKORC1* variants, such as rs61742245 (D36Y), have been linked to warfarin resistance and much higher WSD requirements [28].

The expression of *VKORC1* is under epigenetic regulation. *VKORC1* contains a conserved binding site for the micro-RNA, miR-133a [29]; miR-133a can interact with *VKORC1* mRNA to decrease *VKORC1* mRNA dose-dependently and so human hepatic levels of miR-133a and *VKORC1* mRNA are inversely correlated [30]. Interestingly, patients carrying the minor A allele of rs45547937 (G>A) within *MIR133A2* were found to have significantly higher WSD requirements than wild-type patients [29], but this is one study and needs replicating.

Table 5.1 Anticoagulant pharmacogenomics and clinical outcomes

Clinical outcome	Study	Ethnicity	Locus/ gene	Variant(s)	Effect[a]	References
Warfarin						
Replicated variants						
Dose requirement	MA	AA, A, C	*VKORC1*	-1639G>A	AA vs. GG: ~2–3 mg/day reduction	[32, 38]
	TarSeq	AA		rs61162043 (-8191A>G)	Per minor allele: ~0.8 mg/day increase	[27]
	MA	C	*CYP2C9*	*2	*1/*2 vs. *1/*1: ~1 mg/day reduction	[32]
					*2/*2 vs. *1/*1: ~1.5 mg/day reduction	[32]
	MA	AA, A,C		*3	*1/*3 vs. *1/*1: ~1.5 mg/day reduction	[32, 38]
					*3/*3 vs. *1/*1: ~2.5 mg/day reduction	[32]
	CG	AA		*8	*8 carriers vs. *1/*1: ~1 mg/day reduction	[35, 36, 38, 294, 295]
	TarSeq	AA		rs7089580 (2313A>T)	Per T allele: ~0.5 mg/day increase	[27]
	GWAS	A, C	*CYP4F2*	1297G>A (V433M)	A allele carriers vs. GG: ~0.2 mg/day increase	[40, 41]
	GWAS	AA	*CYP2C* cluster	rs12777823 (G>A)	AG vs. GG: ~1 mg/day reduction	[39]
					AA vs. GG: ~1.5 mg/day reduction	[39]
	ES	AA	*FPGS*	rs7856096 (A>G)	AG: ~1 mg/day reduction	[45]
					GG: ~1.5 mg/day reduction	[45]
	CG	AA	*CALU*	rs339097 (A>G)	A allele carriers vs. GG: ~1 mg/day increase	[38, 46]
Bleeding	MA	AA, A, C	*CYP2C9*	*3	*1/*3 vs. *1/*1: HR 2.05 (95% CI 1.36, 3.10)	[25]
					*3/*3 vs. *1/*1: HR 4.87 (95% CI 1.38, 17.14)	[25]
Over-anticoagulation (INR>4)	MA	AA, A, C	*CYP2C9*	*2	*2 vs. *1: HR 1.52 (95% CI 1.11, 2.09)	[25]
				*3	*3 vs. *1: HR 2.37 (95% CI 1.46, 3.83)	[25]
	MA	AA, A, C	*VKORC1*	-1639G>A	GA vs. GG: HR 1.49 (95% CI 1.15, 1.92)	[25]

(continued)

Table 5.1 (continued)

Clinical outcome	Study	Ethnicity	Locus/ gene	Variant(s)	Effect[a]	References
Candidate genes/variants						
Dose requirement	CG	AA	*CYP2C9*	*6	*6 carriers vs. *1/*1: ~23%/week reduction	[38]
	CG	AA		*5, *6, *11	*2, *3, *5, *6 or *11 carriers vs. *1/*1: ~1 mg/day reduction	[35]
	CG	A (Korean)	*c-MYC*	rs4645974 (C>T) rs4645943 (C>T)	rs4645974 T carriers vs. CC: ~0.5–1 mg/ day decrease rs4645943 T carriers vs. CC: ~0.5 mg/day increase	[51]
	GWAS	C	*DDHD1*	rs17126068	Minor allele: 0.8 mg/ week reduction (square root scale)	[59]
	CG	A (Han Chinese)	*EPHX1*	rs1877724 (C>T)	TT vs. CC: ~0.3 mg/ day decrease	[52]
	CG	A (Korean)	*GATA4*	rs867858 (G>T) + rs10090884 (A>C)	GG/AA vs. all other genotype combinations: ~1 mg/ day reduction	[53]
				rs2645400 (G>T) + rs4841588 (G>T)	GG/GT,TT vs. all other genotype combinations: ~2 mg/ day reduction	[53]
	GWAS	C	*NEDD4*	rs2288344 (A>C)	Per minor (C) allele: 0.2 mg/week increase (square root scale)	[59]
	CG	A (Korean)	*NQO1*	rs10517 (C>T)	rs105R 17 T carriers vs. CC: ~0.4 mg/day increase	[54]
	CG	A (Chinese)	*ORM1*	rs17650 (*F1>*S)	*S/*F1 vs. *F1/*F1: ~0.3 mg/day decrease *S/*S vs. *F1/*F1: ~0.5 mg/day decrease	[55]
	CG	A (Han Chinese)	*POR*	*37 (C>T)	T carriers vs. CC: ~0.4 mg/day increase	[56]
	CG	C	*POR*	rs2868177 -173C>A -208C>T	rs2868177 (additive): ~0.3 mg/day increase 173 CA vs. CC: ~0.7 mg/day decrease 208C>T (additive): ~0.5 mg/day decrease	[57]
	CG	A (Han Chinese)	*PROC*	rs5936 (T>G)	GG vs. TT: ~0.5 mg/ day decrease	[52]
	CG	C		rs2069919 (G>A)	Accounted for 9% of observed warfarin dose variability	[58]

Table 5.1 (continued)

Clinical outcome	Study	Ethnicity	Locus/ gene	Variant(s)	Effect[a]	References
TTR	GWAS	C	*ASPH*	rs4379440 (C>A)	Decrease TTR by 6.8% (95% CI 4.4–9.3%) per minor allele	[59]
Dabigatran						
Bleeding	GWAS	C	*CES1*	rs2244613 (C>A)	Per minor (A) allele: Any bleeding: OR 0.67 (95% CI 0.55, 0.82) ($p = 7 \times 10^{-5}$) Major bleeding: OR 0.66 (95% CI 0.43, 1.01) (NS)	[64]

A Asian (in ethnicity column), *AA* African American, *C* Caucasian (in ethnicity column), *CG* candidate gene study, *GWAS* genome-wide association study, *HR* hazard ratio, *INR* international normalized ratio, *MA* meta-analysis, *NS* not statistically significant, *OR* odds ratio, *TarSeq* targeted re-sequencing, *TTR* time in therapeutic range

[a]All effects are statistically significant unless otherwise stated

5.2.3 Cytochrome P450

5.2.3.1 CYP2C9

Cytochrome P450 (CYP) 2C9 (CYP2C9) metabolises the more potent S-warfarin enantiomer. *CYP2C9*2* and **3* represent non-synonymous reduction-of-function (ROF) variants with minor allele frequencies (MAFs) in Caucasians of 13% and 7%, respectively. *CYP2C9*3* is rare (MAF 4%) in Asians and *2 very rare, whilst both are rare or absent in African populations (MAFs of 0–3.6% for *2, and 0.3–2% for **3*) [12]. *CYP2C9*2* and **3* reduce S-warfarin metabolism by ~30–40% and ~80–90% [31], respectively, prolong S-warfarin half-life, reduce WSD requirements and explain ~15% of WSD variability in Caucasians [17]. They are associated with over-anticoagulation, and importantly **3* is associated with bleeding [25, 32]. The hazard ratios (HRs) for bleeding determined by meta-analysis for **1/*3* and **3/*3* patients, compared to wild-type **1/*1* patients, were 2.05 (95% confidence interval (CI) 1.36, 3.10) and 4.87 (95% CI 1.38, 17.14), respectively, indicating a gene-dose effect [25]. Therefore, it is plausible that the lady in the clinical case carried *CYP2C9*3* ± *VKORC1* -1639A alleles. Interestingly, a drug-drug-gene interaction has been identified; concomitant simvastatin has little impact on WSD in *CYP2C9 *1/*1* patients, but in **1/*3* patients, simvastatin was associated with a further ~21% reduction in WSD, and a suggestive gene-dose trend was evident [33].

In African populations *CYP2C9*5*, **6*, **8* and **11* are prevalent, with a collective frequency of ~20% [34]. *CYP2C9*5*, **8* and **11* represent ROF variants; **6* is a single exonic nucleotide deletion that results in a frame shift and loss of function [34]. In African-Americans, *CYP2C9*8* is the most common haplotype [35, 36] and is associated with both a 30% reduction in S-warfarin clearance [37] and lower WSD requirements [35, 38]. Similarly, *CYP2C9*6* alone [38], *CYP2C9*11* alone [39], and *CYP2C9*2*, **3*, **5*, **6* and **11* collectively [35], are associated with decreased WSD. Targeted re-sequencing has also reported that African-American patients carrying the *CYP2C9* novel SNP, rs7089580, require a modestly higher WSD [27].

5.2.3.2 CYP4F2

GWA-studies that adjusted for *VKORC1* and *CYP2C9* have identified the minor allele of rs2108622 (1297G>A, V433M) to be associated with increased WSD in Asian [40] and Caucasian [41] patients, explaining ~1–7% of WSD variability [40–42]. *CYP4F2* removes active (reduced) vitamin K from the vitamin K cycle, and rs2108622 A allele correlates with lower hepatic CYP4F2 [43]. In African-American patients however, *CYP4F2* rs2108622 has not been associated with WSD [39, 44].

5.2.4 Other Warfarin Pharmacogenomic Genes

In African-American patients, variants in additional genes associated with WSD have been identified and replicated, including within the *CYP2C* gene cluster, in *FPGS* and in *CALU*:

1. rs12777823 (G>A) is a novel noncoding SNP located upstream of *CYP2C18* within the *CYP2C* cluster, which was identified in a recent GWAS and reported to be independent of known *CYP2C9* variants [39]. The minor rs12777823 A allele was associated with reduced WSD requirements. Interestingly, although rs12777823 is present in other ethnicities, it has only been linked to WSD in African-Americans. This suggests it is in linkage disequilibrium (LD) with an African-specific as-yet unidentified causal variant [39].
2. rs7856096 (A>G) is a population-specific regulatory SNP in folylpolyglutamate synthase (*FPGS*), which is a gene encoding a mitochondrial enzyme involved in folate sequestration. rs7856096 was identified by comparing the exome sequences of African-American patients with extremely high or low WSD requirements [45]. The rs7856096 G allele is associated with reduced *FPGS* expression and lower WSD [45]. However, the role of folate homeostasis in warfarin response is currently unknown.
3. rs339097 (A>G) is an intronic variant in *CALU*, and the minor G allele is associated with increased WSD [38, 46]. *CALU* encodes the molecular chaperone calumenin, and is thought to regulate the vitamin K gamma-carboxylation system [46–48]. The impact of *CALU* variation in Caucasian patients remains unresolved [49].

Several candidate associations with WSD have also been identified (Table 5.1). These include variants in *GGCX* [50], *c-MYC* [51], *EPHX1* [52], *GATA4* [53], *NQO1* [54], *ORM1* [55], *POR* [56, 57] and *PROC* [52, 58]. In addition, a recent GWAS has identified novel associations between WSD and variation in *DDHD1* (rs17126068) and *NEDD4* (rs2288344) [59]. *DDHD1* encodes DDHD domain containing 1 protein, *NEDD4* encodes an E3-ubiquitin ligase, and both explained an additional ~1% of the observed WSD variability [59]. Furthermore, the first GWAS to investigate warfarin TTR identified rs4379440 (C>A) within *ASPH* (encoding aspartate beta-hydroxylase), which was associated with reduced TTR (-6.8% per minor allele) [59]. Interestingly, an association between circulating levels of miR-548a-3p and warfarin dose variability has also been recently identified, and coagulation pathway genes are associated with miR-548a-3p [60]. These candidate findings require replication.

5.2.5 Direct-Acting Oral Anticoagulants

The last eight years have seen the emergence of direct-acting oral anticoagulants (DOACs) as warfarin alternatives, and there has been a rapid increase in DOAC prescribing. DOACs reversibly inhibit thrombin (dabigatran) or clotting factor Xa (rivaroxaban, apixaban and edoxaban). Each DOAC has a limited number of fixed dose prescriptions available, they are prescribed without laboratory monitoring, have a rapid onset of action, a wide therapeutic index, few food and drug interactions, and remain on patent. In AF, a meta-analysis has confirmed that DOACs are collectively associated with decreased stroke and systemic embolism, all-cause mortality and intracranial haemorrhage compared to warfarin [61]. However, with the exception of apixaban, they are associated with increased gastrointestinal bleeding [62]. In acute VTE, it has been shown by meta-analysis that DOACs are collectively non-inferior to warfarin, and associated with reduced major bleeding [63].

A GWA sub-study of participants from the principal dabigatran etexilate (DE) RCT, RE-LY, has been performed (Table 5.1) [64]. Interestingly, it identified that each minor allele of rs2244613, an intronic SNP within *CES1*, was associated with both a 15% decrease in dabigatran trough levels and a 33% lower risk of any bleeding in DE-treated patients [64]. Importantly, rs2244613 minor allele carriers experienced decreased bleeding events compared to patients on warfarin, but there was no difference in bleeding rates between the two drugs in non-carriers. Furthermore, the minor allele of rs8192935, within the *CES1* locus, and rs4148738 within *ABCB1*, were associated with a 12% decrease or increase in peak dabigatran concentrations, respectively [64]; these SNPs were not, however, associated with clinical endpoints [64]. In a recent small (n = 92) candidate gene study of these three variants, rs8192935 was associated with trough dabigatran levels, but no associations were found for *CES1* rs2244613 or *ABCB1* rs4148738 [65]. Additional adequately powered studies are needed to determine the generalizability of the GWAS findings.

CES1 encodes liver carboxylesterase 1 (CES1), which is involved in the hydrolysis of multiple ester- and amide bond-containing drugs [64]. The sequential biotransformation of the ingested prodrug, DE, into active dabigatran, is mediated by intestinal CES2 and then hepatic CES1 [66]. *In vitro* functional work has shown that DE activation is reduced by the known rare ROF non-synonymous *CES1* variant, rs71647871 (G143E), but interestingly neither rs2244613 nor rs8192935 are associated with *in vitro* dabigatran production [67]. The loci of these SNPs contain a cluster of *CES* genes (e.g. *CES4*, *CES7*) [64] in addition to *CES1*, and so further research is required to understand their putative roles.

ABCB1 encodes P-glycoprotein (P-gp), an adenosine triphosphate-dependent xenobiotic efflux pump of broad substrate specificity with a role in eliminating substrates into the intestine, bile and urine. Intestinal P-gp activity modulates net absorption of DOACs, including DE (but not active dabigatran) [68], and P-gp inhibitors (e.g. amiodarone, verapamil) increase dabigatran bioavailability by ~10–20% [69]. *ABCB1* is polymorphic with three common SNPs, rs1128503 (1236C-T), rs2032582 (2677G-T) and rs1045642 (3435C-T), which are in strong LD. Furthermore, rs4148738 is in modest LD with rs1045642 ($r^2 = 0.51$) [64].

Our understanding of the pharmacogenomics of anti-Xa DOACs remains relatively rudimentary. However aanalogous to dabigatran and *CES1*, patients carrying the warfarin-sensitive *VKORC1* and *CYP2C9* variants have been reported to have a significantly higher risk of bleeding on warfarin compared to edoxaban, with no difference in bleeding events between treatments in *VKORC1* and *CYP2C9* wild-type homozygotes [70].

5.2.6 Clinical Utility

There is compelling evidence that pharmacogenomics influence WSD requirements [34]. The FDA introduced a dosing table into the warfarin drug label in 2010 based on *VKORC1* and *CYP2C9* genotype combinations [71]; an extended dosing table including nine variants in *VKORC1*, *CYP2C9* and *CYP4F2* has since been developed [72]. Several multivariable algorithms have been assembled to predict optimal warfarin dose when starting treatment (days 1–3) [24]; a few algorithms are available for revising the dose once the day three INR is available (e.g. on days 4–5) [73, 74]. These algorithms are based on clinical and genetic (mainly *VKORC1*, *CYP2C9* ± *CYP4F2* variants) factors, although most are derived from small cohorts. The International Warfarin Pharmacogenetics Consortium (IWPC) algorithm is notable for being developed from 4043 patients and for significantly outperforming its clinical factors-only algorithm (no genetic variants included) in the 46.2% of the population requiring ≤21 mg or ≥49 mg of warfarin/week [75]. The IWPC [75] algorithm, and the Gage [76] algorithm, are high-performing validated algorithms freely available for clinical use at http://www.warfarindosing.org [31] and recommended by the Clinical Pharmacogenetics Implementation Consortium (CPIC) guidelines.

In 2013, two multicentre warfarin pharmacogenomic RCTs were published, with contrasting results. EU-PACT recruited participants from the UK and Sweden (n = 455), compared a pharmacogenomic algorithm to standard dosing, and reported that the TTR for the first 12 weeks of warfarin treatment was significantly better in the pharmacogenomic (67.4%) compared to the standard dosing arm (60.3%, $p < 0.001$) [77]. COAG was US-based (n = 1015), compared pharmacogenomic and clinical algorithms, and found no difference in TTR up to four weeks (45.2% and 45.4% respectively, $p = 0.91$) [21].

Several reasons have been proposed to explain these contrasting results [17]. Notably, whilst EU-PACT recruited predominantly Caucasian patients, COAG was more heterogeneous consisting of ~30% African-American and ~6% Hispanic patients [21]. Importantly, the African-American subgroup had a lower TTR and higher frequency of INRs >3 with pharmacogenomic dosing compared to the clinical algorithm arm [21]. Subsequently, it has been shown that omission of ethnicity-specific variants adversely affects IWPC algorithm performance [78] and an African-American-specific algorithm with superior precision has been developed [79].

The headline results of the Genetic Informatics Trial (GIFT) of warfarin therapy in patients undergoing elective hip or knee replacement surgery have recently been released. This is the largest pharmacogenomic RCT to date (n = 1597) and was powered for clinical endpoints. Importantly, dosing warfarin using a pharmacogenomic algorithm (including clinical factors, *CYP2C9*2*, **3*, *VKORC1* and *CYP4F2* genotypes) led to a significant 27% relative risk reduction in the primary composite endpoint compared to dosing using an algorithm that considers clinical (non-genetic) factors only. The primary composite endpoint included death, confirmed VTE, INR $\geq$ 4 and major bleeding; the pharmacogenomic-mediated reduction appears to have been driven through reducing instances of INR $\geq$ 4 [80].

Warfarin is inexpensive, clinicians are accustomed to it, and it remains the principal oral anticoagulant for patients with mechanical heart valves because dabigatran was associated with increased bleeding and thromboembolic events in these patients [81]. Therefore, it is likely that warfarin will remain a commonly prescribed drug for the foreseeable future. Importantly, data from EU-PACT show that a pharmacogenomic-guided warfarin dosing strategy is cost effective in both the UK, and to a lesser extent, in Sweden [82]. The recent data from GIFT show that genotype-guided dosing of warfarin has clinical utility. Clearly the DOACs are an important innovation, but their cost is a major impediment to their use. Therefore, an integrated overarching clinical and cost-effective approach that appropriately stratifies DOAC and warfarin treatments for AF/VTE patients could be advantageous. There appears to be no differential bleeding risk between DOACs and warfarin if centre-based TTR is ≥66%, as determined by meta-analysis [61]. Therefore, an approach that stratifies patients based on warfarin risk alleles (e.g. ROF variants in *CYP2C9* and *VKORC1*), potentially alongside DOAC-specific risk variants, appears pragmatic and appealing.

Overall, warfarin multivariable models account for ~60% of WSD variability [18]. The ongoing micro-RNA investigations [60], novel findings regarding the influence of circulating clotting factor levels [19], and further research should provide insight into the ~40% unaccounted variability. Further research into the pharmacogenomics of dabigatran and other DOACs, along with studies integrating a novel biomarker-based bleeding risk score (incorporating growth differentiation factor-15, high-sensitivity troponin T and haemoglobin) [83] are also warranted to maximise the benefit: risk profile of oral anticoagulation.

5.3 Statins

5.3.1 Case Study

A 50-year old female Asian office administrator attends a National Health Service (NHS, UK) appointment, instigated by her because her 55-year old brother had recently suffered a myocardial infarction. She has hypertension, treated with ramipril 10 mg daily and amlodipine 5 mg daily, but no known ischaemic heart disease. She is a non-smoker and teetotal. On examination, she is overweight (BMI

27) with a blood pressure of 145/82 mmHg. Subsequent blood results show a cholesterol/high-density lipoprotein (HDL) ratio of 5, but normal renal, liver, thyroid and HbA1c results. Her 10-year risk of CVD is calculated to be 21%, and so, following consultation with her GP, she starts atorvastatin 20 mg daily, and a 24-h ambulatory blood pressure check is arranged. Two weeks later she returns to her GP complaining of non-specific muscle aches, and her statin is switched to simvastatin 40 mg after a one-week washout period. Two weeks later, she returns with muscle heaviness, particularly in her thighs. Urine dipstick shows no 'red blood cells'; serum biochemistry results subsequently show that her creatine kinase (CK) is 5× the upper limit of normal (ULN), although renal function is preserved. Her statin therapy is discontinued for now with a plan to review the decision in one month.

5.3.2 Overview

Statins are hypolipidaemic drugs indicated for both the primary and secondary prevention of CVD. RCT evidence demonstrates that for every one mmol/L reduction in low-density lipoprotein (LDL) cholesterol (LDL-C) during statin therapy, there is an associated 25% reduction in cardiovascular events for each year of treatment (after the first treatment year) [84]. Overall, statins lower LDL-C by 30–63% [85] and reduce cardiovascular events by 20–30% [86]. In the UK, atorvastatin 20 mg daily is indicated for patients with a 10% or greater 10-year risk of cardiovascular disease for primary prevention, and atorvastatin 80 mg daily is first line secondary prevention therapy [87]. Statins are amongst the most commonly prescribed classes of medication worldwide, and in the UK, ~11–12 million people are estimated to be eligible for statin therapy [88, 89]. There are seven currently licensed statins worldwide: atorvastatin, fluvastatin, lovastatin, pitavastatin, pravastatin, rosuvastatin and simvastatin.

The main mechanism of statin action is competitive inhibition of 3-hydroxy-3-methylglutaryl-coenzyme A reductase (HMGCR), the rate limiting enzyme in *de novo* cholesterol synthesis (Fig. 5.3). In turn, this leads to an upregulation of hepatic LDL receptors, which increases hepatic LDL-C influx further decreasing circulating LDL-C [90]. In addition, it is expected that inhibition of HMGCR leads to a reduction in all downstream end-products, including prenylated proteins and coenzyme Q_{10} (CoQ_{10}, also known as ubiquinone), as well as cholesterol (Fig. 5.3) [91]. Several pleiotropic properties have been ascribed to statins, including anti-inflammatory and immune-modulatory effects [92–95], and improved endothelial function [95–97].

Although generally well tolerated, statins have been associated with a range of ADRs including gastro-intestinal disturbances, abnormal liver function tests, depression, fatigue, incident diabetes mellitus, and likely haemorrhagic stroke [84]. However, the most commonly reported statin ADR is statin-associated myotoxicity (SAM), which is thought to comprise two-thirds of all statin ADRs [98]. SAM encompasses a spectrum of presentations (Fig. 5.4) including common muscular symptoms (myalgias, aches, cramps and/or weakness) with no elevation in serum CK, asymptomatic elevations in CK above the upper limit of normal, symptomatic myopathies with elevated CKs of increasing severity, rare but potentially life-threatening rhabdomyolysis, and very rare autoimmune-mediated statin myopathy that persists despite statin cessation [99].

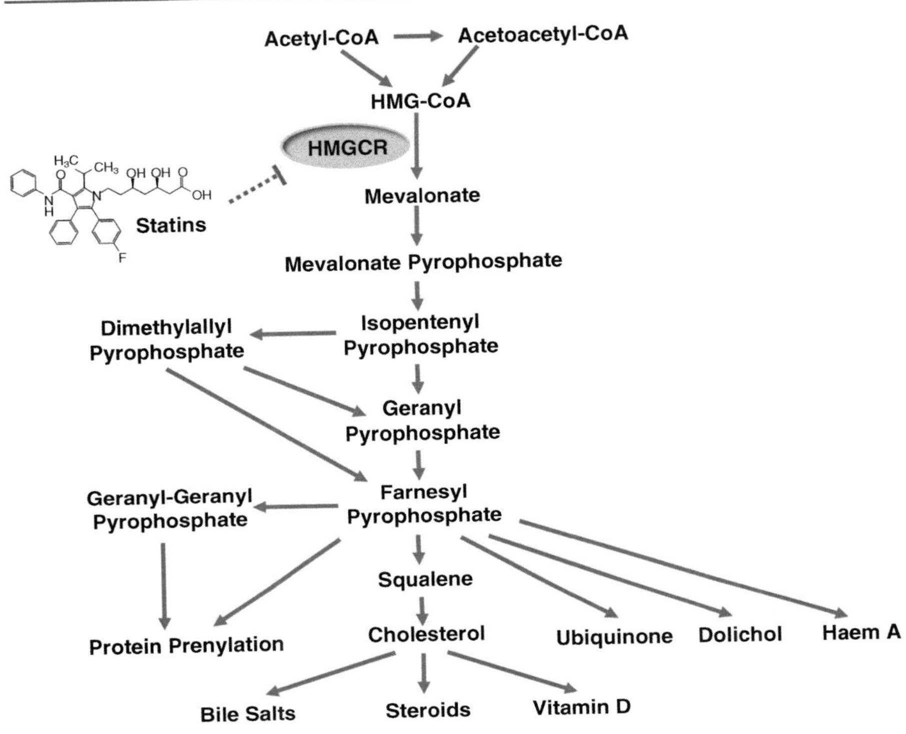

Fig. 5.3 Statin inhibition of the mevalonate pathway. HMGCR=3-hydroxy-3-methyl-glutaryl-coenzyme A (CoA) reductase

The true incidence of SAM is uncertain, occurring in 1.5–5% of participants in RCTs (relative to placebo groups) [100], compared to 10–15% in observational studies [101]. Therefore the underlying benefit: risk profile of statins, particularly in patients at the lower end of the CVD risk spectrum, has been a recent source of controversy [102]. Nevertheless, there is consensus that statins definitely do increase the risk of the more severe forms of myotoxicity, including severe myopathy and rhabdomyolysis [84]. Importantly, cerivastatin was voluntarily withdrawn in 2001 because of 52 cases of fatal rhabdomyolysis [103]. The greater difficulty lies in correctly assigning the aetiology of the commoner milder musculoskeletal symptoms, and in particular whether they are attributable to statin therapy and/or to other conditions (e.g. increased exercise or viral illnesses). Interestingly, a recent six-month RCT conducted in 420 healthy volunteers administered either atorvastatin 80 mg daily or placebo found an increased rate of myalgia amongst the subjects on atorvastatin compared to the placebo group (9.4% vs. 4.6%, respectively, $p = 0.05$) [104], which suggests that myalgias may be caused by intensive atorvastatin therapy in ~5% of people. Furthermore, recent N-of-1 (single-patient) placebo-controlled trials involving patients with a prior history of SAM have reported that ~30–40% subsequently experience muscle-related events only on statin and not placebo [105, 106].

Clinical SAM risk factors include higher statin dose, older age, female gender, low BMI, uncontrolled hypothyroidism, liver disease, intense physical exertion,

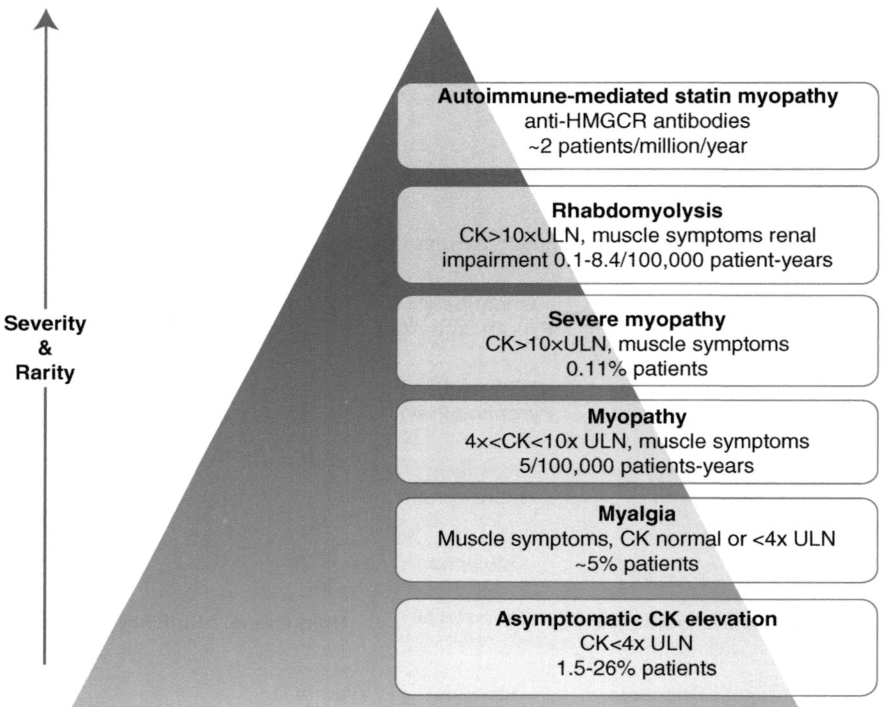

Fig. 5.4 Statin-associated myotoxicity phenotype spectrum. Classification and estimated frequencies are based on Alfirevic *et al.*, 2014 [99], except for myalgia frequency which is derived from Parker et al. [104]

Asian or African ancestry, drug-drug interactions [107, 108], and perhaps low vitamin D levels [91]. High statin equivalent dose increases the risk of severe myopathy by ~six-fold compared to low statin doses [108]. Atorvastatin, lovastatin and simvastatin are CYP3A4 substrates. Concomitant use of CYP3A4-inhibiting drugs, such as itraconazole and clarithromycin, significantly increases the systemic exposure of CYP3A4-metabolised statins [109–111] and are associated with an increased risk of SAM [112]. Therefore, the product labels of these CYP3A4-metabolised statins contraindicate [113, 114] or advocate caution and reduced statin doses [115] to mitigate CYP3A4-mediated interactions. Grapefruit juice has also been associated with increased systemic exposures of atorvastatin [116, 117], lovastatin [118], and simvastatin [119]. Drugs with established significant interactions listed for all seven statins include cyclosporine and gemfibrozil [113–115, 120–123]. In recognition of the importance of statin-drug interactions, recommendations for the management of clinically significant interactions have been recently published [124].

5.3.2.1 SLCO1B1

In 2008, a seminal GWAS reported a strong association between simvastatin myopathy and *SLCO1B1* (Table 5.2) [125]. Briefly, a case-control sub-study of the

Table 5.2 Pharmacogenomics of statin-associated myotoxicity

Study	Locus/ Gene	Variant(s)	Statin	Myotoxicity Phenotype	Effect[a]	References
Replicated variants						
GWAS	*SLCO1B1*	rs4149056 (521 T>C, V174A)	SVT	Mild (CK >3× ULN) & severe myopathy (CK>10× ULN)	(a) 80 mg SVT/day: – Per C allele: OR 4.5 (95% CI 2.6, 7.7) – CC vs. TT: OR 16.9 (95% CI 4.7, 61.1) (b) 40 mg SVT/day: – Per C allele: OR 2.6 (95% CI 1.3, 5.0),	[125]
CG			SVT, ATV	-All myopathy (CK >4× ULN). -Severe myopathy (CK >10× ULN or rhabdomyolysis)	(a) SVT all myopathy: – Per C allele: OR 2.13 (95% CI 1.29, 3.54) (b) SVT severe myopathy: – Per C allele: OR 4.97 (95% CI 2.16, 11.43) (c) rs4149056 NS for all/ severe myopathy in patients only on ATV	[127]
CG			CVT	Severe myopathy (CK >10× ULN)	Per C allele: OR 1.89 (95% CI 1.40, 2.56)	[130]
CG			SVT, ATV,	Severe myopathy (CK >10× ULN)	CC/CT vs. TT: – SVT: OR 3.2 (95% CI 0.83, 11.96), – ATV: NS	[126]
CG			ATV, SVT, PVT	Discontinuation, myalgia, and/or CK >3× ULN	– OR 1.7 (95% CI 1.04–2.8) – Gene-dose trend observed. – Risk highest in patients on SVT – A (non-significant) trend for increased risk in patients on ATV – No increased risk for PVT with rs4149056 C allele	[129]
CG			Mainly SVT	A relevant prescribing change with CK testing/ high ALT	CC/CT vs. TT: OR 2.05 (95% CI 1.02, 4.09)	[128]
CG			ATV, RVT	Muscular intolerance	– ATV: OR 2.7 (95% CI 1.3, 4.9) – RVT NS	[132]
CG			RVT	Muscle symptoms, myopathy, rhabdomyolysis	NS	[131]

(continued)

Table 5.2 (continued)

Study	Locus/ Gene	Variant(s)	Statin	Myotoxicity Phenotype	Effect[a]	References
HLA typing	*HLA-*	*DRB1*11*	Not detailed	anti-HMGCR antibody positive myopathy (symptoms persist after statin discontinuation)	(a) *HLA-DRB1*11* (recognised by HLA-DR11 serotype) significantly more frequent in anti-HMGCR positive white or black myopathy patients than normal controls (b) OR for the presence of *HLA-DRB1*11:01* in anti-HMGCR positive myopathy patients vs. controls is ~24.5 (white patients) and ~56.5 (black patients)	[156]
CG			Not detailed	anti-HMGCR antibodies in patients with IIM or IMNM	In myopathy patients, *HLA-DRB1*11* is more frequent in those positive than those negative for anti-HMGCR antibodies: OR 56.1 (95% CI 5.0–7739), (c) Three myopathy anti-HMGCR positive myopathy patients had high resolution typing and all carried *HLA-DRB1*11:01*	[155]
Candidate PK variants						
CG	*ABCB1*	1236C>T, 2677G>A/T, 3435C>T	ATV, RVT, SVT	CK >3× ULN	1236C>T TT vs. CT/CC: – OR 4.5 (95% CI 1.4, 14.7),	[163]
CG			SVT	Myalgia	Significantly increased risk of endpoint with *ABCB1* variant alleles	[164]
CG			ATV	Muscle symptoms	Increased risk in patients carrying 3435 T compared to 3435C allele (p = 0.043)	[165]
CG			SVT, ATV	Prescribing changes	NS	[166]
Candidate muscle-related variants						
GWAS	*RYR2*	rs2819742 (1559G>A)	CVT	Severe myopathy (CK >10× ULN)	Per A allele: OR 0.48 (95% CI 0.36, 0.63)	[130]
CG	*RYR1*	34 *RYR1* mutations or variants	Not detailed	Mild & severe myopathy	Disease causing mutations or variants in *RYR1* identified in: – 3 of 197 severe statin myopathy cases – 1 of 163 mild myopathy cases – 0 of 133 in statin-tolerant controls	[170]
In vitro eQTL analysis + CG	*GATM*	rs1719247	SVT	Mild (CK >3× ULN) & severe myopathy (CK>10× ULN)	Decreased risk with *GATM* rs1719247 minor allele: – OR 0.60 (95% CI 0.45, 0.81),	[296]

Table 5.2 (continued)

Study	Locus/ Gene	Variant(s)	Statin	Myotoxicity Phenotype	Effect[a]	References
CG	*CPT2*	P50H, S113 L, Q413fs, G549D, R503C, R631C	ATV, CVT, LVT, SVT	Muscle symptoms. Symptoms commonly persist after therapy cessation	A fourfold increase in the number of mutant alleles (in *AMPD1* > *CPT2*/*PYGM*) in the cases compared to the statin-tolerant controls	[167]
	PYGM	R49X, G204S				
	AMPD1	Q12X, P48L, K287I				
CG	*COQ2*	rs4693075 (1022C>G)	ATV, RVT	Muscular intolerance	G minor allele: – RVT: OR 2.6 (95% CI 1.7, 4.4) – Increased risk of muscular symptoms and CK increase with ATV: OR 3.1 (95% CI 1.9, 6.4),	[132]
CG			ATV, RVT	Myopathy	GG vs. CG/CC: – OR 2.33 (95% CI 1.13, 4.81),	[175]
CG			SVT, ATV	Myopathy	NS	[127]

ATV atorvastatin, *ALT* alanine aminotransferase, *CG* candidate gene study, *CK* creatine kinase, *CVT* cerivastatin, *eQTL* expression quantitative trait loci, *GWAS* genome-wide association study, *IIM* idiopathic inflammatory myositis, *IMNM* immune-mediated necrotizing myopathy, *LVT* lovastatin, *NS* not statistically significant, *OR* odds ratio, *PVT* pravastatin, *RVT* rosuvastatin, *SVT* simvastatin

[a]All effects are statistically significant unless otherwise stated

SEARCH RCT compared 85 myopathy cases (CK>3× ULN) to 90 controls, all of whom were prescribed simvastatin 80 mg daily [125]. The GWAS identified a single genome-wide significant signal, which was rs436365, an intronic SNP within *SLCO1B1*. Regional analysis found rs4363657 to be in almost complete linkage disequilibrium with the non-synonymous *SLCO1B1* variant, rs4149056 (531T>C, V174A). The odds ratio (OR) of myopathy in CC versus TT wild-type homozygotes was 16.9 (95% CI 4.7, 61.1); furthermore a gene-dose trend was evident with an OR of 4.5 (95% CI: 2.6, 7.7) per copy of the C allele [125]. This association between simvastatin myopathy and rs4149056 has been replicated [125–127] and confirmed in meta-analysis [127]. However, the OR for the myopathy association is reduced with lower simvastatin doses [125]. Furthermore, rs4149056 has been associated with milder composite adverse outcomes encompassing myalgia, prescription reductions and/or of minor biochemical (e.g. CK) elevations suggestive of simvastatin intolerance [128, 129].

Interestingly, an analysis of historical cases of cerivastatin-related rhabdomyolysis similarly reported a gene-dose risk association with rs4149056 (OR 1.89, 9% CI 1.40, 2.56 per additional C allele) [130]. However, to date, *SLCO1B1* rs4149056 has not been associated with pravastatin [129] or rosuvastatin [131, 132] myotoxicity. Whilst an association between rs4149056 and atorvastatin myotoxicity has been suggested [129, 133] or reported [132] in some studies, several others have found no evidence [126, 127, 134, 135]. Therefore, the influence of rs4149056 on atorvastatin myotoxicity remains unclarified.

SLCO1B1 encodes organic anion-transporting polypeptide 1B1 (OATP1B1), a hepatocyte-specific sinusoidal xenobiotic influx transporter. Mechanistically, rs4149056 is thought to reduce intrinsic OATP1B1 transport given that it does not cause OATP1B1 mis-localisation [136]. PK studies have demonstrated that the variant allele of rs4149056 (encoding 174A) is associated with significantly elevated systemic exposures to all currently available statins, except fluvastatin (Table 5.3) [137–141], and in general the homozygote CC subjects have greater exposure relative to heterozygotes. Importantly, the area under the concentration-time curve for simvastatin acid was 221% larger in rs4149056 CC homozygotes compared to TT wild-type subjects [141], which was the largest increase for any statin. This observation may account for why rs4149056 appears to be a simvastatin-specific myotoxicity risk factor. However, it is also worth noting that simvastatin has traditionally been very commonly prescribed, and so the majority of SAM cases included into studies have been related to simvastatin exposure. Therefore, it is hypothesized that factors that increase systemic statin exposure, including both clinical (e.g. low BMI) and genetic (*SLCO1B1* rs4149056 for simvastatin), lead to elevated muscle statin exposure, which predisposes to myotoxicity through poorly elucidated downstream mechanisms. One unresolved observation is that, whilst rs4149056 C allele increases the simvastatin acid major metabolite, it does not significantly increase parent simvastatin lactone (Table 5.3), and yet the lactone forms of statins are considered more myotoxic [142–145].

The reasons for the uncertainty regarding any atorvastatin myotoxicity rs4149056 association include: fewer atorvastatin cases in studies [127], atorvastatin appears

Table 5.3 The effect of *SLCO1B1* rs4149056 on statin exposure

Statin	AUC (CC vs. TT)[a]	References
Atorvastatin	↑ 2.45-fold (+145%)	[137]
Fluvastatin	↑ 1.19-fold (+19%, NS)	[138]
Lovastatin	↓to 84% (−16%, NS)	[139]
Lovastatin acid	↑2.86-fold (+186%)	[139]
Pitavastatin	↑ 3.08-fold (+208%)	[140]
Pravastatin	↑1.91-fold (+91%)	[138]
Rosuvastatin	↑1.62-fold (+62%)	[137]
Simvastatin	↑ 1.43-fold (+43%, NS)	[141]
Simvastatin acid	↑3.21-fold (+221%)	[141]

Extended from Elsby et al. [157]

[a]The area under the statin plasma concentration time curve (AUC) of subjects homozygous for the *SLCO1B1* rs4149056 minor allele (521 T>C, V174A) compared to subjects homozygous for the rs4149056 wild-type allele. All effects are statistically significant unless otherwise stated. *NS* not statistically significant

less intrinsically myotoxic than simvastatin [142], and the smaller impact of rs4149056 on atorvastatin exposure [137] (Table 5.3) likely because atorvastatin is transported into hepatocytes by OATP1B3, 2B1 and 1A2 as well as OATP1B1 [146]. Nevertheless, an interesting drug-drug-gene has been identified in a PK study where the extent of increase in atorvastatin exposure due to concomitant rifampicin varied by rs4149056 genotype [147].

Therefore, in the clinical case, it is plausible that she had the *SLCO1B1* rs4149056 CC genotype. This genotype potentially exacerbated an interaction between amlodipine (mild CYP3A4 inhibitor) and simvastatin, especially because she was prescribed 40 mg and not 20 mg simvastatin daily, which is now recommended with amlodipine [148].

5.3.2.2 HLA-DRB1*11:01

In the causality assessment of an adverse event, the observation that the event improves when a drug is stopped or its dose reduced is one indication that the adverse event is likely an ADR [149]. Interestingly, several research groups previously noted that the symptoms and CK elevation of a few patients with SAM persist or even progress after statin discontinuation, and these patients response positively to immunosuppressive therapy [150–152]. These features suggest an autoimmune phenomenon, and in 2011 it was reported that these patients, as well as a minority without prior statin exposure (less than 10% in myopathy patients 50 or older), are positive for anti-HMGCR autoantibodies (Table 5.2) [153]. Muscle biopsies of patients with anti-HMGCR antibodies often show necrotizing myopathy with minimal lymphocytic infiltration, although histological features indicative of other conditions (e.g. poly/dermatomyositis) can occur [154, 155]. Pharmacogenomic studies have provided further evidence of an autoimmume aetiology. In white myopathy patients with anti-HMGCR, the HLA class II combination of HLA-DR11; DQA5; DQB7 is significantly overrepresented compared to either controls (statin exposure unknown) or statin intolerant subjects [156]. In black anti-HMGCR myopathy patients, HLA-DR11 alone is markedly elevated compared to black controls [156]. When analysing just myopathy cases, HLA-DR11 is strongly associated with anti-HMGCR [155]. HLA-DR11 is a serotype that recognises alleles *HLA-DRB1*11:01-*11:10*; high resolution typing has revealed that *HLA-DRB1*11:01* is significantly associated with anti-HMGCR positive myopathy [156], and the ORs for the presence of *HLA-DRB1*11:01* in anti-HMGCR myopathy white or black patients, compared to controls, have been estimated to be ~25 and ~57, respectively [156]. *HLA-DRB1*11:01* has been associated with the development of anti-Ro antibodies in neonatal lupus. However, similarly to other drug hypersensitivity reactions, the underlying aetiology remains elusive.

5.3.3 Other Candidate Genes

Variants in both phase I and II genes have been associated with altered statin PK. These include *ABCG2* (encoding breast cancer resistance protein, BCRP), *CYP3A4*22* and *UGT1A3* (encoding uridine diphosphate (UDP)-glucuronosyltransferase 1A3). *ABCG2* rs2231142 (421C>A, Q141K) is associated with increased exposure of atorvastatin, fluvastatin, rosuvastatin and simvastatin [157]. *CYP3A4*22* is associated with increased simvastatin [158] concentrations and a decreased 2-hydroxyatorvastatin metabolite to atorvastatin ratio [159], and the *2 haplotype of *UGT1A3* is associated with elevated atorvastatin lactone metabolite levels [160, 161]. Nevertheless, these PK variants have not been established as SAM risk factors.

The TTT/TTT haplotype of the common *ABCB1* variants, 1236C>T, 2677G>T and 3435C>T, is associated with increased atorvastatin and simvastatin acid exposures compared to subjects with the CGC/CGC haplotype [162]. Furthermore, these variants have been associated with symptom-independent elevated CK levels [163] and muscle symptoms [164, 165] in some candidate gene studies, but not with prescribing changes suggestive of statin intolerance [166].

Muscle-related candidate variants have also been identified. The frequency of patients with lipid lowering (predominantly statin)-induced myopathy carrying aberrant metabolic myopathy genes, including *CPT2* (encoding carnitine palmitoyltransferase 2) and *PYGM* (encoding the muscle isoform of glycogen phosphorylase, which underlies McArdle disease) is higher compared to asymptomatic treated controls [167]. Interestingly, *in vitro* transcriptomics has demonstrated that *CPT2* is amongst the top 1% of genes whose mRNA levels are perturbed by 75 rhabdomyolysis-inducing drugs [168].

RYR1 encodes ryanodine receptor 1, which mediates the release of stored calcium ions from the sarcoplasmic reticulum of skeletal muscle. Deleterious *RYR1* variants are associated with anaesthesia-induced malignant hyperthermia and central core disease [169], and disease-causing mutations or variants in *RYR1* appear to be more frequent in statin myopathy patients than controls [170]. Interestingly, the second major published statin GWAS identified an intronic variant, rs2819742 (1559G>A), in the ryanodine receptor 2 gene (*RYR2*) to be associated with cerivastatin severe myopathy (CK>10× the upper limit of normal) [130]. An additional copy of the minor A allele was associated with reduced myopathy risk (OR 0.48, 95% CI 0.36, 0.63) [130]. However unlike RYR1, RYR2 is expressed mainly in cardiac muscle tissue where it facilitates cardiac calcium-induced calcium release, and deleterious *RYR2* mutations are associated with ventricular arrhythmias [171].

As stated earlier, statin-mediated competitive inhibition of HMGCR leads to the decreased synthesis of coenzyme Q_{10} by interfering with mevalonate production (Fig. 5.3). CoQ_{10} is an important cofactor in mitochondrial respiration [172]. Primary CoQ_{10} deficiency is a clinically and genetically heterogeneous condition, considered to be inherited in an autosomal recessive manner, and has been associated with isolated myopathy, encephalopathy, nephrotic syndrome, cerebellar ataxia and severe infantile multisystemic disease [173]. In patients on statins, reduced circulating CoQ_{10} is routinely observed and some studies have reported a decrease in muscle CoQ_{10} [172]. *COQ2* encodes para-hydroxybenzoate-polyprenyl transferase and defective *COQ2* has been associated with primary CoQ_{10}, which can improve with early CoQ_{10} supplementation [174]. *COQ2* variants, and in particular rs4693075 (1022C>G), have been investigated in relation to SAM with some candidate gene studies [132, 175], but not others [127], finding evidence of an association.

Importantly though, a recent meta-analysis of RCTs found that CoQ_{10} supplementation likely does not reduce SAM, although larger trials are required to confirm this conclusion [176]. One possible biological explanation is that the Q_0 site of mitochondrial complex III, which is involved in transferring electrons from CoQ_{10} to cytochrome *c*, is thought to be an off-target binding site for statin lactones [143], and so CoQ_{10} supplementation alone may not surmount this disruption to mitochondrial electron flow.

5.3.4 Statin Efficacy

The magnitude of lipid-lowering response to a given statin varies between patients; the genetic basis for this heterogeneous efficacy response to statins has been extensively studied, and over 40 candidate genes described [177]. Importantly, a recent meta-analysis of statin efficacy GWAS' that included eight RCTs and 11 prospective observational studies split into discovery (n = 18,596) and replication (n = 22,318) datasets, and a final combined meta-analysis, was undertaken [178]. The included studies contained patients on all statins except pitavastatin, although the most prevalent statins were atorvastatin, pravastatin, rosuvastatin and simvastatin. The analyses were controlled for age, sex and off-treatment LDL-C level. This study confirmed previously identified associations for *APOE* and *LPA* loci with on-statin LDL-C reduction, and identified two novel loci, *SLCO1B1* and *SORT1/CELSR2/PSRC1*, which had not previously been identified in GWAS, with on-statin LDL-C reduction (Table 5.4). The minor alleles of the lead SNPs for *APOE* and *SORT1/CELSR2/PSRC1* were associated with a larger response to statin treatment, and for *LPA* and *SLCO1B1* a smaller statin response. A related genome-wide conditional analysis identified 14 SNPs, which together accounted for ~5% of the observed variation in LDL-C response to statin therapy [178].

APOE encodes apolipoprotein E (apoE), which is present in chylomicrons, very low-density lipoprotein (VLDL), intermediate-density lipoprotein (IDL) and HDL particles [179]. In the periphery, apoE is predominantly synthesised in the liver. *APOE* has two common non-synonymous SNPs, rs429358 (C112R) and rs7412 (R158C), resulting in three apoE isoforms: ε2 (C112, 158C), ε3 (C112, R158) and ε4 (112R, R158). ε3 is considered the 'normal' form. The ε2/ ε2 genotype is

Table 5.4 Validated pharmacogenomic variants associated with differential LDL-C lowering response to statin therapy

Gene	Lead variant	% extra LDL-C lowering (carriers vs. non-carriers)	p-value
APOE	rs445925	5.1	8.52×10^{-29}
LPA	rs10455872	−5.2	7.41×10^{-44}
SLCO1B1	rs2900478	−1.6	1.22×10^{-9}
SORT1/CELSR2/PSRC1	rs646776	1.3	1.05×10^{-9}

These results are derived from a meta-analysis of GWAS data in Postmus et al., 2014 [178]

associated with type III hyperlipoproteinaemia (familial dysbetalipoproteinaemia) with elevated total cholesterol and triglyceride levels, although incomplete genotype-to-phenotype penetrance is observed; ε4 is associated with both Alzheimer's and CVD [179]. In the GWAS meta-analysis, the minor allele of the lead SNP (rs445925) was a proxy for the ε2 allele [178, 180]. ε2 protein is associated with increased hepatic cholesterol synthesis, and so may predispose to greater statin-mediated inhibition of cholesterol synthesis [180, 181].

LPA encodes apolipoprotein(a). Lipoprotein(a) (Lp(a)) is a plasma lipoprotein consisting of an LDL-like particle (cholesterol rich and incorporating a single apolipoprotein B (apoB) molecule) alongside apolipoprotein(a). Circulating Lp(a) levels are significantly more variable than LDL-C levels, and Lp(a) is associated with CVD [182]. The lead SNP, rs10455872, is strongly associated with the *LPA* kringle IV type 2 (KIV-2) copy number variant (CNV); the G allele of rs10455872 is associated with elevated Lp(a) [180] and rs10455872 accounts for ~30% of observed Lp(a) level variability in Caucasians [183]. The association between the rs10455872, Lp(a) level and attenuated response to statin treatment is thought to originate from the methods used in estimating LDL-C levels. Both conventional laboratory LDL-C assays and the Friedewald formula for estimating LDL-C include cholesterol within Lp(a) particles in their LDL-C assessment. However, statins have little impact on circulating Lp(a) [180]. Therefore, patients with the Lp(a)-raising rs10455872 G allele have a greater proportion of circulating cholesterol contained within statin non-responsive Lp(a) particles, relative to statin response LDL particles, and so the total LDL-C reduction observed with statin treatment for these patients is modestly attenuated [180].

The lead GWAS meta-analysis *SLCO1B1* SNP, rs2900478, is in linkage disequilibrium with rs4149056 (531T>C, V174A), and was associated with a marginally smaller LDL-C reduction in response to statin therapy [178]. A PK-PD model simulation has reported that the rs4149056 minor C allele leads to modestly reduced predicted hepatic unbound intracellular statin concentrations, which is in keeping with the meta-analysis results [184]. Therefore, the impact of the rs4149056 C allele includes both substantially elevated plasma statin exposures, and modestly reduced intrahepatic levels.

The mechanisms underlying the association between the minor allele of the *SORT1/CELSR2/PSRC1* locus and the larger reduction in LDL-C in response to statin treatment remain incompletely determined. However, *SORT1* encodes sortilin, an intracellular trafficking protein that can bind to apoB, which is present in LDL-C particles [185]. Therefore, sortilin is implicated in reducing circulating LDL-C by both reducing the hepatic secretion of apoB-containing precursors, and increasing the hepatic influx of LDL-C by binding to sortilin present on the hepatocyte surface [185].

5.3.5 Clinical Utility

It is clear that at the population level, the overall benefits of statin therapy outweigh the risks [84]. However, for individual patients, extreme SAM leads to hospitalisation.

Furthermore, ~10–30% of patients are non-adherent or discontinue statin therapy within a year [186, 187], SAM is more frequent in these patients [188], and statin underutilisation is associated with increased cardiovascular events and mortality [189], underscoring the importance of minimising SAM. In 2011 the FDA revised the simvastatin product label to curtail the use of simvastatin 80 mg because of the elevated myotoxicity risk [190]. CPIC guidelines have been published regarding simvastatin myotoxicity and *SLCO1B1* [107]. Specifically, CPIC advocate that for patients already known to be carry at least one risk allele, a lower starting dose of simvastatin or an alternative statin is prescribed, and routine CK surveillance can be considered [107]. However, clinical uptake has been poor. Specific implementation barriers include: the general trend towards prescribing atorvastatin rather than simvastatin in both primary and secondary prevention settings, the rarity of statin-associated extreme myotoxicity (e.g. rhabdomyolysis) limiting awareness of individual clinicians to the problem, and the controversy regarding the frequency and aetiology of statin-associated mild myotoxicity. A QStatin risk score has been developed to predict statin myopathy, based on clinical risk factors and is of borderline clinical utility [191]. Therefore, it will be important to integrate *SLCO1B1* genotype into this model to improve its predictive capability [192]. However, the positive predictive value of *SLCO1B1* alone for simvastatin myopathy is only ~4% [192], and so further biomarker research is needed.

Although variants have been strongly associated with statin efficacy and have furthered mechanistic understanding, their individual and combined effect sizes are small. Furthermore, the ease of phenotyping lipid profiles and the current trend away from treating to lipid targets mean that they are unlikely to be of clinical utility until/unless such variants (likely with PK variants) can stratify patients according to the statin drug(s) predicted to give them the greatest LDL-C reduction.

5.4 Clopidogrel

5.4.1 Case Study

A 62-year old male Caucasian lorry driver is taken by ambulance to his local accident and emergency department, with a five-hour history of central, dull chest pain. The ECG performed on route showed ST-depression, which was confirmed in the anterolateral leads of his admission 12-lead ECG. He has a background of hypertension and a diagnosis of type II diabetes within the last year. He takes metformin 1500 mg, gliclazide 160 mg, felodipine 5 mg, perindopril 10 mg, and simvastatin 40 mg total daily. His high sensitivity troponin T (TrT) is substantially elevated and a diagnosis of non-ST elevation myocardial infarction is made. Early inpatient coronary angiography shows an occluded left anterior descending artery, which is successfully re-perfused and stented. He is subsequently discharged on dual antiplatelet therapy (DAPT) of aspirin 75 mg and clopidogrel 75 mg daily, alongside other secondary prevention medications (bisoprolol 5 mg daily and his simvastatin is switched for atorvastatin 80 mg).

Two weeks later he represents with crushing central chest pain; his TrT is high and coronary angiography demonstrates stent thrombosis (ST).

5.4.2 Overview

Clopidogrel is a second generation thienopyridine indicated to prevent atherothrombotic events in peripheral arterial disease (PAD), and following an ischaemic stroke, acute coronary syndrome (ACS) or percutaneous coronary intervention (PCI). Clopidogrel is a prodrug; ~15% of absorbed clopidogrel is oxidised in a two-step process involving CYP1A2, CYP3A4/5, CYP2B6, CYP2C9 and CYP2C19 via an intermediate, 2-oxo-clopidogrel. The resultant 5-thiol active species irreversibly inhibits platelet purinergic $P2Y_{12}$ receptors leading to reduced adenosine diphosphate (ADP)-mediated platelet aggregation [193]. The remaining ~85% of absorbed clopidogrel is hydrolysed by CES1 into an inactive metabolite [193]. Despite standard DAPT, ~10% of ACS patients undergoing PCI suffer a recurrent cardiovascular event within one year [194], and up to ~25% are considered clopidogrel resistant according to experimental *ex vivo* platelet function testing [195]. Although definitions of *ex vivo* high on-treatment platelet reactivity (HTPR) vary between studies, persistent HTPR in coronary artery disease (CAD) patients has been consistently associated with adverse cardiovascular outcomes [196, 197]. Clinical factors associated with HTPR include older age, increased BMI, diabetes mellitus, and renal failure [197, 198]. In contrast, the utility of platelet function testing for aspirin remains unclear [199]. The main clopidogrel pharmacogenes are *CYP2C19*, *CES1* and *ABCB1* (Table 5.5).

5.4.2.1 CYP2C19

CYP2C19 appears the dominant CYP responsible for clopidogrel bioactivation. *CYP2C19*2* (rs4244285, c.681G>A, I331V) is the most common ROF allele, with a frequency of up to 35% in Asians and ~15% in Africans and Caucasians [200]. *CYP2C19*3* (rs4986893, c.636G>A) is also relatively common in Asians, with a MAF of up to 9% [200]. At least 33 other *CYP2C19* alleles have been described, but the majority are rare and/or of unknown functional significance [201]. *CYP2C19*2* leads to a cryptic splice variant, and *CYP2C19*3* encodes a premature stop codon [198]. *CYP2C19* ROF alleles have been frequently associated with increased HTPR compared to wild-type (**1/*1*) patients, and account for ~5–12% of observed variability in ADP-induced platelet aggregation [198], which is higher than for any other single known factor. *CYP2C19*17* (rs12248560, c.-806C>T) is another allele common in Africans and Caucasians, but less so in East Asians, with MAFs of ~24, 22 and 1%, respectively. *CYP2C19*17* is associated with increased *CYP2C19* transcription, a modest gain-of-function [198], and has been associated with reduced HTPR [14]. CYP2C19 metabolizer phenotype is categorised into: extensive (normal, **1/*1*), intermediate (ROF heterozygotes), poor (ROF homozygotes/compound heterozygotes) and ultra-rapid (*CYP2C19*17* carriers with no ROF allele).

Table 5.5 Clopidogrel pharmacogenomics and clinical outcomes

Clinical Outcome	Study	Locus/Gene	Variant(s)	Effect[a]	References
Replicated variants:					
Stent thrombosis	MA	*CYP2C19*	*2, *3, *4 - *8	ROF alleles present vs. non-carriers: HR 2.81 (95% CI 1.81, 4.37)	[209]
				1 ROF allele vs. non-carriers: HR 2.67 (95% CI 1.69, 4.22)	[209]
				2 ROF alleles vs. non-carriers: HR 3.97 (95% CI 1.75, 9.02)	[209]
Candidate gene/variants:					
MACE in patients at high risk of MACE (e.g. requiring PCI)	MA	*CYP2C19*	*2, *3, *4 - *8	ROF alleles present vs. non-carriers: HR 1.57 (95% CI 1.13, 2.16)	[209]
				1 ROF allele vs. non-carriers: HR 1.55 (95% CI 1.11, 2.27)	[209]
				2 ROF alleles vs. non-carriers: HR 1.76 (95% CI 1.24, 2.50)	[209]
MACE	MA	*CYP2C19*	*17	HR 0.82 (95% CI 0.72, 0.94)	[297]
	MA	*ABCB1*	3435C>T	Early MACE T vs. C: OR 1.34 (95% CI 1.10, 1.62) Long term MACE in patients on clopidogrel 300 mg daily T vs. C: OR 1.28 (95% CI 1.10, 1.48)	[214]
	CG	*CES1*	rs71647871 (G143E)	After one year, 47 of 344 143GG patients and 0 of 6 143GE patients on clopidogrel had suffered MACE (NS)	[211]

(continued)

Table 5.5 (continued)

Clinical Outcome	Study	Locus/Gene	Variant(s)	Effect[a]	References
Re-stenosis/ occlusion of PAD lesion	MA[b]	*CYP2C19*	*2	*2 vs. non-carriers; OR 5.40 (95% 2.30, 12.70)	[202]
	CG	*ABCB1*	3435C>T	TT vs. CT/CC: OR 3.79 (95% CI 1.03, 13.93)	[202]

CG candidate gene study, *HR* hazard ratio, *MA* meta-analysis, *MACE* major adverse cardiovascular event, *NS* not statistically significant, *OR* odds ratio, *PAD* peripheral artery disease, *PCI* percutaneous coronary intervention, *ROF* reduction-of-function allele/haplotype

[a]All effects are statistically significant unless otherwise stated.

[b]The association between *CYP2C19*2* and re-stenosis/occlusion of treated peripheral lesions has been identified [203], replicated [202] and shown in meta-analysis [202]. However, due to the overall low number of patients in the two studies (n = 122 patients), it has been classified as a candidate association.

Clinically, two small studies and a combined meta-analysis have reported that, in patients with PAD on clopidogrel, carrying *CYP2C19*2* is associated with an increased risk of re-stenosis or occlusion of treated lesions [202, 203]. In stroke medicine, carrying *CYP2C19* ROF alleles (**2* ± **3*) has been associated with an increased risk of stroke recurrence in white patients with an index subcortical stroke (but not African-American or Spanish patients) [204], an increased risk of major adverse cardiovascular events (MACE) in Chinese stroke patients [205], and an increased risk of stroke and MACE in patients with an initial transient ischaemic attack or minor stroke [206]. However, in symptomatic intracranial atherosclerotic disease, *CYP2C19* ROF alleles protected against MACE, which is the opposite direction of effect to what was expected [207].

Most primary clopidogrel-*CYP2C19* studies to date though have focussed on cardiac disease and patients undergoing PCI. Within a 24 month period, 11 discordant overlapping meta-analyses were published, leading to a recent systematic interrogation of the meta-analyses themselves [208]. Importantly, all 11 meta-analyses reported a statistically significant increased risk of ST with *CYP2C19* ROF alleles, although publication bias could not be ruled out in the three meta-analyses that examined it. For illustration, the Mega *et al.* meta-analysis found the HR of ST to be 1.55 (95% CI 1.11, 2.27) and 1.76 (95% CI 1.24, 2.50) in carriers of one or two *CYP2C19* ROF alleles, respectively, suggesting a gene-dose trend [209]. However, there are contrasting results between meta-analyses for the risk of MACE associated with *CYP2C19* ROF alleles, predominantly due to differences in how between-study heterogeneity and bias have been managed [208]. However, a narrative assessment of some of the meta-analyses has led to the plausible observation that *CYP2C19* genotype is likely relevant to clinical events in high risk patients (e.g. ACS patients undergoing PCI) but is clinically insignificant in lower risk groups (e.g. AF patients) [210]. Given the concerns over small-sample and publication biases [208], this hypothesis requires prospective validation. For *CYP2C19*17*, it is not associated with ST and has been inconsistently linked with increased bleeding

[12]. In terms of the clinical case, it is plausible that the patient carried *CYP2C19* ROF alleles, increasing his risk of HTPR and ST with clopidogrel.

5.4.2.2 CES1

CES1 hydrolyses not only ~85% of absorbed clopidogrel, but also both the 2-oxo-clopidogrel intermediate metabolite and the active species, all into inactive metabolites [193]. Carrying the rare 143E variant of *CES1* rs71647871 (G143E) has been associated with impaired *in vitro* hydrolysis of clopidogrel and 2-oxo-clopidogrel [193], increased levels of circulating clopidogrel active metabolite in volunteers, reduced *ex vivo* ADP-induced platelet aggregation in volunteers and patients with CAD on clopidogrel, and a trend for reduced cardiovascular events, albeit in an underpowered comparison [211].

5.4.2.3 ABCB1

The TT genotype of the common synonymous *ABCB1* variant rs1045642 (3435C>T) is associated with lower clopidogrel, 2-oxo-clopidogrel and active metabolite systemic levels, due to increased intestinal efflux [212, 213]. In PAD, after controlling for the presence of *CYP2C19* ROF alleles, 3435TT patients had an increased risk of re-stenosis or occlusion of the treated lesions [202]. A meta-analysis of patients with CAD has indicated that the T allele of *ABCB1* 3435C>T may be associated with an increased risk of MACE, but no associations were detected for ST or HTPR [214].

5.4.3 Newer $P2Y_{12}$ Antagonists

Prasugrel is a third generation thienopyridine indicated in the prevention of atherothrombotic events in patients with ACS undergoing PCI, alongside aspirin. Prasugrel is a prodrug hydrolysed initially by carboxylesterases to thiolactone [215], and then undergoes a single hepatic CYP-mediated oxidative step to form the active metabolite, which irreversibly inhibits $P2Y_{12}$ receptors [216]. The CYP metabolism is mainly by CYP3A4/CYP2B6 and to a lesser degree by CYP2C9/CYP2C19 [198]. Prasugrel consistently produces greater inhibition of platelet aggregation than clopidogrel [217]. Neither common *CYP* variants [218] nor *ABCB1* 3435C>T [219] have been associated with prasugrel active metabolite levels or cardiovascular events. Furthermore, no association between the rs662 (Q192R) variant of *PON1*, which encodes paraoxonase 1, and prasugrel levels or clinical outcomes have been found [220]. These observations mirror the confirmed lack of influence of *PON1* Q192R on clopidogrel interindividual variability [220].

There are different laboratory techniques to determine platelet function; the platelet reactivity index vasodilator-stimulated phosphoprotein (PRI VASP) assay is a novel and highly specific test for $P2Y_{12}$ inhibition [221]. Interestingly, unlike other assays, *CYP2C19*2* and **17* are associated with HTPR and low on-treatment platelet reactivity (LTPR), respectively, in prasugrel-treated patients when measured by PRI VASP [217, 221]. Furthermore, an increased risk of bleeding was associated with prasugrel LTPR [217, 221]. Although these findings require replication by a different research team, they highlight the discordance between platelet function assays and the need for standardisation.

Ticagrelor is a novel cyclopentyltriazolopyrimidine antiplatelet drug indicated with aspirin for the prevention of atherothrombotic events in patients after an ACS. Ticagrelor reversibly and non-competitively inhibits $P2Y_{12}$ receptors without requirement for bioactivation. CYP3A4/5 convert ticagrelor to its major active metabolite, AR-C124910XX (ARC) [222, 223]. Candidate gene analysis in the PLATO RCT genetic sub-study confirmed that *CYP2C19* ROF alleles, **17*, and *ABCB1* 3435C>T do not influence ticagrelor efficacy [224]. However, a recent GWAS involving the ticagrelor-treated patients within this PLATO sub-study has implicated *SLCO1B1*, the *CYP3A4* region and *UGT2B7* [223]. The *SLCO1B1* SNP, rs113681054, surpassed the genome-wide significance threshold in relation to ARC plasma levels and is in LD with non-synonymous *SLCO1B1* rs4149056 (V174A); the minor alleles of both SNPs were found alongside increased circulating ARC and ticagrelor. A rare *UGT2B7* variant, rs61361928 (137T>C, L46P) was significantly associated with higher levels of ARC, but not ticagrelor, by GWAS. Finally, GWAS identified SNPs in the *CYP3A4* locus associated with elevated ticagrelor, but not ARC, concentrations [223]. However, none of these PK variants were associated with MACE, or the ticagrelor ADRs of bleeding or dyspnoea [223].

Cangrelor is a recently licensed intravenous reversible $P2Y_{12}$ antagonist indicated in DAPT in patients with CAD undergoing PCI in whom oral $P2Y_{12}$ antagonists have not been administered and are unsuitable. Currently, little is known regarding cangrelor pharmacogenomics.

5.4.4 Clinical Utility

Clopidogrel is an ideal candidate for pharmacogenomics intervention because it has several indications and is widely used, the atherothrombotic consequences of ineffective clopidogrel can be permanent and life-threatening, and alternative antiplatelet agents exist. Furthermore, the alternative oral drugs (prasugrel, ticagrelor) are more expensive, associated with increased bleeding compared to clopidogrel [222], and their superior effectiveness in ACS patients appears to be reduced in *CYP2C19* extensive metabolisers [200, 225]. Therefore, stratification of antiplatelet therapy will likely improve the benefit: risk profile of antiplatelet therapy.

In 2010, the FDA added a boxed warning to the clopidogrel drug label stating that clopidogrel has decreased effectiveness in *CYP2C19* poor metabolisers and alternative treatments should be considered [226]. Joint guidelines from the American College of Cardiology (ACC) and the American Heart Association (AHA) have addressed the *CYP2C19*-clopidogrel interaction; the guideline for PCI advises against routine *CYP2C19* genotyping, but suggests a potential role for genetic testing in patients undergoing high risk elective procedures (e.g. complex atherosclerotic disease) [227]. The CPIC guidelines recommend that in ACS/PCI patients, in whom *CYP2C19* genotype is already known, an alternative antiplatelet agent is prescribed in intermediate and poor *CYP2C19* metabolisers [200].

Overall, the evidence associating *CYP2C19* genotype with ST in clopidogrel-treated patients is strong, but the association with MACE remains disputed. At least one RCT investigating the controlled, prospective, clinical utility of genotype-informed antiplatelet prescribing in higher- risk patients (Tailored Antiplatelet Therapy Following PCI [TAILOR-PCI]), is ongoing [228]. This RCT is powered for clinical outcomes, and in the intervention arm, patients with *CYP2C19*2* or **3* receive ticagrelor in place of clopidogrel. Interestingly, a recent algorithm has been published that integrates *CYP2C19* genotype and CYP2C19 metabolised co-medications to predict optimal clopidogrel doses [229], which may further help drug selection. Further research into the clinical impacts of *CES1*, *ABCB1* and *CYP2C19*17* is warranted.

5.4.5 Beta-Blockers

Beta-adrenoreceptor (β-AR) antagonists (βBs) are indicated in multiple CVDs including hypertension, angina pectoris, ACS, chronic heart failure and arrhythmias. The pharmacogenomics of βBs in hypertension is highlighted here (Table 5.6). Hypertension is both the most common modifiable risk factor for global disease burden and the most common chronic condition for which drugs are prescribed [230]. Antihypertensive drugs significantly reduce morbidity and mortality [230]. However, only ~50% of patients reach appropriate blood pressure control [231]. Multiple therapeutic drug classes are available to manage hypertension, although the choice of drug and dose is generally through empirical trial-and-error, which can demotivate patients [230]. Except for select populations (e.g. women of child-bearing potential), βBs are not preferred initial therapy for hypertension and are currently fourth-line drugs [232], largely due to efficacy and safety concerns

Table 5.6 Beta blocker pharmacogenomics and clinical outcomes in hypertensive patients

Study	Locus/gene	Variant(s)	Beta blocker	Clinical outcome	Effect[a]	References
Top associations:						
CVD gene array	*SIGLEC12* *A1BG* *F5*	rs16982743 (Q29Stop) rs893184 (H54R) rs4525 (H865R)	Atenolol	MACE	A genetic risk score was constructed and replicated. One point was given for each genotype associated with a higher risk of MACE with CCBs vs. βBs. – With low (0,1) scores, CCBs had a lower risk of MACE vs. βBs: OR 0.60 (95% CI 0.42, 0.86); – With higher scores [2, 3], CCBs had an increased risk of MACE vs. βBs: OR 1.31 (95% CI 1.08, 1.59)	[255]

(continued)

Table 5.6 (continued)

Study	Locus/gene	Variant(s)	Beta blocker	Clinical outcome	Effect[a]	References
CG	*ADRB1*	rs1801253 (1165G>C, R389G), rs1801252 (145A>G, S49G)	Metoprolol	BP	(a) RR389 had 8.6 mmHg greater metoprolol-induced reduction in DBP than 389G carriers (b) S49-R389/S49-R389 had 14.7 mmHg metoprolol-induced DBP reduction vs. 0.5 mmHg in 49G-R389/S49-389G	[233]
CG			Carvedilol	BP	(a) RR389 had 10.61 mmHg carvedilol-induced DBP reduction vs. 2.62 mmHg in 389GG (b) 49G-R389/S49-R389 had 16.11 mmHg carvedilol-induced DBP reduction vs. 2.83 mmHg in S49-389G/S49-389G	[234]
CG			Atenolol	Death	Increased risk of mortality in S49-R389 carriers: – on verapamil: OR 8.58 (95% CI 2.06, 35.8, p = 0.003) – NS on atenolol: OR 2.31 (95% CI 0.82, 6.55, p = 0.11)	[238]
CG	*GRK4*	rs1024323 (C>T, A142V)	Metoprolol	BP	With each 142 V variant allele, there was an increased likelihood of reaching a metoprolol-induced MAP of ≤107 mmHg in African-American men: HR 1.54 (95% CI 1.11, 2.44)	[244]
CG		rs2960306 (G>A, R65L), rs1024323 (C>T, A142V)	Atenolol	BP	– 0, 1 and 2 copies of the variant 65 L-142 V haplotype had atenolol-induced reductions in DBP of 9.1, 6.8 and 5.3 mmHg, respectively. – The 65 L-142 V haplotype was not associated with BP reduction in hydrochlorothiazide-treated patients	[243]
CG			Antihyper-tensive drugs	BP	Increased number of antihypertensive drugs required in 65 L/65 L-142 V/142 V patients to reach the same MAP compared to other haplotypes	[246]

Table 5.6 (continued)

Study	Locus/gene	Variant(s)	Beta blocker	Clinical outcome	Effect[a]	References
Candidate gene/variants:						
GWAS	*ACY3*	3 SNPs in locus. Top SNP is rs2514036 (G>A)	Bisoprolol	BP	For each minor allele, there was a 5.4 mmHg reduction in 24-hour ambulatory SBP on bisoprolol	[253]
CG	*CYP2D6*	*4	Metoprolol	Heart rate	*4/*4 had 8.5 beats/min lower heart rate than *1/*1	[247]
			Metoprolol	BP	*4/*4 had 5.4 mmHg lower DBP than *1/*1	
			Metoprolol	Bradycardia	*4/*4 vs. *1/*1: OR 3.86 (95% CI 1.68, 8.86)	
CG		PM (any 2 of: *3, *4, *5, *6)	Metoprolol	Adverse events	Metoprolol-treated patients experiencing adverse events were ~5× more likely to be a CYP2D6 PM than the general public	[250]
CG	*NR1H3*	rs2279238 (C>T)	Atenolol	MACE	In minor T allele carriers, increased risk of MACE with verapamil, but not with atenolol	[254]

BP blood pressure, *CG* candidate gene study, *CVD* cardiovascular disease, *DBP* diastolic blood pressure, *GWAS* genome-wide association study, *HR* hazard ratio, *MACE* major adverse cardiovascular event, *MAP* mean arterial pressure, *NS* not statistically significant, *OR* odds ratio, *PM* poor metabolizer, *SBP* systolic blood pressure
[a]All effects are statistically significant unless otherwise stated

originating from atenolol trials. However, the high prevalence of hypertension and multi-drug strategies often required for adequate blood pressure control mean that βB treatment for hypertension still occurs, and thus remains clinically relevant.

5.4.5.1 ADRB1

ADRB1 encodes the β_1-AR, which is the predominant cardiomyocyte β-AR subtype and mediates the physiological response to noradrenaline, and to a lesser extent adrenaline [230]. The majority of βBs used in hypertension preferentially inhibit the β_1-AR (e.g. atenolol, bisoprolol, metoprolol), although non-selective β_1 /β_2-AR inhibitors (e.g. propranolol, carvedilol) are also used. *ADRB1* has two common non-synonymous polymorphisms, which are considered functional: rs1801252 (145A>G, S49G) and rs1801253 (1165G>C, R389G). Some studies [233–236], but not all [237], have found that hypertensive patients with the RR389 genotype, or R389-S49 haplotype, have greater βB-mediated blood pressure reductions. Furthermore, patients with hypertension and CAD carrying the R389-S49 haplotype have an increased risk of mortality, which is statistically significant in patients on verapamil but not for those on atenolol, suggesting a βB protective influence [238].

RR389 human non-failing left ventricular membranes have a higher affinity for noradrenaline than membranes expressing the 389G β_1-AR [239]. The R389 β_1-AR is also associated with enhanced agonist-mediated coupling to the second messenger, adenylyl cyclase, and greater downstream signalling [240]. The S49 allele is associated with reduced receptor internalisation, compared to 49G, resulting in increased signalling [241]. However, R389G has a larger effect and may abstruse S49G [241]. A large GWAS meta-analysis has confirmed that R389G contributes to blood pressure traits, with the R389 allele linked to higher blood pressure and increased frequency of hypertension [242]. Therefore it is biologically plausible that the impact of βBs will be greater in patients with wild-type R389, and perhaps S49, because these alleles exhibit enhanced agonist sensitivity [230].

5.4.5.2 GRK4

GRK4 encodes guanine nucleotide-binding protein (G protein)-coupled receptor kinase 4, which targets activated G protein–coupled receptors (GPCRs) for phosphorylation, including the dopamine receptor and potentially the β_1-AR, in order to inactivate them [243]. The variant alleles of the non-synonymous *GRK4* SNPs, rs2960306 (R65L), rs1024323 (A142V) and rs1801058 (A486V) are in moderate LD [244]; they exhibit a gain-of-function and so enhance GRK4-mediated GPCR desensitization [245], which plausibly could diminish the likelihood of hypertension but also βB efficacy. 65L and 142V have been associated with reduced atenolol-induced diastolic blood pressure (DBP) lowering, and furthermore there is a gene-dose trend with increasing copies of the 65L-142V haplotype incrementally reducing DBP response to atenolol [243]. 65L, 142V and 486V are all associated with increased MACE [243]. Although this association was independent of treatment for 65L and 142V, 486V carried a significantly increased MACE risk in patients on verapamil, but not those on atenolol [243]. A potential interaction between *ADRB1* R389G and *GRK4* variants has also been suggested [243], and patients double homozygous for 65L and 142V appear to require a larger number of antihypertensive drugs [246]. In contrast though, another study found that 142V was associated with an improved proportion of African-American men on metoprolol reaching a target mean arterial pressure ($\leq$107 mmHg) [244].

5.4.5.3 CYP2D6

The racemate βB, metoprolol, is metabolized by polymorphic CYP2D6. *CYP2D6*4* (rs3892097, 1846G>A) is the most common non-functional allele, and results from a splicing defect, although several other non-functional *CYP2D6* alleles have also been identified (e.g. **3*, **5*, **6*) [247]. Approximately ~2–5% of African-Americans, <1% of Asians and ~6–10% of Caucasians are poor metabolizers [248]. Poor, and to a lesser extent intermediate metabolizers have increased systemic exposure to both metoprolol enantiomers [249]. However, whilst some studies have reported that *CYP2D6* poor metabolizers have a lower DBP [247] and an increased risk of bradycardia [247] and adverse events [250] on metoprolol, other studies have found no association [235, 251].

5.4.6 Clinical Utility

There is relatively strong evidence for a pharmacogenomic association between *ADRB1* R389G and βB response in hypertension. The metoprolol drug label highlights the impact of *CYP2D6* genotype on metoprolol PK, although currently it considers CYP2D6-dependent metabolism to have little or no effect on metoprolol efficacy or tolerability [252]. Other candidate pharmacogenomic genes that require (drug-specific) replication have been identified, including *ACY3* [253] and *NR1H3* [254] (Table 5.6). Overall though, hypertension pharmacogenomics studies to date have had small to moderate sample sizes, selected different endpoints (e.g. systolic/diastolic/mean blood pressure), often included multiple drugs, and produced inconsistent results. One interesting recent development is the identification and replication of a pharmacogenomic risk score, based on three non-synonymous novel hypertension pharmacogenomic SNPs: rs16982743 (*SIGLEC12*, sialic acid binding Ig-like lectin 12), rs893184 (*A1BG*, alpha-1-B glycoprotein) and rs4525 (*F5*, coagulation factor V) [255]. One point was given for each genotype associated with a higher risk of MACE in patients treated with a calcium channel blocker compared to a βB. Consequently, the risk of MACE was significantly lower in patients with a higher genetic risk score treated with a βB rather than a calcium channel blocker [255]. Further research is required to confirm or refute candidate signals, prospectively test this genetic risk score or subsequent iteration, and to integrate βB hypertension pharmacogenomics with the ongoing pharmacogenomics research of other antihypertensive drugs, including diuretics and ACEIs [256].

5.5 Antiarrhythmics

5.5.1 Atrial Fibrillation

AF is the most prevalent sustained cardiac arrhythmia requiring treatment, and has a substantial socioeconomic impact [257]. Despite advances in catheter-mediated ablation and pacemakers, drugs remain the mainstay of therapy. Both rate and rhythm pharmacological control methods are used; overall these strategies appear equivalently effective [258]. However, a rhythm control strategy using antiarrhythmic drugs is often required in patients with intolerable AF symptoms, and may be more widely applicable because sinus rhythm itself is associated with an improved prognosis [257]. On the other hand, rhythm control is also associated with more adverse events, which may offset at the population level any beneficial antiarrhythmic drug effects [259]. Identification of patient subgroups most likely to benefit from an antiarrhythmic drug strategy would improve AF management.

A recent candidate gene study identified and confirmed that the wild-type allele of rs10033464, a SNP at chromosome locus 4q25, is predictive of maintaining successful rhythm control [260]. Furthermore, rs10033464 wild-type homozygotes had better AF rhythm control with Vaughan Williams class III antiarrhythmic drugs (e.g. amiodarone), whereas variant allele carriers responded better to class I drugs (e.g.

flecainide), suggesting a potential pharmacogenomics effect [260]. Variants at the 4q25 locus have also been associated with AF recurrence after direct current cardioversion [261], and both AF recurrence and AF/atrial tachycardia recurrence after catheter ablation [262, 263]. In GWAS', the strongest signals consistently associated with AF itself are from the 4q25 locus. Although its functional role remains unclear, 4q25 may encompass cis-regulatory elements involved in regulating nearby genes including *PITX2* [264]. *PITX2* encodes paired-like homeodomain transcription factor 2. It has been shown to have a role in embryonic left-right asymmetry and cardiac development including the development of the pulmonary vein myocardium, which is a major source for arrhythmogenic AF foci [265]. Interestingly, a rare *PITX2* mutation (Q102L) has also recently been associated with congenital heart diseases, including tetralogy of Fallot [266, 267].

5.5.2 Torsade de Pointes

Drug-induced symptomatic ventricular arrhythmias are unpredictable, rare, life threatening and a leading cause of drug withdrawal from the market. The long QT syndrome (LQTS) is asymptomatic, results from cardiac repolarization prolongation, is diagnosed by ECG, and importantly can descend into Torsade de Pointes (TdP). Both congenital (cLQTS) and acquired causes for LQTS exist, and the latter includes drug-induced LQTS (DiLQTS). The cardiac repolarization prolongation in most DiLQTS results from drug-induced disruption to the I_{Kr} current, through blockade of its requisite cardiac Kv11.1 potassium channel, whose subunits are encoded by *KCNH2* (also termed *HERG*) [268]. TdP is a rare complication of LQTS, is a stereotyped polymorphic ventricular tachycardia, and is potentially fatal. Most drug-induced TdP (DiTdP) is related to antiarrhythmic drugs (e.g. procainamide, disopyramide, and quinidine). Multiple non-cardiovascular drugs have also been associated with LQTS, although only a minority lead to DiTdP (e.g. domperidone, erythromycin). Although risk of DiTdP can be dose-dependent (e.g. with sotalol), for several drugs it occurs at low concentrations unpredictably (e.g. with quinidine) [269]. For antiarrhythmic drugs, DiTdP is thought to occur in ~1–3% of (hospitalised) patients, but the risk is dramatically lower for QT-prolonging non-cardiovascular drugs [269, 270]. Clinical LQTS risk factors include electrolyte imbalances (e.g. hypokalaemia), female sex, increasing age and structural heart disease.

The most common causes of cLQTS are due to mutations in *KCNQ1* (encoding the Kv7.1 potassium channel subunit), *KCNH2* and *SCN5A* (encoding the $Na_v1.5$ cardiac sodium channel). However, the mutations are incompletely penetrant, and cases of family members harbouring these mutations but not developing TdP until after drug exposure are known [271]. Therefore the concept of a 'reduced repolarization reserve' has been proposed. This theorem suggests that cardiac repolarisation has inbuilt redundancy and so an individual's risk of DiLQTS (and DiTdP) is determined by their combination of genetic, clinical and drug risk factors, which summate to overwhelm this redundancy [268, 272].

A large candidate gene pharmacogenomics study found a suggestive association between rs1805128 (D85N) in *KCNE1* and an increased risk of DiTdP in patients taking a QT-prolonging medication, compared to drug-tolerant and population controls [273]. *KCNE1* rs1805128 has a MAF of ~1–2% in Caucasians, but is less frequent in other ethnicities. Rare *KCNE1* mutations cause ~1% of cLQTS [274], KCNE1 modulates the activity of KCNQ1, and 85N is expected to reduce I_{Ks} and so decrease repolarization reserve [268]. A large GWAS meta-analysis has identified 35 loci that collectively account for ~8–10% of observed QT-interval variability in the general population; the two loci associated with the largest QT-interval increases were *KCNE1* and *NOS1AP* [275]. NOS1AP encodes nitric oxide synthase 1 adapter protein. Although its role in cardiac electrophysiology remains unclear, common variants in *NOS1AP* have been associated with amiodarone-related LQTS/TdP in Caucasians by candidate gene analysis (Caucasian MAFs ~18–30%) [276]. However, a subsequent GWAS in Caucasians found no genome-wide significant signals associated with DiTdP [277]. This DiTdP GWAS had an 80% power to detect a variant at genome-wide significance with a MAF of 10% and OR of ≥2.7, which contests that common variants do not contribute substantively to DiTdP across multiple drugs, at least in Caucasians [277].

A NGS study has found an increased prevalence of novel rare variants within 22 congenital arrhythmia genes, including the 13 identified cLQTS genes, in Caucasian DiTdP patients [278]. Most recently, Caucasian DiLQTS/TdP patients and drug-tolerant controls have been compared using whole-exome sequencing with rare variant bioinformatics [279]. The analyses implicated rare variants within *KCNE1* and *ACN9* in DiLQTS, validated *KCNE1* D85N, and determined that DiLQTS patients have an increased burden of rare non-synonymous variants within a pre-defined set of seven cLQTS potassium channel and channel modulatory genes [279]. *ACN9* is thought to be involved in gluconeogenesis, but its functional relationship to DiLQTS/TdP remains unknown.

In African-American patients, rs7626962 (S1103Y) in *SCN5A* has been implicated by candidate gene analysis in arrhythmias including DITdP [280]. S1103Y has a MAF ~5–10% in those of African descent, but is rare in other ethnicities.

5.5.3 Clinical Utility

The pharmacogenomic variants associated with AF and DiLQTS/TdP remain largely in the discovery stage, and require further validation and investigations with patients of different ethnicities. Whilst common variation may be involved in AF pharmacogenomics, low frequency and rare variants in cardiac electrophysiology genes have been implicated as DiLQTS/TdP genetic susceptibility factors. Importantly, clinical decision support systems are being pioneered that utilise electronic health record clinical information to reduce prescriptions of known QT-prolonging drugs in patients identified at risk of DiLQTS/TdP [281, 282]. As patient sequencing becomes more commonplace, it is conceivable that a patient's rare variant (predicted) deleterious burden within implicated genes could be integrated into these support systems to refine DiLQTS/TdP risk predictions.

5.6 Renin-Angiotensin System Inhibitors

ACEIs antagonise the renin-angiotensin-aldosterone system (RAAS) by inhibiting the conversion of angiotensin I to angiotensin II, and are used in hypertension, ACS, chronic heart failure, diabetic nephropathy, and scleroderma with renal involvement. In patients intolerant to ACEIs, angiotensin II receptor blockers (ARBs) are an alternative.

The most commonly studied ACEI/ARB candidate variant is the 287-base pair Alu repeat insertion/deletion element within the *ACE* gene (rs4646994, *ACE* I/D); the D allele is associated with increased ACE activity. The role of *ACE* I/D in ACEI/ARB pharmacogenomics is disputed though due to conflicting results. On the one hand, for example, a recent non-randomized candidate gene study of CAD patients in Taiwan with 12 years of follow up reported that the *ACE* D allele is associated with an increased risk of MACE, and a pharmacogenomic interaction with ACEIs was detected [283]. Furthermore, a pharmacogenomic risk score composed of *ACE* I/D and rs5186 (1166A>C) in *AGTR1*, which encodes the angiotensin II type I receptor, could categorise patients according to ACEI treatment response [283]. On the other hand, a candidate genetic RCT sub-study found no association between *ACE* I/D and MACE during 4.2 years of follow up in stable CAD Caucasian patients on perindopril [284]. However, they also developed a pharmacogenomic risk score for MACE constructed from three SNPs (rs275651 and rs5182 in *AGTR1*, and rs12050217 in *BK1*). Similarly, this risk score could stratify treatment response [284]. *BK1* encodes the bradykinin type I receptor and is involved in the kallikrein-bradykinin pathway. Furthermore, this latter risk score has recently been used alongside a clinical risk score to further sub-categorize response to perindopril [285]. Overall, these advances are promising, but require external validation. Additional large studies that give consideration for ethnicity, the specific ACEI/ARB investigated, and employ whole genome agnostic approaches are needed to clarify the role of *ACE* I/D and identify new variants.

Notable ADRs associated with ACEIs are a dry cough, and angioedema, which is rare but serious. No association was found in a meta-analysis between *ACE* I/D and ACEI cough [286]. A recent GWAS identified no genome-wide significant signals with ACEI angioedema [287]. However, two SNPs (rs500766 in *PRKCQ*, and rs2724635 in *ETV6*) modestly associated with ACEI angioedema were replicated in a separate cohort [287]. *PRKCQ* and *ETV6* encode protein kinase C θ and transcription factor ETV6, respectively, and both are involved in immune regulation [287].

Conclusion

Intensive research, fuelled by advances in technical and bioinformatic capabilities and increased international collaborative working, has greatly increased our understanding of CVD genomics and cardiovascular drug pharmacogenomics over the last decade. The evidence underpinning the clinical utility of warfarin pharmacogenomics, at least in Caucasian patients in European healthcare settings, is strong. Ongoing pharmacogenomic trials with warfarin [288] and clopidogrel [228] powered for clinical endpoints are expected to provide further clarity. The validated simvastatin myotoxicity-*SLCO1B1* rs4149056 association has already led to a change in practice through reduced simvastatin 80 mg prescribing. However, it is unlikely alone to be sufficiently predictive for clinical adoption. Further research is required to validate and determine the clinical utility of identified pharmacogenomic variants associated with DOACs, βBs, antiarrhythmics and ACEIs.

Although widespread uptake of cardiovascular pharmacogenomics has yet to occur, early adopter sites, principally in the US, have implemented specific cardiovascular drug-gene associations into practice [289, 290]. The solutions they have used to straddle the implementation hurdles and the ensuing long term real world results will provide additional experience and data. If the results are favourable and generalizable, broader adoption of pharmacogenomics is likely. In Europe, a study is underway to implement pre-emptive pharmacogenomics testing via a panel of 50 variants to guide the prescribing of 42 drugs, including cardiovascular prescriptions. This study will assess the impact of this intervention on the collective incidence and severity of subsequent ADRs (http://upgx.eu/).

Moving forward, the integration of multi-omics data alongside genomics information is anticipated to both increase our understanding of drug mechanisms of action and further parse interindividual drug response variability. Most cardiovascular drugs are administered orally. It is already known that the inactivation of digoxin is influenced by gut flora [291], and a gut flora derived metabolite, trimethylamine N-oxide (TMAO), has been recently associated with increased MACE risk [292]. Therefore, it is anticipated that cardiovascular drug-gut microbiome interactions are likely to be increasingly recognised, characterised, and potentially integrated with genomic and other predictors of drug response variability. Furthermore, although not covered here, a pharmacogenomic RCT (Genetically Targeted Therapy for the Prevention of Symptomatic Atrial Fibrillation in Patients With Heart Failure (GENETIC-AF [GENETIC-AF]) is currently recruiting participants to assess whether a novel beta blocker drug, bucindolol, is effective at reducing atrial arrhythmias and mortality in a genetically determined subset of heart failure patients [293]. Therefore, pharmacogenomics is beginning to shape both the clinical use of established cardiovascular drugs and cardiovascular drug development. It is an exciting time, although there remains much to do.

References

1. World Health Organisation. The top 10 causes of death. 2014. http://www.who.int/mediacentre/factsheets/fs310/en/. Accessed 04 May 2016.
2. Laslett LJ, Alagona P, Clark BA, et al. The worldwide environment of cardiovascular disease: prevalence, diagnosis, therapy, and policy issues: a report from the American College of Cardiology. J Am Coll Cardiol. 2012;60(25_S):S1–S49.
3. QuintilesIMS. IMS health forecasts global drug spending to increase 30 percent by 2020, to $1.4 trillion, as medicine use gap narrows. 2015. http://www.imshealth.com/en/about-us/news/ims-health-forecasts-global-drug-spending-to-increase-30-percent-by-2020. Accessed 15 Feb 2017.

4. statista. Global spending on medicines from 2010 to 2020 (in billion U.S. dollars). 2016. https://www.statista.com/statistics/280572/medicine-spending-worldwide/. Accessed 9 Nov 2016.
5. Clinical Gene Networks. Market analysis. 2012. http://cgnetworks.se/page/market/. Accessed 9 Nov 2016.
6. Spear BB, Heath-Chiozzi M, Huff J. Clinical application of pharmacogenetics. Trends Mol Med. 2001;7(5):201–4.
7. Pirmohamed M, James S, Meakin S, et al. Adverse drug reactions as cause of admission to hospital: prospective analysis of 18 820 patients. BMJ. 2004;329(7456):15–9.
8. Davies EC, Green CF, Taylor S, Williamson PR, Mottram DR, Pirmohamed M. Adverse drug reactions in hospital in-patients: a prospective analysis of 3695 patient-episodes. PLoS One. 2009;4(2):e4439.
9. World Health Organisation. WHO technical report no. 498. International drug monitoring: the role of national centres. 1972. http://www.who-umc.org/graphics/24756.pdf. Accessed 9 Nov 2016.
10. Food and Drug Administration. Table of pharmacogenomic biomarkers in drug labeling. 2016. http://www.fda.gov/drugs/scienceresearch/researchareas/pharmacogenetics/ucm083378.htm. Accessed 9 Nov 2016.
11. Martin MA, Kroetz DL. Abacavir pharmacogenetics—from initial reports to standard of care. Pharmacotherapy. 2013;33(7):765–75.
12. Turner RM, Pirmohamed M. Cardiovascular pharmacogenomics: expectations and practical benefits. Clin Pharmacol Ther. 2014;95(3):281–93.
13. van der Graaf PH, Benson N. Systems pharmacology: bridging systems biology and pharmacokinetics-pharmacodynamics (PKPD) in drug discovery and development. Pharm Res. 2011;28(7):1460–4.
14. Johnson JA, Cavallari LH. Pharmacogenetics and cardiovascular disease—implications for personalized medicine. Pharmacol Rev. 2013;65(3):987–1009.
15. Dean L. Warfarin therapy and the genotypes CYP2C9 and VKORC1 2012 Mar 8 [Updated 2016 Jun 8]. Medical Genetics Summaries [Internet]. Bethesda (MD): National Center for Biotechnology Information (US); 2016.
16. Owen RP, Gong L, Sagreiya H, Klein TE, Altman RB. VKORC1 pharmacogenomics summary. Pharmacogenet Genomics. 2010;20(10):642–4.
17. Pirmohamed M, Kamali F, Daly AK, Wadelius M. Oral anticoagulation: a critique of recent advances and controversies. Trends Pharmacol Sci. 2015;36(3):153–63.
18. Jorgensen AL, Hughes DA, Hanson A, et al. Adherence and variability in warfarin dose requirements: assessment in a prospective cohort. Pharmacogenomics. 2013;14(2):151–63.
19. Bourgeois S, Jorgensen A, Zhang EJ, et al. A multi-factorial analysis of response to warfarin in a UK prospective cohort. Genome Med. 2016;8(1):2.
20. Caraco Y, Blotnick S, Muszkat M. CYP2C9 genotype-guided warfarin prescribing enhances the efficacy and safety of anticoagulation: a prospective randomized controlled study. Clin Pharmacol Ther. 2008;83(3):460–70.
21. Kimmel SE, French B, Kasner SE, et al. A pharmacogenetic versus a clinical algorithm for warfarin dosing. N Engl J Med. 2013;369(24):2283–93.
22. Marie I, Leprince P, Menard JF, Tharasse C, Levesque H. Risk factors of vitamin K antagonist overcoagulation. QJM. 2012;105(1):53–62.
23. Jones M, McEwan P, Morgan CL, Peters JR, Goodfellow J, Currie CJ. Evaluation of the pattern of treatment, level of anticoagulation control, and outcome of treatment with warfarin in patients with non-valvar atrial fibrillation: a record linkage study in a large British population. Heart. 2005;91(4):472–7.
24. Lee MT, Klein TE. Pharmacogenetics of warfarin: challenges and opportunities. J Hum Genet. 2013;58(6):334–8.
25. Yang J, Chen Y, Li X, et al. Influence of CYP2C9 and VKORC1 genotypes on the risk of hemorrhagic complications in warfarin-treated patients: a systematic review and meta-analysis. Int J Cardiol. 2013;168(4):4234–43.

26. Yuan HY, Chen JJ, Lee MT, et al. A novel functional VKORC1 promoter polymorphism is associated with inter-individual and inter-ethnic differences in warfarin sensitivity. Hum Mol Genet. 2005;14(13):1745–51.
27. Perera MA, Gamazon E, Cavallari LH, et al. The missing association: sequencing-based discovery of novel SNPs in VKORC1 and CYP2C9 that affect warfarin dose in African Americans. Clin Pharmacol Ther. 2011;89(3):408–15.
28. Loebstein R, Dvoskin I, Halkin H, et al. A coding VKORC1 Asp36Tyr polymorphism predisposes to warfarin resistance. Blood. 2007;109(6):2477–80.
29. Ciccacci C, Rufini S, Politi C, Novelli G, Forte V, Borgiani P. Could MicroRNA polymorphisms influence warfarin dosing? A pharmacogenetics study on mir133 genes. Thromb Res. 2015;136(2):367–70.
30. Perez-Andreu V, Teruel R, Corral J, et al. miR-133a regulates vitamin K 2,3-epoxide reductase complex subunit 1 (VKORC1), a key protein in the vitamin K cycle. Mol Med. 2012;18:1466–72.
31. Johnson JA, Gong L, Whirl-Carrillo M, et al. Clinical pharmacogenetics implementation consortium guidelines for CYP2C9 and VKORC1 genotypes and warfarin dosing. Clin Pharmacol Ther. 2011;90(4):625–9.
32. Jorgensen AL, FitzGerald RJ, Oyee J, Pirmohamed M, Williamson PR. Influence of CYP2C9 and VKORC1 on patient response to warfarin: a systematic review and meta-analysis. PLoS One. 2012;7(8):e44064.
33. Andersson ML, Eliasson E, Lindh JD. A clinically significant interaction between warfarin and simvastatin is unique to carriers of the CYP2C9*3 allele. Pharmacogenomics. 2012;13(7):757–62.
34. Johnson JA, Cavallari LH. Warfarin pharmacogenetics. Trends Cardiovasc Med. 2015;25(1):33–41.
35. Cavallari LH, Langaee TY, Momary KM, et al. Genetic and clinical predictors of warfarin dose requirements in African Americans. Clin Pharmacol Ther. 2010;87(4):459–64.
36. Scott SA, Jaremko M, Lubitz SA, Kornreich R, Halperin JL, Desnick RJ. CYP2C9*8 is prevalent among African-Americans: implications for pharmacogenetic dosing. Pharmacogenomics. 2009;10(8):1243–55.
37. Liu Y, Jeong H, Takahashi H, et al. Decreased warfarin clearance associated with the CYP2C9 R150H (*8) polymorphism. Clin Pharmacol Ther. 2012;91(4):660–5.
38. Ramirez AH, Shi Y, Schildcrout JS, et al. Predicting warfarin dosage in European-Americans and African-Americans using DNA samples linked to an electronic health record. Pharmacogenomics. 2012;13(4):407–18.
39. Perera MA, Cavallari LH, Limdi NA, et al. Genetic variants associated with warfarin dose in African-American individuals: a genome-wide association study. Lancet. 2013;382(9894):790–6.
40. Cha PC, Mushiroda T, Takahashi A, et al. Genome-wide association study identifies genetic determinants of warfarin responsiveness for Japanese. Hum Mol Genet. 2010;19(23):4735–44.
41. Takeuchi F, McGinnis R, Bourgeois S, et al. A genome-wide association study confirms VKORC1, CYP2C9, and CYP4F2 as principal genetic determinants of warfarin dose. PLoS Genet. 2009;5(3):e1000433.
42. Borgiani P, Ciccacci C, Forte V, et al. CYP4F2 genetic variant (rs2108622) significantly contributes to warfarin dosing variability in the Italian population. Pharmacogenomics. 2009;10(2):261–6.
43. McDonald MG, Rieder MJ, Nakano M, Hsia CK, Rettie AE. CYP4F2 is a vitamin K1 oxidase: An explanation for altered warfarin dose in carriers of the V433M variant. Mol Pharmacol. 2009;75(6):1337–46.
44. Bress A, Patel SR, Perera MA, Campbell RT, Kittles RA, Cavallari LH. Effect of NQO1 and CYP4F2 genotypes on warfarin dose requirements in Hispanic-Americans and African-Americans. Pharmacogenomics. 2012;13(16):1925–35.
45. Daneshjou R, Gamazon ER, Burkley B, et al. Genetic variant in folate homeostasis is associated with lower warfarin dose in African Americans. Blood. 2014;124(14):2298–305.

46. Voora D, Koboldt DC, King CR, et al. A polymorphism in the VKORC1 regulator calumenin predicts higher warfarin dose requirements in African Americans. Clin Pharmacol Ther. 2010;87(4):445–51.
47. Wajih N, Hutson SM, Wallin R. siRNA silencing of calumenin enhances functional factor IX production. Blood. 2006;108(12):3757–60.
48. Wallin R, Hutson SM, Cain D, Sweatt A, Sane DC. A molecular mechanism for genetic warfarin resistance in the rat. FASEB J. 2001;15(13):2542–4.
49. Glurich I, Berg RL, Burmester JK. Does CALU SNP rs1043550 contribute variability to therapeutic warfarin dosing requirements? Clin Med Res. 2013;11(2):73–9.
50. Kamali X, Wulasihan M, Yang YC, Lu WH, Liu ZQ, He PY. Association of GGCX gene polymorphism with warfarin dose in atrial fibrillation population in Xinjiang. Lipids Health Dis. 2013;12:149.
51. Lee KE, Chang BC, Park S, Gwak HS. Effects of single nucleotide polymorphisms in c-Myc on stable warfarin doses in patients with cardiac valve replacements. Pharmacogenomics. 2015;16(10):1101–8.
52. Lee MT, Chen CH, Chou CH, et al. Genetic determinants of warfarin dosing in the Han-Chinese population. Pharmacogenomics. 2009;10(12):1905–13.
53. Jeong E, Lee KE, Jeong H, Chang BC, Gwak HS. Impact of GATA4 variants on stable warfarin doses in patients with prosthetic heart valves. Pharmacogenomics J. 2015;15(1):33–7.
54. Chung JE, Chang BC, Lee KE, Kim JH, Gwak HS. Effects of NAD(P)H quinone oxidoreductase 1 polymorphisms on stable warfarin doses in Korean patients with mechanical cardiac valves. Eur J Clin Pharmacol. 2015;71(10):1229–36.
55. Wang LS, Shang JJ, Shi SY, et al. Influence of ORM1 polymorphisms on the maintenance stable warfarin dosage. Eur J Clin Pharmacol. 2013;69(5):1113–20.
56. Zeng WT, Xu Q, Li CH. Influence of genetic polymorphisms in cytochrome P450 oxidoreductase on the variability in stable warfarin maintenance dose in Han Chinese. Eur J Clin Pharmacol. 2016;72(11):1327–34.
57. Zhang X, Li L, Ding X, Kaminsky LS. Identification of cytochrome P450 oxidoreductase gene variants that are significantly associated with the interindividual variations in warfarin maintenance dose. Drug Metab Dispos. 2011;39(8):1433–9.
58. Wadelius M, Chen LY, Eriksson N, et al. Association of warfarin dose with genes involved in its action and metabolism. Hum Genet. 2007;121(1):23–34.
59. Eriksson N, Wallentin L, Berglund L, et al. Genetic determinants of warfarin maintenance dose and time in therapeutic treatment range: a RE-LY genomics substudy. Pharmacogenomics. 2016;17(13):1425–39.
60. Zhang JE, Russomanno G, Wattanachai N, Alfirevic A, Pirmohamed M. Investigating the role of microRNA on warfarin response. Abstract at the British Pharmacological Society Annual Conference. London; 2015.
61. Ruff CT, Giugliano RP, Braunwald E, et al. Comparison of the efficacy and safety of new oral anticoagulants with warfarin in patients with atrial fibrillation: a meta-analysis of randomised trials. Lancet. 2014;383(9921):955–62.
62. Loffredo L, Perri L, Violi F. Impact of new oral anticoagulants on gastrointestinal bleeding in atrial fibrillation: a meta-analysis of interventional trials. Dig Liver Dis. 2015;47(5):429–31.
63. van der Hulle T, Kooiman J, den Exter PL, Dekkers OM, Klok FA, Huisman MV. Effectiveness and safety of novel oral anticoagulants as compared with vitamin K antagonists in the treatment of acute symptomatic venous thromboembolism: a systematic review and meta-analysis. J Thromb Haemost. 2014;12(3):320–8.
64. Pare G, Eriksson N, Lehr T, et al. Genetic determinants of dabigatran plasma levels and their relation to bleeding. Circulation. 2013;127(13):1404–12.
65. Dimatteo C, D'Andrea G, Vecchione G, et al. Pharmacogenetics of dabigatran etexilate interindividual variability. Thromb Res. 2016;144:1–5.
66. Laizure SC, Parker RB, Herring VL, Hu ZY. Identification of carboxylesterase-dependent dabigatran etexilate hydrolysis. Drug Metab Dispos. 2014;42(2):201–6.

67. Shi J, Wang X, Nguyen JH, et al. Dabigatran etexilate activation is affected by the CES1 genetic polymorphism G143E (rs71647871) and gender. Biochem Pharmacol. 2016;119:76–84.
68. Stangier J, Stähle H, Rathgen K, Roth W, Reseski K, Körnicke T. Pharmacokinetics and pharmacodynamics of dabigatran etexilate, an oral direct thrombin inhibitor, with coadministration of digoxin. J Clin Pharmacol. 2012;52(2):243–50.
69. Liesenfeld KH, Lehr T, Dansirikul C, et al. Population pharmacokinetic analysis of the oral thrombin inhibitor dabigatran etexilate in patients with non-valvular atrial fibrillation from the RE-LY trial. J Thromb Haemost. 2011;9(11):2168–75.
70. Mega JL, Walker JR, Ruff CT, et al. Genetics and the clinical response to warfarin and edoxaban: findings from the randomised, double-blind ENGAGE AF-TIMI 48 trial. Lancet. 2015;385(9984):2280–7.
71. Bristol-Myers Squibb Pharma Company. COUMADIN- warfarin sodium tablet) [package insert]. 2016. https://www.ncbi.nlm.nih.gov/books/NBK84174/. Accessed 31 Oct 2016.
72. Shahabi P, Scheinfeldt LB, Lynch DE, et al. An expanded pharmacogenomics warfarin dosing table with utility in generalised dosing guidance. Thromb Haemost. 2016;116(2): 337–48.
73. Lenzini P, Wadelius M, Kimmel S, et al. Integration of genetic, clinical, and INR data to refine warfarin dosing. Clin Pharmacol Ther. 2010;87(5):572–8.
74. Verhoef TI, Redekop WK, Daly AK, van RMF S, de Boer A, Maitland-van der Zee A-H. Pharmacogenetic-guided dosing of coumarin anticoagulants: algorithms for warfarin, acenocoumarol and phenprocoumon. Br J Clin Pharmacol. 2014;77(4):626–41.
75. Klein TE, Altman RB, Eriksson N, et al. Estimation of the warfarin dose with clinical and pharmacogenetic data. N Engl J Med. 2009;360(8):753–64.
76. Gage BF, Eby C, Johnson JA, et al. Use of pharmacogenetic and clinical factors to predict the therapeutic dose of warfarin. Clin Pharmacol Ther. 2008;84(3):326–31.
77. Pirmohamed M, Burnside G, Eriksson N, et al. A randomized trial of genotype-guided dosing of warfarin. N Engl J Med. 2013;369(24):2294–303.
78. Drozda K, Wong S, Patel SR, et al. Poor warfarin dose prediction with pharmacogenetic algorithms that exclude genotypes important for African Americans. Pharmacogenet Genomics. 2015;25(2):73–81.
79. Hernandez W, Gamazon ER, Aquino-Michaels K, et al. Ethnicity-specific pharmacogenetics: the case of warfarin in African Americans. Pharmacogenomics J. 2014;14(3):223–8.
80. American College of Cardiology. Genetically guided warfarin dosing lowers risk of some adverse events. 2017. https://www.sciencedaily.com/releases/2017/03/170320091104.htm. Accessed 19 Apr 2017.
81. Eikelboom JW, Connolly SJ, Brueckmann M, et al. Dabigatran versus warfarin in patients with mechanical heart valves. N Engl J Med. 2013;369(13):1206–14.
82. Verhoef TI, Redekop WK, Langenskiold S, et al. Cost-effectiveness of pharmacogenetic-guided dosing of warfarin in the United Kingdom and Sweden. Pharmacogenomics J. 2016;16(5):478–84.
83. Hijazi Z, Oldgren J, Lindback J, et al. The novel biomarker-based ABC (age, biomarkers, clinical history)-bleeding risk score for patients with atrial fibrillation: a derivation and validation study. Lancet. 2016;387(10035):2302–11.
84. Collins R, Reith C, Emberson J, et al. Interpretation of the evidence for the efficacy and safety of statin therapy. Lancet. 2016;388(10059):2532–61.
85. Rosenson RS. Statins: actions, side effects, and administration. 2016. https://www.uptodate.com/contents/statins-actions-side-effects-and-administration. Accessed 11 Nov 2016.
86. Cholesterol Treatment Trialists' (CTT) Collaboration. Efficacy and safety of more intensive lowering of LDL cholesterol: a meta-analysis of data from 170 000 participants in 26 randomised trials. Lancet. 2010;376(9753):1670–81.
87. NICE Guidance. Cardiovascular disease: risk assessment and reduction, including lipid modification. 2014. https://www.nice.org.uk/guidance/cg181/chapter/1-recommendations?unlid=7811231172015112612221 3. Accessed 19 Oct 2016.

88. NHS Choices. NICE publishes new draft guidelines on statins use. 2014. http://www.nhs.uk/news/2014/02February/Pages/NICE-publishes-new-draft-guidelines-on-statins-use.aspx. Accessed 19 Oct 2016.
89. NICE. Wider use of statins could cut deaths from heart disease. 2014. https://www.nice.org.uk/news/article/wider-use-of-statins-could-cut-deaths-from-heart-disease. Accessed 19 Oct 2016.
90. Goldstein JL, Brown MS. The LDL receptor. Arterioscler Thromb Vasc Biol. 2009;29(4):431–8.
91. Moßhammer D, Schaeffeler E, Schwab M, Mörike K. Mechanisms and assessment of statin-related muscular adverse effects. Br J Clin Pharmacol. 2014;78(3):454–66.
92. Diomede L, Albani D, Sottocorno M, et al. In vivo anti-inflammatory effect of statins is mediated by nonsterol mevalonate products. Arterioscler Thromb Vasc Biol. 2001;21(8):1327–32.
93. Kwak BR, Mach F. Statins inhibit leukocyte recruitment: new evidence for their anti-inflammatory properties. Arterioscler Thromb Vasc Biol. 2001;21(8):1256–8.
94. Almog Y. Statins, inflammation, and sepsis: hypothesis. Chest. 2003;124(2):740–3.
95. Tousoulis D, Antoniades C, Bosinakou E, et al. Effects of atorvastatin on reactive hyperemia and inflammatory process in patients with congestive heart failure. Atherosclerosis. 2005;178(2):359–63.
96. Kaesemeyer WH, Caldwell RB, Huang J, Caldwell RW. Pravastatin sodium activates endothelial nitric oxide synthase independent of its cholesterol-lowering actions. J Am Coll Cardiol. 1999;33(1):234–41.
97. Strey CH, Young JM, Molyneux SL, et al. Endothelium-ameliorating effects of statin therapy and coenzyme Q10 reductions in chronic heart failure. Atherosclerosis. 2005;179(1):201–6.
98. Raju SB, Varghese K, Madhu K. Management of statin intolerance. Indian J Endocrinol Metab. 2013;17(6):977–82.
99. Alfirevic A, Neely D, Armitage J, et al. Phenotype standardization for statin-induced myotoxicity. Clin Pharmacol Ther. 2014;96(4):470–6.
100. Kashani A, Phillips CO, Foody JM, et al. Risks associated with statin therapy: a systematic overview of randomized clinical trials. Circulation. 2006;114(25):2788–97.
101. Abd TT, Jacobson TA. Statin-induced myopathy: a review and update. Expert Opin Drug Saf. 2011;10(3):373–87.
102. Godlee F. Statins BMJ. 2014;349. (http://www.w3.org/1999/xhtml">Statins; The BMJ).
103. Furberg CD, Pitt B. Withdrawal of cerivastatin from the world market. Curr Control Trials Cardiovasc Med. 2001;2(5):205–7.
104. Parker BA, Capizzi JA, Grimaldi AS, et al. Effect of statins on skeletal muscle function. Circulation. 2013;127(1):96–103.
105. Taylor BA, Lorson L, White CM, Thompson PD. A randomized trial of coenzyme Q10 in patients with confirmed statin myopathy. Atherosclerosis. 2015;238(2):329–35.
106. Nissen SE, Stroes E, Dent-Acosta RE, et al. Efficacy and tolerability of evolocumab vs. ezetimibe in patients with muscle-related statin intolerance: the GAUSS-3 randomized clinical trial. JAMA. 2016;315(15):1580–90.
107. Ramsey LB, Johnson SG, Caudle KE, et al. The clinical pharmacogenetics implementation consortium guideline for SLCO1B1 and simvastatin-induced myopathy: 2014 update. Clin Pharmacol Ther. 2014;96(4):423–8.
108. McClure DL, Valuck RJ, Glanz M, Murphy JR, Hokanson JE. Statin and statin-fibrate use was significantly associated with increased myositis risk in a managed care population. J Clin Epidemiol. 2007;60(8):812–8.
109. Jacobson TA. Comparative pharmacokinetic interaction profiles of pravastatin, simvastatin, and atorvastatin when coadministered with cytochrome P450 inhibitors. Am J Cardiol. 2004;94(9):1140–6.
110. Neuvonen PJ, Jalava KM. Itraconazole drastically increases plasma concentrations of lovastatin and lovastatin acid. Clin Pharmacol Ther. 1996;60(1):54–61.

111. Mazzu AL, Lasseter KC, Shamblen EC, Agarwal V, Lettieri J, Sundaresen P. Itraconazole alters the pharmacokinetics of atorvastatin to a greater extent than either cerivastatin or pravastatin. Clin Pharmacol Ther. 2000;68(4):391–400.
112. Neuvonen PJ, Niemi M, Backman JT. Drug interactions with lipid-lowering drugs: mechanisms and clinical relevance. Clin Pharmacol Ther. 2006;80(6):565–81.
113. Merck & Co I. Zocor (simvastatin) tablets - highlights of prescribing information. 2015. https://www.merck.com/product/usa/pi_circulars/z/zocor/zocor_pi.pdf. Accessed 7 July 2016.
114. Merck & Co I. Mevacor (lovastatin) tablets description. 2014. https://www.merck.com/product/usa/pi_circulars/m/mevacor/mevacor_pi.pdf Accessed 7 July 2016.
115. Pfizer Inc. LIPITOR- atorvastatin calcium trihydrate tablet, film coated. Highlights of prescribing information. 2015. http://labeling.pfizer.com/ShowLabeling.aspx?id=587. Accessed 7 July 2016.
116. Ando H, Tsuruoka S, Yanagihara H, et al. Effects of grapefruit juice on the pharmacokinetics of pitavastatin and atorvastatin. Br J Clin Pharmacol. 2005;60(5):494–7.
117. Fukazawa I, Uchida N, Uchida E, Yasuhara H. Effects of grapefruit juice on pharmacokinetics of atorvastatin and pravastatin in Japanese. Br J Clin Pharmacol. 2004;57(4):448–55.
118. Rogers JD, Zhao J, Liu L, et al. Grapefruit juice has minimal effects on plasma concentrations of lovastatin-derived 3-hydroxy-3-methylglutaryl coenzyme A reductase inhibitors. Clin Pharmacol Ther. 1999;66(4):358–66.
119. Lilja JJ, Neuvonen M, Neuvonen PJ. Effects of regular consumption of grapefruit juice on the pharmacokinetics of simvastatin. Br J Clin Pharmacol. 2004;58(1):56–60.
120. AstraZeneca. Crestor (rosuvastatin calcium tablets) - highlights of prescribing information. 2010. http://www.accessdata.fda.gov/drugsatfda_docs/label/2010/021366s016lbl.pdf. Accessed 7 July 2016.
121. Novartis. Lescol (fluvastatin dosium)—highlights of prescribing information. 2012. https://www.pharma.us.novartis.com/sites/www.pharma.us.novartis.com/files/Lescol.pdf. Accessed 7 July 2016.
122. Kowa Pharmaceuticals. Livalo (pitavastatin) tablet - highlights of prescribing information. 2012. http://www.accessdata.fda.gov/drugsatfda_docs/label/2012/022363s008s009lbl.pdf . Accessed 7 July 2016.
123. Bristol-Myers Squibb Company. Pravachol (pravastatin) tablets - highlights of prescribing information. 2013. http://packageinserts.bms.com/pi/pi_pravachol.pdf. Accessed 7 July 2016.
124. Wiggins BS, Saseen JJ, Page RL 2nd, et al. Recommendations for management of clinically significant drug-drug interactions with statins and select agents used in patients with cardiovascular disease: a scientific statement from the American Heart Association. Circulation. 2016;134(21):e468–95.
125. Link E, Parish S, Armitage J, et al. SLCO1B1 variants and statin-induced myopathy—a genomewide study. N Engl J Med. 2008;359(8):789–99.
126. Brunham LR, Lansberg PJ, Zhang L, et al. Differential effect of the rs4149056 variant in SLCO1B1 on myopathy associated with simvastatin and atorvastatin. Pharmacogenomics J. 2012;12(3):233–7.
127. Carr DF, O'Meara H, Jorgensen AL, et al. SLCO1B1 genetic variant associated with statin-induced myopathy: a proof-of-concept study using the clinical practice research datalink. Clin Pharmacol Ther. 2013;94(6):695–701.
128. Donnelly LA, Doney AS, Tavendale R, et al. Common nonsynonymous substitutions in SLCO1B1 predispose to statin intolerance in routinely treated individuals with type 2 diabetes: a go-DARTS study. Clin Pharmacol Ther. 2011;89(2):210–6.
129. Voora D, Shah SH, Spasojevic I, et al. The SLCO1B1*5 genetic variant is associated with statin-induced side effects. J Am Coll Cardiol. 2009;54(17):1609–16.
130. Marciante KD, Durda JP, Heckbert SR, et al. Cerivastatin, genetic variants, and the risk of rhabdomyolysis. Pharmacogenet Genomics. 2011;21(5):280–8.

131. Danik JS, Chasman DI, MacFadyen JG, Nyberg F, Barratt BJ, Ridker PM. Lack of association between SLCO1B1 polymorphisms and clinical myalgia following rosuvastatin therapy. Am Heart J. 2013;165(6):1008–14.
132. Puccetti L, Ciani F, Auteri A. Genetic involvement in statins induced myopathy. Preliminary data from an observational case-control study. Atherosclerosis. 2010;211(1):28–9.
133. de Keyser CE, Peters BJ, Becker ML, et al. The SLCO1B1 c.521T>C polymorphism is associated with dose decrease or switching during statin therapy in the Rotterdam Study. Pharmacogenet Genomics. 2014;24(1):43–51.
134. Santos PC, Gagliardi AC, Miname MH, et al. SLCO1B1 haplotypes are not associated with atorvastatin-induced myalgia in Brazilian patients with familial hypercholesterolemia. Eur J Clin Pharmacol. 2012;68(3):273–9.
135. Hubacek JA, Dlouha D, Adamkova V, et al. SLCO1B1 polymorphism is not associated with risk of statin-induced myalgia/myopathy in a Czech population. Med Sci Monit. 2015;21:1454–9.
136. Nies AT, Niemi M, Burk O, et al. Genetics is a major determinant of expression of the human hepatic uptake transporter OATP1B1, but not of OATP1B3 and OATP2B1. Genome Med. 2013;5(1):1.
137. Pasanen MK, Fredrikson H, Neuvonen PJ, Niemi M. Different effects of SLCO1B1 polymorphism on the pharmacokinetics of atorvastatin and rosuvastatin. Clin Pharmacol Ther. 2007;82(6):726–33.
138. Niemi M, Pasanen MK, Neuvonen PJ. SLCO1B1 polymorphism and sex affect the pharmacokinetics of pravastatin but not fluvastatin. Clin Pharmacol Ther. 2006;80(4):356–66.
139. Tornio A, Vakkilainen J, Neuvonen M, Backman JT, Neuvonen PJ, Niemi M. SLCO1B1 polymorphism markedly affects the pharmacokinetics of lovastatin acid. Pharmacogenet Genomics. 2015;25(8):382–7.
140. Ieiri I, Suwannakul S, Maeda K, et al. SLCO1B1 (OATP1B1, an uptake transporter) and ABCG2 (BCRP, an efflux transporter) variant alleles and pharmacokinetics of pitavastatin in healthy volunteers. Clin Pharmacol Ther. 2007;82(5):541–7.
141. Pasanen MK, Neuvonen M, Neuvonen PJ, Niemi M. SLCO1B1 polymorphism markedly affects the pharmacokinetics of simvastatin acid. Pharmacogenet Genomics. 2006;16(12):873–9.
142. Skottheim IB, Gedde-Dahl A, Hejazifar S, Hoel K, Asberg A. Statin induced myotoxicity: the lactone forms are more potent than the acid forms in human skeletal muscle cells in vitro. Eur J Pharm Sci. 2008;33(4–5):317–25.
143. Schirris TJ, Renkema GH, Ritschel T, et al. Statin-induced myopathy is associated with mitochondrial complex III inhibition. Cell Metab. 2015;22(3):399–407.
144. Skottheim IB, Bogsrud MP, Hermann M, Retterstol K, Asberg A. Atorvastatin metabolite measurements as a diagnostic tool for statin-induced myopathy. Mol Diagn Ther. 2011;15(4):221–7.
145. Hermann M, Bogsrud MP, Molden E, et al. Exposure of atorvastatin is unchanged but lactone and acid metabolites are increased several-fold in patients with atorvastatin-induced myopathy. Clin Pharmacol Ther. 2006;79(6):532–9.
146. Generaux GT, Bonomo FM, Johnson M, Doan KM. Impact of SLCO1B1 (OATP1B1) and ABCG2 (BCRP) genetic polymorphisms and inhibition on LDL-C lowering and myopathy of statins. Xenobiotica. 2011;41(8):639–51.
147. He YJ, Zhang W, Chen Y, et al. Rifampicin alters atorvastatin plasma concentration on the basis of SLCO1B1 521T>C polymorphism. Clin Chim Acta. 2009;405(1–2):49–52.
148. Medicines and Healthcare products Regulatory Agency (MHRA). Simvastatin: updated advice on drug interactions. 2012. https://www.gov.uk/drug-safety-update/simvastatin-updated-advice-on-drug-interactions. Accessed 10 Nov 2016.
149. Gallagher RM, Kirkham JJ, Mason JR, et al. Development and inter-rater reliability of the Liverpool adverse drug reaction causality assessment tool. PLoS One. 2011;6(12):e28096.

150. Needham M, Fabian V, Knezevic W, Panegyres P, Zilko P, Mastaglia FL. Progressive myopathy with up-regulation of MHC-I associated with statin therapy. Neuromuscul Disord. 2007;17(2):194–200.
151. Grable-Esposito P, Katzberg HD, Greenberg SA, Srinivasan J, Katz J, Amato AA. Immune-mediated necrotizing myopathy associated with statins. Muscle Nerve. 2010;41(2):185–90.
152. Christopher-Stine L, Casciola-Rosen LA, Hong G, Chung T, Corse AM, Mammen AL. A novel autoantibody recognizing 200-kd and 100-kd proteins is associated with an immune-mediated necrotizing myopathy. Arthritis Rheum. 2010;62(9):2757–66.
153. Mammen AL, Chung T, Christopher-Stine L, Rosen P, Rosen A, Casciola-Rosen LA. Autoantibodies against 3-hydroxy-3-methylglutaryl-coenzyme a reductase (HMGCR) in patients with statin-associated autoimmune myopathy. Arthritis Rheum. 2011;63(3):713–21.
154. Mammen AL. Statin-associated autoimmune myopathy. N Engl J Med. 2016;374(7):664–9.
155. Limaye V, Bundell C, Hollingsworth P, et al. Clinical and genetic associations of autoantibodies to 3-hydroxy-3-methyl-glutaryl-coenzyme a reductase in patients with immune-mediated myositis and necrotizing myopathy. Muscle Nerve. 2015;52(2):196–203.
156. Mammen AL, Gaudet D, Brisson D, et al. Increased frequency of DRB1*11:01 in anti-hydroxymethylglutaryl-coenzyme A reductase-associated autoimmune myopathy. Arthritis Care Res. 2012;64(8):1233–7.
157. Elsby R, Hilgendorf C, Fenner K. Understanding the critical disposition pathways of statins to assess drug-drug interaction risk during drug development: it's not just about OATP1B1. Clin Pharmacol Ther. 2012;92(5):584–98.
158. Kitzmiller JP, Luzum JA, Baldassarre D, Krauss RM, Medina MW. CYP3A4*22 and CYP3A5*3 are associated with increased levels of plasma simvastatin concentrations in the cholesterol and pharmacogenetics study cohort. Pharmacogenet Genomics. 2014;24(10):486–91.
159. Klein K, Thomas M, Winter S, et al. PPARA: a novel genetic determinant of CYP3A4 in vitro and in vivo. Clin Pharmacol Ther. 2012;91(6):1044–52.
160. Riedmaier S, Klein K, Hofmann U, et al. UDP-glucuronosyltransferase (UGT) polymorphisms affect atorvastatin lactonization in vitro and in vivo. Clin Pharmacol Ther. 2010;87(1):65–73.
161. Cho SK, Oh ES, Park K, Park MS, Chung JY. The UGT1A3*2 polymorphism affects atorvastatin lactonization and lipid-lowering effect in healthy volunteers. Pharmacogenet Genomics. 2012;22(8):598–605.
162. Keskitalo JE, Kurkinen KJ, Neuvoneni PJ, Niemi M. ABCB1 haplotypes differentially affect the pharmacokinetics of the acid and lactone forms of simvastatin and atorvastatin. Clin Pharmacol Ther. 2008;84(4):457–61.
163. Ferrari M, Guasti L, Maresca A, et al. Association between statin-induced creatine kinase elevation and genetic polymorphisms in SLCO1B1, ABCB1 and ABCG2. Eur J Clin Pharmacol. 2014;70(5):539–47.
164. Fiegenbaum M, da Silveira FR, Van der Sand CR, et al. The role of common variants of ABCB1, CYP3A4, and CYP3A5 genes in lipid-lowering efficacy and safety of simvastatin treatment. Clin Pharmacol Ther. 2005;78(5):551–8.
165. Hoenig MR, Walker PJ, Gurnsey C, Beadle K, Johnson L. The C3435T polymorphism in ABCB1 influences atorvastatin efficacy and muscle symptoms in a high-risk vascular cohort. J Clin Lipidol. 2011;5(2):91–6.
166. Becker ML, Visser LE, van Schaik RH, Hofman A, Uitterlinden AG, Stricker BH. Influence of genetic variation in CYP3A4 and ABCB1 on dose decrease or switching during simvastatin and atorvastatin therapy. Pharmacoepidemiol Drug Saf. 2010;19(1):75–81.
167. Vladutiu GD, Simmons Z, Isackson PJ, et al. Genetic risk factors associated with lipid-lowering drug-induced myopathies. Muscle Nerve. 2006;34(2):153–62.
168. Hur J, Liu Z, Tong W, Laaksonen R, Bai JP. Drug-induced rhabdomyolysis: from systems pharmacology analysis to biochemical flux. Chem Res Toxicol. 2014;27(3):421–32.
169. Robinson R, Carpenter D, Shaw MA, Halsall J, Hopkins P. Mutations in RYR1 in malignant hyperthermia and central core disease. Hum Mutat. 2006;27(10):977–89.

170. Vladutiu GD, Isackson PJ, Kaufman K, et al. Genetic risk for malignant hyperthermia in non-anesthesia-induced myopathies. Mol Genet Metab. 2011;104(1–2):167–73.
171. Laitinen PJ, Brown KM, Piippo K, et al. Mutations of the cardiac ryanodine receptor (RyR2) gene in familial polymorphic ventricular tachycardia. Circulation. 2001;103(4):485–90.
172. Deichmann R, Lavie C, Andrews S. Coenzyme Q10 and statin-induced mitochondrial dysfunction. Ochsner J. 2010;10(1):16–21.
173. Quinzii CM, Hirano M. Primary and secondary CoQ(10) deficiencies in humans. Biofactors. 2011;37(5):361–5.
174. Montini G, Malaventura C, Salviati L. Early coenzyme Q10 supplementation in primary coenzyme Q10 deficiency. N Engl J Med. 2008;358(26):2849–50.
175. Oh J, Ban MR, Miskie BA, Pollex RL, Hegele RA. Genetic determinants of statin intolerance. Lipids Health Dis. 2007;6:7.
176. Banach M, Serban C, Sahebkar A, et al. Effects of coenzyme Q10 on statin-induced myopathy: a meta-analysis of randomized controlled trials. Mayo Clin Proc. 2015;90(1):24–34.
177. Verschuren JJ, Trompet S, Wessels JA, et al. A systematic review on pharmacogenetics in cardiovascular disease: is it ready for clinical application? Eur Heart J. 2012;33(2):165–75.
178. Postmus I, Trompet S, Deshmukh HA, et al. Pharmacogenetic meta-analysis of genome-wide association studies of LDL cholesterol response to statins. Nat Commun. 2014;5:5068.
179. Phillips MC. Apolipoprotein E isoforms and lipoprotein metabolism. IUBMB Life. 2014;66(9):616–23.
180. Deshmukh HA, Colhoun HM, Johnson T, et al. Genome-wide association study of genetic determinants of LDL-c response to atorvastatin therapy: importance of Lp(a). J Lipid Res. 2012;53(5):1000–11.
181. Thompson JF, Hyde CL, Wood LS, et al. Comprehensive whole-genome and candidate gene analysis for response to statin therapy in the Treating to New Targets (TNT) cohort. Circ Cardiovasc Genet. 2009;2(2):173–81.
182. Marcovina SM, Koschinsky ML, Albers JJ, Skarlatos S. Report of the national heart, lung, and blood institute workshop on lipoprotein(a) and cardiovascular disease: recent advances and future directions. Clin Chem. 2003;49(11):1785–96.
183. Lanktree MB, Anand SS, Yusuf S, Hegele RA. Comprehensive analysis of genomic variation in the LPA locus and its relationship to plasma lipoprotein(a) in South Asians, Chinese, and European Caucasians. Circ Cardiovasc Genet. 2010;3(1):39–46.
184. Rose RH, Neuhoff S, Abduljalil K, Chetty M, Rostami-Hodjegan A, Jamei M. Application of a physiologically based pharmacokinetic model to predict OATP1B1-related variability in pharmacodynamics of rosuvastatin. CPT Pharmacometrics Syst Pharmacol. 2014;3:e124.
185. Musunuru K, Strong A, Frank-Kamenetsky M, et al. From noncoding variant to phenotype via SORT1 at the 1p13 cholesterol locus. Nature. 2010;466(7307):714–9.
186. Kamal-Bahl SJ, Burke T, Watson D, Wentworth C. Discontinuation of lipid modifying drugs among commercially insured United States patients in recent clinical practice. Am J Cardiol. 2007;99(4):530–4.
187. Rasmussen JN, Chong A, Alter DA. Relationship between adherence to evidence-based pharmacotherapy and long-term mortality after acute myocardial infarction. JAMA. 2007;297(2):177–86.
188. Wei MY, Ito MK, Cohen JD, Brinton EA, Jacobson TA. Predictors of statin adherence, switching, and discontinuation in the USAGE survey: understanding the use of statins in America and gaps in patient education. J Clin Lipidol. 2013;7(5):472–83.
189. De Vera MA, Bhole V, Burns LC, Lacaille D. Impact of statin adherence on cardiovascular disease and mortality outcomes: a systematic review. Br J Clin Pharmacol. 2014;78(4):684–98.
190. Food and Drug Administration. FDA: limit use of 80 mg Simvastatin. 2011. http://www.fda.gov/ForConsumers/ConsumerUpdates/ucm257884.htm. Accessed 28 Oct 2016.
191. Collins GS, Altman DG. Predicting the adverse risk of statin treatment: an independent and external validation of Qstatin risk scores in the UK. Heart. 2012;98(14):1091–7.
192. Stewart A. SLCO1B1 polymorphisms and statin-induced myopathy. PLoS Curr. 2013;5. https://doi.org/10.1371/currents.eogt.d21e7f0c58463571bb0d9d3a19b82203 PMCI.

193. Zhu HJ, Wang X, Gawronski BE, Brinda BJ, Angiolillo DJ, Markowitz JS. Carboxylesterase 1 as a determinant of clopidogrel metabolism and activation. J Pharmacol Exp Ther. 2013;344(3):665–72.
194. Mehta SR, Yusuf S, Peters RJ, et al. Effects of pretreatment with clopidogrel and aspirin followed by long-term therapy in patients undergoing percutaneous coronary intervention: the PCI-CURE study. Lancet. 2001;358(9281):527–33.
195. Matetzky S, Shenkman B, Guetta V, et al. Clopidogrel resistance is associated with increased risk of recurrent atherothrombotic events in patients with acute myocardial infarction. Circulation. 2004;109(25):3171–5.
196. Garabedian T, Alam S. High residual platelet reactivity on clopidogrel: its significance and therapeutic challenges overcoming clopidogrel resistance. Cardiovasc Diagn Ther. 2013;3(1):23–37.
197. Spiliopoulos S, Pastromas G. Current status of high on-treatment platelet reactivity in patients with coronary or peripheral arterial disease: Mechanisms, evaluation and clinical implications. World J Cardiol. 2015;7(12):912–21.
198. Trenk D, Hochholzer W. Genetics of platelet inhibitor treatment. Br J Clin Pharmacol. 2014;77(4):642–53.
199. Aradi D, Storey RF, Komocsi A, et al. Expert position paper on the role of platelet function testing in patients undergoing percutaneous coronary intervention. Eur Heart J. 2014;35(4):209–15.
200. Scott SA, Sangkuhl K, Stein CM, et al. Clinical Pharmacogenetics Implementation Consortium guidelines for CYP2C19 genotype and clopidogrel therapy: 2013 update. Clin Pharmacol Ther. 2013;94(3):317–23.
201. The Human Cytochrome P450 (CYP) Allele Nomenclature Committee. The Human Cytochrome P450 (CYP) Allele Nomenclature Database - CYP2C19 allele nomenclature. 2015. http://www.cypalleles.ki.se/cyp2c19.htm. Accessed 01 Nov 2016.
202. Diaz-Villamarin X, Davila-Fajardo CL, Martinez-Gonzalez LJ, et al. Genetic polymorphisms influence on the response to clopidogrel in peripheral artery disease patients following percutaneous transluminal angioplasty. Pharmacogenomics. 2016;17(12):1327–38.
203. Guo B, Tan Q, Guo D, Shi Z, Zhang C, Guo W. Patients carrying CYP2C19 loss of function alleles have a reduced response to clopidogrel therapy and a greater risk of in-stent restenosis after endovascular treatment of lower extremity peripheral arterial disease. J Vasc Surg. 2014;60(4):993–1001.
204. McDonough CW, McClure LA, Mitchell BD, et al. CYP2C19 metabolizer status and clopidogrel efficacy in the Secondary Prevention of Small Subcortical Strokes (SPS3) study. J Am Heart Assoc. 2015;4(6):e001652.
205. Sun W, Li Y, Li J, et al. Variant recurrent risk among stroke patients with different CYP2C19 phenotypes and treated with clopidogrel. Platelets. 2015;26(6):558–62.
206. Wang Y, Zhao X, Lin J, et al. Association between CYP2C19 loss-of-function allele status and efficacy of clopidogrel for risk reduction among patients with minor stroke or transient ischemic attack. JAMA. 2016;316(1):70–8.
207. Hoh BL, Gong Y, McDonough CW, et al. CYP2C19 and CES1 polymorphisms and efficacy of clopidogrel and aspirin dual antiplatelet therapy in patients with symptomatic intracranial atherosclerotic disease. J Neurosurg. 2016;124(6):1746–51.
208. Osnabrugge RL, Head SJ, Zijlstra F, et al. A systematic review and critical assessment of 11 discordant meta-analyses on reduced-function CYP2C19 genotype and risk of adverse clinical outcomes in clopidogrel users. Genet Med. 2015;17(1):3–11.
209. Mega JL, Simon T, Collet JP, et al. Reduced-function CYP2C19 genotype and risk of adverse clinical outcomes among patients treated with clopidogrel predominantly for PCI: a meta-analysis. JAMA. 2010;304(16):1821–30.
210. Cavallari LH, Duarte JD. Clopidogrel pharmacogenetics: from evidence to implementation. Futur Cardiol. 2016;12(5):511–4.
211. Lewis JP, Horenstein RB, Ryan K, et al. The functional G143E variant of carboxylesterase 1 is associated with increased clopidogrel active metabolite levels and greater clopidogrel response. Pharmacogenet Genomics. 2013;23(1):1–8.

212. Taubert D, von Beckerath N, Grimberg G, et al. Impact of P-glycoprotein on clopidogrel absorption. Clin Pharmacol Ther. 2006;80(5):486–501.
213. Stokanovic D, Nikolic VN, Konstantinovic SS, et al. P-glycoprotein polymorphism C3435T is associated with dose-adjusted clopidogrel and 2-Oxo-clopidogrel concentration. Pharmacology. 2016;97(3–4):101–6.
214. Su J, Xu J, Li X, et al. ABCB1 C3435T polymorphism and response to clopidogrel treatment in coronary artery disease (CAD) patients: a meta-analysis. PLoS One. 2012;7(10):e46366.
215. Yang Y, Lewis JP, Hulot J-S, Scott SA. The pharmacogenetic control of antiplatelet response: candidate genes and CYP2C19. Expert Opin Drug Metab Toxicol. 2015;11(10):1599–617.
216. Ferri N, Corsini A, Bellosta S. Pharmacology of the new P2Y12 receptor inhibitors: insights on pharmacokinetic and pharmacodynamic properties. Drugs. 2013;73(15):1681–709.
217. Grosdidier C, Quilici J, Loosveld M, et al. Effect of CYP2C19*2 and *17 genetic variants on platelet response to clopidogrel and prasugrel maintenance dose and relation to bleeding complications. Am J Cardiol. 2013;111(7):985–90.
218. Mega JL, Close SL, Wiviott SD, et al. Cytochrome P450 genetic polymorphisms and the response to prasugrel: relationship to pharmacokinetic, pharmacodynamic, and clinical outcomes. Circulation. 2009;119(19):2553–60.
219. Mega JL, Close SL, Wiviott SD, et al. Genetic variants in ABCB1, CYP2C19, and cardiovascular outcomes following treatment with clopidogrel and prasugrel. Lancet. 2010;376(9749):1312–9.
220. Mega JL, Close SL, Wiviott SD, et al. PON1 Q192R genetic variant and response to clopidogrel and prasugrel: pharmacokinetics, pharmacodynamics, and a meta-analysis of clinical outcomes. J Thromb Thrombolysis. 2016;41(3):374–83.
221. Cuisset T, Loosveld M, Morange PE, et al. CYP2C19*2 and *17 alleles have a significant impact on platelet response and bleeding risk in patients treated with prasugrel after acute coronary syndrome. JACC Cardiovasc Interv. 2012;5(12):1280–7.
222. Teng R. Ticagrelor: Pharmacokinetic, Pharmacodynamic and Pharmacogenetic Profile: An Update. Clin Pharmacokinet. 2015;54(11):1125–38.
223. Varenhorst C, Eriksson N, Johansson A, et al. Effect of genetic variations on ticagrelor plasma levels and clinical outcomes. Eur Heart J. 2015;36(29):1901–12.
224. Wallentin L, James S, Storey RF, et al. Effect of CYP2C19 and ABCB1 single nucleotide polymorphisms on outcomes of treatment with ticagrelor versus clopidogrel for acute coronary syndromes: a genetic substudy of the PLATO trial. Lancet. 2010;376(9749):1320–8.
225. Sorich MJ, Vitry A, Ward MB, Horowitz JD, McKinnon RA. Prasugrel vs. clopidogrel for cytochrome P450 2C19-genotyped subgroups: integration of the TRITON-TIMI 38 trial data. J Thromb Haemost. 2010;8(8):1678–84.
226. Holmes DR Jr, Dehmer GJ, Kaul S, Leifer D, O'Gara PT, Stein CM. ACCF/AHA clopidogrel clinical alert: approaches to the FDA "boxed warning": a report of the American College of Cardiology Foundation Task Force on clinical expert consensus documents and the American Heart Association endorsed by the Society for Cardiovascular Angiography and Interventions and the Society of Thoracic Surgeons. J Am Coll Cardiol. 2010;56(4):321–41.
227. Levine GN, Bates ER, Blankenship JC, et al. 2011 ACCF/AHA/SCAI Guideline for Percutaneous Coronary Intervention: A Report of the American College of Cardiology Foundation/American Heart Association Task Force on Practice Guidelines and the Society for Cardiovascular Angiography and Interventions. J Am Coll Cardiol. 2011;58(24):e44–e122.
228. Mayo Clinic. Tailored antiplatelet therapy following PCI (TAILOR-PCI). 2012. https://clinicaltrials.gov/ct2/show/NCT01742117. Accessed 9 Nov 2016.
229. Saab YB, Zeenny R, Ramadan WH. Optimizing clopidogrel dose response: a new clinical algorithm comprising CYP2C19 pharmacogenetics and drug interactions. Ther Clin Risk Manag. 2015;11:1421–7.
230. Cooper-DeHoff RM, Johnson JA. Hypertension pharmacogenomics: in search of personalized treatment approaches. Nat Rev Nephrol. 2016;12(2):110–22.
231. Egan BM, Zhao Y, Axon RN. US trends in prevalence, awareness, treatment, and control of hypertension, 1988-2008. JAMA. 2010;303(20):2043–50.

232. National Institute for Health and Care Excellence (NICE). Hypertension in adults: diagnosis and management. 2011. https://www.nice.org.uk/guidance/cg127/chapter/1-Guidance#choosing-antihypertensive-drug-treatment-2. Accessed 9 Nov 2016.
233. Johnson JA, Zineh I, Puckett BJ, McGorray SP, Yarandi HN, Pauly DF. Beta 1-adrenergic receptor polymorphisms and antihypertensive response to metoprolol. Clin Pharmacol Ther. 2003;74(1):44–52.
234. Si D, Wang J, Xu Y, Chen X, Zhang M, Zhou H. Association of common polymorphisms in beta1-adrenergic receptor with antihypertensive response to carvedilol. J Cardiovasc Pharmacol. 2014;64(4):306–9.
235. Wu D, Li G, Deng M, et al. Associations between ADRB1 and CYP2D6 gene polymorphisms and the response to beta-blocker therapy in hypertension. J Int Med Res. 2015;43(3): 424–34.
236. Liu J, Liu ZQ, Yu BN, et al. beta1-Adrenergic receptor polymorphisms influence the response to metoprolol monotherapy in patients with essential hypertension. Clin Pharmacol Ther. 2006;80(1):23–32.
237. O'Shaughnessy MV, Fu B, Dickerson C, Thurston D, Brown MJ. The gain-of-function G389R variant of the β1-adrenoceptor does not influence blood pressure or heart rate response to β-blockade in hypertensive subjects. Clin Sci. 2000;99:233–8.
238. Pacanowski MA, Gong Y, Cooper-Dehoff RM, et al. beta-adrenergic receptor gene polymorphisms and beta-blocker treatment outcomes in hypertension. Clin Pharmacol Ther. 2008;84(6):715–21.
239. O'Connor CM, Fiuzat M, Carson PE, et al. Combinatorial pharmacogenetic interactions of bucindolol and beta1, alpha2C adrenergic receptor polymorphisms. PLoS One. 2012;7(10):e44324.
240. Johnson JA. Advancing management of hypertension through pharmacogenomics. Ann Med. 2012;44(0 1):S17–22.
241. Zhang F, Steinberg SF. S49G and R389G polymorphisms of the beta(1)-adrenergic receptor influence signaling via the cAMP-PKA and ERK pathways. Physiol Genomics. 2013;45(23):1186–92.
242. Johnson AD, Newton-Cheh C, Chasman DI, et al. Association of hypertension drug target genes with blood pressure and hypertension in 86,588 individuals. Hypertension. 2011;57(5):903–10.
243. Vandell AG, Lobmeyer MT, Gawronski BE, et al. G protein receptor kinase 4 polymorphisms: beta-blocker pharmacogenetics and treatment-related outcomes in hypertension. Hypertension. 2012;60(4):957–64.
244. Bhatnagar V, O'Connor DT, Brophy VH, et al. G-protein-coupled receptor kinase 4 polymorphisms and blood pressure response to metoprolol among African Americans: sex-specificity and interactions. Am J Hypertens. 2009;22(3):332–8.
245. Felder RA, Jose PA. Mechanisms of disease: the role of GRK4 in the etiology of essential hypertension and salt sensitivity. Nat Clin Pract Nephrol. 2006;2(11):637–50.
246. Muskalla AM, Suter PM, Saur M, Nowak A, Hersberger M, Krayenbuehl PA. G-protein receptor kinase 4 polymorphism and response to antihypertensive therapy. Clin Chem. 2014;60(12):1543–8.
247. Bijl MJ, Visser LE, van Schaik RH, et al. Genetic variation in the CYP2D6 gene is associated with a lower heart rate and blood pressure in beta-blocker users. Clin Pharmacol Ther. 2009;85(1):45–50.
248. Ma MK, Woo MH, Mcleod HL. Genetic basis of drug metabolism. 2009. http://www.medscape.com/viewarticle/444804_5. Accessed 8 Nov 2016.
249. Sharp CF, Gardiner SJ, Jensen BP, et al. CYP2D6 genotype and its relationship with metoprolol dose, concentrations and effect in patients with systolic heart failure. Pharmacogenomics J. 2009;9(3):175–84.
250. Wuttke H, Rau T, Heide R, et al. Increased frequency of cytochrome P450 2D6 poor metabolizers among patients with metoprolol-associated adverse effects. Clin Pharmacol Ther. 2002;72(4):429–37.

251. Zineh I, Beitelshees AL, Gaedigk A, et al. Pharmacokinetics and CYP2D6 genotypes do not predict metoprolol adverse events or efficacy in hypertension. Clin Pharmacol Ther. 2004;76(6):536–44.
252. Novartis Pharmaceuticals Corporation. LOPRESSOR (metoprolol tartrate) tablet prescribing information. 2008. https://www.accessdata.fda.gov/drugsatfda_docs/label/2008/017963s062,018704s021lbl.pdf. Accessed 9 Nov 2016.
253. Hiltunen TP, Donner KM, Sarin AP, et al. Pharmacogenomics of hypertension: a genome-wide, placebo-controlled cross-over study, using four classes of antihypertensive drugs. J Am Heart Assoc. 2015;4(1):e001521.
254. Price ET, Pacanowski MA, Martin MA, et al. LIVER X receptor alpha gene polymorphisms and variable cardiovascular outcomes in patients treated with antihypertensive therapy: results from the invest-genes study. Pharmacogenet Genomics. 2011;21(6):333–40.
255. McDonough CW, Gong Y, Padmanabhan S, et al. Pharmacogenomic association of nonsynonymous SNPs in SIGLEC12, A1BG, and the selectin region and cardiovascular outcomes. Hypertension. 2013;62(1):48–54.
256. Fontana V, Luizon MR, Sandrim VC. An update on the pharmacogenetics of treating hypertension. J Hum Hypertens. 2015;29(5):283–91.
257. Darbar D. The role of pharmacogenetics in atrial fibrillation therapeutics: is personalized therapy in sight? J Cardiovasc Pharmacol. 2016;67(1):9–18.
258. Wyse DG, Waldo AL, DiMarco JP, et al. A comparison of rate control and rhythm control in patients with atrial fibrillation. N Engl J Med. 2002;347(23):1825–33.
259. Corley SD, Epstein AE, DiMarco JP, et al. Relationships between sinus rhythm, treatment, and survival in the Atrial Fibrillation Follow-Up Investigation of Rhythm Management (AFFIRM) Study. Circulation. 2004;109(12):1509–13.
260. Parvez B, Vaglio J, Rowan S, et al. Symptomatic response to antiarrhythmic drug therapy is modulated by a common single nucleotide polymorphism in atrial fibrillation. J Am Coll Cardiol. 2012;60(6):539–45.
261. Parvez B, Shoemaker MB, Muhammad R, et al. Common genetic polymorphism at 4q25 locus predicts atrial fibrillation recurrence after successful cardioversion. Heart Rhythm. 2013;10(6):849–55.
262. Husser D, Adams V, Piorkowski C, Hindricks G, Bollmann A. Chromosome 4q25 variants and atrial fibrillation recurrence after catheter ablation. J Am Coll Cardiol. 2010;55(8):747–53.
263. Shoemaker MB, Muhammad R, Parvez B, et al. Common atrial fibrillation risk alleles at 4q25 predict recurrence after catheter-based atrial fibrillation ablation. Heart Rhythm. 2013;10(3):394–400.
264. Aguirre LA, Alonso ME, Badía-Careaga C, et al. Long-range regulatory interactions at the 4q25 atrial fibrillation risk locus involve PITX2c and ENPEP. BMC Biol. 2015;13:26.
265. Mommersteeg MT, Brown NA, Prall OW, et al. Pitx2c and Nkx2-5 are required for the formation and identity of the pulmonary myocardium. Circ Res. 2007;101(9):902–9.
266. Zhao C-M, Peng L-Y, Li L, et al. PITX2 loss-of-function mutation contributes to congenital endocardial cushion defect and Axenfeld-Rieger syndrome. PLoS One. 2015;10(4):e0124409.
267. Sun YM, Wang J, Qiu XB, et al. PITX2 loss-of-function mutation contributes to tetralogy of Fallot. Gene. 2016;577(2):258–64.
268. Roden DM. Predicting drug-induced QT prolongation and torsades de pointes. J Physiol. 2016;594(9):2459–68.
269. Roden DM. Long QT syndrome: reduced repolarization reserve and the genetic link. J Intern Med. 2006;259(1):59–69.
270. Behr ER, Roden D. Drug-induced arrhythmia: pharmacogenomic prescribing? Eur Heart J. 2013;34(2):89–95.
271. Donger C, Denjoy I, Berthet M, et al. KVLQT1 C-terminal missense mutation causes a forme fruste long-QT syndrome. Circulation. 1997;96(9):2778–81.
272. Roden DM. Taking the "idio" out of "idiosyncratic": predicting torsades de pointes. Pacing Clin Electrophysiol. 1998;21(5):1029–34.

273. Kaab S, Crawford DC, Sinner MF, et al. A large candidate gene survey identifies the KCNE1 D85N polymorphism as a possible modulator of drug-induced torsades de pointes. Circ Cardiovasc Genet. 2012;5(1):91–9.
274. Abbott GW. KCNE genetics and pharmacogenomics in cardiac arrhythmias: much ado about nothing? Expert Rev Clin Pharmacol. 2013;6(1):49–60.
275. Arking DE, Pulit SL, Crotti L, et al. Genetic association study of QT interval highlights role for calcium signaling pathways in myocardial repolarization. Nat Genet. 2014;46(8):826–36.
276. Jamshidi Y, Nolte IM, Dalageorgou C, et al. Common variation in the NOS1AP gene is associated with drug-induced QT prolongation and ventricular arrhythmia. J Am Coll Cardiol. 2012;60(9):841–50.
277. Behr ER, Ritchie MD, Tanaka T, et al. Genome wide analysis of drug-induced torsades de pointes: lack of common variants with large effect sizes. PLoS One. 2013;8(11):e78511.
278. Ramirez AH, Shaffer CM, Delaney JT, et al. Novel rare variants in congenital cardiac arrhythmia genes are frequent in drug-induced torsades de pointes. Pharmacogenomics J. 2013;13(4):325–9.
279. Weeke P, Mosley JD, Hanna D, et al. Exome sequencing implicates an increased burden of rare potassium channel variants in the risk of drug-induced long QT interval syndrome. J Am Coll Cardiol. 2014;63(14):1430–7.
280. Splawski I, Timothy KW, Tateyama M, et al. Variant of SCN5A sodium channel implicated in risk of cardiac arrhythmia. Science (New York, NY). 2002;297(5585):1333–6.
281. Tisdale JE, Jaynes HA, Kingery JR, et al. Effectiveness of a clinical decision support system for reducing the risk of QT interval prolongation in hospitalized patients. Circ Cardiovasc Qual Outcomes. 2014;7(3):381–90.
282. Sorita A, Bos JM, Morlan BW, Tarrell RF, Ackerman MJ, Caraballo PJ. Impact of clinical decision support preventing the use of QT-prolonging medications for patients at risk for torsade de pointes. J Am Med Inform Assoc. 2015;22(e1):e21–7.
283. Lee JK, Wu CK, Tsai CT, et al. Genetic variation-optimized treatment benefit of angiotensin-converting enzyme inhibitors in patients with stable coronary artery disease: a 12-year follow-up study. Pharmacogenet Genomics. 2013;23(4):181–9.
284. Brugts JJ, Isaacs A, Boersma E, et al. Genetic determinants of treatment benefit of the angiotensin-converting enzyme-inhibitor perindopril in patients with stable coronary artery disease. Eur Heart J. 2010;31(15):1854–64.
285. Oemrawsingh RM, Akkerhuis KM, Van Vark LC, et al. Individualized angiotensin-converting enzyme (ACE)-inhibitor therapy in stable coronary artery disease based on clinical and pharmacogenetic determinants: The PERindopril GENEtic (PERGENE) risk model. J Am Heart Assoc. 2016;5(3):e002688.
286. Mahmoudpour SH, Leusink M, van der Putten L, et al. Pharmacogenetics of ACE inhibitor-induced angioedema and cough: a systematic review and meta-analysis. Pharmacogenomics. 2013;14(3):249–60.
287. Pare G, Kubo M, Byrd JB, et al. Genetic variants associated with angiotensin-converting enzyme inhibitor-associated angioedema. Pharmacogenet Genomics. 2013;23(9):470–8.
288. Do EJ, Lenzini P, Eby CS, et al. Genetics informatics trial (GIFT) of warfarin to prevent deep vein thrombosis (DVT): rationale and study design. Pharmacogenomics J. 2012;12(5):417–24.
289. Dunnenberger HM, Crews KR, Hoffman JM, et al. Preemptive clinical pharmacogenetics implementation: current programs in five US medical centers. Annu Rev Pharmacol Toxicol. 2015;55:89–106.
290. Relling MV, Evans WE. Pharmacogenomics in the clinic. Nature. 2015;526(7573):343–50.
291. Haiser HJ, Seim KL, Balskus EP, Turnbaugh PJ. Mechanistic insight into digoxin inactivation by Eggerthella lenta augments our understanding of its pharmacokinetics. Gut Microbes. 2014;5(2):233–8.
292. Tang WH, Wang Z, Levison BS, et al. Intestinal microbial metabolism of phosphatidylcholine and cardiovascular risk. N Engl J Med. 2013;368(17):1575–84.
293. ClinicalTrials.gov. Genetically targeted therapy for the prevention of symptomatic atrial fibrillation in patients with heart failure (GENETIC-AF). ARCA Biopharma, Inc. 2014.

https://www.clinicaltrials.gov/ct2/show/study/NCT01970501?term=bucindolol&rank=1. Accessed 27 Jan 2015.

294. Mitchell C, Gregersen N, Krause A. Novel CYP2C9 and VKORC1 gene variants associated with warfarin dosage variability in the South African black population. Pharmacogenomics. 2011;12(7):953–63.
295. Nagai R, Ohara M, Cavallari LH, et al. Factors influencing pharmacokinetics of warfarin in African-Americans: implications for pharmacogenetic dosing algorithms. Pharmacogenomics. 2015;16(3):217–25.
296. Mangravite LM, Engelhardt BE, Medina MW, et al. A statin-dependent QTL for GATM expression is associated with statin-induced myopathy. Nature. 2013;502(7471):377–80.
297. Li Y, Tang HL, Hu YF, Xie HG. The gain-of-function variant allele CYP2C19*17: a double-edged sword between thrombosis and bleeding in clopidogrel-treated patients. J Thromb Haemost. 2012;10(2):199–206.

Congenital Cardiovascular Disorders

6

Dirk G. Wilson

Abstract
Congenital heart disease (CHD) is defined as an abnormality of cardiovascular development leading to structural and/or functional problems that can affect the individual at any stage from fetal to adult life. It also encompasses abnormalities encountered in postnatal adaptation, such as persistence of the ductus arteriosus. Cardiovascular abnormalities, as a group, are the most common cause of congenital anomaly and account for around 1% of live births.

Keywords
Congenital heart disease • Genetic testing • Fluorescent in-situ hybridisation
Array comparative genomic hybridisation • Genetic assessment

6.1 Introduction

Congenital heart disease (CHD) is defined as an abnormality of cardiovascular development leading to structural and/or functional problems that can affect the individual at any stage from fetal to adult life. It also encompasses abnormalities encountered in postnatal adaptation, such as persistence of the ductus arteriosus. Cardiovascular abnormalities, as a group, are the most common cause of congenital anomaly and account for around 1% of live births [1, 2]. If bicuspid aortic valve is included as a CHD condition the incidence rises to around 2% [3]. CHD in its most severe forms has a significant disease burden. It is implicated in 10% of stillbirths [4], and, apart from prematurity, CHD is the leading cause of neonatal death,

D.G. Wilson
Children's Heart Unit for Wales and Adult Congenital Heart Disease Unit, University Hospital of Wales, Cardiff and Vale NHS Trust, Cardiff, UK
e-mail: dirk.wilson@wales.nhs.uk

D. Kumar, P. Elliott (eds.), *Cardiovascular Genetics and Genomics*,
https://doi.org/10.1007/978-3-319-66114-8_6

Table 6.1 Environmental risk factors for CHD [9–11]

Infectious agents	Rubella
Maternal drug exposure (non-prescribed)	Alcohol, cannabis/marijuana, cocaine, tobacco
Maternal drug exposure (prescribed)	Anti-epileptic medication, anti-retroviral medication, isotretinoin, lithium
Maternal health problems	Non-gestational diabetes, stress and bereavement, underweight, obesity ± hypercholesterolaemia, phenylketonuria
Maternal toxin exposure	Dioxins, industrial chemicals and solvents, pesticides, polychlorinated biphenyls, proximity to waste site
Paternal drug exposure (non-prescribed)	Cannabis/marijuana, cocaine, tobacco
Paternal toxin exposure	Industrial chemicals and solvents, proximity to waste site

accounting for 4.2% of cases [5]. Nearly half of deaths due to CHD occur during the first year of life [6]. For individuals born with critical CHD, the 1-year survival is estimated at 75%, whereas 97% of infants with non-critical CHD survive the first year [7]. Advances in the diagnosis and management this group of conditions have meant that over 85% of babies born with CHD will now survive to adult life [8]. This has implications for health care professionals caring for this rising cohort of survivors, most of whom will go on to have children of their own.

Various studies have attempted to determine the aetiology of CHD, and, although most cases are sporadic, a variety of environmental risk factors are recognised (Table 6.1). Genetic factors have also been implicated. Developments in molecular techniques and sequencing of the human genome have provided more advanced insights into genetic aetiology of CHD. Animal models have helped to elucidate some of the structural genes that are critical to cardiac development. Along with this, a variety of transcriptional regulators and signalling molecules have been identified. In humans the precise role of these genes and their associated molecular regulators is still under investigation. It is likely the environmental factors identified in the aetiology of CHD are having their influence through an effect on subcellular mechanisms that affect cardiac development.

In this chapter there will be a simple overview of the known genetic causes and associations in CHD. These will include conditions with abnormal numbers of chromosomes (aneuploidy), the microdeletion syndromes with known cardiac implications, and conditions where point mutations are associated with structural heart disease in the young. The role of copy number variants, single nucleotide polymorphisms and epigenetics in the aetiology of CHD will be touched upon. There will also be an exploration of the approach to the clinical and genetic assessment of a patient with CHD.

6.2 Genetic Testing

The techniques for assessing for genetic abnormalities include cytogenetics, DNA mutation analysis, exome sequencing and whole genome sequencing. Cytogenetic techniques include karyotyping, high resolution banding, fluorescent in-situ hybridisation

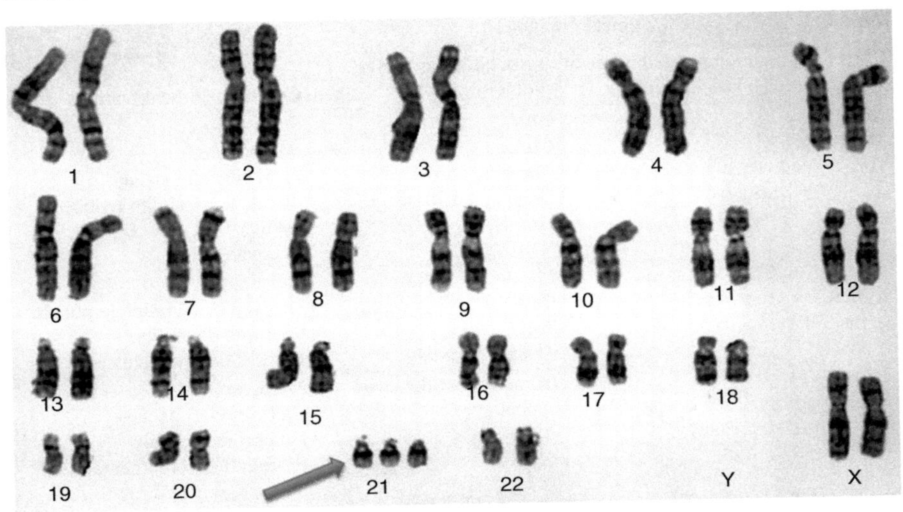

Fig. 6.1 Female karyotype in a child with Down syndrome showing (arrow) aneuploidy of chromosome 21 (Trisomy 21). Courtesy of the All-Wales Genetics Laboratory

(FISH), subtelomeric FISH, and comparative genomic hybridisation (known as array CGH). DNA mutation analysis is available for a select number of conditions. More recently, whole exome and whole genome sequencing are moving from being a research tool to tests used more widely in the clinical arena.

6.2.1 Aneuploidy and Karyotyping

For many years, karyotyping was one of the few tools available to assess the genetic causes of CHD. Aneuploidy is the presence of an abnormal number of chromosomes in a cell, i.e. a chromosome is missing or an extra copy or copies are present. Aneuploidy may be identified using standard karyotyping (Fig. 6.1). The resolution of karyotype is low and structural abnormalities in the chromosome of less than 5–10 Mb in size are not normally identified. Karyotyping is therefore of limited value in trying to ascertain the genetic cause of CHD. The common clinical features and cardiac problems seen in human aneuploidy are set out in Tables 6.2 and 6.3.

6.2.2 Fluorescent In-Situ Hybridisation (FISH)

More than two decades ago FISH analysis was introduced into clinical practice. This permitted assessment of the presence of submicroscopic structural chromosomal abnormalities using targeted probes (Fig. 6.2). Because of the targeted nature of the probes employed, there needed to be a fairly accurate clinical assessment of the likely problem, however, this technique has allowed clinicians to make a molecular diagnosis for a small number of microdeletion and microduplication syndromes associated

Table 6.2 Aneuploidy in clinical practice[a]

Chromosome anomaly and name of syndrome (CHD incidence)	Associated cardiac problems	Common clinical features
XO Monosomy X Turner syndrome (Up to 25% affected)	BAV CoA Thoracic aortic aneurysm ± dissection HLHS	Short stature Webbed neck Fetal cystic hygroma Streak ovaries with reduced fertility Lymphoedema
XXY Klinefelter syndrome (Up to 50% affected)	MVP PDA ToF Ebstein anomaly	Tall stature Delayed or incomplete puberty Learning disability Behavioural problems
Trisomy 13 Patau syndrome (Up to 100% affected)	Isomerism of the atrial appendages ASD VSD TGA PDA	Microcephaly Cleft lip/cleft palate Holoprosencephaly Profound developmental delay Severely reduced life expectancy
Trisomy 18 Edward syndrome (Up to 100% affected)	ASD VSD Polyvalvar disease (thickened, dysplastic)	History of polyhydramnios Overlapping fingers Rockerbottom feet Profound developmental delay Severely reduced life expectancy
Trisomy 21 Down syndrome (40–50% affected)	AVSD ASD VSD PDA ToF (usually with AVSD)	Hypotonia and developmental delay Flat facial features, small ears Upward slant to the eyes with epicanthic folds Single palmar crease Early onset dementia

[a]See Table 6.3 for glossary of terms and abbreviations in this table

Table 6.3 Glossary of terms and abbreviations

Abbreviation	Full name and description
ASD	Atrial septal defect: a defect usually situated in the central portion of the dividing wall between the atriums
APVD	Anomalous pulmonary venous drainage – the pulmonary veins drain to the right side of the heart; this may be partial or complete (PAPVD vs TAPVD)
AVSD	Atrioventricular septal defect – and abnormality of the atrio-ventricular junction characterised in the complete form by a low ASD, a defect in the ventricular septum and an abnormal arrangement of the atrioventricular valves; also known as atrioventricular canal defect or endocardial cushion defect
BAV	Bicuspid aortic valve – the aortic valve has two functioning leaflets; often associated with aortopathy, where the ascending aorta is dilated with an increased risk of dissection
CoA	Coarctation of the aorta – a narrowing in the distal aortic arch in the region of the insertion of the ductus arteriosus
DORV	Double outlet right ventricle – there is a VSD and both great vessels are predominately associated with the right ventricle
HCM	Hypertrophic cardiomyopathy – heart muscle thickening associated with myocyte fibre disarray on histology

Table 6.3 (continued)

Abbreviation	Full name and description
HLHS	Hypoplastic left heart syndrome – severe underdevelopment of the left heart structures and aortic arch
IAA	Interrupted aortic arch – a PDA-dependent lesion where there is a gap in the aorta
LVNC	LV non-compaction cardiomyopathy – developmental abnormality associated with spongy myocardium
MV	Mitral valve
MVP	Mitral valve prolapse – backward movement of the mitral valve leaflet(s), often associated with valve regurgitation
PAH	Pulmonary arterial hypertension – raised pressure in the pulmonary artery due to elevated pulmonary vascular resistance
PDA	Persistent ductus arteriosus – non-closure of the arterial duct after birth
PS	Pulmonary stenosis – narrowed pulmonary valve; peripheral PS refers to narrowing in the pulmonary artery branches
SVAS	Supra-valvar aortic stenosis – narrowing in the ascending aorta
TAAD	Thoracic aortic aneurysm with dissection
TGA	Transposition of the great arteries – the left ventricle gives rise to the pulmonary artery and the right ventricle gives rise to the aorta
ToF	Tetralogy of Fallot – large VSD, aorta overriding the ventricular septum, obstruction to right ventricular outflow and compensatory right ventricular hypertrophy
Truncus	Truncus arteriosus or common arterial trunk – large VSD with single outlet vessel from the heart that divides into aorta and pulmonary arteries
TV	Tricuspid valve
VSD	Ventricular septal defect – a hole in the dividing wall between the ventricles

with CHD (Fig. 6.3). In most cases with multiple clinical features, the critical genomic region includes a number of genes that are associated with CHD. Notable examples include supravalvar aortic stenosis in Williams syndrome with 7q microdeletion (Fig. 6.4) and the DiGeorge/Velo-Cardio-Facial syndrome with 22q microdeletion (Fig. 6.5). The generic term 'contiguous gene syndrome' is commonly referred to such clinical examples of genomic imbalance (Table 6.4).

6.2.3 Array Comparative Genomic Hybridisation (aCGH)

Many laboratories now use genomic microarrays as their first-line diagnostic test for copy number variation (CNV) detection. DNA is fluorescently labelled and co-hybridised with normal control DNA to mapped DNA sequences that are spotted onto a glass slide surface. These clones contain DNA which represent the human DNA sequences, and are regularly spaced across the whole genome. The fluorescent intensities of the DNA hybridised to the spotted clones is measured. If there is more signal from the sample relative to the control then there is likely to be a gain of that genomic region; conversely, if there is less sample relative to the control, then there is a loss of that region. Gains and losses of clones are detected and expressed as a ratio that is plotted against genomic position (Fig. 6.6). The advantage is that this gives the ability to detect simultaneously on any locus: aneuploidies, deletions, duplications and amplifications. This is equivalent to thousands of FISH studies being performed simultaneously and allows the detection of submicroscoptic chromosomal abnormalities.

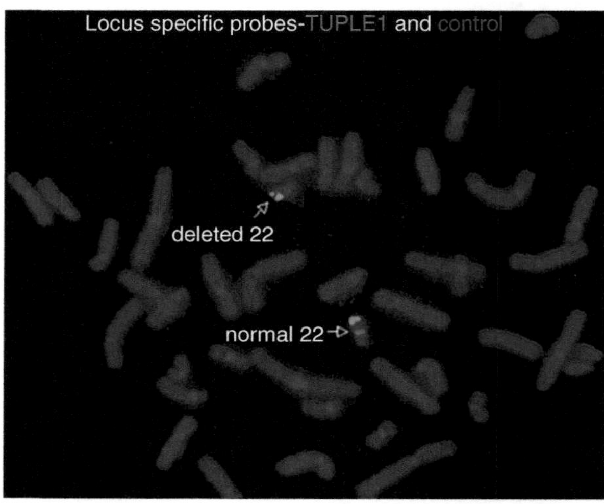

Fig. 6.2 Microdeletion 22q11 in a child with velo-cardio-facial syndrome–note deleted chromosome 22 (top) compared to normal chromosome 22 (bottom). Courtesy of the All-Wales Genetics Laboratory

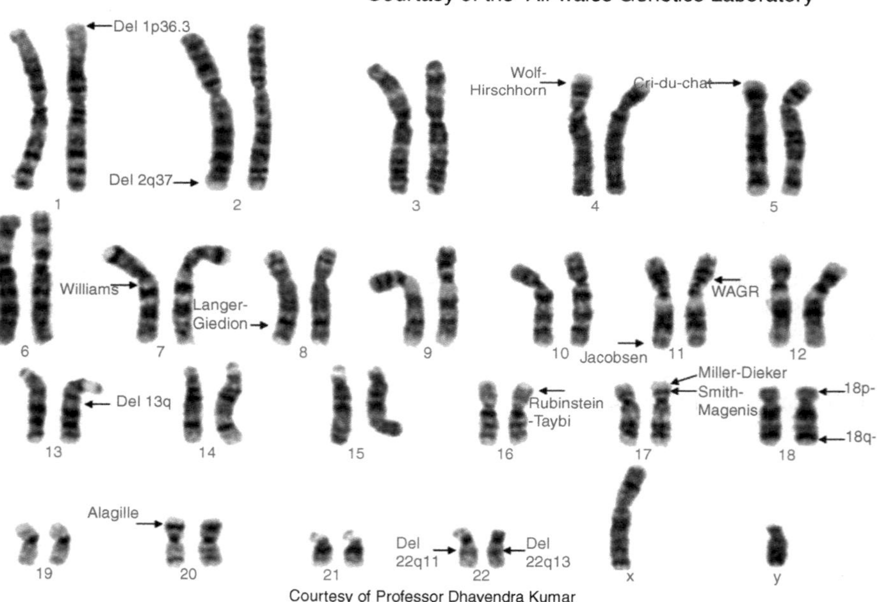

Fig. 6.3 Microdeletion syndromes associated with congenital heart disease (see Table 6.4). Courtesy of Professor Dhavendra Kumar

6.2.4 DNA Point Mutations

A point mutation is a change within a gene in which one base pair of a DNA sequence is altered. These may have one of three outcomes: (1) no effect because the mutated codon still codes for the same amino acid; (2) a change in the encoded amino acid—this may have variable clinical effects; (3) a stop codon may be formed,

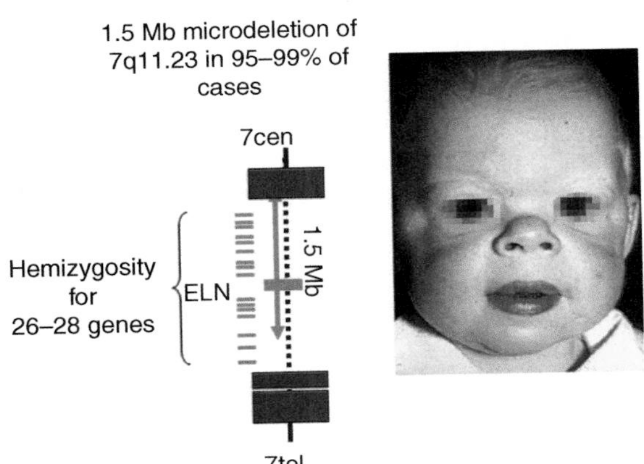

Fig. 6.4 Microdeletion in a child with clinical features of Williams syndrome. Courtesy of Professor Dhavendra Kumar

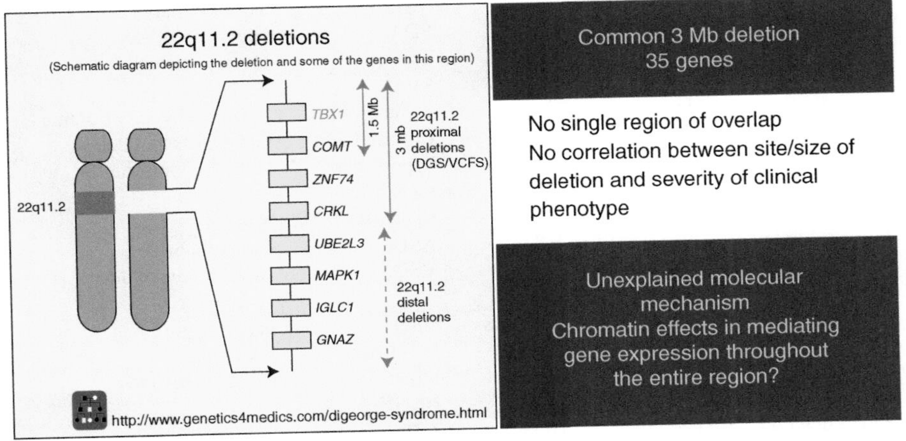

Fig. 6.5 Microdeletion encompassing TBX1 and several other morbid genes: an example of the contiguous gene syndrome

which leads to truncation of the encoded protein, which will usually have altered function [see Chaps. 1 and 2]. In many individuals with complex multiple congenital malformations, mutation in a single gene might present with overlapping clinical features including intellectual difficulties, metabolic abnormality and neuro-psychiatric features ([12], Fig. 6.7). In the case of the Ras-MAP kinase pathway, DNA point mutations in several genes are associated with syndromes with overlapping clinical features, including Noonan, cardiofaciocutaneous and Costello syndromes. Point mutations associated with syndromic CHD are shown in Table 6.5.

Table 6.4 Microdeletion syndromes and CHD (see Table 6.3)

Syndrome and associated microdeletion (CHD incidence)	Inheritance	Implicated cardiac gene	Cardiovascular features	Common clinical features
1p36 deletion (up to 70% affected)	Theoretically AD, but most arise de novo	DVL1	PDA LVNC	Facial features Microcephaly Developmental delay
2q37 deletion (under 20% affected)	Theoretically AD, but most arise de novo	HDAC4	ASD VSD PDA	Facial features Developmental delay Autism spectrum Obesity
Wolf-Hirschhorn 4p16.3 deletion (up to 45% affected)	Theoretically AD, but most arise de novo	Possibly MSX1	ASD VSD PDA ToF DORV	Ataxia Reduced muscle mass and tone Long head with frontal bossing Downslanted palpebral fissures and epicanthic folds Developmental delay
Cri-du-chat 5p15.2 deletion (up to 50% affected)	Theoretically AD, but most arise de novo	CTNND2	ASD VSD PDA ToF	Facial features Microcephaly High-pitched cry Developmental delay
Williams(-Beuren) 7q11.23 deletion (up to 80% affected)	Theoretically AD, but most arise de novo	ELN	SVAS, peripheral PS, CoA and aortic hypoplasia, renal artery stenosis, HCM	Facial features Neonatal hypercalcaemia Developmental delay Outgoing personality
Langer-Giedion 8q4.1 deletion (uncommon)	Theoretically AD, but most arise de novo	EXT1	ASD VSD	Facial features Developmental delay Coloboma
Jacobsen 11q24.1 deletion (around 50% affected)	Theoretically AD, but most arise de novo	FRA11B	VSD Left heart obstruction HLHS	Facial features Austism Bleeding disorder
13q14 deletion (up to 36%)	Theoretically AD, but most arise de novo	Unknown	ASD VSD PDA PS ToF CoA	Facial features Brain malformation Gastro-intestinal problems Retinoblastoma
Rubinstein-Taybi 16p13.3 deletion (up to 33% affected)	Theoretically AD, but most arise de novo	CREBBP EP300	ASD VSD BAV PS CoA PDA	Facial features Broad thumbs and first toes Developmental delay Eye problems Increased risk with anaesthesia

Table 6.4 (continued)

Syndrome and associated microdeletion (CHD incidence)	Inheritance	Implicated cardiac gene	Cardiovascular features	Common clinical features
Miller-Dieker 17p13.3 deletion (uncommon)	Theoretically AD, but most arise de novo	?LIS1	ASD VSD DORV ToF	Facial features Cerebral anomalies including lissencephaly Developmental delay Growth retardation Reduced life expectancy
Smith-Megenis 17p11.2 deletion (25–50% affected)	Theoretically AD, but most arise de novo	RAI1	ASD VSD TAPVD Valve lesions ToF	Facial features Hypotonia and failure to thrive in infancy Developmental delay Short fingers Eye and larynx abnormalities Behavioural problems
18p deletion (<10% affected)	Theoretically AD, but most arise de novo	?LAMA1		Facial and ear features Short fingers and toes Developmental delay
Distal 18q deletion (25–35% affected)	Theoretically AD, but most arise de novo	SMAD4	ASD VSD Valve disease APVD	Mild facial features Cleft palate Hypotonia Short stature Hearing loss Lower limb problems (club and rockerbottom feet) Reduced life expectancy
Alagille 20p12 deletion (up to 90% affected) See also Table 6.5	AD and de novo	JAG1	ASD PS (valve and branches) ToF PDA	Facial features Biliary hypoplasia Butterfly vertebrae Renal problems
DiGeorge 22q11 (up to 80% affected)	AD and de novo	TBX1	VSD Truncus IAA type B	Facial features and palatal abnormalities Thymic hypoplasia with immune deficit Parathyroid hypoplasia Developmental delay Mental health problems
Phelan-McDermid 22q13.3 deletion (around 25% affected)	Theoretically AD, but most arise de novo	?SHANK3	ASD TV dysplasia PDA TAPVD	Minor facial features Developmental delay Autism spectrum behaviours Fleshy hands Dysplastic toenails

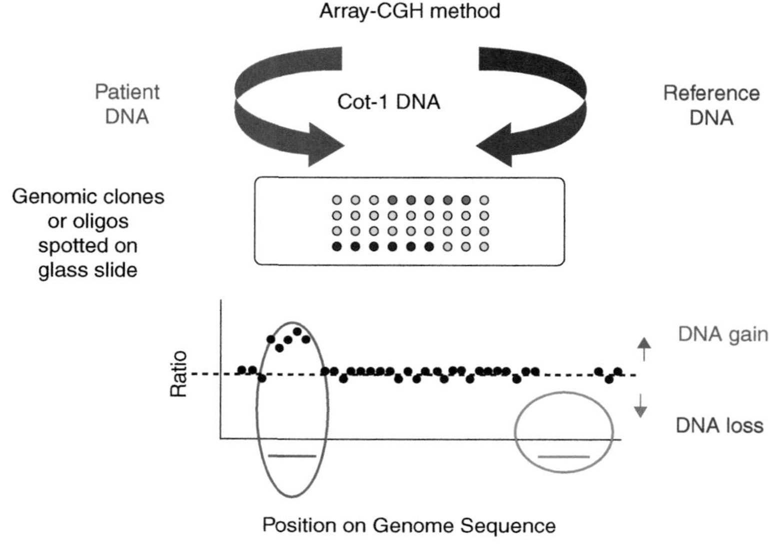

Fig. 6.6 Main steps in the technique of array comparative genomic hybridization (aCGH). Courtesy of Sian Morgan, Principle Scientist, All-Wales Genetics Laboratory

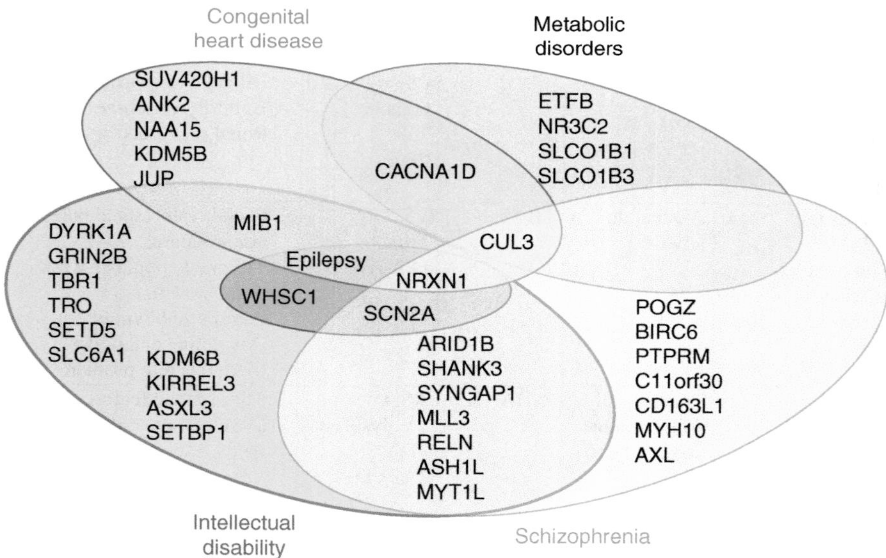

Fig. 6.7 Overlapping multisystem clinical manifestations of DNA point mutations in selected genes associated with CHD. From De Rubeis et al. [12]; with permission

Table 6.5 Point mutations associated with CHD (see Table 6.3)

Gene mutation and associated syndrome (CHD incidence)	Inheritance	Associated gene mutation	Cardiovascular features	Common Clinical features
Alagille (up to 90% affected)	AD	JAG1, NOTCH2	ASD PS and peripheral PS ToF PDA	Facial features Biliary hypoplasia Butterfly vertebrae Renal problems
Cardiofaciocutaneous (up to 70% affected) [RASopathy spectrum]	AD	BRAF, KRAS, MAP2K1 and 2	ASD PS HCM	Facial features Developmental delay
Char (up to 100% affected)	AD	TFAP2b	PDA	Facial features Limb defomity
CHARGE (up to 85% affected)	AD	CHD7, SEMA3E	ASD VSD ASVD ToF spectrum Truncus	Choanal atresia Eye coloboma Developmental delay
Costello (up to 65% affected) [RASopathy spectrum]	AD	HRAS	Atrial arrhythmia HCM PS	Facial features Lax skin Feeding difficulties Sparse or curly hair Developmental delay
Ellis-van Creveld (up to 60% affected)	AR	EVC, EVC2	ASD Common atrium	Dysplastic nails and teeth Short limbs Post-axial polydactyly
Holt-Oram (up to 80% affected)	AD	TBX5	ASD VSD PDA	Upper limb deformity
Kabuki (around 50% affected)	AD	MLL2	ASD VSD TGA ToF CoA MV abnormalities	Facial and eyelid features Scoliosis Developmental delay
Noonan (up to 80% affected) [Rasopathy spectrum]	AD	BRAF, CBL, HRAS, KRAS, MEK1, NF1, NRAS, PTPN11, RAF1, SHOC2, SOS1	ASD PS and peripheral PS HCM PDA	Facial features Short stature Pectus excavatum Webbed neck Cubitus valgus
Okihiro (up to 33% affected) [Clinical overlap with Holt-Oram syndrome]	AD	SALL4	ASD	Eye features Bilateral deafness Radial and thumb anomalies

AD autosomal dominant, *AR* autosomal recessive

Table 6.6 Non-syndromic CHD associated with single gene defects (see Table 6.3)

Gene	Cardiac anomaly
ALK2	AVSD
BMPR2	Septal defect with associated PAH
CRELD1	AVSD
GATA4	ASD, VSD
MYH6	ASD, HCM
NKX2.5	ASD, ToF, TV dysplasia, conduction defects
NOTCH1	BAV, calcific aortic valve disease
PROSIT-240	TGA

6.2.5 Genomic Sequencing

This subject is discussed in detail in Chap. 4. Whole exome sequencing permits the detection of point mutations and small insertion-deletions. The technique is increasingly being offered as a diagnostic test for heterogeneous disorders. A number of DNA point mutations have been identified in a number of non-syndromic forms of CHD (Table 6.6).

Whole genome sequencing allows the characterisation of CNVs to very high levels of accuracy. Utilisation of these techniques has allowed characterisation of several number single nucleotide polymorphisms (SNPs). SNPs are changes in single nucleotides found throughout the genome including coding and non-coding regions. SNPs do not necessarily alter gene function; however, they may influence an organism's response to environmental factors. SNPs that influence the development of CHD have been identified through focusing on candidate genes thought to be involved in the development of CHD. In one study, 20% of individuals with CHD and other anomalies had detectable CNV in the form of deletions and duplications when genome-wide assessment was undertaken. The CNV contained up to 55 genes. Duplications were observed in the long arms of chromosomes 3 and 5 and the short arms of chromosomes 18 and 20 [13].

Vascular endothelial growth factor (VEGF) activity is important in normal heart development. SNPs of VEGF and its promoters have been implicated in increased risk of ToF [14] and AVSD [15]. Polymorphism of the VEGF promoter C-634G has been shown to be protective against isolated VSD [16]. GATA4 sequence variants are associated with ASD, VSD and ToF [17].

Assessment of a cohort from the Baltimore-Washington Infant Study showed 33 SNPs in selected forms of CHD. These included genes controlling folate metabolism, nitric oxide synthase activity, cell-cell interaction, and the regulation of inflammation and blood pressure. Maternal smoking was found to be associated with a higher risk of CHD with certain SNPs [18].

6.3 Epigenetics and Congenital Heart Disease

Epigenetic mechanisms contribute to the regulation of multiple physiological processes during the development and maturation of an individual. DNA methylation occurs via the addition of a methyl group in the 5′ carbon of cytosine on to the DNA molecule. This may result in altered transcription and so alter the pattern of gene expression. DNA methylation abnormalities in genes involved in growth regulation, apoptosis and folate metabolism (GATA4, MSX1 and MTHFS) have been shown to be associated with CHD in Down syndrome and isolated CHD [19].

6.4 Clinical Approach to Genetic Assessment of CHD

6.4.1 Fetal Life

In the UK and other countries with advanced health care systems, antenatal care should include assessment of risk factors for congenital anomalies from early pregnancy. Ultrasonic fetal anomaly surveillance starts with the assessment of nuchal translucency during the first trimester. Increased nuchal translucency is associated with chromosomal aneuploidy, congenital heart disease and other congenital malformations. Its presence highlights the need for increased vigilance during the second trimester [20] and it forms part of the antenatal assessment of the risk of Down syndrome.

Fetal anomaly scanning is undertaken at around 20 weeks of gestation. The cardiac component of this scan consists of assessment of the 4-chamber view, the ventricular outflow tracts and the 3-vessel trachea view. Fetal echocardiography now permits the antenatal diagnosis of >50% of critical CHD.

Up to one third of critical fetal CHD is associated with aneuploidy, therefore, where there is the finding of a critical form of CHD, with or without other associated anomalies, amniocentesis should be offered after appropriate counselling. If a chromosome anomaly is found, ideally there should be joint consideration between the affected couple and Fetal Medicine, Fetal Cardiology and Clinical Genetics regarding the best way forward in the pregnancy. Where the choice is made to continue the pregnancy, multidisciplinary care should continue throughout the pregnancy and into the newborn period.

6.4.2 Neonate and Infant

When there is the finding of CHD in a newborn baby or infant, the assessing clinician should take steps to explore the possible genetic associations. The following should be ascertained:

- Maternal history
  - Age
  - Occupation
  - Drug history (prescribed and non-prescribed)
  - Smoking history
  - Maternal medical conditions (e.g. non-gestational diabetes)
- Family history of CHD or other heart problems
- Consideration of TORCH screen if there are indications that congenital infection may be a possibility

- Paternal history
  - Age
  - Occupation
  - Drug history (prescribed and non-prescribed)
  - Smoking history
  - Paternal medical conditions
- Evidence of dysmorphism in either parent or in siblings
- History of familial or genetic disease
- A full clinical assessment should be undertaken, including plotting of length, weight and head circumference.
- Assessment of presence/absence of dysmorphism
- Type of CHD—is this a cardiac lesion known to be associated with a genetic origin?
- Where there are indications that genetic disease is a possibility, a referral to medical genetics should be made.
- Consider array CGH testing if there is CHD, dysmorphism ± developmental delay, or if the lesion is highly associated with microdeletion (e.g. ToF, truncus arteriosus and other related outflow tract anomalies)
- If a genetic problem is diagnosed, the implications for the parents and any siblings needs to be considered – is there a need for genetic assessment and cardiac surveillance in first degree relatives?

6.4.3 Older Child/Young Person

Most individuals with CHD will present in infancy, although some lesions, such as ASD and BAV are commonly diagnosed in later life. Where a new diagnosis is made the same assessment as that set out above for neonates and infants should be undertaken. The likelihood of a genetic association should be assessed and an appropriate referral to Medical Genetics made. If a genetic association is found, there should be a strategy of disclosure to the young person. The concept of genetic transmissibility should be introduced in a sensitive manner at an appropriate time. This disclosure would ideally be undertaken during teenage years and certainly well in advance of a pregnancy. Assessment of other family members should be carried out if this is indicated.

6.4.4 Adult

In adults with known genetically-associated CHD conditions, the following should be thought about:

- Are all the cardiac problems affected by the condition being assessed appropriately (e.g. long-term aortic surveillance in Turner syndrome)?

- Are all the non-cardiac problems affected by the condition being assessed appropriately (e.g. immune status and mental health problems in DiGeorge syndrome)? Are all relevant health care professionals involved?
- Has appropriate reproductive health advice been given—for women, is the choice of contraception safe and appropriate for the cardiac lesion? What is the medical risk of pregnancy?
- What is the recurrence risk in any offspring? For sporadic CHD with no other family member affected the risk is in the region of 1–6%. Where there is an associated DNA mutation in a parent with CHD, the recurrence risk may be as high as 50%.

Conclusions

CHD lesions are the most common forms of congenital anomaly. Certain CHD lesions are associated with a high morbidity and mortality. Known chromosomal, syndromic, and environmental causes account for around 20% of CHD lesions. The aetiology of the majority of CHD lesions is unknown. Future advances in genomics and epigenetics are likely to provide insights into the aetiological origins of congenital heart defects.

References

1. Botto LD, Correa A, Erickson JD. Racial and temporal variations in the prevalence of heart defects. Pediatrics. 2001;107:e32.
2. Hoffman JI, Kaplan S. The incidence of congenital heart disease. J Am Coll Cardiol. 2002;39(12):1890–900.
3. Gray GW, Salisbury DA, Gulino AM. Echocardiographic and color flow Doppler findings in military pilot applicants. Aviat Space Environ Med. 1995;66:32–4.
4. Hoffman JI. Incidence of congenital heart disease: II. Prenatal incidence. Pediatr Cardiol. 1995;16:155–65.
5. Petrini JR, Gilboa SM, Lee KA, et al. Racial differences by gestational age in neonatal deaths attributable to congenital heart defects—United States, 2003—2006. CDC Weekly. 2010;59(37):1208–11.
6. Gilboa SM, Salemi JL, Nembhard WN, et al. Mortality resulting from congenital heart disease among children and adults in the United States, 1999 to 2006. Circulation. 2010;122:2254–63.
7. Oster ME, Lee KA, Honein MA, et al. Temporal trends in survival among infants with critical congenital heart defects. Pediatrics. 2013;131(5):e1502–8.
8. Warnes CA, Liberthson R, Danielson GK, et al. Task Force 1: the changing profile of congenital heart disease in adult life. J Am Coll Cardiol. 2001;37(5):1170–5.
9. Ewing CK, Loffredo CA, Beaty TH. Paternal risk factors for isolated membranous ventricular septal defects. Am J Med Genet. 1997;71(1):42–6.
10. Cresci M, Foffa I, Ait-Ali L, et al. Maternal and paternal environmental risk factors, metabolizing GSTM1 and GSTT1 polymorphisms, and congenital heart disease. Am J Cardiol. 2011;108(11):1625–31.
11. Feng Y, Yu D, Yang L, et al. Maternal lifestyle factors in pregnancy and congenital heart defects in offspring: review of the current evidence. Ital J Pediatr. 2014;40:85.
12. De Rubeis S, He X, Goldberg AP, et al. Synaptic, transcriptional and chromatin genes disrupted in autism. Nature. 2014;515:209–15.

13. Goldmuntz E, Palru P, Glessner J, et al. Microdeletions and microduplications in patients with congenital heart disease and multiple congenital anomalies. Congenit Heart Dis. 2011;6(6):592–603.
14. Lambrechts D, Devriendt K, Driscoll DA, et al. Low expression VEGF haplotype increases the risk for tetralogy of Fallot: a family based association study. J Med Genet. 2005;42(6):519–22.
15. Smedts HPM, Isaacs A, de Costa D, et al. VEGF polymorphisms are associated with endocardial cushion defects: a family-based case-control study. Pediatr Res. 2010;67:23–8.
16. Xie J, Yi L, ZF X, et al. VEGF C-634G polymorphism is associated with protection from isolated ventricular septal defect: case-control and TDT studies. Eur J Hum Genet. 2007;15(12):1246–51.
17. Tomita-Mitchell A, Maslen CL, Morris CD, et al. GATA4 GATA4 sequence variants in patients with congenital heart disease. J Med Genet. 2007;12:779–83.
18. Kuehl K, Loffredo C, Lammer E, et al. Association of congenital cardiovascular malformations with 33 single nucleotide polymorphisms of selected cardiovascular disease-related genes. Birth Defects Res A Clin Mol Teratol. 2010;88(2):101–10.
19. Serra-Juhe C, Cusco I, Homs A, et al. DNA methylation abnormalities in congenital heart disease. Epigenetics. 2015;10(2):167–77.
20. Guraya SS. The associations of nuchal translucency and fetal abnormalities; significance and implications. J Clin Diagn Res. 2013;7(5):936–41.

Inherited Cardiovascular Metabolic Disorders

7

Elaine Murphy and Oliver Watkinson

Abstract

Cardiovascular involvement is a recognised feature of more than 50 different inherited disorders of metebolism. Most frequently cardiovascular disease associated with inherited disorders of metabolism presents as part of multisystem disease, but on occasion it may be the most significant (e.g., Infantile Pompe disease, Danon disease) or only (e.g., Fabry disease, Glycogen storage disease XV) presenting feature, and a high index of suspicion is needed to reach the correct diagnosis. Diagnosis is important because many of these disorders (partly) respond to treatments such as dietary modification, co-factor administration, enzyme replacement therapy, or haematopoietic stem cell transplantation.

Keywords

Glycogen storage disorders • Polyglucosan body storage disorders • Carnitine transport defects • Fatty acid oxidation disorders • Propionic academia • Lysosomal storage disorders • Mucopolysaccharidosis • Fabry disease • *Mitochondrial disease* • Congenital disorders of glycosylation • Haemochromatosis Alkaptonuria Homocystinuria • Sitosterolemia

E. Murphy (✉)
Charles Dent Metabolic Unit, National Hospital for Neurology and Neurosurgery, London, UK
e-mail: Elaine.Murphy@uclh.nhs.uk

O. Watkinson
Department of Inherited Cardiovascular Disease, St Bartholomew's Hospital, London, UK
e-mail: oliver.watkinson@nhs.net

D. Kumar, P. Elliott (eds.), *Cardiovascular Genetics and Genomics*,
https://doi.org/10.1007/978-3-319-66114-8_7

7.1 Introduction

Inherited metabolic diseases (IMD) are individually rare, clinically widely heterogeneous, and typically, but not always, associated with abnormal biochemical tests (usually specialist rather than routine biochemistry) [1]. Broadly speaking they can be divided into three groups:

1. Disorders of intoxication—these disorders of intermediary metabolism give rise to an acute or progressive intoxication secondary to the accumulation of toxic compounds proximal to a metabolic block. Examples include the organic acidurias, such as propionic acidemia.
2. Disorders of energy metabolism—these give rise to their symptoms chiefly because of an energy deficient in tissues such as liver, muscle, brain or heart. Examples include the mitochondrial respiratory chain defects defects, fatty acid oxidation defects and glycogen storage disorders.
3. Disorders of complex molecules—these involve disturbance in the synthesis or catabolism of complex molecules. Symptoms tend to be progressive and not dependent on dietary/energy intake. Examples include the lysosomal storage disorders and the peroxisomal disorders.

Cardiovascular involvement is a recognised feature of more than 50 different inherited disorders of metebolism. Most frequently cardiovascular disease associated with inherited disorders of metabolism presents as part of multisystem disease, but on occasion it may be the most significant (e.g., Infantile Pompe disease, Danon disease) or only (e.g., Fabry disease, Glycogen storage disease XV) presenting feature, and a high index of suspicion is needed to reach the correct diagnosis. Table 7.1 summarises the inheritance, pattern of cardiovascular involvement, other clinical features, diagnostic investigations and potential treatment options for some of the more prevalent inherited disorders of metabolism. Diagnosis is important because many of these disorders (partly) respond to treatments such as dietary modification, co-factor administration, enzyme replacement therapy, or haematopoietic stem cell transplantation.

Clincial presentation can occur at any age, from the neonatal period to late adulthood, with more severe, and sometimes fatal disease, tending to present in early childhood. Factors including improved medical care, increased awareness of metabolic conditions and newborn screening with early treatment, have led to an increased number of patients with inherited metabolic disease surviving to adulthood and these factors, together with improved access to genetic testing, mean that both paediatric and adult cardiologists need to consider this group of disorders in the differential of unexplained cardiovascular disease. Cardiologists also have an important role in monitoring and managing cardiac disease secondary to known disorders of metabolism.

Table 7.1 Summary of inherited metabolic disorders associated with cardiovascular disease

Condition	Gene (inheritance)	Incidence	Cardiac involvement	Supportive clinical features	(Non-genetic) diagnostic tests	Treatment options
Glycogen storage disorders (GSD): See Table 7.2						
Disorders of fatty acid metabolism						
Carnitine transport defects						
Carnitine deficiency, systemic primary (#212140)	*SLC22A5* (AR)	1:20,000 to 1:70,000. 1 in 300 in the Faroe Islands	Dilated/hypertrophic cardiomyopathy. Cardiac failure. Arrhythmias. Long QT syndrome	Episodes of metabolic decompensation, skeletal myopathy, hypoketotic hypoglycemia	Plasma carnitine levels. Urine organic acids	Carnitine supplementation
Carnitine-acylcarnitine translocase (CACT) deficiency (#212138)	*SLC25A20* (AR)	<100 cases reported	Cardiac arrhythmia, cardiomyopathy, heart block	Hyperammonemia, liver dysfunction, hypoketotic hypoglycemia	Plasma acylcarnitine profile. Urine organic acids. Fibroblast studies	Avoid prolonged fasting. Dietary modification. Medium chain triglyceride supplementation. (Possibly carnitine supplementation)
Carnitine palmitoyltransferase II (CPT2) deficiency (#255110)	*CPT2* (AR)	<500 cases reported	Hypertrophic/dilated cardiomyopathy. Cardiac arrhythmias. Sudden death	Exercise intolerance, myalgia, rhabdomyolysis, acute renal failure	Creatine kinase. Plasma acylcarnitine profile. Urine organic acids. Fibroblast studies	Avoid prolonged fasting. Dietary modification. Medium chain triglyceride supplementation. Triheptanoin

(continued)

Table 7.1 (continued)

Condition	Gene (inheritance)	Incidence	Cardiac involvement	Supportive clinical features	(Non-genetic) diagnostic tests	Treatment options
Fatty acid oxidation defects						
Very long-chain acyl-CoA dehydrogenase (VLCAD) deficiency (#201475)	*ACADVL* (AR)	1:30,000	Hypertrophic/dilated cardiomyopathy	Exercise intolerance, myalgia, rhabdomyolysis, acute renal failure, liver dysfunction, hypoketotic hypoglycemia	Creatine kinase. Plasma acylcarnitine profile. Urine organic acids. Fibroblast studies	Avoid prolonged fasting. Dietary modification. Medium chain triglyceride supplementation. Triheptanoin
Long chain 3-hydroxyacyl-CoA dehydrogenase (LCHAD) deficiency (#609016)	*HADHA* (AR)	1:250,000	Hypertrophic/dilated cardiomyopathy	Muscle weakness, exercise intolerance, progressive axonal sensorimotor peripheral neuropathy, retinopathy, ataxic gait, episodic rhabdomyolysis, acute renal failure	Creatine kinase. Plasma acylcarnitine profile. Urine organic acids. Fibroblast studies	Avoid prolonged fasting. Dietary modification. Medium chain triglyceride supplementation
Mitochondrial trifunctional protein (MTP) deficiency (#609015)	*HADHA* or *HADHB* (AR)	NR				
Mitochondrial electron transfer defects						
Multiple acyl-CoA dehydrogenase (MADD) deficiency (also known as glutaric aciduria II) (#231680)	*ETFA* or *ETFB* or *ETFDH* (AR)	<500 cases reported	Hypertrophic/dilated cardiomyopathy	Muscle symptoms predominate—weakness, exercise intolerance. Risk of episodic vomiting, ketoacidosis/loss of appetite, acute encephalopathy. Facial and cerebral malformations	Plasma acylcarnitine profile. Urine organic acids. Fibroblast studies	Riboflavin supplementation

Organic acidemias						
Propionic acidemia (#606054)	*PCCA or PCCB* (AR)	1:50,000 to 1:100,000	Cardiomyopathy. Arrhythmias. Sudden cardiac death	Metabolic decompensation: ketoacidosis, hypoglycemia, hyperammonemia, pancytopenia, pancreatitis (+/– neurological sequelae), optic atrophy, hearing impairment, renal failure	Plasma acylcarnitine profile. Urine organic acids. PCC enzyme activity	Avoid catabolism. Dietary modification. Carnitine supplementation
Lysosomal storage disorders						
MPS I (Hurler, Scheie disease) (#607,015)	*IDUA* (AR)	1:100,000 (severe from) to 1:500,000 (attenuated form)	Cardiac valve thickening (more severe for left-sided than right-sided valves). Hypertrophy. Conduction abnormalities. Coronary artery disease. Large vessel arterial narrowing/ dilation. Hypertension	Dysostosis multiplex (arthropathy). Carpel tunnel syndrome. Hepatosplenomegaly. Corneal clouding. Hearing impairment. Herniae	Urine glycosaminoglycans. α-L-iduronidase enzyme activity	Hematopoietic stem cell transplantation. ERT for systemic features but does not affect CNS disease

(continued)

Table 7.1 (continued)

Condition	Gene (inheritance)	Incidence	Cardiac involvement	Supportive clinical features	(Non-genetic) diagnostic tests	Treatment options
MPS II (Hunter disease)(309,900)	*IDS* (XL)	1:100,000 to 170,000 (males). Some symptomatic females also reported	Cardiac valve thickening (more severe for left-sided than right-sided valves). Hypertrophy. Conduction abnormalities. Coronary artery disease. Large vessel arterial narrowing/dilation. Hypertension	Dysostosis multiplex. Short stature. Hepatosplenomegaly. Herniae. Global developmental delay	Urine glycosaminoglycans. Iduronate 2-sulfatase enzyme activity	ERT for systemic features but does not affect CNS disease. Hematopoietic stem cell transplantation
MPS IV (Morquio disease)(#253,000)	MPS IVA—*GALNS*(AR) MPS IVB—*GLB1* (AR)	MPS IVA 1:599,000 (UK). MPS IVB 1:1,000,000	Similar to other MPS disorders but prevalence of cardiac involvement is lower	Normal intellect. Short stature. Dysostosis multiplex. Restrictive lung disease. Corneal clouding. Hearing impairment	Urine glycosaminoglycans. N-acetylgalactosamine 6-sulfatase enzyme activity	ERT (for MPS IVA)
MPS VI (Maroteaux-Lamy disease) (#253,200)	*ARSB* (AR)	23 in 10,000,000 (Germany). 40 in 10,000,000 (Australia)	Cardiac valve thickening (more severe for left-sided than right-sided valves). Hypertrophy. Conduction abnormalities. Coronary artery disease	Normal intellect. Short stature. Dysostosis multiplex	Urine glycosaminoglycans. N-acetylgalactosamine-4-sulphatase enzyme activity	ERT

Mucolipidosis II/III (#252500, #252600, #252605)	*GNPTAB* (AR); *GNPTG* (AR)	<1:100,000	Valvular disease. Left and/or right ventricular hypertrophy. Pulmonary hypertension	ML II—onset at birth and more severe course. ML III—later onset. Joint stiffness, dysostosis multiplex. Short stature. Restrictive lung disease	Urine oligosaccharides. Plasma acid hydrolase activities. *N*-acetylglucosamine-1-phosphotransferase enzyme activity	Supportive
Lysosomal acid lipase deficiency (#278000)	*LIPA* (AR)	1:350,000 (severe infantile form). 1:50,000 (late onset form)	Atherosclerosis	Infantile: failure to thrive, hepatomegaly, liver failure, adrenal calcification. Late-onset: dyslipidemia, hepatic fibrosis/cirrhosis, atherosclerosis	Lipid profile. Lysosomal acid lipase enzyme activity	ERT. Liver transplant
Fabry disease (#301500)	*GLA* (XL)	1:50,000 to 1:117,000 males	Cardiomyopathy. Stroke	Renal impairment. Acroparathesia. Angiokeratomota	GLA enzyme activity (men)	ERT. Chaperone therapy
Others						
Mitochondrial disorders (see Chap. 10)	Multiple genes (both nuclear DNA and mitochondrial DNA encoded) (Maternal, AD, AR)	1:5000	Cardiomyopathy (hypertrophic, dilated, LV noncompaction), heart failure, ventricular tachyarrhythmia, sudden cardiac death	Multisystem involvement—neuromuscular, renal, endocrinopathy, retinitis pigmentosa, sensorineural hearing loss	Lactate (Blood/CSF). Supportive features on muscle biopsy. Mitochondrial respiratory chain enzyme activity	Largely supportive

(continued)

Table 7.1 (continued)

Condition	Gene (inheritance)	Incidence	Cardiac involvement	Supportive clinical features	(Non-genetic) diagnostic tests	Treatment options
Congenital disorders of N-glycosylation	Multiple genes (>40)	NR	(Dilated) cardiomyopathy	Developmental delay, hypotonia, multisystem involvement	Transferrin electrophoresis	Largely supportive
Haemachromotosis (#235200) (see Chap. 10)	*HFE* (AR) *TFR2* (AR)	HFE—1:200 to 1:400 (but has low clinical penetrance). TFR2—very rare	Congestive heart failure. Arrhythmias	Arthropathy. Skin pigmentation. Diabetes mellitus, liver fibrosis/ cirrhosis, hypogonadism	Ferritin. Transferrin saturation. Liver function tests	Phlebotomy
Alkaptonuria (#203500)	*HGD* (AR)	1:250,000	Aortic valve disease. Coronary artery calcification	Arthropathy. Ochronosis (blue-black pigmentation of connective tissue). Renal stones	Urine homogentisic acid	NTBC (nitisinone). Restricted protein diet
Homocystinuria (#236200)	*CBS* (AR)	1:200,000 to 1:335,000. 1 in 65,000 in Ireland	Cardiovascular disease (thromboembolism, stroke, dissection)	Marfanoid habitus. Occular lens dislocation. Reduced bone mineral density. Learning difficulties	Plasma amino acids	Restricted protein diet. Methionine-free amino acid supplementation. Betaine. Pyridoxine (vitamin B6)
Sitosterolemia (#210250)	*ABCG5* or *ABCG8* (AR)	NR	Atherosclerosis.	Xanthomata	Plasma sterols	Dietary modification. Ezetimibe

Primary hyperoxaluria (#259900)	*AGXT* (AR)	1–3:1,000,000	Arrhythmias, heart block, atherosclerosis, left ventricular hypertrophy	Renal stones, fractures, Visual impairment	24-hour urine oxalate	High fluid intake. Pyridoxine
Refsum disease (#266500)	*PHYH* (AR)	1:1,000,000 (UK)	Arrhythmia, cardiomyopathy, heart failure	Anosmia, retinitis pigmentosa, ataxia, polyneuropathy, hearing loss	Phytanic acid levels	Dietary restriction of phytanic acid. Plasmaphoresis or lipid apheresis

ERT enzyme replacement therapy, *NR* not reported

The pattern of presentation varies between disorders but includes:

- Cardiomyopathy—5–13.5% of paediatric cardiomyopathies are reported to be caused by an inherited disorder of metabolism [2–4]. Data on the prevelance of inherited metabolic disease in adults with cardiomyopathy are very limited. Hypertrophic, dilated, restrictive, and ventricular noncompaction cardiomyopathies have all been described in association with inherited metabolic disorders. Hypertrophic cardiomyopathy associated with ventricular pre-excitation (VPE) or the Wolff–Parkinson–White (WPW) syndrome suggests a metabolic disorder.
- Arrthythmias—ventricular arrhythmias and sudden cardiac death may relate to toxic metabolites (e.g., fatty acid oxidation defects, organic acidemias), or to structural abnormalities of the cardiac muscle (e.g., glycogen storage disorders, lysosomal storage disorders, congenital disorders of glycosylation).
- Valvular disease—is a significant feature of some mucopolysaccharidoses and mucolipidoses, as well as alkaptonuria.
- Atherosclerosis—may occur secondary to inherited disorder of sterol metabolism (e.g., sitosterolemia).
- Structural cardiac defects—are not frequently associated with inherited disorders of metabolism. Exceptions include disorders of cholesterol biosynthesis (e.g., Smith–Lemli–Opitz syndrome).

7.2 Investigations

Figure 7.1 provides an algorithm for investigation should a cardiologist suspect an inherited disorder of metabolism. Table 7.3 lists some "red-flags" which may suggest an underlying disorder of metabolism. The approach to diagnosis depends on the disorder that is suspected and may include:

- ECG—ventricular pre-excitation (VPE) is a common feature of storage disease (Pompe, Danon, PRKAG2 syndrome) and mitochondrial disorders. A short PR interval without pre-excitation is a common feature in Fabry disease.
- Echocardiogram
- Exercise testing
- Cardiac MRI
- CT angiogram
- Routine biochemistry
- Specialist biochemistry—note enzyme activity is labile, correct sampling conditions are critical.
- Biopsy with histology and immunohistochemistry—skin, liver, muscle, heart as indicated.
- Genetic testing—focused gene panels are increasingly used for disorders with clinical overlap e.g., glycogen or polyglucosan body storage disorders, fatty acid oxidation disorders.

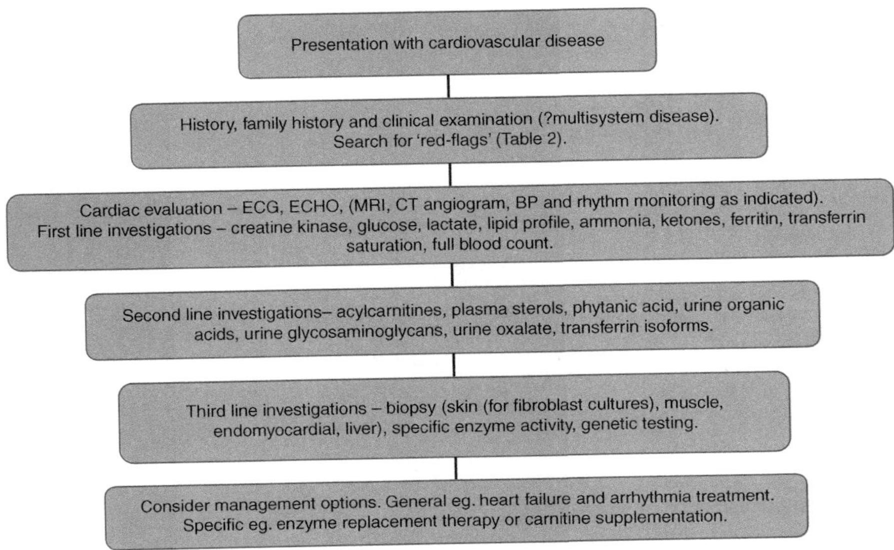

Fig. 7.1 An algorithm for the role of the cardiologist in the investigation and management of cardiovascular disease suspected to be secondary to inherited metabolic disease

Clinical case report 1: Glycogen storage disease IIIa (GSD IIIa)

A 23 year old woman was noted to have severe left ventricular hypertrophy with maximal wall thickness of 3.8 cm [5]. She had been diagnosed with glycogen storage disease type IIIa in childhood. On cardio-pulmonary exercise (CPEX) testing her peak VO_2 was 19.6 mL/kg/min (61% predicted). She was subsequently lost to follow-up and had an uncomplicated pregnancy, with delivery of a healthy infant, at 28 years. By 34 years she was NHYA class 2. Transthoracic echocardiogram (TTE) showed similar severe LVH (MWT 4.0 cm) and a peak VO_2 of 18.3 ml/kg/min (63% predicted).

During a second pregnancy, a TTE at 22 weeks gestation showed LV wall thinning with a MWT of 1.4 cm and impairment of systolic function. By 32 weeks there was LV dilation and a further reduction in MWT to 1.1 cm, with an ejection fraction of 35%. She reported postural dizziness, but no postural drop in BP (88/52 mmHg sitting, 86/52 mmHg standing). She had no symptoms of hypoglycemia during either pregnancy, but did not attend for regular metabolic clinic follow-up. A normal baby was born at term.

Six days following delivery of this child, she developed congestive cardiac failure and required hospitalisation. She repsonded to medical treatment and was commenced on an ACE inhibitor. However, over the next three years, her LV dilated further with a decline in ejection fraction to 30%. By 39 years she was NYHA class III with a peak VO_2 of 8.3 ml/kg/min (Fig. 7.2). Aged 40 years a biventricular implantable cardioverter-defibrillator was inserted and she agreed to be referred for cardiac transplant but died suddenly while on the waiting list.

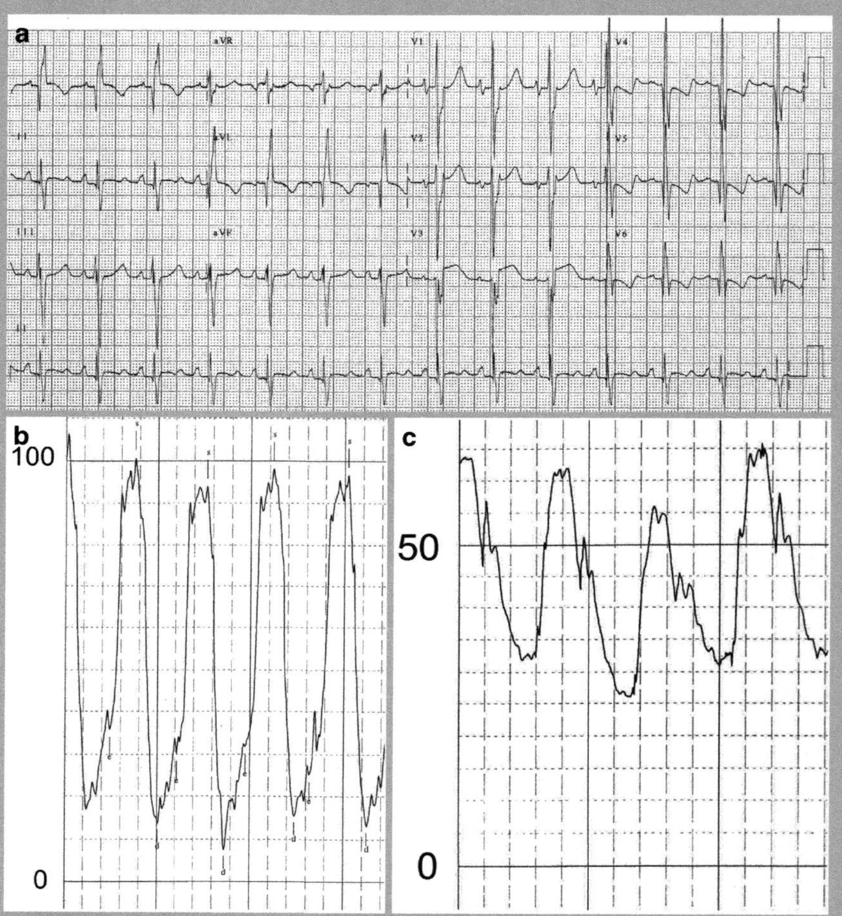

Fig. 7.2 Clinical case report 1: Glycogen storage disease IIIa (GSDIIIa). (**a**) ECG showing a broad QRS complex with increased amplitude and widespread repolarisation changes, suggestive of widespread myocardial disease. (**b**) Left ventricular pressure trace showing low systolic pressure and elevated end diastolic pressure consistent with advanced heart failure. Scale in mmHg. (**c**) Pulmonary artery pressure trace demonstrating elevated pressure caused by left heart failure. Scale in mmHg

Clinical case report 2: Glycogen storage disease IIIa (GSD IIIa)

An 30 year old man presented with breathlessness on walking up hills and going up steps, with associated palpitations. He had been diagnosed with glycogen storage disease type IIIa in childhood. He also reported occasional early morning hypoglycaemia and had proximal skeletal muscle myopathy principally affecting the pelvic girdle.

An ECG showed sinus rhythm with a normal axis and inferolateral T wave inversion with LVH by voltage criteria. A 44-hour rhythm tape showed isolated ventricular ectopics with no significant arrhythmias or pauses. His echocardiogram revealed mild LVH, mainly affecting the anterior septal wall. The MWT was 1.4–1.6 cm in the basal region. Turbulent flow was noted from the apex to mid cavity and to the LVOT with a maximum gradient of 50–60 mmHg at rest (Fig. 7.3). Overall, LV systolic function was good with an ejection fraction estimated at 65–70% but with impaired diastolic function (E/A ratio 0.9).

Age 32 years a pacemaker was inserted. On review age 35 years he reported early morning tiredness and headaches. Medications at this time included Disopyramide 200 mg twice daily, Verapamil 160 mg and 120 mg daily, Aspirin 75 mg daily, Atorvastatin 20 mg daily and Ezetimibe 10 mg daily. Heart sounds were normal, there was a widespread 2/6 systolic murmur, JVP was normal and there were no signs of peripheral or pulmonary oedema. His ECG showed dual-chamber pacing with a ventricular rate of 64 bpm. PR interval was 96 ms, QRS duration 182 ms, QTc 546 ms and QRS axis −89°. His pacemaker check showed a normal pacemaker function within programme parameters. No arrhythmia was identified. He was unable to complete exercise stress testing due to left hip arthritis.

In view of his ongoing symptoms an overnight sleep study was performed. This indicated mild hypercapnia, indicative of respiratory muscle hypoventilation. Overnight non-invasive ventilation (NIV, BiPAP) was commenced. Symptoms improved significantly and 1 year later he remains stable.

The glycogen storage disorders (GSDs)

The GSDs are a group of disorders associated with an inherited defect of glycogen mobilisation or glycogen utilization. Glycogen is a multibranched glucose polymer with a protein core that serves as a form of energy storage. It is stored in all cells but is most abundant in liver and muscle. Liver glycogen maintains blood glucose between meals. Muscle glycogen is the primary source of energy for muscle contraction at the start of exercise. In some disorders, an abnormal form of glycogen, called polyglucosan bodies is stored.

GSDs are generally categorized by the organ or tissue most affected by the underlying defect, namely,

1. disorders affecting mainly muscle (cardiac and skeletal) e.g., GSD II and V.
2. disorders affecting mainly the liver e.g., GSD I, III, VI, and IX.
3. disorders affecting the brain e.g., GSD IV.

Cardiac involvement is a well-known feature in several GSDs and polyglucosan body storage disorders, as summarized in Table 7.2.

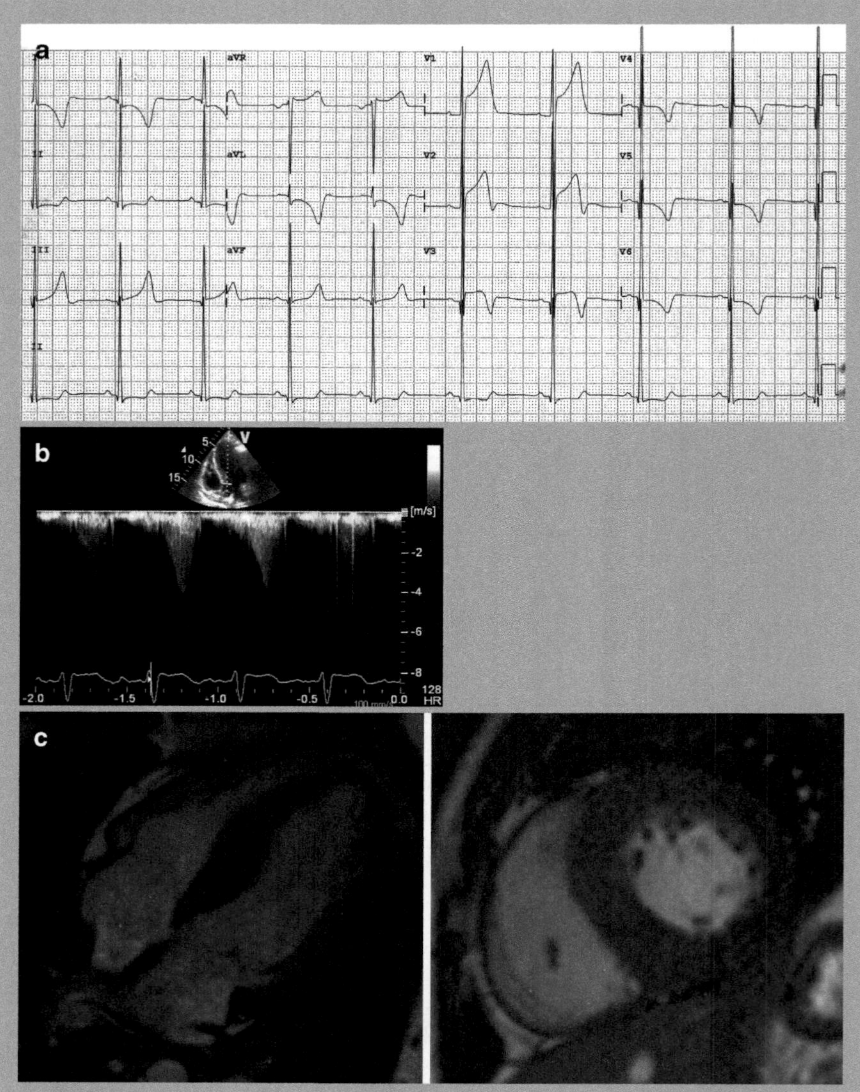

Fig. 7.3 Clinical case report 2: Glycogen storage disease IIIa (GSDIIIa). (**a**) ECG demonstrating changes of widespread left ventricular hypertrophy with very large amplitude QRS complexes throughout, with repolarisation changes. (**b**) Pulse wave Doppler tracing from the apical 5 chamber view showing left ventricular outflow tract obstruction. (**c**) 4 Chamber and short axis MRI images demonstrating concentric left ventricular hypertrophy

Table 7.2 Glycogen storage disorders and polyglucosan body storage disorders associated with cardiac involvement

Disease	Enzyme/protein	Gene (inheritance)	Incidence	Cardiac involvement	Skeletal myopathy	Other supportive clinical features	Diagnostic tests	Treatment options
Glycogen storage disorders								
II (Pompe)	Acid maltase	*GAA* (AR)	1:100,000 (infantile); 1:60,000 (late onset)	Short PR, wide QRS, cardiomegaly, LVOTO	Yes	Hypotonia. Macroglossia. Feeding difficulties	GAA enzyme activity	Enzyme replacement therapy
IIb (Danon)	LAMP-2	*LAMP2* (XL)	NR	Left ventricular hypertrophy. Ventricular preexcitation. Ventricular arrhythmias	Yes	Retinal dystrophy	Immunohistochemistry (biopsy)	Supportive. Cardiac transplant
IIIa (Cori-Forbes)	Glycogen debranching enzyme	*AGL* (AR)	1:100,000	Hypertrophic cardiomyopathy. Cardiac failure. Sudden death	Yes	Hypoglycemia. Hepatomegaly	AGL enzyme activity	Avoid hypoglycemia. High protein diet
V (McArdle)	Myophosphorylase	*PYGM* (AR)	1:100,000	Coronary artery disease	Yes	Exercise intolerance, myalgia, rhabdomyolysis	PYGM mutation analysis. Flat lactate curve on non-ischemic lactate forearm test. (Muscle myophosphorylase activity)	Training to achieve second-wind phenomenon

(continued)

Table 7.2 (continued)

Disease	Enzyme/protein	Gene (inheritance)	Incidence	Cardiac involvement	Skeletal myopathy	Other supportive clinical features	Diagnostic tests	Treatment options
Polyglucosan body storage (PGB) disorders								
PRKAG2	gamma subunit of AMP-kinase	*PRKAG2* (AD)	NR	Ventricular pre-excitation	Yes (rare)	No	Cardiac biopsy	Supportive. Cardiac transplant
RBCK1	RanBP-type and C3HC4-type zinc finger-containing 1	*RBCK1* (AR)	NR	Cardiac failure	Yes	Skeletal myopathy. Autoimmunity. Recurrent infections	Cardiac or skeletal muscle biopsy	Supportive. Cardiac transplant
GYG1	Glycogenin-1	*GYG1* (AR)	NR	(Dilated) cardiomyopathy. Cardiac failure	Yes	Skeletal myopathy	Cardiac or skeletal muscle biopsy	Supportive. Cardiac transplant
GSD IV	Glycogen branching enzyme	*GBE* (AR)	1:600,000–1:800,000	Hypertrophic/dilated cardiomyopathy	Yes (rare)	Hypotonia. Neurologic disease. Liver disease	GBE enzyme activity	Supportive
GSD VII (Tarui)	Phosphofructokinase	*PFKM* (AR)	NR	Valve disease. Hypertrophic cardiomyopathy	Yes	Haemolytic anemia. Exercise intolerance, myalgia, rhabdomyolysis	PFK staining of muscle biopsy	Exercise advice

NR not reported

Table 7.3 "Red-flag" clinical findings which may indicate that cardiovascular disease is secondary to an inherited disorder of metabolism

Red flag	Comment	Disorder
Cardiomyopathy with hypoglycemia	Suggestive of defect in energy production	Fatty acid oxidation defects
		Glycogen storage disorders
Cardiomyopathy with hypotonia (feeding difficulties, respiratory distress)	Suggestive of systemic skeletal muscle disease	Pompe disease
		Mitochondrial disease
		Congenital disorders of glycosylation
Cardiomyopathy with hepatomegaly	Suggestive of a storage disorder	Mucopolysaccharidoses
Cardiomyopathy with dysmorphic features		Mucopolysaccharidoses
		Congenital disorders of glycosylation
Cardiomyopathy with joint contractures/dysostosis		Mucopolysaccharidoses
		Mucolipidoses
Cardiomyopathy presenting after acute metabolic stress	e.g., fasting, fever, intercurrent illness, surgery	Fatty acid oxidation defects
		Propionic acidemia
Hypertrophic cardiomyopathy with ventricular pre-excitation (VPE) or the Wolff–Parkinson–White (WPW) syndrome	Suggestive of a storage disorder	Lysosomal storage disorders
		Glycogen storage disorders
		Mitochondrial disorders

Glycogen storage disease type III

GSDIII (OMIM #232400) is an autosomal recessive condition due to deficiency of glycogen debrancher enzyme, amylo-1,6 glucosidase, and caused by mutations in the *AGL* gene. Two distinct phenotypes exist, IIIa and IIIb. GSDIIIa occurs more frequently (85% of reported cases), causing liver disease and other complications including skeletal myopathy and cardiomyopathy. GSDIIIb is a purely hepatic form.

In patients with GSDIII, during fasting only a limited fraction of glucose stored in the liver as glycogen is readily available for glucose homeostasis. Affected individuals usually present in childhood with hypoglycemia and/or hepatomegaly. Gluconeogenesis and fatty acid oxidation are not impaired and can partially compensate for defects in glycogenolysis.

Diagnosis is usually suspected by findings of hepatomegaly and ketotic hypoglycemia in the setting of elevated serum concentrations of transaminases and creatine kinase in childhood. It can be confirmed by measurement of glycogen debrancher enzyme activity and mutation analysis of the *AGL* gene. Mutations in exon 3 are associated with GSDIIIb, but aside from this there are no clear genotype-phenotype correlations in GSDIII.

Data from an international study on GSDIII describe 175 patients, from 147 families, 91 of whom were followed into adulthood [6]. Cardiac involvement was reported in 58% (87/151), usually first noted in childhood. LVH was most common—found in more than two-thirds of patients on ECG and/or echocardiogram. The remaining patients had other forms of cardiac hypertrophy, including isolated septal, right ventricular or biventricular hypertrophy. Clinically symptomatic cardiomyopathy appeared rare, and the majority of patients seemed to remain stable over time. No patient in this series had a heart transplant.

However, some patients do develop symptomatic disease. A detailed cardiac pathology examination of three patients, from a single centre—one of whom died from sudden cardiac death and another who required cardiac transplantation for end-stage heart failure with severe hypertrophic cardiomyopathy, found evidence of cardiac fibrosis, myocyte vacuolation, and glycogen accumulation in the AV node and smooth muscle of the myocardial arteries [7].

Management

Treatment in childhood includes regular meals, the use of uncooked cornstarch (UCCS, as a source of slow release glucose), higher dietary protein intake to stimulate gluconeogenesis, ± overnight nasogastric feeds to minimise hypoglycemia. Energy and glucose demands fall with age, and not all adults with GSDIII require specific therapy.

There is some evidence that cardiomyopathy can be improved with high-protein diet and avoidance of excessive carbohydrate intake [8].

In common with other women with preexisting cardiac disease, women with GSDIIIa and cardiomyopathy are at risk of cardiac decompensation during pregnancy, and may not be able to adapt to the changes in cardiac and haemodynamic function that are designed to ensure adequate blood supply to the fetus, including increased circulating volume, cardiac output, stroke volume and decreased peripheral resistance and blood pressure. These women therefore need specialist pre-pregnancy counselling, assessment, cardiac surveillance and care throughout pregnancy.

7.2.1 PRKAG2 Syndrome

Figure 7.4 shows typical ECG and cardiac MRI findings from individuals with PRKAG2 mutations. The PRKAG2 gene encodes the gamma 2 subunit of 5′-AMP-activated protein kinase (AMPK), a sensor of cellular energy balance. Mutations of PRKAG2 (OMIM #600858) cause an autosomal dominant disorder characterised by hypertrophic cardiomyopathy, ventricular pre-excitation (VPE) and progressive

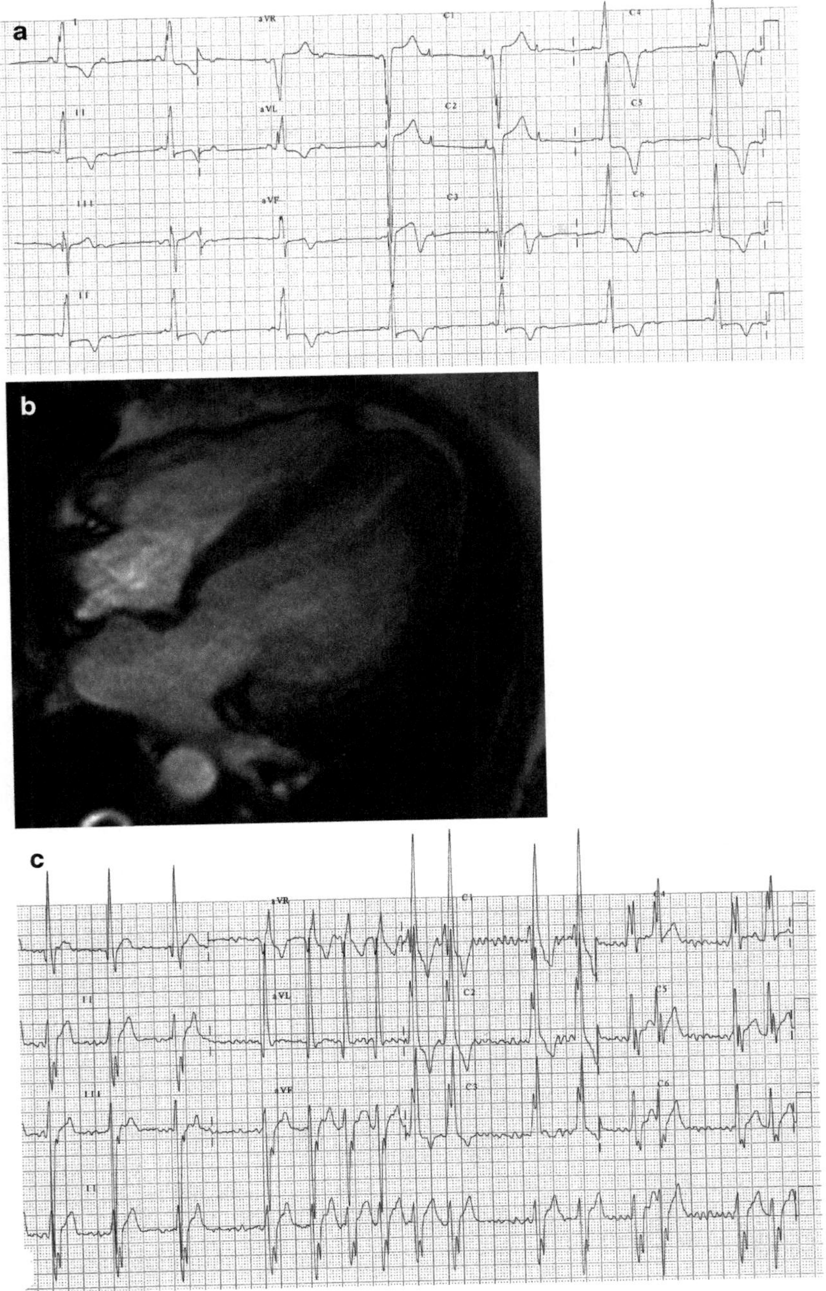

Fig. 7.4 ECG and echocardiogram findings in individuals with a PRKAG2 mutation. (**a**) (*S Patel*) ECG showing 2:1 heart block with atrial abnormalities and changes of left ventricular hypertrophy. (**b**) (Shilpaben Patel) Cardiac MRI 4 chamber view demonstrating left ventricular hypertrophy with an apical distribution. (**c**) (*C Taylor*) ECG with atrial fibrillation, and a broad QRS complex with increased amplitude and left axis deviation. On ECHO this patient had moderate concentric left ventricular hypertrophy with severe impairment of systolic function

heart block [9, 10]. Many patients have isolated cardiac disease, but some also have myopathic symptoms, including myalgia and exercise intolerance.

A short PR interval is common, but the hypertrophy can be variable and includes asymmetric left ventricle hypertrophy, apical hypertrophy or biatrial hypertrophy. A significant proportion of patients progress to severe dilated hypokinetic cardiomyopathy. Endomyocardial biopsy shows non-lysosomal glycogen accumulation.

A common mutation p.Arg302Gln is reported in approximately 50% of cases to date, with the remainder of mutations being largely private. The development of complications (hypertrophic cardiomyopathy [HCM] 61%, VPE 70%, conduction block 22%, by age 40 years) and overall survival rate appear similar between patients carrying the common mutation and others [11].

7.2.2 Management

Patients appear to be at high risk of iatrogenic AV conduction block following ablation procedures, and these should therefore be considered carefully [11]. Pacemaker or defibrillator implantation are reported frequently. A small number of patients have undergone cardiac transplant.

Clinical Case Report 3: Glycogen Storage Disease XV (GSDXV)

A 52-year-old man presented at age 46 years with left-sided weakness [12]. He had a background history of hypertension and dyslipidemia. A right middle cerebral artery infarct was diagnosed. He was treated with thrombolysis and made a good recovery. An echocardiogram at the time showed a thickened interventricular septum (1.3 cm), a mildly dilated LV, and impaired systolic function with an estimated ejection fraction of 40–50%.

There were no other specific medical issues and he remained well until aged 50 years when he developed palpitations, sweatiness and chest pain whilst driving. He was found to have ventricular tachycardia with presyncope and ECG showed sinus rhythm with markedly poor lateral R wave progression (Fig. 7.5). An echocardiogram showed severe left ventricular dilatation. Systolic function was severely impaired with an estimated ejection fraction of 30–35%. There was akinesis of the inferolateral wall and apical lateral wall and hypokinesis of the anterolateral and anterior wall. There was severe left ventricular diastolic dysfunction and moderate left atrial dilatation with mild mitral regurgitation. Left ventricular end diastolic volume was measured at 277 ml, with a posterior wall thickness of 1.0 cm and a septal wall thickness of 1.6 cm. Cardiac MRI confirmed that the left ventricle was severely dilated with a large area of thinning and akinesis affecting the entire lateral wall from base to apex (anterolateral, anterior and inferolateral walls). Other regions were hypertrophied with preserved systolic function. Late enhancement following gadolinium contrast was seen in the entire thinned region.

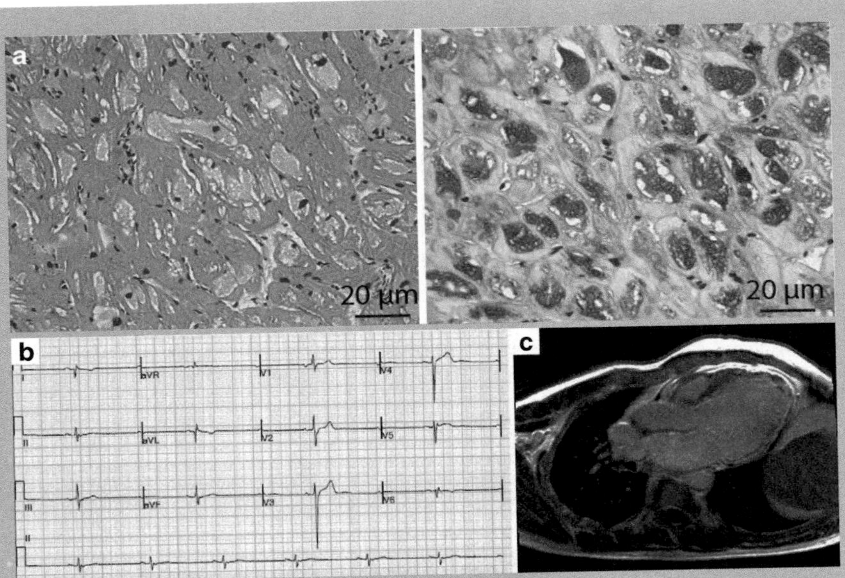

Fig. 7.5 Clinical case report 3: (**a**) Histology, (**b**) ECG and (**c**) MRI findings in an individual with GSDXV; (**a**) An endomyocardial biopsy showed abnormal hypertrophied myocytes with extensive vacuolation replacing most of the cell. There was no evidence of inflammation, no vasculitis and no abnormal infiltrates. PAS-staining was positive with partial removal by diastase. Electron microscopy was not done. (**a-1**) hematoxylin and eosin staining. (**a-2**) the vacuoles show storage of PAS positive material. (**b**) ECG demonstrating sinus rhythm with very poor R wave progression in the lateral leads. (**c**) Cardiac MRI demonstrating a mark- edly dilated left ventricle with thin lateral wall with late gadolinium contrast enhancement

Skeletal muscle strength and an EMG were normal. He did not have hepatomegaly. Blood glucose, lactate, creatine kinase levels, red blood cell and lymphocyte glycogen content were all normal. Genetic testing revealed that he was homozygous for a c.304G > C, p.Asp102His mutation in exon 3 of the *GYG1* gene.

He remained symptomatic with shortness of breath on exertion. A coronary angiogram was normal. An ICD was inserted aged 49 years and a left ventricular assist device aged 51 years. Orthotopic cardiac transplant was performed aged 52 years. Initial post-operative course was complicated by renal impairment requiring haemofiltration. He remains well 1 year post-transplant.

Glycogen storage disease type XV, Glycogenin-1 defects

GSD XV (OMIM #616199) is a rare autosomal recessive disorder caused by mutations in the *GYG1* gene, which encodes the protein glycogenin-1. Most individuals typically present with a late onset skeletal myopathy without cardiomyopathy [13–15]. A few individuals have presented with isolated adult-onset cardiomyopathy, without skeletal muscle involvement [12]. Cellular overload of storage material leading to cell death and secondary fibrosis results in cardiac failure.

Patients with glycogenin-1 deficiency and cardiomyopathy demonstrate extensive late gadolinium enhancement by cardiac MRI. An endomyocardial biopsy will demonstrate glycogen storage, and the diagnosis can be confirmed by *GYG1* gene analysis.

Both normal as well as abnormal glycogen forming amorphous or fibrillar material in the myocardium are seen on biopsy. The accumulated glycogen is partly alpha-amylase resistant and has a partly filamentous structure compatible with amylopectin-like material or polyglucosan bodies. Polyglucosan body storage is also found in other inherited metabolic disorders affecting the heart including deficiency of branching enzyme (GSD IV) and phosphofructokinase (GSD VII), as well as RBCK1 and PRKAG2 defects [16]. These are summarized in Table 7.2.

7.2.3 Pompe Disease (Glycogen Storage Disease Type II)

Pompe disease (OMIM #232300) is a lysosomal storage disorder caused by mutations in the *GAA* gene, resulting in deficiency of the enzyme acid α-glucosidase [17]. Glycogen accumulates in lysosomes resulting in progressive cardiac and skeletal myopathy.

Typically, infants present within the first few months of life, with cardiorespiratory distress, hypotonia and failure to thrive [18]. Without treatment, the condition is rapidly progressive with a median age of death of less than 1 year. Gross hypertrophy of the heart occurs, progressing to left ventricular outflow obstruction. Children may present with congestive cardiac failure due to impaired myocardial relaxation. Enlargement of the heart can also result in diminished lung volumes, atelectasis, and bronchial compression. Progressive deposition of glycogen results in conduction defects, with shortening of the PR interval on ECG. The ECG will also show very large QRS complexes, as well as other features typical of HCM. CXR shows cardiomegaly and sometimes pulmonary oedema. Echocardiogram show severely increased left ventricular mass, usually fairly concentric.

Late-onset Pompe disease in contrast can present at various ages, throughout childhood and adulthood, and is predominantly characterized by skeletal muscle weakness and respiratory insufficiency. Presentation in late childhood to adolescence is typically not associated with heart complications, although some adults with late onset disease have been found to have arteriopathy, with ectasia of the basilar and internal carotid arteries and dilation of the ascending thoracic aorta [19]. Clinically relevant cardiomyopathy is uncommon in late-onset disease and in the occasional adult patient with non-specific cardiac findings, other risk factors such as hypertension, dyslipidemia etc. should be sought [20].

Diagnosis is now frequently done non-invasively by measurement of GAA enzyme activity from dried blood spots. Inheritance is autosomal recessive. Pathogenic variants that introduce mRNA instability, such as nonsense variants, are also more commonly seen in the infantile form as they result in nearly complete absence of GAA enzyme activity. Missense and splicing variants may result in either complete or partial absence of GAA enzyme activity and therefore may be seen in both infant-onset and late-onset Pompe disease.

- Two mutations p.Glu176ArgfsTer45 (c.525delT) and deletion of exon 18 (p.Gly828_Asn882del; c.2482_2646del) are particularly common variants among the Dutch [21]. They result in negligible GAA enzyme activity and are associated with the severe infantile form of the disease.
- c.336-13T>G is seen in 36–90% of cases of late-onset Pompe disease [22, 23]. The variant leads to a leaky splice site resulting in greatly diminished, but not absent, GAA enzyme activity.
- The variant p.Asp645Glu, is found among a high proportion of infant-onset cases in Taiwan and China [24].

7.2.4 Management

Regular intravenous enzyme replacement therapy (ERT) with recombinant GAA (rhGAA) has significantly altered the prognosis of some infants with Pompe disease, with overall survival increasing to about 60%, and ventilator-free survival to 40% [25–27].

Response to ERT in infants depends largely on the child's cross-reactive immunologic material (CRIM) status. CRIM-positive patients produce some protein that is immunologically similar to rhGAA [28]. CRIM-negative children who have infant-onset Pompe disease are likely to have two null variants and produce no protein, or a very truncated GAA [29]. CRIM-negative patients will therefore produce antibodies to ERT that significantly diminish its effectiveness, and may require treatment with additional immunomodulatory therapy in an attempt to mitigate this [30].

In ERT-responsive patients both the septal and posterior wall thicknesses decline rapidly, within weeks [31]. LV size decreases dramatically and the mass-to-volume ratio falls quickly in most patients. With the start of therapy, some patients may experience a decline in indices of systolic function, ejection fraction and the shortening fraction. These improve with ongoing treatment. Left ventricular outflow tract obstruction and symptoms of cardiac failure usually resolve. However, long-term, skeletal and respiratory muscle involvement may not respond so effectively, and significant disability may persist.

7.2.5 Danon Disease

Danon disease (OMIM #300257) is caused by mutations in the lysosome-associated membrane protein-2 (*LAMP2*) gene, a structural protein involved in autophagy [32, 33]. Mutations lead to disruption of intracytoplasmic trafficking and accumulation of autophagic material and glycogen in skeletal and cardiac muscle cells. There are

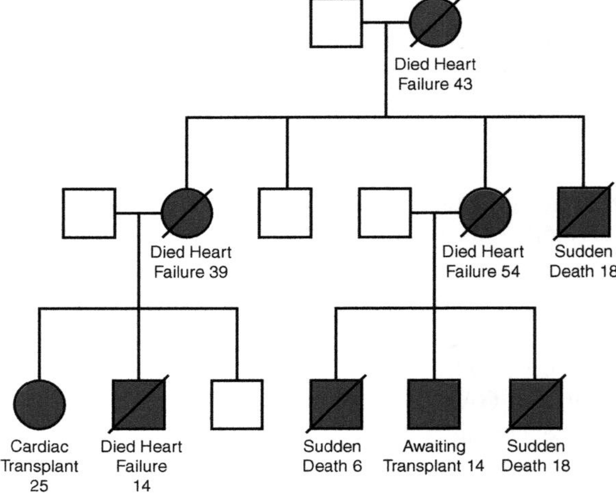

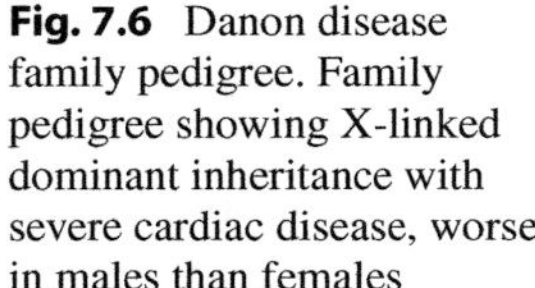

Fig. 7.6 Danon disease family pedigree. Family pedigree showing X-linked dominant inheritance with severe cardiac disease, worse in males than females

three LAMP2 protein isoforms, LAMP-2A, LAMP-2B, and LAMP-2C, which differ only at the carboxy-terminal lysosomal transmembrane domain and at their short cytosolic tail [34]. While LAMP-2A is more ubiquitously expressed, LAMP-2B is expressed at a higher level in the heart, skeletal muscle and brain [35].

The characteristic clinical triad of this X-linked disease is cardiomegaly, proximal muscle weakness and (mild) learning difficulties. Additional features such as retinopathy, pulmonary, gastrointestinal and hepatic disease may also be present [36].

Males tend to present in their teens with symptoms of either skeletal or cardiac myopathy (Fig. 7.6). Cardiomyopathy is progressive and without cardiac transplantation, morbidity, by the age of 25 years, is high [37, 38]. Hypertrophic cardiomyopathy predominates initially, with progressive to dilated cardiomyopathy later in the course of the disease. Atrial and ventricular arrthymias may occur. Cardiac ablation procedures and defibrillator implantation are frequently required. Death may be caused by either cardiac failure or sudden cardiac death.

The most common ECG finding is a Wolff-Parkinson-White syndrome pattern. As WPW is present in nearly 70% of affected males, Danon disease should be excluded in any young male who presents with WPW and cardiomyopathy.

In general, women are less severely affected. The WPW pattern is less frequently seen (27%), and cardiac transplantation is required less often (18%) [36, 37]. Other systemic features also tend to be milder, and less prevalent.

Diagnosis is generally confirmed by genetic testing firstline in those individuals for whom there is a suspicion of the condition. Histology of muscle biopsy typically shows a vacuolar myopathy with small basophilic granules within the myofibers, highlighted with acid phosphatase. Immunohistochemistry reveals LAMP2 protein deficiency.

Genotype-phenotype data indicate that nonsense, frameshift and large deletion/duplication mutations in the *LAMP2* gene are associated with an earlier age of onset. Splicing mutations show a trend towards a later onset, while missense mutations have the latest onset of all mutation types [38, 39]. The exon 7-skipping mutation c.928G > A is the most frequently reported mutation. The vast majority of *LAMP2* mutations affect all three isoforms and to-date isoform-specific mutations have only been reported for the LAMP-2B isoform. These mutations restricted to the LAMP-2B isoform have been reported to cause Danon disease, but with a predominant skeletal muscle weakness.

7.2.5.1 Management

Management includes regular cardiac evaluation, optimising treatment for cardiac failure, with early consideration of ICD implantation for symptomatic arrhythmias. Prompt consideration for cardiac transplantation should be given to patients with progressive symptoms or significant decrease in LVEF.

7.2.6 Disorders of Fatty Acid Metabolism

This group of disorders includes carnitine transport defects, fatty acid oxidation defects and mitochondrial electron transfer defects (see Table 7.1). Mitochondrial fatty acid metabolism (Fig. 7.7) is an important pathway for energy production, particularly during situations of increased metabolic demand such as fasting, febrile illness or exertion. Carnitine transfers long-chain fatty acids as acylcarnitine esters across the inner mitochondrial membrane for β-oxidation, and preserves the cellular CoA homeostasis [40]. Carnitine balance in humans is maintained by dietary sources, endogenous carnitine biosynthesis and efficient renal reabsorption of carnitine.

Most patients with a fatty acid metabolism defect present in childhood, but presentation in adulthood is also recognised. Broadly speaking, earlier onset clinical presentation is associated with more severe, multisystem disease, involving liver, heart and skeletal muscle. Cardiac manifestations include cardiomyopathy, arrhythmias, conduction abnormalities, pericardial effus ion, cardiogenic shock and sudden death. Early-onset cardiomyoapthy is associated with a high mortality. Later–onset disease is more often characterized by exercise-induced muscle pain and weakness, sometimes associated with myoglobinuria and rhabdomyolysis. Cardiac involvement is less prevalent in adult presentations. The majority of heterozygotes are asymptomatic, but some reports of heterozygotes with symptoms have been published.

Tandem mass spectrometric measurement of serum/plasma acylcarnitines is the initial screening test. Definitive diagnosis of fatty acid oxidation disorders is usually made by demonstration of reduced fatty acid oxidation (in cultured fibroblasts) alongside reduced enzyme activity. Histopathological studies of the heart have shown cytoplasmic vacuolation with fatty infiltration [41].

All fatty acid metabolism disorders are autosomal recessively inherited. Increasingly, these genes are included in next-generation sequencing panels for investigation of adults who present with rhabdomyolysis. Prevalent or "common" mutations have been identified in a number of conditions. There is some recognized genotype-phenotype correlation for a number of disorders:

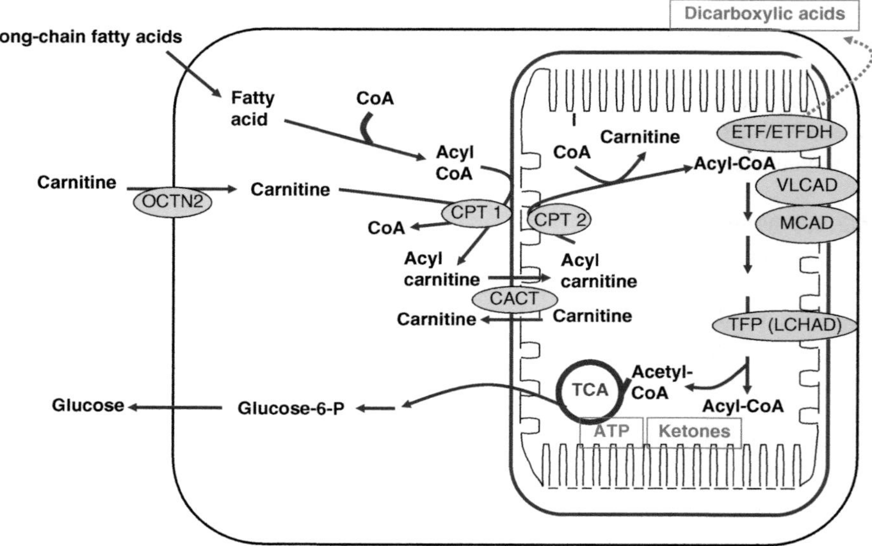

Fig. 7.7 Carnitine transport and fatty acid oxidation. Transfer of carnitine across the cell membrane requires a high-affinity transporter, OCTN2, present in the heart, skeletal muscle and kidney. Long-chain fatty acids are transported across the mitochondrial membrane by a process mediated by acylcarnitine translocase and carnitine palmitoyltransferases 1 and 2. Once inside the mitochondria, the carnitine is recycled to the cytoplasm and the acyl-CoA esters enter the β-oxidation pathway. Each β-oxidation cycle shortens the acyl chain by two carbon atoms and results in the production of one molecule of acetyl-CoA which can then enter the tricarboxylic acid (TCA) cycle ultimately delivering electrons to the mitochondrial respiratory chain to produce energy in the form of ATP or, in the liver, be used to generate ketone bodies

- The homozygous mutation c.95A>G (p.N32S) is associated with a severe genotype and very low levels of free carnitine in individuals from the Faroe Islands [42].
- *CPT2*—the S113L mutation accounts for approximately 60% of mutant alleles in Caucasians with myopathic CPT II deficiency [43]. The P50H mutation is also associated with myopathic disease. These mutations are not associated with cardiac involvement. The following pathogenic variants are associated with the severe infantile hepatocardiomuscular form: p.Tyr120Cys, p.Arg151Gln, p. Asp328Gly, p.Arg382Lys, p.Arg503Cys, p.Tyr628Ser, and p.Arg631Cys. The lethal neonatal form is associated with severe pathogenic variants including p. Lys414ThrfsTer7.
- *ACADVL*—the V243A mutation is associated with mild or asymptomatic disease [44].
- *HADHA*—most Caucasian patients with isolated LCHAD deficiency are homozygous for the G1528C mutation in the *HADHA* gene [45].

7.2.6.1 Management

Carnitine Supplementation

Individuals with primary carnitine deficiency respond well if oral L-carnitine supplementation is started before irreversible organ damage occurs. Doses of 100–400 mg/kg/day, divided in three doses are usually given [46].

Dietary Modifications

A major goal of treatment is to provide a sufficient source of energy, particularly during times of increased demand e.g., intercurrent infection, fever, peri-operatively, during exercise etc. Depending on the disorder, a number of different dietary modifications are suggested and specialist metabolic dietitian support is advised. Most of the evidence for dietary recommendations comes from the paediatric literature and there is little to strongly support regular dietary modifications in newly-presenting adults with for example, myopathic CPT II or VLCAD deficiencies [47, 48] (Fig. 7.8).

In general, prolonged fasting should be avoided in all fatty acid metabolism defects to reduce the risk of acute decompensation. In young children (<1 year) or in those with severe disorders, overnight fasting may need to be avoided, and managed with uncooked cornstarch or continuous overnight pump feeding. Long-chain fat is restricted in patients with severe long-chain FAODs e.g., CPT IA, CACT, CPT II, LCHAD, MTP and VLCAD deficiencies. Replacement medium-chain fats are used as they can enter the mitochondria independently of carnitine and also bypass the long-chain beta oxidation enzymes. Some adults may follow a normal diet when well, but dietary modification (with intravenous dextrose if needed) may be advisable during periods of metabolic stress e.g., intercurrent illness, surgery.

Most adults with CPT II or VLCAD deficiencies, who present with late-onset muscle symptoms only, will follow a normal/low-fat diet with minimal modification when well.

In any patient on a fat-restricted diet consideration should be given to supplementation with essential fatty acids e.g., with walnut, soy or wheatgerm oil.

Supplementation of MCT and carbohydrate 20 min prior to exercise may improve the ability of patients with myopathic long-chain FAODs to exercise [49]. In general exercise is not contraindicated in otherwise well adults with myopathic disease, but they should be advised to take regular rest periods and stay hydrated. Some patients will not be able to tolerate prolonged exercise.

Triheptanoin is an ester of three C7 (odd-chain) fatty acids. Oxidation of triheptanoin generates both propionyl-CoA and acetyl Co-A, and as such is thought to be more effective than conventional MCT in replenishing tricarboxylic acid cycle intermediates. It has been used and recommended in a number of long-chain FAOD, including VLCAD and CPT II deficiencies [50–52].

Many patients with MADD deficiency respond to riboflavin supplementation (usually 100 mg/day) [53, 54].

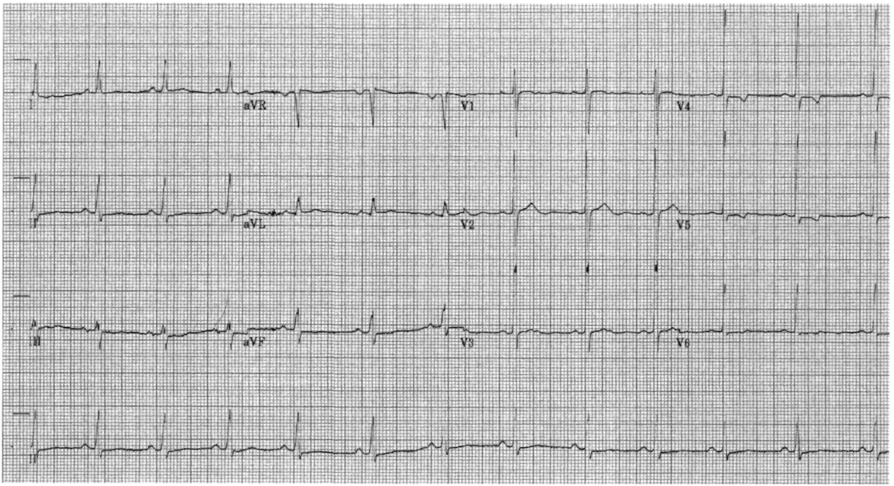

Fig. 7.8 ECG from an individual with very long chain acyl-CoA dehydrogenase (VLCAD) deficiency. ECG showing nonspecific abnormalities of a notched QRS complex and infero-lateral T wave changes

7.2.7 Acute Decompensation

Precipitants of acute decompensation should be avoided/treated promptly if possible e.g., fever, intercurrent illness, prolonged fasting due to surgery or illness, or prolonged physical exertion. Some patients may also experience episodes of decompensation around periods of mental stress e.g., examinations. Symptoms/signs of cardiac involvement should be actively sought during episodes of acute decompensation, particularly in young children.

Patients should have advice regarding starting an appropriate high-carbohydrate oral or intravenous regimen if indicated. The aim is to provide sufficient glucose to stimulate insulin secretion and suppress lipolysis. Hypoglycemia in an adult patient with an FAOD is a late event, and additional glucose should be started without delay, *before* the blood glucose level falls. Essential supplements such as carnitine (in primary carnitine deficiency) or riboflavin (in MADD) should be continued, if necessary by nasogastric tube, particularly in the event of intercurrent illness. In the UK, guidelines for the emergency management of many disorders of fatty acid oxidation are available on the British Inherited Metabolic Disease Group Website at www.BIMDG.org.uk.

Extracorporeal membrane oxygenation (ECMO) has been used in a small number of individuals with decompensated cardiomyopathy, with variable success [55].

Clinical Case Report 4: Propionic Acidemia

A 17 year old male presented with a 6 week history of increasing lethargy and reduced appetite with a severe decompensated cardiomyopathy [56]. He was the eldest child of Pakistani consanguineous parents and had been diagnosed with propionic acidemia (PA) at 18 months of age, having presented with recurrent episodes of ketoacidosis and severe dehydration during intercurrent illness. At 15 years, on routine monitoring, a mild dilated left ventricle, with no haemodynamic consequences was noted.

At this presentation, he was hyperammonemic (ammonia 161 μmol/L). Chest X-Ray showed cardiomegaly. An echocardiogram revealed left ventricle dilation (diastolic left ventricle internal diameter 7.2 cm), mitral regurgitation, apical thrombus, and a shortening fraction of 12%.

A cardiac biopsy was performed which revealed endocardial fibrosis and enlarged mitochondria with atypical cristae on ultrastructural examination. Propionylcarnitine was markedly increased (9.177 nmol/mg, RR: 0.021–0.203) and myocardial CoQ_{10} was markedly decreased (224 pmol/mg, RR: 942–2738).

Treatment from admission consisted of: dietary protein restriction for 5 days, ammonia scavengers, adequate caloric intake, hydroxybutyrate, riboflavin, thiamine, L-carnitine, metronidazole and CoQ10. Inotropic, diuretic and ventilatory support was required. Continuous veno-venous filtration was needed from days 7 to 18. A ventricular assist device (Berlin Heart EXCOR, Berlin Heart AG, Germany) was implanted at day 8. Heart failure slowly improved and the assist device was removed at day 67. He was discharged home at day 95 (shortening fraction 32% at discharge). Medications on discharge included carvedilol 3.125 mg twice daily, spironolactone 25 mg daily, aspirin 75 mg daily and Lisinopril 7.5 mg daily. He remained well for several months.

On follow-up he had ongoing issues with medication compliance. One year after discharge his left ventricular end diastolic measurement was 61 mm (Z-score 5.6) with a fractional shortening of 13%. Two months later, now aged 19 years, this had worsened to LV ED of 69 mm (Z-score 8.6), with an increase in the left atrial area (Z-score 8.7). There was moderate mitral and tricuspid regurgitation, with diastolic dysfunction. There was no pericardial effusion or intracardiac thrombus. The importance of medication adherence was emphasised and carvedilol was increased to 6.25 mg twice daily. Two months after this he re-presented in cardiac failure and was admitted to hospital. Treatment as above was unsuccessful, and he died during this admission.

Propionic acidemia:
The organic acidemia, propionic acidemia (OMIM #606054) is an autosomal recessive condition caused by deficiency of the enzyme propionyl-CoA carboxylase (PCC). PCC is a biotin-dependent enzyme, located in the mitochondrial matrix and involved in the metabolism of propionate, an intermediary metabolite formed from the metabolism of four essential amino acids (methionine, threonine, valine, isoleucine), odd-chain fatty acids and the side chain of cholesterol. Presentation is typically either in the neonatal period with severe ketoacidosis, hyperammonemia, pancytopenia and residual neurological sequelae in survivors or later-onset with recurrent episodes of ketoacidosis triggered by catabolic stress (e.g., fasting, infection or surgery). Treatment includes avoidance of catabolism, adequate calories, reduction in dietary protein intake (to reduce propiogenic precursors), carnitine supplementation and management of acidosis.

Cardiomyopathy has been recognised as a complication of PA since 1993, although there are fewer than 30 reported cases in the literature [56]. The age of diagnosis of PA, degree of metabolic control, or amount of residual enzyme activity do not seem to modify the risk for cardiomyopathy, which has been reported in otherwise well individuals without metabolic decompensation. Cardiomyopathy is most frequently dilated in nature, though hypertrophic disease has also been reported [57]. More than a third of reported patients with cardiomyopathy have died. Figure 7.9 shows ECG and echocardiogram findings in an 10 year old male with cardiomyopathy secondary to PA.

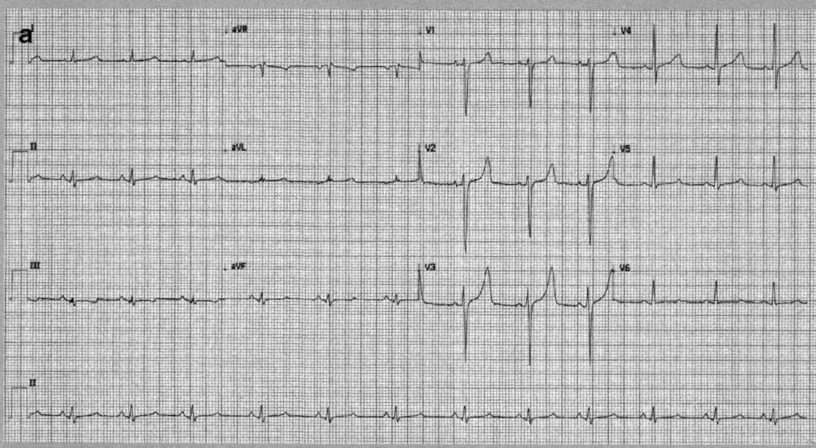

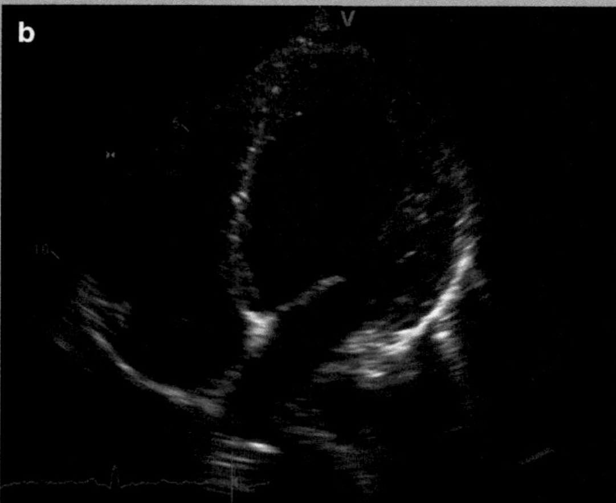

Fig. 7.9 ECG and echocardiogram findings in an individual with propionic acidemia (A Rizvi). (**a**) ECG with reduced QRS amplitude in the limb leads, and infero-lateral T wave changes caused by dilated cardiomyopathy. (**b**) Four chamber image showing left ventricular dilation. Systolic function was severely impaired

The pathogenesis in uncertain but may include direct toxicity of propionyl-carnitine (either acute and/or cumulative long-term) and/or mitochondrial dysfunction (low complex I, III, IV and CoQ10 levels have been reported) [57, 58]. PA-related cardiomyopathy has been reported to be reversible after orthotopic liver transplantation and it has been suggested that liver transplantation could be considered after recovery of cardiac decompensation to prevent further relapses [59–61].

Clinical Case Report X: Mucopolysaccharidosis I (MPS I)(Hurler-Scheie Disease)

A 30 male, diagnosed with an attenuated form of mucopolysaccharidosis type I (MPS I) aged 20 years, presented with increasing breathlessness, and an episode of sudden exertional syncope [62].

An echocardiogram showed thickening of the aortic valve leaflets, with restricted leaflet motion (Fig. 7.10a). He had LVH at the basal septum with a MWT of 1.3 cm. The peak Doppler-derived gradient across the aortic valve was 58 mmHg with a mean gradient of 36 mmHg. Planimetry measurement of the aortic valve area was 0.8 cm^2. CT coronary angiogram was normal.

His other complications of MPS I included: short stature, typical facies, reduced nocturnal oxygen saturation (nadir 60%) and spinal stenosis on MRI (from the cranio-cervical junction to C4/C5) with associated (asymptomatic) cord compression. He had started treatment with enzyme replacement therapy (ERT), laronidase (Aldurazyme®) one year previously.

Following an elective tracheostomy, a transcatheter aortic valve (Edwards Sapien XT 26 mm) (TAV) was inserted under general anaesthesia without complications (Fig. 7.10b). The patient recovered well with resolution of his exertional symptoms.

The mucopolysaccharidososes

The mucopolysaccharidoses (OMIM #252700) are a group of lysosomal storage disorders caused by deficiencies in specific lysosomal enzymes involved in the sequential degradation of glycosaminoglycans (GAGs: dermatan, heparan, keratan and chondroitin sulphates), leading to substrate accumulation in the lysosomes of various cells and tissues, and progressive multi-organ dysfunction. Most patients appear unaffected at birth, but with time develop typical clinical features. Seven disorders (MPS I, II, III, IV, VI, VII and IX), caused by 11 different enzyme deficiencies are described. All, apart from MPS II (X-linked), are autosomal recessive in inheritance. The age at presentation and the severity of phenotype of most disorders is variable but typical

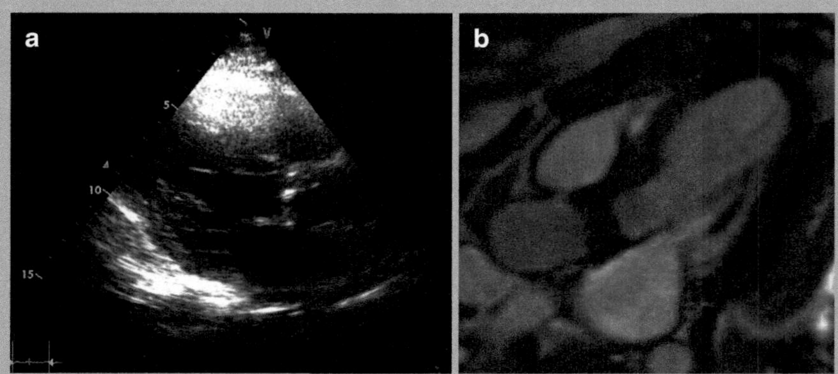

Fig. 7.10 Clinical case report X: Echocardiogram and MRI of an individual with mucopolysaccharidosis I (MPSI) (Z Khan). (**a**) Pre-operative echocardiogram—parasternal long axis image showing diffuse thickening of the aortic valve. (**b**) Post-operative cardiac MRI demonstrating the TAVI in place

complications include: coarse facial features, frequent ear infections and hearing impairment, restrictive pulmonary disease, herniae, hepatosplenomegaly, skeletal and joint involvement (dysostosis multiplex), ocular problems, cardiac disease and (in types I, II, III, VII) intellectual impairment. Those with severe disease present in early childhood, whereas those with attenuated forms may not present until adulthood.

Cardiac problems are reported in all MPS types, and are thought to result from GAG accumulation in the myointima of coronary arteries, myocardium and spongiosa of cardiac valves. This results in cardiac valve thickening, valvular regurgitation and stenosis, and cardiac hypertrophy. Other reported cardiovascular complications include hypertension, heart failure, myocardial infarction, stroke, heart block and sudden death. The prevalence of cardiovascular disease is high, occurring in 60–100% of those with MPS I, II or VI and up to 40% of those with MPS IV [63, 64].

Dermatan sulphate GAGs constitute around 20% of the GAGs in normal heart valves and so cardiac valvular disease is particularly common in those MPS disorders in which dermatan sulphate accumulates, i.e., MPS I, II, and VI (Fig. 7.11). Left-sided valves are more commonly affected and thickening and stiffening of the valve leaflets can lead to mitral and aortic regurgitation and/or stenosis.

Initial cardiac assessment including physical examination, ECG, echocardiogram and Holter monitoring is recommended. Depending on clinical need, this should be repeated every 1–3 years. Bacterial endocarditis prophylaxis is also advised. Treatment options for MPS include hematopoietic stem cell transplantation (MPS I) or ERT (MPS I, II, IVA, VI). Both have been reported to improve cardiomyopathic parameters of disease, but cardiac valve disease

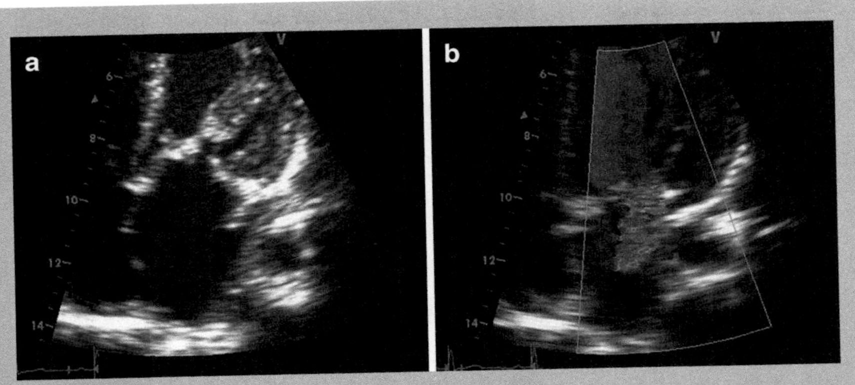

Fig. 7.11 Echocardiogram of an individual with mucopolysaccharidosis VI (MPSVI). Echocardiogram—2d and colour flow mapping images showing diffuse mitral valve thickening with reduced leaflet excursion in systole and moderate regurgitation

appears to be less responsive [65]. Valve replacement may be indicated [66]. Determining timing of surgery may be difficult, as patients with limited mobility may have few symptoms despite significant echocardiogram findings. Most valve replacements to date have been with mechanical valves and the durability of biological valves and TAVI is unknown in this patient group.

Due to the multi-system nature of MPS, operative risks may be higher and involvement of a specialist team is advised with potential airway and intubation issues, spinal cord stenosis, restrictive pulmonary disease, skeletal dysostosis and the short stature of patients to be considered pre-operatively. In addition, valve surgery may be technically difficult due to small, fibrotic valve annuli.

7.2.8 The Mucolipidoses

Figure 7.12 shows an echocardiogram from an individual with mucolipidosis (ML) type III and valve disease. The mucolipidoses combine clinical features of the mucopolysaccharidoses (above) and the sphingolipidoses [67]. Sphingolipids are major components of cellular membranes. Mucolipidosis type II (OMIM #252500) and type III (OMIM #252600) are autosomal recessive conditions caused by deficiency of the enzyme N-acetylglucosamine-1-phosphotransferase, a hexamer (ααββγγ). Mutations in *GNPTAB* (encoding the alpha and beta subunits) cause ML II/III; mutations in *GNPTG* (encoding the gamma subunit) cause ML III. ML II is a more severe phenotype, associated with death in childhood.

Gradual thickening and subsequent insufficiency of the mitral valve and the aortic valve are common from late childhood onward [67–69]. Left and/or right ventricular hypertrophy is often found in older individuals. Pulmonary hypertension may occur in some older individuals. Rapid progression of cardiac disease is rarely

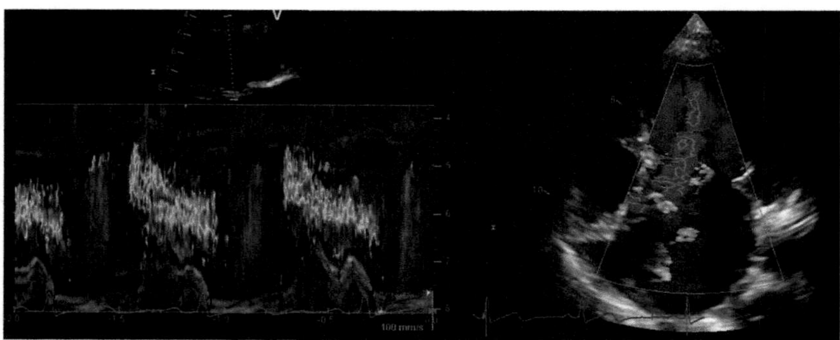

Fig. 7.12 Echocardiogram of an individual with mucolipidosis III. Echocardiogram: M-mode colour flow mapping parasternal long axis view and apical 5 chamber colour flow mapping images showing severe aortic regurgitation

observed in ML III. Cardiorespiratory complications are common causes of death, typically in early to middle adulthood.

Diagnosis is by measurement of the enzyme deficiency in fibroblasts, confirmed by genetic testing. Supportive biochemical findings include increased urinary excretion of oligosaccharides, and that the activity of nearly all lysosomal hydrolases is up to tenfold higher in plasma and other body fluids than in normal controls because of inadequate targeting to lysosomes. Urinary GAGs excretion is normal.

Homozygous and compound heterozygous genotypes that produce no or nearly no functional enzyme activity (caused by premature translation termination and/or frameshift effects) result in the ML II phenotype [70]. Missense mutations, and most of the splice-site variants, that result in up to 10% of residual enzyme activity, cause the more slowly evolving ML III phenotype.

7.2.8.1 Management

Current management options are supportive/symptomatic.

7.2.9 Fabry Disease

Fabry disease (OMIM #301500) is a X-linked lysosomal storage disorder resulting from deficient activity of the enzyme α-galactosidase (α-Gal A) and progressive lysosomal accumulation of globotriaosylceramide (Gb_3) in cells throughout the body [71].

The classic form, occurring in males with less than 1% α-Gal A enzyme activity, usually has its onset in childhood or adolescence with periodic crises of severe pain in the extremities (acroparesthesias), the appearance of vascular cutaneous lesions (angiokeratomas), sweating abnormalities (anhydrosis, hypohydosis, or rarely hyperhidrosis), characteristic corneal and lenticular opacities, and proteinuria.

Gradual deterioration of renal function to end-stage renal disease usually occurs in men in the third to fifth decade. Cardiac and/or cerebrovascular disease, is also a major cause of morbidity and mortality.

Heterozygous females typically have milder symptoms at a later age of onset than males. Rarely, they may be relatively asymptomatic with a normal life span or they may have symptoms as severe as those observed in males with the classic phenotype.

Cardiac involvement in Fabry disease includes a progressive, infiltrative hypertrophic cardiomyopathy with predominantly left ventricular wall-thickening without cavity dilatation, structural changes in the mitral and aortic valves, hypertension, myocardial scarring, progression to heart failure and conduction abnormalities with increased risk of arrhythmias and sudden death. Progressive Gb_3 accumulation and fibrosis are thought to be the major mechanisms underlying these abnormalities.

ECG changes including ST segment changes, T-wave inversion, and dysrhythmias such as a short PR interval and intermittent supraventricular tachycardias may be caused by infiltration of the conduction system (Fig. 7.13). Left ventricular hypertrophy, often associated with hypertrophy of the interventricular septum and appearing similar to hypertrophic cardiomyopathy (HCM), is progressive and occurs earlier in males than females.

Magnetic resonance studies using gadolinium demonstrate late enhancement areas, corresponding to myocardial fibrosis and associated with decreased regional functioning as assessed by strain and strain-rate imaging [72, 73]. T_1 mapping illustrates intramural fat deposition and posterior wall fibrosis [74].

7.2.10 Cardiac Variant Fabry Disease

Men with greater than 1% α-Gal A activity may have a cardiac variant phenotype that usually presents in the sixth to eighth decade with left ventricular hypertrophy, mitral insufficiency and/or cardiomyopathy, and proteinuria, but without significant renal disease. Magnetic resonance imaging of the heart typically shows late enhancement of the posterior wall with gadolinium reflecting posterior wall fibrosis [72]. Clinical manifestations of the cardiac variant of Fabry disease are found in women as well as men.

7.2.10.1 Genotype-Phenotype Correlations

Private mutations are common in families with Fabry disease making prediction of genotype-phenotype associations difficult.

- Affected males with frameshift and nonsense variants typically present with classic Fabry disease; males with missense pathogenic variants can present with either classic or atypical phenotypes [75]. Individuals with later-onset atypical variants (renal, cardiac, or cerebrovascular disease) tend to have missense or splicing mutations that express residual α-Gal A enzyme activity [76].

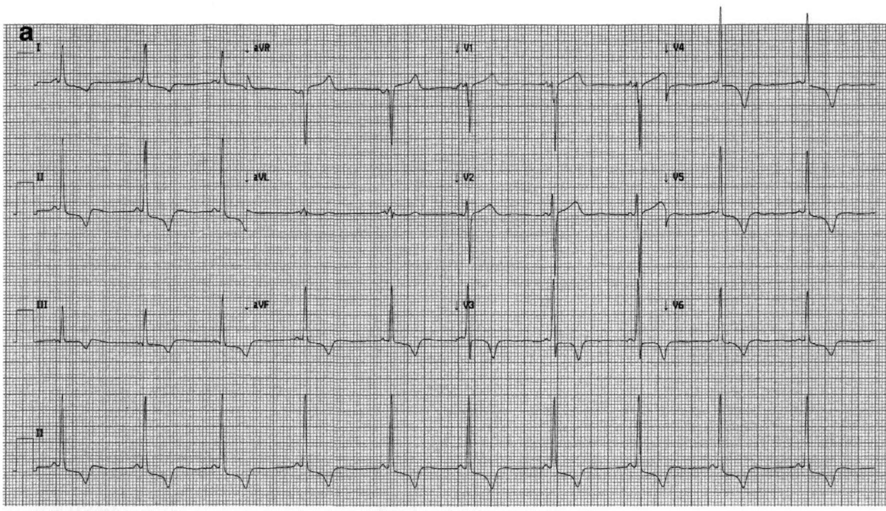

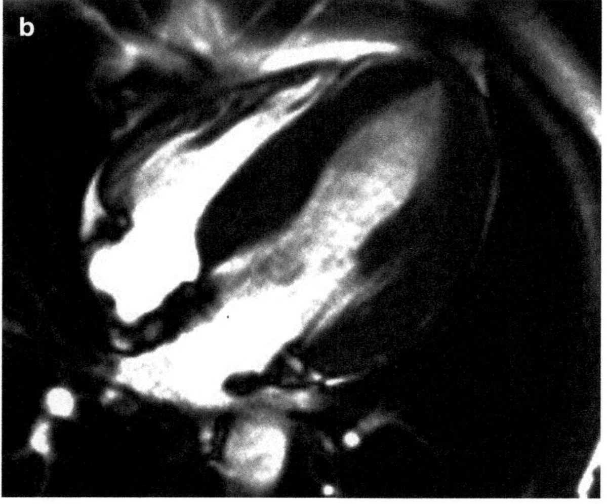

Fig. 7.13 ECG and MRI findings in Fabry disease. (**a**) The ECG shows changes of LV hypertrophy and a short PR interval. (**b**) The cardiac MRI shows concentric left ventricular hypertrophy with diffuse late gadolinium enhancement

- A number of mutations including (p.Arg112His, p.Arg301Gln, and p.Gly328Arg) have been identified in individuals with both the classic phenotype and the cardiac variant phenotype, suggesting that other modifying factors may be involved in disease expression [77].
- Disease manifestations in individuals with the p.Asn215Ser mutation are reported to be less severe than those in age-matched individuals with classic Fabry disease [78].
- Newborn screening in Taiwan has revealed a high prevalence (~1:1600 males) of individuals with the IVS4+919G>A mutation which is associated with late-onset cardiac features [79].

7.2.10.2 Management

There are a number of available licensed treatments for Fabry disease including two intravenous enzyme replacement therapies (agalsidase alfa (Replagal®) and agalsidase beta (Fabrazyme®)) and Migalastat (Galafold®), an orally administered molecule that binds with and refolds the faulty α-Gal A enzyme to restore its activity. This allows it to enter the lysosome and to break down Gb_3.

ERT is reported to slow the progression to LVH, and to reduce or stabilize LVMI in patients with LVH at initiation of treatment, but may not be able to reverse or stabilize cardiac disease in older patients with more severe disease [80–82]. A meta-analysis of effect of ERT on LVM (in which the longest follow-up period was 5.5 years) showed that in men with LVH at baseline ERT stabilizes the increase in LVM. In men without LVH at baseline, LVM showed a slight increase during ERT, but this increase was lower than that in an untreated group [83]. In women with LVH at baseline there was a decrease in LVM with ERT, and stabilization in those without LVH. A 10-year follow-up study of 45 patients on ERT with agalsidase alfa, showed that no patients without LVH at treatment initiation developed LVH, and that no patients with LVH at treatment initiation showed an increase in LVM [81]. At treatment initiation 14 of these individuals had New York Heart Association, NYHA class symptoms ≥II and 11 had anginal symptoms (Canadian Cardiovascular Society, CCS score ≥ 2). Two individuals improved and one worsened their NYHA score, while the others remained stable. All eleven individuals improved their CCS score.

Early data suggests that Migalastat, the oral pharmacological chaperone that stabilises specific mutant (amenable) forms of α-Gal to facilitate normal lysosomal trafficking, may be a viable alternative to intravenous ERT [84].

Although disease-specific evidence is lacking general preventive measures such as weight management, stopping smoking and use of antithrombotic, antihypertensive and lipid-lowering agents are recommended in individuals with symptoms of cardiac ischemia.

7.2.11 Mitochondrial Diseases

Mitochondrial diseases are discussed in detail in Chap. 10, mitochondrial cardiovascular disorders.

7.2.12 Congenital Disorders of Glycosylation

Congenital disorders of glycosylation (CDG) are a group of disorders caused by defects in the synthesis and processing of the glycan moiety of glycoproteins and glycolipids [85]. Glycan chains may be either N-linked (via the "N" atom of a particular amino acid) or O-linked (via the "O" atom of a particular amino acid) to a protein. Glycosylation is essential to result in the unique structure that gives a glycoprotein its distinct structure, solubility and stability, ensuring that the final protein is localized correctly and functionally intact.

CDGs are in general multisystem diseases, most often presenting in childhood, though milder cases have been diagnosed in adulthood. They are divided into four groups: disorders of protein N-glycosylation, O-glycosylation, lipid glycosylation and disorders of other glycosylation pathways and multiple glycosylation pathways. They are named by their gene symbol, followed by –CDG. The majority have involvement of the central nervous system. There is wide clinical variability, but symptoms include psychomotor retardation, ataxia, polyneuropathy, epilepsy, endocrine abnormalities, growth retardation, visual and hearing loss, cardiac, renal, hepatic and gastrointestinal involvement. Both hypertrophic and dilated cardiomyopathy have been described [86–93].

Protein N-glycosylation disorders are the most prevalent and, by far, the most common disorder is PMM2-CDG which typically presents in early childhood with hypotonia, strabismus, inverted nipples, dysmorphic facial features, failure to thrive and cardiac involvement (cardiomyopathy or pericardial effusions). Dilated cardiomyopathy has also been described in patients with ALG6-CDG, DPM3-CDG, and DOLK-CDG.

DOLK-CDG is a disorder with dilated cardiomyopathy with ichthyosiform skin abnormalities and hypotonia, with a highly variable outcome. Children with predominant cardiac involvement, without significant multisystem organ disease have been reported [94]. Several have received a cardiac transplant for symptomatic disease, which may be precipitated by intercurrent infection. Patients with CDG may be at risk of disordered coagulation, the potential for imbalance of the level of both pro- and anticoagulant factors may lead to either bleeding or thrombosis. During catabolic states (e.g., infection, fever) therefore careful attention needs to be given to prevention of bleeding, thrombosis, and stroke like-episodes in those with cardiomyopathy, particularly if surgery is required. Prolonged immobilization and dehydration should also be avoided.

There are characteristic laboratory features which may support a diagnosis of a CDG, including decreased factor IX, XI, AT-III, protein C, protein S, albumin and caeruloplasmin. Liver function tests may be abnormal and there may be associated anemia, thrombocytopenia and endocrine abnormalities. Serum transferrin glycoform analysis by isoelectric focusing or mass spectrometry is used as a simple screening tool for CDG. The activity of the PMM2-CDG (phosphomannomutase) enzyme can be measured directly in leucocytes.

Inheritance is mostly autosomal recessive, sometimes autosomal dominant or (very rarely) in an X-linked pattern. Molecular testing approaches can include single-gene testing, a multi-gene panel, or more comprehensive exome/genome testing.

With regard to PMM2-CDG, three pathogenic variants are common in individuals of European ancestry and may be included on carrier screening panels:

- The pathogenic variant p.Arg141His is found in the compound heterozygous state in approximately 40% of individuals. It is never found in the homozygous state.
- The pathogenic variant p.Phe119Leu is frequently found in northern Europe, where the genotype [p.Arg141His]+[p.Phe119Leu] makes up a majority of all pathogenic variants [95]. This [p.Arg141His]+[p.Phe119Leu] genotype represents the severe end of the clinical spectrum of PMM2-CDG.

- The pathogenic variants p.Val231Met (associated with high early mortality) and p.Pro113Leu are common all over Europe.

Treatment options are limited and largely supportive in nature. No specific treatment is available for PMM2-CDG, but monosaccharide supplementation has been shown to be useful in a number of other CDGs.

7.2.13 Alkaptonuria

Alkaptonuria (OMIM #203500) is caused by deficiency of homogentisate 1,2-dioxygenase, an enzyme involved in tyrosine metabolism. In alkaptonuria, homogentisic acid accumulates, is oxidised to a melanin-like polymer that binds to and damages connective tissue, producing a characteristic dark pigment, ochronosis.

The diagnosis is made about 20% of the time in children under 1 year when the dark urine is noticed in their nappies [96]. HGA in the urine darkens upon standing or exposure to light. The remaining individuals are not usually diagnosed until the third or fourth decade of adulthood. The main presenting complaint is initially of back and later large joint pain, but as the disease progresses it becomes more multisystem, with involvement of the skin, cardiac, and genitourinary systems.

Cardiovascular disease becomes evident in patients in their 50s and 60s. Features include valvular disease and vascular calcification. Pigment deposition, followed by calcification is most common in the aortic valve. In one series of patients over 65 years, 25% had developed aortic sclerosis, 25% aortic stenosis and 25% had undergone a valve replacement [97]. The mitral, tricuspid and pulmonary valves were infrequently affected.

In addition, calcification of the coronary arteries and aorta occurs frequently. Of 40 patients who underwent a CT scan, 65% had significant aortic calcification, with increasing frequency in older age [97].

The diagnosis can be confirmed by measurement of increased HGA excretion in the urine. Mutation analysis of the *HGD* gene is not required to confirm the diagnosis—but a database of known sequence variants is available at http://hgddatabase.vctisr.sk.

7.2.13.1 Management

Routine annual echocardiograms are recommended after age 40 years, or more frequently if clinically indicated, to monitor for aortic valve disease.

Treatment aims to reduce the concentration of HGA. Nitisinone (NTBC; 2-(2-nitro-4-fluromethylbenzoyl)-1,3-cyclohexanedione) is an inhibitor of the tyrosine catabolic pathway, which reduces HGA production [96]. Long term (3 year) reduction of urine and plasma HGA can be achieved with a low dose of nitisinone [98]. It is not yet known whether this will lead to a reduction in clinical progression of the disease, and patient trials are currently underway. Nitisinone causes a rise in plasma tyrosine concentration, which has been associated with eye complications (photophobia, pain, keratopathy) in some patients. A low protein diet is therefore also advised to minimise the elevation in plasma tyrosine.

7.2.14 Homocystinuria

Homocystinuria (HCU, OMIM #236200) is an autosomal recessive condition caused by deficiency of the enzyme cystathione β-synthase, and characterized biochemically by significant elevation of the plasma amino acid, homocysteine (typically >150 μmol/L on diagnosis). Classical clinical manifestations involve the eye, skeleton, central nervous and vascular systems but age of onset and severity vary widely among affected individuals. Based mainly on genotype, a subset of patients respond to pyridoxine (vitamin B6), these patients tend to present later, and with a milder phenotype [99].

Vascular abnormalities, are well recognized in HCU [99, 100]. Most commonly they consist of deep venous thrombosis with/without pulmonary embolism, less frequently stroke (due to sagittal sinus thrombosis or carotid disease), and myocardial infarction. Occlusive vascular disease may result in cognitive decline and is associated with significant morbidity and mortality.

In the large international study of the natural history of HCU, just over a third of patients had suffered a thromboembolic event—with cerebrovascular accidents accounting for a third of these [99]. The chance of having any thromboembolic event was about 25% by age 16 and 50% by age 29 years. Treatment for B6-responsive patients significantly reduced the occurrence of thromboembolism but patients who had an event remained at higher risk for a recurrent episode. Thromboembolism was a causative or contributory factor in nearly 80% of the 64 patients in the study who had died.

158 patients from another multicentre study were followed for 2841 patient-years of treatment [100]. Among the vascular events documented were: cerebrovascular accident, transient ischemic attack, saggital sinus thrombosis, pulmonary embolism, myocardial infarction, deep vein thrombosis and abdominal aortic aneurysm. There was a highly significant (85%) risk reduction in expected vascular events among treated patients. This reduction in risk occurs despite the fact that treatment of HCU often does not result in normal levels of homocysteine and most patients still have hyperhomocysteinuria.

The diagnosis of classic homocystinuria is by measurement of amino acids in plasma, assay of cystathionine β-synthase (CBS) enzyme activity in cultured fibroblasts, or molecular genetic testing of the *CBS* gene.

The two most common *CBS* pathogenic variants, p.Ile278Thr and p.Gly307Ser, are found in exon 8.

- p.Ile278Thr is pan ethnic; overall, it accounts for nearly 25% of all pathogenic variants, including 29% of the variant alleles in the UK and 18% in the US [101] [Moat et al 2004]. Presence of a p.Ile278Thr allele predicts B_6 responsiveness.
- In some populations specific mutations have been repeatedly detected such as the c.919G>A (p.G307S) in the Irish, the c.572C>T (p.T191M) in Spanish, Portuguese and South Americans and the c.1006C>T (p.R336C) in the Qatari population, all causing a severe pyridoxine non-responsive form of disease when inherited in the homozygous state [102–104].

7.2.14.1 Management

The aim of treatment is to reduce total homocysteine levels to at least less than 100 μmol/L and preferably to as close to normal as possible [105]. Adequate B12 and folate should be ensured for all patients (with supplementation if needed).

In those countries where patients are identified by newborn screening then a natural protein restricted diet supplemented by a synthetic methionine-free, cystine-supplemented amino acid mixture is introduced. However, starting a low protein diet is often unpalatable and unacceptable to older children and adult-diagnosed patients and many of these are not on a protein-restricted diet and are treated with medications alone. Betaine is a methyl donor which has been shown to reduce homocysteine by increasing homocysteine methylation via betaine-homocysteine methyltransferase.

Pyridoxine (vitamin B6) is a co-factor .for the enzyme cystathionine beta-synthase that converts homocysteine to cystathionine. Approximately 50% of patients with homocystinuria respond to B6 therapy though responsiveness is not uniform and not all patients will completely normalise their biochemistry [99].

Some clinicians use oral anti-coagulant treatment on a routine basis to further reduce the risk of thrombotic episodes though the long term benefits of this are unproven. Pregnancy is a particular time of risk for a thrombotic event in women with homocystinuria and prophylactic anti-coagulation, continued for the first 6 weeks post-partum, is recommended.

7.2.15 Sitosterolemia

Sitosterolemia (also known as phytosterolemia, OMIM #210250) is a very rare autosomal recessive condition caused by mutations in the *ABCG5* and *ABCG8* genes [106]. It is characterized biochemically by an increased concentration of plant sterols [107].

Clinically patients present with:

- Tendon xanthomas or tuberous xanthomas that can occur in childhood and in unusual locations,
- Premature atherosclerosis (angina, aortic valve involvement, myocardial infarction, and sudden death),
- Hemolytic anemia, abnormally shaped erythrocytes (stomatocytes), and large platelets (macrothrombocytopenia).

Sitosterolemia is likely to be underdiagnosed. Plant sterols are not detected by standard laboratory measurements of cholesterol, and total cholesterol concentration can be variable—ranging from normal to values similar to that seen in homozygous familial hypercholesterolemia. If the diagnosis is suspected then specialist analysis will show elevation of the plant sterols (sitosterol, campesterol, and stigmasterol). Shellfish sterols may also be increased.

Sterolin-1 (encoded by *ABCG5*) and sterolin-2 (encoded by *ABCG8*) form a heterodimer transporter; thus, affected individuals have biallelic pathogenic variants of either *ABCG5* or *ABCG8*. Asians primarily have pathogenic variants in *ABCG5* and whites primarily have pathogenic variants in *ABCG8*.

7.2.15.1 Management

Sitosterolemia does not respond to standard statin treatment. Treatment aims to reduce plasma concentration of plant sterols to as close as possible to normal concentrations (reductions of 10–50% with treatment are reported).

A diet low in shellfish sterols and plant sterols (i.e., avoidance of vegetable oils, margarine, nuts, seeds, avocados, chocolate, and shellfish) is recommended. Margarines and other products containing stanols are contraindicated as they can exacerbate plant stanol accumulation [108]. Dietary advice is usually combined with the sterol absorption inhibitor ezetimibe, and if needed, a bile acid sequestrant such as cholestryramine [109]. Partial or complete ileal bypass surgery has also been shown to reduce sterol levels [110].

7.2.16 Genetic Counselling for Inherited Disorders of Metabolism

The majority of inherited disorders of metabolism are autosomal recessively inherited and so the following risks to other family members apply:

Parents of a proband

- The parents of an affected individual are obligate heterozygotes and therefore carry one mutated allele.

Siblings of a proband

- At conception, each sibling of an affected individual has a 25% chance of being affected, a 50% chance of being a carrier, and a 25% chance of being unaffected and not a carrier.
- Once an at-risk sibling is known to be unaffected, the risk of his/her being a carrier is 2/3.

Offspring of a proband.

- Offspring are obligate heterozygotes (carriers) and therefore carry one mutated allele.

Heterozygotes (carriers) are generally asymptomatic. However, in the case of fatty acid oxidation disorders potential manifesting heterozygotes have been reported [111].

The small number of X-linked disorders include mucopolysaccharidosis type II (Hunter disease), Danon disease and Fabry disease. In MPS II the following risks apply:

Parents of a proband

- The father of an affected male will not have the disease nor will he be a carrier of the pathogenic variant.

- In a family with more than one affected individual, the mother of an affected male may be an obligate carrier. Rarely, some heterozygous females manifest findings of MPS II. This is thought to result from skewed inactivation of the normal paternally inherited X chromosome and expression of the maternally inherited mutated *IDS* allele [112].
- If a woman has more than one affected son and the pathogenic variant cannot be detected in DNA extracted from her leukocytes, she has germline mosaicism.
- If pedigree analysis reveals that the proband is the only affected family member, the mother may be a carrier or the pathogenic variant in the affected male may be de novo, in which case the mother is not a carrier.
- When an affected male is the only affected individual in the family, there are several possibilities regarding his mother's carrier status:
  - He has a de novo pathogenic variant and his mother is not a carrier.
  - His mother has a de novo pathogenic variant either (a) as a "germline mutation" (i.e., present at the time of her conception and therefore in every cell of her body); or (b) as "germline mosaicism" (i.e., present in some of her germ cells only). Germline mosaicism for an *IDS* pathogenic variant has been observed in MPS II [113]. Thus, even if the pathogenic variant has not been identified in leukocyte DNA from the mother, siblings of the proband are still at increased risk of inheriting the pathogenic variant.
  - His mother has a pathogenic variant that she inherited from a maternal female ancestor.

Siblings of a proband

- The risk to siblings depends on the carrier status of the mother.
- If the mother of the proband has the pathogenic variant identified in her son, the chance of transmitting it in each pregnancy is 50%. Male siblings who inherit the pathogenic variant will be affected; female siblings who inherit the pathogenic variant will be carriers.

Offspring of a proband.

- Affected males will pass the pathogenic variant to all of their daughters and none of their sons.

In Danon disease hemizygous men are more severely affected than women, but many women also experience symptoms, including both dilated and hypertrophic cardiomyopathy [37].

For autosomal dominantly inherited conditions, such as cardiomyopathy caused by *PRKAG2* mutations, each child of an individual with a familial mutation has a 50% chance of inheriting the pathogenic variant and therefore being at risk for developing the disease.

7.2.17 Prenatal Testing and Preimplantation Genetic Diagnosis

Once the pathogenic variant has been identified in an affected family member, prenatal testing for a pregnancy at increased risk and preimplantation genetic diagnosis is possible.

References

1. Sanderson S, Green A, Preece MA, Burton H. The incidence of inherited metabolic disorders in the West Midlands, UK. Arch Dis Child. 2006;91(11):896–9.
2. Cox GF. Diagnostic approaches to pediatric cardiomyopathy of metabolic genetic etiologies and their relation to therapy. Prog Pediatr Cardiol. 2007;24(1):15–25.
3. Byers SL, Ficicioglu C. Infant with cardiomyopathy: when to suspect inborn errors of metabolism? World J Cardiol. 2014;6(11):1149–55.
4. Badertscher A, Bauersfeld U, Arbenz U, Baumgartner MR, Schinzel A, Balmer C. Cardiomyopathy in newborns and infants: a broad spectrum of aetiologies and poor prognosis. Acta Paediatr. 2008;97(11):1523–8.
5. Ramachandran R, Wedatilake Y, Coats C, et al. Pregnancy and its management in women with GSD type III—a single centre experience. J Inherit Metab Dis. 2012;35(2):245–51.
6. Sentner CP, Hoogeveen IJ, Weinstein DA, et al. Glycogen storage disease type III: diagnosis, genotype, management, clinical course and outcome. J Inherit Metab Dis. 2016;39(5):697–704.
7. Austin SL, Proia AD, Spencer-Manzon MJ, Butany J, Wechsler SB, Kishnani PS. Cardiac pathology in glycogen storage disease type III. JIMD Rep. 2012;6:65–72.
8. Sentner CP, Caliskan K, Vletter WB, Smit GP. Heart failure due to severe hypertrophic cardiomyopathy reversed by low calorie, high protein dietary adjustments in a glycogen storage disease type IIIa patient. JIMD Rep. 2012;5:13–6.
9. Gollob MH. Glycogen storage disease as a unifying mechanism of disease in the PRKAG2 cardiac syndrome. Biochem Soc Trans. 2003;31(Pt 1):228–31.
10. Gollob MH, Green MS, Tang AS, et al. Identification of a gene responsible for familial Wolff-Parkinson-White syndrome. N Engl J Med. 2001;344(24):1823–31.
11. Thevenon J, Laurent G, Ader F, et al. High prevalence of arrhythmic and myocardial complications in patients with cardiac glycogenosis due to PRKAG2 mutations. Europace. 2017;19(4):651–9.
12. Hedberg-Oldfors C, Glamuzina E, Ruygrok P, et al. Cardiomyopathy as presenting sign of glycogenin-1 deficiency-report of three cases and review of the literature. J Inherit Metab Dis. 2017;40(1):139–49.
13. Colombo I, Pagliarani S, Testolin S, et al. Longitudinal follow-up and muscle MRI pattern of two siblings with polyglucosan body myopathy due to glycogenin-1 mutation. J Neurol Neurosurg Psychiatry. 2016;87(7):797–800.
14. Luo S, Zhu W, Yue D, et al. Muscle pathology and whole-body MRI in a polyglucosan myopathy associated with a novel glycogenin-1 mutation. Neuromuscul Disord. 2015;25(10):780–5.
15. Malfatti E, Nilsson J, Hedberg-Oldfors C, et al. A new muscle glycogen storage disease associated with glycogenin-1 deficiency. Ann Neurol. 2014;76(6):891–8.
16. Oldfors A, DiMauro S. New insights in the field of muscle glycogenoses. Curr Opin Neurol. 2013;26(5):544–53.
17. Hers HG. alpha-Glucosidase deficiency in generalized glycogenstorage disease (Pompe's disease). Biochem J. 1963;86:11–6.
18. Byrne BJ, Kishnani PS, Case LE, et al. Pompe disease: design, methodology, and early findings from the Pompe Registry. Mol Genet Metab. 2011;103(1):1–11.

19. El-Gharbawy AH, Bhat G, Murillo JE, et al. Expanding the clinical spectrum of late-onset Pompe disease: dilated arteriopathy involving the thoracic aorta, a novel vascular phenotype uncovered. Mol Genet Metab. 2011;103(4):362–6.
20. Boentert M, Florian A, Drager B, Young P, Yilmaz A. Pattern and prognostic value of cardiac involvement in patients with late-onset pompe disease: a comprehensive cardiovascular magnetic resonance approach. J Cardiovasc Magn Reson. 2016;18(1):91.
21. Van der Kraan M, Kroos MA, Joosse M, et al. Deletion of exon 18 is a frequent mutation in glycogen storage disease type II. Biochem Biophys Res Commun. 1994;203(3):1535–41.
22. Hermans MM, van Leenen D, Kroos MA, et al. Twenty-two novel mutations in the lysosomal alpha-glucosidase gene (GAA) underscore the genotype-phenotype correlation in glycogen storage disease type II. Hum Mutat. 2004;23(1):47–56.
23. Montalvo AL, Bembi B, Donnarumma M, et al. Mutation profile of the GAA gene in 40 Italian patients with late onset glycogen storage disease type II. Hum Mutat. 2006;27(10):999–1006.
24. Shieh JJ, Lin CY. Frequent mutation in Chinese patients with infantile type of GSD II in Taiwan: evidence for a founder effect. Hum Mutat. 1998;11(4):306–12.
25. Broomfield A, Fletcher J, Davison J, et al. Response of 33 UK patients with infantile-onset Pompe disease to enzyme replacement therapy. J Inherit Metab Dis. 2016;39(2):261–71.
26. Hahn A, Praetorius S, Karabul N, et al. Outcome of patients with classical infantile Pompe disease receiving enzyme replacement therapy in Germany. JIMD Rep. 2015;20:65–75.
27. Kishnani PS, Corzo D, Nicolino M, et al. Recombinant human acid [alpha]-glucosidase: major clinical benefits in infantile-onset Pompe disease. Neurology. 2007;68(2):99–109.
28. Banugaria SG, Prater SN, Ng YK, et al. The impact of antibodies on clinical outcomes in diseases treated with therapeutic protein: lessons learned from infantile Pompe disease. Genet Med. 2011;13(8):729–36.
29. Bali DS, Goldstein JL, Banugaria S, et al. Predicting cross-reactive immunological material (CRIM) status in Pompe disease using GAA mutations: lessons learned from 10 years of clinical laboratory testing experience. Am J Med Genet C Semin Med Genet. 2012;160C(1):40–9.
30. Kishnani PS, Goldenberg PC, DeArmey SL, et al. Cross-reactive immunologic material status affects treatment outcomes in Pompe disease infants. Mol Genet Metab. 2010;99(1):26–33.
31. Levine JC, Kishnani PS, Chen YT, Herlong JR, Li JS. Cardiac remodeling after enzyme replacement therapy with acid alpha-glucosidase for infants with Pompe disease. Pediatr Cardiol. 2008;29(6):1033–42.
32. Danon MJ, SJ O, DiMauro S, et al. Lysosomal glycogen storage disease with normal acid maltase. Neurology. 1981;31(1):51–7.
33. Nishino I, Fu J, Tanji K, et al. Primary LAMP-2 deficiency causes X-linked vacuolar cardiomyopathy and myopathy (Danon disease). Nature. 2000;406(6798):906–10.
34. Majer F, Pelak O, Kalina T, et al. Mosaic tissue distribution of the tandem duplication of LAMP2 exons 4 and 5 demonstrates the limits of Danon disease cellular and molecular diagnostics. J Inherit Metab Dis. 2014;37(1):117–24.
35. Konecki DS, Foetisch K, Zimmer KP, Schlotter M, Lichter-Konecki U. An alternatively spliced form of the human lysosome-associated membrane protein-2 gene is expressed in a tissue-specific manner. Biochem Biophys Res Commun. 1995;215(2):757–67.
36. Sugie K, Yamamoto A, Murayama K, et al. Clinicopathological features of genetically confirmed Danon disease. Neurology. 2002;58(12):1773–8.
37. Boucek D, Jirikowic J, Taylor M. Natural history of Danon disease. Genet Med. 2011;13(6):563–8.
38. D'Souza RS, Levandowski C, Slavov D, et al. Danon disease: clinical features, evaluation, and management. Circ Heart Fail. 2014;7(5):843–9.
39. van der Kooi AJ, van Langen IM, Aronica E, et al. Extension of the clinical spectrum of Danon disease. Neurology. 2008;70(16):1358–9.
40. Rebouche CJ. Kinetics, pharmacokinetics, and regulation of L-carnitine and acetyl-L-carnitine metabolism. Ann N Y Acad Sci. 2004;1033:30–41.

41. Singla M, Guzman G, Griffin AJ, Bharati S. Cardiomyopathy in multiple Acyl-CoA dehydrogenase deficiency: a clinico-pathological correlation and review of literature. Pediatr Cardiol. 2008;29(2):446–51.
42. Rasmussen J, Nielsen OW, Janzen N, et al. Carnitine levels in 26,462 individuals from the nationwide screening program for primary carnitine deficiency in the Faroe Islands. J Inherit Metab Dis. 2014;37(2):215–22.
43. Carnitine WT, Palmitoyltransferase II. Deficiency. In: Pagon RA, Adam MP, Ardinger HH, et al., editors. GeneReviews(R). Seattle, WA: University of Washington; 1993.
44. Goetzman ES, Wang Y, He M, Mohsen AW, Ninness BK, Vockley J. Expression and characterization of mutations in human very long-chain acyl-CoA dehydrogenase using a prokaryotic system. Mol Genet Metab. 2007;91(2):138–47.
45. IJ L, Ruiter JP, Hoovers JM, Jakobs ME, Wanders RJ. Common missense mutation G1528C in long-chain 3-hydroxyacyl-CoA dehydrogenase deficiency. Characterization and expression of the mutant protein, mutation analysis on genomic DNA and chromosomal localization of the mitochondrial trifunctional protein alpha subunit gene. J Clin Invest. 1996;98(4):1028–33.
46. Magoulas PL, El-Hattab AW. Systemic primary carnitine deficiency: an overview of clinical manifestations, diagnosis, and management. Orphanet J Rare Dis. 2012;7:68.
47. Spiekerkoetter U, Lindner M, Santer R, et al. Treatment recommendations in long-chain fatty acid oxidation defects: consensus from a workshop. J Inherit Metab Dis. 2009;32(4):498–505.
48. Spiekerkoetter U, Lindner M, Santer R, et al. Management and outcome in 75 individuals with long-chain fatty acid oxidation defects: results from a workshop. J Inherit Metab Dis. 2009;32(4):488–97.
49. Gillingham MB, Scott B, Elliott D, Harding CO. Metabolic control during exercise with and without medium-chain triglycerides (MCT) in children with long-chain 3-hydroxy acyl-CoA dehydrogenase (LCHAD) or trifunctional protein (TFP) deficiency. Mol Genet Metab. 2006;89(1–2):58–63.
50. Roe CR, Sweetman L, Roe DS, David F, Brunengraber H. Treatment of cardiomyopathy and rhabdomyolysis in long-chain fat oxidation disorders using an anaplerotic odd-chain triglyceride. J Clin Invest. 2002;110(2):259–69.
51. Roe CR, Yang BZ, Brunengraber H, Roe DS, Wallace M, Garritson BK. Carnitine palmitoyltransferase II deficiency: successful anaplerotic diet therapy. Neurology. 2008;71(4): 260–4.
52. Vockley J, Burton B, Berry GT, et al. UX007 for the treatment of long chain-fatty acid oxidation disorders: safety and efficacy in children and adults following 24weeks of treatment. Mol Genet Metab. 2017;120(4):370–7.
53. Olsen RK, Olpin SE, Andresen BS, et al. ETFDH mutations as a major cause of riboflavin-responsive multiple acyl-CoA dehydrogenation deficiency. Brain J Neurol. 2007;130(Pt 8):2045–54.
54. Grunert SC. Clinical and genetical heterogeneity of late-onset multiple acyl-coenzyme A dehydrogenase deficiency. Orphanet J Rare Dis. 2014;9:117.
55. Katz S, Landau Y, Pode-Shakked B, et al. Cardiac failure in very long chain acyl-CoA dehydrogenase deficiency requiring extracorporeal membrane oxygenation (ECMO) treatment: a case report and review of the literature. Mol Genet Metab Rep. 2017;10:5–7.
56. Baruteau J, Hargreaves I, Krywawych S, et al. Successful reversal of propionic acidaemia associated cardiomyopathy: evidence for low myocardial coenzyme Q10 status and secondary mitochondrial dysfunction as an underlying pathophysiological mechanism. Mitochondrion. 2014;17:150–6.
57. Mardach R, Verity MA, Cederbaum SD. Clinical, pathological, and biochemical studies in a patient with propionic acidemia and fatal cardiomyopathy. Mol Genet Metab. 2005;85(4):286–90.
58. de Keyzer Y, Valayannopoulos V, Benoist JF, et al. Multiple OXPHOS deficiency in the liver, kidney, heart, and skeletal muscle of patients with methylmalonic aciduria and propionic aciduria. Pediatr Res. 2009;66(1):91–5.

59. Ameloot K, Vlasselaers D, Dupont M, et al. Left ventricular assist device as bridge to liver transplantation in a patient with propionic acidemia and cardiogenic shock. J Pediatr. 2011;158(5):866–7. Author reply 867.
60. Romano S, Valayannopoulos V, Touati G, et al. Cardiomyopathies in propionic aciduria are reversible after liver transplantation. J Pediatr. 2010;156(1):128–34.
61. Sato S, Kasahara M, Fukuda A, et al. Liver transplantation in a patient with propionic acidemia requiring extra corporeal membrane oxygenation during severe metabolic decompensation. Pediatr Transplant. 2009;13(6):790–3.
62. Felice T, Murphy E, Mullen MJ, Elliott PM. Management of aortic stenosis in mucopolysaccharidosis type I. Int J Cardiol. 2014;172(3):e430–1.
63. Braunlin E, Wang R. Cardiac issues in adults with the mucopolysaccharidoses: current knowledge and emerging needs. Heart. 2016;102(16):1257–62.
64. Braunlin EA, Harmatz PR, Scarpa M, et al. Cardiac disease in patients with mucopolysaccharidosis: presentation, diagnosis and management. J Inherit Metab Dis. 2011;34(6):1183–97.
65. Lin HY, Chuang CK, Chen MR, et al. Cardiac structure and function and effects of enzyme replacement therapy in patients with mucopolysaccharidoses I, II, IVA and VI. Mol Genet Metab. 2016;117(4):431–7.
66. Rocha RV, Alvarez RJ, Bermudez CA. Valve surgery in a mucopolysaccharidosis type I patient: early prosthetic valve endocarditis. Eur J Cardiothorac Surg. 2012;41(2):448–9.
67. Cathey SS, Leroy JG, Wood T, et al. Phenotype and genotype in mucolipidoses II and III alpha/beta: a study of 61 probands. J Med Genet. 2010;47(1):38–48.
68. Steet RA, Hullin R, Kudo M, et al. A splicing mutation in the alpha/beta GlcNAc-1-phosphotransferase gene results in an adult onset form of mucolipidosis III associated with sensory neuropathy and cardiomyopathy. Am J Med Genet A. 2005;132A(4):369–75.
69. Leroy JG, Cathey SS, Friez MJ. Mucolipidosis III Alpha/Beta. In: Pagon RA, Adam MP, Ardinger HH, et al., editors. GeneReviews(R). Seattle, WA: University of Washington; 1993.
70. Tappino B, Chuzhanova NA, Regis S, et al. Molecular characterization of 22 novel UDP-N-acetylglucosamine-1-phosphate transferase alpha- and beta-subunit (GNPTAB) gene mutations causing mucolipidosis types IIalpha/beta and IIIalpha/beta in 46 patients. Hum Mutat. 2009;30(11):E956–73.
71. Mehta A, Hughes DA. Fabry disease. In: Pagon RA, Adam MP, Ardinger HH, et al., editors. GeneReviews(R). Seattle, WA: University of Washington; 1993.
72. Moon JC, Sachdev B, Elkington AG, et al. Gadolinium enhanced cardiovascular magnetic resonance in Anderson-Fabry disease. Evidence for a disease specific abnormality of the myocardial interstitium. Eur Heart J. 2003;24(23):2151–5.
73. Weidemann F, Breunig F, Beer M, et al. The variation of morphological and functional cardiac manifestation in Fabry disease: potential implications for the time course of the disease. Eur Heart J. 2005;26(12):1221–7.
74. Sado DM, White SK, Piechnik SK, et al. Identification and assessment of Anderson-Fabry disease by cardiovascular magnetic resonance noncontrast myocardial T1 mapping. Circ Cardiovasc Imaging. 2013;6(3):392–8.
75. Pan X, Ouyang Y, Wang Z, et al. Genotype: a crucial but not unique factor affecting the clinical phenotypes in Fabry disease. PLoS One. 2016;11(8):e0161330.
76. Rolfs A, Bottcher T, Zschiesche M, et al. Prevalence of Fabry disease in patients with cryptogenic stroke: a prospective study. Lancet. 2005;366(9499):1794–6.
77. Ashton-Prolla P, Tong B, Shabbeer J, Astrin KH, Eng CM, Desnick RJ. Fabry disease: twenty-two novel mutations in the alpha-galactosidase A gene and genotype/phenotype correlations in severely and mildly affected hemizygotes and heterozygotes. J Investig Med. 2000;48(4):227–35.
78. Schaefer E, Mehta A, Gal A. Genotype and phenotype in Fabry disease: analysis of the Fabry Outcome Survey. Acta Paediatr Suppl. 2005;94(447):87–92. Discussion 79.
79. Lin HY, Chong KW, Hsu JH, et al. High incidence of the cardiac variant of Fabry disease revealed by newborn screening in the Taiwan Chinese population. Circ Cardiovasc Genet. 2009;2(5):450–6.

80. Kampmann C, Linhart A, Devereux RB, Schiffmann R. Effect of agalsidase alfa replacement therapy on Fabry disease-related hypertrophic cardiomyopathy: a 12- to 36-month, retrospective, blinded echocardiographic pooled analysis. Clin Ther. 2009;31(9):1966–76.
81. Kampmann C, Perrin A, Beck M. Effectiveness of agalsidase alfa enzyme replacement in Fabry disease: cardiac outcomes after 10 years' treatment. Orphanet J Rare Dis. 2015;10:125.
82. Weidemann F, Breunig F, Beer M, et al. Improvement of cardiac function during enzyme replacement therapy in patients with Fabry disease: a prospective strain rate imaging study. Circulation. 2003;108(11):1299–301.
83. Rombach SM, Smid BE, Linthorst GE, Dijkgraaf MG, Hollak CE. Natural course of Fabry disease and the effectiveness of enzyme replacement therapy: a systematic review and meta-analysis: effectiveness of ERT in different disease stages. J Inherit Metab Dis. 2014;37(3):341–52.
84. Hughes DA, Nicholls K, Shankar SP, et al. Oral pharmacological chaperone migalastat compared with enzyme replacement therapy in Fabry disease: 18-month results from the randomised phase III ATTRACT study. J Med Genet. 2017;54(4):288–96.
85. Scott K, Gadomski T, Kozicz T, Morava E. Congenital disorders of glycosylation: new defects and still counting. J Inherit Metab Dis. 2014;37(4):609–17.
86. Clayton PT, Winchester BG, Keir G. Hypertrophic obstructive cardiomyopathy in a neonate with the carbohydrate-deficient glycoprotein syndrome. J Inherit Metab Dis. 1992;15(6):857–61.
87. Garcia Silva MT, de Castro J, Stibler H, et al. Prenatal hypertrophic cardiomyopathy and pericardial effusion in carbohydrate-deficient glycoprotein syndrome. J Inherit Metab Dis. 1996;19(2):257–9.
88. Malhotra A, Pateman A, Chalmers R, Coman D, Menahem S. Prenatal cardiac ultrasound finding in congenital disorder of glycosylation type 1a. Fetal Diagn Ther. 2009;25(1):54–7.
89. Footitt EJ, Karimova A, Burch M, et al. Cardiomyopathy in the congenital disorders of glycosylation (CDG): a case of late presentation and literature review. J Inherit Metab Dis. 2009;32(Suppl 1):S313–9.
90. Marquardt T, Hulskamp G, Gehrmann J, Debus V, Harms E, Kehl HG. Severe transient myocardial ischaemia caused by hypertrophic cardiomyopathy in a patient with congenital disorder of glycosylation type Ia. Eur J Pediatr. 2002;161(10):524–7.
91. Kranz C, Jungeblut C, Denecke J, et al. A defect in dolichol phosphate biosynthesis causes a new inherited disorder with death in early infancy. Am J Hum Genet. 2007;80(3):433–40.
92. Al-Owain M, Mohamed S, Kaya N, Zagal A, Matthijs G, Jaeken J. A novel mutation and first report of dilated cardiomyopathy in ALG6-CDG (CDG-Ic): a case report. Orphanet J Rare Dis. 2010;5:7.
93. Lefeber DJ, Schonberger J, Morava E, et al. Deficiency of Dol-P-Man synthase subunit DPM3 bridges the congenital disorders of glycosylation with the dystroglycanopathies. Am J Hum Genet. 2009;85(1):76–86.
94. Kapusta L, Zucker N, Frenckel G, et al. From discrete dilated cardiomyopathy to successful cardiac transplantation in congenital disorders of glycosylation due to dolichol kinase deficiency (DK1-CDG). Heart Fail Rev. 2013;18(2):187–96.
95. Jaeken J, Matthijs G. Congenital disorders of glycosylation. Annu Rev Genomics Hum Genet. 2001;2:129–51.
96. Phornphutkul C, Introne WJ, Perry MB, et al. Natural history of alkaptonuria. N Engl J Med. 2002;347(26):2111–21.
97. Hannoush H, Introne WJ, Chen MY, et al. Aortic stenosis and vascular calcifications in alkaptonuria. Mol Genet Metab. 2012;105(2):198–202.
98. Introne WJ, Perry MB, Troendle J, et al. A 3-year randomized therapeutic trial of nitisinone in alkaptonuria. Mol Genet Metab. 2011;103(4):307–14.
99. Mudd SH, Skovby F, Levy HL, et al. The natural history of homocystinuria due to cystathionine beta-synthase deficiency. Am J Hum Genet. 1985;37(1):1–31.
100. Yap S, Boers GH, Wilcken B, et al. Vascular outcome in patients with homocystinuria due to cystathionine beta-synthase deficiency treated chronically: a multicenter observational study. Arterioscler Thromb Vasc Biol. 2001;21(12):2080–5.

101. Moat SJ, Bao L, Fowler B, Bonham JR, Walter JH, Kraus JP. The molecular basis of cystathionine beta-synthase (CBS) deficiency in UK and US patients with homocystinuria. Hum Mutat. 2004;23(2):206.
102. Cozar M, Urreizti R, Vilarinho L, et al. Identification and functional analyses of CBS alleles in Spanish and Argentinian homocystinuric patients. Hum Mutat. 2011;32(7):835–42.
103. Alcaide P, Krijt J, Ruiz-Sala P, et al. Enzymatic diagnosis of homocystinuria by determination of cystathionine-ss-synthase activity in plasma using LC-MS/MS. Clin Chim Acta. 2015;438:261–5.
104. Gan-Schreier H, Kebbewar M, Fang-Hoffmann J, et al. Newborn population screening for classic homocystinuria by determination of total homocysteine from Guthrie cards. J Pediatr. 2010;156(3):427–32.
105. Morris AA, Kozich V, Santra S, et al. Guidelines for the diagnosis and management of cystathionine beta-synthase deficiency. J Inherit Metab Dis. 2017;40(1):49–74.
106. Berge KE, Tian H, Graf GA, et al. Accumulation of dietary cholesterol in sitosterolemia caused by mutations in adjacent ABC transporters. Science. 2000;290(5497):1771–5.
107. Bhattacharyya AK, Connor WE. Beta-sitosterolemia and xanthomatosis. A newly described lipid storage disease in two sisters. J Clin Invest. 1974;53(4):1033–43.
108. Connor WE, Lin DS, Pappu AS, Frohlich J, Gerhard G. Dietary sitostanol and campestanol: accumulation in the blood of humans with sitosterolemia and xanthomatosis and in rat tissues. Lipids. 2005;40(9):919–23.
109. Salen G, von Bergmann K, Lutjohann D, et al. Ezetimibe effectively reduces plasma plant sterols in patients with sitosterolemia. Circulation. 2004;109(8):966–71.
110. Nguyen LB, Shefer S, Salen G, Tint SG, Batta AK. Competitive inhibition of hepatic sterol 27-hydroxylase by sitosterol: decreased activity in sitosterolemia. Proc Assoc Am Physicians. 1998;110(1):32–9.
111. Anichini A, Fanin M, Vianey-Saban C, et al. Genotype-phenotype correlations in a large series of patients with muscle type CPT II deficiency. Neurol Res. 2011;33(1):24–32.
112. Jurecka A, Krumina Z, Zuber Z, et al. Mucopolysaccharidosis type II in females and response to enzyme replacement therapy. Am J Med Genet A. 2012;158A(2):450–4.
113. Froissart R, Da Silva IM, Maire I. Mucopolysaccharidosis type II: an update on mutation spectrum. Acta Paediatr. 2007;96(455):71–7.

Mitochondrial Cardiovascular Diseases

8

Michael J. Keogh, Hannah E. Steele, and Patrick F. Chinnery

Abstract

Primary disorders of mitochondrial dysfunction due to mutations in nuclear genes or mitochondrial DNA can present with cardiac phenotypes, either in isolation or within the context of a multi-system mitochondrial encephalomyopathy. Hypertrophic cardiomyopathy and conduction defects are common, but other cardiac manifestations have been described. A systematic approach to the biochemical and/or genetic evaluation of these patients will usually identify the underlying cause, enabling genetic counseling and supportive management of both the cardiac and extra-cardiac features.

Keywords

Mitochondria • Mitochondrial encephalomyopathy • mtDNA • Metabolic cardiomyopathy • Hypertrophic cardiomyopathy • Conduction defect • Kearns-Sayer syndrome • Barth syndrome

M.J. Keogh
Department of Clinical Neuroscience, Cambridge Biomedical Campus, Cambridge, Cambridgeshire, UK
e-mail: mjk72@cam.ac.uk

H.E. Steele
Neurology Department, The Newcastle Upon Tyne Hospitals NHS Trust, Institute of Genetic Medicine, Newcastle University, Newcastle Upon Tyne, Tyne and Wear, UK
e-mail: Hannah.Steele@ncl.ac.uk

P.F. Chinnery (✉)
Department of Clinical Neurosciences, Addenbrooke's Hospital, University of Cambridge, Cambridge Biomedical Campus, Cambridge, UK
e-mail: pfc25@medschl.cam.ac.uk

D. Kumar, P. Elliott (eds.), *Cardiovascular Genetics and Genomics*,
https://doi.org/10.1007/978-3-319-66114-8_8

8.1 General Introduction

The myocardium and the cardiac conduction system are highly energy dependent. Mitochondria are the principal source of intracellular energy, in the form of adenosine triphosphate (ATP), so it comes as no surprise that mitochondrial dysfunction can lead to cardiovascular disease. Mitochondrial mechanisms have been implicated in most common cardiac disorders, from ischaemic heart disease through to idiopathic dilated cardiomyopathy. However, this chapter will focus on genetic disorders of mitochondrial function that cause cardiovascular disease. Although isolated cardiomyopathy or hypertension have been described in patients with genetically-determined mitochondrial dysfunction, in most instances, the cardiovascular features are part of a multisystem disorder affecting other organs and tissues that are dependent on oxidative metabolism. When taken together, cardiac abnormalities affect up to 65% of patients with primary mitochondrial disorders [1]. This equates to a population prevalence of cardiac dysfunction secondary to a mitochondrial disease of ~1/10,000 [2], therefore affecting ~6500 individuals in the UK, and ~30,000 in the USA.

8.2 Mitochondrial Biology and the Genetic Basis of Mitochondrial Disease

Mitochondria are subcellular organelles composed of ~1500 proteins and are found in all nucleated mammalian cells. Mitochondria have several functions, including calcium signaling, and a role in apoptosis, but a key role is their involvement in metabolism, cellular respiration, and the generation of ATP. This is achieved by a group of proteins assembled into five multimeric complexes on the inner mitochondrial membrane—the mitochondrial respiratory chain complexes I–IV, and complex V, the linked ATP synthase (Fig. 8.1). The metabolism of carbohydrates, amino acids, and fatty acids generates the reduced cofactors NADH, NADPH, and $FADH_2$ that transfer electrons to complex I and II before being passed through to IV of the respiratory chain, pumping protons out of the mitochondrial matrix into the intermembrane space. This creates an electrochemical gradient that is harnessed by complex V (ATP synthase) to generate ATP from ADP. This machinery has a dual genetic origin, with 13 peptides synthesized within the mitochondrial matrix from the 16.5 Kb mitochondrial DNA (mtDNA), and the remainder synthesized in the cytoplasm from nuclear gene transcripts [3].

MtDNA (Fig. 8.2) codes for seven complex I subunits (NADH-ubiquinone oxidoreductase), one of the complex III subunits (ubiquinol-cytochrome *c* oxidoreductase), three of the complex IV (cytochrome *c* oxidase) subunits, and the ATPase 6 and ATPase 8 subunits of complex V. In addition, two ribosomal RNA genes (12S and 16S rRNA), and 22 transfer RNA genes provide the necessary RNA components for the mitochondrial translation machinery. The remaining polypeptides, including all of the complex II subunits, are synthesized from nuclear gene transcripts within the cytosol. These are subsequently imported into the mitochondria through the inner and outer

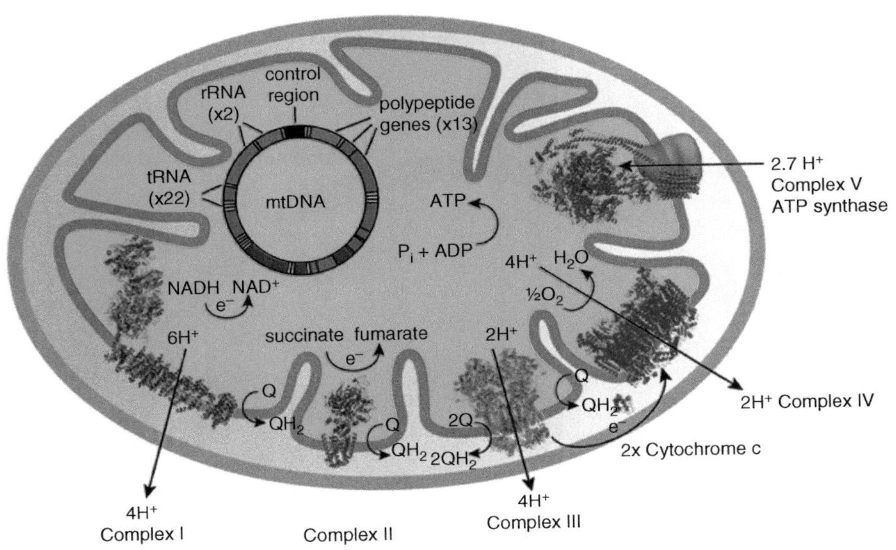

Fig. 8.1 Mitochondrial respiratory chain and mitochondrial DNA. The mitochondrial respiratory chain consists of 5 enzyme complexes that use the products of intermediary metabolism (of proteins, carbohydrates and fats) to synthesise adenosine triphosphate (ATP). MtDNA is maintained by a number of nuclear encoded factors. Nuclear factors also regulate the transcription of mtDNA (forming a messenger RNA template) and the translation of the transcripts into proteins within the mitochondrion. Nuclear DNA also codes for most of the respiratory chain subunits and the complex assembly factors. MtDNA codes for 13 essential respiratory chain subunits and part of the machinery needed for protein synthesis within the mitochondrial matrix. Q = co-enzyme Q10 (ubiquinone). H+ = protons

membrane translocation complexes. There are many additional nuclear-encoded proteins that are essential for mitochondrial function including chaperones involved in the assembly of the respiratory chain, the mtDNA polymerase ϒ, and proteins involved in the maintenance of mtDNA, mitochondrial transcription and protein translation. Mutations in nuclear and mtDNA genes can therefore cause mitochondrial cardiovascular disease.

Cardiac cells cell contains >1000 copies of mtDNA. Individuals with mtDNA disease often harbour a mixture of mutated and wild-type (normal) mtDNA—a situation called heteroplasmy [3]. Single cells only express a respiratory chain defect when the proportion of mutated mtDNA exceeds a critical threshold with low levels of wild type mtDNA. Different organs, and even adjacent cells within the same organ, may contain different amounts of mutated mtDNA. This variability, coupled with tissue-specific differences in the threshold and the varied dependence of different organs on oxidative metabolism, explains in part why certain tissues are preferentially affected in patients with mtDNA disease. In general, post-mitotic (non-dividing) tissues such as cardiomyocytes and the cardiac conduction system typically contain much higher levels of mutated mtDNA, in contrast to rapidly dividing tissues such as the blood, which contain lower levels of mutant mtDNA.

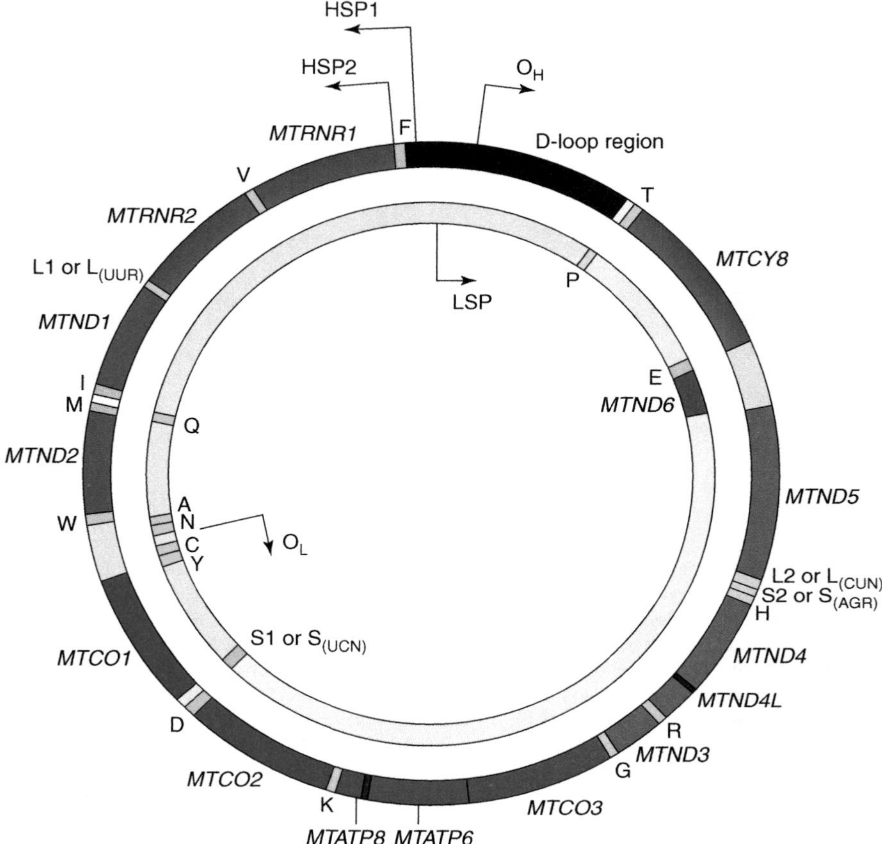

Fig. 8.2 Human mitochondrial DNA. The 16,569 base pair human mitochondrial genome (mtDNA) include an inner 'light' (L)-strand and an outer 'heavy' (H)-strand reflecting the increased guanine content. Structurakl genes include 13 ubunits of the mitochondrial respiratory chain for *MTND1–MTND6* and *MTND4L* (complex I); *MTCYB* (complex III); *MTCO1–3* (complex IV); and *MTATP6* and *MTATP8* (complex V). The 22 tRNA and 2 rRNA genes are interspersed between the peptide-encoding genes. MtDNA replication is carried out by mtDNA polymerase gamma (pol γ), in partnership with a helicase Twinkle, topoisomerase I, mtDNA single-stranded binding protein and others. Two models of mtDNA replication have been proposed. In the 'strand-displacement' or 'asynchronous' model. Replication is initiated by transcription within the noncoding mtDNA displacement (D) loop and proceeds clockwise from the origin of heavy-strand replication (O_H, also known as OriH) until the origin of light-strand replication (O_L) is exposed, allowing light-strand synthesis to proceed clockwise until the entire molecule is copied. Alternatively, symmetric strand-coupled replication might occur in certain circumstances; where replication is initiated from multiple origins distributed across a 4 kb fragment 3′ from the D loop, and proceeds in both directions in replication 'bubbles'. Replication is arrested at O_H, allowing the remainder of the molecule to be copied in one direction. Human mtDNA has three transcription promoters: Hsp1 enables transcription of the two ribosomal RNAs; Hsp2 promotes transcription of the rest of the heavy strand as a large polycystronic transcript, which is subsequently spliced into functional tRNA, rRNA and mRNAs; and L promotes transcription of the light strand as either one long transcript or as several small primer transcripts by RNase mitochondrial RNA processing (MRP). Transcription initiation involves the mitochondrial RNA polymerase and the mitochondrial transcription factors A and B2

MtDNA is transmitted exclusively down the maternal line. Deleted molecules are rarely transmitted from clinically affected females to their offspring (risk ~1 in 24). By contrast, a female harboring a heteroplasmic mtDNA point mutation, or mtDNA duplications, may transmit a variable amount of mutated mtDNA to her children. Early during development of the female germ line, the number of mtDNA molecules within each oocyte is drastically reduced before being subsequently amplified to reach a final number ~500,000 in each mature oocyte. This restriction and amplification (also called the mitochondrial 'genetic bottleneck') contributes to the variability between individual oocytes, and the different levels of mutant mtDNA seen in the offspring of a heteroplasmic mother female [3].

8.3 Clinical Evaluation of Mitochondrial Disease

Mitochondrial disease is clinically and genetically variable, and can present at any age. The same clinical syndrome can be caused by different genetic defects affecting either nuclear or mitochondrial genes, and the same genetic defect may present in a variety of different ways. It is often possible to identify well-defined clinical syndromes but many patients present with a collection of clinical features that are highly suggestive of respiratory chain disease but do not fit into a discrete clinical category [4]. Table 8.1 summarises the classical clinical syndromes of mitochondrial disease and Fig. 8.3 shows the approach to the clinical evaluation of mitochondrial diseases. Clinical syndromes with prominent cardiac features are discussed in detail below.

The assessment of mitochondrial disorders involved a detail history, including a family history, followed by a systematic clinical examination to identify the multisystem features of mitochondrial disease. Clinical investigations fall into two main groups: clinical investigations used to characterize the pattern and nature of the different organs involved, and specific investigations to identify the biochemical or genetic abnormality.

8.3.1 General Clinical Investigations

Given the prevalence of cardiac features, routine clinical investigation includes a cardiac assessment (ECG and echocardiography, ± cardiac MRI), and an endocrine assessment (oral glucose tolerance test, HbA1c, thyroid function tests, alkaline phosphatase, fasting calcium, and parathyroid hormone levels). The organic and amino acids in urine may prove informative, but are often normal. Blood and cerebrospinal fluid lactate levels are more helpful in the investigation of children than adults, but the results should be interpreted carefully because there are many causes of blood and cerebrospinal fluid lactic acidosis, including fever, sepsis, dehydration, seizures, and stroke. The cerebrospinal fluid protein may be elevated in some mitochondrial disorders. The serum creatine kinase level may be raised but is often normal. Neurophysiological studies may identify a myopathy or neuropathy. Electroencephalography may reveal diffuse slow-wave activity consistent with a

Table 8.1 Clinical syndromes of mitochondrial disease

Clinical syndrome	Clinical features	Age of onset	Genetic basis
Alpers-Huttenlocher syndrome; childhood myocerebral hepatopathy syndrome	Seizures, developmental delay, hypotonia, hepatic failure	Infancy/ childhood/ early adult life	Recessive mutations in *POLG*
Barth syndrome	Cardiomyopathy, neutropenia, myopathy	Infancy/ childhood/ early adult life	X-linked mutations in *TAZ*
Chronic progressive external ophthalmoplegia (CPEO)	Ptosis, ophthalmoparesis. Proximal myopathy often present. Various other clinical features variably present	Any age of onset. Typically more severe phenotype with younger onset	mtDNA single deletions mtDNA point mutations (including m.3243A>G, m.8344A>G) nDNA mutations (*POLG1*, *POLG2*, *SLC25A4*, *C10orf2*, *RRM2B*, *TK2*, and *OPA1*)
Kearns-Sayre syndrome (KSS)	PEO, ptosis, pigmentary retinopathy, cardiac conduction abnormality, ataxia, CSF elevated protein, diabetes mellitus, sensorineural hearing loss, myopathy	<20 years	mtDNA single deletions
Leber hereditary optic neuropathy (LHON)	Subacute painless bilateral visual failure Males:females approx. 4:1 Dystonia Cardiac pre-excitation syndromes	Median age of onset 24 years	mtDNA point mutations (m.11778G>A, m.14484T>C, m.3460A>G)
Mitochondrial encephalopathy, lactic acidosis, stroke like episodes (MELAS)	Stroke-like episodes with encephalopathy, migraine, seizures. Variable presence of myopathy, cardiomyopathy, deafness, endocrinopathy, ataxia. A minority of patients have PEO	Typically <40 years of age but childhood more common	mtDNA point mutations (m.3243A>G in 80%, m.3256C>T, m.3271T>C, m.4332G>A, m.13513G>A, m.13514A>G)
Mitochondrial neurogastrointestinal encephalopathy (MNGIE)	PEO, ptosis, GI dysmotility, proximal myopathy, axonal polyneuropathy, leukodystrophy	Childhood to early adulthood	nDNA mutations in *TYMP*; MNGIE-like syndromes may occur due to nDNA gene mutations with PEO
Myoclonus, epilepsy, and ragged-red fibres (MERRF)	Stimulus sensitive myoclonus, generalized seizures, ataxia, cardiomyopathy. A minority of patients have PEO	Teenage or early adult life	mtDNA point mutations (m.8344A>G most common; m.8356T>C, m.12147G>A)

Table 8.1 (continued)

Clinical syndrome	Clinical features	Age of onset	Genetic basis
Neurogenic weakness with ataxia and retinitis pigmentosa (NARP)	Ataxia, pigmentary retinopathy, weakness	Childhood or early adult life	*MTATP6* mutation (usually at m.8993)
POLG-related Ataxia neuropathy syndromes (ANS): Including MIRAS, SCAE, SANDO, MEMSA	SANDO: PEO, dysarthria, sensory neuropathy, cerebellar ataxia Other ANS: Sensory axonal neuropathy with variable degrees of sensory and cerebellar ataxia. Epilepsy, dysarthria, or myopathy are present in some	Teenage or adult life	nDNA mutations (*POLG, C10orf2, OPA1*)
Senger syndrome	Hypotonia, myopathy, congenital Cataract, cardiomyopathy	Neonatal or infancy	Recessibe mutations *AGK*

MIRAS mitochondrial recessive ataxia syndrome, *SCAE* spinocerebellar ataxia with epilepsy, *SANDO* sensory ataxia with dysphagia and ophthalmoplegia, *MEMSA* myoclonic epilepsy myopathy sensory ataxia

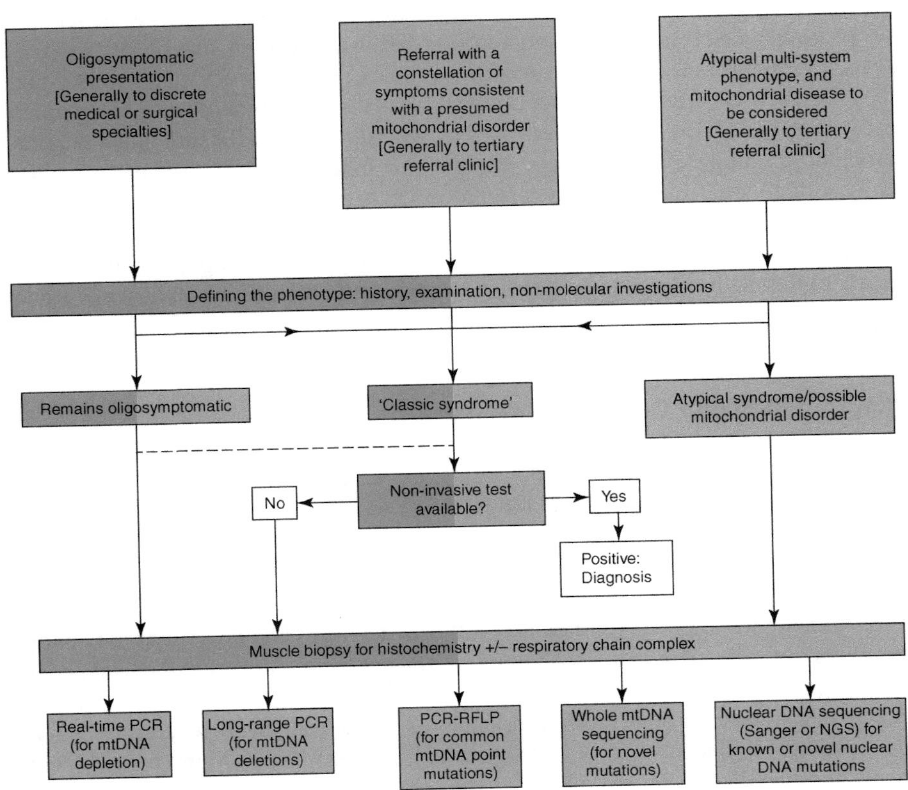

Fig. 8.3 Clinical approach to the investigation of suspected mitochondrial disorders

subacute encephalopathy, or evidence of seizure activity. Cerebral imaging may be abnormal, showing lesions of the basal ganglia, high signal in the cortex of deep white matter, or focal stroke-like lesions which cross vascular territories.

8.3.2 Specific Investigations for Mitochondrial Disease

In some patients, a defined clinical syndrome may indicate a specific molecular genetic blood test leading to the diagnosis (e.g. LHON, or *POLG* diseases). In others, a systematic approach is needed, guided by the clinical evaluation. The primary aim is to identify evidence of mitochondrial dysfunction in a clinically affected tissue. In adults this usually involves a skeletal muscle biopsy. In children the biopsy may be taken from another affected organ (e.g. the liver), or investigations carried out on skin fibroblasts. The muscle biopsy is initially analysed histochemically, revealing subsarcolemmal accumulation of mitochondria (so-called 'ragged red' fibres), or cytochrome *c* oxidase deficiency. A mosaic of cytochrome *c* oxidase-positive and cytochrome *c* oxidase-negative muscle fibres suggests an underlying primary mtDNA defect or a secondary defect of mtDNA as seen in patients with mutations in the nuclear gene *POLG* or *OPA1*. Patients who have cytochrome *c* oxidase deficiency due to a nuclear genetic defect usually have a global deficiency of this enzyme affecting all muscle fibres. Electron microscopy may identify paracrystalline inclusions in the inter-membrane space, but these are non-specific and may be seen in other non mitochondrial disorders. Respiratory chain complex assays can be carried out on various tissues. Measurement of the individual respiratory chain complexes determines whether an individual has multiple complex defects that would suggest an underlying mtDNA defect, involving either a tRNA gene or a large deletion, or a nuclear genetic defect affecting protein translation within mitochondria. Isolated complex defects may be due to point mutations in either mitochondrial or nuclear genes. Co-enzyme Q_{10} can be measured directly in affected tissues.

8.3.3 Molecular Genetic Investigations

The molecular genetic investigation of mitochondrial disease involves: (a) the targeted analysis of candidate genes for specific mutations based on the clinical presentation; (b) the systematic evaluation of mtDNA or specific nuclear genes guided by the laboratory investigations; and (c) larges-scale screening of nuclear candidate genes using multi-gene panels, exome sequencing, or whole genome sequencing. For some mtDNA defects (particularly mtDNA deletions and depletion) the abnormality is not detectable in a DNA sample extracted from blood, and the analysis of DNA extracted from muscle is essential to establish the diagnosis. Urinary epithelium can also be used in some circumstances as a surrogate due to its predilection to accumulate a greater degree of mtDNA mutations than blood. Many patients with mitochondrial disease have a previously unrecognized mtDNA defect and it is necessary to sequence directly the mitochondrial genome. If a novel base change is heteroplasmic, this suggests that it is of relatively recent onset. Family, tissue segregation, and single cell studies may show that higher levels of the mutation are associated with mitochondrial dysfunction and disease, which strongly suggests that the mutation is causing the disease. Nuclear genetic mitochondrial disorders are highly heterogeneous. Although there are some common candidates (eg *POLG*, *SPG7*, *OPA1*), novel mutations and novel disease genes are still being identified. This is particularly the case in children with autosomal recessive mitochondrial disease. Trio sequencing is a valuable strategy because *de novo* dominant mutations are now well recognised (eg *ANT1*).

8.4 Clinical Management of Mitochondrial Diseases

There is currently no definitive treatment for patients with mitochondrial disease, and clinical management focuses on minimizing disability, preventing complications, and genetic counseling. Supportive care is best provided by the integrated multidisciplinary team involving the primary physician, other specialist physicians (ophthalmology, diabetes specialists, cardiology), specialist nurses, physiotherapists, and speech therapists. The primary aim is the early detection of treatable complications, with a strong emphasis on cardiac surveillance for the reasons outlined below.

Using current investigations, a genetic diagnosis is possible in the majority of patients, enabling reliable genetic counseling. Nuclear genetic disorders can be autosomal dominant, autosomal recessive, or X-linked; and de novo dominant disorders are now well recognized. For patients with mtDNA mutations, males cannot transmit pathogenic mtDNA defects, and mtDNA deletions are rarely transmitted. Women harboring heteroplasmic pathogenic mtDNA point mutations may transmit the genetic defect to their offspring. The mitochondrial genetic 'bottleneck' leads to a variation in the proportion of mutated mtDNA that is transmitted to any offspring, meaning that a female to have mildly affected as well as severely affected children. The risk of having affected offspring varies from mutation to mutation, and although there does appear to be a relationship between the level of mutated mtDNA in the mother and the risk of affected offspring. Mitochondrial donation offers the hope of prevention for some women at risk of transmitting mtDNA mutations.

With the exception of idebenone, which has been approved for licensing by the European Medicines Agency for LHON [5], there are no established treatments for mitochondrial disorders [6]. Anecdotal reports describe benefits from ubiquinone (coenzyme Q_{10}) in patients with disorders of coenzyme Q_{10} biogenesis, and some patients have a riboflavin-responsive disorder. Several clinical trials are currently evaluating the effects of novel treatment approaches in patients with mitochondrial disease. Stem cell transplantation is effective in patients with very rare autosomal recessive enzyme defects (MNGIE, caused my mutations in *TP*) [7]. Dichloracetate can be used to reduce lactic acid levels but may cause an irreversible toxic neuropathy and is therefore not used in adults. Aerobic exercise is important for patients with mtDNA disease, and isometric muscle contraction may lead to an improvement in muscle strength.

8.5 Cardiac Features of Mitochondrial Disease

8.5.1 Hypertrophic Cardiomyopathy

Hypertrophic cardiomyopathy is present in ~40% of patients with mitochondrial disorders [8, 9], usually as part of a multisystem disorder. Occasionally the cardiac hypertrophy can be the presenting feature, particularly in mildly affected relatives with mtDNA mutations detected through cardiac surveillance (e.g. m.3243A<G). Many patients remain asymptomatic from the cardiac perspective, but some develop severe left ventricular dysfunction or present with sudden cardiac death. The clinical features include exercise intolerance and dyspnea [8]. However, given the co-existence of cognitive and physical impairment due to neuromuscular disease, or breathlessness linked to exercise due to lactic acidosis, in many patients the cardiac features can be overlooked.

In a small number of families, an isolated cardiomyopathy resulting from a homoplasmic mutation (m.4300A>G) in mt-tRNA^{Ile} (*MTTI*) has been described [10]. However, these isolated cardiac syndromes are rare, and mtDNA mutations causing cardiac hypertrophy are usually heteroplasmic, including m.3243A>G, first described in Mitochondrial Encephalomyopathy with Lactic Acidosis (MELAS), and m.8344A>G first described in Myoclonic Epilepsy with Ragged Red Fibres (MERRF). Although robust epidemiological data is lacking, it does appear that mutations in non mt-tRNA genes (eg mt-rRNAs and protein coding genes) are significantly less likely to result in cardiac involvement. Cardiac MRI (CMR) in patients with the m.3243A>G mtDNA mutation shows a specific pattern including concentric hypertrophy and patchy intramural late-gadolinium-enhancement (LGE) in the myocardium (Fig. 8.4 and MR video) [9], differing to that seen in patients with Chronic Progressive External Ophthalmoplegia (CPEO). For patients with the m.3243A>G mutation a positive correlation between skeletal muscle heteroplasmy levels and left ventricular mass [11] was noted, and over a 7 year follow up period there was an

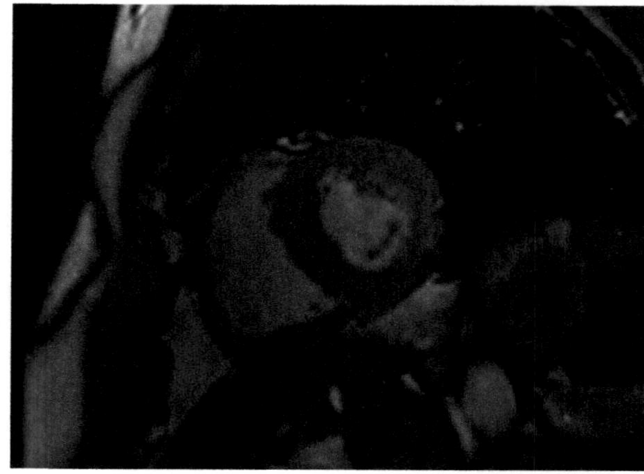

Fig. 8.4 Cardiac imaging showing concentric hypertrophy in a m.3243A>G mutation carrier (and linked MR video, both adapted from Ref. [37])

inverse correlation between the degree of LVH and systolic function [12]. Taken together, these data suggest that the burden of heteroplasmy is likely to be the main determinant of the severity of cardiac sequelae following diagnosis in m.3243A>G. Left-ventricular outflow obstruction (LVOTO) seems to be a rare complication of mitochondrial HCM, in contrast to non-mitochondrial cardiomyopathies [12].

Approximately 60% of patients with KSS or CPEO develop left ventricular hypertrophy (LVH), with intramural late-gadolinium-enhancement (LGE) in the basal and LV inferolateral wall and evidence of concentric remodelling on cardiac MR, which is distinct from the cardiac manifestations seen in m.3243A>G carriers [9].

8.5.2 Dilated Cardiomyopathy

Dilated cardiomyopathy (DCM) is characterized by an enlarged and weakened left ventricle, and is an uncommon features of mitochondrial diseases [13]. Where present, DCM appears to develop as a secondary consequence of pre-existing hypertrophic cardiomyopathy. However, the observation of DCM at diagnosis in some patients with high levels of cardiac heteroplasmy (90–95% mutant load) [14] suggests that particularly high heteroplasmy levels may favor the development of a DCM rather than LVH.

8.5.3 Left Ventricular Non-Compaction

Left ventricular non-compaction (LVNC) has been associated with mitochondrial disorders in three contexts three observations: Barth syndrome (see below), a small number of cases of Leber hereditary optic neuropathy (LHON, m. 3460A>G), and the heteroplasmic m.3243A>G mtDNA mutation. Further evidence of a link with mitochondrial dysfunction comes from the observation of decreased mtDNA copy number and low-level rare (presumed somatic) heteroplasmic mtDNA point mutations in cardiac muscle from patients with idiopathic forms of LVNC [15].

8.5.4 Electropathies

8.5.4.1 Bradyarrhythmias

The majority of bradyarrhythmias in mitochondrial disorders stem from disruption of the cardiac conduction system, with varying forms of atrio-ventricular block observed, although a small number of patients have been described with a bradyarrythmia secondary to cardiovascular autonomic impairment [16]. Cardiac conduction defects are common in patients with Kearns-Sayre syndrome (KSS) due to a single large-scale deletion, affecting up to 90% of patients with PR-interval prolongation, 2nd or 3rd degree AV block, His-Ventricular interval prolongation (due to distal disease) and Stokes Adams attacks [17]. KSS falls at one end of a spectrum of mitochondrial disease caused by single large-scale deletions of mtDNA, with isolated Chronic Progressive Ophthalmoplegia (CPEO) at the other extreme. Patients with CPEO are therefore at risk of developing cardiac conduction defects, and should also undergo regular ECG monitoring. MtDNA point mutations and nuclear-genetic mitochondrial disorders are a less frequent cause of bradyarrhythmias. When they occur, this is usually in association with LVH [18].

8.5.4.2 Tacchyarrythmias

Wolff–Parkinson–White (WPW) syndrome is the most common form of tachyarrhythmia observed in mitochondrial disorders, seen in around ~15% of patients with the m.8344A>G mutation in one series [19], and a similar proportion with the m.3243A>G mutation [1]. The WPW syndrome usually develops before 40 years of age, and may precede the development of symptoms in other organ systems by over a decade [20], and does not appear to correlate with skeletal muscle heteroplasmy. Patients with Leber's hereditary optic neuropathy (LHON) have also been described to have an increased risk of WPW [21], although several small case series have failed to observe this association [22]. Finally, a small number of cases of ventricular pre-excitation syndromes, such as ventricular tachycardia (VT), have been observed in patients with both mtDNA deletions and mtDNA point mutations.

8.6 Cardiac Manifestations in Common Mitochondrial Syndromes

8.6.1 Kearns-Sayre Syndrome (KSS)

The Kearns-Sayre Syndrome (KSS) is characterized by: (1) symptom onset before 20 years, (2) a pigmentary retinopathy, and (3) an ophthalmoplegia; often in association with cerebellar ataxia, deafness, dementia, a raised CSF protein and a cardiac conduction defect. The cardiac conduction defects range from PR prolongation through to 2nd and 3rd degree block, His-Ventricular block, DCM, or Stoke-Adams attacks (Fig. 8.5). The progression to 3rd degree heart block (complete heart block) can be rapid and explain why sudden death occurs in ~10% of patients with KSS [23]. Regular (12 monthly) ECG monitoring is mandatory, and there should be a low threshold for pacemaker implantation. However, this may precipitate Torsade de points [24], so a preventative implantable cardiac defibrillator (ICD) placement has been proposed by some centers.

8.6.2 m.3243A>G

The m.3243 mtDNA mutation was first described in mitochondrial encephalopmyopathy with lactic acidosis and stroke-like episodes (MELAS). The 'full blown' syndrome is a multisystem disorder which also includes seizures, (dementia, and a proximal myopathy, but most patients with m.3243A>G do not have such an

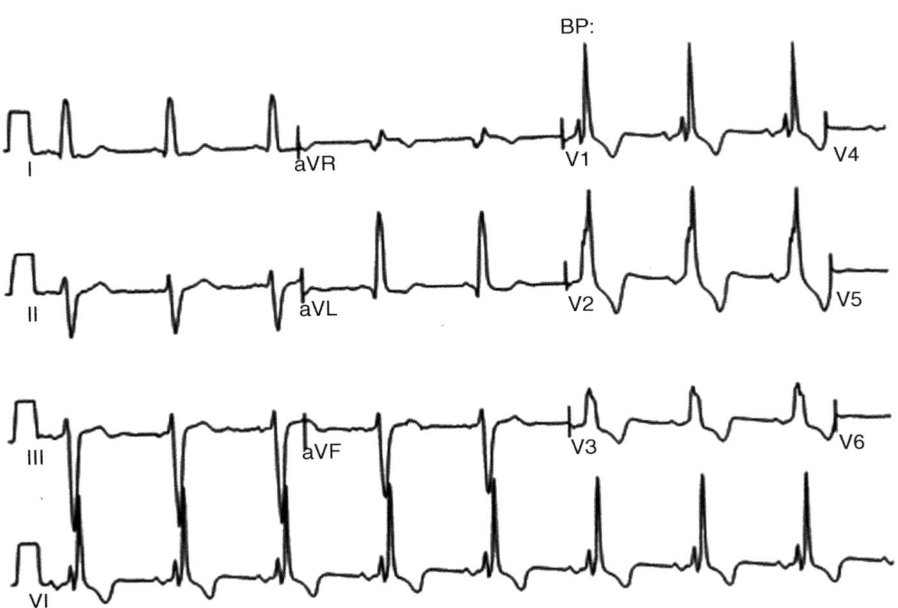

Fig. 8.5 12-lead electrocardiogram in the Kearns-Sayre syndrome caused by a single large heteroplasmic mtDNA deletion (adapted from J Med Genet 1999)

extensive phenotype, and many have isolated diabetes and deafness. Cardiac features are extremely common in m.3243A>G carriers, with approximately 50% of patients developing a cardiac abnormality (Fig. 8.4 and MR video). The most common cardiac complication is a hypertrophic cardiomyopathy without left ventricular outflow obstruction (LVOTO), which may later develop into a dilated cardiomyopathy. It appears that both the risk and severity of the cardiomyopathy is related to the level of the m.3243A>G mutation in the myocardium. WPW has been described in ~15% of patients, without clear association to underlying myocardial heteroplasmy level.

8.6.3 m.8344A>G

The m.8344A>G mutation was first described in patients with myoclonus, epilepsy and ragged red fibres observed in a skeletal muscle biopsy (MERRF). The cardiac features are similar to those observed in m.3243A>G carriers, and present in ~40% of patients. These include a cardiomyopathy and WPW in roughly equal proportions, with other cardiac abnormalities such as incomplete left bundle branch block also described [19]. The level of heteroplasmy required to cause a cardiomyopathy may be relatively low, so it is important for clinicians to remain vigilant in known cases and their potentially affected maternal relatives [25].

8.6.4 m.8993T>G/C

The m.8993A>G/C mutation was first described in patients with neuropathy, ataxia and retinitis pigmentosa (NARP), although the same two mtDNA mutations (m.8993T>G and m.8993T>C) also cause Leigh syndrome. Given the rarity of the disorder, accurate quantification of the prevalence and phenotype of cardiac symptoms is difficult to determine. However, cardiac failure remains a common cause of death in infants with Leigh syndrome [26] but is rare in patients with NARP [27].

8.6.5 LHON

Leber's Hereditary Optic Neuropathy (LHON) is a common mitochondrial disorder caused by homoplasmic point mutations that usually causes isolated dysfunction of the retinal ganglion cells (Table 8.1). The vast majority of patients only develop a sub-acute irreversible optic neuropathy, but 'LHON plus' syndromes (LHON with additional non-ophthalmological symptoms) have been described, including cardiac manifestations such as myocardial hypertrophy, unexplained left ventricular dilatation [28], or ventricular pre-excitation disorders [21]. Notably however, these studies are from geographically isolated regions or single large extended pedigrees, raising the possibility that environmental or nuclear genetic modifiers may contribute to these findings [22].

8.6.6 Barth Syndrome

Barth syndrome is a rare multisystem mitochondrial disorder characterized by a dilated cardiomyopathy, skeletal myopathy, neutropenia and short stature due to mutations in *TAZ* gene on the X-chromosome. The disorder exclusively affects in males with a frequency of ~1 in 400,000 [29], and presents at birth or in early infancy with hypotonia and growth delay. Around 70% of affected individuals also develop a cardiomyopathy within the first year of life, most commonly within the first six months [30]. The most common form of cardiomyopathy is a dilated cardiomyopathy which is often accompanied by endocardial fibroelastosis (EFE) [31], and 50% have prominent left ventricular trabeculations in-keeping with Left Ventricular Non-Compaction (LVNC). Hypertrophic cardiomyopathy appears to be rare in patients Barth syndrome. Barth Syndrome accounts for ~5% of all forms of cardiomyopathy diagnosed in male infants, and can be diagnosed by measuring the MLCL:L4-CL ratio on dried bloodspot cards [32].

The clinical management of Barth syndrome involves standard medical therapy for heart failure, though there are no systematic studies of any particular treatment regime. Around 50% of boys will normalize their ejection fraction and left diastolic volumes with treatment [33]. Long-term surveillance for cardiac arrhythmias should also be undertaken, with a low threshold for Implantable Cardiac Defibrillators (ICDs) where symptomatology or electrophysiological investigations suggest a possible ventricular arrhythmia. Around 1 in 7 children with Barth Syndrome will require a cardiac transplantation, generally with good results [34], though a considered approach to immunosuppression must be undertaken given the co-existent neutropenia.

8.6.7 Sengers Syndrome

Sengers Syndrome is a rare autosomal recessive multisystem mitochondrial disorder characterized by congenital cataracts, a hypertrophic cardiomyopathy, mitochondrial myopathy and an exertional lactic acidosis, and occurs due to mutations in the mitochondrial acylglycerol kinase gene *AGK* [35]. The disorder can manifest either as a severe neonatal form caused by homozygous nonsense mutations in *AGK*, which is invariably fatal due to a dilated cardiomyopathy; or with a more benign clinical course due to at least one mutation in a splice-site or start codon of *AGK* [36]. The cardiac phenotype of individuals with the milder phenotype is typically involves a hypertrophic cardiomyopathy rather than a dilated cardiomyopathy.

8.7 Cardiac Investigations in Mitochondrial Diseases

All patients with any form of suspected or confirmed mitochondrial disease should have cardiac screening as part of their diagnostic evaluation, and annually throughout follow-up (Fig. 8.5).

8.7.1 Initial Screening

Where a mitochondrial disease is confirmed or suspected, affected individuals and potential carriers should undergo a standard 12-lead electrocardiogram (ECG) and 2D–echocardiography (ECHO) to enable a baseline functional and structural cardiac assessment (Fig. 8.6). Where there is a phenotype with high risk of cardiac conduction defect (such as KSS), or in cases where WPW is possible (eg m.3243A>G and m.8344A>G), careful assessment of the ECG should be undertaken as emerging abnormalities may be subtle. Furthermore, given that ECHO is highly operator dependent, we would advise that it be undertaken in tertiary centers familiar with atypical cardiomyopathies.

8.7.2 Advanced Imaging Techniques

Cardiac MR and magnetic resonance spectroscopy (MRS) have largely been used in a research context, although clinical experience is growing. Established findings include: concentric LV hypertrophy; cardiac remodeling (increased torsion and longitudinal fibre shortening) [37] and impaired tissue bio-energetics (reduced PCr/ATP ratio) [38]. Abnormalities of myocardial function are also emerging in asymptomatic individuals with normal 12-lead ECG and ECHO who carry the m.3243A>G mutation [39]. Cardiac MR offers an increased ability to detect structural abnormalities that may be missed with echocardiography (such as left ventricular non-compaction), and bio-energetic abnormalities of the myocardium that may act as diagnostic markers of mitochondrial disorders. More frequently at present, CMR is used to further define abnormalities identified using echocardiography. The improved sensitivity of CMR permits identification of characteristic cardiomyopathy patterns indicative of alternative genetic causes [40].

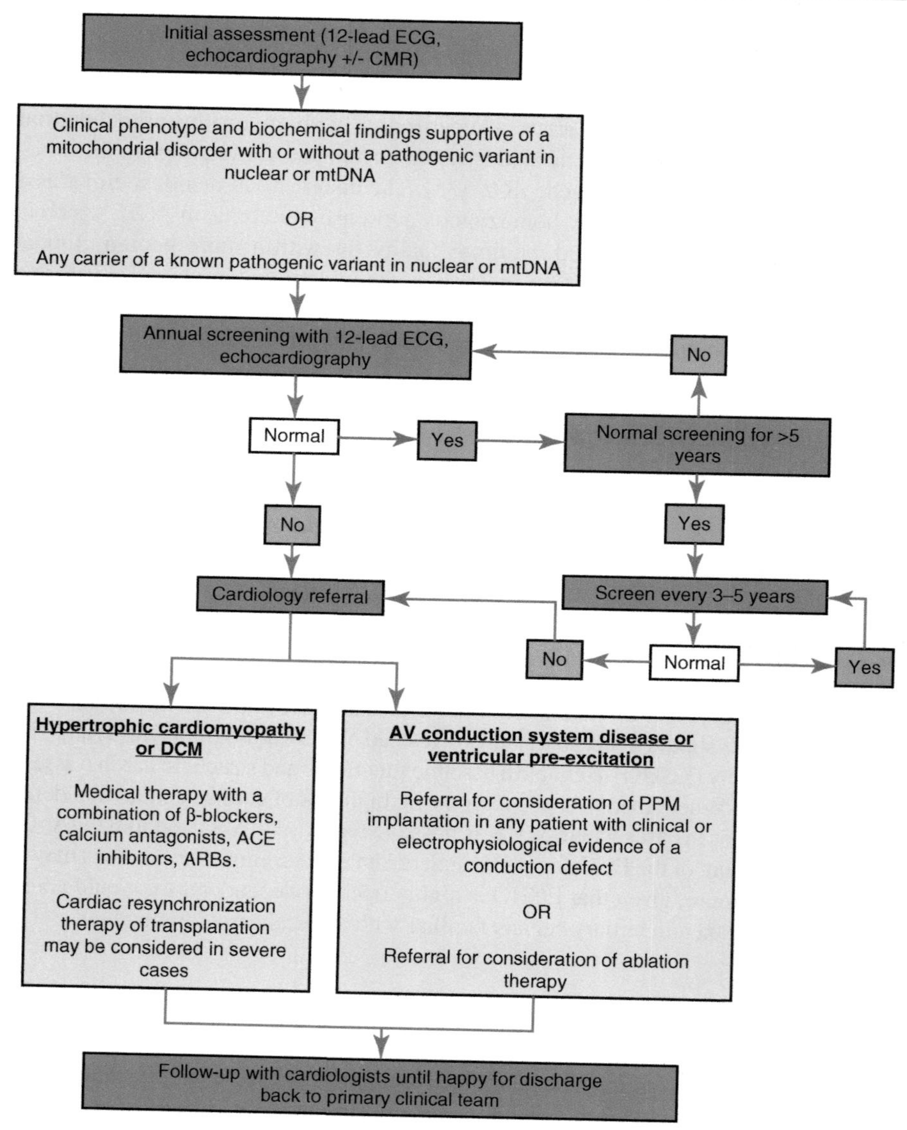

Fig. 8.6 Cardiac investigations and surveillance in patients with mitochondrial disorders. Blue boxes represent screening or clinical sessions. Yellow boxes indicate key moments of clinical decision making. Key. *CMR* cardiac MRI, *DCM* Dilated cardiomyopathy, *AV* atrioventricular, *PPM* permanent pacemaker, *ACE* angiotensin converting enzyme, *ARB* angiotensin receptor blocker

8.7.3 Cardiac Biopsy

Cardiac biopsy is another potentially valuable investigation for select patients., However as the risk of serious complication from cardiac biopsy is around 1%, this must be balanced against likely diagnostic yield. Therefore, as the molecular etiology in most patients with a phenotype suggestive of a mitochondrial disease will arise from (a) a pathogenic homoplasmic point mutation that is detectable in blood; (b) a nuclear DNA mutation that is detectable in blood; or (c) a heteroplasmic point mutation that is detectable in urine, skeletal muscle or blood, alternative less invasive investigative strategies are usually more appropriate.

In contrast, a cardiac biopsy may be useful in cases of isolated undiagnosed cardiomyopathies in which a mitochondrial diagnosis had not previously been considered. In these cases a combination of mitochondrial proliferation and evidence of impaired cytochrome c oxidase (COX) or succinate dehydrogenase (SDH) activity may be observed and prompt further investigation for a mitochondrial aetiology. In our experience however, this type of presentation is rare.

8.7.4 Cardiac Surveillance

Assuming that the initial screening investigations are normal in a patient, how often should they continue to undergo cardiac surveillance? Whilst there are no specific guidelines, we advocate an approach similar to that suggested by Bates et al. [2] with annual follow-up for at least 5 years, extending to every 3–5 years where investigations (ECG & ECHO) are normal. When an abnormality is detected - either at baseline or during follow-up—the patient should be referred to a cardiologist with a sub-specialty interest in mitochondrial disease for consideration of further investigation, pharmacological therapy, or intervention as indicated (Fig. 8.6).

8.8 Treatment of Mitochondrial Cardiac Disease

8.8.1 Cardiomyopathies

Treatment paradigms for mitochondrial cardiomyopathies typically follow those employed for other causes of HCM without LVOTO [2, 41], including a combination of diuretics, B-blockers, angiotensin-converting (ACE) inhibitors, and angiotensin receptor blockers (ARB) for patients with a low ejection fraction (<50%). It should be stressed that there is limited follow-up data available from patients with mitochondrial disorders, so the long-term benefits of these treatments have yet to be established. Given the lack of specific evidence, implantable cardioverter defibrillator (ICD) devices and cardiac resynchronization therapy should be used in line with standard guidelines [41].

8.8.2 Electrophysiological Management of Arrhythmias and Conduction Defects

There is some controversy over the management of arrhythmias and conduction defects arising in patients with mitochondrial disease. It has been suggested that permanent pacemaker (PPM) placement be undertaken in patients with mitochondrial disorders as soon as any evidence of atrioventricular block is observed (even first degree heart block) [2]—especially in disorders such as KSS/CPEO where progressive AV nodal disease is common and can progress rapidly. However, others suggest that conventional pacing/ICD implantation guidelines be followed [42]. The treatment of supra-ventricular tachyarrythmias mirrors standard practice and incorporates both pharmacological and, where required, electrophysiological approaches.

8.8.3 Transplantation

Cardiac transplantation is predominantly reserved for young patients with end-stage cardiomyopathy and little of no evidence of non-cardiac involvement of their mitochondrial disease. However, in many patients is not easy to give a confident long-term view on the risk of developing progressive neurological features, and there is a lack of long-term follow up data.

8.9 Summary and Future Developments

Disorders of mitochondrial dysfunction may result from either due to mutations in nuclear genes or mitochondrial DNA. In addition to many energy dependent organs and systems, these often present with cardiac phenotypes, either in isolation or within the context of a multi-system mitochondrial encephalomyopathy. Hypertrophic cardiomyopathy and conduction defects are common, but other cardiac manifestations have been described. A systematic approach to the biochemical and/or genetic evaluation of these patients will usually identify the underlying cause, enabling genetic counseling and supportive management of both the cardiac and extra-cardiac features.

In most cases, there is no specific treatment for mitochondrial dysfunction. Traditionally, mitochondrial disease has been treated with so-called “mitochondrial cocktails,” containing different vitamins, co-factors, and nutritional supplements, but these usually lack a major therapeutic impact. A number of new therapeutic approaches for mitochondrial disorders are under development.

One major development is heteroplasmy shifting, where the focus is to reduce the ratio of mutant to healthy mitochondria inside cells by selectively inhibiting the multiplication of mutated mitochondria. Another approach focuses on restoring or bypassing enzymes that are defective in mitochondrial disease; for example, coenzyme Q10 and riboflavin supplements to treat mitochondrial disease caused by defect in the biosynthesis of coenzyme Q10 and riboflavin transporter disorders, respectively.

Stem cell therapy and gene therapy techniques are being investigated, but these are still in early pre-clinical stage development. Several clinical trials are underway for assessing efficacy of new drugs for restoring the mitochondrial dysfunction using a number of complex molecular systems.

Probably the most dramatic therapeutic approach in the field of mitochondrial disease has been mitochondrial donation IVF, so called ‘three parents offspring’. Although it cannot treat people with mitochondrial disease, it can offer women with the disease the option of having children who will not be affected by it. This technique is performed using a donor egg cell, containing healthy mitochondria. The egg nucleus is removed and replaced with that of the mother, who has mitochondrial disease and the egg is then fertilized with the father's sperm. This technique was unanimously approved by the UK Parliament and is fast emerging as a major treatment approach for mitochondrial disease. However, it is not applicable to mitochondrial disease caused by nuclear DNA mutation.

References

1. Anan R, Nakagawa M, Miyata M, et al. Cardiac involvement in mitochondrial diseases. A study on 17 patients with documented mitochondrial DNA defects. Circulation. 1995;91(4):955–61.
2. Bates MG, Bourke JP, Giordano C, d'Amati G, Turnbull DM, Taylor RW. Cardiac involvement in mitochondrial DNA disease: clinical spectrum, diagnosis, and management. Eur Heart J. 2012;33(24):3023–33.
3. Stewart JB, Chinnery PF. The dynamics of mitochondrial DNA heteroplasmy: implications for human health and disease. Nat Rev Genet. 2015;16(9):530–42.
4. Gorman GS, Chinnery PF, DiMauro S, et al. Mitochondrial diseases. Nat Rev Dis Primers. 2016;2:16080.
5. Klopstock T, Yu-Wai-Man P, Dimitriadis K, et al. A randomized placebo-controlled trial of idebenone in Leber's hereditary optic neuropathy. Brain. 2011;134(Pt 9):2677–86.
6. Pfeffer G, Horvath R, Klopstock T, et al. New treatments for mitochondrial disease-no time to drop our standards. Nat Rev Neurol. 2013;9(8):474–81.
7. Halter JP, Michael W, Schupbach M, et al. Allogeneic haematopoietic stem cell transplantation for mitochondrial neurogastrointestinal encephalomyopathy. Brain. 2015;138(Pt 10):2847–58.
8. Limongelli G, Tome-Esteban M, Dejthevaporn C, Rahman S, Hanna MG, Elliott PM. Prevalence and natural history of heart disease in adults with primary mitochondrial respiratory chain disease. Eur J Heart Fail. 2010;12(2):114–21.
9. Florian A, Ludwig A, Stubbe-Drager B, et al. Characteristic cardiac phenotypes are detected by cardiovascular magnetic resonance in patients with different clinical phenotypes and genotypes of mitochondrial myopathy. J Cardiovasc Magn Reson. 2015;17:40.
10. Taylor RW, Giordano C, Davidson MM, et al. A homoplasmic mitochondrial transfer ribonucleic acid mutation as a cause of maternally inherited hypertrophic cardiomyopathy. J Am Coll Cardiol. 2003;41(10):1786–96.
11. Vydt TC, de Coo RF, Soliman OI, et al. Cardiac involvement in adults with m.3243A>G MELAS gene mutation. Am J Cardiol. 2007;99(2):264–9.
12. Okajima Y, Tanabe Y, Takayanagi M, Aotsuka H. A follow up study of myocardial involvement in patients with mitochondrial encephalomyopathy, lactic acidosis, and stroke-like episodes (MELAS). Heart. 1998;80(3):292–5.
13. Tveskov C, Angelo-Nielsen K. Kearns-Sayre syndrome and dilated cardiomyopathy. Neurology. 1990;40(3 Pt 1):553–4.
14. Stalder N, Yarol N, Tozzi P, et al. Mitochondrial A3243G mutation with manifestation of acute dilated cardiomyopathy. Circ Heart Fail. 2012;5(1):e1–3.
15. Tang S, Batra A, Zhang Y, Ebenroth ES, Huang T. Left ventricular noncompaction is associated with mutations in the mitochondrial genome. Mitochondrion. 2010;10(4):350–7.
16. Di Leo R, Musumeci O, de Gregorio C, et al. Evidence of cardiovascular autonomic impairment in mitochondrial disorders. J Neurol. 2007;254(11):1498–503.
17. Young TJ, Shah AK, Lee MH, Hayes DL. Kearns-Sayre syndrome: a case report and review of cardiovascular complications. Pacing Clin Electrophysiol. 2005;28(5):454–7.
18. Majamaa-Voltti K, Peuhkurinen K, Kortelainen ML, Hassinen IE, Majamaa K. Cardiac abnormalities in patients with mitochondrial DNA mutation 3243A>G. BMC Cardiovasc Disord. 2002;2:12.
19. Wahbi K, Larue S, Jardel C, et al. Cardiac involvement is frequent in patients with the m.8344A>G mutation of mitochondrial DNA. Neurology. 2010;74(8):674–7.
20. Sproule DM, Kaufmann P, Engelstad K, Starc TJ, Hordof AJ, De Vivo DC. Wolff-Parkinson-White syndrome in patients with MELAS. Arch Neurol. 2007;64(11):1625–7.

21. Nikoskelainen EK, Savontaus ML, Huoponen K, Antila K, Hartiala J. Pre-excitation syndrome in Leber's hereditary optic neuropathy. Lancet. 1994;344(8926):857–8.
22. Kirkman MA, Yu-Wai-Man P, Korsten A, et al. Gene-environment interactions in Leber hereditary optic neuropathy. Brain. 2009;132(Pt 9):2317–26.
23. Khambatta S, Nguyen DL, Beckman TJ, Wittich CM. Kearns-Sayre syndrome: a case series of 35 adults and children. Int J Gen Med. 2014;7:325–32.
24. Subbiah RN, Kuchar D, Baron D. Torsades de pointes in a patient with Kearns-Sayre syndrome: a fortunate finding. Pacing Clin Electrophysiol. 2007;30(1):137–9.
25. DiMauro S, Hirano M. Merrf. In: Pagon RA, Adam MP, Ardinger HH, et al., editors. GeneReviews(R). Seattle, WA: University of Washington; 1993.
26. Thorburn DR, Rahman S. Mitochondrial DNA-associated leigh syndrome and NARP. In: Pagon RA, Adam MP, Ardinger HH, et al., editors. GeneReviews(R). Seattle, WA: University of Washington; 1993.
27. Rawle MJ, Larner AJ. NARP syndrome: a 20-year follow-up. Case Rep Neurol. 2013; 5(3):204–7.
28. Sorajja P, Sweeney MG, Chalmers R, et al. Cardiac abnormalities in patients with Leber's hereditary optic neuropathy. Heart. 2003;89(7):791–2.
29. Dudek J, Maack C. Barth syndrome cardiomyopathy. Cardiovasc Res. 2017. https://doi.org/10.1093/cvr/cvx014. [Epub ahead of print].
30. Roberts AE, Nixon C, Steward CG, et al. The Barth Syndrome Registry: distinguishing disease characteristics and growth data from a longitudinal study. Am J Med Genet A. 2012;158A(11):2726–32.
31. Clarke SL, Bowron A, Gonzalez IL, et al. Barth syndrome. Orphanet J Rare Dis. 2013;8:23.
32. Kulik W, van Lenthe H, Stet FS, et al. Bloodspot assay using HPLC-tandem mass spectrometry for detection of Barth syndrome. Clin Chem. 2008;54(2):371–8.
33. Spencer CT, Bryant RM, Day J, et al. Cardiac and clinical phenotype in Barth syndrome. Pediatrics. 2006;118(2):e337–46.
34. Mangat J, Lunnon-Wood T, Rees P, Elliott M, Burch M. Successful cardiac transplantation in Barth syndrome--single-centre experience of four patients. Pediatr Transplant. 2007;11(3): 327–31.
35. Mayr JA, Haack TB, Graf E, et al. Lack of the mitochondrial protein acylglycerol kinase causes Sengers syndrome. Am J Hum Genet. 2012;90(2):314–20.
36. Haghighi A, Haack TB, Atiq M, et al. Sengers syndrome: six novel AGK mutations in seven new families and review of the phenotypic and mutational spectrum of 29 patients. Orphanet J Rare Dis. 2014;9:119.
37. Hollingsworth KG, Gorman GS, Trenell MI, et al. Cardiomyopathy is common in patients with the mitochondrial DNA m.3243A>G mutation and correlates with mutation load. Neuromuscul Disord. 2012;22(7):592–6.
38. Lodi R, Rajagopalan B, Blamire AM, Crilley JG, Styles P, Chinnery PF. Abnormal cardiac energetics in patients carrying the A3243G mtDNA mutation measured in vivo using phosphorus MR spectroscopy. Biochim Biophys Acta. 2004;1657(2–3):146–50.
39. Bates MG, Hollingsworth KG, Newman JH, et al. Concentric hypertrophic remodelling and subendocardial dysfunction in mitochondrial DNA point mutation carriers. Eur Heart J Cardiovasc Imaging. 2013;14(7):650–8.
40. Partington SL, Givertz MM, Gupta S, Kwong RY. Cardiac magnetic resonance aids in the diagnosis of mitochondrial cardiomyopathy. Circulation. 2011;123(6):e227–9.
41. Authors/Task Force members, Elliott PM, Anastasakis A, et al. 2014 ESC Guidelines on diagnosis and management of hypertrophic cardiomyopathy: the Task Force for the Diagnosis and Management of Hypertrophic Cardiomyopathy of the European Society of Cardiology (ESC). Eur Heart J. 2014;35(39):2733–79.
42. Brignole M, Auricchio A, Baron-Esquivias G, et al. 2013 ESC Guidelines on cardiac pacing and cardiac resynchronization therapy: the Task Force on cardiac pacing and resynchronization therapy of the European Society of Cardiology (ESC). Developed in collaboration with the European Heart Rhythm Association (EHRA). Eur Heart J. 2013;34(29):2281–329.

Inherited Cardiac Muscle Disorders: Hypertrophic and Restrictive Cardiomyopathies

9

Mohammed Majid Akhtar, Juan Pablo Kaski, and Perry Elliott

Abstract

Inherited cardiomyopathies as a collective group, are relatively common cardiac disorders. Individuals can present with symptoms of chest pain, dyspnoea, palpitations, syncope and with progressive heart failure or sudden cardiac death. Genetic mutations are the commonest cause of these disorders; having implications for both the affected proband and their extended family. Early identification of the disease process can allow institution of treatment with pharmacological and non-pharmacological therapy to ameliorate symptoms, retard disease progression and in some cases prolong life by changing the natural course of the disease. An appreciation of the underlying genetics is essential to understand the molecular basis of disease as well as to help identify other individuals at risk of developing the disease phenotype. The following chapter provides insight into the genetic aetiology underlying these diverse disease processes and the clinical management of these inherited cardiomyopathies.

M.M. Akhtar
Barts Heart Centre, Department of Inherited Cardiovascular Diseases, St Bartholomew's Hospital, London, UK

J.P. Kaski
Paediatric Inherited Cardiovascular Diseases, Centre for Inherited Cardiovascular Diseases, Great Ormond Street Hospital, London, UK

P. Elliott, MBBS, MD, FRCP, FESC, FACC (✉)
Barts Heart Centre, Department of Inherited Cardiovascular Diseases, St Bartholomew's Hospital, London, UK

Cardiovascular Medicine, University College London, London, UK

Clinical Research, UCL Institute of Cardiovascular Science, London, UK
e-mail: perry.elliott@ucl.ac.uk

D. Kumar, P. Elliott (eds.), *Cardiovascular Genetics and Genomics*,
https://doi.org/10.1007/978-3-319-66114-8_9

Keywords
Hypertrophic cardiomyopathy • Dilated cardiomyopathy • Restrictive cardiomyopathy • Metabolic cardiomyopathy • Sarcomere

9.1 Introduction

Cardiomyopathies are defined as myocardial disorders in which the heart is structurally and functionally abnormal, in the absence of coronary artery disease, valvular heart disease, hypertension or congenital heart disease sufficient to cause the observed myocardial abnormality [1]. Cardiomyopathies are classified into four main subtypes based on ventricular morphology and physiology: hypertrophic cardiomyopathy (HCM); dilated cardiomyopathy (DCM, Chap. 10); restrictive cardiomyopathy (RCM); and arrhythmogenic right ventricular cardiomyopathy (ARVC, Chap. 11). Cases that do not readily fit into these subtypes are termed “unclassified cardiomyopathies”, and include left ventricular non-compaction (see Chap. 12), endocardial fibroelastosis and Takotsubo cardiomyopathy. Each subtype of cardiomyopathy is subdivided into familial (genetic) and non-familial (acquired) forms [1].

9.2 Hypertrophic Cardiomyopathy

Hypertrophic cardiomyopathy (HCM) is defined as left ventricular hypertrophy in the absence of abnormal loading conditions (valve disease, hypertension, congenital heart defects) sufficient to explain the degree of hypertrophy [1]. Studies in North America, Europe, Japan and China consistently report a prevalence of unexplained left ventricular (LV) hypertrophy of approximately 1 in 500 adults [2–7]. The prevalence of HCM in children is unknown, but population-based studies have reported an annual incidence of 0.3–0.5 per 100,000 [8, 9].

9.2.1 Etiology

In most adolescents and adults, HCM is inherited as an autosomal dominant trait caused by mutations in cardiac sarcomere protein genes [10–12]. In less than 10% of infants and children, and in an even smaller proportion of adults, HCM can be associated with inborn errors of metabolism, neuromuscular disorders and malformation syndromes [1, 13–17]. Patients with cardiomyopathy associated with metabolic disorders or malformation syndromes are often diagnosed earlier in life (infancy or early childhood), whereas those with neuromuscular diseases tend to be diagnosed as teenagers [15]. Children with HCM associated with an inborn error of metabolism or malformation syndrome have a significantly worse survival than patients with HCM associated with sarcomeric mutations [18].

9.2.2 Cardiac Pathology in HCM

The most common pattern of myocardial hypertrophy in sarcomeric HCM is asymmetric septal hypertrophy [19, 20]. However, other patterns also occur, including concentric, mid-ventricular (sometimes associated with a left ventricular apical aneurysm [21]) and apical patterns of hypertrophy [22–25]. Coexistent right ventricular hypertrophy is common but rarely, if ever, occurs in isolation [19]. The papillary muscles are often displaced anteriorly and may have abnormal insertion into the mitral valve which predisposes to systolic anterior motion of the mitral valve and outflow tract obstruction [26]. The mitral valve itself is often structurally abnormal with an elongated anterior mitral valve leaflet allowing sufficient mobility for systolic anterior motion [27]. Myocardial bridging of the left anterior descending coronary artery has been observed in adults and children with HCM [28, 29].

Histologically, familial HCM is characterised by a triad of myocyte hypertrophy, myocyte disarray (architectural disorganisation of the myocardium, with adjacent myocytes aligned obliquely or perpendicular to each other in association with increased interstitial collagen) and interstitial fibrosis [19, 20] (Fig. 9.1). Although myocyte disarray occurs in many pathologies, the presence of extensive disarray (more than 10% of the ventricular myocardium) is generally thought to be a highly

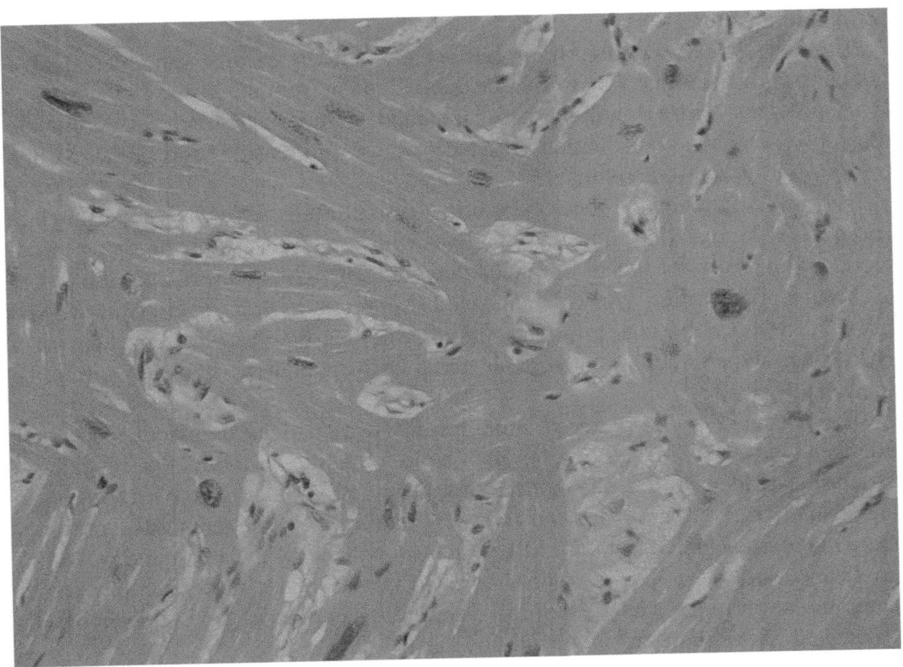

Fig. 9.1 High power hematoxylin and eosin sections of ventricular myocardium showing the typical swirling and splayed pattern of myocytes in myocyte disarray. The enlarged and hyperchromatic nuclei indicate myocyte hypertrophy. There is an increase in interstitital fibrous tissue. *Courtesy of Dr Michael Ashworth, Great Ormond Street Hospital, London, UK*

specific marker for HCM [19, 20]. Small intramural coronary arteries are often dysplastic and narrowed due to wall thickening by smooth muscle cell medial wall hyperplasia and are one of the potential mechanisms of chest pain in the presence of unobstructed epicardial coronary arteries [30].

Patients with HCM often have concomitant diastolic dysfunction which affects both the passive and active phase of diastole. The chamber hypertrophy and consequent stiffness result in impaired passive filling of the ventricles and raised filling pressures which can also impair coronary blood flow. Interstitial fibrosis, often found in the areas of maximal hypertrophy, contributes to diastolic LV impairment.

9.2.3 Sarcomere Protein Disease

The cardiac sarcomere consists of thin and thick filaments and associated proteins. Each myosin thick filament molecule consists of two myosin heavy chains, two essential myosin light chains and two regulatory myosin light chain complexes. There is one myosin-binding protein C (MYBPC3) molecule for every ten myosin molecules. Actin forms the thin filament and has binding sites involved in actin-myosin crossbridge formation. The troponin complex (formed of troponin C, troponin I and troponin T) and tropomyosin have important regulatory roles in exposing actin binding sites [31].

Titin, the largest sarcomeric protein, spans half the cardiac sarcomere and is bound to myosin along its length on the thick filament from the Z-disk to the M-line. It also interacts with actin along the I band and has important structural (sarcomere assembly), mechanotransduction (passive stiffness and tension) and cell signalling roles (via titin-kinase domains) [32].

Recently, mutations in genes encoding z-disc proteins have also been shown to cause HCM in a small proportion of patients who do not carry more common sarcomeric mutations. The genes implicated include myozenin (*MYOZ2*), telethonin (*TCAP*), alpha-actinin-2 (*ACTN2*), muscle LIM protein (*CRP3*) and nexilin (*NEXN*) [33–37]. Some mutations in Z-disc proteins have a pleotropic effect, causing a HCM phenotype in certain individuals and a DCM phenotype in others within the same family [38].

The presence of a sarcomeric mutation in HCM patients is associated with a younger age of disease onset; higher likelihood of familial disease; higher incidence of familial sudden cardiac death; more significant left ventricular hypertrophy and a higher incidence of cardiovascular mortality than in HCM patients who are sarcomere mutation negative [39–42]. Although most patients with pathogenic mutations are heterozygotes, in as many as 5% of cases, patients have more than one pathogenic mutation in the same gene or in a different sarcomeric gene, a phenomenon associated with a more severe phenotype and worse outcomes [11].

Mutations in *βMYH7* and *MYBPC3* account for 60–70% of HCM patients identified to possess a pathogenic mutation [32, 43]. Pathogenic mutations in *MYH7* are predominantly missense, with single nucleotide-base substitution resulting in a non-synonymous single amino acid substitution. The majority of mutations in *MYBPC3* however, are nonsense mutations due to insertion/deletions, splice-site variants or premature stop codons resulting in a truncated protein transcript [32, 44].

There is considerable genetic heterogeneity in HCM, with thousands of different mutations identified to date; many are unique or private within families. Some mutations also show marked variation in disease penetrance and clinical expression [45, 46]. Given the large size of individual cardiac sarcomere genes, and the random nature of mutational events, it is logical that sarcomeric genes are prone to de-novo mutational events [47].

9.2.4 Cellular Mechanisms and Pathways

The mechanisms by which mutations in sarcomeric protein genes result in the characteristic pathophysiological features of hypertrophic cardiomyopathy are incompletely understood.

The majority of missense mutations, such as those in *MYH7*, are believed to have a dominant negative effect, acting as a "poison polypeptide" on sarcomere function, i.e. the mutant protein is incorporated into the sarcomere, but its interaction with the normal wild-type protein disrupts normal sarcomeric assembly and function. These mutations may involve a change in an amino acid in a highly-conserved residue, changes in an important kinase domain (affecting ligand interaction) or in a surface-exposed portion of the molecule affecting protein-protein interaction. Missense mutations can also cause protein misfolding and accelerated removal by ubiquitin-proteasomal surveillance pathways.

In truncating mutations, as in the case of many pathogenic *MYBPC3 variants*, haploinsufficiency is postulated as a mechanism for disease pathogenesis. The reported absence of detectable truncated myosin binding protein c in western-blot analysis of myectomy specimens of patients with this mutation has been suggested to be due to nonsense mediated mRNA decay of abnormal transcripts or ubiquitin-mediated proteasomal degradation of aberrant truncated protein [48–51].

Allelic heterogeneity may be explained by the effect of different mutations on the structure and function of the complete peptide. *β*-myosin heavy chain, for example, consists of a globular head, an α-helical rod and a hinge region. The globular head contains binding sites for ATPase and actin as well as interaction sites for regulatory and essential light chains in the head-rod region. The majority of disease-causing *β*-myosin heavy chain mutations are found in one of four locations: the actin binding site, the nucleotide binding pocket, the hinge region adjacent to the binding site for two reactive thiols and in the α-helix close to the essential light chain interaction site. Therefore, depending on the position of the mutation, different changes might be expected in ATPase activity, actin-myosin interaction and protein conformation during contraction.

It has been previously speculated that the HCM disease phenotype results from reduced contractile function caused by altered actin-myosin interactions, and consequent inappropriate compensatory hypertrophic remodelling. This theory has also been supported by transgenic murine models (with *MYBPC3* mutations) showing disarray of the sarcomere on a cellular level [52], reduced myocyte contractile power as well as reduced rates of actin-myosin cross-bridge detachment in various assays [53].

However, studies of myocyte function in patients who harbour sarcomeric mutations are inconsistent as some *MYH7* mutations are associated with increased cardiomyocyte mechanical contractile forces in vitro [54, 55]. Biophysical studies of HCM mutant proteins have shown an increase in calcium sensitivity, leading to increases in tension generation and ATPase activity [56–72]. Animal studies have also confirmed altered calcium homeostasis as a key contributor to the pathophysiological processes that lead to the development of LV hypertrophy.

Murine models of sarcomeric HCM demonstrate increased calcium sensitivity and altered calcium cycling between the sarcomere and the sarcoplasmic reticulum. In vitro studies using purified myosin filaments and skinned papillary muscle from mice with the Arg403Gly mutation in the *MYH6* gene demonstrated increased calcium sensitivity of force development, predicted to cause impaired ventricular relaxation in vivo [73, 74]. Similarly, several studies in murine models of *TNNT2* and *TPM1* disease have demonstrated an increase in calcium sensitivity [75–81].

TNNT2 mouse models show varying degrees of myocyte disarray and fibrosis with minimal LVH, in common with *TNNT2* disease expression in humans [77, 80–82]. Troponin-mutated mice exhibit severely impaired myocardial relaxation, independent of the degree of fibrosis, and consistent with the finding of increased calcium sensitivity at a myofilament level [77, 80, 81]. Abnormal calcium kinetics may also contribute to the higher incidence of sudden death in patients with *TNNT2* mutations. In support of this, ventricular myocytes from mice harbouring the I79N mutation in *TNNT2* have a shorter effective refractory period with a lower terminal repolarization phase of the action potential and slowed decay kinetics, significantly increased diastolic calcium concentrations with isoproterenol, and stress-induced ventricular tachycardia [83].

Impaired calcium homeostasis and cellular signalling may result in an upregulation of myocyte hypertrophy via CaMKII (calcium/calmodulin-dependent protein kinase 2) phosphorylation, which in turn, induces factors such as myocyte enhancer factor 2. This has also been shown to be associated with focal myocardial scarring resulting from cellular death of stressed HCM myocytes [84]. Transcriptional analysis of ventricular myocytes prior to the advent of LVH in animal models, demonstrates an upregulation of periostin, transforming growth factor ß and other pro-fibrotic and proliferative intracellular signals to induce pathological remodelling in HCM. The administration of TGF-ß neutralizing antibodies in this murine model prevented non-myocyte proliferation and fibrosis. Chronic administration of an angiotensin II type 1 receptor antagonist also prevented the onset of LVH in mutation positive but phenotypic negative mice [85].

Some HCM mutations may result in inefficient ATP usage at the myofilament level, suggesting that cardiac myocytes in HCM have greater energy requirements than normal cells [86]. This is supported by findings from murine models of HCM, where mutations in *MYH6*, *MYBPC3*, *TNNT2*, and *TNNI3* result in increased contractility but at the expense of inefficient ATP utilization [55, 73, 76, 87, 88].

Furthermore, mice harbouring the Arg403Gly mutation in *MYH6* have reduced basal energy stores and abnormal ATP/ADP ratios [54, 55, 67, 89]. This inefficient utilization of ATP is also seen in metabolic disorders or mitochondrial cytopathies, which can produce a pattern of LV hypertrophy similar to that in sarcomeric HCM.

9.2.5 Phenotypic Variability

There is a substantial variation in the expression of identical mutations indicating that other genetic and possibly environmental factors influence disease expression. The effect of age is perhaps the best characterized factor, most patients developing ECG and echocardiographic manifestations of the disease after puberty and before the age of thirty [90]. Gender also appears to influence disease expression in sarcomere protein disease. Studies on the Arg403Gly *MYH6* mouse model show the development of left ventricular dilatation and systolic impairment in male but not female mice [91], and there is evidence to suggest that, in humans, males are at greater risk of developing end stage disease than females [92]. Other potential modifying factors include renin-angiotensin-aldosterone system gene polymorphism, and the occurrence of homozygosity and compound heterozygosity [93, 94].

9.2.6 Childhood Onset-HCM

The importance of sarcomeric protein gene mutations in childhood hypertrophic cardiomyopathy is unknown. The observation that the development of left ventricular hypertrophy in individuals with familial disease often occurs during the period of somatic growth in adolescence [95, 96] has led to the suggestion that sarcomeric protein disease in very young children is rare [97]. However, recent studies of children with HCM have shown that, like in adults, sarcomeric protein gene mutations account for approximately 50% of cases of idiopathic HCM, even in infants and young children [98, 99] (Table 9.1).

9.2.7 Clinical Presentation of HCM

9.2.7.1 Symptoms

Many individuals with HCM have few, if any, symptoms. The initial diagnosis is often made during family screening or following the incidental detection of a heart murmur or via an abnormal routine ECG. The most common symptoms are dyspnoea and chest pain, which are commonly exertional, but may also occur at rest or following large meals. Syncope is a relatively common symptom and is caused by multiple mechanisms including left ventricular outflow tract obstruction (LVOTO), abnormal vascular responses and atrial and ventricular arrhythmias [13, 100, 101]. Unexplained or exertional syncope is associated with an increased risk of sudden death in children and adolescents. Infants can present with symptoms of heart

Table 9.1 Classification and etiology of hypertrophic cardiomyopathy

Familial	Non-familial
Familial, unknown gene **Sarcomeric protein genes:** β myosin heavy chain Cardiac myosin binding protein c Cardiac troponin I Troponin T α-tropomyosin Essential myosin light chain Regulatory myosin light chain Cardiac actin Titin Troponin C Muscle LIM protein FHL-1 **Glycogen storage disease:** e.g. GSD II (Pompe's disease); GSD III (Forbes' disease), AMP kinase/PRKAG2 (WPW, HCM, conduction disease) Danon disease (LAMP2 gene) **Lysosomal storage diseases** (e.g. Anderson-Fabry disease, Hurler's syndrome) **Disorders of Fatty Acid Metabolism** **Carnitine deficiency** **Phosphorylase B kinase deficiency** **Mitochondrial cytopathies** (e.g. MELAS, MERRF, LHON) **Syndromic HCM** • Noonan syndrome • LEOPARD syndrome • Friedreich's ataxia • Beckwith-Wiedemann syndrome • Swyer syndrome (pure gonadal dysgenesis) • Costello syndrome **Other:** • Phospholamban promoter • Familial Transthyretin Amyloidosis	**Obesity** **Infants of diabetic mothers** **Athletic training** **Amyloid (AL/TTR)** **Hypertension** **Drug-Induced (Tacrolimus, Steroids)**

Data from Elliott et al. (2008) "Classification of the cardiomyopathies: a position statement from the European Society of Cardiology working group on myocardial and pericardial diseases" Eur Heart J *29*, 270–276

FHL-1 four and a half LIM domains protein 1, *GSD* glycogen storage disease, *AMP kinase* 5′ adenosine monophosphate-activated protein kinase, *PRKAG2* 5′-AMP-activated protein kinase subunit gamma-2, *WPW* Wolff-Parkinson-White syndrome, *HCM* hypertrophic cardiomyopathy, *LAMP2* lysosome-associated membrane protein 2, *MELAS* mitochondrial encephalomyopathy, lactic acidosis, and stroke-like episodes, *MERRF* myoclonic epilepsy with ragged-red fibers, *LHON* leber hereditary optic neuropathy, *LEOPARD* lentigines, ECG abnormalities, ocular hypertelorism, pulmonary stenosis, abnormal genitalia, retardation of growth and sensorineural deafness, *AL amyloid* amyloid light-chain, *TTR amyloid* transthyretin amyloidosis

failure, such as breathlessness, poor feeding, excessive sweating and failure to thrive [102–106]. These symptoms usually occur in the presence of apparently normal left ventricular ejection fraction and are often caused by outflow tract obstruction, mid-cavity gradient or diastolic dysfunction.

9.2.7.2 Clinical Examination

General examination may provide important diagnostic clues in patients with syndromic or metabolic phenocopies of sarcomeric HCM. Patients with HCM phenocopies may have other clinical features or diagnostic 'red flags' not associated with sarcomeric HCM such as cataracts, cognitive deficit, or skin rashes (such as in Anderson-Fabry Disease or LEOPARD syndrome) [16].

Paradoxically, the cardiovascular examination is often normal, but in patients with left ventricular outflow tract obstruction, the arterial pulse may have a bisferiens character. The jugular venous pulsation may have a prominent 'a' wave, caused by reduced right ventricular compliance. Palpation of the precordium may reveal a sustained, or double, apical pulsation, reflecting an atrial impulse followed by LV contraction; rarely, an additional late systolic impulse, resulting in a triple apex beat, may be felt. Auscultatory findings in patients with obstructive HCM include an ejection systolic murmur at the left lower sternal edge radiating to the right upper sternal edge and apex, but usually not to the carotid arteries or axilla. This murmur may be associated with a palpable precordial thrill. As the obstruction in HCM is a dynamic phenomenon, the intensity of the murmur is increased by manoeuvres that reduce the preload or afterload, such as standing from a squatting position or the valsalva manoeuvre. Most patients with LV outflow tract obstruction also have mitral regurgitation (caused by abnormal coaptation of the mitral valve leaflets during systole).

9.2.8 Natural History

HCM can present at any age, from infancy to advanced age [107]. Many patients follow a stable and benign course, with a low risk of adverse events, but a large number experience progressive symptoms caused by a gradual deterioration in left ventricular systolic and diastolic function and atrial arrhythmias. A proportion of individuals die suddenly from ventricular arrhythmias, whereas others may die from progressive heart failure, thromboembolism, and rarely, infective endocarditis.

Recent studies in adults with HCM report annual sudden death rates of 1% or less in adults [107, 108] and 1–1.5% per year in children and adolescents. Progression to a "burnt out" phase [92, 109–121], has a reported prevalence ranging from 2 to 15% in adults [92, 117, 120]. This stage is characterized by progressive left ventricular dilatation, wall thinning and systolic impairment [122–124] and is associated with a poor prognosis [120], with an overall mortality rate of up to 11% per year [92]. Presentation in infancy can also be associated with severe and intractable heart failure [104–106, 125].

Atrial fibrillation (AF) is the commonest sustained arrhythmia in HCM, occurring in up to 25% of patients [126–128]. Its development is related to left atrial dilatation, and its incidence increases with age [129, 130]. Although well tolerated in many cases, AF can result in acute and severe haemodynamic deterioration and is associated with a high risk of thromboembolism.

9.2.9 Investigations

9.2.9.1 Electrocardiography

The resting 12-lead ECG is abnormal in 95% of individuals with HCM. Common features include large voltage QRS complexes, repolarization abnormalities (with ST segment elevation or depression), pathological Q waves (most frequently in the inferolateral leads) and left atrial enlargement. Voltage criteria for LV hypertrophy alone is not specific for HCM, and is often seen in normal, healthy teenagers and young adults. In infants, right ventricular hypertrophy on the ECG is commonly found. Giant negative T waves in the mid-precordial leads are characteristic of apical HCM [131].

Some patients have a short PR interval or a slurred upstroke to the QRS (not associated with an accessory pathway). Patients that have HCM secondary to mutations in the AMP kinase pathway, often have pre-excitation on their ECG together with LVH.

Atrioventricular conduction delay (including first-degree block) is rare except in particular subtypes of hypertrophic cardiomyopathy (e.g. in association with mutations in *PRKAG2* and mitochondrial disease) [132, 133]. Conduction abnormalities should prompt consideration of a potential HCM phenocopy such as cardiac amyloidosis or Anderson-Fabry disease [134]. In first-degree relatives of HCM, the ECG sometimes shows subtle abnormalities without echo features of hypertrophy.

The frequency of supraventricular and ventricular arrhythmias in HCM increases with age [127, 135–137]. Ambulatory ECG monitoring reveals supraventricular arrhythmias in 30–50% and non-sustained ventricular tachycardia (NSVT) in 25–30% of individuals [138]. Most episodes of NSVT are relatively slow, asymptomatic, and occur during periods of increased vagal tone. Sustained ventricular tachycardia is uncommon, but may occur in association with apical aneurysms [139].

9.2.9.2 Echocardiography

HCM is identified by the presence on echocardiography of LV wall thickness greater than two standard deviations above the body surface area-corrected mean in any myocardial segment (see also Chap. 8). In a proband with suspected HCM, a wall thickness >=15 mm is usually required or >=13 mm in a first degree relative of a patient with HCM [14]. Any pattern of LV hypertrophy is consistent with the diagnosis of HCM, including concentric (equal hypertrophy across all segments of the left ventricle), eccentric (with the lateral and posterior walls more affected than the septum), distal (distal segments more affected than basal segments), and apical (hypertrophy confined to the left ventricular apex) [25, 140–142] patterns.

Approximately 25% of patients have LVOTO at rest, and as many as 70% may have latent, or provocable LVOTO, caused by contact between the anterior mitral valve leaflet or chordae and the ventricular septum during systole [143, 144]. Most patients with systolic anterior motion of the mitral valve and LVOTO have a posteriorly directed jet of mitral regurgitation. In some patients, systolic obliteration of the left ventricular cavity may produce a high velocity gradient in the mid-ventricle and consequent midcavity obstruction [145]. Right ventricular outflow tract obstruction may be seen in infants with HCM, and in older children and adults with cardiomyopathy associated with Noonan syndrome and some metabolic disorders.

Left ventricular global systolic function, as assessed by changes in ventricular volume during the cardiac cycle, is typically increased. However, regional and long-axis function on tissue Doppler or strain deformation analysis is often reduced, and cardiac output responses during exercise may be impaired [146–148]. Diastolic function is often impaired in patients with HCM. Characteristically, patients with diastolic left ventricular impairment demonstrate reduced early diastolic (Ea) velocities in the mitral annulus and septum, and a reversal of the ratio of early to late diastolic velocities (Ea/Aa). In addition, the ratio of mitral inflow E wave to annular early diastolic velocity (E/Ea) can be used as a measure of left ventricular end-diastolic pressure, and predicts exercise capacity in adults [149] and children [150] with HCM. Tissue Doppler imaging may be useful in detecting mild disease in otherwise phenotypically normal gene carriers [151, 152].

9.2.9.3 Cardiopulmonary Exercise Testing

Individuals with HCM usually have a reduced peak oxygen consumption during exercise testing compared with healthy age-matched controls, even when asymptomatic [153, 154]. This can help from a diagnostic perspective in differentiation of patients with HCM from those with an athlete's heart where athletic individuals quite often have a supranormal peak oxygen consumption.

In addition, one quarter of adults with HCM have an abnormal blood pressure response to exercise, with the blood pressure falling or failing to rise by more than 20–25 mmHg from baseline [155, 156]. This results from abnormal vasodilatation of the non-exercising vascular beds, possibly triggered by inappropriate firing of left ventricular baroreceptors [100] and impaired cardiac output responses [157]. CPEX can also provide useful prognostic information in HCM patients. Exercise parameters such as ventilatory efficiency, anaerobic threshold and peak oxygen consumption may predict mortality from heart failure [158].

9.2.9.4 Cardiac Magnetic Resonance Imaging

Cardiac magnetic resonance imaging is used to evaluate the distribution and severity of LV hypertrophy and can provide functional measurements of systolic and diastolic function (see Chap. 7). It is particularly useful for assessing the degree of apical hypertrophy and the presence of apical aneurysms in the distal variant of HCM which may be sometimes sub-optimally assessed on TTE. In addition, magnetic resonance imaging can be used to assess myocardial tissue characteristics in vivo with gadolinium contrast agents. Many patients with HCM have areas of patchy gadolinium hyperenhancement particularly in the regions of maximal hypertrophy and studies suggest that the extent of gadolinium enhancement correlates with risk factors for sudden death and with progressive left ventricular remodelling [159, 160]. Adenosine induced stress perfusion MRI can be used to look for areas of reduced perfusion on stress that may be due to concomitant epicardial coronary artery disease or due to microvascular dysfunction. [161, 162].

9.2.10 Clinical Management

9.2.10.1 Symptoms

Patients with LVOTO require lifestyle advice including remaining adequately hydrated, avoiding excess ethanol intake, optimising body mass index and avoiding large heavy meals. β-adrenergic receptor blockers are recommended first line in patients with symptomatic obstructive HCM. β-blockers can reduce symptoms of chest pain, dyspnoea and presyncope on exertion. Studies using very large doses of propranolol in children and adolescents have reported improved long-term survival [163], but side-effects are common, as they can affect growth and school performance in young children or trigger depression [107].

In adults, the addition of the class I antiarrhythmic disopyramide can also reduce obstruction and improve symptoms [164–167], an effect exerted through its negative inotropic and peripheral vasoconstriction action. Disopyramide dose uptitration is limited by its anticholinergic side-effects including constipation, urinary retention, dry eyes and dry mouth resulting in it being contraindicated in patients with glaucoma or prostatic symptoms. In addition, disopyramide causes prolongation of the QT interval and so the ECG must be monitored regularly and other drugs that prolong the QT interval should be avoided.

Calcium antagonists, verapamil or diltiazem, may be used as an alternative to beta-blockers, to improve LVOTO symptoms by relieving myocardial ischaemia and reducing myocardial contractility [168, 169]. Verapamil has negative chronotropic, negative inotropic and positive lusitropic (improves diastolic filling) actions. However, in patients with severe symptoms caused by large (>100 mmHg) gradients and pulmonary hypertension, verapamil can cause rapid haemodynamic deterioration [170, 171] and therefore must be used with caution in this group. Spironolactone may be used to improve symptoms related to diastolic dysfunction or raised LV filling pressures.

Candidates for invasive management of LV outflow tract symptoms include those with NYHA class 3–4 symptoms on maximal tolerated medical therapy with an LVOT gradient >=50 mmHg and or recurrent exertional syncope [14]. The reference standard therapy [172–176] is septal myectomy, in which a trough of muscle is removed from the interventricular septum through an aortic incision. In the hands of experienced surgeons, the peri-operative mortality is <1% and the success rate is high, with long-term abolition of outflow gradient, resulting in a marked improvement in symptoms and exercise capacity in over 90% of patients [14]. Complications include complete heart block requiring permanent pacemaker insertion in less than 5% of patients and ventricular septal defect. Post-myectomy, patients may develop a mild degree of aortic insufficiency which may progress slowly over time [177, 178]. As many as 20% of patients undergoing myectomy, require mitral valve intervention as well via an Alfieri stitch or MV replacement.

Alcohol septal ablation (ASA) of the interventricular septum is an alternative procedure in which 95% alcohol is injected into a septal perforator of the left anterior descending coronary artery branch using a small over the wire balloon catheter located in one of the first or second septal perforators to produce an area of localized myocardial necrosis within the basal septum and induce septal hypokinesis [179–181]. Myocardial damage is kept to a minimum by visualizing the area supplied by the perforator branch using echocardiographic visualization of intra-coronary contrast injection. The incidence of permanent pacing is upto 15% given the risk of transient or permanent AV block.

Pacing of the right ventricular apex has been suggested to provide beneficial haemodynamic effects in patients with LVOTO. Pacing causes paradoxical septal motion away from systolic anterior motion of the mitral valve and contributes to reduced LV inotropy and reduced degrees of outflow tract obstruction [182]. The response of pacing with a short AV delay to manage LVOTO is variable [182–185] and is usually reserved for those that have conduction disease and are likely to require pacing or in those not amenable to myectomy or ASA.

In patients without LVOTO, chest pain and dyspnoea are usually caused by LV diastolic impairment and myocardial ischaemia. Treatment in this group of patients is empiric and often suboptimal. Both β-blockers and calcium antagonists can ameliorate symptoms by improving LV relaxation and filling, reducing LV contractility and relieving myocardial ischaemia. 25% of patients with mid-cavity obstruction go on to develop LV apical aneurysms. In some cases, patients can develop LV thrombus within the aneurysm, which would mandate anticoagulation. LV aneurysms may also act as a substrate for monomorphic ventricular tachycardia.

Individuals who develop end-stage disease should receive conventional heart failure treatment, and if appropriate, be considered for device therapy (CRT) or for cardiac transplantation [186]. A recent study suggested that biventricular pacing improved heart failure symptoms and resulted in reverse atrial and ventricular remodelling in up to 40% of patients with end-stage HCM [187].

A select subgroup of patients with HCM and refractory symptoms despite optimal management should be considered for referral for cardiac transplantation.

9.2.11 Sudden Cardiac Death

Although, the overall risk of sudden death in patients with HCM is low, at less than 1% per annum, a minority of individuals have a much greater risk of ventricular arrhythmia and sudden death [188, 189]. The most reliable predictor of sudden cardiac death in HCM is a history of previous cardiac arrest [190, 191]. In patients without such a history, the most clinically useful markers of risk are: a family history of sudden cardiac death [192, 193]; unexplained syncope (unrelated to neurocardiogenic mechanisms); an abnormal blood pressure response to upright exercise particularly if under the age of 40 [156, 194, 195]; non-sustained ventricular tachycardia on ambulatory electrocardiographic monitoring or during exercise [135, 194, 196]; and left ventricular wall thickness of 30 mm or more [197, 198]. Patients with none of these features have a low risk of sudden death (less than 1% per year), whereas those with two or more risk factors are at substantially higher risk of dying suddenly. A recent retrospective, multi-centred analysis resulted in the formulation of the HCM risk-SCD score to estimate annual mortality rates and help guide defibrillator therapy [199]. This scoring system incorporates variables including age, maximum wall thickness, left atrial dimension, LV outflow tract gradient [200], presence of NSVT, family history of sudden cardiac death and unexplained syncope and takes into account the incremental impact continuous variables such as larger LV wall thickness have on the risk of SCD, rather than absolute 'cut-offs' that the older conventional algorithms utilise [199].

In patients considered to be at high risk of sudden death, insertion of an implantable cardioverter-defibrillator (ICD) should be considered [107]. Retrospective registry data demonstrate that ICDs prevent sudden death in patients with HCM, with annual appropriate discharge rates of 11% in secondary prevention patients (those with a history of prior cardiac arrest or sustained ventricular arrhythmia) and 3–5% in the primary prevention group [201, 202]. In children with HCM, appropriate discharge rates are higher in the secondary prevention group [203, 204].

9.3 Metabolic Cardiomyopathies

A number of inheritable inborn errors of metabolism are associated with left ventricular hypertrophy (Table 9.1) (see also Chap. 7).

9.3.1 Anderson-Fabry Disease (AFD)

Anderson-Fabry disease (AFD) is a lysosomal storage disorder caused by mutations in the α-galactosidase A gene. It is inherited as an X-linked dominant trait and the resultant enzyme deficiency causes progressive accumulation of glycosphingolipid in the skin, nervous system, kidneys and most commonly, the heart [205, 206]. Cardiac manifestations include progressive left ventricular hypertrophy (which can be a sarcomeric HCM phenocopy), valve disease, conduction abnormalities, supraventricular and ventricular arrhythmias. AFD is associated with a high burden of cardiovascular morbidty and mortality with one cohort study identifying 10% of patients developing severe heart failure; 6% of patients requiring bradycardia pacing and 3% with cardiovascular mortality [207]. Disease expression begins after adolescence in males and females [206, 208–210] with males generally more severely affected than their female counterparts due to the X-linked pattern of inheritance. Treatment with recombinant α-galactosidase A improves renal and neurological manifestations as well as quality of life, but its effect on the cardiac manifestations is still not determined [206]. Studies involving small number of patients have suggested that in patients without myocardial fibrosis, enzyme replacement therapy results in a reduction in LV mass and improvement in myocardial function although this effect is only minimal once patients have mild or more advanced myocardial fibrosis [211].

9.3.2 Danon Disease

Danon disease is an X-linked lysosomal storage disorder, characterised clinically by cardiomyopathy, skeletal myopathy and developmental delay. It is caused by mutations in the gene encoding lysosome-associated membrane protein-2 (LAMP-2) [212] and results in intra-cytoplasmic accumulation of autophagic material and glycogen within vacuoles in cardiac and skeletal myocytes [213]. Males develop symptoms during childhood and adolescence, whereas female carriers usually develop hypertrophic or dilated cardiomyopathy during adulthood [214]. The prognosis is generally poor, with most patients dying from cardiac failure, although sudden death is also reported, even in female carriers [214]. It has been identified as a relatively common cause of unexplained left ventricular hypertrophy in paediatric populations, accounting for 6% of cases in a cohort of 136 paediatric patients with HCM [215]. The average age of symptom onset in males is 12.1 years, cardiac transplantation at 17.9 years and mortality at 19 years; which is over a decade earlier than their female counterparts [216]. Other features of Danon disease include Wolff-Parkinson-White syndrome, elevated serum creatine kinase and retinitis pigmentosa [217].

9.3.3 *Pompe Disease* (Glycogen Storage Disease Type IIa)

Pompe disease (glycogen storage disease type IIa) is an autosomal recessive disorder caused by a deficiency in the enzyme acid maltase. Infantile, juvenile and adult variants are recognised, differing in their age of onset, rate of disease progression and organ involvement. The infantile and childhood forms are characterized by myocardial glycogen deposition, massive cardiac hypertrophy and heart failure. The infantile form presents in the first few months of life with severe skeletal muscle hypotonia, progressive weakness, cardiomegaly, hepatomegaly and macroglossia and is usually fatal before 2 years of age due to cardiorespiratory failure. The ECG typically shows broad high-voltage QRS complexes and ventricular pre-excitation. In the juvenile and adult onset variants, disease is usually limited to skeletal muscle, with a slowly progressive proximal myopathy and respiratory muscle weakness. Recombinant enzyme replacement in the infantile and childhood forms appears to cause regression of left ventricular hypertrophy and is associated with improved survival [218–220].

9.3.4 Wolff-Parkinson-White syndrome

Mutations in the gene encoding the γ_2 *subunit of the adenosine monophosphate-activated protein kinase* (*PRKAG2*) [221, 222] are responsible for a syndrome of hypertrophic cardiomyopathy, conduction abnormalities and Wolff-Parkinson-White syndrome and are inherited in an autosomal dominant fashion. The majority of these patient have the missense mutation p.Arg302Gln, in the *PRKAG2* gene

[223]. This 'gain of function' mutation in basal AMP kinase activity results in excessive myocardial glucose uptake and pathological glycogen storage within cardiomyocytes [224, 225]. Histologically, there is an accumulation of glycogen within cardiac myocytes and the conduction tissue. A skeletal myopathy is present in many individuals and skeletal muscle biopsy shows excess mitochondria and ragged red fibres [226]. Patients develop progressive conduction disease, often requiring a pacemaker by their fourth or fifth decade in life, and left ventricular hypertrophy and atrial arrhythmias are common [225, 227]. The left ventricular hypertrophy may be asymmetric left ventricular hypertrophy, apical hypertrophy or even biventricular hypertrophy [223]. Electrocardiographic expression is universal by the age of 18 years [226]. Disease-related mortality is related to thromboembolic stroke (resulting from atrial fibrillation) and sudden cardiac death [226]. In a cohort analysis of 34 patients with *PRKAG2* mutations, 61% developed a HCM phenotype, 22% developed conduction block and 20% had sudden cardiac death by the age of 40 [223]. Recent studies suggest that *PRKAG2* mutations account for no more than 1% of cases of HCM [226].

9.3.5 Mitochondrial Cardiomyopathies

Primary mitochondrial disorders are caused by sporadic or inherited mutations in nuclear or mitochondrial DNA that are transmitted as autosomal dominant, autosomal recessive, X-linked or maternal traits (see also Chap. 8). The most frequent abnormalities occur in genes that encode the respiratory chain protein complexes, leading to impaired oxygen utilization and reduced energy production. The clinical presentation of mitochondrial disease is variable in age at onset, symptoms, and the range and severity of organ involvement. Cardiac involvement is a feature in up to 40% of mitochondrial encephalomyopathies [228], and usually takes the form of a hypertrophic cardiomyopathy [229–231], although other cardiomyopathies, including dilated cardiomyopathy and left ventricular non-compaction are reported [228]. Children with mitochondrial disease and cardiac involvement present earlier than those with non-cardiac disease [228, 229] and have a much worse prognosis [228]. The cardiac phenotype is usually concentric LV hypertrophy without outflow tract obstruction, and rapid progression to left ventricular dilatation, systolic impairment and heart failure is described [228, 229]. Sudden arrhythmic death has also been reported [228, 229]. Complications such as heart failure and ventricular arrhythmias can be exacerbated by a metabolic crisis precipitated by febrile illness or surgery. Some of the mitochondrial disorders include MELAS (Mitochondrial Encephalomyopathy, Lactic Acidosis and Stroke-like episodes), MERRF (Myoclonic Epilepsy with Ragged Red Fibres), MIDD (Maternally Inherited Deafness and Diabetes), LHON (Leber Hereditary Optic Neuropathy), Leigh Syndrome, Barth Syndrome and Kearns-Sayre Syndrome [232]. In a case series of patients with MERRF, early age of disease onset was the only factor associated with the occurrence of myocardial disease [233].

9.3.6 Friedreich's Ataxia

Friedreich's ataxia is an autosomal recessive condition caused by mutations in the frataxin gene. Cardiac involvement is very common, and is usually (but not exclusively) characterized by concentric LV hypertrophy without LV outflow tract obstruction [234]. Patients are usually asymptomatic from a cardiac viewpoint, but progression to LV dilatation and heart failure is described [235]. As many as 60% of patients with Friedreich's ataxia die from cardiac causes [236].

9.4 Malformation Syndromes Associated with LV Hypertrophy

A number of malformation syndromes, most of which present in childhood, are associated with HCM (see also Chap. 6).

9.4.1 Noonan Syndrome

Noonan syndrome is characterized by short stature, dysmorphic facies, skeletal malformations and a webbed neck [237–239]. Cardiac involvement is present in up to 90% of patients with Noonan syndrome and most commonly takes the form of pulmonary valve stenosis and HCM [240]. Some cases present with congestive cardiac failure in infancy and may be associated with biventricular hypertrophy and bilateral ventricular outflow tract obstruction [240]. The cardiac histological findings in Noonan syndrome are indistinguishable from idiopathic HCM [241]. Noonan syndrome is inherited as an autosomal dominant trait with variable penetrance and expression. Mutations in the *PTPN11* gene, encoding the protein tyrosine phosphatase SHP-2 (a protein with a critical role in RAS-ERK-mediated intracellular signal transduction pathways controlling diverse developmental processes [242]), have been shown to cause Noonan syndrome [243]. To date, at least 39 different mutations have been identified, accounting for approximately 50% of cases of Noonan syndrome [239]. Other genes implicated in Noonan syndrome include *SOS1* [244] (encoding a RAS-specific guanine nucleotide exchange factor), which accounts for up to 28% of cases [245, 246]; *KRAS* (which encodes a GTP-binding protein in the RAS-ERK pathway) in less than 5% of cases [247]; and *RAF1* (a downstream effector of RAS) [248, 249]. Only 5–9% of all individuals with mutations in the *PTPN11* gene have hypertrophic cardiomyopathy [250, 251]. In one longitudinal study of 74 patients with Noonan syndrome and HCM, affected individuals were more likely to present at an earlier age (before 6 months of age) and with congestive cardiac failure when compared to children with sarcomeric HCM. They also had a significant early mortality of 22% at 1 year [252].

9.4.2 LEOPARD Syndrome

LEOPARD syndrome (Lentigines, ECG abnormalities, Ocular hypertelorism, Pulmonary stenosis, Abnormalities of the genitalia, Retardation of growth, and Deafness) shares many phenotypic features with Noonan syndrome, and recent studies have shown that most patients with LEOPARD syndrome also have mutations in the *PTPN11* gene [253]. HCM in patients with LEOPARD syndrome is usually asymmetric LVH and is generally found in as many as 80% of patients with cardiac defects. Patients may also develop significant LV outflow tract obstruction in upto 40% of cases [254]. The HCM usually precedes the lentigine formation and it can worsen with the appearance of lentigines [255]. Sudden death has also been reported in patients with LEOPARD syndrome and HCM [256].

Key Points

- Hypertrophic cardiomyopathy is a heterogeneous condition that can affect patients at any age
- Most cases are caused by autosomal dominant mutations in cardiac sarcomere protein genes
- Other causes include inherited errors of metabolism, mitochondrial disease, malformation syndromes and neuromuscular disorders
- The management of hypertrophic cardiomyopathy includes evaluation of family members, symptom management, and identification and prevention of disease-related complications, including sudden cardiac death, heart failure and thromboembolism

9.5 Dilated Cardiomyopathy

Dilated cardiomyopathy (DCM) is a myocardial disorder characterized by the presence of LV dilatation and LV systolic impairment in the absence of abnormal loading conditions or coronary artery disease sufficient to cause global systolic dysfunction [1]. Right ventricular dilatation and dysfunction may also be present. There are also overlapping phenotypes with arrhythmogenic cardiomyopathy or LV non-compaction. The prevalence of DCM is thought to be in the range of 1 in 2500 adults, with an annual incidence of between 5 and 8 per 100,000 [2]. Familial DCM accounts for between 20–48% of cases of DCM [257]. In children, the incidence is much lower (0.5–0.8 per 100,000 per year), but DCM is the commonest cardiomyopathy in the paediatric population [8, 9].

9.5.1 Etiology

DCM can be caused by toxins, neuromuscular disorders, inborn errors of metabolism and malformation syndromes (Table 9.2), but in the majority of patients, no identifiable cause is found ('idiopathic DCM') [58, 194]. Up to 25% of individuals

Table 9.2 Classification and etiology of dilated cardiomyopathy

Familial	Non-familial
Familial, unknown gene **Sarcomeric protein mutations** • MYH7 (β myosin heavy chain) • MYBPC3 (Cardiac myosin binding protein c) • TNNT2 (Troponin T) • TNNI3 (Troponin I) • TTN (Titin) **Z band and associated proteins:** • ZASP • Muscle LIM protein • TCAP • BAG3 (Bcl2-Associated Athanogene) • FLNC (Filamin C) **Cytoskeletal genes:** • Dystrophin • Desmin • Metavinculin • Sarcoglycan complex • CRYAB • Epicardin Nuclear membrane • Lamin A/C • Emerin **Intercalated disc protein mutations** • Desmoplakin **Mitochondrial cytopathy**	**Myocarditis** (infective/toxic/immune) **Kawasaki disease** **Eosinophilic** (Churg Strauss syndrome) **Viral persistence e.g. Retroviral disease (HIV)** **Drugs e.g. Anthracycline induced cardiomyopathy; Cocaine** **Pregnancy and Peri-partum cardiomyopathy** **Endocrine e.g. Thyroid dysfunction** **Nutritional**—thiamine, carnitine, selenium, hypophosphataemia, hypocalcaemia **Alcohol** **Tachycardia-induced cardiomyopathy**

Data from Elliott et al. (2008) "Classification of the cardiomyopathies: a position statement from the European Society of Cardiology working group on myocardial and pericardial diseases" Eur Heart J *29*, 270–276
ZASP ZO-2 associated speckle protein, *TCAP* titin-cap, *CRYAB* crystallin alpha B

with DCM have familial disease, in which at least one other first-degree relative is affected [258], and a further 20% of family members have isolated LV enlargement with preserved systolic function, a proportion (up to 10%) of whom subsequently develop overt DCM [259, 260]. Genetic causes of DCM may result in a purely isolated cardiac phenotype or also result in a peripheral skeletal myopathy.

9.5.2 Familial/Genetic DCM

A number of genetic mutations can cause DCM [86]. In the majority of cases, these are transmitted as an autosomal dominant trait, but other forms of inheritance, including autosomal recessive, X-linked (e.g. dystrophin, tafazzin or emerin) and matrilinear inheritance are also recognized. The mutations implicated in DCM are heterogeneous and involve genes encoding proteins in various cellular structures such as nuclear envelope, cytoskeleton, cardiac sarcomere, mitochondrial and calcium handling transporters [261, 262].

Genes implicated in isolated DCM include cytoskeletal (δ-sarcoglycan [263], β-sarcoglycan [264] and desmin) and sarcomere protein genes (including Titin [265], α-cardiac actin [266], troponin T [267], β-myosin heavy chain [267], troponin C [268, 269] and α-tropomyosin [270]). Many of these are non-synonymous missense mutations or involve insertion-deletions or substitutions resulting in protein truncation (via a premature stop codon).

The pathophysiological mechanisms by which cytoskeletal mutations cause DCM include impaired transmission of contractile force generated by the sarcomere. In many cases, sarcomeric protein gene mutations associated with DCM are located in functional domains involved in force propagation, suggesting a common pathophysiological mechanism with cytoskeletal mutations [261]. As in HCM, altered myocyte bioenergetic processes also play a role in the development of DCM associated with sarcomeric and cytoskeletal mutations. Troponin T mutations, for example, can cause DCM by altering calcium sensitivity and cell contractility.

Titin is the largest sarcomere protein encompassing almost half of the sarcomere. It plays an important organisational and anchoring role, regulating sarcomere length within the cardiac myocyte. Recently, the role of Titin (*TTN*) mutations in the pathogenesis of DCM has been identified, accounting for as many as 35% of sarcomeric mutations implicated in DCM. Truncating TTN mutations are associated with DCM and cluster in the A band of the Titin molecule. In one analysis of a DCM cohort, 54 out of 312 DCM patients had nonsense, frame-shift or splice-site affecting mutations that truncated the titin molecule [265].

Mutations in other genes including Troponin C (*TNNC1*), Troponin T (*TNNT2*), Tropomyosin (*TPM1*), Myosin Heavy Chain (*MYH7*) or Myosin Binding Protein C (*MYBPC3*) can also cause the onset of a DCM phenotype. For example, a lysine base-pair deletion at position 210 of the troponin T gene results in a gain of function of the coded mutant protein which in turn disrupts inter-molecular interaction within the sarcomere between troponin T and tropomysosin capitulating the DCM phenotype [271, 272].

Tropomyosin mutations cause DCM as well as LV non-compaction. A D230N mutation in the *TPM1* gene was previously described in two different large cohorts [273]. This mutation reduces the calcium sensitivity of actinin-activated myosin ATPase and is associated with a heterogeneous DCM phenotype from DCM onset in childhood to mild LV dilatation.

Specific mutations (e.g. S532P and F764 L) in the *MYH7* gene are associated with familial DCM and LVNC [274]. These mutations affect the myosin head and actin binding, resulting in reduced sarcomere energy efficiency.

Mutations in genes that encode costamere proteins also cause DCM. These proteins link the cytoskeleton to the cell membrane as well as to the extracellular matrix. The dystrophin complex, which is linked to cytoplasmic proteins and to integrin, talin and vinculin, all protect against contraction injury to the striated muscle [275]. Loss of function mutations in these integral structures in the dystrophin complex render the cardiomyocyte susceptible to contraction damage [276].

Mutations in proteins in the Z band of the cardiac sarcomere have also been identified in the pathogenesis of DCM. The Z band is the electron microscopic dense region where thin filaments and titin molecules anchor. Mutations in cardiac ankyrin repeat protein (*CARP*), *TCAP*, alpha-actinin 2 (*ACTN2*) and muscle lim protein (*MLP*) have been identified.

Several genes are also associated with isolated DCM and conduction disease [86, 277], but only one, lamin A/C which encodes a nuclear envelope intermediate filament protein, has been identified. Lamins A and C together with other lamin associated proteins form part of the LINC complex and are located in the nucleoplasm as well as the nuclear membrane. Lamins A and C are differently spliced proteins encoded by the *LMNA* gene. Mutations in lamin A/C result in atrial arrhythmia and progressive atrioventricular conduction disease that frequently precedes the development of LV dilatation and systolic dysfunction by several years [278–280] (see also Chap. 10). Some mutations in lamin A/C result in DCM and conduction disease alone [279], whereas others lead to juvenile-onset muscular dystrophies (including Emery-Dreiffus muscular dystrophy) [281, 282] or familial partial lipodystrophy with insulin resistant diabetes [283]. Over 200 mutations in the *LMNA* gene have been identified; the majority are autosomal dominant, although recessive variants have also been identified. In one study of familial DCM and concomitant conduction tissue disease, 33% of patients had a mutation in the *LMNA* gene [284]. Pathogenic mutations, particularly frameshift mutations, in the *LMNA* gene also increase the risk of ventricular dysrhythmias [285]. The pathophysiological mechanisms underlying disease in Lamin A/C remain poorly understood, but several hypotheses have been proposed. These include nuclear fragility with disruption of the nuclear architecture; alterations in cellular signalling or gene expression, resulting in abnormal interaction between lamins and other nuclear proteins such as desmin; and interference with the processing of pre-lamin A, which results in abnormal lamin function and nuclear abnormalities [286, 287]. Cardiac myocytes from mice deficient in lamin A/C have abnormalities of the nucleus and desmin cytoskeletal network and impaired mechanotransduction and activation of transcriptional programmes in response to mechanical stress [288–290].

Recently, mutations in the Filamin C (*FLNC*) gene, have been identified as a cause of DCM or arrhythmogenic cardiomyopathy. Filamin C is a protein that attaches the cardiac sarcomere to the cellular membrane and mutations in this gene can also be associated with myofibrillar myopathy. Truncating mutations in *FLNC* are associated with ventricular dilatation and dysfunction; myocardial fibrosis, ventricular arrhythmias and sudden cardiac death with >97% penetrance by 40 years of age [291].

X-linked inheritance accounts for between 2–5% of familial cases of DCM [292–295]. Most cases are caused by Duchenne, Becker and Emery-Dreifuss muscular dystrophies. Isolated X-linked DCM, also caused by mutations in the dystrophin gene, was first described in 1987 in young males with severe disease and rapid progression of congestive cardiac failure to death or transplantation [296]. The condition is characterized by raised serum creatine kinase muscle isoforms, but does not result in the clinical features of muscular dystrophy seen in Duchenne or Becker muscular dystrophies. Female carriers of Duchenne and Becker muscular dystrophies, as well as female carriers of X-linked DCM, develop DCM later in life, usually in their 50s, that is milder in severity than that in their male counterparts. Cardiac muscle biopsies in female carriers show a mosaic pattern of dystrophin expression [297].

Barth syndrome (DCM, skeletal myopathy and neutropenia) is an X-linked disorder cause by mutations in the G4.5 gene, which encodes the protein tafazzin [298, 299]. The condition typically presents in male neonates or young infants with congestive heart failure, neutropenia and 3-methylgutaconic aciduria. Although some children die in infancy (due to progressive heart failure, sudden death or sepsis), most survive into childhood and beyond, but the DCM persists. Mutations in the G4.5 gene also cause isolated DCM, endocardial fibroelastosis and LV noncompaction, with or without the other features of Barth syndrome [300, 301].

9.5.3 Non-familial/Non-genetic DCM

While numerous causes of non-familial DCM are recognized (Table 9.2), in most patients, no obvious environmental or endogenous trigger for disease is found. Non-familial causes should prompt a search for autoimmune, toxin, infective and metabolic aetiologies [302].

Acute or chronic myocarditis may result in a dilated cardiomyopathy phenotype. In animal models, acute myocarditis caused by viral infection results in an initial phase of myocyte necrosis and macrophage activation, which in turn results in the release of numerous cytokines including interleukin-1, tumour necrosis factor and interferon gamma. These stimulate the infiltration of mononuclear cells and production of neutralizing antibodies, resulting in viral clearance [303]. Following this viral clearance phase, the heart may recover completely or may enter a chronic phase secondary to activation of neuro-humoral systems, resulting in ongoing fibrosis, LV dilatation and heart failure.

Myocarditis is often a difficult diagnosis as it encompasses a variety of clinical presentations such as acute coronary syndrome, arrhythmic presentation and congestive heart failure. The gold standard for diagnosis is an invasive endomyocardial biopsy to demonstrate active myocardial inflammation however there is significant variability in the utilisation of this technique [304, 305]. Increasingly, non-invasive imaging modalities such as CMRI are being used to confirm the diagnosis.

Many studies have examined the prevalence of myocardial inflammation and viral particles in DCM. Studies using immunocytochemical techniques to detect myocardial inflammation show that up to two-thirds of patients have an inflammatory cardiomyopathy [306, 307]. This is associated with increased expression of HLA class II major histo-compatibility antigens as well as cell adhesion molecules [307].

The underlying cause of the inflammation seen in DCM remains incompletely understood. There is circumstantial evidence that some of the inflammation relates to auto-immune processes: there is an association between DCM and HLA-DR4 antigen; many patients have elevated levels of circulating cytokines and cardiac-specific antibodies; there is evidence for familial aggregation of auto-immune diseases in some individuals with DCM; and relatives of patients with DCM also have increased levels of circulating cytokines and anti-heart antibodies [308–311].

A second hypothesis is that the inflammation is secondary to the persistence of viral particles in the myocardium. Studies in children suggest that 20% of patients with DCM have evidence for viral persistence compared to 1.4% of normal controls [312]. In adults, the prevalence varies from 0% to as many as 80% of patients [313–315]. There are several reasons for the variability, including differences related to the size and number of the biopsy samples or to laboratory technique and processing.

9.5.4 Other Causes of Dilated Cardiomyopathy in Childhood

Inborn errors of metabolism account for only 4% of cases of DCM. Of these, mitochondrial disorders are the commonest (46% of cases), followed by Barth syndrome (24%) and primary or systemic carnitine deficiency (11%) [295]. Patients with DCM in association with metabolic disease typically present in infancy and there is a male predominance. Malformation syndromes are rarely associated with DCM in 1% of cases [295]. Hypocalcaemic rickets can present as an isolated DCM in infancy [316–321].

9.5.5 Pathology

The characteristic macroscopic features of DCM are the presence of a globular shaped heart with ventricular (and often also atrial) chamber dilatation and diffuse endocardial thickening [322]. Thrombus may be present in the atrial appendages and within the ventricular cavity. Overall, myocardial mass is increased, but ventricular wall thickness is reduced. The histological features of DCM are non-specific and include myocyte degeneration, interstitial fibrosis, myocyte nuclear hypertrophy and pleomorphism (Fig. 9.2). There is often extensive myofibrillary loss, resulting in a vacuolated appearance of the myocytes. In addition, there is frequently an increase in interstitial T lymphocytes and focal accumulation of macrophages associated with individual myocyte death [322].

9.5.6 Clinical Presentation

The symptoms and signs associated with DCM are highly variable and dependent on the degree of left ventricular dysfunction. Whilst sudden cardiac death or a

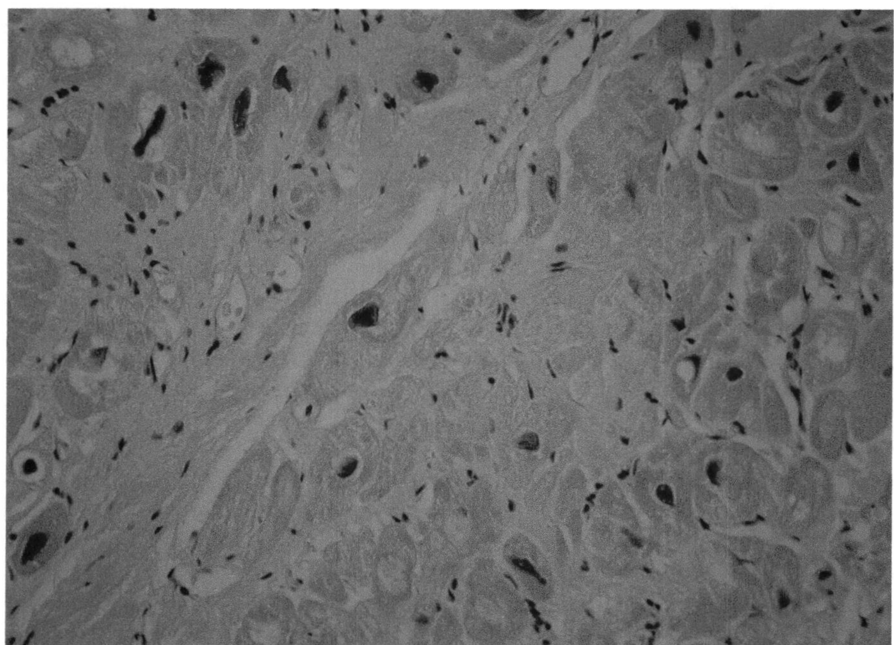

Fig. 9.2 Histology of dilated cardiomyopathy: This section shows myocyte morphology in dilated cardiomyopathy, individual myocytes showing hypertrophy with some vacuolation and enlarged, irregular hyperchormatic dark blue nuclei. Some myocytes are trapped in fibrous tissue [light pink]. *Courtesy of Dr Margaret Burke, Harefield Hospital, London, UK*

thromboembolic event may be the initial presentation, the majority of patients present with symptoms of high pulmonary venous pressure, arrhythmias (such as atrial fibrillation) and/or low cardiac output. This presentation can be acute (often precipitated by intercurrent illness or arrhythmia [58, 194, 323]) or chronic, with symptoms preceding the diagnosis by many months or years. Increasingly, DCM is diagnosed incidentally in asymptomatic individuals as a result of familial screening or routine medical assessment.

9.5.6.1 Symptoms

Older children and adults often present initially with reduced exercise tolerance and dyspnoea on exertion. As LV function deteriorates, dyspnoea at rest, orthopnoea, paroxysmal nocturnal dyspnoea, peripheral oedema and ascites may develop. Infants with DCM typically present with poor feeding, tachypnoea, respiratory distress, diaphoresis during feeding and failure to thrive. In children, symptoms related to mesenteric ischaemia may occur, such as abdominal pain after meals, nausea, vomiting and anorexia. Symptoms related to arrhythmia such as palpitation, presyncope and syncope occur at any age.

9.5.6.2 Physical Examination

Multisystem examination is important in patients with DCM, as it may direct towards underlying aetiology. Examination of the neuromuscular system may reveal features of mild or subclinical skeletal myopathy and ophthalmological examination may identify pigmentary retinopathy in mitochondrial disorders. Features of low cardiac output include persistent sinus tachycardia, cool peripheries, weak peripheral pulses and, in advanced disease, hypotension. The jugular venous pressure may be elevated. There may also be signs of respiratory distress, particularly in infants and younger children. Palpation of the precordium usually reveals a displaced apical impulse. Hepatomegaly and ascites are common in patients with congestive cardiac failure. Peripheral and sacral oedema may also be seen. Auscultation of the heart may reveal the presence of a third (and sometimes fourth) heart sound resulting in a gallop rhythm. There may be a pansystolic murmur at the apex radiating to the axilla caused by functional mitral regurgitation. Auscultation of the chest may also reveal basal crackles; infants may present with wheeze that is difficult to distinguish from asthma or bronchiolitis.

9.5.7 Natural History

The prognosis of DCM is variable and depends on the presentation and aetiology. Early survival studies suggested a mortality in symptomatic adults with idiopathic DCM approaching 25% at 1 year and 50% at 5 years [324]. More recent reports have shown better outcomes, with 5-year mortality rates of approximately 20%, perhaps reflecting earlier disease recognition and treatment, and advances in medical therapy. Most patients die of progressive congestive cardiac failure, but thromboembolism and sudden cardiac death are also important. In children, actuarial rates of freedom from death or transplantation range from 70 to 80% at 1 year and 55 to 65% at 5 years [295, 325, 326], including patients with viral myocarditis. In the paediatric population, predictors of poor outcome include older age at diagnosis, reduced fractional shortening (expressed as a function of body surface area or age), congestive cardiac failure at presentation and familial, idiopathic or neuromuscular disease [295, 326].

9.5.8 Investigations

9.5.8.1 Electrocardiography

The 12-lead ECG in DCM may be normal, but can show sinus tachycardia and non-specific ST segment and T wave changes (usually in the inferior and lateral leads). In patients with extensive LV fibrosis, abnormal Q waves (particularly in the septal leads) may be present as may poor R wave progression in the precordial leads. Evidence of atrial enlargement and voltage criteria for ventricular hypertrophy (usually left, but occasionally bilateral ventricular hypertrophy) is common. All degrees of atrioventricular block may be seen, and should raise the possibility of mutations in the lamin A/C gene. Supraventricular (particularly atrial fibrillation) and ventricular arrhythmias are common in DCM. Studies have shown a prevalence of non-sustained ventricular tachycardia in adults as high as 43% [327]; in the pediatric population, ventricular tachycardia is less common, occurring in 9.5% of cases [328]. Prolonged QRS duration, particularly in the context of LBBB represents a degree of interventricular dysynchrony and suggests a role for biventricular pacing in the management of some DCM patients.

9.5.8.2 Echocardiography

In general, the presence of a LV end-diastolic dimension greater than two standard deviations above body surface area-corrected means (or greater than 112% of predicted dimension) and fractional shortening less than 25% (ejection fraction less than 55%) are sufficient to make the diagnosis of DCM [329–331]. The presence and severity of functional mitral (and tricuspid) regurgitation due to annular dilatation can be assessed using colour flow Doppler. In addition, pulsed-wave and continuous wave Doppler can be used to estimate pulmonary artery systolic pressures. Although primarily regarded as a disease of impaired systolic LV function, patients with DCM also frequently have abnormalities of diastolic LV function. A restrictive physiology (grade 3 diastolic dysfunction) with raised atrial filling pressures is associated with higher mortality rates in DCM cohorts compared to those that have pseudonormal or impaired relaxation patterns of mitral inflow.

Echocardiography may identify regional wall motion abnormalities, which together with the clinical history may be used to assess the likelihood of ischaemic cardiomyopathy. Regional wall motion abnormalities can also occur in infiltrative and inflammatory causes of DCM such as sarcoidosis [323, 332]. Serial echocardiography over time can also provide an assessment of the progression or regression of LV dilatation and impairment on medical therapy.

9.5.8.3 Cardiac Biomarkers

Levels of serum creatine kinase should be measured in all patients with DCM, as this may provide important clues to the aetiology of the condition (elevated in patients with dystrophin and Lamin A/C mutations). Other cardiac biomarkers, such as Troponin I and Troponin T, may also be elevated in DCM. Plasma B-type natriuretic peptide levels are elevated in children and adults with chronic heart failure and predict survival, hospitalization rates and listing for cardiac transplantation [323, 333]. Worsening renal function in patients with advanced cardiac disease may suggest the onset of a cardio-renal syndrome and is a marker of poor outcome and need for advance heart failure therapies.

9.5.8.4 Exercise Testing

Symptom limited exercise testing combined with respiratory gas analysis is a useful technique to assess functional limitation and disease progression. Typically, patients with DCM have lower exercise duration, peak oxygen consumption and systolic blood pressure at peak exercise than normal controls [334]. The detection of respiratory markers of severe lactic acidaemia during metabolic exercise testing can point towards mitochondrial or metabolic causes for the DCM. CPEX assessment is used in patients being considered for transplantation to assess their VO_2 max and to ensure cardiac limitation to exercise. Outcomes of CPEX correlate with prognosis in DCM [335].

9.5.8.5 Cardiac Catheterization

Cardiac catheterization can be useful to exclude significant coronary arterial disease and to monitor pulmonary arterial pressures. Endomyocardial biopsy (EMB) is a useful adjunct in the investigation of some patients with DCM and may be diagnostic for myocarditis and for some metabolic or mitochondrial disorders [336]. EMB often identifies non-specific abnormalities such as interstitial fibrosis and increased nuclei with myocyte hypertrophy. Where patients are being evaluated for the aetiology of suspected chronic myocarditis then viral PCR can be used to look for persisting viral genome. International guidelines recommend that endomyocardial biopsy should be performed in the setting of new onset unexplained heart failure of less than 2 weeks duration with normal or enlarged left ventricular dimensions and hemodynamic compromise, or between 2 weeks and 3 months in the presence of left ventricular dilatation and ventricular arrhythmias or higher degree heart block [337].

9.5.8.6 Cardiac Magnetic Resonance Imaging

Cardiac magnetic resonance imaging is a useful alternative imaging technique in patients with poor echocardiographic windows and is the gold standard for measurement of volumes and ventricular ejection fraction [323]. In addition, the detection of fibrosis with gadolinium contrast enhancement may provide an imaging-guided method to improve the diagnostic yield of endomyocardial biopsies [338]. Late gadolinium enhancement may be distributed at the RV insertion points and in a mid-wall pattern suggestive of underlying myopathic disease. Subepicardial LGE however, is more suggestive of myocarditis and together with T2-STIR mapping (reflecting oedema) may suggest active myocardial inflammation.

Serial cardiac MRI can be used to monitor for progression in the pattern or extent of fibrosis and to monitor resolution of myocardial inflammation. Early gadolinium enhancement sequences can also be used to look for and characterise LV thrombus.

9.5.8.7 Holter Analysis

Holter monitors may be used to look for evidence of atrial fibrillation or non-sustained VT. Reduced heart rate variability in patients with DCM is associated with a worse prognosis.

9.5.9 Management

Therapy aims to improve symptoms and prevent disease progression and complications such as progressive cardiac failure, sudden cardiac death and thromboembolism. Loop and thiazide diuretics are used in all heart failure patients with fluid retention to achieve a euvolaemic state. However, they should not be used as monotherapy as they exacerbate neurohormonal activation, which may contribute to disease progression. Spironolactone, a specific aldosterone antagonist, reduces relative mortality by 30% in adults with severe heart failure (NYHA class IV and ejection fraction less than 35%) [339]. Side-effects include hyperkalaemia (although this is infrequent in the presence of normal renal function) and gynaecomastia. Epleronone, a drug with an identical mechanism of action can be used instead, particularly if gynaecomastia becomes a problem [340].

9.5.9.1 Angiotensin Converting Enzyme (ACE) Inhibitors and Angiotensin Receptor Blockers

Activation of the renin-angiotensin-aldosterone system is central to the pathophysiology of heart failure, regardless of the underlying aetiology [329, 341]. Numerous randomised trials have shown that ACE inhibitors improve symptoms, reduce hospitalisations and reduce cardiovascular mortality in adults with heart failure [342–345]. They also reduce the rate of disease progression in asymptomatic patients. Most patients tolerate ACE inhibitors well. The most common side-effects are a dry cough and symptomatic hypotension (particularly following the initial dose), which can be prevented with careful dose uptitration.

Angiotensin receptor blockers block the cell surface receptor for angiotensin II, and have similar haemodynamic effects to ACE inhibitors but with a better side-effect profile. Angiotensin receptor blockers are currently recommended in adults who do not tolerate ACE inhibitors [346–349].

9.5.9.2 β-Blockers

Excess sympathetic activity contributes to heart failure, and multicentred, placebo controlled trials, using carvedilol [350–352], metoprolol [353] and bisoprolol [354] have shown substantial reductions in mortality (from sudden death and progressive heart failure) in adults with predominantly NYHA class II and III heart failure symptoms. β-blockers are usually well tolerated; side-effects include bradycardia, hypotension and fatigue.

9.5.9.3 Digoxin

Digoxin improves symptoms in patients with heart failure [355], but no survival benefit has been demonstrated in large study cohorts [341]. Supra-therapeutic serum digoxin levels may be associated with increased mortality in some patients [356]. Although digoxin is still widely used to treat heart failure in infants and children, there remains limited data on its efficacy in paediatric populations [357].

9.5.9.4 Ivabradine

Ivabradine is a negative chronotrope and a selective inhibitor of the I_f channel located in the sino-atrial node. In one randomized, placebo-controlled trial in patients with impaired LV systolic function, ivabradine therapy was associated with a reduction in hospital admission and mortality from heart failure [358]. Ivabradine can be used alone or in conjunction with beta-blockers, in particular if beta-blocker dose uptitration is limited by hypotension.

9.5.9.5 Entresto (Sacubitril/Valsartan)

Entresto is a combination drug that provides combined inhibition of the renin-angiotensin-aldosterone (RAAS) system (valsartan) and of neprilysin (sacubitril). This results in an increase of vasoactive natriuretic peptides and increases natriuresis, aldosterone suppression, vasodilation and inhibition of fibrosis. A single multi-centred, randomized controlled trial (PARADIGM-HF) demonstrated that Entresto is superior to ACE inhibition alone in individuals with chronic heart failure [359]. There is limited knowledge on whether these results are transferable to patients with idiopathic or familial dilated cardiomyopathy as the majority of patients (60%) recruited into this study had ischaemic cardiomyopathy.

9.5.9.6 Anticoagulation

The annual risk of thromboembolism in patients with dilated cardiomyopathy is between 1.5–3.5% per year [360]. Anticoagulation with warfarin is advised in patients in whom an intracardiac thrombus is identified echocardiographically and in those with a history of thromboembolism or atrial fibrillation. There is no trial data to recommend prophylactic anticoagulation in DCM [361], but some patients with severe ventricular dilatation and moderate to severe LV systolic impairment may benefit from empirical warfarin therapy [362].

9.5.9.7 Treatment of Arrhythmia in DCM

The overall risk of sudden cardiac death in DCM is low in patients receiving optimal medical therapy but individuals with some sub-types of disease, for example caused by *LMNA* and *FLNC* mutations, are more prone to ventricular arrhythmia. Whilst the indications for secondary prevention ICD in DCM, are unequivocal in survivors of aborted SCD or patients presenting with haemodynamically unstable sustained VT, the role of a primary prevention ICD in DCM is less clear. The pivitol Sudden Cardiac Death in Heart Failure Trial (SCD-HeFT), showed no survival benefit of amiodarone therapy (compared with a 23% reduction in overall mortality with implantable cardioverter-defibrillator implantation) [363]. Similar findings were demonstrated in the recent multi-centred, randomized controlled DANISH trial (Defibrillator implantation in Patients with Nonischemic Systolic Heart Failure); which demonstrated that ICD implantation was not associated with an overall survival benefit in terms of all-cause mortality or cardiovascular mortality in patients with nonischemic cardiomyopathy although there was a significant reduction in the incidence of sudden cardiac death in those that received ICD. Sub-group analysis also identified that all-cause mortality was also reduced in the ICD cohort in patients below the age of 59 years [364].

AF is the commonest sustained rhythm abnormality in patients with heart failure [365]. In a previous single centred study of patients with idiopathic DCM, 5.7% of patients developed AF on long-term follow-up (90 ± 58 months). Dilated left atrium and a lower LV ejection fraction were predictors of new onset AF with those developing AF having a higher rate of mortality or cardiac transplantation compared to those that remained in sinus rhythm over the follow-up duration [366].

9.5.9.8 Non-pharmacological Treatment of Advanced DCM

Cardiac transplantation remains the mainstay of management of children and adults with intractable heart failure symptoms and end stage disease. However, its use is limited by a shortage of donor organs and the development of graft vasculopathy. Therefore, a number of other approaches aimed at improving symptoms and stabilizing the disease or delaying transplantation have emerged. In some cases, mechanical assist devices, such as left ventricular assist devices (LVAD), the Berlin heart, or extracorporeal membrane oxygenation (ECMO) may be required [367–369]. Studies in children have shown good results with aggressive management of end-stage dilated cardiomyopathy, including bridging to recovery [370].

9.5.9.9 Cardiac Resynchronisation Therapy (CRT)

Many patients with DCM have abnormal LV activation that in turn results in prolonged and incoordinate ventricular relaxation. Cardiac resynchronization therapy (biventricular or multisite pacing) attempts to re-establish synchronous atrioventricular, interventricular and intraventricular contraction to maximize ventricular efficiency. Studies in adults with severe heart failure and left bundle branch block have shown marked symptomatic improvement [371], and reduced mortality from heart failure or sudden death [372–374]. DCM is a predictor of positive response to cardiac resynchronization. Patients with DCM have a greater improvement in LV systolic function and improved reverse remodelling with reduction in LV end-diastolic volumes than patients with ischaemic cardiomyopathy after CRT implantation [375].

9.5.10 Prognosis

DCM is a heterogeneous group of disorders and so prognosis is difficult to characterise for a particular group of patients. Generally, prognosis is worse for those that have an ongoing damaging stimulus to the heart such as ongoing persistence of myocardial inflammation or ongoing ethanol abuse. A subgroup of patients, despite being on optimal medical therapy will continue to progress to end-stage heart failure and cardiogenic shock requiring LVAD support or cardiac transplantation for survival.

9.5.11 Summary and Key Points

Dilated cardiomyopathy is characterised by the presence of left ventricular dilatation and systolic dysfunction (Box 13.2). Despite a thorough search for underlying aetiology, most cases remain idiopathic. As genetic causes account for a significant proportion of individuals, a detailed family pedigree and potential familial screening to identify other individuals at-risk is important. Advances in pharmacological, device and advanced heart failure therapy have improved survival and quality of life, but the prognosis in many cases remains poor. Novel pharmacological and device therapies may provide further improvements in long-term outcome.

Key Points

- Most cases of dilated cardiomyopathy are idiopathic
- Familial disease occurs in up to 35% of individuals
- Inheritance can be autosomal dominant, autosomal recessive, X-linked or mitochondrial
- Genes implicated in familial disease include myocardial cytoskeletal, sarcomere protein and nuclear envelope genes
- Advances in pharmacologic and non-pharmacologic therapy have improved survival and quality of life, but the prognosis in many cases remains poor

9.6 Restrictive Cardiomyopathy

Restrictive cardiomyopathy (RCM) is characterised by an abnormal pattern of ventricular filling in which increased myocardial stiffness causes a precipitous increment in ventricular pressure with only small increases in ventricular volume in the presence of normal or reduced diastolic volumes of one or both ventricles, normal or reduced systolic volumes and normal ventricular wall thickness [1]. Restrictive ventricular *physiology* can also occur in HCM and DCM. RCM is the least common of all the cardiomyopathies.

9.6.1 Etiology

Restrictive cardiomyopathy is associated with several conditions (Table 9.3), including infiltrative and storage disorders, familial and endomyocardial disease [376]. In adults, RCM is most commonly caused by cardiac amyloidosis in the Western world, while in the tropics, endomyocardial fibrosis is the commonest cause in

Table 9.3 Classification and etiology of restrictive cardiomyopathy

Familial	Non-familial
Familial, unknown gene	**Amyloid (AL/TTR)**
Sarcomeric protein mutations:	**Scleroderma**
• Troponin I (RCM ± HCM)	**Endomyocardial fibrosis**
• Essential light chain of myosin	• Hypereosinophilic syndrome
Familial Amyloidosis	• Idiopathic
• Transthyretin (RCM + neuropathy)	• Drugs: (serotonin, methysergide, ergotamine, mercurial agents, busulfan)
• Apolipoprotein (RCM + nephropathy)	**Carcinoid heart disease**
Desminopathy (desmin gene mutation)—associated with skeletal myopathy	**Metastatic cancers**
Pseudoxanthoma elasticum	**Radiation**
Hereditary Haemochromatosis	**Drugs: Anthracycline**
Anderson-Fabry disease	
Glycogen storage disease	

Data from Elliott et al. (2008) "Classification of the cardiomyopathies: a position statement from the European Society of Cardiology working group on myocardial and pericardial diseases" Eur Heart J 29, 270–276

adults and probably also in children [376]. Outside of the tropics, most cases of RCM in children are idiopathic [376].

9.6.1.1 Idiopathic Restrictive Cardiomyopathy

Many cases of RCM in adults, and the majority in children, remain idiopathic. Familial disease is described in approximately 30% of patients with RCM [377]. Little is known about the role of genetic mutations in idiopathic RCM due to the rarity of the condition, as well as because most studies to date have only included small patient cohorts undergoing limited genetic panels. Autosomal dominant, autosomal recessive, X-linked and matrilinear patterns of inheritance have been demonstrated.

Mutations in cardiac sarcomere genes have been implicated in the pathogenesis of RCM with one study identifying mutations in the cardiac troponin I gene in over 50% of adults with idiopathic restrictive cardiomyopathy [378]. Subsequently, mutations in β-myosin heavy chain gene were identified in adults with familial HCM with a restrictive phenotype and little or no hypertrophy. An I79N mutation in the TNNT2 gene has been shown to be accountable for divergent phenotypes of RCM, HCM and DCM within the same family [379].

In a recent study of 32 probands with end-stage idiopathic RCM, a pathogenic mutation was identified in 60% of cases; involving *MYH7*, *DES*, *FLNC*, *MYBPC3*, *LMNA*, *TCAP*, *TNNI3*, *TNNT2*, *TPM1* and *LAMP2* genes [380]. Another study involving next-generation sequencing of 24 patients with idiopathic RCM, identified pathogenic or likely-pathogenic variants in 54% with mutations occurring in genes encoding sarcomeric, cystoskeletal and Z-disk associated proteins [381].

In children with idiopathic RCM, mutations in the genes encoding troponin I, troponin T, α-cardiac actin and β-myosin heavy chain have also been reported [378, 382–384].

Mutations in the gene encoding desmin (an intermediate filament protein with key structural and functional roles within skeletal and cardiac myocyte myofibrils) causes RCM associated with skeletal myopathy and cardiac conduction system abnormalities [385]. Desmin mutations are inherited in an autosomal dominant manner, but sporadic mutations are not infrequent [385]. The presence of a desmin mutation should lower the threshold for consideration for prophylactic defibrillator implantation, particularly in the presence of conduction disease [386].

The finding that mutations in sarcomere protein genes cause restrictive cardiomyopathy has provided new insights into the pathophysiology of restrictive left ventricular physiology. In vitro studies have suggested that troponin I mutations that cause RCM have a greater increase in calcium ion sensitivity than those that cause HCM, resulting in more severe diastolic dysfunction and potentially accounting for the restrictive phenotype in humans [387, 388]. In addition, the hearts of troponin I-mutated transgenic mice show increased contractility and impaired relaxation [389]. Similar findings have been observed in mice with disease-causing alpha-myosin heavy chain mutations [55]. These results suggest that altered calcium sensitivity may play a role in the development of RCM. However, the fact that the same mutation within the same family can result in both restrictive and hypertrophic phenotypes suggests that other genetic and environmental factors are likely to also be involved in the pathogenesis of restrictive cardiomyopathy [390].

9.6.1.2 Endomyocardial Fibrosis and Eosinophilic Cardiomyopathy

Restrictive ventricular physiology can be caused by endocardial pathology (fibrosis, fibroelastosis and thrombosis). These disorders are sub-classified according the presence of eosinophilia into endomyocardial diseases with hypereosinophilia (hypereosinophilic syndromes (HES)) and endomyocardial disease without hypereosinophilia (e.g. endomyocardial fibrosis). Parasitic infection, drugs such as methysergide, inflammatory and nutritional factors are implicated in acquired forms of endomyocardial fibrosis.

The acute variant of eosinophilic cardiomyopathy is known as Loffler's endocarditis whereas the chronic variant is known as endomyocardial fibrosis. In Loffler's endocarditis, there is an acute inflammatory process and eosinophilia which results in myocardial tissue infiltration classically involving one or both ventricular apex, chordae tendinae and ventricular inflow tract. This results in valvular regurgitation and impaired diastolic filling.

Endomyocardial fibrosis onset is usually insidious, with progressive biventricular failure in most cases. The overall prognosis is poor, with a 44% mortality rate at 1 year, increasing to nearly 90% at 3 years [391]. Typically, fibrous endocardial lesions in the right and/or left ventricular inflow tract cause incompetence of the atrioventricular valves leading to pulmonary congestion and right heart failure. Endomyocardial fibrosis involves both ventricles in the majority of cases but there are variants in which only the LV (40%) or only the RV (10%) is involved. Patients with endomyocardial fibrosis may remain stable with chronic symptoms for decades prior to a rapid decline.

9.6.2 Pathology

The macroscopic features of restrictive cardiomyopathy include biatrial dilatation in the presence of normal heart weight, a small ventricular cavity and no left ventricular hypertrophy. However, the morphologic spectrum of primary restrictive cardiomyopathy includes mild ventricular hypertrophy with increased heart weight and mild ventricular dilatation without hypertrophy [392]. In many hearts, there is thrombus in the atrial appendages and patchy endocardial fibrosis [376].

The histological features of idiopathic restrictive cardiomyopathy are classically non-specific with patchy interstitial fibrosis, which may range in extent from very mild to severe [376]. There may also be fibrosis of the sinoatrial and atrioventricular nodes [393]. Myocyte disarray is not uncommon in patients with pure restrictive cardiomyopathy, even in the absence of macroscopic ventricular hypertrophy [392]. In patients with infiltrative and metabolic cardiomyopathies, there will be specific findings appropriate to the disorder [322].

9.6.3 Clinical Features

9.6.3.1 Symptoms

The presentation of restrictive cardiomyopathy is usually with symptoms and signs of cardiac failure and arrhythmia. In children, disease progression is rapid, with over 50% of children dying within 2 years of diagnosis and most children requiring cardiac transplantation within 4 years [394, 395]. The presentation and natural history in adults is more variable. Common symptoms include dyspnoea on exertion, recurrent respiratory tract infections, and general fatigue and weakness. This may progress rapidly to dyspnoea at rest, orthopnoea and paroxysmal nocturnal dyspnoea. Symptoms related to increased right-sided pressures may include peripheral oedema and abdominal distension due to ascites. Many patients complain of chest pain and symptoms suggestive of arrhythmia such as palpitation. Syncope is a presenting symptom in 10% of children with restrictive cardiomyopathy [396, 397]. Rarely, sudden death may be the initial manifestation of the disease.

9.6.3.2 Physical Examination

Clinical examination typically reveals signs of left and right-sided cardiac failure. Tachypnoea, signs of respiratory distress and failure to thrive are seen in infants and young children. In older children and adults, the jugular venous pressure is elevated, with a prominent y descent, and a JVP that fails to fall (or may even rise) during inspiration (Kussmaul's sign). Peripheral oedema, ascites and hepatomegaly are common. The apical impulse is usually normal. Cardiac auscultation reveals a normal first heart sound and normal splitting of the second heart sound. The pulmonary component of the second heart sound may be loud, if pulmonary vascular resistance is high. There is usually a third heart sound (and occasionally a fourth heart sound) giving rise to a gallop rhythm. The murmurs of atrioventricular valve regurgitation may be heard.

Depending on the aetiology of the restrictive cardiomyopathy, other clinical signs may be elicited such as conjunctival pallor, petechiae, skin bruising and carpal tunnel syndrome in some patients with amyloidosis [134, 398]. Skin pigmentation and peripheral arthropathy may be found in patients with underlying haemochromatosis and cardiac MRI can be used to assess iron loading and monitor response to therapy. A peripheral subtle skeletal muscle phenotype such as weakness may be found in patients with desmin mutations.

9.6.4 Investigations

9.6.4.1 Electrocardiography

The resting 12-lead electrocardiogram is abnormal in most patients with restrictive cardiomyopathy. The most frequent abnormalities include p-mitrale and p-pulmonale, non-specific ST segment and T wave abnormalities, ST segment depression and T wave inversion, usually in the inferolateral leads. Voltage criteria for left and right ventricular hypertrophy may also be present, although in patients with amyloidosis, low voltage QRS complexes are seen despite the presence of

LVH. Conduction abnormalities, including intraventricular conduction delay, AV block, poor R wave progression in the anterior precordial leads and abnormal Q waves may also be seen. In RCM, due to elevated LA pressures and LA dilatation, there is a higher incidence of AF, which may be seen on the ECG. Sarcoidosis may present with AV block [332]. Desmin mutations are also associated with AV block.

9.6.4.2 Echocardiography

Typically, there is marked dilatation of both atria, often dwarfing the size of the ventricles, in the presence of normal or mildly reduced systolic function, and a non-hypertrophied, non-dilated left ventricle. In children, severe impairment of left ventricular systolic function (fractional shortening less than 25%) may develop in as many as 30% of cases [396, 399–401]. Many patients with a clinical label of restrictive cardiomyopathy also have mild left ventricular hypertrophy [396, 399–402], which may represent part of the spectrum of sarcomere protein disease.

The pattern of mitral inflow pulsed-wave Doppler velocities in restrictive cardiomyopathy is typically one of increased early diastolic filling velocity, decreased atrial filling velocity, an increased ratio of early diastolic filling to atrial filling, a decreased E wave deceleration time, and a decreased isovolumic relaxation time. Pulmonary vein and hepatic vein pulsed-wave Doppler velocities demonstrate higher diastolic than systolic velocities, increased atrial reversal velocities, and an atrial reversal duration greater than mitral atrial filling duration. Tissue Doppler imaging shows reduced diastolic annular velocities, and an increased ratio of early diastolic tissue Doppler annular velocity to mitral early diastolic filling velocity, reflecting elevated left ventricular end-diastolic pressures.

9.6.4.3 Cardiopulmonary Exercise Testing

Symptom-limited exercise testing with respiratory gas analysis provides a useful objective measure of exercise limitation, which can help in symptom management and is an important component of the pre-transplantation assessment. Peak oxygen consumption is usually reduced. Exercise testing may also reveal ischaemic electrocardiographic changes at higher heart rates, which may correlate with symptoms such as chest pain in children [377, 397].

9.6.4.4 Cardiac Catheterization

The characteristic hemodynamic feature on cardiac catheterization is a deep and rapid early decline in ventricular pressure at the onset of diastole, with a rapid rise to a plateau in early diastole, the so-called dip-and-plateau or square root sign [376]. Left ventricular end-diastolic, left atrial and pulmonary capillary wedge pressures are markedly elevated, and usually 5 mmHg or more greater than right atrial and right ventricular end-diastolic pressures. Volume loading and exercise accentuate the difference between left and right-sided pressures. Cardiac catheterisation is also useful to differentiate constrictive pericarditis from restrictive cardiomyopathy where there is a discordance in diastolic ventricular pressures between the LV and RV in RCM compared to constrictive pericarditis where there is a concordance. Apical obliteration may be demonstrated on LV/RV angiography or on 2-D echocardiography.

In children, pulmonary hypertension is frequently present during initial cardiac catheterisation. Elevated pulmonary vascular resistance indices are commonly found, and tend to progress during follow-up [394, 401, 403]. Elevated pulmonary vascular resistance may initially be reversible with nitric oxide or prostacyclin [394, 403], but it is usually not possible to predict the development of fixed pulmonary vascular resistance [401].

9.6.5 Management

9.6.5.1 Symptomatic Therapy

Diuretics are useful in patients with symptoms and signs of pulmonary or systemic venous congestion. Over-diuresis, however should be avoided as it may result in excessive preload reduction and haemodynamic collapse. Careful fluid management is an important aspect of the treatment of patients with restrictive cardiomyopathy. In view of atrial enlargement and propensity to atrial arrhythmia, prophylactic anticoagulation with warfarin or antiplatelet agents is recommended. As the atrial contribution to ventricular filling in patients with restrictive cardiomyopathy is important, efforts to maintain sinus rhythm with ß-blockers and amiodarone may be appropriate. Treatment with afterload-reducing agents, such as angiotensin-converting enzyme inhibitors, calcium channel blockers and nitrates rarely improves symptoms and can cause deterioration [404]. In patients with atrial dysrhythmias, control of ventricular rate is important and digoxin may play a role in ventricular rate control as do the other negative chronotropes.

9.6.5.2 Optimisation of Haemodynamics Prior to Transplantation

Transplantation is the only definitive treatment for children with restrictive cardiomyopathy, and for adults with advanced disease that is unresponsive to medical therapy. In children, whilst fixed, irreversible elevations in pulmonary vascular resistance preclude orthotopic cardiac transplantation [401], short-term pre-transplantation treatment with prostacyclin has been shown to reduce transpulmonary gradients sufficiently to allow orthotopic heart transplantation in most children with restrictive cardiomyopathy [394]. Patients should undergo serial holter monitoring; implantable cardioverter-defibrillators may be offered to patients with evidence of ventricular arrhythmia as a bridge to transplantation.

9.6.6 Summary and Key Points

Restrictive cardiomyopathy (RCM) is uncommon but a large proportion of cases may be familial due to diverse genetic aetiology. Adequate symptom control frequently requires diuretic therapy. Patients are closely monitored for raised pulmonary arterial pressures which may prompt referral for advanced heart failure strategies. Prognosis is variable but in particular, poor in infants and children, where cardiac transplantation may be helpful.

Key Points

- Restrictive cardiomyopathy is the rarest of the cardiomyopathies
- Most cases are idiopathic
- Familial disease is recognised in up to 50% of individuals with idiopathic restrictive cardiomyopathy
- Genes implicated in idiopathic restrictive cardiomyopathy include sarcomere protein genes and desmin
- Other causes include infiltrative and storage disorders
- Prognosis is poor, especially in infants and children, in whom transplantation is usually the only therapeutic option.

References

1. Elliott P, Anderson B, Arbustini E, Bilinska Z, Cecchi F, Charron P, Dubourg O, Kuhl U, Maisch B, McKenna WJ, et al. Classification of the cardiomyopathies: a position statement from the European Society of Cardiology Working Group on Myocardial and Pericardial Diseases. Eur Heart J. 2008;29:270–6.
2. Codd MB, Sugrue DD, Gersh BJ, Melton LJ 3rd. Epidemiology of idiopathic dilated and hypertrophic cardiomyopathy. A population-based study in Olmsted County, Minnesota, 1975-1984. Circulation. 1989;80:564–72.
3. Hada Y, Sakamoto T, Amano K, Yamaguchi T, Takenaka K, Takahashi H, Takikawa R, Hasegawa I, Takahashi T, Suzuki J, et al. Prevalence of hypertrophic cardiomyopathy in a population of adult Japanese workers as detected by echocardiographic screening. Am J Cardiol. 1987;59:183–4.
4. Maron BJ, Peterson EE, Maron MS, Peterson JE. Prevalence of hypertrophic cardiomyopathy in an outpatient population referred for echocardiographic study. Am J Cardiol. 1994;73:577–80.
5. Maron BJ, Gardin JM, Flack JM, Gidding SS, Kurosaki TT, Bild DE. Prevalence of hypertrophic cardiomyopathy in a general population of young adults. Echocardiographic analysis of 4111 subjects in the CARDIA Study. Coronary Artery Risk Development in (Young) Adults. Circulation. 1995;92:785–9.
6. Morita H, Larson MG, Barr SC, Vasan RS, O'Donnell CJ, Hirschhorn JN, Levy D, Corey D, Seidman CE, Seidman JG, et al. Single-gene mutations and increased left ventricular wall thickness in the community: the Framingham Heart Study. Circulation. 2006;113:2697–705.
7. Zou Y, Song L, Wang Z, Ma A, Liu T, Gu H, Lu S, Wu P, Zhang dagger Y, Shen dagger L, et al. Prevalence of idiopathic hypertrophic cardiomyopathy in China: a population-based echocardiographic analysis of 8080 adults. Am J Med. 2004;116:14–8.
8. Lipshultz SE, Sleeper LA, Towbin JA, Lowe AM, Orav EJ, Cox GF, Lurie PR, McCoy KL, McDonald MA, Messere JE, et al. The incidence of pediatric cardiomyopathy in two regions of the United States. N Engl J Med. 2003;348:1647–55.
9. Nugent AW, Daubeney PE, Chondros P, Carlin JB, Cheung M, Wilkinson LC, Davis AM, Kahler SG, Chow CW, Wilkinson JL, et al. The epidemiology of childhood cardiomyopathy in Australia. N Engl J Med. 2003;348:1639–46.
10. Marian AJ, Roberts R. The molecular genetic basis for hypertrophic cardiomyopathy. J Mol Cell Cardiol. 2001;33:655–70.
11. Richard P, Charron P, Carrier L, Ledeuil C, Cheav T, Pichereau C, Benaiche A, Isnard R, Dubourg O, Burban M, et al. Hypertrophic cardiomyopathy: distribution of disease genes, spectrum of mutations, and implications for a molecular diagnosis strategy. Circulation. 2003;107: 2227–32.

12. Seidman JG, Seidman C. The genetic basis for cardiomyopathy: from mutation identification to mechanistic paradigms. Cell. 2001;104:557–67.
13. Elliott P, McKenna WJ. Hypertrophic cardiomyopathy. Lancet. 2004;363:1881–91.
14. Elliott RM, Anastasakis A, Borger MA, Borggrefe M, Cecchi F, Charron P, Hagege AA, Lafont A, Limongelli G, Mahrholdt H, McKenna WJ, Mogensen J, Nihoyannopoulos P, Nistri S, Pieper PG, Pieske B, Rapezzi C, Rutten FH, Tillmanns C, Watkins H. 2014 ESC guidelines on diagnosis and management of hypertrophic cardiomyopathy. Eur Heart J. 2014;35: 3733–2779.
15. Nugent AW, Daubeney PE, Chondros P, Carlin JB, Colan SD, Cheung M, Davis AM, Chow CW, Weintraub RG. Clinical features and outcomes of childhood hypertrophic cardiomyopathy: results from a national population-based study. Circulation. 2005;112:1332–8.
16. Rapezzi C, Arbustini E, Caforio AL, Charron P, Gimeno-Blanes J, Helio T, Linhart A, Mogensen J, Pinto Y, Ristic A, Seggewiss H, Sinagra G, Tavazzi L, Elliott PM. Diagnostic work-up in cardiomyopathies: bridging the gap between clinical phenotypes and final diagnosis. A position statement from the ESC Working Group on Myocardial and Pericardial Diseases. Eur Heart J. 2013;34(19):1448–58.
17. Schwartz ML, Cox GF, Lin AE, Korson MS, Perez-Atayde A, Lacro RV, Lipshultz SE. Clinical approach to genetic cardiomyopathy in children. Circulation. 1996;94:2021–38.
18. Colan SD, Lipshultz SE, Lowe AM, Sleeper LA, Messere J, Cox GF, Lurie PR, Orav EJ, Towbin JA. Epidemiology and cause-specific outcome of hypertrophic cardiomyopathy in children: findings from the Pediatric Cardiomyopathy Registry. Circulation. 2007;115(6):773–81.
19. Davies MJ, McKenna WJ. Hypertrophic cardiomyopathy—pathology and pathogenesis. Histopathology. 1995;26:493–500.
20. Hughes SE. The pathology of hypertrophic cardiomyopathy. Histopathology. 2004;44:412–27.
21. Maron BJ, Hauser RG, Roberts WC. Hypertrophic cardiomyopathy with left ventricular apical diverticulum. Am J Cardiol. 1996;77:1263–5.
22. Maron BJ, Bonow RO, Seshagiri TN, Roberts WC, Epstein SE. Hypertrophic cardiomyopathy with ventricular septal hypertrophy localized to the apical region of the left ventricle (apical hypertrophic cardiomyopathy). Am J Cardiol. 1982;49:1838–48.
23. Sperling RT, Parker JA, Manning WJ, Danias PG. Apical hypertrophic cardiomyopathy: clinical, electrocardiographic, scintigraphic, echocardiographic, and magnetic resonance imaging findings of a case. J Cardiovasc Magn Reson. 2002;4:291–5.
24. Webb JG, Sasson Z, Rakowski H, Liu P, Wigle ED. Apical hypertrophic cardiomyopathy: clinical follow-up and diagnostic correlates. J Am Coll Cardiol. 1990;15:83–90.
25. Wigle ED, Sasson Z, Henderson MA, Ruddy TD, Fulop J, Rakowski H, Williams WG. Hypertrophic cardiomyopathy. The importance of the site and the extent of hypertrophy. A review. Prog Cardiovasc Dis. 1985;28:1–83.
26. Silbiger JJ. Abnormalities of the mitral apparatus in hypertrophic cardiomyopathy: echocardiographic, pathophysiologic, and surgical insights. J Am Soc Echocardiogr. 2016;29(7): 622–39.
27. Klues HG, Maron BJ, Dollar AL, Roberts WC. Diversity of structural mitral valve alterations in hypertrophic cardiomyopathy. Circulation. 1992;85:1651–60.
28. Kitazume H, Kramer JR, Krauthamer D, El Tobgi S, Proudfit WL, Sones FM. Myocardial bridges in obstructive hypertrophic cardiomyopathy. Am Heart J. 1983;106:131–5.
29. Yetman AT, McCrindle BW, MacDonald C, Freedom RM, Gow R. Myocardial bridging in children with hypertrophic cardiomyopathy—a risk factor for sudden death. N Engl J Med. 1998;339:1201–9.
30. Maron BJ, Wolfson JK, Epstein SE, Roberts WC. Intramural ("small vessel") coronary artery disease in hypertrophic cardiomyopathy. J Am Coll Cardiol. 1986;8:545–57.
31. Lopes LR, Elliott PM. A straightforward guide to the sarcomeric basis of cardiomyopathies. Heart. 2014;100:1916–23.
32. Harris SP, Lyons RG, Bezold KL, Robbins J, Seidman C, Watkins H. In the thick of it. HCM-causing mutations in myosin binding proteins of the thick filament. Circ Res. 2011;108: 751–64.

33. Bos JM, Poley RN, Ny M, Tester DJ, Xu X, Vatta M, Towbin JA, Gersh BJ, Ommen SR, Ackerman MJ. Genotype-phenotype relationships involving hypertrophic cardiomyopathy-associated mutations in titin, muscle LIM protein, and telethonin. Mol Genet Metab. 2006;88: 78–85.
34. Chiu C, Bagnall RD, Ingles J, Yeates L, Kennerson M, Donald JA, Jormakka M, Lind JM, Semsarian C. Mutations in alpha-actinin-2 cause hypertrophic cardiomyopathy: a genome-wide analysis. J Am Coll Cardiol. 2010;55:1127–35.
35. Geier C, Perrot A, Ozcelik C, Binner P, Counsell D, Hoffmann K, Pilz B, Martiniak Y, Gehmlich K, van der Ven PF, Furst DO, Vornwald A, von Hodenberg E, Numberg P, Scheffold T, Dietz R, Osterziel KJ. Mutations in the human muscle LIM protein gene in families with hypertrophic cardiomyopathy. Circulation. 2003;107(10):1390–5.
36. Osio A, Tan L, Chen SN, Lombardi R, Nagueh SF, Shete S, Roberts R, Willerson JT, Marian AJ. Myozenin 2 is a novel gene for human hypertrophic cardiomyopathy. Circ Res. 2007; 100:766–8.
37. Wang H, Li Z, Wang J, Sun K, Cui Q, Song L, Zou Y, Wang X, Liu X, Hui R, Fan Y. Mutations in NEXN, a Z-disc gene, are associated with hypertrophic cardiomyopathy. Am J Hum Genet. 2010;87(5):687–93.
38. Ackerman MJ, Bos JM. Z-Disc genes in Hypertrophic cardiomyopathy—stretching the cardiomyopathies? JACC. 2010;55(11):1136–8.
39. Lopes LR, Rahman MS, Elliott PM. A systematic review and meta-analysis of genotype-phenotype associations in patients with hypertrophic cardiomyopathy caused by sarcomeric protein mutations. Heart. 2013;99(24):1800–11.
40. Lopes LR, Zekvati A, Syrris P, Hubank M, Giambartolomei C, Dalageorgou C, Jenkins S, McKenna W, Plagnol V, Elliott PM, UK10k Consortium. Genetic complexity in hypertrophic cardiomyopathy revealed by high-throughput sequencing. J Med Genet. 2013;50(4):228–39.
41. Lopes LR, Syrris P, Guttmann OP, O'Mahony C, Tang HC, Dalageorgou C, Jenkins S, Hubank M, Monserrat L, McKenna WJ, Plagnol V, Elliott PM. Novel genotype-phenotype associations demonstrated by high-throughput sequencing in patients with hypertrophic cardiomyopathy. Heart. 2015;101(4):294–301.
42. Lopes LR, Murphy C, Syrris P, Dalageorgou C, McKenna WJ, Elliott PM, Plagnol V. Use of high-throughput targeted exome-sequencing to screen for copy number variation in hypertrophic cardiomyopathy. Eur J Med Genet. 2015;58(11):611–6.
43. Xu Q, Dewey S, Nguyen S, Gomes AV. Malignant and benign mutations in familial cardiomyopathies: insights into mutations linked to complex cardiovascular phenotypes. J Mol Cell Cardiol. 2010;48:899–909.
44. Bonne G, Carier L, Bercovici J, Cruaud C, Richard P, Hainque B, Gautel M, Labeit S, James M, Beckmann J, Weissenbach J, Vosberg H, Fiszman M, Komajda M, Schwarts K. Cardiac myosin binding protein-C gene splice acceptor site mutation is associated with familial hypertrophic cardiomyopathy. Nat Genet. 1995;11:438–40.
45. Arad M, Seidman JG, Seidman CE. Phenotypic diversity in hypertrophic cardiomyopathy. Hum Mol Genet. 2002;11:2499–506.
46. Ho CY, Landstrom AP, Ackerman MJ. Genetics and clinical destiny: improving care in hypertrophic cardiomyopathy. Circulation. 2010;122:2430–40.
47. Seidman CE, Seidman JG. Identifying sarcomere gene mutations in hypertrophic cardiomyopathy: a personal history. Circ Res. 2011;108:743–50.
48. Carrier L, Schlossarek S, Willis MS, Eschenhagen T. The ubiquitin-proteasome system and nonsense-mediated mRNA decay in hypertrophic cardiomyopathy. Cardiovasc Res. 2010;85:330–8.
49. Marston S, Copeland O, Jacques A, Livesey K, Tsang V, McKenna WJ, Jalilzadeh S, Carballo S, Redwood C, Watkins H. Evidence from human myectomy samples that MYBPC3 mutations cause hypertrophic cardiomyopathy through haploinsufficiency. Circ Res. 2009;105(3):219–22.
50. Sarikas A, Carrier L, Schenke C, Doll D, Flavigny J, Lindenberg KS, Eschenhagen T, Zolk O. Impairment of the ubiquitin-proteasome system by truncated cardiac myosin binding protein C mutants. Cardiovasc Res. 2005;66(1):33–44.

51. Van Dijk SJ, Dooijes D, dos Remedios C, Michels M, Lamers JM, Winegrad S, Schlossarek S, Carrier L, ten Cate FJ, Stienen GJ, van der Velden J. Cardiac myosin-binding protein C mutations and hypertrophic cardiomyopathy: haploinsufficiency, deranged phosphorylation, and cardiomyocyte dysfunction. Circulation. 2009;119(11):1473–83.
52. Yang Q, Sanbe A, Osinska H, Hewett TE, Klevitsky R, Robbins J. In vivo modeling of myosin binding protein C familial hypertrophic cardiomyopathy. Circ Res. 1999;85:841–7.
53. Razumova MV, Shaffer JF, Tu AY, Flint GV, Regnier M, Harris SP. Effects of the N-terminal domains of myosin binding protein-C in an in vitro motility assay: evidence for long-lived cross-bridges. J Biol Chem. 2006;281:35846–54.
54. Redwood CS, Moolman-Smook JC, Watkins H. Properties of mutant contractile proteins that cause hypertrophic cardiomyopathy. Cardiovasc Res. 1999;44:20–36.
55. Tyska MJ, Hayes E, Giewat M, Seidman CE, Seidman JG, Warshaw DM. Single-molecule mechanics of R403Q cardiac myosin isolated from the mouse model of familial hypertrophic cardiomyopathy. Circ Res. 2000;86:737–44.
56. Bing W, Knott A, Redwood C, Esposito G, Purcell I, Watkins H, Marston S. Effect of hypertrophic cardiomyopathy mutations in human cardiac muscle alpha-tropomyosin (Asp175Asn and Glu180Gly) on the regulatory properties of human cardiac troponin determined by in vitro motility assay. J Mol Cell Cardiol. 2000;32:1489–98.
57. Deng Y, Schmidtmann A, Redlich A, Westerdorf B, Jaquet K, Thieleczek R. Effects of phosphorylation and mutation R145G on human cardiac troponin I function. Biochemistry. 2001;40:14593–602.
58. Elliott K, Watkins H, Redwood CS. Altered regulatory properties of human cardiac troponin I mutants that cause hypertrophic cardiomyopathy. J Biol Chem. 2000;275:22069–74.
59. Harada K, Takahashi-Yanaga F, Minakami R, Morimoto S, Ohtsuki I. Functional consequences of the deletion mutation deltaGlu160 in human cardiac troponin T. J Biochem. 2000;127:263–8.
60. Harada K, Potter JD. Familial hypertrophic cardiomyopathy mutations from different functional regions of troponin T result in different effects on the pH and Ca2+ sensitivity of cardiac muscle contraction. J Biol Chem. 2004;279:14488–95.
61. Heller MJ, Nili M, Homsher E, Tobacman LS. Cardiomyopathic tropomyosin mutations that increase thin filament Ca2+ sensitivity and tropomyosin N-domain flexibility. J Biol Chem. 2003;278:41742–8.
62. Kobayashi T, Dong WJ, Burkart EM, Cheung HC, Solaro RJ. Effects of protein kinase C dependent phosphorylation and a familial hypertrophic cardiomyopathy-related mutation of cardiac troponin I on structural transition of troponin C and myofilament activation. Biochemistry. 2004;43:5996–6004.
63. Kohler J, Chen Y, Brenner B, Gordon AM, Kraft T, Martyn DA, Regnier M, Rivera AJ, Wang CK, Chase PB. Familial hypertrophic cardiomyopathy mutations in troponin I (K183D, G203S, K206Q) enhance filament sliding. Physiol Genomics. 2003;14:117–28.
64. Lang R, Gomes AV, Zhao J, Housmans PR, Miller T, Potter JD. Functional analysis of a troponin I (R145G) mutation associated with familial hypertrophic cardiomyopathy. J Biol Chem. 2002;277:11670–8.
65. Michele DE, Albayya FP, Metzger JM. Direct, convergent hypersensitivity of calcium-activated force generation produced by hypertrophic cardiomyopathy mutant alpha-tropomyosins in adult cardiac myocytes. Nat Med. 1999;5:1413–7.
66. Morimoto S, Lu QW, Harada K, Takahashi-Yanaga F, Minakami R, Ohta M, Sasaguri T, Ohtsuki I. Ca(2+)-desensitizing effect of a deletion mutation Delta K210 in cardiac troponin T that causes familial dilated cardiomyopathy. Proc Natl Acad Sci U S A. 2002;99:913–8.
67. Palmer BM, Fishbaugher DE, Schmitt JP, Wang Y, Alpert NR, Seidman CE, Seidman JG, VanBuren P, Maughan DW. Differential cross-bridge kinetics of FHC myosin mutations R403Q and R453C in heterozygous mouse myocardium. Am J Physiol. 2004;287:H91–9.
68. Redwood C, Lohmann K, Bing W, Esposito GM, Elliott K, Abdulrazzak H, Knott A, Purcell I, Marston S, Watkins H. Investigation of a truncated cardiac troponin T that causes familial

hypertrophic cardiomyopathy: Ca(2+) regulatory properties of reconstituted thin filaments depend on the ratio of mutant to wild-type protein. Circ Res. 2000;86:1146–52.
69. Roopnarine O. Mechanical defects of muscle fibers with myosin light chain mutants that cause cardiomyopathy. Biophys J. 2003;84:2440–9.
70. Szczesna D, Zhang R, Zhao J, Jones M, Guzman G, Potter JD. Altered regulation of cardiac muscle contraction by troponin T mutations that cause familial hypertrophic cardiomyopathy. J Biol Chem. 2000;275:624–30.
71. Szczesna D, Ghosh D, Li Q, Gomes AV, Guzman G, Arana C, Zhi G, Stull JT, Potter JD. Familial hypertrophic cardiomyopathy mutations in the regulatory light chains of myosin affect their structure, Ca2+ binding, and phosphorylation. J Biol Chem. 2001;276:7086–92.
72. Westfall MV, Borton AR, Albayya FP, Metzger JM. Myofilament calcium sensitivity and cardiac disease: insights from troponin I isoforms and mutants. Circ Res. 2002;91:525–31.
73. Blanchard E, Seidman C, Seidman JG, LeWinter M, Maughan D. Altered crossbridge kinetics in the alpha MHC403/+ mouse model of familial hypertrophic cardiomyopathy. Circ Res. 1999;84:475–83.
74. Palmiter KA, Tyska MJ, Haeberle JR, Alpert NR, Fananapazir L, Warshaw DM. R403Q and L908V mutant beta-cardiac myosin from patients with familial hypertrophic cardiomyopathy exhibit enhanced mechanical performance at the single molecule level. J Muscle Res Cell Motil. 2000;21:609–20.
75. Michele DE, Gomez CA, Hong KE, Westfall MV, Metzger JM. Cardiac dysfunction in hypertrophic cardiomyopathy mutant tropomyosin mice is transgene-dependent, hypertrophy-independent, and improved by beta-blockade. Circ Res. 2002;91:255–62.
76. Miller T, Szczesna D, Housmans PR, Zhao J, de Freitas F, Gomes AV, Culbreath L, McCue J, Wang Y, Xu Y, et al. Abnormal contractile function in transgenic mice expressing a familial hypertrophic cardiomyopathy-linked troponin T (I79N) mutation. J Biol Chem. 2001;276:3743–55.
77. Oberst L, Zhao G, Park JT, Brugada R, Michael LH, Entman ML, Roberts R, Marian AJ. Dominant-negative effect of a mutant cardiac troponin T on cardiac structure and function in transgenic mice. J Clin Invest. 1998;102:1498–505.
78. Prabhakar R, Boivin GP, Grupp IL, Hoit B, Arteaga G, Solaro JR, Wieczorek DF. A familial hypertrophic cardiomyopathy alpha-tropomyosin mutation causes severe cardiac hypertrophy and death in mice. J Mol Cell Cardiol. 2001;33:1815–28.
79. Prabhakar R, Petrashevskaya N, Schwartz A, Aronow B, Boivin GP, Molkentin JD, Wieczorek DF. A mouse model of familial hypertrophic cardiomyopathy caused by a alpha-tropomyosin mutation. Mol Cell Biochem. 2003;251:33–42.
80. Tardiff JC, Factor SM, Tompkins BD, Hewett TE, Palmer BM, Moore RL, Schwartz S, Robbins J, Leinwand LA. A truncated cardiac troponin T molecule in transgenic mice suggests multiple cellular mechanisms for familial hypertrophic cardiomyopathy. J Clin Invest. 1998;101:2800–11.
81. Tardiff JC, Hewett TE, Palmer BM, Olsson C, Factor SM, Moore RL, Robbins J, Leinwand LA. Cardiac troponin T mutations result in allele-specific phenotypes in a mouse model for hypertrophic cardiomyopathy. J Clin Invest. 1999;104:469–81.
82. Watkins H, McKenna WJ, Thierfelder L, Suk HJ, Anan R, O'Donoghue A, Spirito P, Matsumori A, Moravec CS, Seidman JG, et al. Mutations in the genes for cardiac troponin T and alpha-tropomyosin in hypertrophic cardiomyopathy. N Engl J Med. 1995;332(16):1058–64.
83. Knollmann BC, Kirchhof P, Sirenko SG, Degen H, Greene AE, Schober T, Mackow JC, Fabritz L, Potter JD, Morad M. Familial hypertrophic cardiomyopathy-linked mutant troponin T causes stress-induced ventricular tachycardia and Ca2+–dependent action potential remodeling. Circ Res. 2003;92:428–36.
84. Konno T, Chen D, Wang L, Wakimoto H, Teekakirikul P, Nayor M, Kawana M, Eminaga S, Gorham JN, Pandya K, Smithies O, Naya FJ, Olson EN, Seidman JG, Seidman CE. Heterogeneous myocyte enhancer factor-2 (Mef2) activation in myocytes predicts focal scarring in hypertrophic cardiomyopathy. Proc Natl Acad Sci U S A. 2010;107:18097–102.

85. Teekakirikul P, Eminaga S, Toka O, Alcai R, Wang L, Wakimoto H, Nayor M, Konno T, Gorham JM, Wolf CM, Kim JB, Schmitt JP, Molkentin JD, Norris RA, Tager AM, Hoffman SR, Markwald RR, Seidman CE, Seidman JG. Cardiac fibrosis in mice with hypertrophic cardiomyopathy is mediated by non-myocyte proliferation and required Tgf- ß. J Clin Invest. 2010;120(10):3520–9.
86. Ahmad F, Seidman JG, Seidman CE. The genetic basis for cardiac remodelling. Annu Rev Genomics Hum Genet. 2005;6:185–216.
87. Chandra M, Rundell VL, Tardiff JC, Leinwand LA, De Tombe PP, Solaro RJ. Ca(2+) activation of myofilaments from transgenic mouse hearts expressing R92Q mutant cardiac troponin T. Am J Physiol. 2001;280:H705–13.
88. Crilley JG, Boehm EA, Blair E, Rajagopalan B, Blamire AM, Styles P, McKenna WJ, Ostman-Smith I, Clarke K, Watkins H. Hypertrophic cardiomyopathy due to sarcomeric gene mutations is characterized by impaired energy metabolism irrespective of the degree of hypertrophy. J Am Coll Cardiol. 2003;41:1776–82.
89. Spindler M, Saupe KW, Christe ME, Sweeney HL, Seidman CE, Seidman JG, Ingwall JS. Diastolic dysfunction and altered energetics in the alpha MHC403/+ mouse model of familial hypertrophic cardiomyopathy. J Clin Invest. 1998;101:1775–83.
90. Michels M, Soliman OI, Phefferkom J, Hoedemaekers YM, Kofflard MJ, Dooijes D, Majoor-Krakauer D, Ten Cate FJ. Disease penetrance and risk stratification for sudden cardiac death in asymptomatic hypertrophic cardiomyopathy mutation carriers. Eur Heart J. 2009;30(21):2593–8.
91. Olsson MC, Palmer BM, Leinwand LA, Moore RL. Gender and aging in a transgenic mouse model of hypertrophic cardiomyopathy. Am J Physiol. 2001;280:H1136–44.
92. Harris KM, Spirito P, Maron MS, Zenovich AG, Formisano F, Lesser JR, Mackey-Bojack S, Manning WJ, Udelson JE, Maron BJ. Prevalence, clinical profile, and significance of left ventricular remodeling in the end-stage phase of hypertrophic cardiomyopathy. Circulation. 2006;114:216–25.
93. Lechin M, Quinones MA, Omran A, Hill R, Yu QT, Rakowski H, Wigle D, Liew CC, Sole M, Roberts R, et al. Angiotensin-I converting enzyme genotypes and left ventricular hypertrophy in patients with hypertrophic cardiomyopathy. Circulation. 1995;92:1808–12.
94. Marian AJ, Yu QT, Workman R, Greve G, Roberts R. Angiotensin-converting enzyme polymorphism in hypertrophic cardiomyopathy and sudden cardiac death. Lancet. 1993;342:1085–6.
95. Jensen MK, Havndrup O, Christiansen M, Andersen PS, Diness B, Axelsson A, Skovby F, Kober L, Bundgaard H. Penetrance of hypertrophic cardiomyopathy in children and adolescents. Circulation. 2013;127:48–54.
96. Maron BJ, Spirito P, Wesley Y, Arce J. Development and progression of left ventricular hypertrophy in children with hypertrophic cardiomyopathy. N Engl J Med. 1986;315:610–4.
97. Maron BJ. Hypertrophic cardiomyopathy in childhood. Pediatr Clin North Am. 2004;51:1305–46.
98. Kaski JP, Syrris P, Tome Esteban MT, Jenkins S, Pantazis A, Deanfield JE, McKenna WJ, Elliot PM. Prevalence of sarcomere protein gene mutations in preadolescent children with hypertrophic cardiomyopathy. Circ Cardiovasc Genet. 2009;2:436–41.
99. Morita H, Rehm HL, Menesses A, McDonough B, Roberts AE, Kucherlapati R, Towbin JA, Seidman JG, Seidman CE. Shared genetic causes of cardiac hypertrophy in children and adults. N Engl J Med. 2008;358:1899–908.
100. Counihan PJ, Frenneaux MP, Webb DJ, McKenna WJ. Abnormal vascular responses to supine exercise in hypertrophic cardiomyopathy. Circulation. 1991;84:686–96.
101. Tome Esteban MT, Kaski JP. Hypertrophic cardiomyopathy in children. Paediatr Child Health. 2007;17:19–24.
102. Bruno E, Maisuls H, Juaneda E, Moreyra E, Alday LE. Clinical features of hypertrophic cardiomyopathy in the young. Cardiol Young. 2002;12:147–52.
103. Maron BJ, Henry WL, Clark CE, Redwood DR, Roberts WC, Epstein SE. Asymetric septal hypertrophy in childhood. Circulation. 1976;53:9–19.

104. Maron BJ, Tajik AJ, Ruttenberg HD, Graham TP, Atwood GF, Victorica BE, Lie JT, Roberts WC. Hypertrophic cardiomyopathy in infants: clinical features and natural history. Circulation. 1982;65:7–17.
105. Schaffer MS, Freedom RM, Rowe RD. Hypertrophic cardiomyopathy presenting before 2 years of age in 13 patients. Pediatr Cardiol. 1983;4:113–9.
106. Skinner JR, Manzoor A, Hayes AM, Joffe HS, Martin RP. A regional study of presentation and outcome of hypertrophic cardiomyopathy in infants. Heart (British Cardiac Society). 1997;77:229–33.
107. Maron MS, Olivotto I, Betocchi S, Casey SA, Lesser JR, Losi MA, Cecchi F, Maron BJ. Effect of left ventricular outflow tract obstruction on clinical outcome in hypertrophic cardiomyopathy. N Engl J Med. 2003;348:295–303.
108. Maron BJ, Casey SA, Poliac LC, Gohman TE, Almquist AK, Aeppli DM. Clinical course of hypertrophic cardiomyopathy in a regional United States cohort. JAMA. 1999;281:650–5.
109. Beder SD, Gutgesell HP, Mullins CE, McNamara DG. Progression from hypertrophic obstructive cardiomyopathy to congestive cardiomyopathy in a child. Am Heart J. 1982;104:155–6.
110. Biagini E, Coccolo F, Ferlito M, Perugini E, Rocchi G, Bacchi-Reggiani L, Lofiego C, Boriani G, Prandstraller D, Picchio FM, et al. Dilated-hypokinetic evolution of hypertrophic cardiomyopathy: prevalence, incidence, risk factors, and prognostic implications in pediatric and adult patients. J Am Coll Cardiol. 2005;46:1543–50.
111. Bingisser R, Candinas R, Schneider J, Hess OM. Risk factors for systolic dysfunction and ventricular dilatation in hypertrophic cardiomyopathy. Int J Cardiol. 1994;44:225–33.
112. Fighali S, Krajcer Z, Edelman S, Leachman RD. Progression of hypertrophic cardiomyopathy into a hypokinetic left ventricle: higher incidence in patients with midventricular obstruction. J Am Coll Cardiol. 1987;9:288–94.
113. Fujiwara H, Onodera T, Tanaka M, Shirane H, Kato H, Yoshikawa J, Osakada G, Sasayama S, Kawai C. Progression from hypertrophic obstructive cardiomyopathy to typical dilated cardiomyopathy-like features in the end stage. Jpn Circ J. 1984;48:1210–4.
114. Hecht GM, Klues HG, Roberts WC, Maron BJ. Coexistence of sudden cardiac death and end-stage heart failure in familial hypertrophic cardiomyopathy. J Am Coll Cardiol. 1993;22:489–97.
115. Maron BJ, Spirito P. Implications of left ventricular remodeling in hypertrophic cardiomyopathy. Am J Cardiol. 1998;81:1339–44.
116. Seiler C, Jenni R, Vassalli G, Turina M, Hess OM. Left ventricular chamber dilatation in hypertrophic cardiomyopathy: related variables and prognosis in patients with medical and surgical therapy. Br Heart J. 1995;74:508–16.
117. Spirito P, Maron BJ, Bonow RO, Epstein SE. Occurrence and significance of progressive left ventricular wall thinning and relative cavity dilatation in hypertrophic cardiomyopathy. Am J Cardiol. 1987;60:123–9.
118. ten Cate FJ, Roelandt J. Progression to left ventricular dilatation in patients with hypertrophic obstructive cardiomyopathy. Am Heart J. 1979;97:762–5.
119. Thaman R, Gimeno JR, Reith S, Esteban MT, Limongelli G, Murphy RT, Mist B, McKenna WJ, Elliott PM. Progressive left ventricular remodeling in patients with hypertrophic cardiomyopathy and severe left ventricular hypertrophy. J Am Coll Cardiol. 2004;44:398–405.
120. Thaman R, Gimeno JR, Murphy RT, Kubo T, Sachdev B, Mogensen J, Elliott PM, McKenna WJ. Prevalence and clinical significance of systolic impairment in hypertrophic cardiomyopathy. Heart (British Cardiac Society). 2005;91:920–5.
121. Yutani C, Imakita M, Ishibashi-Ueda H, Hatanaka K, Nagata S, Sakakibara H, Nimura Y. Three autopsy cases of progression to left ventricular dilatation in patients with hypertrophic cardiomyopathy. Am Heart J. 1985;109:545–53.
122. Cohn JN, Ferrari R, Sharpe N. Cardiac remodeling—concepts and clinical implications: a consensus paper from an international forum on cardiac remodeling. Behalf of an International Forum on Cardiac Remodeling. J Am Coll Cardiol. 2000;35:569–82.
123. McKenna WJ, Behr ER. Hypertrophic cardiomyopathy: management, risk stratification, and prevention of sudden death. Heart (British Cardiac Society). 2002;87:169–76.

124. Rosmini S, Biagini E, O'Mahony C, Bulluck H, Ruozi N, Lopes LR, Guttmann O, Reant P, Quarta CC, Pantazis A, Tome-Esteban M, McKenna WJ, Rapezzi C, Elliott PM. Relationship between aetiology and left ventricular systolic dysfunction in hypertrophic cardiomyopathy. Heart. 2017;103(4):300–6.
125. Maron BJ, Edwards JE, Henry WL, Clark CE, Bingle GJ, Epstein SE. Asymmetric septal hypertrophy (ASH) in infancy. Circulation. 1974;50:809–20.
126. Olivotto I, Cecchi F, Casey SA, Dolara A, Traverse JH, Maron BJ. Impact of atrial fibrillation on the clinical course of hypertrophic cardiomyopathy. Circulation. 2001;104:2517–24.
127. Robinson K, Frenneaux MP, Stockins B, Karatasakis G, Poloniecki JD, McKenna WJ. Atrial fibrillation in hypertrophic cardiomyopathy: a longitudinal study. J Am Coll Cardiol. 1990;15:1279–85.
128. Spirito P, Lakatos E, Maron BJ. Degree of left ventricular hypertrophy in patients with hypertrophic cardiomyopathy and chronic atrial fibrillation. Am J Cardiol. 1992;69:1217–22.
129. Guttmann OP, Rahman MS, O'Mahony C, Anastasakis A, Elliott PM. Atrial fibrillation and thromboembolism in patients with hypertrophic cardiomyopathy: systematic review. Heart. 2014;100(6):465–72.
130. Guttmann OP, Pavlou M, O'Mahony C, Monserrat L, Anastasakis A, Rapezzi C, Biagini E, Gimeno JR, Limongelli G, Garcia-Pavia P, McKenna WJ, Omar RZ, Elliott PM, Hypertrophic Cardiomyopathy Outcomes Investigators. Prediction of thrombo-embolic risk in patients with hypertrophic cardiomyopathy (HCM Risk-CVA). Eur J Jeart Fail. 2015;17(8):837–45.
131. Yamaguchi H, Ishimura T, Nishiyama S, Nagasaki F, Nakanishi S, Takatsu F, Nishijo T, Umeda T, Machii K. Hypertrophic nonobstructive cardiomyopathy with giant negative T waves (apical hypertrophy): ventriculographic and echocardiographic features in 30 patients. Am J Cardiol. 1979;44:401–12.
132. Fananapazir L, Tracy CM, Leon MB, Winkler JB, Cannon RO 3rd, Bonow RO, Maron BJ, Epstein SE. Electrophysiologic abnormalities in patients with hypertrophic cardiomyopathy. A consecutive analysis in 155 patients. Circulation. 1989;80:1259–68.
133. Krikler DM, Davies MJ, Rowland E, Goodwin JF, Evans RC, Shaw DB. Sudden death in hypertrophic cardiomyopathy: associated accessory atrioventricular pathways. Br Heart J. 1980;43:245–51.
134. Bennani Smires Y, Victor G, Ribes D, Berry M, Cognet T, Mejean S, Huart A, Roussel M, Petermann A, Roncalli J, Carrie D, Rousseau H, Berry I, Chauveau D, Galinier M, Lairez O. Pilot study for left ventricular imaging phenotype of patients over 65 years old with heart failure and preserved ejection fraction: the high prevalence of amyloid cardiomyopathy. Int J Cardiovasc Imaging. 2016;32(9):1403–13.
135. Maron BJ, Savage DD, Wolfson JK, Epstein SE. Prognostic significance of 24 hour ambulatory electrocardiographic monitoring in patients with hypertrophic cardiomyopathy: a prospective study. Am J Cardiol. 1981;48:252–7.
136. McKenna WJ, England D, Doi YL, Deanfield JE, Oakley C, Goodwin JF. Arrhythmia in hypertrophic cardiomyopathy: influence on prognosis. Br Heart J. 1981;46:168–72.
137. McKenna WJ, Franklin RC, Nihoyannopoulos P, Robinson KC, Deanfield JE. Arrhythmia and prognosis in infants, children and adolescents with hypertrophic cardiomyopathy. J Am Coll Cardiol. 1988;11:147–53.
138. Adabag AS, Casey SA, Kuskowski MA, Zenovich AG, Maron BJ. Spectrum and prognostic significance of arrhythmias on ambulatory Holter electrocardiogram in hypertrophic cardiomyopathy. J Am Coll Cardiol. 2005;45(5):697–704.
139. Alfonso F, Frenneaux MP, McKenna WJ. Clinical sustained uniform ventricular tachycardia in hypertrophic cardiomyopathy: association with left ventricular apical aneurysm. Br Heart J. 1989;61:178–81.
140. Klues HG, Schiffers A, Maron BJ. Phenotypic spectrum and patterns of left ventricular hypertrophy in hypertrophic cardiomyopathy: morphologic observations and significance as assessed by two-dimensional echocardiography in 600 patients. J Am Coll Cardiol. 1995;26:1699–708.

141. Maron BJ, Gottdiener JS, Epstein SE. Patterns and significance of distribution of left ventricular hypertrophy in hypertrophic cardiomyopathy. A wide angle, two dimensional echocardiographic study of 125 patients. Am J Cardiol. 1981;48:418–28.
142. Shapiro LM, McKenna WJ. Distribution of left ventricular hypertrophy in hypertrophic cardiomyopathy: a two-dimensional echocardiographic study. J Am Coll Cardiol. 1983;2: 437–44.
143. Maron MS, Olivotto I, Zenovich AG, Link MS, Pandian NG, Kuvin JT, Nistri S, Cecchi F, Udelson JE, Maron BJ. Hypertrophic cardiomyopathy is predominantly a disease of left ventricular outflow tract obstruction. Circulation. 2006;114:2232–9.
144. Shah JS, Tome Esteban MT, Thaman R, Sharma R, Mist B, Pantazis A, Ward D, Kohli SK, Page SP, Demetrescu C, et al. Prevalence of exercise induced left ventricular outflow tract obstruction in symptomatic patients with non-obstructive hypertrophic cardiomyopathy. Heart (British Cardiac Society). 2007;94:1288–94.
145. Minami Y, Kajimoto K, Terajima Y, Yashiro B, Okayama D, Haruki S, Nakajima T, Kawashiro N, Kawana M, Hagiwara N. Clinical implications of midventricular obstruction in patients with hypertrophic cardiomyopathy. J Am Coll Cardiol. 2011;57(23):2346–55.
146. Okeie K, Shimizu M, Yoshio H, Ino H, Yamaguchi M, Matsuyama T, Yasuda T, Taki J, Mabuchi H. Left ventricular systolic dysfunction during exercise and dobutamine stress in patients with hypertrophic cardiomyopathy. J Am Coll Cardiol. 2000;36:856–63.
147. Perrone-Filardi P, Bacharach SL, Dilsizian V, Panza JA, Maurea S, Bonow RO. Regional systolic function, myocardial blood flow and glucose uptake at rest in hypertrophic cardiomyopathy. Am J Cardiol. 1993;72:199–204.
148. Tabata T, Oki T, Yamada H, Abe M, Onose Y, Thomas JD. Subendocardial motion in hypertrophic cardiomyopathy: assessment from long- and short-axis views by pulsed tissue Doppler imaging. J Am Soc Echocardiogr. 2000;13:108–15.
149. Matsumura Y, Elliott PM, Virdee MS, Sorajja P, Doi Y, McKenna WJ. Left ventricular diastolic function assessed using Doppler tissue imaging in patients with hypertrophic cardiomyopathy: relation to symptoms and exercise capacity. Heart (British Cardiac Society). 2002; 87:247–51.
150. McMahon CJ, Nagueh SF, Pignatelli RH, Denfield SW, Dreyer WJ, Price JF, Clunie S, Bezold LI, Hays AL, Towbin JA, et al. Characterization of left ventricular diastolic function by tissue Doppler imaging and clinical status in children with hypertrophic cardiomyopathy. Circulation. 2004;109:1756–62.
151. Nagueh SF, Bachinski LL, Meyer D, Hill R, Zoghbi WA, Tam JW, Quinones MA, Roberts R, Marian AJ. Tissue Doppler imaging consistently detects myocardial abnormalities in patients with hypertrophic cardiomyopathy and provides a novel means for an early diagnosis before and independently of hypertrophy. Circulation. 2001;104:128–30.
152. Poutanen T, Tikanoja T, Jaaskelainen P, Jokinen E, Silvast A, Laakso M, Kuusisto J. Diastolic dysfunction without left ventricular hypertrophy is an early finding in children with hypertrophic cardiomyopathy-causing mutations in the beta-myosin heavy chain, alpha-tropomyosin, and myosin-binding protein C genes. Am Heart J. 2006;151:725.
153. Jones S, Elliott PM, Sharma S, McKenna WJ, Whipp BJ. Cardiopulmonary responses to exercise in patients with hypertrophic cardiomyopathy. Heart (British Cardiac Society). 1998;80:60–7.
154. Sharma S, Elliott P, Whyte G, Jones S, Mahon N, Whipp B, McKenna WJ. Utility of cardiopulmonary exercise in the assessment of clinical determinants of functional capacity in hypertrophic cardiomyopathy. Am J Cardiol. 2000;86:162–8.
155. Olivotto I, Maron BJ, Montereggi A, Mazzuoli F, Dolara A, Cecchi F. Prognostic value of systemic blood pressure response during exercise in a community-based patient population with hypertrophic cardiomyopathy. J Am Coll Cardiol. 1999;33:2044–51.
156. Sadoul N, Prasad K, Elliott PM, Bannerjee S, Frenneaux MP, McKenna WJ. Prospective prognostic assessment of blood pressure response during exercise in patients with hypertrophic cardiomyopathy. Circulation. 1997;96:2987–91.

157. Ciampi Q, Betocchi S, Lombardi R, Manganelli F, Storto G, Losi MA, Pezzella E, Finizio F, Cuocolo A, Chiariello M. Hemodynamic determinants of exercise-induced abnormal blood pressure response in hypertrophic cardiomyopathy. J Am Coll Cardiol. 2002;40:278–84.
158. Coats CJ, Rantell K, Bartnik A, Patel A, Mist B, McKenna WJ, Elliott PM. Cardiopulmonary exercise testing and prognosis in hypertrophic cardiomyopathy. Circ Heart Fail. 2015;8(6):1022–31.
159. Choudhury L, Mahrholdt H, Wagner A, Choi KM, Elliott MD, Klocke FJ, Bonow RO, Judd RM, Kim RJ. Myocardial scarring in asymptomatic or mildly symptomatic patients with hypertrophic cardiomyopathy. J Am Coll Cardiol. 2002;40:2156–64.
160. Moon JC, McKenna WJ, McCrohon JA, Elliott PM, Smith GC, Pennell DJ. Toward clinical risk assessment in hypertrophic cardiomyopathy with gadolinium cardiovascular magnetic resonance. J Am Coll Cardiol. 2003;41:1561–7.
161. Gyllenhammar T, Fernlund E, Jablonowski R, Jogi J, Engblom H, Liuba P, Arheden H, Carlsson M. Young patients with hypertrophic cardiomyopathy, but not subjects at risk, show decreased myocardial perfusion reserve quantified with CMR. Eur Heart J Cardiovasc Imaging. 2014;15(12):1350–7.
162. Ismail TF, Hsu LY, Greve AM, Goncalves C, Jabbour A, Gulati A, Hewins B, Mistry N, Wage R, Roughton M, Ferreira PF, Gatehouse P, Firmin D, O'Hanlon R, Pennell DJ, Prasad SK, Arai AE. Coronary microvascular ischemia in hypertrophic cardiomyopathy—a pixel-wise quantitative cardiovascular magnetic resonance perfusion study. J Cardiovasc Magn Reson. 2014;16:49.
163. Ostman-Smith I, Wettrell G, Riesenfeld T. A cohort study of childhood hypertrophic cardiomyopathy: improved survival following high-dose beta-adrenoceptor antagonist treatment. J Am Coll Cardiol. 1999;34:1813–22.
164. Pollick C. Disopyramide in hypertrophic cardiomyopathy. II. Noninvasive assessment after oral administration. Am J Cardiol. 1988;62:1252–5.
165. Pollick C, Kimball B, Henderson M, Wigle ED. Disopyramide in hypertrophic cardiomyopathy. I. Hemodynamic assessment after intravenous administration. Am J Cardiol. 1988;62:1248–51.
166. Sherrid M, Delia E, Dwyer E. Oral disopyramide therapy for obstructive hypertrophic cardiomyopathy. Am J Cardiol. 1988;62:1085–8.
167. Sherrid MV, Barac I, McKenna WJ, Elliott PM, Dickie S, Chojnowska L, Casey S, Maron BJ. Multicenter study of the efficacy and safety of disopyramide in obstructive hypertrophic cardiomyopathy. J Am Coll Cardiol. 2005;45:1251–8.
168. Bonow RO, Dilsizian V, Rosing DR, Maron BJ, Bacharach SL, Green MV. Verapamil-induced improvement in left ventricular diastolic filling and increased exercise tolerance in patients with hypertrophic cardiomyopathy: short- and long-term effects. Circulation. 1985;72:853–64.
169. Udelson JE, Bonow RO, O'Gara PT, Maron BJ, Van Lingen A, Bacharach SL, Epstein SE. Verapamil prevents silent myocardial perfusion abnormalities during exercise in asymptomatic patients with hypertrophic cardiomyopathy. Circulation. 1989;79:1052–60.
170. Epstein SE, Rosing DR. Verapamil: its potential for causing serious complications in patients with hypertrophic cardiomyopathy. Circulation. 1981;64:437–41.
171. Wigle ED, Rakowski H, Kimball BP, Williams WG. Hypertrophic cardiomyopathy. Clinical spectrum and treatment. Circulation. 1995;92:1680–92.
172. Morrow AG, Reitz BA, Epstein SE, Henry WL, Conkle DM, Itscoitz SB, Redwood DR. Operative treatment in hypertrophic subaortic stenosis. Techniques, and the results of pre and postoperative assessments in 83 patients. Circulation. 1975;52:88–102.
173. Ommen SR, Maron BJ, Olivotto I, Maron MS, Cecchi F, Betocchi S, Gersh BJ, Ackerman MJ, McCully RB, Dearani JA, et al. Long-term effects of surgical septal myectomy on survival in patients with obstructive hypertrophic cardiomyopathy. J Am Coll Cardiol. 2005;46:470–6.
174. Schulte HD, Bircks WH, Loesse B, Godehardt EA, Schwartzkopff B. Prognosis of patients with hypertrophic obstructive cardiomyopathy after transaortic myectomy. Late results up to twenty-five years. J Thorac Cardiovasc Surg. 1993;106:709–17.

175. Theodoro DA, Danielson GK, Feldt RH, Anderson BJ. Hypertrophic obstructive cardiomyopathy in pediatric patients: results of surgical treatment. J Thorac Cardiovasc Surg. 1996;112:1589–97. discussion 1597–1589
176. Williams WG, Wigle ED, Rakowski H, Smallhorn J, LeBlanc J, Trusler GA. Results of surgery for hypertrophic obstructive cardiomyopathy. Circulation. 1987;76:V104–8.
177. Seiler CH, Hess OM, Schoenbeck M, et al. Long term follow-up of medical versus surgical therapy for hypertrophic cardiomyopathy: a retrospective study. J Am Coll Cardiol. 1991;17:634–42.
178. Woo A, Williams WG, Choi R, et al. Clinical and echocardiographic determinants of long-term survival after surgical myectomy in obstructive hypertrophic cardiomyopathy. Circulation. 2005; 111:2033–41.
179. Faber L, Seggewiss H, Gleichmann U. Percutaneous transluminal septal myocardial ablation in hypertrophic obstructive cardiomyopathy: results with respect to intraprocedural myocardial contrast echocardiography. Circulation. 1998;98:2415–21.
180. Knight C, Kurbaan AS, Seggewiss H, Henein M, Gunning M, Harrington D, Fassbender D, Gleichmann U, Sigwart U. Nonsurgical septal reduction for hypertrophic obstructive cardiomyopathy: outcome in the first series of patients. Circulation. 1997;95:2075–81.
181. Lakkis NM, Nagueh SF, Dunn JK, Killip D, Spencer WH 3rd. Nonsurgical septal reduction therapy for hypertrophic obstructive cardiomyopathy: one-year follow-up. J Am Coll Cardiol. 2000;36:852–5.
182. Mohiddin SA, Page S. Long-term benefits of pacing in obstructive hypertrophic cardiomyopathy. Heart. 2010;96:328–30.
183. Fananapazir L, Epstein ND, Curiel RV, Panza JA, Tripodi D, McAreavey D. Long-term results of dual-chamber (DDD) pacing in obstructive hypertrophic cardiomyopathy. Evidence for progressive symptomatic and hemodynamic improvement and reduction of left ventricular hypertrophy. Circulation. 1994;90:2731–42.
184. Maron BJ, Nishimura RA, McKenna WJ, Rakowski H, Josephson ME, Kieval RS. Assessment of permanent dual-chamber pacing as a treatment for drug-refractory symptomatic patients with obstructive hypertrophic cardiomyopathy. A randomized, double-blind, crossover study (M-PATHY). Circulation. 1999;99:2927–33.
185. Nishimura RA, Trusty JM, Hayes DL, Ilstrup DM, Larson DR, Hayes SN, Allison TG, Tajik AJ. Dual-chamber pacing for hypertrophic cardiomyopathy: a randomized, double-blind, crossover trial. J Am Coll Cardiol. 1997;29:435–41.
186. Brignole M, Auricchio A, Baron-Esquivias G, Bordachar P, Boriani G, Breithardt OA, Cleland J, Deharo JC, Delgado V, Elliott PM, Gorenek B, Israel CW, Leclercq C, Linde C, Mont L, Padletti L, Sutton R, Vardas PE. 2013 ESC guidelines on cardiac pacing and cardiac resynchronization therapy. The Task Force on cardiac pacing and resynchronization therapy of the European Society of Cardiology (ESC). Developed in collaboration with the European Heart Rhythm Association (EHRA). Eur Heart J. 2013;34:2281–329.
187. Rogers DP, Marazia S, Chow AW, Lambiase PD, Lowe MD, Frenneaux M, McKenna WJ, Elliott PM. Effect of biventricular pacing on symptoms and cardiac remodelling in patients with end-stage hypertrophic cardiomyopathy. Eur J Heart Fail. 2008;10:507–13.
188. Maron BJ. Hypertrophic cardiomyopathy: a systematic review. JAMA. 2002;287:1308–20.
189. Maron BJ, McKenna WJ, Danielson GK, Kappenberger LJ, Kuhn HJ, Seidman CE, Shah PM, Spencer WH 3rd, Spirito P, Ten Cate FJ, et al. American College of Cardiology/European Society of Cardiology Clinical Expert consensus document on hypertrophic cardiomyopathy. A report of the American College of Cardiology Foundation Task Force on clinical expert consensus documents and the European Society of Cardiology Committee for practice guidelines. Eur Heart J. 2003;24:1965–91.
190. Cecchi F, Maron BJ, Epstein SE. Long-term outcome of patients with hypertrophic cardiomyopathy successfully resuscitated after cardiac arrest. J Am Coll Cardiol. 1989;13:1283–8.
191. Elliott PM, Sharma S, Varnava A, Poloniecki J, Rowland E, McKenna WJ. Survival after cardiac arrest or sustained ventricular tachycardia in patients with hypertrophic cardiomyopathy. J Am Coll Cardiol. 1999;33:1596–601.

192. Maron BJ, Lipson LC, Roberts WC, Savage DD, Epstein SE. "Malignant" hypertrophic cardiomyopathy: identification of a subgroup of families with unusually frequent premature death. Am J Cardiol. 1978;41:1133–40.
193. McKenna W, Deanfield J, Faruqui A, England D, Oakley C, Goodwin J. Prognosis in hypertrophic cardiomyopathy: role of age and clinical, electrocardiographic and hemodynamic features. Am J Cardiol. 1981;47:532–8.
194. Elliott PM, Poloniecki J, Dickie S, Sharma S, Monserrat L, Varnava A, Mahon NG, McKenna WJ. Sudden death in hypertrophic cardiomyopathy: identification of high risk patients. J Am Coll Cardiol. 2000;36:2212–8.
195. Frenneaux MP, Counihan PJ, Caforio AL, Chikamori T, McKenna WJ. Abnormal blood pressure response during exercise in hypertrophic cardiomyopathy. Circulation. 1990;82: 1995–2002.
196. Monserrat L, Elliott PM, Gimeno JR, Sharma S, Penas-Lado M, McKenna WJ. Non-sustained ventricular tachycardia in hypertrophic cardiomyopathy: an independent marker of sudden death risk in young patients. J Am Coll Cardiol. 2003;42:873–9.
197. Elliott PM, Gimeno Blanes JR, Mahon NG, Poloniecki JD, McKenna WJ. Relation between severity of left-ventricular hypertrophy and prognosis in patients with hypertrophic cardiomyopathy. Lancet. 2001;357:420–4.
198. Spirito P, Bellone P, Harris KM, Bernabo P, Bruzzi P, Maron BJ. Magnitude of left ventricular hypertrophy and risk of sudden death in hypertrophic cardiomyopathy. N Engl J Med. 2000;342:1778–85.
199. O'Mahony C, Jichi F, Pavlou M, Monserrat L, Asatasakis A, Rapezzi C, Biagini E, Gimeno JR, Limongelli G, McKenna WJ, Omar RZ, Elliott PM. A novel clinical risk prediction model for sudden cardiac death in hypertrophic cardiomyopathy (HCM Risk-SCD). Eur Heart J. 2013;35(30):2010–20.
200. Elliott PM, Gimeno JR, Tome MT, Shah J, Ward D, Thaman R, Mogensen J, McKenna WJ. Left ventricular outflow tract obstruction and sudden death risk in patients with hypertrophic cardiomyopathy. Eur Heart J. 2006;27:1933–41.
201. Maron BJ, Shen WK, Link MS, Epstein AE, Almquist AK, Daubert JP, Bardy GH, Favale S, Rea RF, Boriani G, et al. Efficacy of implantable cardioverter-defibrillators for the prevention of sudden death in patients with hypertrophic cardiomyopathy. N Engl J Med. 2000;342: 365–73.
202. Maron BJ, Spirito P, Shen WK, Haas TS, Formisano F, Link MS, Epstein AE, Almquist AK, Daubert JP, Lawrenz T, et al. Implantable cardioverter-defibrillators and prevention of sudden cardiac death in hypertrophic cardiomyopathy. JAMA. 2007;298:405–12.
203. Kaski JP, Tome Esteban MT, Lowe M, Sporton S, Rees P, Deanfield JE, McKenna WJ, Elliott PM. Outcomes after implantable cardioverter-defibrillator treatment in children with hypertrophic cardiomyopathy. Heart (British Cardiac Society). 2007;93:372–4.
204. Silka MJ, Kron J, Dunnigan A, Dick M 2nd. Sudden cardiac death and the use of implantable cardioverter-defibrillators in pediatric patients. The Pediatric Electrophysiology Society. Circulation. 1993;87:800–7.
205. Favalli V, Disabella E, Molinaro M, Tagliani M, Scarabotto A, Serio A, Grasso M, Narula N, Giorgianni C, Caspani C, Concardi M, Agozzino M, Giordano C, Smirmova A, Kodama T, Giuliani L, Antoniazzi E, Borroni RG, Vassallo C, Mangione F, Scelsi L, Ghio S, Pellegrini C, Zedde M, Fancellu L, Sechi G, Ganau A, Piga S, Colucci A, Concolino D, Di Mascio MT, Toni D, Diomedi M, Rapezzi C, Biagini E, Marini M, Rasura M, Melis M, Nucera A, Guidetti D, Mancuso M, Scoditti U, Cassini P, Narula J, Tavazzi L, Arbustini E. Genetic screening of Anderson-Fabry disease in probands referred from multispeciality clinics. J Am Coll Cardiol. 2016;68(10):1037–50.
206. Linhart A, Elliott PM. The heart in Anderson-Fabry disease and other lysosomal storage disorders. Heart (British Cardiac Society). 2007;93:528–35.
207. Patel V, O'Mahony C, Hughes D, Rahman MS, Coats C, Murphy E, Lachmann R, Mehta A, Elliott PM. Clinical and genetic predictors of major cardiac events in patients with Anderson-Fabry disease. Heart. 2015;101(12):961–6.

208. Linhart A, Palecek T, Bultas J, Ferguson JJ, Hrudova J, Karetova D, Zeman J, Ledvinova J, Poupetova H, Elleder M, et al. New insights in cardiac structural changes in patients with Fabry's disease. Am Heart J. 2000;139:1101–8.
209. Mehta A, Ricci R, Widmer U, Dehout F, Garcia de Lorenzo A, Kampmann C, Linhart A, Sunder-Plassmann G, Ries M, Beck M. Fabry disease defined: baseline clinical manifestations of 366 patients in the Fabry Outcome Survey. Eur J Clin Invest. 2004;34:236–42.
210. Shah JS, Hughes DA, Sachdev B, Tome M, Ward D, Lee P, Mehta AB, Elliott PM. Prevalence and clinical significance of cardiac arrhythmia in Anderson-Fabry disease. Am J Cardiol. 2005;96:842–6.
211. Weidemann F, Niemann M, Breunig F, Herrmann S, Beer M, Stork S, Voelker W, Ertl G, Wanner C, Stratmann J. Long-term effects of enzyme replacement therapy on fabry cardiomyopathy. Circulation. 2009;119:524–9.
212. Nishino I, Fu J, Tanji K, Yamada T, Shimojo S, Koori T, Mora M, Riggs JE, Oh SJ, Koga Y, et al. Primary LAMP-2 deficiency causes X-linked vacuolar cardiomyopathy and myopathy (Danon disease). Nature. 2000;406:906–10.
213. Danon MJ, Oh SJ, DiMauro S, Manaligod JR, Eastwood A, Naidu S, Schliselfeld LH. Lysosomal glycogen storage disease with normal acid maltase. Neurology. 1981;31:51–7.
214. Sugie K, Yamamoto A, Murayama K, Oh SJ, Takahashi M, Mora M, Riggs JE, Colomer J, Iturriaga C, Meloni A, et al. Clinicopathological features of genetically confirmed Danon disease. Neurology. 2002;58:1773–8.
215. Fu L, Luo S, Cai S, Hong W, Guo Y, Wu J, Liu T, Zhao C, Li F, Huang H, Huang M, Wang J. Identification of LAMP2 mutations in early-onset Danon disease with hypertrophic cardiomyopathy by targeted next-generation sequencing. Am J Cardiol. 2016;118(6):888–94.
216. Boucek D, Jirikowic J, Taylor M. Natural history of Danon disease. Genet Med. 2011;13:563–8.
217. Prall FR, Drack A, Taylor M, Ku L, Olson JL, Gregory D, Mestroni L, Mandava N. Ophthalmic manifestations of Danon disease. Ophthalmology. 2006;113:1010–3.
218. Del Rizzo M, Fanin M, Cerutti A, Cazzorla C, Milanesi O, Nascimbeni AC, Angelini C, Giordano L, Bordugo A, Burlina AB. Long-term follow-up results in enzyme replacement therapy for Pompe disease: a case report. J Inherit Metab Dis. 2010;33(Suppl 3):S389–93.
219. Klinge L, Straub V, Neudorf U, Schaper J, Bosbach T, Gorlinger K, Wallot M, Richards S, Voit T. Safety and efficacy of recombinant acid alpha-glucosidase (rhGAA) in patients with classical infantile Pompe disease: results of a phase II clinical trial. Neuromuscul Disord. 2005;15:24–31.
220. Limongelli G, Fratta F. S1.4 cardiovascular involvement in Pompe disease. Acta Myol. 2011;30(3):202–3.
221. Blair E, Redwood C, Ashrafian H, Oliveira M, Broxholme J, Kerr B, Salmon A, Ostman-Smith I, Watkins H. Mutations in the gamma (2) subunit of AMP-activated protein kinase cause familial hypertrophic cardiomyopathy: evidence for the central role of energy compromise in disease pathogenesis. Hum Mol Genet. 2001;10:1215–20.
222. Fabris E, Brun F, Porto AG, Losurdo P, Serdoz LV, Zecchin M, Severini GM, Mestroni L, Di Chiara A, Sinagra G. Cardiac hypertrophy, accessory pathway, and conduction system disease in an adolescent—the PRKAG2 cardiac syndrome. JACC. 2013;62(9):e17.
223. Thevenon J, Laurent G, Ader F, Laforet P, Klug D, Duva Pentiah A, Gouya L, Maurage CA, Kacet S, Eicher JC, Albuisson J, Desnos M, Bieth E, Duboc D, Martin L, Reant P, Picard F, Bonithon-Kopp C, Gautier E, Binquet C, Thauvin-Robinet C, Faivre L, Bouvagnet P, Charron P, Richard P. High prevalence of arrhythmic and myocardial complications in patients with cardiac glycogenosis due to PRKAG2 mutations. Europace. 2017;19(4):651–9.
224. Burwinkel B, Scott JW, Buhrer C, van Landeghem FKH, Cox GF, Wilson CJ, Hardie DG, Kilimann MW. Fatal congenital heart glycogenesis caused by a recurrent activating R531Q mutation in the gamma2-subunit of AMP-activated protein kinase (PRKAG2), not by phosphorylase kinase deficiency. Am J Hum Genet. 2005;76:1034–49.
225. Zhang L-P, Hui B, Gao B-R. High risk of sudden death associated with a PRKAG2-related familial Wolff-Parkinson-White syndrome. J Electrocardiol. 2011;44(4):483–6.

226. Murphy RT, Mogensen J, McGarry K, Bahl A, Evans A, Osman E, Syrris P, Gorman G, Farrell M, Holton JL, et al. Adenosine monophosphate-activated protein kinase disease mimicks hypertrophic cardiomyopathy and Wolff-Parkinson-White syndrome: natural history. J Am Coll Cardiol. 2005;45:922–30.
227. Gollob MH. Modulating phenotypic expression of the PRKAG2 Cardiac syndrome. Circulation. 2008;117:134–5.
228. Scaglia F, Towbin JA, Craigen WJ, Belmont JW, Smith EO, Neish SR, Ware SM, Hunter JV, Fernbach SD, Vladutiu GD, et al. Clinical spectrum, morbidity, and mortality in 113 pediatric patients with mitochondrial disease. Pediatrics. 2004;114:925–31.
229. Holmgren D, Wahlander H, Eriksson BO, Oldfors A, Holme E, Tulinius M. Cardiomyopathy in children with mitochondrial disease; clinical course and cardiological findings. Eur Heart J. 2003;24:280–8.
230. Limongelli G, Masarone D, Pacileo G. Mitochondrial disease and the heart. Heart. 2017;103:390–8.
231. Majamaa-Voltti K, Peuhkurinen K, Kortelainen MJ, Hassinen IE, Majamaa K. Cardiac abnormalities in patients with mitochondrial DNA mutation 3243A>G. BMC Cardiovasc Disord. 2002;2:12. https://doi.org/10.1186/1471-2261-2-12.
232. Meyers DE, Basha HI, Koenig MK. Mitochondrial cardiomyopathy—pathophysiology, diagnosis and management. Tex Heart Inst J. 2013;40(4):385–94.
233. Wahbi K, Larue S, Jardel C, Meune C, Stojkovic T, Ziegler F, et al. Cardiac involvement is frequent in patients with the m.8344A>G mutation of mitochondrial DNA. Neurology. 2010;74(8):674–7.
234. Child JS, Perloff JK, Bach PM, Wolfe AD, Perlman S, Kark RA. Cardiac involvement in Friedreich's ataxia: a clinical study of 75 patients. J Am Coll Cardiol. 1986;7:1370–8.
235. Casazza F, Ferrari F, Piccone U, Maggiolini S, Capozi A, Morpurgo M. Progression of cardiopathology in Friedreich ataxia: clinico-instrumental study. Cardiologia (Rome, Italy). 1990;35:423–31.
236. Jensen MK, Bundgaard H. Cardiomyopathy in Friedreich Ataxia—exemplifying the challenges faced by cardiologists in the management of rare diseases. Circulation. 2012;125:1591–3.
237. Noonan JA, Ehmke DA. Associated noncardiac malformations in children with congenital heart disease. J Pediatr. 1963;63:468.
238. Noonan JA. Hypertelorism with Turner phenotype. A new syndrome with associated congenital heart disease. Am J Dis Child. 1968;116:373–80.
239. Tartaglia M, Gelb BD. Noonan syndrome and related disorders: genetics and pathogenesis. Annu Rev Genomics Hum Genet. 2005;6:45–68.
240. Sharland M, Burch M, McKenna WM, Paton MA. A clinical study of Noonan syndrome. Arch Dis Child. 1992;67:178–83.
241. Burch M, Mann JM, Sharland M, Shinebourne EA, Patton MA, McKenna WJ. Myocardial disarray in Noonan syndrome. Br Heart J. 1992;68:586–8.
242. Chen B, Bronson RT, Klaman LD, Hampton TG, Wang JF, Green PJ, Magnuson T, Douglas PS, Morgan JP, Neel BG. Mice mutant for Egfr and Shp2 have defective cardiac semilunar valvulogenesis. Nat Genet. 2000;24:296–9.
243. Tartaglia M, Mehler EL, Goldberg R, Zampino G, Brunner HG, Kremer H, van der Burgt I, Crosby AH, Ion A, Jeffery S, et al. Mutations in PTPN11, encoding the protein tyrosine phosphatase SHP-2, cause Noonan syndrome. Nat Genet. 2001;29:465–8.
244. Tartaglia M, Pennacchio LA, Zhao C, Yadav KK, Fodale V, Sarkozy A, Pandit B, Oishi K, Martinelli S, Schackwitz W, et al. Gain-of-function SOS1 mutations cause a distinctive form of Noonan syndrome. Nat Genet. 2007;39:75–9.
245. Roberts AE, Araki T, Swanson KD, Montgomery KT, Schiripo TA, Joshi VA, Li L, Yassin Y, Tamburino AM, Neel BG, et al. Germline gain-of-function mutations in SOS1 cause Noonan syndrome. Nat Genet. 2007;39:70–4.
246. Zenker M, Horn D, Wieczorek D, Allanson J, Pauli S, van der Burgt I, Doerr HG, Gaspar H, Hofbeck M, Gillessen-Kaesbach G, et al. SOS1 is the second most common Noonan gene but plays no major role in cardio-facio-cutaneous syndrome. J Med Genet. 2007;44:651–6.

247. Schubbert S, Zenker M, Rowe SL, Boll S, Klein C, Bollag G, van der Burgt I, Musante L, Kalscheuer V, Wehner LE, et al. Germline KRAS mutations cause Noonan syndrome. Nat Genet. 2006;38:331–6.
248. Pandit B, Sarkozy A, Pennacchio LA, Carta C, Oishi K, Martinelli S, Pogna EA, Schackwitz W, Ustaszewska A, Landstrom A, et al. Gain-of-function RAF1 mutations cause Noonan and LEOPARD syndromes with hypertrophic cardiomyopathy. Nat Genet. 2007;39:1007–12.
249. Razzaque MA, Nishizawa T, Komoike Y, Yagi H, Furutani M, Amo R, Kamisago M, Momma K, Katayama H, Nakagawa M, et al. Germline gain-of-function mutations in RAF1 cause Noonan syndrome. Nat Genet. 2007;39:1013–7.
250. Tartaglia M, Kalidas K, Shaw A, Song X, Musat DL, van der Burgt I, Brunner HG, Bertola DR, Crosby A, Ion A, et al. PTPN11 mutations in Noonan syndrome: molecular spectrum, genotype-phenotype correlation, and phenotypic heterogeneity. Am J Hum Genet. 2002;70:1555–63.
251. Zenker M, Buheitel G, Rauch R, Koenig R, Bosse K, Kress W, Tietze HU, Doerr HG, Hofbeck M, Singer H, et al. Genotype-phenotype correlations in Noonan syndrome. J Pediatr. 2004;144:368–74.
252. Wilkinson JD, Lowe AM, Salbert BA, Sleeper LA, Colan SD, Cox GF, Towbin JA, Connuck DM, Messere JE, Lipshultz SE. Outcomes in children with Noonan syndrome and hypertrophic cardiomyopathy: a study from the Pediatric Cardiomyopathy Registry. Am Heart J. 2012;164(3):442–8.
253. Digilio MC, Conti E, Sarkozy A, Mingarelli R, Dottorini T, Marino B, Pizzuti A, Dallapiccola B. Grouping of multiple-lentigines/LEOPARD and Noonan syndromes on the PTPN11 gene. Am J Hum Genet. 2002;71:389–94.
254. Limongelli G, Pacileo G, Marino B, Digilio MC, Sarkozy A, Elliott P, Versacci P, Calabro P, De Zorzi A, Di Salvo G, Syrris P, Patton M, McKenna WJ, Dallapiccola B, Calabro R. Prevalence and clinical significance of cardiovascular abnormalities in patients with the LEOPARD syndrome. Am J Cardiol. 2007;100:736–41.
255. Sarkozy A, Digilio MC, Dallapiccola B. Leopard syndrome. Orphanet J Rare Dis. 2008;3:13.
256. Woywodt A, Welzel J, Haase H, Duerholz A, Wiegand U, Potratz J, Sheikhzadeh A. Cardiomyopathic lentiginosis/LEOPARD syndrome presenting as sudden cardiac arrest. Chest. 1998;113:1415–7.
257. Taylor MRG, Carniel E, Mestroni L. Cardiomyopathy, familial dilated. Orphanet J Rare Dis. 2006;1:27.
258. Grunig E, Tasman JA, Kucherer H, Franz W, Kubler W, Katus HA. Frequency and phenotypes of familial dilated cardiomyopathy. J Am Coll Cardiol. 1998;31:186–94.
259. Baig MK, Goldman JH, Caforio AL, Coonar AS, Keeling PJ, McKenna WJ. Familial dilated cardiomyopathy: cardiac abnormalities are common in asymptomatic relatives and may represent early disease. J Am Coll Cardiol. 1998;31:195–201.
260. Mahon NG, Murphy RT, MacRae CA, Caforio AL, Elliott PM, McKenna WJ. Echocardiographic evaluation in asymptomatic relatives of patients with dilated cardiomyopathy reveals preclinical disease. Ann Intern Med. 2005;143:108–15.
261. Bowles NE, Bowles KR, Towbin JA. The “final common pathway” hypothesis and inherited cardiovascular disease. The role of cytoskeletal proteins in dilated cardiomyopathy. Herz. 2000;25:168–75.
262. McNally EM, Golbus JR, Puckelwartz MJ. Genetic mutations and mechanisms in dilated cardiomyopathy. J Clin Invest. 2013;123(1):19–26.
263. Tsubata S, Bowles KR, Vatta M, Zintz C, Titus J, Muhonen L, Bowles NE, Towbin JA. Mutations in the human delta-sarcoglycan gene in familial and sporadic dilated cardiomyopathy. J Clin Invest. 2000;106:655–62.
264. Barresi R, Di Blasi C, Negri T, Brugnoni R, Vitali A, Felisari G, Salandi A, Daniel S, Cornelio F, Morandi L, et al. Disruption of heart sarcoglycan complex and severe cardiomyopathy caused by beta sarcoglycan mutations. J Med Genet. 2000;37:102–7.
265. Herman DS, Lam L, Taylor MR, Wang L, Teekakirikul P, Christodoulou D, Conner L, DePalma SR, McDonough B, Sparks E, Teodorescu DL, Cirino AL, Banner NR, Pennell

DJ, Graw S, Merlo M, Di Lenarda A, Sinagra G, Bos JM, Ackerman MJ, Mitchell RN, Murry CE, Lakdawala NK, Ho CY, Barton PJ, Cook SA, Mestroni L, Seidman JG, Seidman CE. Truncations of titin causing dilated cardiomyopathy. N Engl J Med. 2012;366(7):619–28.
266. Olson TM, Michels VV, Thibodeau SN, Tai YS, Keating MT. Actin mutations in dilated cardiomyopathy, a heritable form of heart failure. Science (New York, NY). 1998;280:750–2.
267. Kamisago M, Sharma SD, DePalma SR, Solomon S, Sharma P, McDonough B, Smoot L, Mullen MP, Woolf PK, Wigle ED, et al. Mutations in sarcomere protein genes as a cause of dilated cardiomyopathy. N Engl J Med. 2000;343:1688–96.
268. Kaski JP, Burch M, Elliott PM. Mutations in the cardiac Troponin C gene are a cause of idiopathic dilated cardiomyopathy in childhood. Cardiol Young. 2007;17:675–7.
269. Mogensen J, Murphy RT, Shaw T, Bahl A, Redwood C, Watkins H, Burke M, Elliott PM, McKenna WJ. Severe disease expression of cardiac troponin C and T mutations in patients with idiopathic dilated cardiomyopathy. J Am Coll Cardiol. 2004;44:2033–40.
270. Olson TM, Kishimoto NY, Whitby FG, Michels VV. Mutations that alter the surface charge of alpha-tropomyosin are associated with dilated cardiomyopathy. J Mol Cell Cardiol. 2001;33: 723–32.
271. Du CK, et al. Knock-in mouse model of dilated cardiomyopathy caused by troponin mutation. Circ Res. 2007;101(2):185–94.
272. Karmisago M, Sharma SD, DePalma SR, Solomon S, Sharma P, McDonough B, Smoot L, Mullen MP, Woolf PK, Wigle ED, Seidman JG, Seidman CE. Mutations in sarcomere protein genes as a cause of dilated cardiomyopathy. N Engl J Med. 2000;343(23):1688–96.
273. Lakdawala NK, Dellefave L, Redwood CS, Sparks E, Cirino AL, Depalma S, Colan SD, Funke B, Zimmerman RS, Robinson P, Watkins H, Seidman CE, Seidman JG, McNally EM, Ho CY. Familial dilated cardiomyopathy caused by an alpha-tropomyosin mutation: the distinctive natural history of sarcomeric dilated cardiomyopathy. J Am Coll Cardiol. 2010;55(4):320–9.
274. Klaassen S, Probst S, Oechslin E, Gerull B, Krings G, Schuler P, Greutmann M, Hurlimann D, Yegitbasi M, Pons L, Gramlich M, Drenckhahn JD, Heuser A, Berger F, Jenni R, Thierfelder L. Mutations in sarcomere protein genes in left ventricular nocompaction. Circulation. 2008;117(22):2893–901.
275. Lapidos KA, Kakkar R, McNally EM. The dystrophin glycoprotein complex: signaling strength and integrity for the sarcolemma. Circ Res. 2004;94(8):1023–31.
276. Yasuda S, Townsend D, Michele DE, Favre EG, Day SM, Metzger JM. Dystrophic heart failure blocked by membrane sealant poloxamer. Nature. 2005;436(7053):1025–9.
277. Towbin JA, Bowles NE. The failing heart. Nature. 2002;415:227–33.
278. Brodsky GL, Muntoni F, Miocic S, Sinagra G, Sewry C, Mestroni L. Lamin A/C gene mutation associated with dilated cardiomyopathy with variable skeletal muscle involvement. Circulation. 2000;101:473–6.
279. Fatkin D, MacRae C, Sasaki T, Wolff MR, Porcu M, Frenneaux M, Atherton J, Vidaillet HJ Jr, Spudich S, De Girolami U, et al. Missense mutations in the rod domain of the lamin A/C gene as causes of dilated cardiomyopathy and conduction-system disease. N Engl J Med. 1999;341:1715–24.
280. Kass S, MacRae C, Graber HL, Sparks EA, McNamara D, Boudoulas H, Basson CT, Baker PB 3rd, Cody RJ, Fishman MC, et al. A gene defect that causes conduction system disease and dilated cardiomyopathy maps to chromosome 1p1-1q1. Nat Genet. 1994;7:546–51.
281. Bonne G, Di Barletta MR, Varnous S, Becane HM, Hammouda EH, Merlini L, Muntoni F, Greenberg CR, Gary F, Urtizberea JA, et al. Mutations in the gene encoding lamin A/C cause autosomal dominant Emery-Dreifuss muscular dystrophy. Nat Genet. 1999;21:285–8.
282. Muchir A, Bonne G, van der Kooi AJ, van Meegen M, Baas F, Bolhuis PA, de Visser M, Schwartz K. Identification of mutations in the gene encoding lamins A/C in autosomal dominant limb girdle muscular dystrophy with atrioventricular conduction disturbances (LGMD1B). Hum Mol Genet. 2000;9:1453–9.
283. Shackleton S, Lloyd DJ, Jackson SN, Evans R, Niermeijer MF, Singh BM, Schmidt H, Brabant G, Kumar S, Durrington PN, et al. LMNA, encoding lamin A/C, is mutated in partial lipodystrophy. Nat Genet. 2000;24:153–6.

284. Arbustini E, Pilotto A, Repetto A, Grasso M, Negri A, Diegoli M, Campana C, Scelsi L, Baldini E, Gavazzi A, Tavazzi L. Autosomal dominant dilated cardiomyopathy with atrioventricular block: a lamin A/C defect-related disease. J Am Coll Cardiol. 2002;39(6):981–90.
285. Van Rijsingen IA, Arbustini E, Elliott PM, Mogensen J, Hermans-van Ast JF, van der Kooi AJ, van Tintelen JP, van den Berg MP, Pilotto A, Pasotti M, Jenkins S, Rowland C, Aslam U, Wilde AA, Perrot A, Pankuweit S, Zwinderman AH, Charron P, Pinto YM. Risk factors for malignant ventricular arrhythmias in lamin a/c mutation carriers a European cohort study. J Am Coll Cardiol. 2012;59(5):493–500.
286. Capell BC, Collins FS. Human laminopathies: nuclei gone genetically awry. Nat Rev. 2006;7:940–52.
287. Worman HJ, Bonne G. "Laminopathies": a wide spectrum of human diseases. Exp Cell Res. 2007;313:2121–33.
288. Broers JL, Peeters EA, Kuijpers HJ, Endert J, Bouten CV, Oomens CW, Baaijens FP, Ramaekers FC. Decreased mechanical stiffness in LMNA−/− cells is caused by defective nucleo-cytoskeletal integrity: implications for the development of laminopathies. Hum Mol Genet. 2004;13:2567–80.
289. Lammerding J, Schulze PC, Takahashi T, Kozlov S, Sullivan T, Kamm RD, Stewart CL, Lee RT. Lamin A/C deficiency causes defective nuclear mechanics and mechanotransduction. J Clin Invest. 2004;113:370–8.
290. Sullivan T, Escalante-Alcalde D, Bhatt H, Anver M, Bhat N, Nagashima K, Stewart CL, Burke B. Loss of A-type lamin expression compromises nuclear envelope integrity leading to muscular dystrophy. J Cell Biol. 1999;147:913–20.
291. Ortiz-Genga MF, Cuenca S, Del Ferro M, Zorio E, Salgado-Arnanda R, Climent V, Padron-Barthe L, Duro-Aguado I, Jimenez-Jaimez J, Hidalgo-Olivares VM, Garcia-Campo E, Lanzillo C, Suarez-Mier P, Yonath H, Marcos-Alonso S, Ochoa JP, Santome JL, Garcia-Giustiniani D, Rodriguez-Garrido JL, Dominguez F, Merlo M, Palomino J, Pena ML, Trujillo JP, Martin-Vila A, Stolfo D, Molina P, Lara-Pezzi E, Calvo-Iglesias FE, Nof E, Calo L, Barriales-Villa R, Gimeno-Blanes JR, Arad M, Garcia-Pavo P, Monserrat L. Truncating FLNC mutations are associated with high-risk dilated and arrhythmogenic cardiomyopathies. J Am Coll Cardiol. 2016;68(22):2440–51.
292. Cohen N, Muntoni F. Multiple pathogenetic mechanisms in X linked dilated cardiomyopathy. Heart (British Cardiac Society). 2004;90:835–41.
293. Muntoni F, Cau M, Ganau A, Congiu R, Arvedi G, Mateddu A, Marrosu MG, Cianchetti C, Realdi G, Cao A, et al. Brief report: deletion of the dystrophin muscle-promoter region associated with X-linked dilated cardiomyopathy. N Engl J Med. 1993;329:921–5.
294. Towbin JA, Hejtmancik JF, Brink P, Gelb B, Zhu XM, Chamberlain JS, McCabe ER, Swift M. X-linked dilated cardiomyopathy. Molecular genetic evidence of linkage to the Duchenne muscular dystrophy (dystrophin) gene at the Xp21 locus. Circulation. 1993;87:1854–65.
295. Towbin JA, Lowe AM, Colan SD, Sleeper LA, Orav EJ, Clunie S, Messere J, Cox GF, Lurie PR, Hsu D, et al. Incidence, causes, and outcomes of dilated cardiomyopathy in children. JAMA. 2006;296:1867–76.
296. Berko BA, Swift M. X-linked dilated cardiomyopathy. N Engl J Med. 1987;316:1186–91.
297. Politano L, Nigro V, Nigro G, Petretta VR, Passamano L, Papparella S, Di Somma S, Comi LI. Development of cardiomyopathy in female carriers of Duchenne and Becker muscular dystrophies. JAMA. 1996;275:1335–8.
298. Barth PG, Scholte HR, Berden JA, Van der Klei-Van Moorsel JM, Luyt-Houwen IE, Van't Veer-Korthof ET, Van der Harten JJ, Sobotka-Plojhar MA. An X-linked mitochondrial disease affecting cardiac muscle, skeletal muscle and neutrophil leucocytes. J Neurol Sci. 1983;62:327–55.
299. Kelley RI, Cheatham JP, Clark BJ, Nigro MA, Powell BR, Sherwood GW, Sladky JT, Swisher WP. X-linked dilated cardiomyopathy with neutropenia, growth retardation, and 3-methylglutaconic aciduria. J Pediatr. 1991;119:738–47.
300. Bleyl SB, Mumford BR, Thompson V, Carey JC, Pysher TJ, Chin TK, Ward K. Neonatal, lethal noncompaction of the left ventricular myocardium is allelic with Barth syndrome. Am J Hum Genet. 1997;61:868–72.

301. D'Adamo P, Fassone L, Gedeon A, Janssen EA, Bione S, Bolhuis PA, Barth PG, Wilson M, Haan E, Orstavik KH, et al. The X-linked gene G4.5 is responsible for different infantile dilated cardiomyopathies. Am J Hum Genet. 1997;61:862–7.
302. Gavazzi A, De Maria R, Parolini M, Porcu M. Alcohol abuse and dilated cardiomyopathy in men. Am J Cardiol. 2000;85(9):1114–8.
303. Feldman AM, McNamara D. Myocarditis. N Engl J Med. 2000;343:1388–98.
304. Caforio ALP, Pankuweit S, Arbustini E, Basso C, Gimeno-Blanes J, Felix SB, Fu M, Helio T, Heymans S, Jahns R, Klingel K, Linhart A, Maisch B, McKenna W, Mogensen J, Pinto YM, Ristic A, Schultheiss HP, Seggewiss H, Tavazzi L, Thiene G, Yilmaz A, Charron P, Elliott PM. Current state of knowledge on aetiology, diagnosis, management, and therapy of myocarditis: a position statement of the European Society of Cardiology Working Group on Myocardial and Pericardial Diseases. Eur Heart J. 2013;34:2636–48.
305. Magnani JW, Dec GW. Myocarditis: current trends in diagnosis and treatment. Circulation. 2006;113:876–90.
306. Maisch B, Richter A, Sandmoller A, Portig I, Pankuweit S. Inflammatory dilated cardiomyopathy (DCMI). Herz. 2005;30:535–44.
307. Noutsias M, Seeberg B, Schultheiss HP, Kuhl U. Expression of cell adhesion molecules in dilated cardiomyopathy: evidence for endothelial activation in inflammatory cardiomyopathy. Circulation. 1999;99:2124–31.
308. Caforio AL, Keeling PJ, Zachara E, Mestroni L, Camerini F, Mann JM, Bottazzo GF, McKenna WJ. Evidence from family studies for autoimmunity in dilated cardiomyopathy. Lancet. 1994;344:773–7.
309. Caforio AL, Goldman JH, Baig MK, Haven AJ, Dalla LL, Keeling PJ, McKenna WJ. Cardiac autoantibodies in dilated cardiomyopathy become undetectable with disease progression. Heart (British Cardiac Society). 1997;77:62–7.
310. Caforio AL, Mahon NJ, Tona F, McKenna WJ. Circulating cardiac autoantibodies in dilated cardiomyopathy and myocarditis: pathogenetic and clinical significance. Eur J Heart Fail. 2002;4:411–7.
311. Mahrholdt H, Wagner A, Deluigi CC, Kispert E, Hager C, Meinhardt G, Vogelsberg H, Fritz P, Dippon J, Bock CT, Klingel K, Kandolf R, Sechtem U. Presentation, patterns of myocardial damage, and clinical course of viral myocarditis. Circulation. 2006;114(15):1581–90.
312. Schowengerdt KO, Ni J, Denfield SW, Gajarski RJ, Bowles NE, Rosenthal G, Kearney DL, Price JK, Rogers BB, Schauer GM, et al. Association of parvovirus B19 genome in children with myocarditis and cardiac allograft rejection: diagnosis using the polymerase chain reaction. Circulation. 1997;96:3549–54.
313. Baboonian C, Treasure T. Meta-analysis of the association of enteroviruses with human heart disease. Heart (British Cardiac Society). 1997;78:539–43.
314. Kuhl U, Pauschinger M, Noutsias M, Seeberg B, Bock T, Lassner D, Poller W, Kandolf R, Schultheiss HP. High prevalence of viral genomes and multiple viral infections in the myocardium of adults with "idiopathic" left ventricular dysfunction. Circulation. 2005;111:887–93.
315. Wessely R, Klingel K, Santana LF, Dalton N, Hongo M, Jonathan Lederer W, Kandolf R, Knowlton KU. Transgenic expression of replication-restricted enteroviral genomes in heart muscle induces defective excitation-contraction coupling and dilated cardiomyopathy. J Clin Invest. 1998;102:1444–53.
316. Abdullah M, Bigras JL, McCrindle BW. Dilated cardiomyopathy as a first sign of nutritional vitamin D deficiency rickets in infancy. Can J Cardiol. 1999;15:699–701.
317. Gulati S, Bajpai A, Juneja R, Kabra M, Bagga A, Kalra V. Hypocalcemic heart failure masquerading as dilated cardiomyopathy. Indian J Pediatr. 2001;68:287–90.
318. Labrune P, Bader B, Devictor D, Madelin JC, Huault G. Hypocalcemia, cardiac failure and ventricular tachycardia in an infant with rickets. Arch Fr Pediatr. 1986;43:413–5.
319. Maiya S, Sullivan I, Allgrove J, Yates R, Malone M, Brain C, Archer N, Mok Q, Daubeney P, Tulloh R, et al. Hypocalcaemia and vitamin D deficiency: an important, but preventable, cause of life-threatening infant heart failure. Heart (British Cardiac Society). 2008;94:581–4.

320. Price DI, Stanford LC Jr, Braden DS, Ebeid MR, Smith JC. Hypocalcemic rickets: an unusual cause of dilated cardiomyopathy. Pediatr Cardiol. 2003;24:510–2.
321. Yaseen H, Maragnes P, Gandon-Laloum S, Bensaid P, N'Guyen B, Ricaud D, Lecacheux C. A severe form of vitamin D deficiency with hypocalcemic cardiomyopathy. Pediatrie. 1993;48:547–9.
322. Hughes SE, McKenna WJ. New insights into the pathology of inherited cardiomyopathy. Heart (British Cardiac Society). 2005;91:257–64.
323. Ponikowski P, Voors AA, Anker SD, Bueno H, Cleland JGF, Coats AJS, Falk V, Gonzalez-Juanatey JR, Harjola VP, Jankowska EA, Jessup M, Linde C, Nihoyannopoulos P, Parissis JT, Pieske B, Riley JP, Rosano GMC, Ruilope LM, Ruschitzka F, Rutten FH, van der Meer P. 2016 ESC guidelines for the diagnosis and treatment of acute and chronic heart failure: the Task Force for the diagnosis and treatment of acute and chronic heart failure of the European Society of Cardiology (ESC) developed with the special contribution of the Heart Failure Association (HFA) of the ESC. Eur Heart J. 2016;37(27):2129–200.
324. Abelmann WH, Lorell BH. The challenge of cardiomyopathy. J Am Coll Cardiol. 1989;13:1219–39.
325. Burch M, Siddiqi SA, Celermajer DS, Scott C, Bull C, Deanfield JE. Dilated cardiomyopathy in children: determinants of outcome. Br Heart J. 1994;72:246–50.
326. Daubeney PE, Nugent AW, Chondros P, Carlin JB, Colan SD, Cheung M, Davis AM, Chow CW, Weintraub RG. Clinical features and outcomes of childhood dilated cardiomyopathy: results from a national population-based study. Circulation. 2006;114:2671–8.
327. Zecchin M, Di Lenarda A, Gregori D, Moretti M, Driussi M, Aleksova A, Chersevani D, Sabbadini G, Sinagra G. Prognostic role of non-sustained ventricular tachycardia in a large cohort of patients with idiopathic dilated cardiomyopathy. Ital Heart J. 2005;6:721–7.
328. Friedman RA, Moak JP, Garson A Jr. Clinical course of idiopathic dilated cardiomyopathy in children. J Am Coll Cardiol. 1991;18:152–6.
329. Elliott P. Cardiomyopathy. Diagnosis and management of dilated cardiomyopathy. Heart (British Cardiac Society). 2000;84:106–12.
330. Henry WL, Gardin JM, Ware JH. Echocardiographic measurements in normal subjects from infancy to old age. Circulation. 1980;62:1054–61.
331. Richardson P, McKenna W, Bristow M, Maisch B, Mautner B, O'Connell J, Olsen E, Thiene G, Goodwin J, Gyarfas I, et al. Report of the 1995 World Health Organization/International Society and Federation of Cardiology Task Force on the definition and classification of cardiomyopathies. Circulation. 1996;93:841–2.
332. Doughan AR, Williams BR. Cardiac sarcoidosis. Heart (British Cardiac Society). 2006;92:282–8.
333. Price JF, Thomas AK, Grenier M, Eidem BW, O'Brian Smith E, Denfield SW, Towbin JA, Dreyer WJ. B-type natriuretic peptide predicts adverse cardiovascular events in pediatric outpatients with chronic left ventricular systolic dysfunction. Circulation. 2006;114:1063–9.
334. Guimaraes GV, Bellotti G, Mocelin AO, Camargo PR, Bocchi EA. Cardiopulmonary exercise testing in children with heart failure secondary to idiopathic dilated cardiomyopathy. Chest. 2001;120:816–24.
335. Gitt AK, Wasserman K, Kilkwski C, et al. Exercise anaerobic threshold and ventilatory efficiency identify heart failure patients for high risk of early death. Circulation. 2002;106:3079–84.
336. Parrillo JE, Aretz HT, Palacios I, Fallon JT, Block PC. The results of transvenous endomyocardial biopsy can frequently be used to diagnose myocardial diseases in patients with idiopathic heart failure. Endomyocardial biopsies in 100 consecutive patients revealed a substantial incidence of myocarditis. Circulation. 1984;69:93–101.
337. Cooper LT, Baughman KL, Feldman AM, Frustaci A, Jessup M, Kuhl U, Levine GN, Narula J, Starling RC, Towbin J, et al. The role of endomyocardial biopsy in the management of cardiovascular disease: a scientific statement from the American Heart Association, the American College of Cardiology, and the European Society of Cardiology endorsed by the Heart Failure Society of America and the Heart Failure Association of the European Society of Cardiology. Eur Heart J. 2007;28:3076–93.

338. De Cobelli F, Pieroni M, Esposito A, Chimenti C, Belloni E, Mellone R, Canu T, Perseghin G, Gaudio C, Maseri A, et al. Delayed gadolinium-enhanced cardiac magnetic resonance in patients with chronic myocarditis presenting with heart failure or recurrent arrhythmias. J Am Coll Cardiol. 2006;47:1649–54.
339. Pitt B, Zannad F, Remme WJ, Cody R, Castaigne A, Perez A, Palensky J, Wittes J. The effect of spironolactone on morbidity and mortality in patients with severe heart failure. Randomized Aldactone Evaluation Study Investigators. N Engl J Med. 1999;341:709–17.
340. Zannad F, McMurray JJV, Krum H, van Veldhuisen DJ, Swedburg K, Shi H, Vincent J, Pocock SJ, Pitt B for the EMPHASIS-HF Study Group. Epleronone in patients with systolic heart failure and mild symptoms. N Engl J Med. 2011;364:11–21.
341. Rosenthal D, Chrisant MR, Edens E, Mahony L, Canter C, Colan S, Dubin A, Lamour J, Ross R, Shaddy R, et al. International Society for Heart and Lung Transplantation: practice guidelines for management of heart failure in children. J Heart Lung Transplant. 2004;23:1313–33.
342. The CONSENSUS Trial Study Group. Effects of enalapril on mortality in severe congestive heart failure. Results of the Cooperative North Scandinavian Enalapril Survival Study (CONSENSUS). N Engl J Med. 1987;316:1429–35.
343. The SOLVD Investigators. Effect of enalapril on survival in patients with reduced left ventricular ejection fraction and congestive heart failure. N Engl J Med. 1991;325:293–302.
344. The SOLVD Investigators. Effect of enalapril on mortality and the development of heart failure in asymptomatic patients with reduced left ventricular ejection fraction. N Engl J Med. 1992;327:685–91.
345. Cohn JN, Johnson G, Ziesche S, Cobb F, Francis G, Tristani F, Smith R, Dunkman WB, Loeb H, Wong M, et al. A comparison of enalapril with hydralazine-isosorbide dinitrate in the treatment of chronic congestive heart failure. N Engl J Med. 1991;325:303–10.
346. Cohn JN, Tognoni G. A randomized trial of the angiotensin-receptor blocker valsartan in chronic heart failure. N Engl J Med. 2001;345:1667–75.
347. Hamroff G, Katz SD, Mancini D, Blaufarb I, Bijou R, Patel R, Jondeau G, Olivari MT, Thomas S, Le Jemtel TH. Addition of angiotensin II receptor blockade to maximal angiotensin-converting enzyme inhibition improves exercise capacity in patients with severe congestive heart failure. Circulation. 1999;99:990–2.
348. McKelvie RS, Yusuf S, Pericak D, Avezum A, Burns RJ, Probstfield J, Tsuyuki RT, White M, Rouleau J, Latini R, et al. Comparison of candesartan, enalapril, and their combination in congestive heart failure: randomized evaluation of strategies for left ventricular dysfunction (RESOLVD) pilot study. The RESOLVD Pilot Study Investigators. Circulation. 1999;100:1056–64.
349. Pfeffer MA, Swedberg K, Granger CB, Held P, McMurray JJ, Michelson EL, Olofsson B, Ostergren J, Yusuf S, Pocock S. Effects of candesartan on mortality and morbidity in patients with chronic heart failure: the CHARM-overall programme. Lancet. 2003;362:759–66.
350. Cleland JG, Charlesworth A, Lubsen J, Swedberg K, Remme WJ, Erhardt L, Di Lenarda A, Komajda M, Metra M, Torp-Pedersen C, et al. A comparison of the effects of carvedilol and metoprolol on well-being, morbidity, and mortality (the "patient journey") in patients with heart failure: a report from the Carvedilol Or Metoprolol European Trial (COMET). J Am Coll Cardiol. 2006;47:1603–11.
351. Packer M, Bristow MR, Cohn JN, Colucci WS, Fowler MB, Gilbert EM, Shusterman NH. The effect of carvedilol on morbidity and mortality in patients with chronic heart failure. U.S. Carvedilol Heart Failure Study Group. N Engl J Med. 1996;334:1349–55.
352. Packer M, Coats AJ, Fowler MB, Katus HA, Krum H, Mohacsi P, Rouleau JL, Tendera M, Castaigne A, Roecker EB, et al. Effect of carvedilol on survival in severe chronic heart failure. N Engl J Med. 2001;344:1651–8.
353. Effect of metoprolol CR/XL in chronic heart failure: Metoprolol CR/XL Randomised Intervention Trial in Congestive Heart Failure (MERIT-HF). Lancet. 1999; 353:2001–7.
354. The Cardiac Insufficiency Bisoprolol Study II (CIBIS-II): a randomised trial. Lancet. 1999; 353:9–13.

355. Packer M, Gheorghiade M, Young JB, Costantini PJ, Adams KF, Cody RJ, Smith LK, Van Voorhees L, Gourley LA, Jolly MK. Withdrawal of digoxin from patients with chronic heart failure treated with angiotensin-converting-enzyme inhibitors. RADIANCE Study. N Engl J Med. 1993;329:1–7.
356. Rathore SS, Curtis JP, Wang Y, Bristow MR, Krumholz HM. Association of serum digoxin concentration and outcomes in patients with heart failure. JAMA. 2003;289:871–8.
357. Jain S, Vaidyanathan B. Digoxin in management of heart failure in children: should it be continued or relegated to the history books? Ann Pediatr Cardiol. 2009;2(2):149–52.
358. Swedberg K, Komajda M, Bohm M, Borer JS, Ford I, Dubost-Brama A, Lerebours G, Tavazzi L on behalf of the SHIFT Investigators. Ivabradine and outcomes in chronic heart failure (SHIFT): a randomised placebo-controlled study. Lancet. 2010;376:875–85.
359. McMurray JJV, Packer M, Desai AS, Gong J, Lefkowitz MP, Rizkala AR, Rouleau JL, Shi VC, Solomon SD, Swedburg K, Zile MR, PARADIGM-HF Investigators and Committees. Angiotensin-neprilysin inhibition versus enalapril in heart failure. N Engl J Med. 2014;371:993–1004.
360. Sirajuddin RA, Miller AB, Geraci SA. Anticoagulation in patients with dilated cardiomyopathy and sinus rhythm: a critical literature review. J Card Fail. 2002;8:48–53.
361. Massie BM, Collins JF, Ammon SE, Armstrong PW, Cleland JGF, Ezekowitz M, Jafri SM, Krol WF, O'Connor CM, Schulman KA, Teo K, Warren SR for the WATCH Trial Investigators. Randomized trial of warfarin, aspirin, and clopidogrel in patients with chronic heart failure. Circulation. 2009;119:1616–24.
362. Koniaris L, Goldhaber S. Anticoagulation in dilated cardiomyopathy. JACC. 1998;31(4):745.
363. Bardy GH, Lee KL, Mark DB, Poole JE, Packer DL, Boineau R, Domanski M, Troutman C, Anderson J, Johnson G, et al. Amiodarone or an implantable cardioverter-defibrillator for congestive heart failure. N Engl J Med. 2005;352:225–37.
364. Kober L, Thune JJ, Nielsen JC, Haarbo J, Videbaek L, Korup E, Jensen G, Hildebrandt P, Steffensen FH, Bruun NE, Eiskjaer H, Brandes A, Thogersen AM, Gustafsson F, Egstrup K, Videbaek R, Hassager C, Svendsen JH, Hofsten DE, Torp-Pedersen C, Pehrson S for the DANISH Investigators. Defibrillator implantation in patients with nonischemic systolic heart failure. N Engl J Med. 2016;375:1221–30.
365. Maisel WH, Stevenson LW. Atrial fibrillation in heart failure: epidemiology, pathophysiology, and rationale for therapy. Am J Cardiol. 2003;91:2D–8D.
366. Aleksova A, Merlo M, Zecchin M, Sabbadini G, Barbati G, Vitrella G, Di Lenarda A, Sinagra G. Impact of atrial fibrillation on outcome of patients with idiopathic dilated cardiomyopathy: data from the heart muscle disease registry of trieste. Clin Med Res. 2010;8(3–4):142–9.
367. Duncan BW, Hraska V, Jonas RA, Wessel DL, Del Nido PJ, Laussen PC, Mayer JE, Lapierre RA, Wilson JM. Mechanical circulatory support in children with cardiac disease. J Thorac Cardiovasc Surg. 1999;117:529–42.
368. Hetzer R, Loebe M, Potapov EV, Weng Y, Stiller B, Hennig E, exi-Meskishvili V, Lange PE. Circulatory support with pneumatic paracorporeal ventricular assist device in infants and children. Ann Thorac Surg. 1998;66:1498–506.
369. Levi D, Marelli D, Plunkett M, Alejos J, Bresson J, Tran J, Eisenring C, Sadeghi A, Galindo A, Fazio D, et al. Use of assist devices and ECMO to bridge pediatric patients with cardiomyopathy to transplantation. J Heart Lung Transplant. 2002;21:760–70.
370. McMahon AM, van DC, Burch M, Whitmore P, Neligan S, Rees P, Radley-Smith R, Goldman A, Brown K, Cohen G, et al. Improved early outcome for end-stage dilated cardiomyopathy in children. J Thorac Cardiovasc Surg. 2003;126:1781–7.
371. Auricchio A, Stellbrink C, Block M, Sack S, Vogt J, Bakker P, Klein H, Kramer A, Ding J, Salo R, et al. Effect of pacing chamber and atrioventricular delay on acute systolic function of paced patients with congestive heart failure. The Pacing Therapies for Congestive Heart Failure Study Group. The Guidant Congestive Heart Failure Research Group. Circulation. 1999;99:2993–3001.
372. Bristow MR, Saxon LA, Boehmer J, Krueger S, Kass DA, De Marco T, Carson P, DiCarlo L, DeMets D, White BG, et al. Cardiac-resynchronization therapy with or without an implantable defibrillator in advanced chronic heart failure. N Engl J Med. 2004;350:2140–50.

373. Cleland JG, Daubert JC, Erdmann E, Freemantle N, Gras D, Kappenberger L, Tavazzi L. The effect of cardiac resynchronization on morbidity and mortality in heart failure. N Engl J Med. 2005;352:1539–49.
374. Cleland JG, Daubert JC, Erdmann E, Freemantle N, Gras D, Kappenberger L, Tavazzi L. Longer-term effects of cardiac resynchronization therapy on mortality in heart failure [the CArdiac REsynchronization-Heart Failure (CARE-HF) trial extension phase]. Eur Heart J. 2006;27:1928–32.
375. McLeod CJ, Shen WK, Rea RF, Friedman PA, Hayes DL, Wokhlu A, Webster TL, Wiste HJ, Hodge DO, Bradley DJ, Hammill SC, Packer DL, Cha YM. Differential outcome of cardiac resynchronization therapy in ischemic cardiomyopathy and idiopathic dilated cardiomyopathy. Heart Rhythm. 2011;8(3):377–82.
376. Kushwaha SS, Fallon JT, Fuster V. Restrictive cardiomyopathy. N Engl J Med. 1997; 336:267–76.
377. Denfield SW. Restrictive cardiomyopathy and constrictive pericarditis. In: Chang AC, Towbin JA, editors. Heart failure in children and young adults: from molecular mechanisms to medical and surgical strategies. Philadelphia: Saunders Elsevier; 2006. p. 264–77.
378. Mogensen J, Kubo T, Duque M, Uribe W, Shaw A, Murphy R, Gimeno JR, Elliott P, McKenna WJ. Idiopathic restrictive cardiomyopathy is part of the clinical expression of cardiac troponin I mutations. J Clin Invest. 2003;111:209–16.
379. Menon S, Michels V, Pellikka P, Ballew J, Karst M, Herron K, Nelson S, Rodeheffer R, Olson T. Cardiac troponin T mutation in familial cardiomyopathy with variable remodeling and restrictive physiology. Clin Genet. 2008;74:445–54.
380. Gallego-Delgado M, Delgado JF, Brossa-Loidi V, Palomo J, Marzoa-Rivas R, Perez-Villa F, Salazar-Mendiguchia J, Ruiz-Canop MJ, Gonzalez-Lopez E, Padron-Barthe L, Bornstein B, Alonso-Pulpon L, Garcia-Pavia P. Idiopathic restrictive cardiomyopathy is primarily a genetic disease. JACC. 2016;67(25):3021–3.
381. Kostareva A, Kiselev A, Gudkova A, Frishman G, Ruepp A, Frishmana D, Smolina N, Tarnovskaya S, Nilsson D, Zlotina A, Khodyuchenko T, Vershinina T, Pervunina T, Klyushina A, Kozlenok A, Sjoberg G, Golovijova I, Sejersen T, Shlyakhto E. Genetic spectrum of idiopathic restrictive cardiomyopathy uncovered by next-generation sequencing. PLoS One. 2016;11:e0163362.
382. Karam S, Raboisson MJ, Ducreux C, Chalabreysse L, Millat G, Bozio A, Bouvagnet P. A de novo mutation of the beta cardiac myosin heavy chain gene in an infantile restrictive cardiomyopathy. Congenit Heart Dis. 2008;3:138–43.
383. Kaski JP, Syrris P, Tome Esteban MT, Fenton MJ, Christensen M, Andersen PS, Sebire N, Ashworth M, Deanfield JE, McKenna WJ, Elliott PM, et al. Idiopathic restrictive cardiomyopathy in children is caused by mutations in cardiac sarcomere protein genes. Heart. 2008;94(11):1478–84.
384. Peddy SB, Vricella LA, Crosson JE, Oswald GL, Cohn RD, Cameron DE, Valle D, Loeys BL. Infantile restrictive cardiomyopathy resulting from a mutation in the cardiac troponin T gene. Pediatrics. 2006;117:1830–3.
385. Dalakas MC, Park KY, Semino-Mora C, Lee HS, Sivakumar K, Goldfarb LG. Desmin myopathy, a skeletal myopathy with cardiomyopathy caused by mutations in the desmin gene. N Engl J Med. 2000;342:770–80.
386. Luethje LGC, Boennemann C, Goldfarb L, Goebel HH, Halle M. Prophylactic implantable cardioverter defibrillator placement in a sporadic desmin related myopathy and cardiomyopathy. PACE. 2004;27(4):559–60.
387. Gomes AV, Liang J, Potter JD. Mutations in human cardiac troponin I that are associated with restrictive cardiomyopathy affect basal ATPase activity and the calcium sensitivity of force development. J Biol Chem. 2005;280:30909–15.
388. Yumoto F, Lu QW, Morimoto S, Tanaka H, Kono N, Nagata K, Ojima T, Takahashi-Yanaga F, Miwa Y, Sasaguri T, et al. Drastic Ca2+ sensitization of myofilament associated with a small structural change in troponin I in inherited restrictive cardiomyopathy. Biochem Biophys Res Commun. 2005;338:1519–26.

389. James J, Zhang Y, Osinska H, Sanbe A, Klevitsky R, Hewett TE, Robbins J. Transgenic modeling of a cardiac troponin I mutation linked to familial hypertrophic cardiomyopathy. Circ Res. 2000;87:805–11.
390. Kubo T, Gimeno JR, Bahl A, Steffensen U, Steffensen M, Osman E, Thaman R, Mogensen J, Elliott PM, Doi Y, et al. Prevalence, clinical significance, and genetic basis of hypertrophic cardiomyopathy with restrictive phenotype. J Am Coll Cardiol. 2007;49:2419–26.
391. Shaper AG, Hutt MS, Coles RM. Necropsy study of endomyocardial fibrosis and rheumatic heart disease in Uganda 1950-1965. Br Heart J. 1968;30:391–401.
392. Angelini A, Calzolari V, Thiene G, Boffa GM, Valente M, Daliento L, Basso C, Calabrese F, Razzolini R, Livi U, et al. Morphologic spectrum of primary restrictive cardiomyopathy. Am J Cardiol. 1997;80:1046–50.
393. Fitzpatrick AP, Shapiro LM, Rickards AF, Poole-Wilson PA. Familial restrictive cardiomyopathy with atrioventricular block and skeletal myopathy. Br Heart J. 1990;63:114–8.
394. Fenton MJ, Chubb H, McMahon AM, Rees P, Elliott MJ, Burch M. Heart and heart-lung transplantation for idiopathic restrictive cardiomyopathy in children. Heart (British Cardiac Society). 2006;92:85–9.
395. Russo LM, Webber SA. Idiopathic restrictive cardiomyopathy in children. Heart (British Cardiac Society). 2005;91:1199–202.
396. Gewillig M, Mertens L, Moerman P, Dumoulin M. Idiopathic restrictive cardiomyopathy in childhood. A diastolic disorder characterized by delayed relaxation. Eur Heart J. 1996;17:1413–20.
397. Rivenes SM, Kearney DL, Smith EOB, Towbin JA, Denfield SW. Sudden death and cardiovascular collapse in children with restrictive cardiomyopathy. Circulation. 2000;102: 876–82.
398. Shah KB, Inoue Y, Mehra MR. Amyloidosis and the heart: a comprehensive review. Arch Intern Med. 2006;166:1805–13.
399. Chen Sc, Balfour IC, Jureidini S. Clinical spectrum of restrictive cardiomyopathy in children. J Heart Lung Transplant. 2001;20:90–2.
400. Denfield SW, Rosenthal G, Gajarski RJ, Bricker JT, Schowengerdt KO, Price JK, Towbin JA. Restrictive cardiomyopathies in childhood. Etiologies and natural history. Tex Heart Inst J. 1997;24:38–44.
401. Weller RJ, Weintraub R, Addonizio LJ, Chrisant MR, Gersony WM, Hsu DT. Outcome of idiopathic restrictive cardiomyopathy in children. Am J Cardiol. 2002;90:501–6.
402. Lewis AB. Clinical profile and outcome of restrictive cardiomyopathy in children. Am Heart J. 1992;123:1589–93.
403. Kimberling MT, Balzer DT, Hirsch R, Mendeloff E, Huddleston CB, Canter CE. Cardiac transplantation for pediatric restrictive cardiomyopathy: presentation, evaluation, and short-term outcome. J Heart Lung Transplant. 2002;21:455–9.
404. Bengur AR, Beekman RH, Rocchini AP, Crowley DC, Schork MA, Rosenthal A. Acute hemodynamic effects of captopril in children with a congestive or restrictive cardiomyopathy. Circulation. 1991;83:523–7.

Inherited Cardiac Muscle Disease: Dilated Cardiomyopathy

10

Eloisa Arbustini, Lorenzo Giuliani, Alessandro Di Toro, and Valentina Favalli

Abstract

Dilated cardiomyopathy (DCM) is a chronic primary heart muscle disease defined by "the presence of unexplained dilatation and systolic impairment of the left or both ventricles". It represents the end-phenotype of heart muscle damage induced by different genetic (>100 known disease genes) and non-genetic causes (inflammatory, toxic, and immune-mediated). In familial genetic DCM, the most common inheritance is autosomal dominant irrespective of the possible complex genetics (> than one mutation) identifiable with the modern massive parallel sequencing of multi-gene panels. The precise diagnosis (identification of the cause) starts with clinical hypothesis that should be generated on the basis of deep phenotyping of the proband and relatives, clinical history and pathology investigations. Genetic tests in probands and cascade family screening in clinically phenotyped families provide the basis for segregation studies that are major contributors to the assignment of a causative role of mutations in families.

Keywords

Genetic dilated cardiomyopathies • DCM clinical cases • Familial • Mutation Lamin • Nebulette • Phospholamban • Dystrophin • Arrhythmogenic Mithocondrial • Myopathy • Peripartum

---

E. Arbustini (✉) • L. Giuliani • A. Di Toro • V. Favalli
IRCCS Foundation Policlinico San Matteo, Center for Inherited Cardiovascular Diseases, Pavia, Italy
e-mail: e.arbustini@smatteo.pv.it; lorenzopaolo.giuliani@gmail.com; alessandro.ditoro@gmail.com; valentinafavalli@gmail.com

D. Kumar, P. Elliott (eds.), *Cardiovascular Genetics and Genomics*,
https://doi.org/10.1007/978-3-319-66114-8_10

10.1 Introduction

Dilated cardiomyopathy (DCM) is a chronic primary heart muscle disease defined by "the presence of unexplained dilatation and systolic impairment of the left or both ventricles". It represents the *end-phenotype* of heart muscle damage induced by different genetic and non-genetic causes. Genetic causes are heterogeneous with more that 100 disease genes described to date as possible cause of DCM phenotype. Non genetic-DCM includes inflammatory, autoimmune and toxic causes. The diagnosis of genetic DCM should be preceded by clinical screening of families to assess the inherited vs. the sporadic status of the disease; in genotyped families, these data constitute the basis for genotype—phenotype correlation and segregation studies. The precise diagnosis of DCM coincides with the identification of the cause of the disease, either genetic or non-genetic. This chapter illustrates cases with familial and apparently sporadic DCM in which genetic testing provided the precise specific diagnosis (pathologic mutation) or genetic make-up of uncertain significance. Each example gives clues and considerations that can be easily translated in the clinical practice. The major message from family studies is clinical: family screening provides the evidence of genetic disease, both presymptomatic and clinically manifest, and in genotyped families, the possibility of preclinical and prenatal diagnosis.

10.2 Dilated Cardiomyopathy-Basic Facts

10.2.1 Definition

Current definitions of Dilated cardiomyopathy (DCM) are based on morpho-functional phenotypic criteria. DCM is a chronic primary heart muscle disease defined by "the presence of unexplained dilatation and systolic impairment of the left or both ventricles" according to the European Society of Cardiology, (ESC) [1] and "by ventricular chamber enlargement and systolic dysfunction with normal LV wall thickness" according to the American Heart Association (AHA) [2]. The last statement of the AHA defines DCM as a spectrum of heterogeneous myocardial disorders that are characterized by ventricular dilation and depressed myocardial performance in the absence of hypertension, valvular, congenital, or ischemic heart disease [3].

DCM represents the *end-phenotype* of heart muscle damage induced by different causes. *Intermediate or early phenotypes* are characterized by borderline but persistent LV (Left Ventricular) dilation and/or mild LV dysfunction and may present with arrhythmias and/or conduction disease; a recent position statement of the ESC Working Group on Myocardial and Pericardial Diseases introduced the Non Dilated Hypokinetic Cardiomyopathy (NDHC) to better describe affected family members recognized by family screening in the early phases of the disease [4]. *Pre-clinical* diagnoses are feasible in genotyped familial DCM when a phenotypically healthy member is carrier of the mutation that is proven to cause the disease in the family. More than 60% of DCMs are familial diseases with identifiable genetic defects [5].

Acquired disorders manifesting with the DCM phenotype (DCM phenocopies) are sporadic and categorized as non-genetic DCM. This distinction separates genetic DCM from acquired, non-genetic, and potentially reversible phenotypes that are induced by protean causes (infectious, autoimmune/immune-mediated, toxic) and is clinically useful because treatments for acquired DCM may differ from those for familial DCM. Therefore DCM can be grouped mechanistically as genetic and non-genetic. This chapter illustrates cases with familial and apparently sporadic DCM in which genetic testing provided either the precise specific diagnosis (pathologic mutation) or a genetic make-up of uncertain significance. Each example gives clues and considerations that can be easily translated in the clinical practice.

10.2.2 Epidemiology

Epidemiology data are old and have been achieved on the basis of the phenotypes. They date back the pre-genetic era: incidence is estimated in 6.0 per 100000 person-years and prevalence is 36.5 in 100000 (about 1:2500) [6]. Early diagnoses, systematic family screening, genetic testing, and advanced diagnostics for non-genetic DCM are expected to provide new epidemiology estimates in the short term [7–14]. In a near future genetic epidemiology will integrate with the phenotype-based epidemiology: when the DCM phenotype will be integrated with the aetiology, as feasible by the novel MOGE(S) nosology [15], the prevalence data of each subtype of DCM will fall under the threshold prevalence of rare diseases (<1:2000): this is anticipated by the genetic heterogeneity, with more than 100 disease and candidate genes identified to date in familial DCM [16]. Cardio-laminopathies are considered a paradigmatic and replicated example [17].

10.2.3 Diagnostic Work-Up

The following work-up applies to all cases of DCM and is structured on the basis of indications of recent guidelines and recommendations of Scientific Societies [1, 18, 19].

DCM clinically manifests with systolic heart failure (HF). Presenting symptoms are often non-specific and includes palpitations, fatigue, breathlessness, and signs of congestion/fluid retention [1]. The diagnosis is based on left ventricular systolic dysfunction (impaired LV ejection fraction measured using 2D echocardiography) and LV dilatation (as defined by Z score > 2 standard deviations) for LV end-diastolic volumes or diameters. Coronary arteries are usually angiographically patent [1, 2]: flow-limiting luminal stenosis in one or more epicardial coronary arteries can exists concurrently and be demonstrated in genetic DCM [20]. Cardiac magnetic resonance (CMR) helps to confirm the diagnosis, adds information on the type and extent of myocardial fibrosis when present [21] and contributes to the evaluation of the trabecular anatomy. Three-dimensional echocardiography can add information on valve anatomy and LV remodelling [22]. Contrast echocardiography increases accuracy to

2D and 3D volume assessment and highlights trabecular anatomy; it may help when the image quality is suboptimal [23]. Myocardial deformation imaging techniques [24] or myocardial tagging by CMR can diagnose "early" DCM [25].

10.2.4 Familial Dilated Cardiomyopathy

The DCM is "familial" (*FDCM*) when two or more members of the same family are affected [1, 18]. The phenotype characterization of the proband requires the exploration of the cardiovascular system as well as the musculoskeletal, ocular, cutaneous, auditory and nervous system [19] because different extra-cardiac traits may occur and characterize DCM caused by defects of the different genes. Each DCM should be considered a potential genetic disease: genetic counselling with pedigree construction and collection of the clinical history of relatives provide a first evaluation of the family context [18]. The key action is clinical family screening, irrespective of genetic testing. The screening recapitulates the work-up in probands: physical examination, electrocardiography (ECG), transthoracic echocardiography (TTE), and biochemical testing, followed by regular monitoring of relatives. After completion of the family screening, the genetic or sporadic origin of the disease is clinically established at baseline and provides information on the pattern of inheritance, which is, by itself, one of the contributors for a pre-genetic test hypothesis. Data collected from family screening are fundamental for geno-phenotype segregation studies after completion of genetic testing in the family [5].

Members of families with genetic DCM can be affected, with or without symptoms, or manifest early signs of LV remodelling and/or borderline dysfunction [1, 4] or demonstrate (1) electrocardiographic abnormalities [such as conduction disease; short PR interval/Wolff-Parkinson-White; prolonged QT interval; T wave abnormalities; early repolarization; abnormal high or low voltages of the QRS]; (2) increased biochemical markers such as serum creatine phosphokinase (sCPK) or lactic acid; (3) extra-cardiac traits such as skeletal muscle disease, auditory defects, ocular abnormalities, gastrointestinal disturbances, renal disease, cutaneous lesions, cognitive impairment, abnormal faces or cryptogenic stroke, can be associated with DCM caused by different disease genes [19]. These traits may occur in probands as well as in relatives. In sporadic DCM relatives are asymptomatic and show normal instrumental features [1, 18, 19].

Monitoring of family members and long-term follow-up provide useful data for the diagnosis of familial disease when one or more family members are unaffected at the first family screening but develop the disease later on in the course of their life. Clinical monitoring further provides reliable data on the natural history of the disease [9, 12]. Therefore clinical family screening and re-screening (or monitoring) are integral and indispensable for the diagnosis of FDCM [18, 19].

Genetic heterogeneity characterizes DCM: more than 100 genes are now included in the list of disease and candidate genes [16]. Disease genes code for different proteins active in structural and functional pathways of the cardiac myocytes and include sarcomeric, nuclear envelope, Z-disk, intermediate filaments, mitochondrial proteins, sarcolemmal proteins, ion channels and proteins of the Golgi apparatus and sarcoplasmic reticulum [4, 26]. The mechanisms through which mutations in different genes cause similar functional and structural cardiac end-phenotype depends on the gene and the role of its product in the myocyte, type of mutation and its effects on the protein expression, epistatic and epigenetic factors. Haploinsufficiency is a common mechanism in dilated cardiolaminopathies and dilated cardiodystrophinopathies [27–30]. Same genes and mutations may be associated with different cardiomyopathy phenotypes in members of same families: hypertrophic cardiomyopathy (HCM), restrictive cardiomyopathy (RCM) and arrhythmogenic right ventricular cardiomyopathy (ARVC). The paradigmatic example is DCM caused by mutations in sarcomeric genes such as *MYH7* [31].

Genetic testing is currently performed using massive parallel sequencing of multigene panels (Next Generation Sequencing, NGS) for both nuclear [32] and MtDNA [33] genes. NGS technologies are faster and cheaper than Sanger-based technologies. Of the large number of known disease and candidate genes for DCM, some are confirmed as disease genes (i.e. *LMNA*, *DYS*, *EMD*, *PLN*, and sarcomere genes) and are now systematically tested in probands/index patients. Other less common genes are still provisional and described in unique or few families. Interpretation of genetic testing is the challenge of the next decade: when testing hundreds of genes including giant genes such as *Titin* (*TTN*), complex genes such as *Duchenne Muscle Dystrophy* (*DMD*) and *Obscurin*, the probability of finding more than one mutation/individual increases [5, 34]. Further developments are needed to generate efficient tools for exploring the functional effects and pathologic role of novel mutations, especially when considering that most heritable DCM are Mendelian diseases transmitted through an autosomal dominant mode, a rule that does not change in families in which more than one mutation is identified. This implies that one major (or leading) mutation, or two mutations co-inherited from the same parent, plays a causative role, with other variants potentially acting as phenotype modifiers. Misinterpretation of the role of the mutation in the pathogenesis of the DCM may have severe implications for the patient and family, especially when procreative plans include prenatal diagnosis.

At present, genetic defects are identified in about 60% of FDCM: additional disease genes will be added to this list in the near future.

The interpretation of the results of NGS-based genetic tests requires bioinformatics pipelines: from raw data that include thousands of genetic variants/patient, the analysis ends with one or a few probable or possible disease mutation(s). The genetic variants can be known and proven to be the cause of the disease, or novel, thus requiring demonstration of their pathogenicity. This means that their effects should be confirmed by functional and pathologic studies in either endomyocardial biopsy (EMB) or by in vitro studies on fibroblasts or induced Pluripotent Stem Cells -derived(iPSC-derived) myocytes obtained form skin fibroblasts or circulating cells of patients who carry the mutation. Segregation studies in families (mutated family members are affected and non-mutated are non-affected) are uniquely important [35]. This latter proof of evidence may require follow-up studies because the segregation may not appear evident at baseline family screening. Table 10.1 summarizes the phases of the diagnostic genetic work-up in cardiomyopathies.

Table 10.1 Criteria and tools for the definition of pathogenic mutations

Steps	Criteria	Information/data	Examples and contributions of the different tools supporting interpretation of the genetic variants/ mutations identified in DCM
Mutation types, protein expression and predicting in silico tools	Non-synonymous genetic mutations/variants	Type of mutation • Missense (up to 80% of all genetic DCM, except DMD) • In-frame ins-del • Nonsense • Frameshift • Splice site • Large gene rearrangements	The prevalence of the different types of mutations differs: e.g. • most mutations in *LMNA* are missense; • most mutations in *MYH7* are missense; • most mutations in *MYBPC3* are frameshift, nonsense or splice-site; • most mutations in *DMD* are large rearrangements (in-frame or out-of-frame deletions);
	Synonymous genetic variants introducing cryptic splice sites	Some genetic variant may introduce cryptic splice sites; the abnormal splicing may affect the structure of the mutated protein	e.g. p.(Lys171Lys) and p.(Gly608Gly) *LMNA* mutations
	Protein expression in target tissue	The candidate protein (gene) is expressed in the myocardium	The gene is expressed (including isoforms: e.g. DMD, LDB3) in the cardiac myocytes
	Mutated residues in the evolutive scale	The affected residue is conserved in different species through evolution	The mutated aminoacid is a key residue for the function of the protein; its loss predicts a derangement of function
	In silico analysis for missense mutations	Tools that provide scores on the possible damaging role of the observed variant. Warning: the combination of these tools ends in a contributory but non-conclusive interpretation	These tools provide support but do not, by themselves, prove pathogenicity; genetic variants can be: probably damaging, possibly damaging, tolerated/benign. A colour code can be assigned
	In silico analysis for splice site mutations	Tools that provide scores on the possible activation of a cryptic splice site	The tools contribute to the interpretation. The final demonstration is obtained with RNA studies showing either insertion or deletions of protein fragments

Table 10.1 (continued)

Steps	Criteria	Information/data	Examples and contributions of the different tools supporting interpretation of the genetic variants/ mutations identified in DCM
Genetic epidemiology	**Control series** • Public DB including large series of "unaffected" anonymized subjects • Local population control series add information on ethnic/ race variability: geographic origin should be considered **Case series** Published series reporting the prevalence of defects in given disease genes. Warning: prevalence data in clinical series that investigated a unique gene may not inform about the pathogenicity of the mutations	The absence of given genetic mutations/variants in a large number of healthy controls, or their presence at a very low minor allele frequency (MAF) demonstrates that: • the mutation/variant is not a common polymorphism • the mutation/variant is a possible candidate • in any case, the mutation/ variant should be considered with caution before either excluding or confirming its potential role in the pathogenesis of the disease	Large databases are available and include data from anonimyzed populations; for cardiomyopathies their reliability is limited by: • The high prevalence of cardiomyopathies such as HCM and therefore of their disease-causing mutations (control series enrolled without imaging do not exclude the erroneous enrolment of HCM asymptomatic cases) • The lack of definition of "control" for *genetic control series* (inclusion does not rely on ECG and echocardiographic exclusion of the disease) • The age-dependence of the cardiomyopathy phenotype (the age of subjects included in CTRL series may limit the values of reported MAF
Family studies	Recurrence of the same variants/mutations in more families sharing similar phenotypes	The demonstration that the same mutation recurs in more unrelated families in which it is associated with the same phenotype, reinforces the pathogenic role	Typical examples are recurrent mutations such as p.(Arg190Trp) or p.(Glu161Lys) in *LMNA* gene or p.(Arg403Trp) in *MYH7* gene, among others
	Segregation studies demonstrating that: • affected family members carry the mutation • healthy family members do not carry the mutation	The segregation of the phenotype with the genotype in the family provides a robust contribution to the interpretation of the role of the mutation in the phenotype. Long-term follow-up may modify the scenario	This assessment can be limited by the small size of the family; or by the non-availability of living relatives to expand the clinical and genetic investigation
	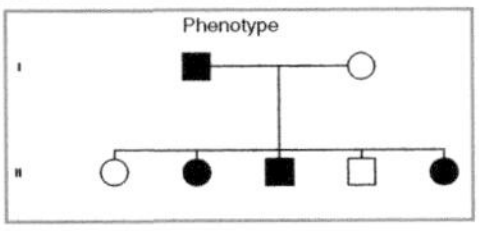 Phenotype	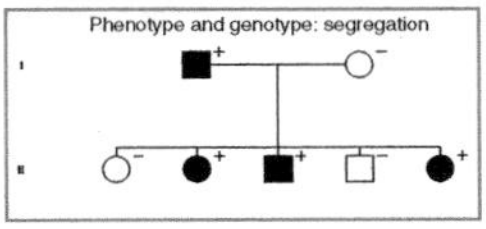 Phenotype and genotype: segregation	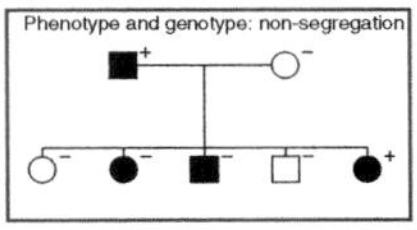 Phenotype and genotype: non-segregation

(continued)

Table 10.1 (continued)

Steps	Criteria	Information/data	Examples and contributions of the different tools supporting interpretation of the genetic variants/ mutations identified in DCM
Pathology	Pathologic studies • Endomyocardial Biopsy • Hearts excised at transplantation • Apex samples from patients implanted with VAD systems • Muscle biopsies	Conventional histopathology provides diagnostic information on myocarditis, intramyocyte storage diseases and infiltration diseases. Immynohistochemistry and protein analysis (from Western blot of a single protein to extensive proteomic and metabolomic studies) may inform on the abnormal, defective expression of the mutated protein in affected myocardium	This type of studies is useful to assess: haploinsufficiency (e.g. *LMNA, DMD*) when the genetic defects are associated with variation in the expression of the mutated protein at the myocardial level; common intermediate or end-stage mechanisms of myocyte damage (e.g. autophagy)
	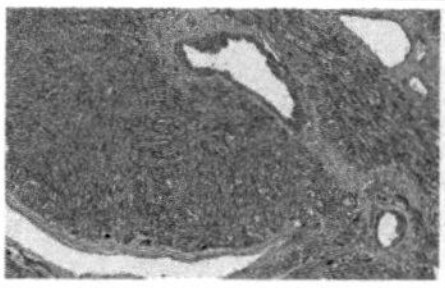	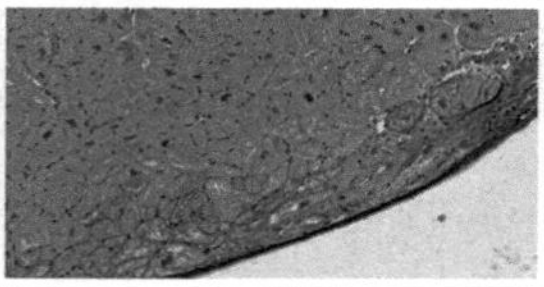	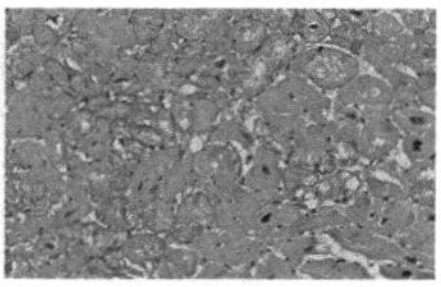
Experi-mental studies	iPSC- derived myocytes (iPSC-CM)	Investigate in vitro the morphofunctional cellular effects of mutations: *Pharmacologic tests* • responsiveness of affected cells to drugs. *Cellular electrophysiology* • mecha nisms of electrical instability and arrhythmogenic potential	The methods are complex and time-consuming but consolidated and feasible. The information achievable with iPSC-CM can contribute to the final interpretation of the pathogenicity and provide in vitro models for functional studies.
	Early iPSC-CM from skin fibroblasts of a DCM patient: • note the position, size and morphology of the central group of cells during contraction and relaxation	Relaxation 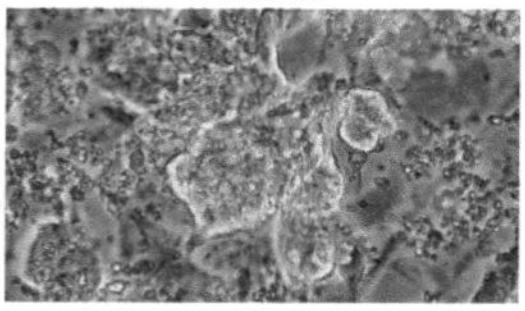	Contraction 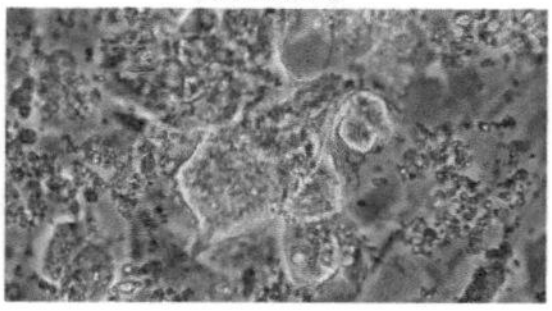
	Animal models	Mouse models offer the possibility of reproducing phenotypes associated with mutations that cause the DCM	Major limitations of the systemic implementation of mouse models: time, facilities and costs. Non-representative of the complex individual genetics

10.3 Clinical Cases: Genetic DCM

The clinical cases selected for this chapter are paradigmatic examples of DCM with identical (same disease gene and mutation), similar (different mutations in the same gene) or different (different disease gene) causes. Each case/family is presented in a figure that includes all key information on phenotype and cause, and is shortly commented in the text that highlights the considerations that can be useful for the clinical evaluation of patients and families.

The ideal diagnostic screening starts with the clinical diagnosis in probands and ends with the identification of the cause of the disease (either genetic or non-genetic) and family screening. Although all DCM phenotypes look alike (LV dilation and dysfunction), each patient/family may demonstrate peculiar clinical profiles that can be sub-grouped on the basis of recurrent traits. The ideal diagnostic and nosology scenario should contribute to distinguish DCM per phenotype and cause. In this chapter, the clinical cases are presented per both phenotype and cause.

10.3.1 Nuclear Envelopathies

Diseases affecting integrity of the nuclear envelope (NE) can manifest with DCM phenotype. The NE is a complex membrane system constituted of nuclear pores, inner (INM) and outer (ONM) nuclear membranes and nuclear lamina. NE contains a large number of different proteins that are involved in chromatin organization and gene regulation [36]. To date, DCM has been associated with mutations in proteins of the

- inner nuclear membrane [Thymopoietin or Lamina-associated polypeptide 2 (LAP2) and Lamina-associated polypeptide 1 (LAP1)].
- outer nuclear membrane (Nesprin 1alpha that binds lamin A/C and is also associated with autosomal dominant Emery-Dreifuss Muscular Dystrophy (EDMD) type 4 and Nesprin 2 that is associated with the autosomal dominant EDMD type 5)].
- nuclear lamina (Lamin A and Lamin C).

The paradigmatic examples of DCM caused by defects in nuclear lamina are *dilated* cardiolaminopathies (6–7% of all DCM in consecutive series) [17, 37] and dilated cardioemerinopathies (<1% in consecutive series): conduction system disease is the phenotypic hallmark of these diseases and occurs in up to 80% of patients with Lamin A/C defects (DCM-CD) and in all patients with EDMD-related gene defects [5]. Data on LAP- and Nesprin-associated DCM are limited but do not demonstrate recurrent conduction disease.

10.3.1.1 Dilated Cardiolaminopathies Without Myopathy

In dilated cardiolaminopathies, the development of conduction system disease usually precedes the appearance of the DCM [17] (Fig. 10.1); the natural history is characterized by progressive prolongation of the PR interval, LV dilation and

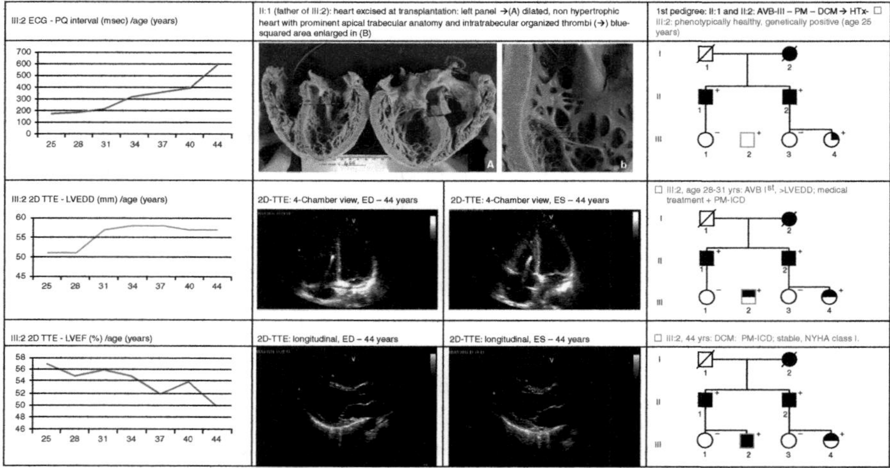

AVB = Atrio-ventricular block; PM = Pace Maker; HTx = Heart transplantation; TTE = Transthoracic Echocardiogram; LVEDD = Left Ventricu;ar End Diastolic Diameter; ICD = Implantable Cardioverter Defibrillator; LV EF = left Ventricular Ejection Fraction; ED = End Diastole; ES = End Systole.

Fig. 10.1 Dilated cardiolaminopathy: *LMNA* (p.Glu111X)

dysfunction. Cardiolaminopathies display high arrhythmogenic potential, both atrial and ventricular arrhythmias; life-threatening ventricular arrhythmias may manifest in mildly dilated and dysfunctioning hearts and can be the first clinical manifestation of the disease [38]. Recent guidelines on the primary prevention of sudden cardiac death (SCD) recommend (Class IIa, Level B) implantable cardioverter defibrillator (ICD) in patients with DCM, a confirmed disease-causing *LMNA* mutation and clinical risk factors [39]: non sustained ventricular tachycardia (NSVT) during ambulatory electrocardiographic monitoring, left ventricular ejection fraction (LVEF) < 45% on initial evaluation, male gender and non-missense mutations (insertion, deletion, truncation or mutations affecting splicing) [39]. These recommendations constitute a step forward gene/disease-specific treatment and therefore precision and personalized medicine in cardiology. *LMNA* gene is now routinely tested in patients with DCM.

More than 500 mutations have been identified to date in *LMNA* gene: missense mutations represent about 80% of all mutations while truncation-predicting mutations (*stop*, *frameshift*, *splice site*) are less common (about 20%) (http://www.umd.be/LMNA/). The majority of mutations are private; however same mutations (http://www.umd.be/LMNA/) have been found in numerous families in which affected members shared similar phenotype (Table 10.2).

10.3.1.2 The Malignant p.Arg190Trp Mutation in *LMNA*

Figure 10.2 summarizes the clinical evolution of the disease in the proband and the early phases of the disease in her son. The p.(Arg190Trp) mutation identified in this family is one of the most common defects affecting Lamin AC, with 47 reports for p.(Arg190Trp) substitution and 4 reports for p.(Arg190Gln) at http://www.umd.be/LMNA/ (Table 10.2). This mutation is confirmed as disease-causing mutation.

Table 10.2 Selected examples of the phenotypes and geographic origin of recurrent mutations (from http://www.umd.be/LMNA/): Key messages

Mutation	Described in	Phenotype
p.(Ser143Pro)	Finland	DCM-CD
p.(Ser143Phe)	Germany	Progeroid syndrome with myopathy and possible AF
p.(Glu161Lys)	France, Italy, S.Korea, USA	DCM-CD
p.(Arg190Trp)	Italy, Germany, Ireland, Spain, Filand, UK, Japan, USA, S.Korea	DCM-CD; (1 case, UK ARVC)
p.(Arg190Gln)	USA	DCM-CD
p.(Glu203Lys)	USA	DCM-CD
p.(Glu203Gly)	Non-specified	DCM-CD
p.(Arg225X)	Italy, Belgium, USA, Japan, China	DCM-CD
p.(Arg225Gln)	Spain	EMDM
p.(Arg249Gln)	France, Germany, Italy, Spain, Russia, Japan, USA, S.Korea	EMDM,LGMD1B; (1 L-DCM)
p.(Arg249Gln)	USA, Argentina, Japan, others non specified	L-CMD, EMDM, Striated muscle laminopathy
p.(Arg298Cys)	Algeria, Marocco	EMDM; AR-CMT2; less common: isolated cardiac disease.
p.(Arg377His)	Netherland, France, Italy, Belgium, Russia, USA, Carrabean	LGMD1B; EMDM; quadricipital myopathy + DCM-CD
p.(Arg377Cys)	France, Japan	LGMD1B; EMDM; striated muscle laminopathy
p.(Arg377Leu)	Italy, Belgium, S.Korea	LGMD1B; EMDM; 1 DCM-CD
p.(Arg453Trp)	UK, Spain, Italy, France, Belgium, Poland, Hungary, Japan, USA	EMDM; LGMD1B; EMDM + FPLD (1 case)
p.(Arg453Trp)	Spain	L-DCM (1 case)
p.(Arg482Trp)	Spain, France, Germany, UK, Portugal, USA, Brazil, India	FPLD; FPLD + LGMD1B;
p.(Arg482Gln)	Germany, Poland, USA	FPLD
p.(Arg482Leu)	Germany; others, non specified	FPLD
p.(Gly608Gly)	Italy, Spain, France, Netheralnd, Turkey, Morocco, Egypt, USA, Canada, S.Korea	Progeria; (1 restrictive dermopathy)
p.(Gly608Ser)	Canada; 1 unspecified	Progeria

(continued)

Table 10.2 (continued)

Mutation	Described in	Phenotype
p.(Arg644Cys)	Italy, Denmark, UK, Netherland; USA, India	DCM-CD; EMDM; LGMD1B; striated muscle myopathy; progeroid syndrome; FPLD; isolated AF; HCM + myopathy; HCM; Aortic valve insufficiency and Aneurysm; HCM; ARVC.
p.(Arg644His)	UK	L-CMD (1 case)

There are mutations such as p.(Arg190Trp) that do not associate with muscle involvement
Mutations such as p.(Glu203Lys) only cause DCM-CD
Mutation as p.(Arg482Gln) only cause FPLD
Mutations such as p.(Gly608Gly) only cause progeria
Mutations such as p.(Arg644Cys) are associated with protean conditions; their pathogenic role should be considered with caution. A second mutation (non-searched for) could be the primary genetic defects causing the phenotype
AF atrial fibrillation, *HCM* hypertrophic cardiomyopathy, *DCM* dilated cardiomyopathy, *DCM-CD* dilated cardiomyopathy with conduction disease, *LGMD* limb girdle muscular dystrophy, *EMDM* Emery Dreiffus muscular dystrophy, *FPLD* familial progeriod lipodystrophy, *L-CMD* Lamin congenital muscular dystrophy

This family provides data for practical comments:

1. The affected members of the first three generations of the family do not provide informations about the natural history of the disease: they were all diagnosed with DCM in the clinically overt phase of the disease (DCM with angiographically normal coronary arteries and conduction disease) and treated according to protocols dating back 20–30 years.
2. The presence of *LMNA* p.(Arg190Trp) mutation in both IV:2 and IV:3 indicates that III:2 and III:3 were obligate carriers of the genetic defect, while no information can be inferred for III:4, who was affected but offspring IV:4 and IV:5 tested negative. Therefore family member III:4 does not fulfil the criteria to be defined obligate carrier.
3. The natural history of the disease in the family can be written for IV:2 and will further enrich of the future follow-up data from V:2, while family member IV:3 was diagnosed when the DCM was clinically manifest.
4. Due to the frequent conduction disease, beta-blockers (BB) can be safely used only in patients who underwent pacemaker (PM) implantation. The choice of BB can be tailored according to the prevalent clinical need: arrhythmias or heart failure (e.g. sotalol vs. metoprolol or carvedilol or bisoprolol).
5. The ESC recommendation for primary prevention do not include malignant missense mutation such as the p.(Arg190Trp) and leave cardiologists to their own expertise and decisions [39]. Therefore, although these guidelines are very recent, they do not address clinical needs in real life.

10.3.1.3 Dilated Cardiolaminopathy: Detection of Proven Pathologic Mutations in Singleton

The clinical histories of the four probands and families shown in Fig. 10.3a–d are similar, all starting from atrioventricular block (AVB) that required PM implantation 7–12 years before the development of DCM phenotype. In the large family

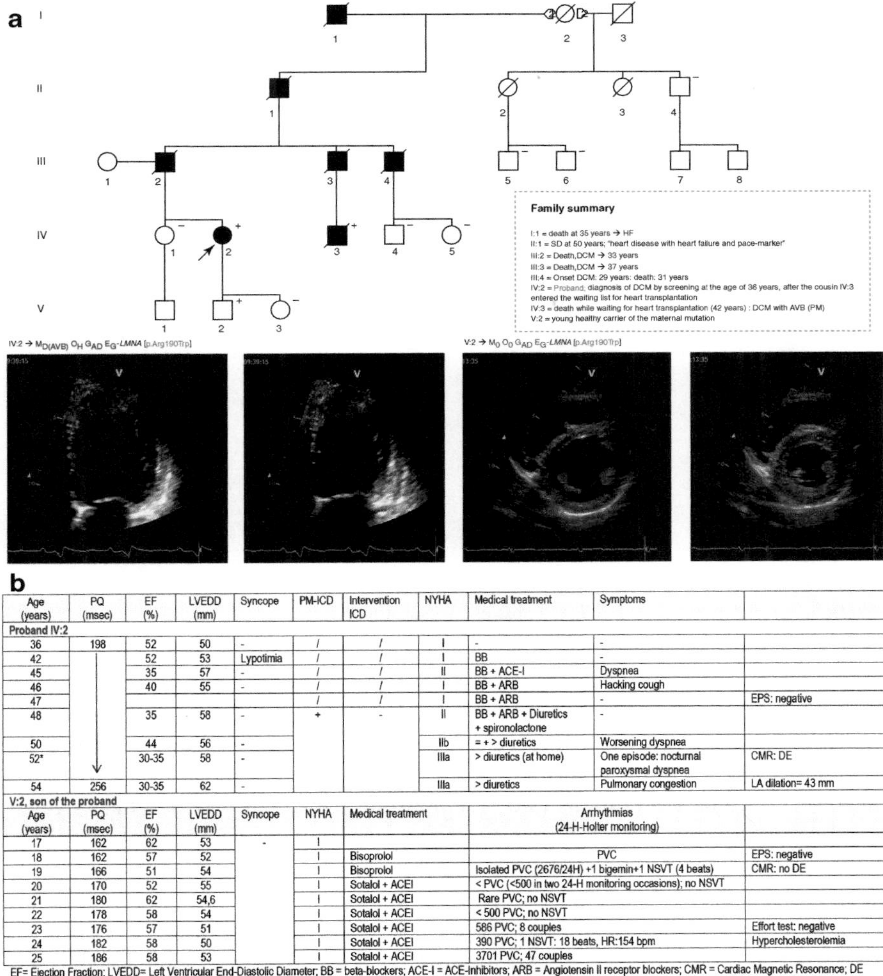
a
I
II
III
IV
V
Family summary
I:1 = death at 35 years → HF
II:1 = SD at 50 years; "heart disease with heart failure and pace-marker"
III:2 = Death,DCM → 33 years
III:3 = Death,DCM → 37 years
III:4 = Onset DCM: 29 years: death: 31 years
IV:2 = Proband; diagnosis of DCM by screening at the age of 36 years, after the cousin IV:3 entered the waiting list for heart transplantation
IV:3 = death while waiting for heart transplantation (42 years) : DCM with AVB (PM)
V:2 = young healthy carrier of the maternal mutation
IV:2 → $M_{D(AVB)}$ O_H G_{AD} E_G-*LMNA* [p.Arg190Trp]
V:2 → M_0 O_0 G_{AD} E_G-*LMNA* [p.Arg190Trp]
V
b

Age (years)	PQ (msec)	EF (%)	LVEDD (mm)	Syncope	PM-ICD	Intervention ICD	NYHA	Medical treatment	Symptoms	
Proband IV:2										
36	198	52	50	-	/	/	I	-	-	
42	↓	52	53	Lypotimia	/	/	I	BB	-	
45		35	57	-	/	/	II	BB + ACE-I	Dyspnea	
46		40	55	-	/	/	I	BB + ARB	Hacking cough	
47					/	/	I	BB + ARB	-	EPS: negative
48		35	58	-	+	-	II	BB + ARB + Diuretics + spironolactone	-	
50		44	56	-			IIb	= + > diuretics	Worsening dyspnea	
52*		30-35	58	-			IIIa	> diuretics (at home)	One episode: nocturnal paroxysmal dyspnea	CMR: DE
54	256	30-35	62	-			IIIa	> diuretics	Pulmonary congestion	LA dilation= 43 mm

Age (years)	PQ (msec)	EF (%)	LVEDD (mm)	Syncope	NYHA	Medical treatment	Arrhythmias (24-H-Holter monitoring)	
V:2, son of the proband								
17	162	62	53	-	I			
18	162	57	52		I	Bisoprolol	PVC	EPS: negative
19	166	51	54		I	Bisoprolol	Isolated PVC (2676/24H) +1 bigemin+1 NSVT (4 beats)	CMR: no DE
20	170	52	55		I	Sotalol + ACEI	< PVC (<500 in two 24-H monitoring occasions); no NSVT	
21	180	62	54,6		I	Sotalol + ACEI	Rare PVC; no NSVT	
22	178	58	54		I	Sotalol + ACEI	< 500 PVC; no NSVT	
23	176	57	51		I	Sotalol + ACEI	586 PVC; 8 couples	Effort test: negative
24	182	58	50		I	Sotalol + ACEI	390 PVC; 1 NSVT: 18 beats, HR:154 bpm	Hypercholesterolemia
25	186	58	53		I	Sotalol + ACEI	3701 PVC; 47 couples	

EF= Ejection Fraction; LVEDD= Left Ventricular End-Diastolic Diameter; BB = beta-blockers; ACE-I = ACE-Inhibitors; ARB = Angiotensin II receptor blockers; CMR = Cardiac Magnetic Resonance; DE = Delayed Enhancement; LA = Left Atrium; EPS = Electrophysiology Study; PVC = Premature Ventricular Contraction; NSVT = Non-Sustained Ventricular Tachycardia.

* indication to heart transplantation: refused by the patient.

Fig. 10.2 Pedigree. Two-dimensional TTE view proband and son carriers of the common p.(Arg190Trp), family summary (**a**) and clinical data (**b**)

shown in Fig. 10.3a, the affected members shared slowly progressing conduction disease and DCM: none of the affected members of the Ist and IInd generations could undergo genetic testing and only three members of the IIIrd generation (A-III:7, A-III:26 and A-III:27) were affected and alive when genetic test for *LMNA* was introduced. The p.(Glu161Lys) mutation in the Lamin AC segregated with the phenotype after screening of affected members of the IV generation: the youngest mutated members of the IVth generation (A-IV:6 and A-IV:9, both under 20 years of age) are still unaffected and undergo regular clinical monitoring. The mutation identified in this family has been reported (http://www.umd.be/LMNA/) as associated with DCM with AVB, without muscle involvement.

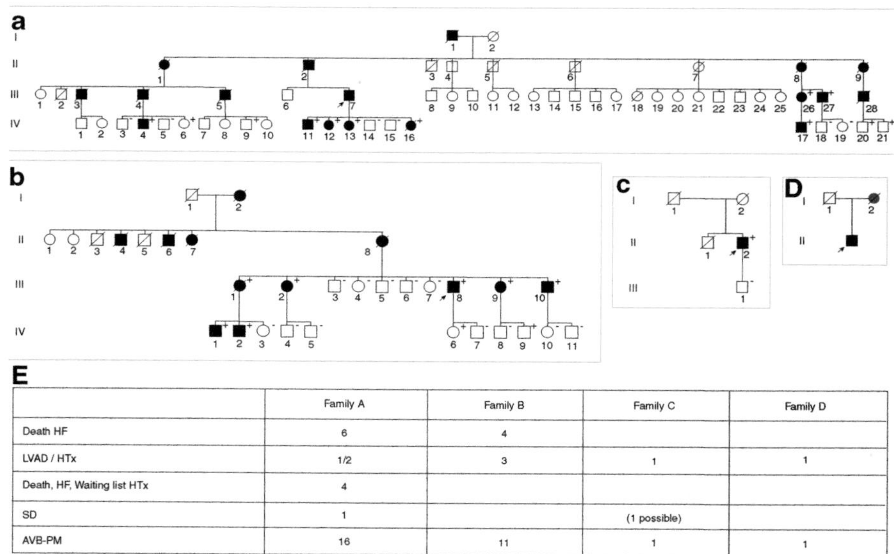

	Family A	Family B	Family C	Family D
Death HF	6	4		
LVAD / HTx	1/2	3	1	1
Death, HF, Waiting list HTx	4			
SD	1		(1 possible)	
AVB-PM	16	11	1	1

Fig. 10.3 Dilated cardiolaminopathy: *LMNA* (p.Glu161Lys). (**a–d**) four pedirees with Lamin mutation. (**e**) summary of main DCM features in 4 families

The clinical history of the family shown in Fig. 10.3b is similar to that of family A. The 50-year-old male proband (B-III:8) first complained fatigue and nocturnal paroxysms of dyspnea. The ECG showed AVB and a few premature ventricular complex (PVC) (<100 in multiple 24-H Holter monitoring occasions). The first cardiologic evaluation demonstrated LV dilation and LVEF = 20% (NYHA functional class IIb). Epicardial coronary arteries were patent. The patient was diagnosed with DCM and entered the diagnostic work-up for stratification of the arrhythmogenic risk. Electrophysiological study (EPS) was negative for inducible arrhythmias. On the basis of the severe LV dysfunction, the patient received an ICD-PM according to guidelines available in 2007. His medical treatment was optimized and adjusted during the course of 9 years, but ended in heart transplantation. The patient was addressed to genetic evaluation. In his family, the mother had died for heart failure at the age of 67 years, after a 15-year history of HF, with PM implantation (complete AVB) at the age of 52 years. Three maternal siblings were affected (DCM with PM). One affected sister (B-III:1) and two of her sons (B-IV:1 and B-IV:2) were equally affected. Genetic testing in the proband identified the p.(Glu161Lys) mutation that was also found in B-III:2,B-III:9 and B-III:10. Siblings B-III:3–7 tested negative. The genetic test was further extended to the two young offspring of B-III:2 (both negative), B-III:8 (one positive and one negative), B-III:9 (one negative and one positive) and B-III:10 (both negative). The young mutation carriers (B-IV:6 and B-IV:9) are undergoing regular clinical monitoring.

The probands of families C (Fig. 10.3c) and D (Fig. 10.3d) presented with apparently sporadic DCM associated with AVB; their clinical history was similar: both underwent PM implantation, upgrading to ICD and successful heart transplantation 13 and 9 years later, respectively. Although family screening and segregation studies were not feasible, the mutation was the same identified in families A and B. Therefore, the identification of the pathogenic mutation p.(Glu161Lys) labels these apparently sporadic DCM as proven genetic disease. Key messages that can be derived from the above four examples are:

1. Segregation studies in large families are essential contributors to the final interpretation of the role of the mutation.
2. The likely obligate carrier status of A-I:1 and B-I:2 can be inferred but not proven because the respective spouse and husband were not tested. Non-tested, but obligate carriers of mutations (e.g. A-III:4) inform on the obligate carrier status of their affected parents (A-II:1); this information is equally reliable for A-II:9 whose son had not genetic testing but both nephews (A-IV:20 and A-IV: 21) are carriers.
3. Inheritance pattern in family B could be either autosomal dominant or matrilineal; the former is clarified by carriers B-IV:6.
4. The genetic disease in probands C-II:2 and D-II:1 is proven by the pathologic mutation and by the typical gene-associated phenotype (CD-DCM).
5. The high number of events in the four families may reflect past late diagnoses and treatment protocols in 1st and 2nd generation of families A and B and can contribute to stratify prognosis in youngest members of the 3rd and 4th generation.

10.3.1.4 Dilated Cardiolaminopathies with Skeletal Muscle Involvement

Cardiolaminopathies can be associated with variable involvement of the skeletal muscle. Affected members of the family shown in Fig. 10.4 demonstrate Emery-Dreifuss muscle dystrophy, DCM and conduction disease. The early clinical manifestation of the disease was characterised by increased levels of sCPK without functional muscle impairment in the proband (III:3) when her older sister was already manifesting clinical signs of muscle dystrophy and atrial arrhythmias. In the two sisters (III:1 and III:3) the clinical phenotype differed, with muscle dystrophy prevailing in III:1 and DCM in III:3. The major difference in the clinical history of the two sisters is that the latter had two pregnancies, both successful but with caesarean section. Their mother was affected by muscle dystrophy: she died suddenly at 42 years. The two young daughters of III:3 are healthy and their levels of sCPK are normal; they are undergoing regular clinical monitoring. The origin of the mutation cannot be established: maternal parents (I:1 and I:2) had died at 70 and 80 years respectively, but there are no available clinical reports documenting their clinical status. The mutation identified in the family is an in-frame insertion of three bases corresponding to the in-frame addition of a unique residue (Leucine).

This family gives the opportunity for highlighting:

1. phenotype heterogeneity in family members who are carriers of the same mutation
2. atrial arrhythmias are a relevant contributor to the cardiac phenotype

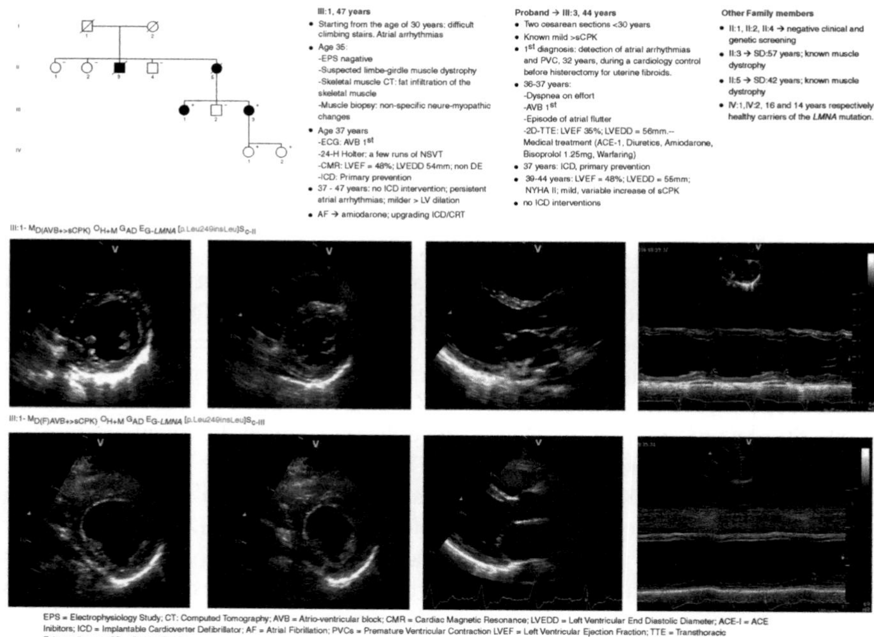

Fig. 10.4 Dilated cardiolaminopathy and myopathy

3. biomarkers such as > sCPK can, by themselves, contribute to the clinical hypothesis
4. open question: could pregnancies in III:3 have influenced the cardiac phenotype?
5. In real life, indications to ICD implantation do not necessarily adhere to guidelines (e.g. III:1); the final decision on how to manage patients with potentially malignant genotypes is part of the responsibilities of cardiologists.

10.3.1.5 Dilated Cardioemerinopathies

Emerin defects typically cause Emery-Dreifuss Muscular Dystrophy (EDMD). The cardiac involvement is characterised by conduction disease either isolated or associated with DCM phenotype [40]. Arrhythmias are common [41]. The inheritance is X-linked recessive and muscle dystrophy is the marker of disease in affected males. Cardiac involvement is common and manifests with palpitations, presyncope and syncope, poor exercise tolerance, and heart failure [40, 41]. The clinical differential diagnosis with autosomal dominant laminopathies is the inheritance pattern and the type of muscle disease. The Fig. 10.5 shows the examples of two families in which probands demonstrated similar phenotypes: early conduction disease, LV dilation and dysfunction and mild muscle dystrophy (A-II:1) vs. increased sCPK without functional impairment (B-II:2). The arrhythmogenic risk in the two conditions can eventually differ: data on laminopathies are robust while those on emerinopathies are still limited. Figure 10.5 illustrates the key differences of the two different conditions.

10.3.2 Dystrophin and Dystrophin Associated Glycoprotein Complex

Dystrophin is a rod-like protein that is located at the inner surface of muscle fibers. Defects in Dystrophin cause Duchenne Muscular Dystrophy (DMD, *MIM#310200*), Becker Muscular Dystrophy (BMD, *MIM#300376*) and X-Linked Dilated Cardiomyopathy [30, 42–44]. Dystrophin is associated with a large oligomeric complex of sarcolemmal proteins and glycoproteins, the dystrophin-glycoprotein complex (DGC), whose protein components can be grouped in the dystroglycan and the sarcoglycan complexes. The DGC couple the sarcolemmal cytoskeleton with the extracellular matrix; loss of this structural link renders the sarcolemma

Diagnostic steps	**Proband A (Dilated Cardio-Emerinopathy) with PM**	***Concepts and deductions***	**Proband B (Dilated Cardio-Laminopathy) with PM**
Step 1: diagnosis in probands	45 years; Proband: DCM (mild) + CD LVEF = 45% LVEDD= 54mm PVCs = 164/24h sCPK = 246, 412, 219 mU; muscle impairment and contractures Comorbidity: hypercholesterolemia	*Clinical concepts and orientation:* *both probands look phenotypically similar*	37 years; Proband: DCM (mild) + CD LVEF = 42% LVEDD = 56mm EVB = 348/24h sCPK = 291 mU max; Comorbidity: thyroid dysfunction
Step 2: **add** gender	Male	*Helping or confounding?*	Male
Step 3: add counselling and family pedigree: **add** possible inheritance	Both parents: unaffected Kids are healthy	*Family history: de novo or XLR, or sporadic DCM in proband A and AD DCM in proband B*	Affected father, healthy mother. One affected sister
Step 4: clinical family screening: **add proven clinical information on relatives**	Mother is non-affected; 61 years. One younger brother is healthy. Two sons and one daughter (10, 8, 5 years respectively) are unaffected.	*Different inheritance is confirmed. Genetic testing planned on the phenotype and inheritance*	The father (→ proband) is affected; one sister (prior athlete, volley) is affected. The son is non-affected (15 years) and one nephew is recognised as affected by DCM at clinical family screening
Pedigree: indicates the inheritance. The two pedigrees in this raw show two adult male probands (→)	I, II, III	*LEFT: apparently sporadic DCM with conduction disease* *RIGHT autsosomal dominant DCM with conduction disease*	I, II, III
Genetic testing highlights rules of X-linked recessive (pink column) and autosomal dominant (light blue column) inheritance	I, II, III	*In XLR diseases, males cannot transmit to males but obligatory transmit to females;* *in AD diseases males transmit to males.*	I, II, III
Step 5: genetic testing: nuclear envelopathies	**Genetic testing: Emerinopathy**	*Similar phenotype; different causes; different diseases*	**Genetic testing: Laminopathy**
Step 6: monitoring of the proband and family. Further 24-H Holter monitoring and biomarkers	Progression with imaging studies→CMR: small area of LGE in the anterior septum; 1 run, NSVT recorded in 24H Holter monitoring.		Progression with imaging studies→CMR: two small areas of LGE in the anterior septum and wall. No significant arrhythmias in 24H Holter monitoring.

DCM = Dilated Cardiomyopathy; PM=Pace-Maker; CD = Conduction Disease; LVEF = Left Ventricular Ejection Fraction; LVEDD = Left Ventricular End-Diastolic Diameter; PVCs = Premature Ventricular Contraction; EVB=Ectopic Ventricular Beats; sCPK = Serum Creatin Phosphokinase; XLR = X-Linked Recessive; AD = Autosomal Dominant; CMR = Cardiac Magnetic Resonance; LGE = Late Gadolinium Enhancement; NSVT = Non-Sustained Ventricular Tachycardia.

Fig. 10.5 The diagnostic steps and the clinical similarities and differences between dilated cardioemerinopathies and dilated cardiolaminopathies

susceptible to damage when exposed to mechanical stress. Defects in genes coding for DGC components cause autosomal recessive muscle dystrophies: DCM is rare.

10.3.2.1 Dilated Cardiodystrophinopathies

Most data on cardiodystrophinopathies have been generated in series of patients with DMD and BMD; single case reports and a few series described patients presenting with DCM phenotype at onset [43, 44]. The precise diagnosis can be missed when non-specifically investigated. Patients with dilated cardiodystrophynopathies can successfully undergo heart transplantation with long-term survival similar to other non-DYS-related DCM. DCM-DYS typically manifests in male patients who carry large DMD gene rearrangements, both in frame and out-of-frame deletions (>80%) [43]; in a minority of cases mutations are either nonsense or missense. DYS mutations are associated with loss of protein expression at the level of the cardiomyocyte sarcolemma (Fig. 10.6). XL-DCM-DYS carries a low arrhythmogenic risk even when patients show severely dilated and dysfunctioning hearts fulfilling criteria for ICD implantation for primary prevention of SCD according to current guidelines. No ICD shock was observed during a median follow-up of 14 months (interquartile range: 5–25 months) in 34 patients with DCM caused by defects of dystrophin [43]. DCM-DMD may show Left Ventricular Non Compaction (LVNC) that occurs in about 30% of cases and is now proposed as a prognostic marker [45].

The pedigree in Fig. 10.6 shows a typical clinical example of X-linked recessive inheritance: the mother (I:2) of the proband (II:2) is the healthy carrier of the mutation (*DYS-Del* [44–47]). The probability of passing the mutation to the offspring is 50% for each pregnancy. Vice versa each affected male passes the mutation to all daughters but not to sons: the sons of affected mutated males (they are obviously all negative) and the daughters (they are all carriers) do not need genetic testing. In case of parental consanguinity, the probability that both parents carry the same DYS mutation should be considered for testing. In this family, the immunohistochemical study of the myocardium showed loss of expression and irregular distribution of the

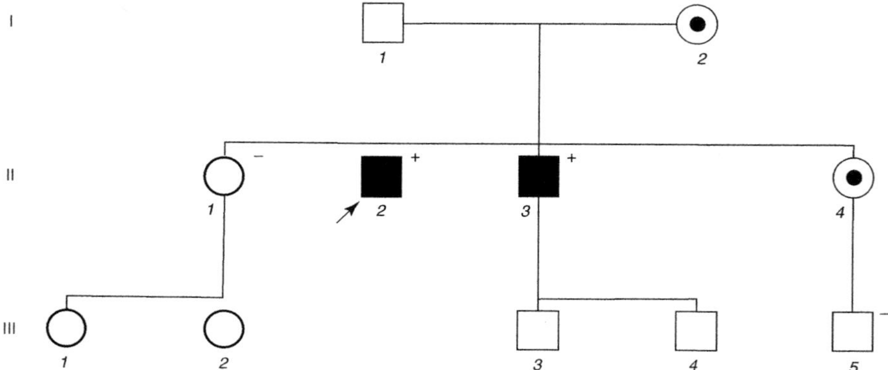

Fig. 10.6 X-linked recessive inheritance in cardiodystrophinopathies

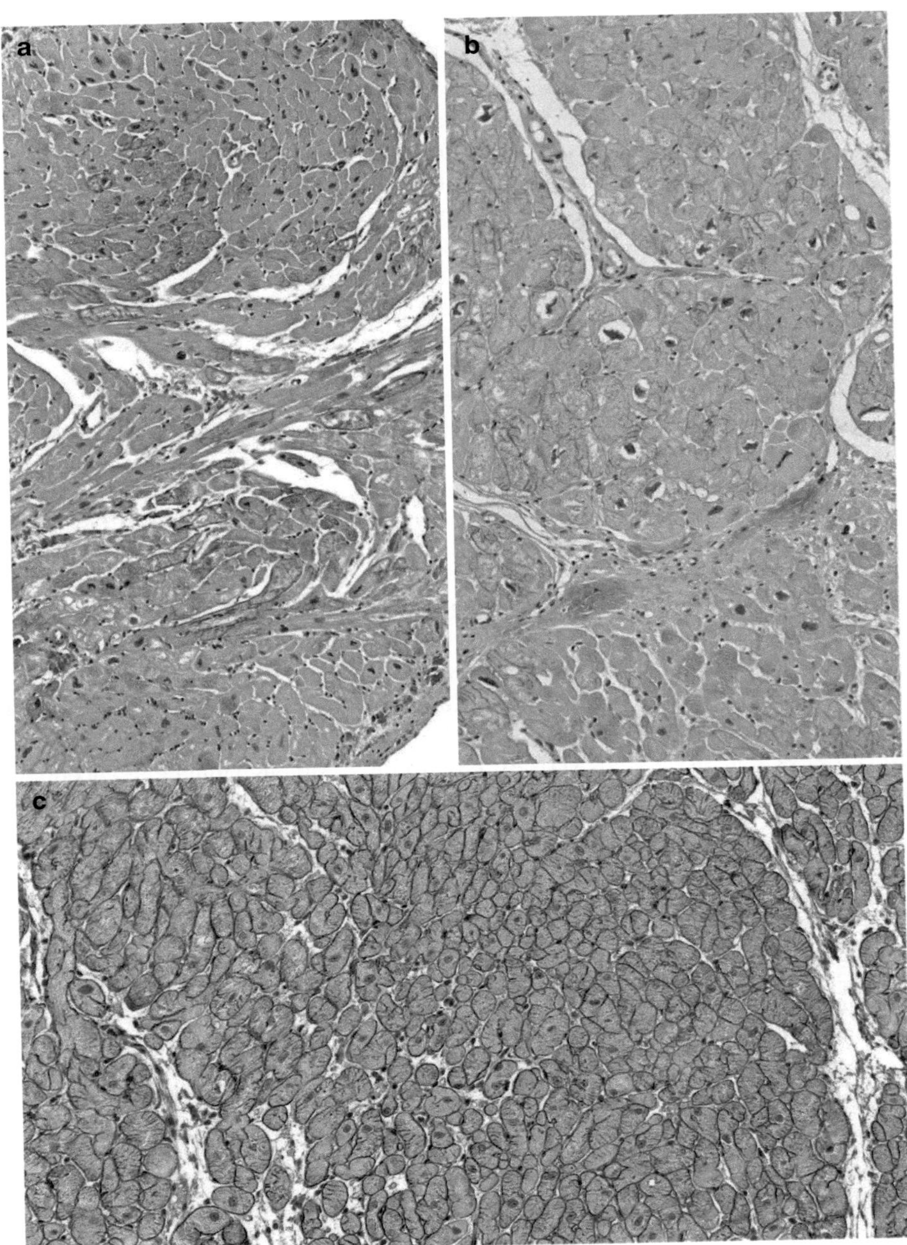

Fig. 10.6 (continued)

protein (Fig. 10.6a, b) compared with myocardium from a patient with DCM and non-mutated *DYS* (Fig. 10.6c). In male patients with DCM and either increased sCPK or traits suggestive of muscle dystrophy, the defective immunostaining with anti-Dystrophin antibodies (the complete set includes antibodies specifically targeting N-terminus, rod domain, and C-terminus) is strongly suggestive for the precise diagnosis of cardiodystrophinopathy, which should confirmed by genetic testing.

In the family shown in Fig. 10.7 the proband presented with sporadic DCM: after completion of family screening, he was the only affected member of the family; his sCPK levels were mildly and inconstantly increased. His grandmother was healthy at the age of 72 years; his mother did not show cardiac or extracardiac traits or markers of disease. The diagnosis in the proband was done on the basis of incidental detection of increased sCPK when he was 12-year-old, asymptomatic and without clinical manifestations of dystrophy. During the course of 9 years of follow-up the boy developed a mild LV dilation and borderline LV dysfunction (50% Ejection Fraction, EF), did not show ventricular arrhythmias and maintained stable in NYHA class I while being treated with ACE-I and BB. The CMR confirmed prominent trabeculations that do not fulfil criteria for the diagnosis of LVNC.

10.3.3 DCM Associated with Mutations in Z-Disk Proteins

The sarcomeric Z-disk anchors thin (actin) filaments and links titin and actin filaments from opposing sarcomere halves. Key molecules identified to date as Z-disk components include, among others, LDB3 (CYPHER-ZASP), NEXN, T-CAP, MYOZ2, VCL, CSRP3, ANKRD1, ACTN2, MYPN. Although mutations encoding these proteins have been reported to cause DCM and HCM current evidence suggests that mutations in Z-disk genes are rare and can be the cause of the disease or more commonly act as modifiers of the DCM phenotype caused by mutations in other disease genes. The two examples shown in Figs. 10.8 and 10.9 support a modifier rather than a causative role for these genes.

10.3.3.1 Dilated Cardiozaspopathies

Defects in *LDB3* (*CYPHER-ZASP*; Zaspopathies) have been associated with DCM with and without LVNC, HCM, and myofibrillar myopathy. The protein interacts with α-actin, α-actinin, and myotilin and is involved in maintainance of the structural integrity of the striated muscle Z-disc in multiple species.

The original interest for *LDB3* mutations was related to their association with adult-onset, isolated, dilated LVNC cardiomyopathy [46] (OMIM*605906.0007). However, the most common "variant" p.(Asp117Asn) or p.(Asp232Asn) (Allele Frequency in Exome Variant Server=AA=0/AG=84/GG=6116, http://evs.gs.washington.edu/EVS/) which had been originally described as disease-causing mutation [46], was recently reported as polymorphism in a Beduin population in which it occurs in 5.2% of non-affected individuals [47]. Other variants are reported in gene-specific variation database (http://www.dmd.nl/nmdb/variants.php?select_db=LDB3&action=view_all). The association of *LDB3* variants with increased trabeculation/LVNC should be matter of further

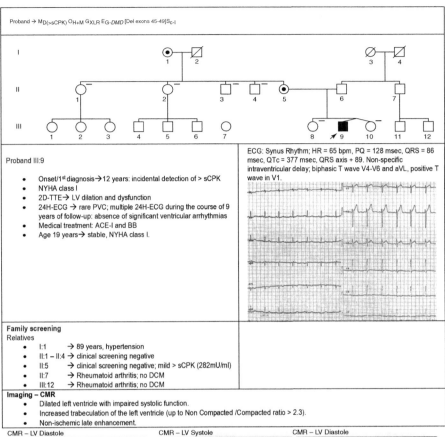

Proband → $M_{D(>sCPK)}$ O_{H+M} G_{XLR} $E_{G\text{-}DMD\,[Del\ exons\ 45\text{-}49]}$ $S_{C\text{-}I}$

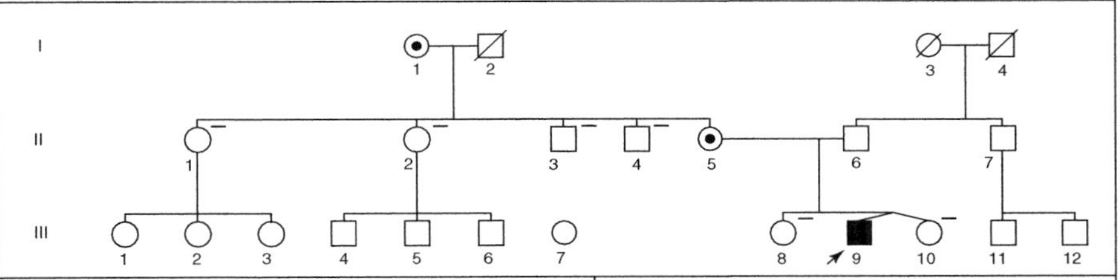

Proband III:9

- Onset/1st diagnosis→12 years: incidental detection of > sCPK
- NYHA class I
- 2D-TTE→ LV dilation and dysfunction
- 24H-ECG → rare PVC; multiple 24H-ECG during the course of 9 years of follow-up: absence of significant ventricular arrhythmias
- Medical treatment: ACE-I and BB
- Age 19 years→ stable, NYHA class I.

ECG: Synus Rhythm; HR = 65 bpm, PQ = 128 msec, QRS = 86 msec, QTc = 377 msec, QRS axis + 89. Non-specific intraventricular delay; biphasic T wave V4-V6 and aVL, positive T wave in V1.

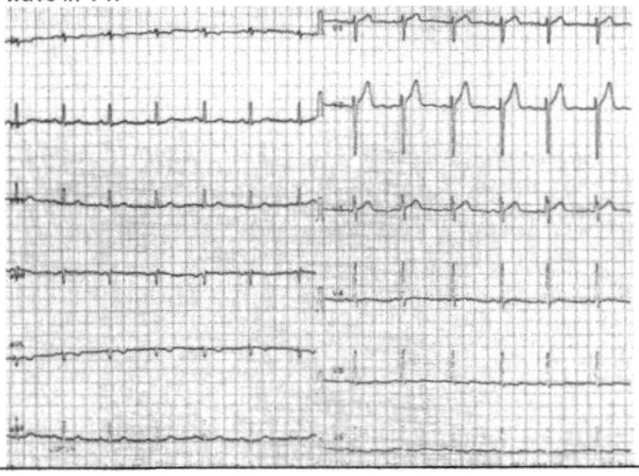

Family screening

Relatives

- I:1 → 89 years, hypertension
- II:1 – II:4 → clinical screening negative
- II:5 → clinical screening negative; mild > sCPK (282mU/ml)
- II:7 → Rheumatoid arthritis; no DCM
- III:12 → Rheumatoid arthritis; no DCM

Imaging – CMR

- Dilated left ventricle with impaired systolic function.
- Increased trabeculation of the left ventricle (up to Non Compacted /Compacted ratio > 2.3).
- Non-ischemic late enhancement.

CMR – LV Diastole

CMR – LV Systole

CMR – LV Diastole

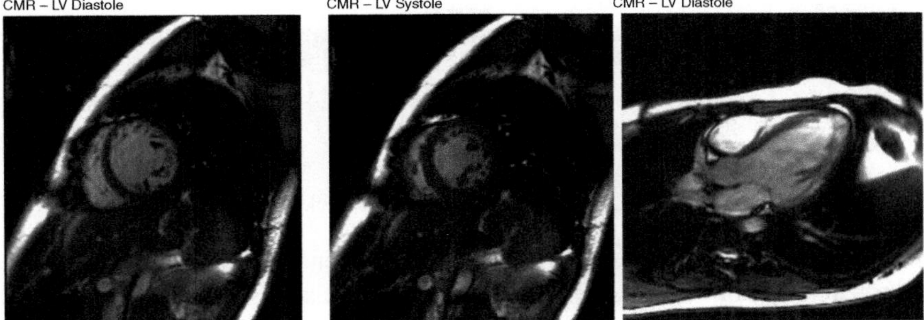

DCM= Dilated Cardiomyopathy; sCPK = Serum Creatin Phosphokinase; XLR = X-Linked Recessive; TTE= Transthoracic Echocardiogram; PVC= Premature Ventricular Contraction; ACE-I= ACE Inibitors; BB= Beta Blockers; LV= Left Ventricle; CMR= Cardiac Magnetic Resonance.

Fig. 10.7 Apparently sporadic, genetic DCM

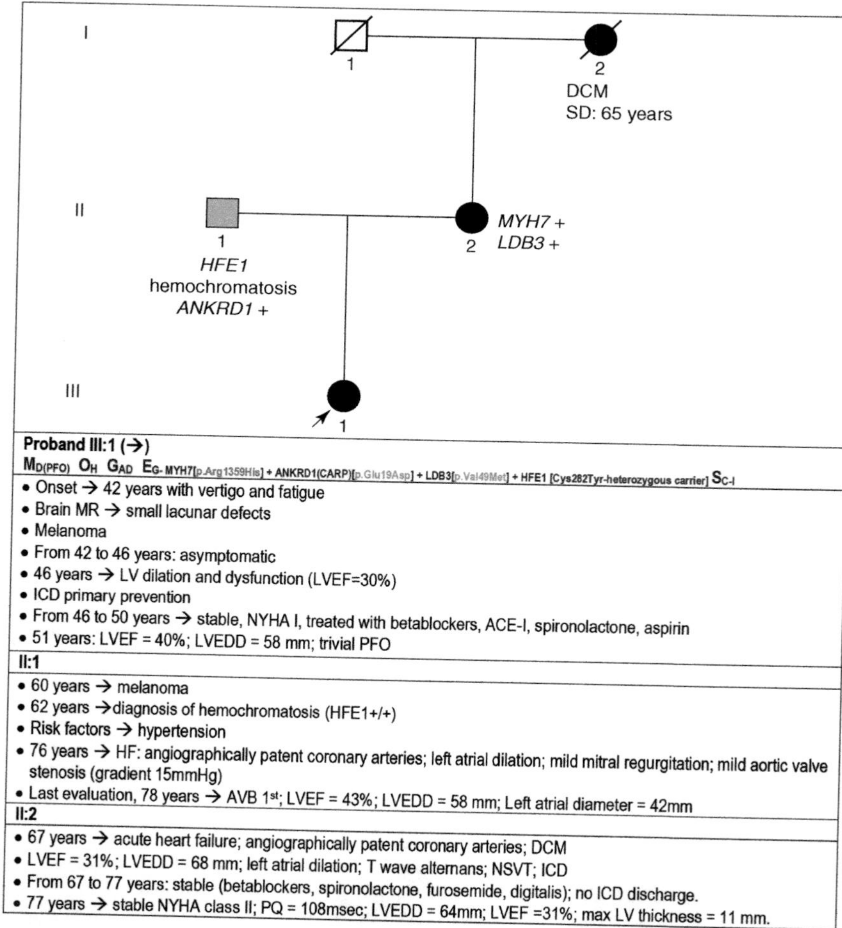

DCM = Dilated Cardiomyopathy; PFO=Patent Foramen Ovale; MR = Magnetic Resonance; AD = Autosomal Dominant; ICD= Implantable Cardioverter Defibrillator; LVEF = Left Ventricular Ejection Fraction; LVEDD = Left Ventricular End-Diastolic Diameter; NSVT = Non-Sustained Ventricular Tachycardia; LV= Left Ventricle.

Fig. 10.8 Autosomal dominant DCM with complex genetic background

investigation to definitely assess its role in the trabecular anatomy of DCM hearts. *LDB3* variants are common: they are frequently found in association with mutations in other disease gene. *The example shown in* Fig. 10.8 demonstrates the complex genetic make-up in a family in which the disease-causing mutation seems to be the p.(Arg1359His) in *MYH7* gene, while the variants p.(Glu19 Asp) in *ANKRD1* gene and the p.(Val49Met) in *LDB3* gene could contribute to the phenotype in the proband, who developed the disease at the age of 42 years. In her mother the disease onset coincided with acute heart failure at the age of 67 years: she does not carry the *ANKRD1* variant. The father is affected by *HFE* hemochromatosis and he only passed one 282 mutated allele to the daughter (healthy carrier) and the *ANKRD1* variant. The course of the disease was characterised

A) The pedigree shows the autosomal dominant DCM; I:2 was proven to be affected but she did not have genetic testing. Her DCM Was not associated with conduction disease. I:1 was described as healthy but he died suddenly at the age of 57.

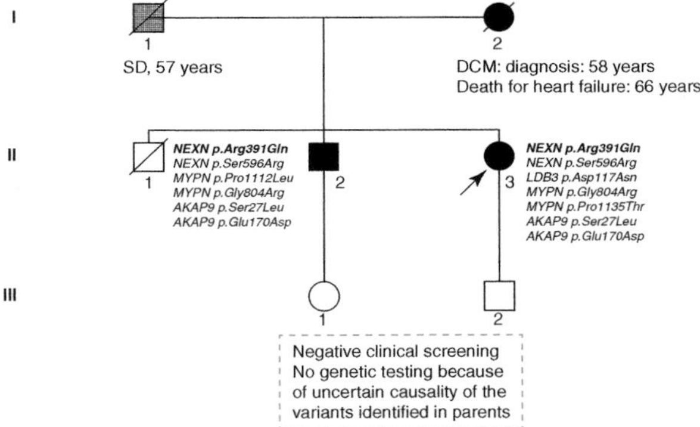

B) The table below shows the stable clinical evolution of the disease in sibs II:2 and II:3. Their cardiac magnetic resonance showed mall DE areas in the basal portion of the free lateral LV wall. Both sibs showed a few PVCs (<500/24 H) in multiple 24–H–Holter.

II:2				
Age	EF (%)	LVEDD (mm)	Treatments	NYHA
47 yrs	22	68	Variably adjusted	III
49 yrs	40	65	• ACEI	II
51 yrs	40	63	• BB	II
52 yrs	40	64	• Diuretics	II
II:3				
Age	EF (%)	LVEDD (mm)	Treatments	NYHA
40 yrs	38	61	Variably adjusted	III
43 yrs	50	59	• ACEI	II b
46	45	60	• BB	II
48	40	58	• Diuretics	II
49	40	60		II
51	40	59		II
54	40	50		II b

SD= Sudden Death; DCM=Dilated Cardiomyopathy; DE=Delayed Enhancement; PVC=Premature Vantricular Contraction; EF= Fiection Fraction I VEDD= Left Ventricle End=Diastolic Diameter ACF–I=ACF Inhibitors BB= Beta Blockers

Fig. 10.9 The figure shows the pedigree **A**) and the results of cardiac review **B**) the uncertain interpretation of genetic results limits the possible interpretation of the results and parents decided not to test their healthy children. *ACE-I* ace inhibitors, *BB* beta blockers, *DCM* dilated cardiomyopathy, *DE* delayed enhancement, *EF* ejection fraction, *LVEDD* left ventricle end-diastolic diameter, *PVC* premature ventricular contraction, *SD* sudden death

by a mild phenotype at onset, transient worsening that led to ICD implantation in primary prevention, and is now stable, NYHA class I, since 5 years in optimal medical treatment, and no appropriate ICD interventions.

Considerations

- The role of mutations in *LDB3* in DCM without LV hyper-trabeculations or LVNC deserves further studies and evidences.
- At present, in our experience, the p.(Asp117Asn) variant in *LDB3* can be considered as potentially influencing LV trabecular anatomy but we have no evidence that, by itself, the variant is the unique cause of the DCM.
- In our early Sanger-based sequencing experience the causal link of *LDB3* variants with DCM was inferred by apparent segregation but later on, with expansion

of the number of tested genes and the number of screened family members, we found *LDB3* variants frequently recurring in patients/families in which mutations in other genes were proven to cause the disease (incomplete genotyping).
- We advice caution before releasing diagnostic conclusive reports on mutations in *LDB3* as unique cause of DCM.

10.3.3.2 Dilated Nexilinopathies

Nexilin (encoded by *NEXN gene*) is a Z-disk protein whose defects cause perturbation of Z-disk stability and heart failure in experimental models and DCM in humans through a dominant-negative effect. A recurrent mutation (founder mutation) causes DCM in 0.6% of consecutive German patients: the mutation consists of the deletion of the evolutionary highly conserved amino acid glycine at position 650 p.(Gly650del). Other missense mutations have been identified and associated with DCM [48]. Variants are common in *NEXN*: the interpretation of their role in the pathogenesis of the DCM requires caution and may remain non-conclusive as in the family shown in Fig. 10.9. In this family the "asymptomatic" father of the proband died suddenly at the age of 57 years and the cause of death remained non-clarified (the autopsy was not performed). The mother had been diagnosed with DCM at the age of 58 years and died for heart failure 8 years later. She did not receive PM or ICD. The affected family members are two siblings, showing similar but non-identical genetic make up. Of the two *NEXN* variants identified in the two sibs, one p.(Arg391Gln), is novel, unreported in existing databases and predicted as potentially pathogenic by in silico tools. The second variant p.(Ser596Arg) is known, rare and predicted as possibly damaging. In both sibs variants with potential modifier effects are equally present with the exception of the p.(Asp117Asn) in *LDB3* gene, which was identified in II:3 but not in II:2. The overall genetic make-up of the two sibs is at present non-conclusive. The immunostaining of the EMB with anti-LDB3 antibodies in the sib carrier of the p.(Asp117Asn) variant in *LDB3* gene was similar to that observed in controls that do not carry this variant. Additional functional studies have not been performed. At present III:1 and III:2, the two young sons of the two sibs, on the basis of the non conclusive genetic data, did not undergo genetic testing: both had negative clinical screening and none of them at present, could contribute to further interpretation of the potential role of variants identified in this family. The risk is labelling the two boys as genetically affected, when, vice versa, the real cause of the disease in the family is not proven. We advise caution against releasing genetic reports that describe variants whose role is not proven by segregation studies and functional data. The table in Fig. 10.9b shows the stable clinical condition of the DCM during the long-term course in optimal medical treatment. No family members manifested conduction disease or required ICD implantation.

10.3.4 Dilated Phospholambanopathies

DCM-PLNs are a distinct group of DCM caused by mutations in the *Phospholamban gene* that encodes a protein expressed in the sarcoplasmic reticulum (SR) membrane. Phospholamban inhibits cardiac muscle sarcoplasmic reticulum Ca(2+)-ATPase (SERCA2a) in the unphosphorylated state. Mutations in *PLN* impair SR calcium homeostasis and cause DCM [49]. Less commonly, mutations in *PLN* cause HCM [50]. The p.(Arg14del) is the most frequently identified mutation in Dutch cardiomyopathy patients (10–15%), both DCM or arrhythmogenic phenotypes [51]. Patients diagnosed with DCM associated with p.(Arg14del) demonstrate high arrhythmogenic risk and sudden cardiac death as first disease presentation [50, 51]. A common ECG pattern in *PLN* mutation carriers is a low-voltage QRS complex and inverted T waves in leads V4–V6 [52]. In non-Dutch patients *PLN* mutations are less common but equally malignant [53, 54]. Therefore, although rare, *PLN* mutations can be clinically suspected in patients with DCM, high arrhythmogenic risk and low voltage on ECG.

10.3.5 Dilated Sarcomeric Cardiomyopathy

10.3.5.1 Dilated Myosinopathies

Mutations in the *MYH7* gene (typically causing HCM) may associate with DCM [31]. Recent experimental studies suggest that loss of function mutations are associated with DCM while mutations causing gain of function are associated with HCM. The reconstitution of the entire contractile system [actin and myosin and Tropomyosin 1, Troponin C, Troponin I, and Troponin T] seems to be necessary to fully understand the effects of *MYH7* mutations in HCM and DCM [55]. Additional explanations include the possibility of compound mutations in *MtDNA* genes and in the *MYH7 gene*: patients who carry the sole *MYH7* mutation demonstrate HCM, while those carrying both *MYH7* and *MtDNA* mutations develop "hypertrophic dilated cardiomyopathy" with an end-phenotype resembling DCM [56]. Yet another explanation is the presence of more than one mutation in the same patient: depending on the mutation, the DCM phenotype could be explained by a complex genetic make-up in which more than one mutation contributes to the final phenotype. Overall, the role of *MYH7* in DCM remains a matter of research and deserves specific investigation for any novel mutation identified in patients with DCM.

The family shown in Fig. 10.10 highlights the problem of complex interpretation of genetic testing when mutations identified in the proband are two (or more) and both are potentially pathogenic. When family segregation cannot be investigated, the assignment of the causal role to one or to the other mutation may remain unfeasible. When family members to be tested are healthy children or adolescent (minors), parents can be reluctant to decide about genetic testing. In this family a key member could have been the mother of the proband, but she died before genetic work-up. Therefore, in complex situations with uncertain interpretation, geneticists and cardiologists should not force interpretations or decisions. Excluding a causative role of the *TTN* missense variant, the possible scenarios for the three clinically healthy kids of the proband include: (1) they may carry only one of the two mutations (either *MYH7* or *MYBPC3*); (2) they may carry both variants. The father would know whether the risk of developing the disease exists or is higher with *MYH7* or

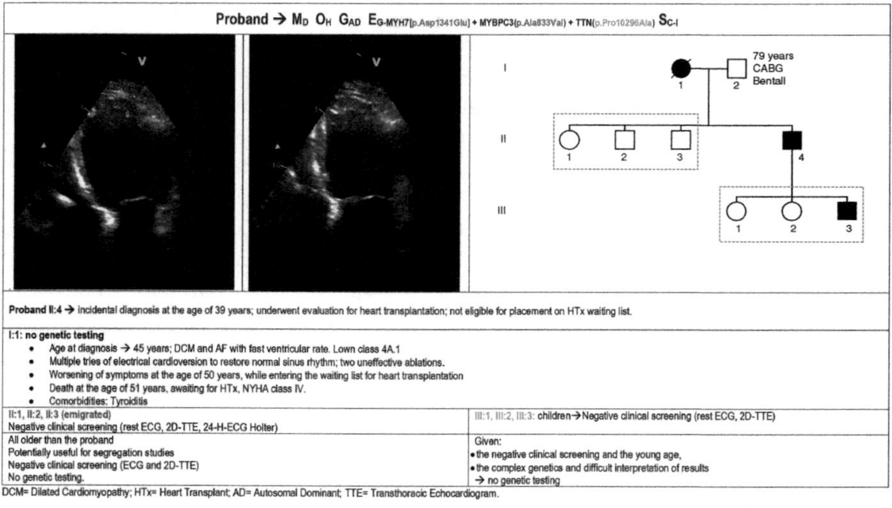

Proband → M_D O_H G_{AD} $E_{G\text{-}MYH7[p.Asp1341Glu] + MYBPC3(p.Ala833Val) + TTN(p.Pro10296Ala)}$ $S_{C\text{-}I}$
V
V
I
II
III
79 years
CABG
Bentall
1
2
1
2
3
4
1
2
3
Proband II:4 → incidental diagnosis at the age of 39 years; underwent evaluation for heart transplantation; not eligible for placement on HTx waiting list.
I:1: no genetic testing
• Age at diagnosis → 45 years; DCM and AF with fast ventricular rate. Lown class 4A.1
• Multiple tries of electrical cardioversion to restore normal sinus rhythm; two uneffective ablations.
• Worsening of symptoms at the age of 50 years, while entering the waiting list for heart transplantation
• Death at the age of 51 years, awaiting for HTx, NYHA class IV.
• Comorbidities: Tyroiditis
II:1, II:2, II:3 (emigrated)
Negative clinical screening (rest ECG, 2D-TTE, 24-H-ECG Holter)
III:1, III:2, III:3: children→Negative clinical screening (rest ECG, 2D-TTE)
All older than the proband
Potentially useful for segregation studies
Negative clinical screening (ECG and 2D-TTE)
No genetic testing.
Given:
• the negative clinical screening and the young age,
• the complex genetics and difficult interpretation of results
→ no genetic testing
DCM= Dilated Cardiomyopathy; HTx= Heart Transplant; AD= Autosomal Dominant; TTE= Transthoracic Echocardiogram.

Fig. 10.10 Sarcomeric DCM. *AD* autosomal dominant, *HTx* heart transplant, *TTE* transthoracic echocardiogram

with *MYBPC3* mutation. Since at present we do not have answer, the genetic basis of the DCM in II:4 should be considered not suitable for conclusive diagnostic interpretation.

This family gives the opportunity for the following considerations:

- The identification of more than one mutation with possible pathologic effect obligates to segregation studies that establish the mono or bi-parental origin of the mutations
- If each mutation is inherited from one of the two parents and the inheritance of the trait is autosomal dominant, one of the two mutations may have a leading role and the one can act as possible modifier of the phenotype.
- The findings are relevant for interpretation of the results of cascade genetic testing in families.

10.3.5.2 Dilated Troponinopathies

The comprehension of mechanisms that cause DCM in patients with mutations in *TNNT2* or *TNNI3* is currently complicated by the different phenotypes associated with these genes, typically RCM, HCM, HCM with restrictive pattern, DCM and hypokinetic without LV dilation. *TNNT2*-related cardiomyopathies are diseases with exclusive cardiac involvement [57].

The proband shown in Fig. 10.11 is a 41-year-old woman who had three uncomplicated pregnancies. Her clinical history started at the age of 36 years when, after a febrile flu, she manifested profound fatigue, cough and palpitations. A cardiologic evaluation demonstrated LV dilation and mild dysfunction (EF = 45%), normal LV thickness (9 mm), normal levels of NTProBNP, rare PVC. Coronary arteries were

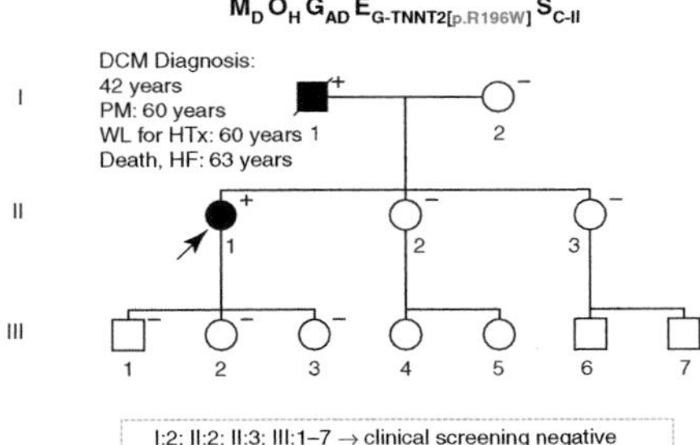

II:1 Age, years	Symptoms
36	Fatigue, cough, palpitations after febrile flu, NYHA II
36	2D-TEE→ LVEF=45%; LVEDD=49mm; IVS=9mm
37	2D-TEE→ LVEF=43%; LVEDD=48mm
38	Syncope with spontanous recovery
	LVEF=45%; LA=30mm, 19/10 cm², 42/22ml
	Further syncope episodes; absence of documented arrhythmias
	EPS → negative; loop-recorder (Reveal)
	Further syncope→ no arrhythmias
	Tilt-test→ no inducible neuro-mediated syncope
	Neurological evaluation including brain magnetic resonance → negative
39	Further syncope episodes → ICD
	Further syncope episodes → no ICD shock
40	LVEF=40%; LVEDD=49mm
	Worsening of fatigue and dyspnea, NYHA III
	ICD→ no shock; several episodes of NSVT
41	LVEF=35%; LVEDD=50mm, NYHA IIIb
	Evaluation for heart transplantation

DCM= Dilated Cardiomyopathy; AD= Autosomal Dominant; PM= Pace-Maker; WL= Waiting List; Htx= Heart Transplant; HF= Heart Failure; TTE= Transthoracic Echocardiogram; LVEF= ;Left Ventricular Ejection Fraction; LVEDD= Left Ventricular End-Diastolic Diamter; IVS= Inter-Ventricular Septum; LA= Left Atrium; EPS= Electrophysiological Study; ICD= Implantable Cardioverter Defibrillator; NSVT= Non-Sustained Ventricular Tachicardia.

Fig. 10.11 Proband of a 41-year-old woman who had three uncomplicated pregnancies. *AD* autosomal dominant, *DCM* dilated cardiomyopathy, *EPS* electrophysiological study, *HF* heart failure, *Htx* heart transplant, *ICD* implantable cardioverter defibrillator, *IVS* interventricular septum, *LA* left atrium, *LVEDD* left ventricular end-diastolic diameter, *LVEF* left ventricular ejection fraction, *NSVT* nonsustained ventricular tachycardia, *PM* pacemaker, *TTE* transthoracic echocardiogram, *WL* waiting list

angiographically patent. CMR demonstrated subepicardial delayed enhancement (DE) of the lateral left ventricular wall and increased apical trabeculation. She was given metoprolol and ACE-I. After one year, clinical controls demonstrated LV EF = 43%; a further CMR questioned the presence of DE (*doubt* DE in the report) and described “dysmorphic right ventricle (RV) apex without evidence of fibro-fatty infiltration, normal RVEF”. A first syncope occurred two years after the diagnosis: the patient described loss of consciousness with spontaneous relapse. The LV was not dilated (48 mm); the left atrium showed normal diameter (30 mm), areas (19/10 cm^2) and volumes (42/22 ml); LVEF was 45%. Further syncope episodes and absence of documented ventricular arrhythmias led to the implantation of a loop-recorder (reveal) after a negative EPS. A tilt test did not induce a neuro-mediated syncope. The recurrence of syncope led to ICD implantation that did not shock when the patient had other syncopal episodes. The neurologic evaluation including brain imaging excluded primary and secondary defects. During the next 2 years the fatigue and dyspnea progressively worsened; the ICD did not intervene but recorded several episodes of NSVT. LVEF decreased from 40% to 35% with normal size. The NYHA class progressed from II to IIIb: the patient underwent evaluation for heart transplant (HTx) with the final diagnosis of hypokinetic LV cardiomyopathy. The family shown in Fig. 10.12 highlights how the health status of the family changed during the course of 12 years.

10.3.5.3 Dilated Cardiotitinopathies

The Titin (TTN) gene encodes the largest human protein and one of the most abundant striated-muscle protein [58]. Truncation predicting mutations have been identified in 25% of familial DCM and in 18% of sporadic DCM [59]. The penetrance of *TTN* truncating mutations was higher than 95% for the patients who were more than 40 years of age. Clinical manifestations, morbidity and mortality were similar to those observed in DCM patients who were non-carriers of *TTN*

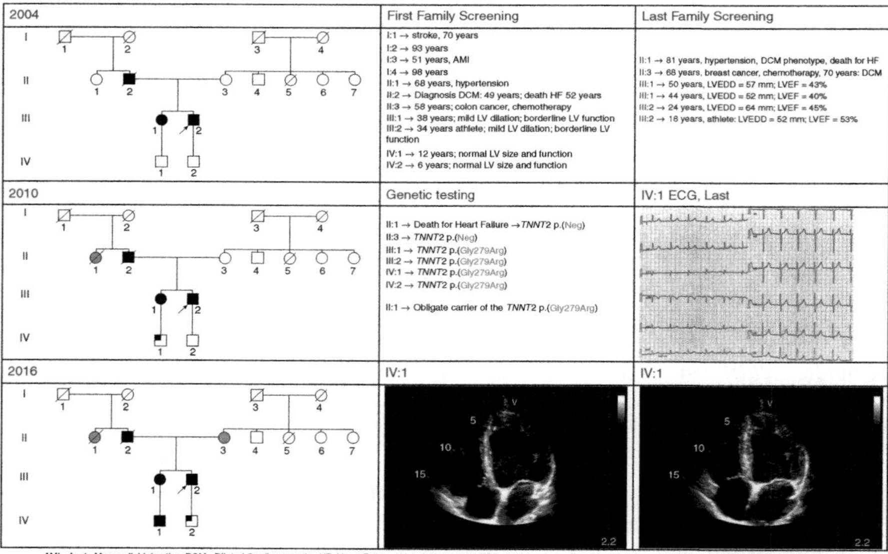

Fig. 10.12 Familial dilated troponinopathy 2: from baseline screening to last follow-up 12 years after the diagnosis. *AMI* acute myocardial infarction, *DCM* dilated cardiomyopathy, *HF* heart failure, *LV* left ventricle, *LVEDD* left ventricular end-diastolic diameter, *LVEF* left ventricular ejection fraction

mutations. DCM was not accompanied by conduction system or skeletal-muscle disease [59]. A further study in women with peripartum cardiomyopathy (PPCM) showed a distribution of truncating variants remarkably similar to that found in patients with DCM [60]. *TTN* mutations have been also associated with hypertrophic cardiomyopathy (*MIM#613765*); muscular dystrophy, limb-girdle, type 2J (LGMD2J–*MIM#608807*); autosomal recessive early onset myopathy with fatal cardiomyopathy (MIM#611705); tardive tibial muscular dystrophy (*MIM#600334*); and proximal myopathy with early respiratory muscle involvement (*MIM#603689*) [61–63]. Since one in 500 individuals in the general population carries a truncation variant in the TTN A-band, the interpretation of such mutations in DCM should be cautious [64]. The relevance of defining the precise role of *TTN* in DCM is now supported by the possibility that antisense mediated exon skipping can be explored as therapeutic strategy [65].

The family shown in Fig. 10.13:

- Highlights the possible segregation of the *TTN* truncation-predicting mutation in the family.
- The second possible mutation in MYH6 is missense and inherited by an healthy young family member who did not, vice versa, inherit the *TTN* mutation (III:5): the question from the affected father was about the risk that his son will develop cardiomyopathy.
- Although this probability is likely low, we do not have the proof that this assertion can be done at the diagnostic level.

10.3.6 Nebulette-DCM

Mutations in the cardio-specific protein nebulette, encoded by the *NEBL gene, have been associated with DCM* [66], *HCM* [67] and *endocardial fibroelastosis* [66]. The protein belongs to the nebulin family of actin-binding proteins that play their role in myofibrillogenesis, Z-line assembly, and interactions with filamin C, myopalladin, α-actinin 2, tropomyosin and troponin T [67]. The prevalence is 1.8% in consecutive series of DCM patients [2]. Functional effects of *NEBL* mutations have been explored in experimental models demonstrating lethal cardiac structural abnormalities in mutant embryonic hearts [68]. In addition, nebulette polymorphisms in the actin-binding motif have been proposed as a genetic marker of susceptibility to nonfamilial idiopathic DCM [66]. Mutations in this gene however have been investigated in series of probands but not in families. The following examples (Fig. 10.14) show that segregation studies in families are essential for interpretation even in case of truncation predicting mutations.

10.3.6.1 Case A

The proband is a 73-year-old man who developed DCM at the age of 50 years. The DCM phenotype was not associated with cardiac or extracardiac markers and did not show arrhythmogenic potential. The heart was markedly enlarged (left ventricular

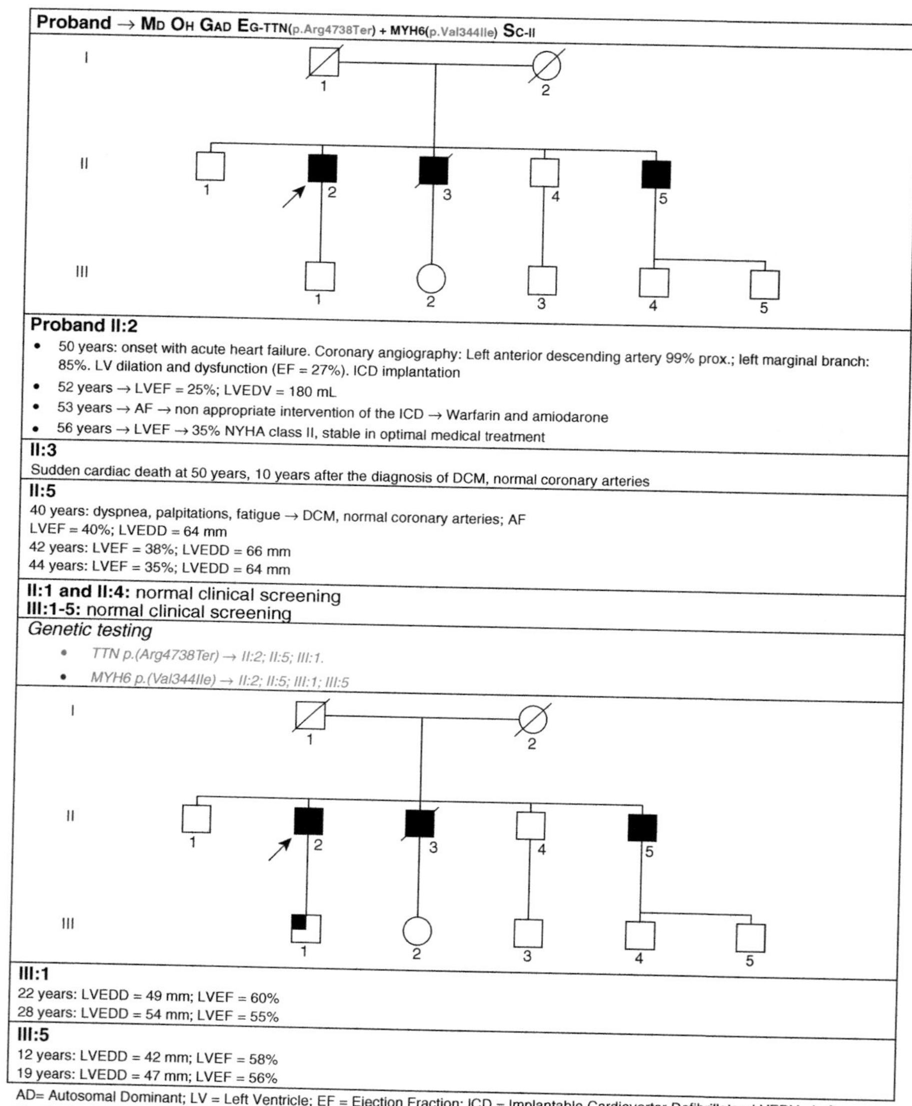

Fig. 10.13 Dilated cardiotitinopathy or myosinopathy? *AD* autosomal dominant, *AF* atrial fibrillation, *DCM* dilated cardiomyopathy, *LV* left ventricle, *EF* ejection fraction, *ICD* implantable cardioverter defibrillator, *LVEDD* left ventricular end-diastolic diameter, *LVEDV* left ventricular end-diastolic volume

end-diastolic diameter–LVEDD = 74 mm) and the LV function severely depressed (LVEF = 22%). He underwent heart transplantation two years after the diagnosis. The two sons underwent clinical screening and regular clinical monitoring: during the course 23 years, one of them developed LV dilation with preserved LV function

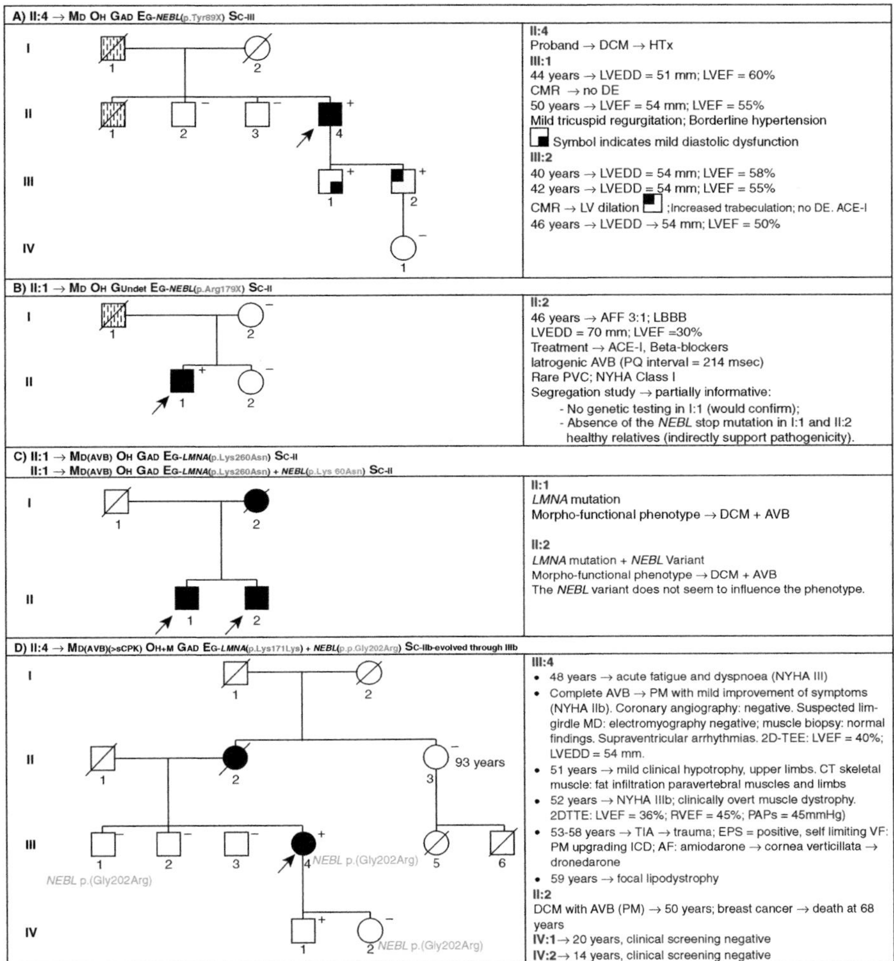

VUS= Variant Unknown Significance; AD= Autosomal Dominant;DCM= Dilated Cardiomyopathy; HTx= Heart Transplantation; LVEDD= Left Ventricular End-Diastolic Diameter; LVEF= Left Ventricular Ejection Fraction; CMR= Cardiac Magnetic Resonance; DE= Delayed Enhancement; ACE-I= ACE Inhibitors; Aff= Atrial Fibrillation/Flutter; AVB= Atrio-Ventricular Block; PVC= Premature Ventricular Complex; LBBB= Left Bundle Branch Block; PM= Pace-Maker; ICD= Implantable Cardioverter Defibrillator; MD= Muscular Dystrophy; TEE= Transthoracic Echocardiography; RVEF= Right Ventricular Ejetion Fraction; PAP= Pulmonary Artery Pression Systolic; TIA= Transient Ischemic Attack; EPS= Electrophysiological Study; VF= Ventricular Fibrillation; AF= Atrial Fibrillation.

Fig. 10.14 Four pedigrees showing families in which mutations in *NEBL* gene has been identified, with (**a**) and (**b**) possible disease-causing mutations and (**c**) and (**d**) showing missense gene VUS

(III:2), starting from the age of 40 years and one developed mild diastolic dysfunction (III:1) with preserved systolic function, starting at the age of 42 years. None of them developed conduction disease; one, III:2, referred an episode of non-witnessed syncope. 24 h ECG monitoring showed PVC (<500/24 h); EPS was negative. Both are now treated with beta-blockers; III:2 is further treated with ACE-I. We identified the p.(Tyr89*) mutation in the proband and in his two sons. We hypothesized that the mutation is associated with a late-onset DCM phenotype. Therefore the possibility that both III:1 and III:2 develop manifest phenotype in the next years cannot be excluded. The interpretation remains non-conclusive.

10.3.6.2 Case B

The proband is a 55-year-old man in which the onset of the symptoms coincided with the perception of profound fatigue that led him to the emergency room where he was diagnosed with atrial flutter (AFL) at the age of 49 years. After pharmacologic restoring of sinus rhythm ECG showed left bundle branch block (LBBB); 2D-TTE demonstrated a markedly enlarged LV (LVEDD = 70 mm) and severely depressed LV function (EF = 30%). Coronary arteries were angiographically normal. He was prescribed BB, ACE-I and aspirin. The patient refused the proposal of ICD implantation and magnetic resonance. After 7 years from onset of symptoms the patient is stable in NYHA class I, with iatrogenic AVB (PQ = 214 ms); EF = 37% and LVEDD = 65 mm. 24 h Holter monitoring showed rare PVC. In this proband we identified the *NEBL* p.(Arg179*) mutation, which was absent in her clinically healthy sister and in his 82-year-old mother. Since the father died at the age of 60 years for lung cancer, segregation of the genotype with the phenotype in the family could not be further explored.

10.3.6.3 Case C

The probands are two sibs [50 (II:1) and 40 (II:2) years, respectively] who were addressed to the clinical attention in the same clinical occasion after the maternal death for HF (I:2); she was affected by ischemic heart disease, hypercholesterolemia, diabetes mellitus and hypertension. They were both diagnosed with DCM, demonstrated normal coronary arteries, absence of conduction disease on baseline ECG and no significant arrhythmias. 24 h ECG Holter monitoring recorded Luciani-Wenckebach nocturnal periodisms in II: 1 but not in II:2. In these two sibs multigene panel analysis demonstrated the p.(Lys260Asn) in *Lamin AC* and the p.(Lys60Asn) in *Nebulette* in only one of the two sibs. This variant has been reported as disease-causing mutation and shown to be associated with profound morphologic changes in cardiac myocytes of experimental mouse model, with founders of the K60N line dying at 1 year of age with severe heart failure [1].

10.3.6.4 Case D

The proband complained transient dyspnoea and palpitations in the last months of both pregnancies (age 34 and 39 years, respectively). She was well until the age of 48 years, when she complained acute fatigue, dyspnoea and palpitations. She was diagnosed with DCM and complete AVB and treated with PM implantation and amiodarone for atrial arrhythmias that were not controlled by BB. Amiodarone was discontinued after a few months for thyroid toxicity and the patient underwent ablation for the atrial arrhythmias. The procedure was unsuccessful. Biochemical tests showed mild increased sCPK. The profound fatigue and dyspnoea suggested a possible myasthenia gravis, which was further excluded with specific tests; several neuromyology evaluations, including electromyography, tested negative. Skeletal muscle biopsy was non-informative. Computerized tomography (CT) of the limb and axial muscles showed focal fat infiltration. The NYHA class progressed from early class II to IIIb: LVEF declined to 36% and the patient developed mild pulmonary hypertension (40–45 mmHg). The PM was upgraded to ICD after a positive EPS. Rhythm control attempts using amiodarone and dronedarone were not feasible for the development of cornea verticillata with visual impairment and acute hepatic toxicity respectively. The patient suffered further progression of her focal lipodystrophy. Fatigue, dyspnoea and walking limitations are progressively worsening in the context of a DCM characterised by very mild LV dilation (LVEDD = 52 mm) and dysfunction (LVEF = 45%). The genetic test identified the known c.513G>A p.(Lys171Lys) mutation in *LMNA* gene [69] and the known p.(Gly202Arg) mutation in *NEBL* [66]. The synonymous *LMNA* change alters mRNA splicing and causes muscular dystrophy, limb-girdle, type 1B (LGMD1B). In this family, the mother was affected by DCM with AVB, treated with PM implantation at the age of 58 years; 10 years later she developed breast cancer that was treated with trastuzumab (see PPCM). Clinical family screening excluded cardiac and muscle phenotypes in other living family members. Segregation studies showed that the p.(Gly202Arg) mutation in *NEBL* is likely a polymorphism given that the older brother (III:1) is carrier and healthy. The same variant has been inherited by the young healthy daughter, but not by the young healthy son who is carrier of the *LMNA* mutation.

10.3.6.5 Practical Considerations

The above-described examples suggest that NEBL-associated DCM is:

- Adult-onset and pure cardiac phenotype (cases A and B); cases reported to date, and our own experience in 500 DCM with 16 mutated probands did not highlight clinical markers (red flags) recurrently associated with the disease.
- Slowly progressing LV dilation and dysfunction in optimal medical treatment.
- Arrhythmogenic risk stratification is limited by the few genetic studies and series on NEBL-associated DCM; the arrhythmogenic risk seems low.
- In patients with clinical markers such as conduction disease, other disease genes should be investigated (see family C).
- Family history is essential for early diagnosis: at the time of first and second pregnancy of the proband III:4 of family D, the mother (II:2) was affected. Family screening, both clinical and genetic, is essential and irreplaceable.
- The role of missense *NEBL* variants should be interpreted cautiously (Families C and D).

10.4 "Arrhythmogenic" Dilated Cardiomyopathy

The diagnosis of DCM does not imply or include the description of the arrhythmogenic characteristics of the disease. The term "arrhythmogenic" typically pertains to the diagnostic definition of arrhythmogenic right ventricular cardiomyopathy (classic form) and to the two variants involving the left ventricle (biventricular and predominantly left). The disease is now termed arrhythmogenic cardiomyopathy

(ACM). Mutations in genes coding for desmosome proteins are one of the major diagnostic criteria of the Task Force 2010 for arrhythmogenic cardiomyopathies (right, biventricular and predominantly left) [70]. However, mutations in desmosome genes can be associated with DCM in patients that do not show functional involvement of the right ventricle or traits recurring in ACM. This is the case of the family shown in Fig. 10.15 that summarizes the clinical history and the genetic

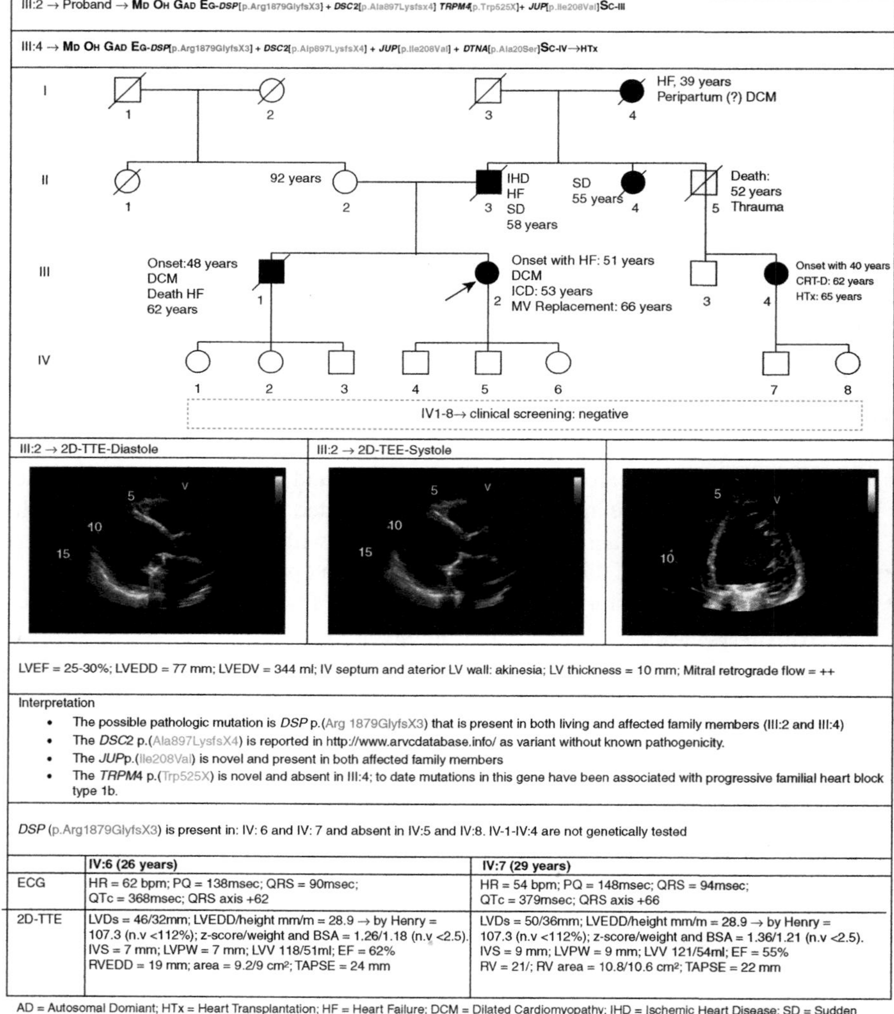

LVEF = 25-30%; LVEDD = 77 mm; LVEDV = 344 ml; IV septum and aterior LV wall: akinesia; LV thickness = 10 mm; Mitral retrograde flow = ++

Interpretation

- The possible pathologic mutation is *DSP* p.(Arg 1879GlyfsX3) that is present in both living and affected family members (III:2 and III:4)
- The *DSC2* p.(Ala897LysfsX4) is reported in http://www.arvcdatabase.info/ as variant without known pathogenicity.
- The *JUP*p.(Ile208Val) is novel and present in both affected family members
- The *TRPM4* p.(Trp525X) is novel and absent in III:4; to date mutations in this gene have been associated with progressive familial heart block type 1b.

DSP (p.Arg1879GlyfsX3) is present in: IV: 6 and IV: 7 and absent in IV:5 and IV:8. IV-1-IV:4 are not genetically tested

	IV:6 (26 years)	**IV:7 (29 years)**
ECG	HR = 62 bpm; PQ = 138msec; QRS = 90msec; QTc = 368msec; QRS axis +62	HR = 54 bpm; PQ = 148msec; QRS = 94msec; QTc = 379msec; QRS axis +66
2D-TTE	LVDs = 46/32mm; LVEDD/height mm/m = 28.9 → by Henry = 107.3 (n.v <112%); z-score/weight and BSA = 1.26/1.18 (n.v <2.5). IVS = 7 mm; LVPW = 7 mm; LVV 118/51ml; EF = 62% RVEDD = 19 mm; area = 9.2/9 cm²; TAPSE = 24 mm	LVDs = 50/36mm; LVEDD/height mm/m = 28.9 → by Henry = 107.3 (n.v <112%); z-score/weight and BSA = 1.36/1.21 (n.v <2.5). IVS = 9 mm; LVPW = 9 mm; LVV 121/54ml; EF = 55% RV = 21/; RV area = 10.8/10.6 cm²; TAPSE = 22 mm

AD = Autosomal Domiant; HTx = Heart Transplantation; HF = Heart Failure; DCM = Dilated Cardiomyopathy; IHD = Ischemic Heart Disease; SD = Sudden Death; ICD = Implantable Cardioverter Defibrillator; MV = Mitral Valve; CRT-D = Cardiac Resynchronization Therapy Device; TTE = Transthoracic Echocardiography; TEE = Transesophageal echocardiography; LVEF = Left Ventricular Ejection Fraction; LVEDD = Left Ventricular End-Diastolic Diameter; LVEDV = Left Ventricular End-Diastolic Volume; LV = Left Ventricle; HR = Heart Rate; LVDs = Left Ventricle Diameter Systolic; BSA = Body Surface Area; IVS = Inter Ventricular Septum; LVPW = Left Ventricle Posterior Wall; LVV = Left Ventricle Volume; EF = Ejection Fraction; RVEDD = Right Ventricle End-Diastolic Diameter; TAPSE = Tricuspid Annular Plane Systolic Excursion; RV = Right Ventricle.

Fig. 10.15 Antirhythmogenic dilated cardiomyopathy

basis of a familial DCM with high arrhythmogenic substrate and exclusive involvement of the left ventricle. The proband is a 69-year-old woman in which the first diagnosis of DCM coincided with acute heart failure 18 years before. During the long course of the disease, the patient underwent ICD implantation in primary prevention, mitral valve replacement and ventricular remodelling. After surgery, she progressively worsened and is now in NYHA class III. Her cousin (III:4) had her first diagnosis of DCM at 40 years of age: the disease progressed slowly during the course of 25 years and she had heart transplantation at the age of 65 years. In the two cousins (III:2 and III:4) we identified two frameshift mutations (one in *DSP* and one in *DSC2*, Fig. 10.15). This implies that their related parents (II:3 and II:5) who could not be tested, were obligate carriers. For many years the disease of the two cousins was considered unrelated because the father of III:2 also had confounding ischemic heart disease (IHD) and the father of III:4 had died for traumatic causes. In addition to these two mutations, III:2 is carrier of a stop mutation in *TRPM4* and a missense variant in *JUP*, while III:4 is carrier of a variant in *DTNA*, a gene known to be associated with LVNC. At present family members of the IV generation are clinically well, not yet convinced to have genetic testing because there is no prevention strategy before early signs of disease manifest.

This family is a paradigmatic example of:

- Underestimation of family risk starting from the grandmother I:4 who died for heart failure (but with limited documented clinical information) after her third delivery, and then progressing with family member III:1 who could not undergo HTx for multiple organ failure (MOF) and liver disease, the confounding history of IHD in II:3 and the SCD in the II:4 who was affected by DCM.
- Limited answer to the question on how to prevent the manifestations of the disease; the only possible suggestion for healthy family members may address life styles; however, the simple switch from the formal diagnosis of DCM to ACM could modify the indication to ICD implantation in primary prevention according to current guidelines. No guideline indicates ICD implantation in healthy relatives of DCM patients.

The open question is whether desmosome diseases should be considered as having identical arrhythmogenic risk, irrespective of the clinical phenotype (ACM or DCM) and whether the phenotypic distinction makes sense once the DCM-associated mutation has been identified and coincides with those recurring in ACM. The diagnostic definition of dilated desmosomalopathy seems to accurately describe the phenotype. The term was proposed by Corrado et al. in 2005 [71] for precise description of ACM with known and typical genetic causes. In their editorial, Authors anticipated the impact of precise diagnosis in the definition and classification of cardiomyopathies. Originally, desmosomalopathies described the classical ARVC caused by mutations in genes coding desmosome proteins (*DSC*, *DSG2*, etc.). The extensive screening of these genes in patients with other cardiomyopathies demonstrated that DCM can be allelic at the same loci identified for ARVC. Later on, the revised task force criteria for ARVC introduced the two novel phenotypes (biventricular and left dominant arrhythmogenic cardiomyopathy) associated with mutations in these genes and genetic testing was included in the list of major diagnostic criteria. In clinical practice the two phenotypes may be difficult to distinguish from DCM, especially when biventricular involvement is present and instrumental markers of classic ARVC are absent.

10.4.1 Dilated Cardiomitomyopathies

In this subgroup of patients, the DCM is usually observed in the context of multiorgan syndromes with a peculiar risk of complications such as cryptogenic strokes and intolerance to several drugs [33, 72]. Mitochondrial cardiomyopathies can be caused by mutations in *MtDNA* genes (maternal inheritance) and in nuclear genes (Mendelian inheritance: no male passes down the disease to children) coding mitochondrial proteins. A third group of mitochondrial disease is represented by iatrogenic phenocopies: mitochondrial toxicity may manifest with deafness, neuropathy, myopathy, cardiomyopathy, hyperlactatemia, lactic acidosis, pancreatitis and lipodystrophy.

The cardiac phenotype is characterized by either non-obstructive hypertrophic phenotype mimicking HCM evolving through LV dilation and dysfunction or by DCM, without significant evidence of LV wall thickening. ECG markers include short PR interval and possible ventricular preexcitation.

The clinical manifestations associated with mutations in mitochondrial DNA genes depend on the grade of heteroplasmy in affected organs. They are commonly observed in families in which mutation carriers also express non-cardiac traits such as hearing loss, palpebral ptosis, myopathy, renal failure, cryptogenic stroke, diabetes, optic neuritis, and/or retinitis pigmentosa. Sequencing of MtDNA, either by Sanger-based techniques or NGS tools, identifies the causative mutation. Nuclear "Mitochondrial" cardiomyopathies are inherited according to Mendelian rules: they can be autosomal dominant or recessive. Typical cardiac phenotypes are primarily DCM such as in the autosomal recessive DCM caused by *ANT1* mutations or in autosomal dominant DCM and progressive external ophthalmoplegia caused by *POLG1* mutations.

10.4.1.1 Mitochondrial DNA Defect Related Cardiomyopathy

The proband is a 50-year-old female with a complex clinical history that started with sensorineural hearing loss since the age of 6 years (Fig. 10.16). Her mother died at the age of 54 years: she suffered hearing loss, diabetes, heart and renal failure.

The patient had one miscarriage and a full-term pregnancy with a male child; she developed hypertension, insulin-dependent diabetes mellitus, dyslipidemia and obesity in her young adulthood. At the age of 45 years her ECG showed inferior Q wave and low progression of R wave in septal leads that were not present in prior ECG. The 2D-TTE did not show significant abnormalities; she refused coronary angiography. During the following months her diabetes rapidly worsened with two

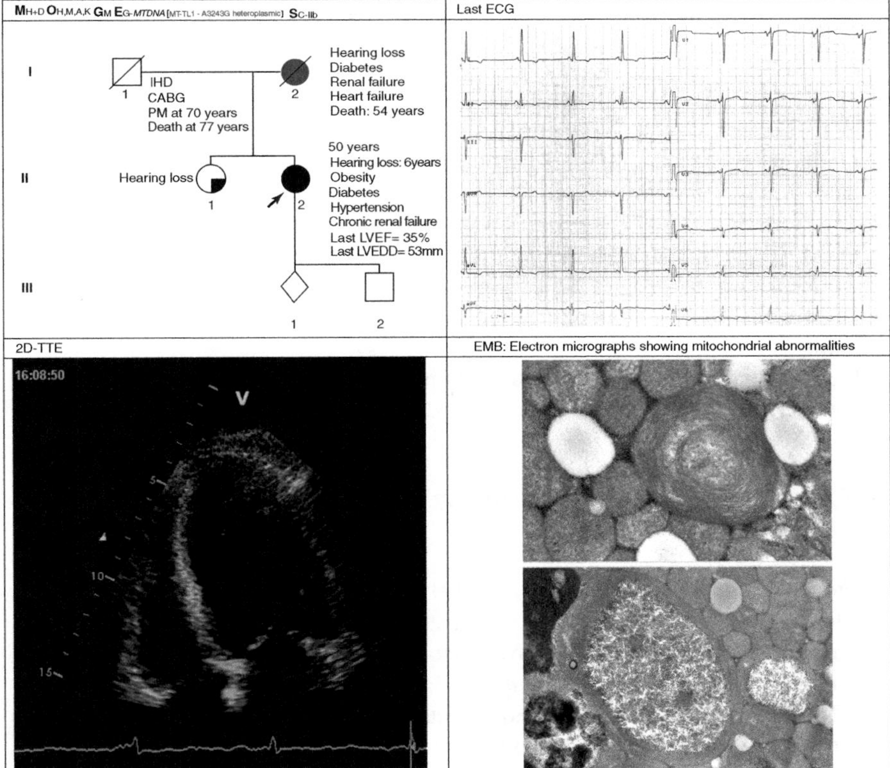

DCM= Dilated Cardiomyopathy; IHD= Ischemic Heart Disease; CABG= Coronary Artery Bypass Graft; TTE= Transthoracic Echocardiography; LVEF= Left Ventricular Ejection Fraction; LVEDD= Left Ventricular End-Diastolic Diameter; EMB= Endomyocardial Biopsy.

Fig. 10.16 Mitochondrial DCM in MELAS

episodes of diabetic coma. She did not complain angina or syncope. She was addressed to our centre for the recent onset dyspnoea on effort (NYHA II). Her ECG showed Q wave in leads D2, D3, aVF, V4–V6 with low progression of R wave from V1 to V6, normal PQ interval (170 ms), slight prolongation of the corrected QT interval (467 ms), and LV overload. Her echocardiogram showed mildly dilated LV (LVEDD = 53 mm), decreased LVEF = 42%, increased LA diameter (45 mm), mild mitral regurgitation, maximal LV thickness = 13 mm; more prominent at the septal level. She was diagnosed with dilated HCM. The genetic testing identified the *MT-TL1*-A3243G heteroplasmic mutation in the mitochondrial DNA. Kidney functional tests demonstrated 2.19 mg/dl creatinin level. Brain Magnetic resonance showed pituitary microadenoma (8 mm): the endocrinologic evaluation excluded functional effects. Coronary angiography showed double vessel disease (ostial left anterior descending artery and 1st marginal branch). The patient is stable in NYHA class IIb. Her son is 18-year-old, asymptomatic, carrier of the maternal mutation with current negative instrumental evaluation.

The above example helps highlighting the key issues in diseases caused by mitochondrial DNA mutations:

- Matrilineal inheritance is characterized by transmission of the *MtDNA* defects from mothers to offspring, both males and females; fathers do not pass down the mutation to offspring. Therefore an *MtDNA* mutation cannot cause cardiomyopathy in a father and his son.
- The phenotype manifestations depend upon the amount of mutated *MtDNA* in the different organs/tissues and by a tissue-specific threshold level, usually around 90%.
- Organs/tissues involvement can vary in different affected members of the same family.
- Prenatal diagnosis is feasible but does not inform about the risk of manifested phenotype.

10.4.2 DCM in Myotonic Dystrophy Type 1 (DM1): Steinert Disease

Myotonic dystrophy type 1 (DM1) (MIM#160900) is the most common adult-onset hereditary muscle disease, with an estimated prevalence around 1:9000 [73]. DM1 is caused by expansion of a CTG trinucleotide repeat in the non-coding region of *Dystrophia Myotonica Protein Kinase* (*DMPK*) *gene*. Myotonic dystrophy type 2 (DM2) is less common and is caused by heterozygous expansion of a CCTG repeat in intron 1 of the zinc finger protein-9 gene (*ZNF9*) (MIM#602668). DM1 is inherited in an autosomal dominant mode. A length exceeding 34 CTG repeats in *DMPK* is abnormal. Molecular genetic testing detects the mutation in nearly 100% of affected individuals. Pathogenic alleles may expand in length during gametogenesis, resulting in the transmission of longer trinucleotide repeat alleles that may be associated with earlier onset and more severe phenotype than that observed in the carrier parent. The carrier parent may not show traits of disease and the DCM can appear as sporadic, especially in small families. Prenatal testing is possible for pregnancies at increased risk when the diagnosis of DM1 has been confirmed by molecular genetic testing in an affected family member. The heart is frequently involved: the most common cardiac manifestation is conduction disease with or without LV dilation and dysfunction. Cardiologists are involved either as consultants in patients with recognised and diagnosed DM1 or as major players in the diagnosis when the disease onset coincides with arrhythmias or AVB and muscle manifestations are still latent or mild and unrecognized.

In the proband shown in Fig. 10.17 the first clinical report is the ECG that was performed at the military service physical exam showing a right bundle branch block (RBBB) (information from the narrative of the patient). During the course of 10 years the patient developed mild muscle weakness, overt signs of myopathy/dystrophy with mild increased sCPK (max = 345 U/L), palpebral ptosis, dysphagia, conduction disease (AVB) and mild DCM. The clinical screening of his relatives

A) "Phenotypically" sporadic, mild DCM with conduction disease	
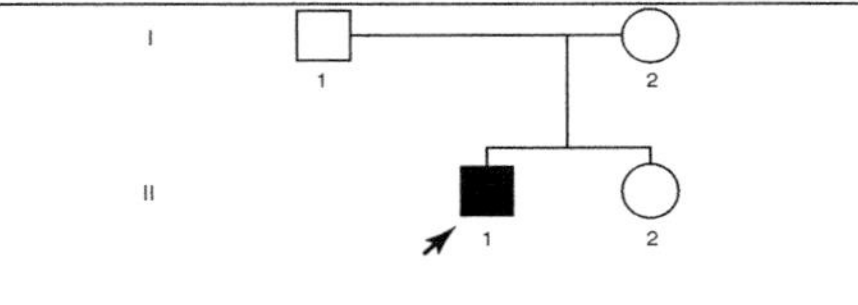 I 1 2 II 1 2	Proband, History • Age = 18 years • First clinical record → military service physical exam: RBBB • 2D-TTE → described as normal
Proband: 28 years → Dysphagia, dysphonia, mildly dilated cardiomyopathy, AVB, muscle weakness; no cataract; premature baldness; no significant endocrine distrurbances; mild increase of sCPK = 252	*DMPK*= E2 allele (500-1000 CTG repeats) *MYH6*[c.4651-3C>A] *KCNA5*[p.Gly63_Pro73del]
Father, 52 years → clinical screening negative; known arterial hypertension; follow-up: LV thickness = 10 mm	*DMPK*= normal allele *MYH6*[c.4651-3C>A]
Mother, 45 years → clinical screening negative; normal sCPK levels; no documented arrhythmias or conduction defects	*DMPK*= ~100-150 CTG repeats) *KCNA5*[p.Gly63_Pro73del]
Sister, 25 years → clinical screening negative	*DMPK*= normal allele *MYH6 and KCNA5 = negative*
Expanded genetic testing: 2 VUS	
$M_{D(AVB)}$ $O_{H,M,GE}$ G_{AD} $E_{G\text{-}DMPK}$ [E2 - 500-1000 CTG]+ *MYH6*[c.4651-3C>A] + *KCNA5*[p.Gly63_Pro73del] $S_{C\text{-}II}$	

RBBB= Right Bundle Branch Block; TTE= Transthoracic Echocardiography; AVB= Atrio-Ventricular Block.

Fig. 10.17 Steinert muscle dystrophy and cardiomyopathy

was negative (both ECG and 2D-TTE); the father was diagnosed with hypertension. The cardiomyopathy looked sporadic. However, genetic testing demonstrated a *DMPK* gene mutation that was inherited from his "phenotypically healthy" mother. Expanded genetic testing identified two additional digenic variants whose impact on the phenotype seemed null, given that both father and mother were phenotypically healthy.

This case gives the opportunity of a few specific considerations:

1. Cardiologists can be involved in the management of the cardiac manifestations in patients with recognized and diagnosed DM1 or when the disease onset coincides with supraventricular and ventricular arrhythmias or AVB and muscular symptoms are still latent or mild and unrecognized.
2. The DCM phenotype can occur as a result of the *DMPK* gene defect or be associated with mutations in genes that typically cause DCM.
3. Both DM1 and DCM are autosomal dominant diseases; genetic testing plays a key role in unravelling the genetic cause of the cardiomyopathy especially when the parent carrier of the expanded allele does not coincide with the one affected by DCM.
4. When *DMPK* defect is isolated, the DCM phenotype usually progresses slowly, and often remains stable for decades. However, the high arrhythmic risk is well known and the ICD implantation for primary prevention of sudden death in DM1 patients is recommended as class IIb, level of evidence B, in 2015 ESC guidelines on primary prevention in cardiomyopathies [39].

10.5 Peripartum Cardiomyopathy (PPCM)

In the Workshop held by the National Heart Lung and Blood Institute and the Office of Rare Diseases (2000) Peripartum cardiomyopathy (PPCM) was defined as a "rare life-threatening cardiomyopathy of unknown cause that occurs in the peripartum period in previously healthy women: diagnosis is confined to a narrow period and requires echocardiographic evidence of LV systolic dysfunction" [74]. According to the ESC, "PPCM is an idiopathic cardiomyopathy presenting with HF secondary to LV systolic dysfunction towards the end of pregnancy or in the months following delivery, where no other cause of HF is found. It is a diagnosis of exclusion". The LV may not be dilated but the ejection fraction is nearly always reduced below 45% [75]. In both definitions the condition is "idiopathic" (no detectable cause of heart failure); the *temporal appearance* is in the last month of pregnancy or during the first 5 months postpartum; *pre-existing known heart disease* is absent; the diagnosis is confirmed by the regression of PPCM within 12 months after delivery [75, 76]. Risk factors for PPCM include advanced age (>30 years), multiparity, African American race, obesity, substance use, preeclampsia, and chronic hypertension [76]. Etiologic hypotheses include familial/genetic predisposition, maladaptive response to hemodynamic stresses of pregnancy, stress-activated cytokines, malnutrition and selenium deficiency, fetal microchimerism, prolactin, and prolonged tocolysis [77]. Genetic hypothesis is supported by a recent study reporting truncation-predicting variants in *Titin* gene in PPCM (15%) (vs. 17% in DCM) [60]. The hemodynamic changes in the last trimester of pregnancy may contribute to unmask an underlying asymptomatic genetic disease, either absent or unrecognized before pregnancy and delivery.

Figure 10.18 shows two paradigmatic examples of women diagnosed with PPCM, all fulfilling current diagnostic criteria for PPCM. The two cases deserve a few and different considerations:

10.5.1 Case A

The proband was incidentally diagnosed with atrial fibrillation (AF) at the age of 34 years. After many unsuccessful attempts to restore sinus rhythm (medical therapy, shocks, ablations) the chronic AF was treated with amiodarone and warfarin. The LV function and dimensions were normal. However, 10 years later she experienced cardiac arrest that was successfully resuscitated. She developed third degree AVB and she underwent PM-ICD implantation. She received an ICD shock in response to ventricular tachycardia. Cardiologic investigations included 2D-TTE that demonstrated severe LV dysfunction and dilation with enlarged left atrium; coronary angiography showed normal coronary arteries. She underwent heart transplantation 11 years after the onset of the first AF episode.

Considerations:

- The maternal history was underestimated. In fact the mother had died at the age of 26 years, 15 days after delivery (die in childbirth), an event that was considered a non-preventable misfortune. The poorly informative medical reports after

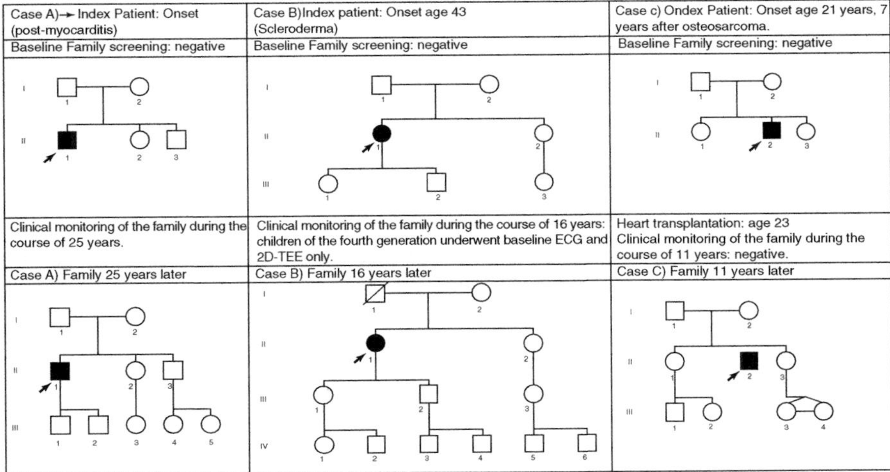

Case A)→ Index Patient: Onset (post-myocarditis)
Baseline Family screening: negative
Case B)Index patient: Onset age 43 (Scleroderma)
Baseline Family screening: negative
Case c) Ondex Patient: Onset age 21 years, 7 years after osteosarcoma.
Baseline Family screening: negative
Clinical monitoring of the family during the course of 25 years.
Case A) Family 25 years later
Clinical monitoring of the family during the course of 16 years: children of the fourth generation underwent baseline ECG and 2D-TEE only.
Case B) Family 16 years later
Heart transplantation: age 23
Clinical monitoring of the family during the course of 11 years: negative.
Case C) Family 11 years later

Fig. 10.18 Peripartum cardiomyopathy: often the pregnancy unmasks pre-existing asymptomatic cardiomyopathy

discharge from the obstetric department only described lower limb oedema that was attributed to the delivery and construed as liable to spontaneous resolution.

- The genetic test performed in the proband demonstrated a truncating protein mutation in the *LMNA* gene. The gene tested negative in the father, who is alive and well. Although likely, we cannot demonstrate that the mother was carrier of the same mutation. The maternal family is small and non-informative thus preventing extension of family screening to maternal relatives.
- The open question is whether an earlier diagnosis could have modified the evolution of the disease. For sure the timely identification of the cardiac laminopathy would have led to ICD implantation before the cardiac arrest.

10.5.2 Case B

After the acute onset of HF a few days after delivery, the LV function partially recovered and the patient was regularly followed-up and optimally treated for 15 years. During this long period of time the clinical conditions were stable. The relapse was with acute pulmonary oedema; the LV function was severely depressed; an ICD was implanted in primary prevention without discharge during the course of 12 months, when no significant improvement of the LV function was achieved and the patient was addressed to HTx.

This case gives a few considerations:

1. The paternal family history was ignored: he suffered chronic renal failure and DCM that was attributed to juvenile malignant arterial hypertension. The paternal uncle (II:2) had died for the consequences of a stroke (probably, but not

proven) triggered by atrial fibrillation; his son had died suddenly, shortly after a medical examination (only including ECG, Chest X-ray and clinical evaluation) for recent palpitations and chest pain attributed to stress and suspected thyroid dysfunction (biochemical tests had been planned but not performed): medical reports describe mildly increased cardiac shadow and a few PVC and RBBB. The cause of death was attributed to acute myocardial infarction but autopsy was not performed.

2. The diagnosis of PPCM in the proband was typical in terms of closeness to delivery, systolic dysfunction and absence of heart disease before pregnancy. A possible genetic cause was not suspected. The baseline cardiac evaluation before pregnancy was not available and the possible presence of asymptomatic DCM is unknown. The only pre-delivery cardiologic test was an ECG that did not show significant abnormalities. The cascade of cardiac events led to heart transplantation 15 years after the onset of symptoms.
3. Today, the increasing awareness of familial DCM would probably modify the interpretation of the cause of the DCM; the family history would be considered as a warning and the patient would undergo cardiology evaluation including ECG and 2D-TTE. This would provide a baseline evaluation that could either demonstrate a clinically silent DCM or a normally sized and functioning LV and therefore support the hypothesis of PPCM.

10.6 Non-Genetic DCM

Non-genetic DCM (Fig. 10.19) includes autoimmune, inflammatory and toxic forms [1–3, 15, 26]. The role of genetic defects should be theoretically excluded. However, the etiologic scenario of the autoimmune and inflammatory diseases is rapidly evolving. In the past, the etiologic basis of non-genetic DCM was considered to be polygenic or multifactorial. However, new discoveries now demonstrate that, in an increasing proportion of these diseases, the causes are genetic frequently affecting the Interleukin pathway [78].

The diagnostic work-up of post-inflammatory and autoimmune/immune-mediated DCM is extensively described in the recent document of the Working Group on Myocardial and Pericardial Diseases of the ESC [79]. The clinical phenotype of patient with DCM phenotype caused by infectious, autoimmune and toxic noxae should be entirely sustained by the given causes. The follow-up of index patients and families is, once again, a robust contributor to the evidence that relatives do not develop the disease. A major confirmatory role of the correct interpretation of the acquired cause of DCM is the long-term follow-up of the families. The three examples in Fig. 10.19 give an immediate view on how the long-term monitoring of the family (demonstrating that the disease does not appear in relatives of the index patient) confirms the non-genetic origin of the disease.

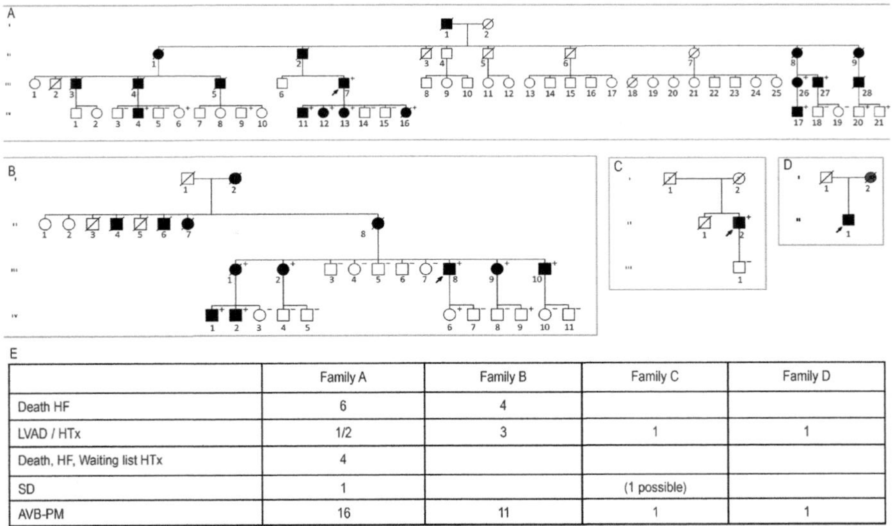

	Family A	Family B	Family C	Family D
Death HF	6	4		
LVAD / HTx	1/2	3	1	1
Death, HF, Waiting list HTx	4			
SD	1		(1 possible)	
AVB-PM	16	11	1	1

Fig. 10.19 Nongenetic DCM: long-term follow-up in families contributes to confirm the nongenetic origin of the DCM

Conclusions

Although DCM can be grouped mechanistically as genetic and non-genetic, most DCMs are familial diseases with heterogeneous genetic causes. Mutations in more than 100 disease genes playing in different pathways are associated with a similar end-cardiac phenotype: LV dilation and dysfunction. The precise diagnosis (identification of the cause) starts with clinical hypothesis that should be generated on the basis of deep phenotyping of the proband and family, clinical history and pathology investigations. Clinical family screening is often sufficient to clinically diagnose familial DCM. Genetic test is first performed in probands and then followed by cascade family screening, when gene mutations or variants are identified. Segregation studies in families are major contributors to the assignment of a causative role of the mutation in the family. Pathologic studies or in vitro tests can further add information on the potential functional effects of the mutations on the expression of the mutated protein.

Acknowledgements Research on heritable cardiomyopathies has been supported by grants from European Union INHERITANCE project #241924 and by the Italian Ministry of Health "Diagnosis and Treatment of Hypertrophic Cardiomyopathies" (#RF-PSM-2008-1145809) to Dr. Arbustini, IRCCS Policlinico San Matteo, Pavia; E-Rare Project 2014 OSM–Dilated Cardiomyopathies to Dr. Serio. Patients and families are supported by the Charity MAGICA (MAlattie GenetIche CArdiovascolari).

References

1. Elliott P, Andersson B, Arbustini E, et al. Classification of the cardiomyopathies: a position statement from the European Society Of Cardiology Working Group on Myocardial and Pericardial Diseases. Eur Heart J. 2008;29:270–6.
2. Maron BJ, Towbin JA, Thiene G, et al. Contemporary definitions and classification of the cardiomyopathies: an American Heart Association Scientific Statement from the Council on Clinical Cardiology, Heart Failure and Transplantation Committee; Quality of Care and Outcomes Research and Functional Genomics and Translational Biology Interdisciplinary Working Groups; and Council on Epidemiology and Prevention. American Heart Association; Council on Clinical Cardiology, Heart Failure and Transplantation Committee; Quality of Care and Outcomes Research and Functional Genomics and Translational Biology Interdisciplinary Working Groups; Council on Epidemiology and Prevention. Circulation. 2006;113: 1807–16.
3. Bozkurt B, Colvin M, Cook J, et al. Current diagnostic and treatment strategies for specific dilated cardiomyopathies: a scientific statement from the American Heart Association. Circulation. 2016;134:579–646.
4. Pinto YM, Elliott PM, Arbustini E, et al. Proposal for a revised definition of dilated cardiomyopathy, hypokinetic non-dilated cardiomyopathy, and its implications for clinical practice: a position statement of the ESC. Eur Heart J. 2016;37:1850–8.
5. Favalli V, Serio A, Grasso M, Arbustini E. Genetic causes of dilated cardiomyopathy. Heart. 2016;102:2004–14.
6. Codd MB, Sugrue DD, Gersh BJ, et al. Epidemiology of idiopathic dilated and hypertrophic cardiomyopathy. A population-based study in Olmsted County, Minnesota, 1975–1984. Circulation. 1989;80:564–72.
7. Morales A, Hershberger RE. Genetic evaluation of dilated cardiomyopathy. Curr Cardiol Rep. 2013;15:375.
8. Baig MK, Goldman JH, Caforio AL, et al. Familial dilated cardiomyopathy: cardiac abnormalities are common in asymptomatic relatives and may represent early disease. J Am Coll Cardiol. 1998;31:195–201.
9. Gruenig E, Tasman JA, Kuecherer H, et al. Frequency and phenotypes of familial dilated cardiomyopathy. J Am Coll Cardiol. 1998;31:186–94.
10. Gavazzi A, Repetto A, Scelsi L, et al. Evidence-based diagnosis of familial non-X-linked dilated cardiomyopathy. Prevalence, inheritance and characteristics. Eur Heart J. 2001;22:73–81.
11. Crispell KA, Hanson EL, Coates K, et al. Periodic rescreening is indicated for family members at risk of developing familial dilated cardiomyopathy. J Am Coll Cardiol. 2002;39: 1503–7.
12. Michels VV, Olson TM, Miller FA, et al. Frequency of development of idiopathic dilated cardiomyopathy among relatives of patients with idiopathic dilated cardiomyopathy. Am J Cardiol. 2003;91:1389–92.
13. Repetto A, Serio A, Pasotti M, et al. Rescreening of "healthy" relatives of patients with dilated cardiomyopathy identifies subgroups at risk of developing the disease. Eur Heart J Suppl. 2004;6:F54–60.
14. Mahon NG, Murphy RT, MacRae CA, et al. Echocardiographic evaluation in asymptomatic relatives of patients with dilated cardiomyopathy reveals preclinical disease. Ann Intern Med. 2005;143:108–15.
15. Arbustini E, Narula N, Dec GW, et al. The MOGE(S) classification for a phenotype-genotype nomenclature of cardiomyopathy: endorsed by the World Heart Federation. J Am Coll Cardiol. 2014;64:304–18.
16. Haas J, Frese KS, Peil B, et al. Atlas of the clinical genetics of human dilated cardiomyopathy. Eur Heart J. 2015;36:1123–35a.
17. Brodt C, Siegfried JD, Hofmeyer M, et al. Temporal relationship of conduction system disease and ventricular dysfunction in LMNA cardiomyopathy. J Card Fail. 2013;19:233–9.

18. Charron P, Arad M, Arbustini E, et al. Genetic counselling and testing in cardiomyopathies: a position statement of the European Society of Cardiology Working Group on Myocardial and Pericardial Diseases. Eur Heart J. 2010;31:2715–26.
19. Rapezzi C, Arbustini E, Caforio ALP, et al. Diagnostic work-up in cardiomyopathies: bridging the gap between clinical phenotypes and final diagnosis. A position statement from the ESC Working Group on Myocardial and Pericardial Diseases. Eur Heart J. 2013;34:1448–58.
20. Repetto A, Dal Bello B, Pasotti M, et al. Coronary atherosclerosis in end-stage idiopathic dilated cardiomyopathy: an innocent bystander? Eur Heart J. 2005;26:1519–27.
21. Barison A, Grigoratos C, Todiere G, Aquaro GD. Myocardial interstitial remodelling in non-ischaemic dilated cardiomyopathy: insights from cardiovascular magnetic resonance. Heart Fail Rev. 2015;20:731–49.
22. Tsuburaya RS, Uchizumi H, Ueda M, et al. Utility of real-time three-dimensional echocardiography for Duchenne muscular dystrophy with echocardiographic limitations. Neuromuscul Disord. 2014;24:402–8.
23. Jenkins C, Moir S, Chan J, Rakhit D, Haluska B, Marwick TH. Left ventricular volume measurement with echocardiography: a comparison of left ventricular opacification, three-dimensional echocardiography, or both with magnetic resonance imaging. Eur Heart J. 2009;30:98–106.
24. Mada RO, Lysyansky P, Daraban AM, Duchenne J, Voigt JU. How to define end-diastole and end-systole?: impact of timing on strain measurements. JACC Cardiovasc Imaging. 2015;8:148–57.
25. Moody WE, Taylor RJ, Edwards NC, et al. Comparison of magnetic resonance feature tracking for systolic and diastolic strain and strain rate calculation with spatial modulation of magnetization imaging analysis. J Magn Reson Imaging. 2015;41:1000–12.
26. Arbustini E, Narula N, Tavazzi L, et al. The MOGE(S) classification of cardiomyopathy for clinicians. J Am Coll Cardiol. 2014;64:304–18.
27. McNally EM, Golbus JR, Puckelwartz MJ. Genetic mutations and mechanisms in dilated cardiomyopathy. J Clin Invest. 2013;123:19–26.
28. Wolf CM, Wang L, Alcalai R, et al. Lamin A/C haploinsufficiency causes dilated cardiomyopathy and apoptosis-triggered cardiac conduction system disease. J Mol Cell Cardiol. 2008;44:293–303.
29. Narula N, Favalli V, Tarantino P, et al. Quantitative expression of the mutated lamin A/C gene in patients with cardiolaminopathy. J Am Coll Cardiol. 2012;60:1916–20.
30. Wahbi K. Cardiac involvement in dystrophinopathies. Arch Pediatr. 2015;22:12S37–41.
31. Moore JR, Leinwand L, Warshaw DM. Understanding cardiomyopathy phenotypes based on the functional impact of mutations in the myosin motor. Circ Res. 2012;111:375–85.
32. Mogensen J, van Tintelen JP, Fokstuen S, et al. The current role of next-generation DNA sequencing in routine care of patients with hereditary cardiovascular conditions: a viewpoint paper of the European Society of Cardiology working group on myocardial and pericardial diseases and members of the European Society of Human Genetics. Eur Heart J. 2015;36:1367–70.
33. Zaragoza MV, Fass J, Diegoli M, Lin D, Arbustini E. Mitochondrial DNA variant discovery and evaluation in human Cardiomyopathies through next-generation sequencing. PLoS One. 2010;5:e12295.
34. Hershberger RE, Hedges DJ, Morales A. Dilated cardiomyopathy: the complexity of a diverse genetic architecture. Nat Rev Cardiol. 2013;10:531–47.
35. Hinson JT, Chopra A, Nafissi N, et al. HEART DISEASE. Titin mutations in iPS cells define sarcomere insufficiency as a cause of dilated cardiomyopathy. Science. 2015;349:982–6.
36. Dobrzynska A, Gonzalo S, Shanahan C, Askjaer P. The nuclear lamina in health and disease. Nucleus. 2016;7:233–48.
37. Parks SB, Kushner JD, Nauman D, Ludwigsen S, Peterson A, Li D, Litt M, Porter CB, Rahko PS. Lamin A/C mutation analysis in a cohort of 324 unrelated patients with idiopathic or familial dilated cardiomyopathy. Am Heart J. 2009;156:161–9.
38. Van Rijsingen IA, Arbustini E, Elliott PM, Mogensen J, Hermans-van Ast JF, van der Kooi AJ, van Tintelen JP, van den Berg MP, Pilotto A, Pasotti M, Jenkins S, Rowland C, Aslam U, Wilde

AA, Perrot A, Pankuweit S, Zwinderman AH, Charron P, Pinto YM. Risk factors for malignant ventricular arrhythmias in lamin a/c mutation carriers a European cohort study. J Am Coll Cardiol. 2012;59:493–500.

39. Priori SG, Blomström-Lundqvist C, Mazzanti A, Blom N, Borggrefe M, Camm J, Elliott PM, Fitzsimons D, Hatala R, Hindricks G, Kirchhof P, Kjeldsen K, Kuck KH, Hernandez-Madrid A, Nikolaou N, Norekvål TM, Spaulding C, Van Veldhuisen DJ. 2015 ESC Guidelines for the management of patients with ventricular arrhythmias and the prevention of sudden cardiac death: The Task Force for the Management of Patients with Ventricular Arrhythmias and the Prevention of Sudden Cardiac Death of the European Society of Cardiology (ESC). Endorsed by: Association for European Paediatric and Congenital Cardiology (AEPC). Eur Heart J. 2015;36:2793–867.
40. Finsterer J, Stöllberger C, Sehnal E, Rehder H, Laccone F. Dilated, arrhythmogenic cardiomyopathy in emery-dreifuss muscular dystrophy due to the emerinsplice-site mutation c.449+1G>A. Cardiology. 2015;130:48–51.
41. Sakata K, Shimizu M, Ino H, Yamaguchi M, Terai H, Fujino N, Hayashi K, Kaneda T, Inoue M, Oda Y, Fujita T, Kaku B, Kanaya H, Mabuchi H. High incidence of sudden cardiac death with conduction disturbances and atrial cardiomyopathy caused by a nonsense mutation in the STA gene. Circulation. 2005;111:3352–8.
42. Kamdar F, Garry DJ. Dystrophin-deficient cardiomyopathy. J Am Coll Cardiol. 2016;67:2533–46.
43. Diegoli M, Grasso M, Favalli V, et al. Diagnostic work-up and risk stratification in X-linked dilated cardiomyopathies caused by dystrophin defects. J Am Coll Cardiol. 2011;58:925–34.
44. Kimura S, Ikezawa M, Ozasa S, et al. Novel mutation in splicing donor of dystrophin gene first exon in a patient with dilated cardiomyopathy but no clinical signs of skeletal myopathy. J Child Neurol. 2007;22:901–6.
45. Knöll R, Buyandelger B, Lab M. The sarcomeric Z-disc and Z-discopathies. J Biomed Biotechnol. 2011;2011:569628.
46. Vatta M, Mohapatra B, Jimenez S, Sanchez X, Faulkner G, Perles Z, Sinagra G, Lin JH, TM V, Zhou Q, Bowles KR, Di Lenarda A, Schimmenti L, Fox M, Chrisco MA, Murphy RT, McKenna W, Elliott P, Bowles NE, Chen J, Valle G, Towbin JA. Mutations in Cypher/ZASP in patients with dilated cardiomyopathy and left ventricular non-compaction. J Am Coll Cardiol. 2003;42:2014–27.
47. Levitas A, Konstantino Y, Muhammad E, et al. D117N in Cypher/ZASP may not be a causative mutation for dilated cardiomyopathy and ventricular arrhythmias. Eur J Hum Genet. 2016;24:666–71.
48. Hassel D, Dahme T, Erdmann J, Meder B, Huge A, Stoll M, Just S, Hess A, Ehlermann P, Weichenhan D, Grimmler M, Liptau H, Hetzer R, Regitz-Zagrosek V, Fischer C, Nürnberg P, Schunkert H, Katus HA, Rottbauer W. Nexilin mutations destabilize cardiac Z-disks and lead to dilated cardiomyopathy. Nat Med. 2009;15:1281–8.
49. Haghighi K, Kolokathis F, Gamolini AO, et al. A mutation in the human phospholamban gene, deleting arginine 14, results in lethal, hereditary cardiomyopathy. Proc Nat Acad Sci. 2006;103:1388–93.
50. Minamisawa S, Sato Y, Tatsuguchi Y, et al. Mutation of the phospholamban promoter associated with hypertrophic cardiomyopathy. Biochem Biophys Res Commun. 2003;304:1–4.
51. Van der Zwaag PA, van Rijsingen IA, Asimaki A, et al. Phospholamban R14del mutation in patients diagnosed with dilated cardiomyopathy or arrhythmogenic right ventricular cardiomyopathy: evidence supporting the concept of arrhythmogenic cardiomyopathy. Eur J Heart Fail. 2012;14:1199–207.
52. Groeneweg JA, van der Zwaag PA, Olde Nordkamp LR, et al. Arrhythmogenic right ventricular dysplasia/cardiomyopathy according to revised 2010 task force criteria with inclusion of non-desmosomal phospholamban mutation carriers. Am J Cardiol. 2013;112:1197–206.
53. Sanoudou D, Kolokathis F, Arvanitis D, et al. Genetic modifiers to the PLN L39X mutation in a patient with DCM and sustained ventricular tachycardia? Glob Cardiol Sci Pract. 2015;2015:29.

54. Liu GS, Morales A, Vafiadaki E, et al. A novel human R25C-phospholamban mutation is associated with super-inhibition of calcium cycling and ventricular arrhythmia. Cardiovasc Res. 2015;107:164–74.
55. Spudich JA, Aksel T, Bartholomew SR, et al. Effects of hypertrophic and dilated cardiomyopathy mutations on power output by human β-cardiac myosin. J Exp Biol. 2016;219:161–7.
56. Arbustini E, Fasani R, Morbini P, et al. Coexistence of mitochondrial DNA and beta myosin heavy chain mutations in hypertrophic cardiomyopathy with late congestive heart failure. Heart. 1998;80:548–58.
57. Daehmlow S, Erdmann J, Knueppel T, Gille C, Froemmel C, Hummel M, Hetzer R, Regitz-Zagrosek V. Novel mutations in sarcomeric protein genes in dilated cardiomyopathy. Biochem Biophys Res Commun. 2002;298:116–20.
58. Chauveau C, Rowell J, Ferreiro A. A rising titan: TTN review and mutation update. Hum Mutat. 2014;35:1046–59.
59. Herman DS, Lam L, Taylor MRG, et al. Truncations of titin causing dilated cardiomyopathy. N Engl J Med. 2012;366:619–28.
60. Ware JS, Li J, Mazaika E, IMAC-2 and IPAC Investigators. Shared genetic predisposition in peripartum and dilated cardiomyopathies. N Engl J Med. 2016;374:233–41.
61. Hackman P, Marchand S, Sarparanta J, et al. Truncating mutations in C-terminal titin may cause more severe tibial muscular dystrophy (TMD). Neuromuscul Disord. 2008;18:922–8.
62. Hackman P, Vihola A, Haravuori H, et al. Tibial muscular dystrophy is a titinopathy caused by mutations in TTN, the gene encoding the giant skeletal-muscle protein titin. Am J Hum Genet. 2002;71:492–500.
63. Carmignac V, Salih MA, Quijano-Roy S, et al. C-terminal titin deletions cause a novel early-onset myopathy with fatal cardiomyopathy. Ann Neurol. 2007;61:340–51.
64. Akinrinade O, Koskenvuo JW, Alastalo TP. Prevalence of titin truncating variants in general population. PLoS One. 2015;10:e0145284.
65. Gramlich M, Pane LS, Zhou Q, et al. Antisense-mediated exon skipping: a therapeutic strategy for titin-based dilated cardiomyopathy. EMBO Mol Med. 2015;7:562–76.
66. Purevjav E, Varela J, Morgado M, et al. Nebulette mutations are associated with dilated cardiomyopathy and endocardial fibroelastosis. J Am Coll Cardiol. 2010;56:1493–502.
67. Perrot A, Tomasov P, Villard E, et al. Mutations in NEBL encoding the cardiac Z-disk protein nebulette are associated with various cardiomyopathies. Arch Med Sci. 2016;12:263–78.
68. Arimura T, Nakamura T, Hiroi S, et al. Characterization of the human nebulette gene: a polymorphism in an actin-binding motif is associated with nonfamilial idiopathic dilated cardiomyopathy. Hum Genet. 2000;107:440–51.
69. Todorova A, Halliger-Keller B, Walter MC, Dabauvalle MC, Lochmüller H, Müller CR. A synonymous codon change in the LMNA gene alters mRNA splicing and causes limb girdle muscular dystrophy type 1B. J Med Genet. 2003;40:e115.
70. Marcus FI, McKenna WJ, Sherrill D, et al. Diagnosis of arrhythmogenic right ventricular cardiomyopathy/dysplasia: proposed modification of the Task Force Criteria. Eur Heart J. 2010;31:806–14.
71. Corrado D, Basso C, Thiene G. Is it time to include ion channel diseases among cardiomyopathies? J Electrocardiol. 2005;38(4 Suppl):81–7.
72. Brunel-Guitton C, Levtova A, Sasarman F. Mitochondrial diseases and cardiomyopathies. Can J Cardiol. 2015;31:1360–76.
73. Hermans MC, Faber CG, Bekkers SC, et al. Structural and functional cardiac changes in myotonic dystrophy type 1: a cardiovascular magnetic resonance study. J Cardiovasc Magn Reson. 2012 Jul 24;14:48.
74. Pearson GD, Veille JC, Rahimtoola S, et al. Peripartum cardiomyopathy: National Heart, Lung, and Blood Institute and Office of Rare Diseases (National Institutes of Health) workshop recommendations and review. JAMA. 2000;283:1183–8.
75. Sliwa K, Hilfiker-Kleiner D, Petrie MC, Heart Failure Association of the European Society of Cardiology Working Group on Peripartum Cardiomyopathy. Current state of knowledge on aetiology, diagnosis, management, and therapy of peripartum cardiomyopathy: a position

statement from the Heart Failure Association of the European Society of Cardiology Working Group on peripartum cardiomyopathy. Eur J Heart Fail. 2010;12:767–78.
76. Kolte D, Khera S, Aronow WS, et al. Temporal trends in incidence and outcomes of peripartum cardiomyopathy in the United States: a nationwide population-based study. J Am Heart Assoc. 2014;3:e001056.
77. Grixti S, Magri CJ, Xuereb R, Fava S. Peripartum cardiomyopathy. Br J Hosp Med (Lond). 2015;76:95–100.
78. Pathak S, McDermott MF, Savic S. Autoinflammatory diseases: update on classification diagnosis and management. J Clin Pathol. 2017;70:1–8.
79. Caforio AL, Pankuweit S, Arbustini E, et al. Current state of knowledge on aetiology, diagnosis, management, and therapy of myocarditis: a position statement of the European Society of Cardiology Working Group on Myocardial and Pericardial Diseases. Eur Heart J. 2013;34:2636–48.

Inherited Cardiac Muscle Disorders: Arrhythmogenic Right Ventricular Cardiomyopathy

11

Kalliopi Pilichou, Barbara Bauce, Gaetano Thiene, and Cristina Basso

Abstract

Arrhythmogenic Cardiomyopathy (AC) is characterized by cardiomyocyte death with fibro-fatty repair, clinically manifesting with palpitations, syncope or cardiac arrest usually in adolescence or young adulthood. AC represents one of the major causes of sudden death in the young and athletes. The estimated prevalence of AC in the general population ranges from 1:2000 to 1:5000. AC affects more frequently males than females (up to 3:1), despite a similar prevalence of carrier status, and due to age-related penetrance becomes clinically overt most often in the second-fourth decade of life.

Keywords

Arrhythmogenic cardiomyopathy • Sudden death • Genetics • Heart failure Implantable cardioverter defibrillator

11.1 Introduction

Arrhythmogenic Cardiomyopathy (AC) is characterized by cardiomyocyte death with fibro-fatty repair, clinically manifesting with palpitations, syncope or cardiac arrest usually in adolescence or young adulthood [1–5]. AC represents one of the major causes of sudden death in the young and athletes [1, 6, 7]. The estimated prevalence of AC in the general population ranges from 1:2000 to 1:5000 [3, 5]. AC

K. Pilichou (✉) • B. Bauce • G. Thiene • C. Basso
Department of Cardiac, Thoracic and Vascular Sciences, Pathological Anatomy-Cardiovascular Pathology, University of Padua Medical School, Padua, Italy

Cardio-Thoracic and Vascular Sciences, Policlinico Universitario di Padova, Padova, Italy
e-mail: kalliopi.pilichou@unipd.it

D. Kumar, P. Elliott (eds.), *Cardiovascular Genetics and Genomics*,
https://doi.org/10.1007/978-3-319-66114-8_11

affects more frequently males than females (up to 3:1), despite a similar prevalence of carrier status, and due to age-related penetrance becomes clinically overt most often in the second-fourth decade of life [3, 5].

Advances in DNA sequencing have led to the identification of more than ten disease-causative genes associated with AC. Nearly half of AC-patients harbor mutations in genes encoding desmosomal proteins and less than 1% carry mutations in non-desmosomal genes [7].

A familial background consistent with an autosomal-dominant trait of inheritance is described in 50% of AC-patients, even if recessive variants have also been reported, either associated or not with palmoplantar keratosis and woolly hair. The inheritance pattern of AC is more complex than previously appreciated, with frequent requirement for more than one mutation for fully penetrant disease. Compound/digenic heterozygosity was identified in up to 25% of AC-causing desmosomal gene mutation carriers, explaining in part the phenotypic variability.

In the era of Next Generation Sequencing (NGS), parallel analysis of thousand genes is feasible and many rare variants can be detected, so the challenge is to distinguish causative mutations from the genetic noise since genetic testing.

11.2 Major Clinical and Pathologic Features

11.2.1 Clinical Case 1

20-year-old soccer player died suddenly while watching a game with friends at home [8]. At annual preparticipation screening, electrocardiogram (ECG) was normal with consequent sport eligibility (Fig. 11.1a). History for juvenile sudden death and hypertrophic cardiomyopathy was reported on the mother's side of the family. Postmortem examination of the heart showed normal dimensions (weight, 347 g; wall thicknesses of left ventricle (LV) and septum 13 mm and right ventricle (RV), 3 mm), in the absence of aneurysms or chamber dilatation; a subepicardial scar-like grey rim was evident in the anterolateral and posterior LV free wall and in the septum (Fig. 11.1b).

Coronary arteries had a normal origin and course, with patent lumen. Histological examination revealed extensive subepicardial and intramural fibrous replacement with scarce fatty tissue infiltration, involving the entire LV circumference and the septum (Fig. 11.1c). Right ventricular involvement was only focally detected, in the anterior wall. The features were in keeping with either chronic myocarditis or left-dominant AC.

At postmortem, molecular pathology investigation by polymerase chain reaction ruled out the presence of viral genomes in the myocardium. Genetic testing of all AC-related genes was performed on DNA isolated from frozen tissue sample. A heterozygous nonsense mutation of desmoplakin (DSP) at position c.448C>T in exon 4, resulting in a premature stop codon and truncation (p.Arg150Stop) at the N-terminal domain of the protein, was detected in the proband (Fig. 11.1d). All family members underwent genetic screening that identified the same DSP mutation in the 54-year-old father and the 19-year old sister. Interestingly, the father appeared to be the first mutation carrier in the family, suggesting a dominant de novo mutation.

The 54-year-old asymptomatic father showed low QRS voltages and a single premature ventricular complex (PVC) with a left bundle branch block (LBBB) pattern at 12-lead ECG; signal-averaged ECG was positive at 2 filters (40 and 80 Hz). Echocardiography was normal, whereas cine cardiac magnetic resonance (CMR) showed anterolateral RV dyskinesia; LV posterolateral late enhancement (LE) was evident on contrast enhanced (CE)–CMR.

The 19-year-old sister has been followed-up since the age of 9 for idiopathic ventricular arrhythmias (PVCs with an LBBB pattern) discovered at preparticipation screening. Pharmacological therapy was undertaken with solatol (50 mg × 2). Low QRS voltage, inverted T wave in lead V1, incomplete right bundle branch block, and a nonpathological Q wave in inferior leads were found; late potentials were absent at all filters. Frequent PVCs (>500/24 h) were detected at Holter monitoring.

Echocardiography was normal; cine-CMR showed subtricuspid and RV outflow tract dyskinesia; CE-CMR revealed circumferential subepicardial LV LE. Both father and sister reached a borderline AC diagnosis according to the 2010 Task Force Criteria-TFC [9]. However, LV LE at CE-CMR and low QRS voltages in the peripheral leads on ECG were highly suggestive for a left-dominant form of AC, and an implantable cardioverter defibrillator was recommended.

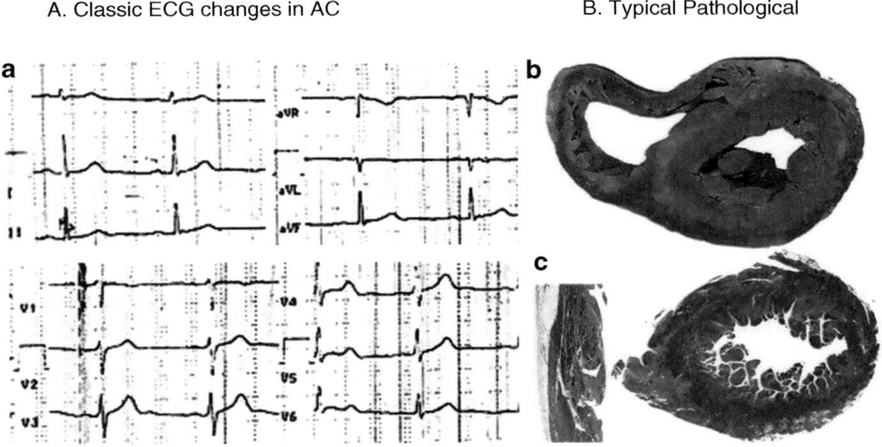

Fig. 11.1 (**a**) Basal 12-lead ECG at annual preparticipation screening showing normal findings. (**b**) Transverse section of the heart showing a subepicardial scar-like grey rim in the anterolateral and posterior LV free wall and in the septum, in the absence of wall thinning and aneurysm formation. (**c**) Histological examination revealed focal RV involvement (on the left) and extensive circumferential, subepicardial, and intramural fibrous replacement of the LV free wall (on the right). LV indicates left ventricle; and RV, right ventricle. (**d**) Family pedigree with autosomal dominant inheritance of the disease of a denovo mutation. Squares = male sex, circles = female sex, arrow = proband. Black squares/circles = mutation carriers, DSP = desmoplakin. PVC = premature ventricular complexes

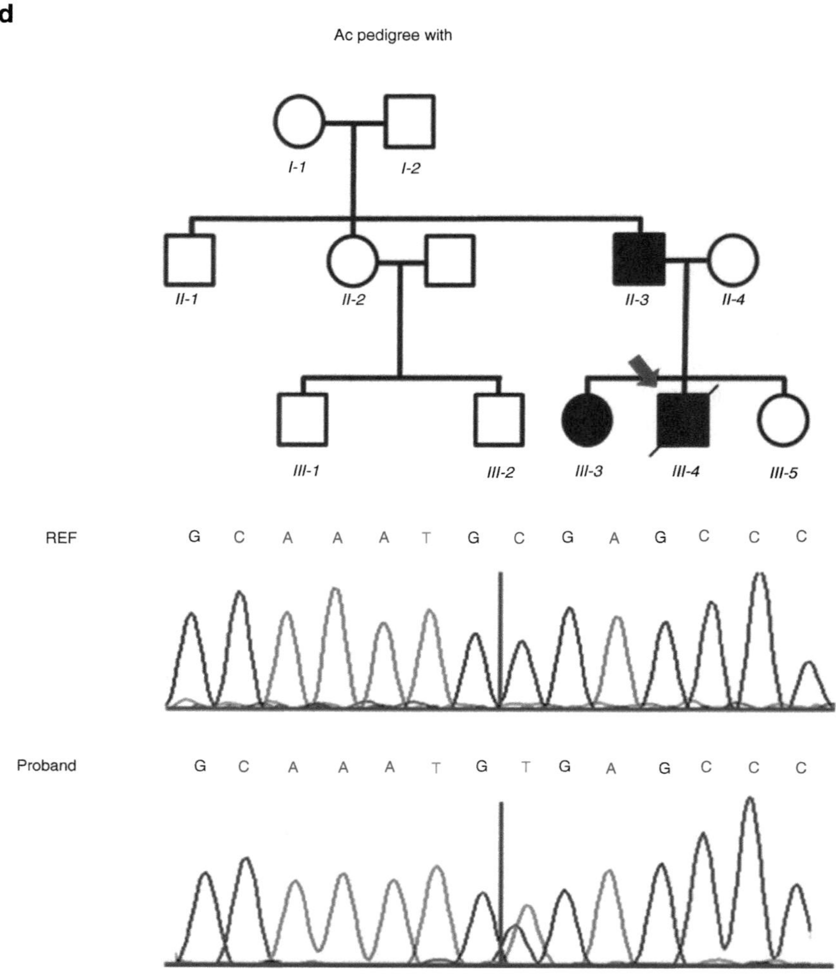

Fig. 11.1 (continued)

Outcome Autopsy including postmortem genetic test allowed a final diagnosis of left-dominant AC as cause of sudden death. As such, it was the starting point for cascade genetic screening of the family members and cardiological workup, including CE-CMR in mutation carriers, despite the absence of morphofunctional abnormalities at 2-dimensional echocardiography. These data further highlight the importance of comprehensive genetic screening, the limitations of 2010 TFC criteria for LV AC and the fundamental role of CE-CMR in achieving the correct diagnosis in gene mutation carriers.

11.2.2 Pathological Features

AC is a "structural" cardiomyopathy characterized by the replacement of the ventricular myocardium by fibro-fatty tissue [1, 2]. Myocardial atrophy occurs progressively with time, starts from the epicardium and eventually extends down to reach the endocardium as to become transmural. This entity should not be confused with Uhl's disease, a congenital heart defect in which the RV myocardium fails to develop during embryonic life [10, 11]. The gross pathognomonic features of AC consist of RV aneurysms, whether single or multiple, located in the so-called "triangle of dysplasia" (i.e. inflow, apex and outflow tract) [2]. Up to 76% of the AC hearts studied at post-mortem revealed isolated or predominant LV involvement, usually limited to the subepicardium or midmural layers of the postero-lateral free wall [2, 4, 12]. Hearts with end-stage disease and congestive heart failure exhibit multiple RV aneurysms, thinning of the RV free wall and huge chamber dilatation, with a high prevalence of biventricular involvement, while the ventricular septum is mostly spared [2].

Histological examination reveals islands of surviving myocytes, interspersed with fibrous and fatty tissue [1, 2]. Fatty infiltration of the RV is not a sufficient morphologic hallmark of AC [13] and replacement-type fibrosis and myocyte degenerative changes should be always searched for. Myocyte necrosis is seldom evident and may be associated with inflammatory infiltrates [2]. Myocardial inflammation has been reported in up to 75% of hearts at autopsy [14]. An apoptotic mechanism of myocyte death has been also proven in humans [15, 16]. Rather than being a continuous ongoing process, disease progression may occur through periodic "acute bursts" of an otherwise stable disease, as to mimic "infarct-like" myocarditis or simulate myocardial infarction. In a desmoglein-2 transgenic animal model, spontaneous myocyte necrosis was demonstrated to be the key initiator of myocardial injury, triggering progressive myocardial damage, followed by an inflammatory response [17]. The detection of viral genomes in humans led to the possibility of an infective viral etiology, but it is most likely that either viruses are innocent bystanders or that myocardial cell degeneration may serve as a milieu favoring viral settlement [18].

11.2.3 Clinical Features and Natural History

Clinical manifestations vary with age and stage of disease [9]. Heart palpitations, syncope, or cardiac arrest are common in young adults or adolescents. However the most common signs of AC are PVCs or ventricular tachycardia (VT) with LBBB morphology and T-wave inversion in V1- V3 on ECG. Less common presentations are RV or biventricular dilatation, with or without heart failure symptoms, mimicking dilated cardiomyopathy and requiring heart transplantation at the end-stage.

Frequent non-specific clinical features comprise myocarditis or a myocardial infarction like-picture with chest pain, dynamic ST-T wave changes on the 12-lead ECG, myocardial enzyme release in the setting of normal coronary arteries [3].

The four phases of RV AC are described in Box 11.1 [19].

Box 11.1 Natural History of the Classic AC Variant:

1. Concealed—with subtle RV structural changes, with or without ventricular arrhythmias, during which sudden death may even be the first disease presentation.
2. Overt electrical disorder—with symptomatic life-threatening ventricular arrhythmias associated with clear-cut RV morpho-functional abnormalities.
3. RV failure—due to progression and extension of the RV disease
4. Biventricular failure—caused also by pronounced LV disease.

Electrical instability that may lead to arrhythmic sudden death can occur at any time during the course of the disease [3, 5, 6, 21, 22]. AC has been reported as the second leading cause of sudden death in the young and the first cause in competitive athletes in the Veneto Region in Italy [1, 6, 21]. The incidence of sudden death ranges from 0.08 to 3.6% per year in adults with AC [3, 5, 22]. While patients with an overt disease phenotype more often experience scar-related re-entrant VT, those with an early stage or "hot phase" of the disease may manifestate with ventricular fibrillation (VF) due to acute myocyte death and reactive inflammation [20]. More recently, gap junction remodeling and sodium channel interference have been advanced in experimental models as an alternative explanation for life-threatening arrhythmias even in the pre-phenotypic disease stage [22, 23].

AC diagnosis requires multiple criteria, combining different sources of diagnostic information, such as morpho-functional (by echocardiography and/ or angiography and/ or CMR), histopathological on endomyocardial biopsy, ECG, arrhythmias and familial history, including genetics. The diagnostic criteria, originally put forward in 1994 [24], were revised in 2010 to improve diagnostic sensitivity, but with the important prerequisite of maintaining diagnostic specificity (Table 11.1) [9]. To this aim, quantitative parameters have been included and abnormalities are defined, based on the comparison with normal subject data. Moreover, T-wave inversion in V_1-V_3, and VT with a LBBB morphology with superior or indeterminate QRS axis (either sustained or no sustained), have become major diagnostic criteria [25]; and T-wave inversion in V_1-V_2 in the absence of right bundle branch block (RBBB), and in V_1-V_4, in the presence of complete RBBB, has been included among the minor criteria. Finally, in the family history category, the confirmation of AC in a first-degree relative, by either meeting current criteria or pathologically (at autopsy or transplantation), and the identification of a pathogenic mutation, categorized as associated or probably associated with AC, are considered major criteria. Because of the diagnostic implications, however, caution is highly recommended since the pathogenic significance of a single mutation is increasingly questioned (see genetic section 11-c-3).

Table 11.1 2010 Revised Task Force Criteria for arrhythmogenic cardiomyopathy

1. Global or Regional dysfunction and structural alterations[a]		
Major	By 2D echo	Regional RV akinesia, dyskinesia, or aneurysm and one of the following (end-diastole):
		• PLAX RVOT ≥32 mm (corrected for body size [PLAX/BSA] ≥19 mm/m^2)
		• PSAX RVOT ≥36 mm (corrected for body size [PSAX/BSA] ≥21 mm/m^2)
		• or fractional area change ≤33%
	By CMR	Regional RV akinesia or dyskinesia or dyssynchronous RV contraction and one of the following:
		• Ratio of RV end-diastolic volume to BSA ≥110 mL/m^2 (male) or ≥100 mL/m^2 (female)
		• or RV ejection fraction ≤40%
	By RV angiography	Regional RV akinesia, dyskinesia, or aneurysm
Minor	By 2D echo	Regional RV akinesia or dyskinesia and one of the following (end diastole):
		• PLAX RVOT ≥29 to <32 mm (corrected for body size [PLAX/BSA] ≥16 to <19 m/m^2)
		• PSAX RVOT ≥32 to <36 mm (corrected for body size [PSAX/BSA] ≥18 to <21 mm/m^2)
		• or fractional area change >33% to ≤40%
	By CMR	Regional RV akinesia or dyskinesia or dyssynchronous RV contraction and one of the following:
		• Ratio of RV end-diastolic volume to BSA ≥100 to <110 mL/m^2 (male) or ≥90 to <100 mL/m^2 (female)
		• or RV ejection fraction >40% to ≤45%
2. Tissue characterization of ventricular wall		
Major	Fibrofatty replacement of myocardium on endomyocardial biopsy	
	Residual myocytes <60% by morphometric analysis (or <50% if estimated), with fibrous replacement of the RV free wall myocardium in ≥1 sample, with or without fatty replacement of tissue on EMB	
Minor	Residual myocytes <60% by morphometric analysis (or <50% if estimated), with fibrous replacement of the RV free wall myocardium in ≥1 sample, with or without fatty replacement of tissue on EMB	
3. Repolarization abnormalities		
Major	• Inverted T waves in right precordial leads (V1, V2, and V3) or beyond in individuals >14 years of age (in the absence of complete RBBB QRS ≥120 ms)	
Minor	• Inverted T waves in leads V1 and V2 in individuals >14 years of age (in the absence of complete RBBB) or in V4, V5, or V6	
	• Inverted T waves in leads V1, V2, V3, and V4 in individuals >14 years of age in the presence of complete RBBB	
4. Depolarization/conduction abnormalities		
Major	• Epsilon wave (reproducible low-amplitude signals between end of QRS complex to onset of the T wave) in the right precordial leads (V1 to V3)	

(continued)

Table 11.1 (continued)

Minor	• Late potentials by SAECG in ≥1 of 3 parameters in the absence of a QRS duration of ≥110 ms on the standard ECG
	• Filtered QRS duration (fQRS) ≥114 ms
	• Duration of terminal QRS <40 μV (low-amplitude signal duration) ≥38 ms
	• Root-mean-square voltage of terminal 40 ms ≤20 μV
	• Terminal activation duration of QRS ≥55 ms measured from the nadir of the S wave to the end of the QRS, including R', in V1, V2, or V3, in the absence of complete RBBB
5. Arrhythmias	
Major	• Nonsustained or sustained VT of LBBB morphology with superior axis (negative or indeterminate QRS in leads II, III, and aVF and positive in lead aVL)
Minor	• Nonsustained or sustained VT of RVOT, LBBB morphology with inferior axis (positive QRS in leads II, III, and aVF and negative in lead aVL) or of unknown axis
	• >500 PVCs per 24 h (Holter)
6. Family history	
Major	• AC confirmed in a first-degree relative who meets current Task Force criteria
	• AC confirmed pathologically at autopsy or surgery in a first-degree relative
	• Identification of a pathogenic mutation[b] categorized as associated or probably associated with AC in the patient under evaluation
Minor	• History of AC in a first-degree relative in whom it is not possible or practical to determine whether the family member meets current Task Force criteria
	Premature sudden death (35 years of age) due to suspected AC in a first-degree relative
	AC confirmed pathologically or by current Task Force Criteria in second-degree relative

Two major, or one major and two minor, or four minor criteria from different categories: definite AC diagnosis. One major and one minor, or three minor criteria: borderline AC diagnosis. One major of two minor criteria: possible AC diagnosis

[a]Hypokinesis is not included in the definition of RV regional wall motion abnormalities in the proposed modified criteria

[b]A pathogenic mutation is a DNA alteration associated with AC that alters or is expected to alter the encoded protein, is unobserved or rare in a large non-AC control population, and either alters or is predicted to alter the structure or function of the protein or has demonstrated linkage to the disease phenotype in a conclusive pedigree

BSA body surface area, *CMR* cardiac magnetic resonance, *EMB* endomyocardial biopsy, *LBBB* left bundle branch block, *PLAX* parasternal long-axis view, *PSAX* parasternal short-axis view, *PVC* premature ventricular complex, *RBBB* right bundle branch block, *RV* right ventricle, *RVOT* RV outflow tract, *VT* ventricular tachycardia

AC diagnosis is exceptionally made below the age of 10, due to absent or limited morpho-functional phenotype age-related [3, 5, 26]. Syncope, palpitations and ventricular arrhythmias are also common in the pediatric age [26]. Adult-based diagnostic criteria are valid in the pediatric age group as well, exception made for inverted T wave in right precordial leads in children <12 years of age, which is often normal [27]. Non-invasive clinical investigation follow-up in children with a family and/ or personal history suspicious for AC or healthy gene carriers, is recommended to monitor the pending disease onset in the pubertal period.

The revised 2010 criteria can easily recognize RV and BV AC but lacks specific diagnostic guidelines for the non-classical LV disease pattern. ECG abnormalities such as lateral or inferolateral T-wave inversion (leads V_5, V_6, L_I, and aVL), low voltage QRS complex on peripheral leads and RBBB/ polymorphic ventricular arrhythmias suggest a left-side involvement [28]. Contrast-enhanced CMR is the more sensitive imaging diagnostic tool to detect LV involvement by non-invasive tissue characterization [29]. LV involvement should be considered a mirror of RV involvement [29, 30]. Late gadolinium enhancement is in fact by far a more-sensitive indicator of even early or minor left-sided disease, and is detected frequently in a segment without a concomitant morphofunctional wall-motion abnormality, thus preceding the onset of LV dysfunction or dilatation. Typically, LV late gadolinium enhancement involves the inferolateral and inferoseptal regions, and affects the subepicardial or midwall layers (so called non-ischemic LV scars). Differential diagnosis with dilated cardiomyopathy and chronic myocarditis is mandatory for risk-stratification and familial-evaluation purposes. The propensity to electrical instability that exceeds the degree of ventricular dysfunction is typical of LV AC, in contrast to dilated cardiomyopathy where life-threatening ventricular arrhythmias usually occur in the setting of systolic dysfunction with low ejection fraction (<35%). Moreover, a regional rather than global involvement is more in keeping with AC, particularly when RV abnormalities are prominent.

11.2.3.1 Differential Diagnosis

Diagnostic dilemmas comprise myocarditis, sarcoidosis, RV infarction, dilated cardiomyopathy, Chagas disease, Brugada syndrome, idiopathic RV outflow tract VT, pulmonary hypertension and congenital heart disease with right chambers overload [3, 31].

Endomyocardial biopsy from the RV free wall, where the fibrofatty replacement is detectable and transmural, is crucial in selected cases to reach the final diagnosis ruling out in vivo the so-called phenocopies, such as myocarditis and sarcoidosis, especially when dealing with probands with sporadic forms, and in the setting of negative or doubtful CMR and/ or electrovoltage mapping [9, 32]. Based on the current endomyocardial biopsy guidelines, fibrous or fibrofatty replacement with <60% residual myocardium in at least one endomyocardial biopsy sample is a major criterion, and 60–75% residual myocardium is a minor criterion for AC. However, quantitative criteria should not exclude qualitative evaluation of the biopsy microscopically. Replacement-type fibrosis including some inflammatory infiltrates, myocyte degeneration, and evidence of adipogenesis are microscopic hallmark of AC [31]. Electrovoltage mapping is an invasive electrophysiological tool that should be performed in selected patients with suspected AC, in the setting of ventricular arrhythmias of RV origin, and/or when CE-CMR is negative or doubtful in terms of RV involvement [32].

One of the main diagnostic clinical challenges remains to differentiate AC from idiopathic RV outflow tract VT, which is usually benign. The absence of ECG repolarization/ depolarization abnormalities and of ventricular structural changes, the recording of a single VT morphology, the non-inducibility at programmed ventricular stimulation and of a normal electroanatomic voltage mapping, together with the non-familial background, support the idiopathic nature of the VT [32]. The abnormal low-voltage areas found in AC patients correspond to the loss of electrically active myocardium caused by fibrofatty replacement ("electrical scars"). Of note, in nonadvanced stages, scar tissue may be confined to epicardial/ midmural layers, sparing (or reaching focally) the endocardial region. Thus, bipolar endocardial voltage mapping of the RV free wall may underestimate or miss nontransmural low-voltage areas [33].

Finally, in athletes the major challenge is to distinguish AC from so-called "athletic heart", i.e. physiological adaptation to training with hemodynamic overload. RV enlargement, ECG abnormalities and arrhythmias are well documented in endurance athletes, reflecting the increased hemodynamic load during exercise [3]. Global RV systolic dysfunction and/ or regional wall motion abnormalities, such as bulgings or aneurysms, are more in keeping with AC rather than physiologic ventricular remodelling. The absence of overt structural changes of the RV, frequent PVBs or inverted T waves in the precordial leads all support a benign nature.

11.2.4 Conventional Therapeutic and Interventional Management

The most important goals of clinical management of AC patients are shown in the Box 11.2.

Box 11.2 Goals of Clinical Management

1. Reduction of mortality, either by arrhythmic sudden death or heart failure
2. Prevention of disease progression leading to RV, LV or biventricular dysfunction
3. Attenuation of symptoms and improvement quality of life by decreasing or suppressing palpitations, VT recurrences or implantable cardioverter defibrillator (ICD) discharges (either appropriate or inappropriate)
4. Reducing heart failure symptoms and increasing exercise capacity [28, 34].

Management options for AC comprise life-style modifications, pharmacologic treatment, catheter ablation, ICD implantation, and exceptionally heart transplantation. Before any therapy is undertaken, life-style modification should be pursued. Sport activity in adolescents and young adults is associated with an increased risk of sudden death, thus supporting the concept that avoiding effort is "per se" lifesaving [1, 6]. Recently, it has been demonstrated that endurance sports and frequent exercise increase age-related penetrance, risk of VTs, and occurrence of heart failure in AC desmosomal gene carriers [20].

Different *antiarrhythmic drugs* have been employed, such as sodium channel blockers, β-blockers, sotalol, amiodarone, verapamil alone or combinations. Although, contradictory data regarding the effectiveness of empiric arrhythmic drugs has been published, showing either a higher efficiency of amiodarone or inefficacy of anti-arrhythmic drugs against sudden death and ICD intervention, co-administration of more than one drug should be avoided [20, 35, 36].

Catheter ablation of the re-entry circuit is a nonpharmacological, interventional therapeutic option for AC patients who have VT. In fact, VT is the result of a scar-related macro-reentry circuit due to RV fibrofatty replacement, which is suitable for mapping and interruption by catheter ablation [37]. Catheter ablation may be guided by either conventional electrophysiological or substrate-based mapping. Linear ablation lesions connecting or encircling ventricular scar areas obtain the isolation of the re-entry circuit. In the presence of a large RV scar burden and/or in patients with VT recurrence, combined endo- and epicardial substrate-based VT ablation, incorporating scar dechanneling technique, would increase the short- and longterm success rate. However, the epicardial approach has a significant procedural complication rate (up to 8%) and should always performed in high volume referral centers [37].

ICD therapy is the first line approach for the highest-risk patients, whose natural history is typically characterized by the risk of sudden death [20, 35, 38, 39]. Data obtained from either primary or secondary prevention studies indicate that ICD therapy improves longterm outcome of selected high-risk AC patients, with significant mortality reduction. Overall, 48–78% of patients received appropriate ICD interventions during the mean follow-up period of 2–7 years after implantation [20, 39]. Different studies on ICD therapy in AC patients have also provided valuable information about the risk predictors for VF or VT triggering appropriate ICD discharges during follow-up. The strongest predictors of a life-saving ICD intervention was aborted sudden death due to VT/VF and syncope. The presence of multiple risk factors increases the likelihood of appropriate ICD therapy. Most importantly, asymptomatic probands and relatives without relevant risk factors as well as healthy gene carriers show a low rate of arrhythmic events over a long-term follow-up, regardless of family history of sudden death. Despite well-known ICD benefit on survival, disadvantages are related to the lead and device-related complications like infectious dislodgement as well as the inappropriate ICD intervention, which occurs in 10–25% of AC patients and is usually caused by sinus tachycardia or atrial tachyarrhythmia [20, 39]. Frequent ICD discharges in AC patients can be reduced by appropriate ICD reprogramming and/ or co-administration of beta-blocker therapy.

Cardiac Transplantation AC patients with severe, refractory biventricular heart failure or unmanageable VTs may become candidates to heart transplantation. The most common indication for cardiac transplantation is heart failure, and, in less than one-third of patients, unbearable ventricular arrhythmias with electric storms [3].

11.2.5 Arrhythmic Risk Stratification

Arrhythmic risk stratification relies on phenotypic predictors such as previous cardiac arrest due to VF, sustained VT, unexplained syncope, severe RV or LV dilatation/ dysfunction, compound and digenic heterozygosity of desmosomal gene mutations, low QRS amplitude, QRS fragmentation, male gender, young age at time of diagnosis, proband status, inducibility at programmed ventricular stimulation, burden of electroanatomic scar and scar-related fractioned electrograms, and extent of T wave inversion across the precordial and inferior leads on ECG. In a recent document on risk stratification and treatment of AC [39], indications for ICD implantation were determined by consensus, taking into account the statistical risk, general health, socioeconomic factors, psychological impact and adverse effects of the device. The flowchart is shown in Fig. 11.2.

It is noteworthy, that these recommendations apply to the classical RV variant of AC and prognostic data are not yet available for the left-dominant one, which is increasingly detected by contrast enhanced CMR.

Pregnancy is generally well tolerated but a cardiological evaluation prior to conception is mandatory for individualized arrhythmic risk stratification and prescription of the best antiarrhythmic therapy [35]. β-blocker treatment is better since no teratogenic effects are known but they may be associated with intrauterine growth retardation and neonatal bradycardia or hypoglycemia [40].

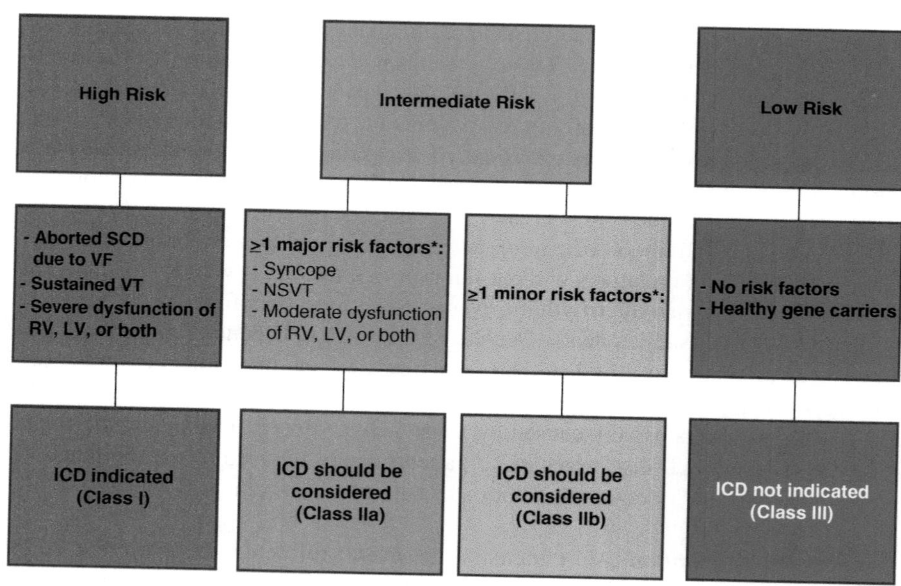

Fig. 11.2 Flow chart of risk stratification and indications for ICD in AC. The estimated risk of major arrhythmic events in the high-risk category is >10%/year, in the intermediate ranges from 1 to 10%/year, and in the low-risk category is <1%/year The high risk category includes patients who experienced cardiac arrest due to VF or sustained VT and most benefit from ICD (estimated annual event rate >10%/year). The low risk category comprises probands and relatives without risk factors as well as healthy gene carriers (estimated annual event rate <1%/year), who do not require any treatment. The intermediate risk category includes AC patients with ≥1 risk factors, except those mentioned in the high risk category (estimated annual event rate between 1 and 10%/year). The decision to implant an ICD in these patients should be made on individual basis. (from Ref. [39]). *SCD* sudden cardiac death, *VF* ventricular fibrillation, *VT* ventricular tachycardia, *RV* right ventricle, *LV* left ventricle

11.3 Genetic Perspectives of Arrhythmic Cardiomyopathy

Although the first description of the inherited nature of arrhythmic cardiomyopathy (AC) as autosomal dominant trait with variable expression and age-related penetrance resides back to the 80s [41], the discovery of disease-causing genes came later on. The plakoglobin gene (JUP) was the first discovered disease gene in a fully penetrant autosomal-recessive form of AC associated with palmoplantar keratosis, also known as Naxos cardiocutaneous syndrome [42, 43]. Subsequently, mutations of the DSP gene were found to cause another autosomal-recessive cardiocutaneous syndrome, i.e. Carvajal syndrome [44]. Soon after, heterozygous mutations in the same gene were identified for the first time in a dominant form of AC without hair/skin abnormalities [45]. To-date, different disease genes have been linked to the classical inheritance pattern of AC, highlighting genetic heterogeneity [7]. Most of mutations in dominant forms have been identified in desmosomal genes including DSP, plakophilin-2 (PKP2), desmoglein-2 (DSG2), desmocollin-2 (DSC2) and JUP [43, 45–49] (Table 11.2). Only isolated reports showed causal mutations in non-desmosome genes, such as transmembrane protein 43 (TMEM43), desmin (DES), titin (TTN), lamin A/C (LMNA), phospholamban (PLN), αT-catenin (CTNNA3), filamin C (FLNC), N-cadherin (CDH2) sometimes with a clinical phenotype similar but not identical to AC, so as to be considered phenocopies or overlap syndromes [50–57]. Moreover, mutations in the regulatory region of transforming growth factor beta-3 gene have also been reported [58], but their pathogenicity is still controversial. Ryanodine receptor 2 gene mutations are nowadays associated with catecholaminergic polymorphic VT (CPVT) rather than AC, as originally considered [59].

Thus, most pathogenic mutations involve structural proteins that contribute in the organization of the intercalated disc. It is noteworthy that these intercalated discs were described as containing a mixed-type junctional structure instead of classical adherens junctions, the so-called area composita) (Fig. 11.3) [60, 61].

Comprehensive exomic sequence analysis of the known desmosomal AC-related genes currently identifies approximately 50% of AC probands [7, 62–66]. The most commonly defective AC gene is PKP2 (10–45%), followed by DSP (10–15%), DSG2 (7–10%) and DSC2, JUP (1–2%). About 10–25% of AC patients are compound, heterozygous mutation carriers [7, 62–65]. Although "private" mutations predominate in AC patients, founder mutations in both desmosomal and extra-desmosomal encoding genes have been reported [7, 66]. Entire PKP2 exons or even whole gene deletions have been even described in AC patients with a frequency of approximately 2% [67]. The sporadic, non-familial forms of AC may represent chronic myocarditis.

11.3.1 Genetic Risk Assessment

Genetic risk assessment constitutes an essential component of genetic counseling for individual and family decision making and should be looked at as an ongoing process of analysis of estimates.

Table 11.2 Genetic background of arrhythmogenic cardiomyopathy

MIM entry	Locus	Disease gene	Gene	Mode of transmission	Author, year (Reference)	Comment
Desmosomal genes						
#611528	17q21.2	Plakoglobin	*JUP*	AD/AR	McKoy et al. [43]	AR form: Cardiocutaneous syndrome
#601214						
#607450	6p24.3	Desmoplakin	*DSP*	AD/AR	Rampazzo et al. [45]	AR form: Cardiocutaneous syndrome
#605676						
#609040	12p11.21	Plakophilin-2	*PKP2*	AD/AR	Gerull et al. [46]	
#610193	18q12.1	Desmoglein-2	*DSG2*	AD/AR	Pilichou et al. [47]	
#610476	18q12.1	Desmocollin-2	*DSC2*	AD/AR	Syrris et al. [48]	
Non-desmosomal genes						
#600996	1q43	Cardiac Ryanodine Receptor	*RYR2*	AD	Tiso et al. [59]	CPVT (AC phenocopy)
#107970	14q24.3	Transforming growth factor-beta-3	*TGFB3*	AD	Beffagna et al. [58]	Modifier?
#604400	3p25.1	Transmembrane Protein 43	*TMEM43*	AD	Merner et al. [50]	
	2q35	Desmin	*DES*	AD	Van Tintelen et al. [51]	Overlap syndrome (DC and HC phenotype, early conduction disease)
	6q22.31	Phospholamban	*PLN*	AD	Van der Zwaag et al. [52]	
	2q31.2	Titin	*TTN*	AD	Taylor et al. [53]	Overlap syndrome (early conduction disease, AF)
	1q22	Lamin A/C	LMNA	AD	Quarta et al. [54]	Overlap syndrome
#615616	10q21.3	alpha-T-catenin	CTNAA3	AD	Van Hengel et al. [55]	
	7q32.1	Filamin C	FLNC	AD	Ortiz-Genga et al. [56]	Overlap syndrome (HC and DC phenotype)
	18q12.1	N-Cadherin	CDH2	AD	Mayosi et al. [57]	

AD autosomal dominant, *AR* autosomal recessive, *CPVT* catecholaminergic ventricular tachycardia, *DC* dilated cardiomyopathy, *HC* hypertrophic cardiomyopathy

Molecular Landscape of AC

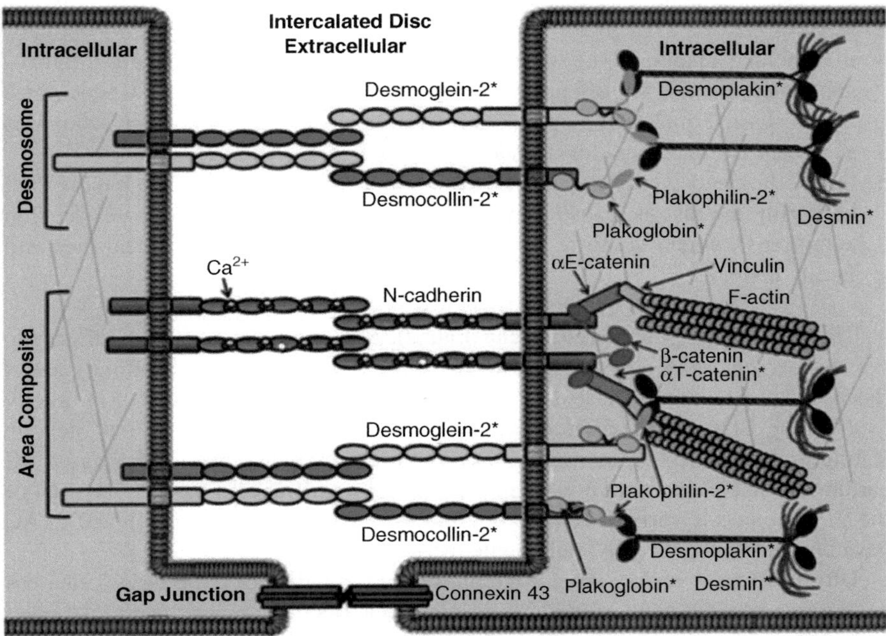

Fig. 11.3 Schematic representation of intercalated discs comprising area composita, desmosomes and gap junctions (data from Ref. [61])

Genotyping success rate in AC varies according to cohort location and ethnicity, sequencing techniques, selection and stringency of criteria by which mutations are considered causative. Moreover, the routine use of Next Generation Sequencing for the analysis of large panels of genes o even the analysis of the whole exome is leading to the identification of a large number of nucleotide variants with uncertain clinical significance.

In order to estimate accurately the genetic risk, the following information at a particular point in time should be considered:

1. the results of genetic testing (causative mutations vs frequent/rare nucleotide variants) in affected patients having clear symptoms/signs of the disease; thus, is of utmost importance to distinguish pathogenic mutations from genetic noise based on the American College of Medical Genetics and Genomics (ACMG) guidelines [68];
2. the genetic risk data obtained from population studies, based on published exome/ whole genome data from a finite number of cases in specific and highly monitored populations (1000 Genome Project, Exome Aggregation Consortium-ExAC, Exome Sequencing Project-ESP, TOPMED, dbSNPs.). In AC mutations with allelic

frequency (MAF, minor allele frequency) less than 0.02–0.05% should be considered pathogenic or likely pathogenic in the context of the disease phenotype;
3. the results of genetic testing on parents, siblings, and close relatives (cascade screening);
4. the prenatal diagnosis (i.e. through amniocentesis or pre-implantation diagnosis), where the risk for offspring can be calculated; however, the low penetrance of the disease makes the application of prenatal diagnosis in many countries subjected to ethical and legal issues;
5. the predictive power of the genetic testing (considering that an at-risk individual harboring the disease-causing mutation/allele, given enough time, will develop symptoms), which is rather low in AC if not integrated with clinical data and family history.

The results from genetic testing can dramatically increase the accuracy of genetic risk assessment. However, analytical or interpretative laboratory errors may affect risk assessment directly (false detection of mutation or polymorphism) or indirectly by altering estimates of allele distribution and carrier frequencies. Thus, genetic testing and its interpretation should be performed by geneticists in dedicated AC cardiogenetic centers, with pre- and post-counseling facilities. Of note, only 364 of the 919 nucleotide variants reported in all desmosome-related genes linked to AC have been considered really pathogenic [65].

Ultimately, to calculate the probability of the individual developing AC, one has to take into account genetic and environmental factors influencing the disease onset and progression such as the number of genes causing or involved in the disease and their associated risk, physical activities, type of work, sex and age-penetrance. However, it remains to be elucidated whether all these factors have the same weight or some are more important to the outcome than others.

11.3.2 Genetic Counseling

Genetic counseling, developed to address the medical and social consequences of Mendelian disorders, has become an integral part of genetic testing. Genetic counseling as currently practiced is focused on the assessment of genetic risk, education of at-risk individuals and family members about the disease management and manifestation as well as about reproductive options, and provision of psychological and emotional support to cope with mostly untreatable diseases.

Pre-test counseling in AC should be offered to all index cases in order to draw family pedigrees by accurately collecting family history information, to aid patients' comprehension regarding genetic test benefits and limitations, consequences in case of a positive genetic test and the possibility/meaning of an uninformative or negative genetic test. Given that the prevalence of causal genes and mutations has yet to be determined, a negative or uninformative genetic test due to the limited diagnostic yield from screening of known causal genes does not exclude a genetic background. A positive genetic test in the affected AC proband is enabling the identification of early asymptomatic carriers through cascade genetic screening of family members but also may serve to re-assure family members negative on cascade screening.

Post counseling is mandatory in order to aid patients understanding about the meaning of the genetic test findings for themselves and their families, and to aid clinicians interpretation in correlation with familial and clinical evidences. Finally, family history is dynamic and should be updated over time, thus it is necessary to work together with patients through genetic counseling helping them to understand the importance in sharing this information with their families in order to enable the detection of asymptomatic family members.

11.4 Genotype-Phenotype Correlation in Desmosomal-Related AC

The significance of genetic testing in developing a clinical strategy is still controversial, since genotype-phenotype correlation in AC patients is limited due to the small population size and the wide heterogeneity both from the clinical and genetical view point.

To-date, despite the similar prevalence of desmosomal mutation carriers in both genders, the clinical expression of the disease is usually more severe in men, with a higher prevalence of male than female patients who fulfil the diagnostic criteria [69].

Most of early genotype–phenotype correlation studies were based on a few families, separately addressed mutations in different desmosomal genes, and compared clinical manifestations of AC mutation carriers versus noncarriers [70, 71]. Although some differences have been reported with regard to a series of clinical, ECG, and morphofunctional RV abnormalities in variables between AC gene-positive and gene-negative patients, detection of AC desmosomal gene mutations was not associated with an enhanced susceptibility to life-threatening arrhythmias and did not predict arrhythmic outcome compared with an unknown genotype.

Few available studies correlating the phenotype to the underlying genotype provided contradictory findings with regard to the association between specific desmosomal genes or mutation and clinical features. A specific trend toward more prevalent LV involvement was attributed to *DSP* mutations by Quarta et al. [72] and to *DSG-2* mutations by Fressart et al. [73], but not always confirmed by others.

In our series of 134 desmosomal gene mutation carriers, disease penetrance was higher in patients with multiple mutations than in those with single mutations and the difference remained statistically significant after adjustment for age and sex [63]. Among patients with single mutation, disease penetrance did not differ according to specific desmosomal genes or to the presence of missense versus non missense mutations. In the subgroup of 61 patients with single mutation who fulfilled the diagnostic criteria for either borderline or definite ARVC, carriers of single non missense mutations significantly more often had right precordial T-wave inversion extending beyond lead V3 and showed a trend toward a lower mean RV fractional area change compared with carriers of single missense mutations. No statistically significant differences in the clinical phenotype were attributable to specific desmosomal genes, with the exception of *DSP* gene mutation carriers who distinctively had more frequent negative T-waves confined to leads V4 to V6, low QRS voltages in limb leads, and LV dysfunction with ejection fraction.

Similar data were reported in the large USA and Dutch AC cohorts, with pathogenic mutations in desmosomal and non-desmosomal genes identified in 577 patients [65]. In fact, individuals with more than one mutation have considerably worse clinical course with significantly earlier onset of symptoms and first sustained arrhythmia, a greater chance of developing sustained VT/VF, and a five-fold increase in the risk of developing LV dysfunction and heart failure than those carrying a single mutation. Among carriers of a single mutation presenting alive, this study demonstrated that the risk of LV involvement and development of heart failure is intrinsically related to the mutated gene. Conversely, carriers of single mutations in all the genes had a high risk of developing a life-threatening arrhythmia, with no significant differences in VT/VF survival among the different genes. PLN mutation carriers had an older age of presentation although they showed a worse long-term prognosis, with more left ventricular dysfunction and heart failure. Also DSP mutation carriers were more likely to develop heart failure and signs of LV involvement, confirming the observation from prior smaller cohorts. These authors also provided evidence that missense variants, defined as pathogenic by predicting algorithms, are associated with a similar prognosis as premature truncating or splice site mutations.

On the basis of these preliminary data, compound or digenic (compound/digenic heterozygosity) desmosomal mutations, which accounts for up to 25% of AC patient in different series, are now considered in the risk stratification for the prevention of sudden cardiac death [39].

Finally, a complete/partial deletion of PKP2 gene has been demonstrated in at least 2% of AC patients carry showing similar phenotypic features with AC patients carrying other desmosomal point mutations [67].

Conclusions

AC is mainly an autosomal dominant cardiac disorder with variable expressivity and age-related penetrance. Genetic screening in AC is a tool able to differentiate patients with overlapping clinical entities as well as to identify AC patients with a broad spectrum of clinical features. The application of genetic testing and the interpretation of genetic variations in AC is still a challenge for the clinicians. Other mechanisms, such as epigenetic factors including MiRNA, could contribute to desmosomal dysfuntion and an AC phenotype and are currently under investigation. Large scale genotype-phenotype correlations studies are still needed to define the role of genetic screening for disease management in the clinical practice.

References

1. Thiene G, Nava A, Corrado D, et al. Right ventricular cardiomyopathy and sudden death in young people. N Engl J Med. 1988;318:129–33.
2. Basso C, Thiene G, Corrado D, et al. Arrhythmogenic right ventricular cardiomyopathy. Dysplasia, dystrophy, or myocarditis? Circulation. 1996;94:983–91.

3. Basso C, Corrado D, Marcus FI, et al. Arrhythmogenic right ventricular cardiomyopathy. Lancet. 2009;373:1289–300.
4. Basso C, Bauce B, Corrado D, et al. Pathophysiology of arrhythmogenic cardiomyopathy. Nat Rev Cardiol. 2011;9:223–33.
5. Nava A, Bauce B, Basso C, et al. Clinical profile and long-term follow-up of 37 families with arrhythmogenic right ventricular cardiomyopathy. J Am Coll Cardiol. 2000;36:2226–33.
6. Corrado D, Basso C, Pavei A, et al. Trends in sudden cardiovascular death in young competitive athletes after implementation of a preparticipation screening program. JAMA. 2006;296:1593–601.
7. Pilichou K, Thiene G, Bauce B, et al. Arrhythmogenic cardiomyopathy. Orphanet J Rare Dis. 2016;11:33.
8. Pilichou K, Mancini M, Rigato I, et al. Nonischemic left ventricular scar: sporadic or familial? Screen the genes, scan the mutation carriers. Circulation. 2014;130:e180–2.
9. Marcus FI, McKenna WJ, Sherrill D, et al. Diagnosis of arrhythmogenic right ventricular cardiomyopathy/dysplasia: proposed modification of the Task Force Criteria. Circulation. 2010;121:1533–41.
10. Basso C, Corrado D, Thiene G. Arrhythmogenic right ventricular cardiomyopathy: what's in a name? From a congenital defect (dysplasia) to a genetically determined cardiomyopathy (dystrophy). Am J Cardiol. 2010;106:275–7.
11. Uhl HS. A previously undescribed congenital malformation of the heart: almost total absence of the myocardium of the right ventricle. Bull Johns Hopkins Hosp. 1952;91:197–209.
12. Marcus FI, Nava A, Thiene G. Arrhythmogenic right ventricular cardiomyopathy/dysplasia – recent advances. Milano: Springer; 2007.
13. Basso C, Burke M, Fornes P, Association for European Cardiovascular Pathology, et al. Guidelines for autopsy investigation of sudden cardiac death. Virchows Arch. 2008;452:11–8.
14. Thiene G. The research venture in arrhythmogenic right ventricular cardiomyopathy: a paradigm of translational medicine. Eur Heart J. 2015;36:837–46.
15. Mallat Z, Tedgui A, Fontaliran F, et al. Evidence of apoptosis in arrhythmogenic right ventricular dysplasia. N Engl J Med. 1996;335:1190–6.
16. Valente M, Calabrese F, Thiene G, et al. In vivo evidence of apoptosis in arrhythmogenic right ventricular cardiomyopathy. Am J Pathol. 1998;152:479–84.
17. Pilichou K, Remme CA, Basso C, et al. Myocyte necrosis underlies progressive myocardial dystrophy in mouse dsg2-related arrhythmogenic right ventricular cardiomyopathy. J Exp Med. 2009;206:1787–802.
18. Calabrese F, Basso C, Carturan E, et al. Arrhythmogenic right ventricular cardiomyopathy/dysplasia: is there a role for viruses? Cardiovasc Pathol. 2006;15:11–7.
19. Thiene G, Nava A, Angelini A, et al. Anatomoclinical aspects of arrhythmogenic right ventricular cardiomyopathy. In: Baroldi G, Camerini F, Goodwin JF, editors. Advances in cardiomyopathies. Berlin: Springer Verlag; 1990. p. 397–408.
20. Basso C, Corrado D, Bauce B, et al. Arrhythmogenic right ventricular cardiomyopathy. Circ Arrhythm Electrophysiol. 2012;5:1233–46.
21. Corrado D, Basso C, Schiavon M, Thiene G. Screening for hypertrophic cardiomyopathy in young athletes. N Engl J Med. 1998;339:364–9.
22. Rizzo S, Lodder EM, Verkerk AO, et al. Intercalated disc abnormalities, reduced Na(+) current density, and conduction slowing in desmoglein-2 mutant mice prior to cardiomyopathic changes. Cardiovasc Res. 2012;95:409–18.
23. Cerrone M, Noorman M, Lin X, et al. Sodium current deficit and arrhythmogenesis in a murine model of plakophilin-2 haploinsufficiency. Cardiovasc Res. 2012;95:460–8.
24. McKenna WJ, Thiene G, Nava A, et al. Diagnosis of arrhythmogenic right ventricular dysplasia/cardiomyopathy. Task Force of the Working Group Myocardial and Pericardial Disease of the European Society of Cardiology and of the Scientific Council on Cardiomyopathies of the International Society and Federation of Cardiology. Br Heart J. 1994;71:215–8.
25. Migliore F, Zorzi A, Michieli P, et al. Prevalence of cardiomyopathy in Italian asymptomatic children with electrocardiographic T-wave inversion at preparticipation screening. Circulation. 2012;125:529–38.

26. Daliento L, Turrini P, Nava A, et al. Arrhythmogenic right ventricular cardiomyopathy in young versus adult patients: similarities and differences. J Am Coll Cardiol. 1995;25:655–64.
27. Bauce B, Basso C, Rampazzo A, et al. Clinical profile of four families with arrhythmogenic right ventricular cardiomyopathy caused by dominant desmoplakin mutations. Eur Heart J. 2005;26:1666–75.
28. Migliore F, Zorzi A, Silvano M, et al. Clinical management of arrhythmogenic right ventricular cardiomyopathy: an update. Curr Pharm Des. 2010;16:2918–28.
29. Perazzolo Marra M, Leoni L, Bauce B, et al. Imaging study of ventricular scar in arrhythmogenic right ventricular cardiomyopathy: comparison of 3D standard electroanatomical voltage mapping and contrast-enhanced cardiac magnetic resonance. Circ Arrhythm Electrophysiol. 2012;5:91–100.
30. di Gioia CR, Giordano C, Cerbelli B, Pisano A, Perli E, De Dominicis E, Poscolieri B, Palmieri V, Ciallella C, Zeppilli P, d'Amati G. Nonischemic left ventricular scar and cardiac sudden death in the young. Hum Pathol. 2016;58:78–89.
31. Basso C, Ronco F, Marcus F, et al. Quantitative assessment of endomyocardial biopsy in arrhythmogenic right ventricular cardiomyopathy/dysplasia: an in vitro validation of diagnostic criteria. Eur Heart J. 2008;29:2760–71.
32. Corrado D, Basso C, Leoni L, et al. Three-dimensional electroanatomical voltage mapping and histologic evaluation of myocardial substrate in right ventricular outflow tract tachycardia. J Am Coll Cardiol. 2008;51:731–9.
33. Migliore F, Zorzi A, Silvano M, et al. Prognostic value of endocardial voltage mapping in patients with arrhythmogenic right ventricular cardiomyopathy/dysplasia. Circ Arrhythm Electrophysiol. 2013;6:167–76.
34. Rigato I, Corrado D, Basso C, et al. Pharmacotherapy and other therapeutic modalities for managing arrhythmogenic right ventricular cardiomyopathy. Cardiovasc Drugs Ther. 2015;29:171–7.
35. Wichter T, Paul TM, Eckardt L, et al. Arrhythmogenic right ventricular cardiomyopathy. Antiarrhythmic drugs, catheter ablation, or ICD? Herz. 2005;30:91–101.
36. Corrado D, Leoni L, Link MS, et al. Implantable cardioverter-defibrillator therapy for prevention of sudden death in patients with arrhythmogenic right ventricular cardiomyopathy/dysplasia. Circulation. 2003;108:3084–91.
37. Garcia FC, Bazan V, Zado ES, et al. Epicardial substrate and outcome with epicardial ablation of ventricular tachycardia in arrhythmogenic right ventricular cardiomyopathy/dysplasia. Circulation. 2009;120:366–75.
38. Corrado D, Calkins H, Link MS, et al. Prophylactic implantable defibrillator in patients with arrhythmogenic right ventricular cardiomyopathy/dysplasia and no prior ventricular fibrillation or sustained ventricular tachycardia. Circulation. 2010;122:1144–52.
39. Corrado D, Wichter T, Link MS, et al. Treatment of arrhythmogenic right ventricular cardiomyopathy/dysplasia: an international task force consensus statement. Circulation. 2015;132:441–53.
40. Bauce B, Daliento L, Frigo G, et al. Pregnancy in women with arrhythmogenic right ventricular cardiomyopathy/dysplasia. Eur J Obstet Gynecol Reprod Biol. 2006;127:186–9.
41. Nava A, Thiene G, Canciani B, et al. Familial occurrence of right ventricular dysplasia: a study involving nine families. J Am Coll Cardiol. 1988;12:1222–8.
42. Protonotarios N, Tsatsopoulou A, Patsourakos P, et al. Cardiac abnormalities in familial palmoplantar keratosis. Br Heart J. 1986;56:321–6.
43. McKoy G, Protonotarios N, Crosby A, et al. Identification of a deletion in plakoglobin in arrhythmogenic right ventricular cardiomyopathy with palmoplantar keratoderma and woolly hair (Naxos disease). Lancet. 2000;355:2119–24.
44. Norgett EE, Hatsell SJ, Carvajal-Huerta L, et al. Recessive mutation in desmoplakin disrupts desmoplakin-intermediate filament interactions and causes dilated cardiomyopathy, woolly hair and keratoderma. Hum Mol Genet. 2000;9:2761–6.
45. Rampazzo A, Nava A, Malacrida S, et al. Mutation in human desmoplakin domain binding to plakoglobin causes a dominant form of arrhythmogenic right ventricular cardiomyopathy. Am J Hum Genet. 2002;71:1200–6.

46. Gerull B, Heuser A, Wichter T, et al. Mutations in the desmosomal protein plakophilin-2 are common in arrhythmogenic right ventricular cardiomyopathy. Nat Genet. 2005;37:106.
47. Pilichou K, Nava A, Basso C, et al. Mutations in desmoglein-2 gene are associated with arrhythmogenic right ventricular cardiomyopathy. Circulation. 2006;113:1171–9.
48. Syrris P, Ward D, Evans A, et al. Arrhythmogenic right ventricular dysplasia/cardiomyopathy associated with mutations in the desmosomal gene desmocollin-2. Am J Hum Genet. 2006;79:978–84.
49. Asimaki A, Syrris P, Wichter T, et al. A novel dominant mutation in plakoglobin causes arrhythmogenic right ventricular cardiomyopathy. Am J Hum Genet. 2007;81:964–73.
50. Merner ND, Hodgkinson KA, Haywood AF, et al. Arrhythmogenic right ventricular cardiomyopathy type 5 is a fully penetrant, lethal arrhythmic disorder caused by a missense mutation in the TMEM43 gene. Am J Hum Genet. 2008;82:809–21.
51. van Tintelen JP, Van Gelder IC, Asimaki A, et al. Severe cardiac phenotype with right ventricular predominance in a large cohort of patients with a single missense mutation in the DES gene. Heart Rhythm. 2009;6:1574–83.
52. van der Zwaag PA, Cox MG, van der Werf C, et al. Plakophilin-2 p.Arg79X mutation causing arrhythmogenic right ventricular cardiomyopathy/dysplasia. Neth Hear J. 2010;18:583–91.
53. Taylor M, Graw S, Sinagra G, et al. Genetic variation in titin in arrhythmogenic right ventricular cardiomyopathy-overlap syndromes. Circulation. 2011;124:876–85.
54. Quarta G, Syrris P, Ashworth M, et al. Mutations in the Lamin A/C gene mimic arrhythmogenic right ventricular cardiomyopathy. Eur Heart J. 2012;33:1128–36.
55. van Hengel J, Calore M, Bauce B, et al. Mutations in the area composita protein αT-catenin are associated with arrhythmogenic right ventricular cardiomyopathy. Eur Heart J. 2013;34:201–10.
56. Ortiz-Genga MF, Cuenca S, Dal Ferro M, et al. Truncating FLNC mutations are associated with high-risk dilated and arrhythmogenic cardiomyopathies. J Am Coll Cardiol. 2016;68:2440–51.
57. Mayosi BM, Fish M, Shaboodien G, et al. Identification of cadherin 2 (CDH2) mutations in arrhythmogenic right ventricular cardiomyopathy. Circ Cardiovasc Genet. 2017;10:e001605.
58. Beffagna G, Occhi G, Nava A, et al. Regulatory mutations in transforming growth factor-beta3 gene cause arrhythmogenic right ventricular cardiomyopathy type 1. Cardiovasc Res. 2005;65:366–73.
59. Tiso N, Stephan DA, Nava A, et al. Identification of mutations in the cardiac ryanodine receptor gene in families affected with arrhythmogenic right ventricular cardiomyopathy type 2 (ARVD2). Hum Mol Genet. 2001;10:189–94.
60. Franke WW, Borrmann CM, Grund C, Pieperhoff S. The area composita of adhering junctions connecting heart muscle cells of vertebrates. I. Molecular definition in intercalated disks of cardiomyocytes by immunoelectron microscopy of desmosomal proteins. Eur J Cell Biol. 2006;85:69–82.
61. Turkowski KL, Tester DJ, Bos JM, Haugaa KH, Ackerman MJ. Whole exome sequencing with genomic triangulation implicates CDH2-encoded N-cadherin as a novel pathogenic substrate for arrhythmogenic cardiomyopathy. Congenit Heart Dis. 2017;12:226–35.
62. Bauce B, Nava A, Beffagna G, et al. Multiple mutations in desmosomal proteins encoding genes in arrhythmogenic right ventricular cardiomyopathy/dysplasia. Heart Rhythm. 2010;7:22–9.
63. Rigato I, Bauce B, Rampazzo A, et al. Compound and digenic heterozygosity predicts lifetime arrhythmic outcome and sudden cardiac death in desmosomal gene-related arrhythmogenic right ventricular cardiomyopathy. Circ Cardiovasc Genet. 2013;6:533–42.
64. Xu T, Yang Z, Vatta M, Multidisciplinary Study of Right Ventricular Dysplasia Investigators, et al. Compound and digenic heterozygosity contributes to arrhythmogenic right ventricular cardiomyopathy. J Am Coll Cardiol. 2010;55:587–97.
65. Lazzarini E, Jongbloed JD, Pilichou K, et al. The ARVD/C genetic variants database: 2014 update. Hum Mutat. 2015;36:403–10.
66. Bhonsale A, Groeneweg JA, James CA, et al. Impact of genotype on clinical course in arrhythmogenic right ventricular dysplasia/cardiomyopathy-associated mutation carriers. Eur Heart J. 2015;36:847–55.

67. Cox MG, van der Zwaag PA, van der Werf C, et al. Arrhythmogenic right ventricular dysplasia/cardiomyopathy: pathogenic desmosome mutations in index-patients predict outcome of family screening: Dutch arrhythmogenic right ventricular dysplasia/cardiomyopathy genotype-phenotype follow-up study. Circulation. 2011;123:2690–700.
68. Richards S, Aziz N, Bale S, ACMG Laboratory Quality Assurance Committee, et al. Standards and guidelines for the interpretation of sequence variants: a joint consensus recommendation of the American College of Medical Genetics and Genomics and the Association for Molecular Pathology. Genet Med. 2015;17:405–24.
69. Xu Z, Zhu W, Wang C, et al. Genotype-phenotype relationship in patients with arrhythmogenic right ventricular cardiomyopathy caused by desmosomal gene mutations: a systematic review and meta-analysis. Sci Rep. 2017;7:41387.
70. Dalal D, James C, Devanagondi R, et al. Penetrance of mutations in plakophilin-2 among families with arrhythmogenic right ventricular dysplasia/cardiomyopathy. J Am Coll Cardiol. 2006;48:1416–24.
71. van Tintelen JP, Entius MM, Bhuiyan ZA, Jongbloed R, Wiesfeld AC, Wilde AA, et al. Plakophilin-2 mutations are the major determinant of familial arrhythmogenic right ventricular dysplasia/cardiomyopathy. Circulation. 2006;113:1650–8.
72. Quarta G, Muir A, Pantazis A, Syrris P, Gehmlich K, Garcia-Pavia P, et al. Familial evaluation in arrhythmogenic right ventricular cardiomyopathy: impact of genetics and revised task force criteria. Circulation. 2011;123:2701–9.
73. Fressart V, Duthoit G, Donal E, Probst V, Deharo JC, Chevalier P, et al. Desmosomal gene analysis in arrhythmogenic right ventricular dysplasia/ cardiomyopathy: spectrum of mutations and clinical impact in practice. Europace. 2010;12:861–8.

Inherited Cardiac Muscle Disorders: Left Ventricular Noncompaction

12

James Marangou, Michael Frenneaux, and Girish Dwivedi

Abstract

Left ventricular noncompaction (LVNC) is a type of structural cardiac abnormality that displays genotypic and phenotypic heterogeneity. Morphologically, it is characterized by prominent ventricular trabeculae and deep intertrabecular recesses. It has traditionally been thought to be related to intrauterine arrest of myocardial development. While it is classified as a primary cardiomyopathy of genetic origin by the American Heart Association, the European Society of Cardiology classification defines it as an unclassified cardiomyopathy. Originally thought to be a rare disease seen mainly in children, there has been increasing identification in adults likely due to increased awareness and advances in cardiovascular imaging. Furthermore, although it is often associated with other congenital cardiac anomalies it can also be seen in association with dilated, hypertrophic and restrictive cardiomyopathies and in the absence of any cardiac defects.

Keywords

Arrhythmia • Embolism • Cardiomyopathy • Heart failure • Noncompaction Trabeculations

J. Marangou
Department of Cardiology, Fiona Stanley Hospital, Perth, WA, Australia
e-mail: james.marangou@health.wa.gov.au

M. Frenneaux
University of East Anglia, Norwich Medical School, Norwich Research Park, Norwich, Norfolk, UK
e-mail: m.frenneaux@uea.ac.uk

G. Dwivedi (✉)
Wesfarmers Chair in Cardiology, Harry Perkins Institute of Medical Research, Nedlands, WA, Australia
e-mail: girish.dwivedi@perkins.uwa.edu.au

D. Kumar, P. Elliott (eds.), *Cardiovascular Genetics and Genomics*,
https://doi.org/10.1007/978-3-319-66114-8_12

12.1 Introduction

Left ventricular noncompaction (LVNC) is a type of structural cardiac abnormality that displays genotypic and phenotypic heterogeneity. Morphologically, it is characterized by prominent ventricular trabeculae and deep intertrabecular recesses [1–3]. It has traditionally been thought to be related to intrauterine arrest of myocardial development [1, 2, 4]. While it is classified as a primary cardiomyopathy of genetic origin by the American Heart Association [3], the European Society of Cardiology classification defines it as an unclassified cardiomyopathy [5]. Originally thought to be a rare disease seen mainly in children, there has been increasing identification in adults likely due to increased awareness and advances in cardiovascular imaging. Furthermore, although it is often associated with other congenital cardiac anomalies [2, 6, 7] it can also be seen in association with dilated, hypertrophic and restrictive cardiomyopathies and in the absence of any cardiac defects [8, 9]. Although there is increasing evidence of various genetic associations, the final common pathway to the disease remains elusive. There is also suggestion of acquired and reversible phenotypes [10, 11]. Clinical manifestations are variable, ranging from no symptoms to disabling congestive heart failure, arrhythmias, and systemic thromboembolism. Echocardiography has been the diagnostic procedure of choice; however the use of cardiac magnetic resonance imaging (MRI) is steadily rising. Treatment centers on the management of heart failure, arrhythmias, and prevention of thromboembolic events.

12.2 Cardiac Embryology and Development

A number of studies have shown that the development of the human heart involves precisely regulated molecular and embryogenetic events [12, 13]. Each event is initiated by a specific signaling molecule and mediated by tissue-specific transcription factor(s). It was initially thought that all the cells that comprise the muscle of the mature heart originate from bilaterally distributed mesodermal fields that were established during early gastrulation [14]. However, it is now known that the cellular components that ultimately develop in to the myocardium have multiple origins [14]. Furthermore, addition of myocardial cells to the developing heart occurs at various stages during embryogenesis [15]. Myocardial development involves the formation of two different myocardial layers within the ventricular wall, the trabecular layer and the subepicardial compact layer. The endocardium constitutes the cellular base of the trabecular layer while the compact layer is formed underneath the epicardium. The process of ventricular trabeculation is considered a highly synchronized developmental process that changes at every stage of cardiac development. Prior to the development of the coronary circulation, the embryonic myocardium consists of a "spongy" meshwork of interwoven myocardial fibers forming trabeculae with deep intertrabecular recesses, which communicate with the left ventricular (LV) cavity [14, 16, 17]. These intertrabecular spaces are responsible for blood supply to the myocardium at this stage of cardiac development. Cardiac trabeculation is dependent on the secretion of various factors during development such as neuregulin, serotonin

2B receptor, vascular endothelial growth factor and angiopoietin [12, 13]. During weeks 5–8 of human fetal development, the ventricular myocardium undergoes a gradual process of compaction, from the epicardium towards endocardium, from base to apex, with transformation of the relatively large intertrabecular spaces into capillaries with gradual disappearance of the large spaces within the trabecular meshwork and completion of compaction [14, 16, 17]. Occurring parallel to this process of compaction of the ventricular myocardium, is the formation of the coronary vessels ending with the establishment of the coronary circulation [14, 16, 17].

12.3 Noncompaction of the Left Ventricular Myocardium

LVNC has traditionally been thought to be the result of arrested endomyocardial morphogenesis [1, 9, 18]. It was first described in association with other congenital anomalies, such as obstruction of the right ventricular (RV) or LV outflow tracts, complex cyanotic congenital heart diseases, and coronary artery anomalies [2, 6, 9] (Table 12.1). Although the abnormal compaction process in these cases is still not completely understood, it has been suggested that pressure overload or myocardial ischemia associated with these conditions prevents regression of the embryonic myocardial sinusoids. Arrest of the regression of the embryonic myocardial sinusoids results in the persistence of deep intertrabecular recesses in communication with both the ventricular cavity and the coronary circulation [19].

Isolated noncompaction of the ventricular myocardium (iNVM) first described by Chin et al. in 1990, is characterized by persistent embryonic myocardial morphology found in the absence of other cardiac anomalies, particularly congenital [1]. The deep recesses in isolated noncompaction communicate only with the ventricular cavity and not with the coronary circulation as can be the case with LVNC associated with congenital cardiac anomalies [20].

Noncompaction of the RV may coexist with LV involvement [6, 9, 19] but due to the difficulty encountered in distinguishing noncompaction from normal RV trabeculations, several authors challenge the existence of isolated RV noncompaction [19, 21].

It should be noted that there has been no definitive proof of an arrest in embryonic endomyocardial morphogenesis. In an interesting series, Bleyl et al. did not find any characteristic features of noncompaction on fetal echocardiography in three infants who were subsequently diagnosed with iNVM [22, 23]. These findings challenge the theory of arrested embryonic development as the pathogenesis of LV noncompaction [22–24] and suggest an acquired condition rather than congenital. Alternatively, these findings may reflect limitations of fetal echocardiography [22, 23]. Other investigators have postulated that other pathogenetic processes could account for noncompaction such as dissection of myocardium, frustrated attempts of myocardial hypertrophy, myocardial tearing caused by dilatation, a metabolic defect, or compensatory hypervascularization [24]. The morphological findings of LVNC have been observed across a spectrum of cardiac diseases including dilated, hypertrophic and restrictive cardiomyopathies, suggesting that it is not a single entity [8]. Cases of acquired LVNC have been described [10, 11, 25], further

Table 12.1 Structural heart diseases associated with left ventricular noncompaction

Absent aortic valve
Anomalous origin of right subclavian artery
Anomalous pulmonary venous return
Aortic stenosis
Aortico-left ventricular tunnel
Arteriovenous block
Atrial isomerism
Atrial septal aneurysm
Atrial septal defect
Atrio-ventricular diverticulum
Bicuspid aortic valve
Coarctation of the aorta
Congenital mitral valve stenosis
Coronary osteal stenosis
Dextrocardia
Double orifice mitral valve
Ebstein's anomaly
Heterotaxy
Histiocyte cardiomyopathy
Hypoplastic left heart syndrome
Hypoplastic right ventricle
Malposed great arteries
Mitral valve cleft
Patent ductus arteriosus
Polyvalvular dysplasia
Pulmonary hypertension
Pulmonary stenosis
Right ventricular muscle bands
Tetralogy of Fallot
Transposition of the great arteries
Ventricular inversion
Ventricular septal defect

Source: Adapted from [118]

challenging the theory that LVNC is purely due to arrested embryonic endomyocardial development.

The nomenclature of noncompaction of the ventricular myocardium (NVM) has been effectively superseded by LVNC. Furthermore iNVM or isolated LVNC may cause confusion, as the majority of LVNC are associated with some other cardiac abnormality, whether functional or structural [e.g. dilated cardiomyopathy (DCM)] [8].

More recently it has been suggested that LVNC be separated in to seven different groups [26]:

- Isolated LVNC (iLVNC); describes the appearance of LVNC in the absence of cardiac dysfunction or clinical symptoms.
- LVNC associated with LV dilatation and dysfunction at the onset, such as seen in association with the X-linked disorder Barth syndrome.

- LVNC in combination with another cardiomyopathy (e.g. DCM or HCM)
- LVNC associated with congenital heart disease
- LVNC associated with a genetic syndrome (e.g. Anderson-Fabry disease)
- Acquired or potentially reversible iLVNC (e.g. athletes, sickle cell anaemia)
- RV noncompaction, either with or without LV involvement

12.4 Pathology

In addition to the first necropsy findings described by Chin et al. [1], many other studies published in cases with LVNC reveal prominent trabecular meshwork and numerous intertrabecular recesses in the ventricular myocardium [2, 4, 9]. The recesses, lined with endothelium in continuity with the ventricular myocardium, have been described to extend deep into the trabecular meshwork, and to end blindly at the compact outer layer, without communication with the coronary circulation [1, 27]. In an autopsy series of 474 normal hearts by Boyd et al., up to 70% had prominent trabeculations in the LV cavity, but only 4% of these had more than three trabeculations [28].

12.5 Pathophysiology

There are no specific abnormal findings on coronary angiography in patients with LVNC [1, 29, 30]. Positron emission tomography has demonstrated a decrease in coronary flow reserve in noncompacted and compacted segments of the LV. It is likely that microcirculatory dysfunction might contribute to LV contractile dysfunction and be responsible for the subendocardial fibrosis found on histology as most of the compacted segments have evidence of reduced coronary flow reserve as demonstrated by wall motion abnormalities [21, 30–32]. A case report showing impaired aerobic fatty acid metabolism in noncompacted ventricular segments support the putative mechanism that in LVNC, myocardial failure and remodeling are the result of ischaemia [33]. Clinical symptoms of cardiac failure which are seen in the majority of the patients with LVNC are probably secondary to both systolic as well as diastolic LV dysfunction. The subendocardial hypoperfusion and microcirculatory dysfunction seen in these patients even in the absence of epicardial coronary artery disease may play important roles in ventricular dysfunction and arrhythmogenesis.

12.6 Genetics of LVNC

Our understanding of the molecular signaling pathways governing the morphogenesis of the cardiovascular system has increased significantly in recent years. A number of candidate genes have been identified that are thought to be involved in myocardial morphogenesis. Indeed, recent studies have suggested that the genetic aetiology underlying previously hitherto considered 'distinct' cardiomyopathies may be shared, with commonality in genetic origin being found in ventricular non-compaction, hypertrophic and dilated cardiomyopathies [34, 35]. However, despite the progress made in genomics the precise mechanisms underlying myocardial noncompaction are unclear.

The inheritance of LVNC may either be sporadic or familial. An autosomal dominant mode of inheritance is considered to be more common than X-linked inheritance for familial cases [22, 23, 36, 37] although autosomal recessive inheritance has also been suggested [38]. Increased occurrence of LVNC in family members of an affected individual has been widely observed since the initial description of LVNC [1, 9]. In two of the largest series of patients with LVNC [37, 39], the frequency of familial noncompaction was found to be 25% and 33%.

There have been more than twenty genes described to be definitely or possibly associated with LVNC, either in isolation or in combination with other forms of cardiomyopathy [40]. Many of these genes have been identified in single case studies and therefore should be considered provisional. Currently the Online Mendelian Inheritance in Man catalog describes ten unique loci and associated LVNC phenotypes (LVNC1, LVNC2 etc). LVNC may also be seen as a cardiac feature in a variety of metabolic diseases and genetic syndromes (Table 12.2).

12.6.1 Genes Linked to Noncompaction

DTNA which is located on 18q12.1 and encodes for dystrobrevin-[alpha], a dystrophin-associated protein involved in maintaining the structural integrity of the

Table 12.2 Syndromes associated with left ventricular noncompaction

Syndrome	Locus	Clinical characteristics
Barth syndrome	Xq28	Dilated cardiomyopathy, neutropenia, skeletal myopathy
Beals syndrome	5q23-q31	Congenital contractures, delayed motor development, marfanoid
Beckers muscular dystrophy	Xp21.2	Muscle wastage, cardiomyopathy, arrhythmias
Charcot Marie Tooth disease type 1A	17p11.2	Peripheral neuropathy, muscle atrophy
Duchennes muscular dystrophy	Xp21.2	Muscle degeneration, cardiomyopathy, arrhythmias
Melnick-Needles sydrome	Xq28	Skeletal abnormalities, craniofacial dysmorphogenesis
Myotonic dystrophy	19q13.2-q13.3	Myotonia, distal weakness, cognitive impairment
Myoadenylate-deaminase deficiency	1p21-p13	Exercise intolerance, myalgia
Nail-patella syndrome	9q34.1	Nail dysplasia, patellar hypoplasia
Noonan syndrome	12q24.1	Failure to thrive, cardiomyopathy, septal defects
Roifman syndrome	X	Dysgammablobulinemia, skeletal dysplasia
Trisomy 13		Cognitive impairment, polydactyly, skeletal abnormalities

Source: Adapted from [41]

muscle membrane [42]. Heterozygous mutations of DTNA cause LVNC. Four different mutations in LDB3 (ZASP), which is located on 10q23.2 and encodes for the LIM domain binding 3 protein (ZASP or Cypher), a muscle sarcomeric Z-band protein, have been identified in four affected families and two sporadic cases (LVNC). Most of these individuals with LDB3 mutations had features of noncompaction and/or DCM [37, 43, 44]. LVNC is also caused by mutation in the ACTC1 on chromosome 15q14, which is also associated with hypertrophic cardiomyopathy (HCM) and atrial septal defect [35]. A heterozygous mutation in the MYH7 gene on chromosome 14q12 has been associated with LVNC, HCM and myosin storage myopathy. The gene TNNT2 encodes cardiac troponin T2 and heterozygous mutation of the gene on chromosome 1q32 is associated with LVNC and DCM [45]. Mutation of the gene MIB1 on chromosome 18q11 was identified in two out of 100 probands with LVNC, one missense and one nonsense mutation respectively [46]. PRDM16 gene on chromosome 1q36 mutation has been associated with both dilated cardiomyopathy and LVNC [47]. Heterozygous missense mutations of the TPM1 gene on chromosome 15q22.1 have been identified in two unrelated families with LVNC and DCM [48]. TPM1 gene encodes for Tropomyosin alpha-1 protein found in striated and smooth muscle. The MYPBC3 gene on chromosome 11p11 encodes for sarcomeric proteins involved in cardiomyocyte contraction. Heterozygous mutations of MYPBC3 have been identified in multiple different families with LVNC [49]. A mutation in LMNA, which is located on 1q22 encoding for lamin A/C, was identified in a single family consisting of an individual with LVNC and three mutation carriers had a DCM or mild LV enlargement [50]. Emery–Dreifuss muscular dystrophy, limb girdle muscular dystrophy1B, Hutchinson–Gilford progeria syndrome and atypical Werner syndrome have also been found to be associated with mutations in LMNA.

TAZ which is located on Xq28 and encodes taffazin (G4.5 protein) involved in the biosynthesis of cardiolipin, an essential component of the mitochondrial inner membrane, was the first locus discovered to be associated with LVNC [22, 23]. Barth syndrome, a metabolic condition characterized by DCM, with or without noncompaction, 3-methylglutaconic aciduria, skeletal myopathy and neutropenia is also described with mutations in TAZ [51]. In total, six different mutations in TAZ have been described in children with LVNC [22, 23, 37, 42, 43, 52]. Large studies screening for mutations in the known loci [9, 37, 52–54] find that most affected individuals do not have mutations detected in either TAZ or DTNA. The contribution of LMNA, SCNA, MYH7 and MYBP3 to the etiology of LVNC is not known. Therefore, it would not be unreasonable to conclude that the genetic etiology of most LVNC is still unknown.

12.6.2 Loci and Chromosomal Regions Associated with LVNC

A newborn girl with facial dysmorphism, multiple ventricular septal defects and epilepsy [55]—array-CGH detected up to a 5.9 Mb terminal deletion at 1p36—was shown to have LVNC. Although, LVNC had not been previously reported in other patients described with 1q43 deletion syndrome, in a recent report, a newborn girl with LVNC, facial dysmorphism, hypotonia, cardiac septal defects was found to have an interstitial 5.4 Mb deletion of 1q43 [56]. The authors contemplated that haploinsufficiency of 1q43 containing the cardiac ryanodine receptor gene is the cause of LVNC. It is possible that chromosome 1 may contain two noncompaction associated loci at 1p36 and 1q43. Patients with 1p36 deletion syndrome can also develop DCM.

NKX2-5 is a potential locus associated with LVNC on the chromosome 5. The NKX2-5 gene encodes for a key transcription factor in cardiogenesis. Mutations of this gene are associated with a variety of congenital heart diseases such as atrial septal defect, double-outlet right ventricle, tetralogy of Fallot, arteriovenous block and Ebstein's anomaly [57, 58]. Deletion of 5q35, which includes the NKX2-5 gene, was detected in a girl with an atrial septal defect, patent ductus arteriosus, minor dysmorphism, developmental delay, heart block, DCM, and LVNC [59]. Furthermore features of LVNC are notable in the NKX2-5 mutant mouse model [60]. These findings add weight, but are not conclusive, of the link between NKX2-5 mutations and LVNC. A full list of gene mutations associated with LVNC can be found in Table 12.3.

Table 12.3 Genes associated with left ventricular noncompaction

Gene	Protein	Inheritance
ABCC9	ATP-binding cassette	AD
ACTC1	Cardiac alpha-actin	AD
ACTN2	Alpha-actinin 2	AD
CASQ2	Calsequestrin 2	AR
DMPK	Dystrophia myotonica protein kinase	AD
DSP	Desmoplakin	AD
DTNA	Dystrobrevin	AD
G4.5	Tafazzin	X-linked
HCN4	Hyperpolarization-activated cyclic nucleotide-gated potassium channel 4	AD
LDB3	Z-band alternatively spliced PDZ motif-containing protein	AD
LMNA	Lamin AC	AD
MIB1	Mindbomd, homolog of Drosophlia	AD
MYBPC3	Myosin-binding protein C	AD
MYH7	Beta-myosin heavy chain 7	AD
PLEKHM2	Pleckstrin homology domain-containing protein	AD
PKP2	Plakophilin 2	AR
PRDM16	PR domain protein 16	AD
RYR2	RYR2	AD
SCN5A	Sodium channel, voltage gated type V, alpha subunit	AD
TNNT2	Cardiac troponin T2	AD
TPM1	Tropomyosin 1	AD

NB: Many of these genes have been identified in single case studies and therefore should be considered provisional

Source: Adapted from [26]

12.7 Metabolic Diseases and Genetic Syndromes Associated with LVNC

Mutations in the Tafazzin gene, an X-linked condition, lead to Barth Syndrome. Tafazzin is a proposed signaling molecule regulating apoptosis and a known component of the inner mitochondrial membrane [61]. Barth syndrome is associated with DCM. However, in a recent publication, Schlame and colleagues described features of LVNC in 15 of the 30 patients with Barth syndrome [61]. Interestingly one child was noted to have LVNC at birth but LVNC disappeared by the age of 6 years [61]. Indeed, it is possible that such remodeling may cause underestimation of the true incidence of LVNC amongst patients with Barth syndrome.

LVNC may also be seen as a feature of mitochondrial diseases. In two large studies of pediatric patients with mitochondrial disorder LVNC was seen as one of the cardiac features [62, 63]. Similarly in adults, out of 62 patients with LVNC, 13 were found to have metabolic myopathy, a condition described with respiratory chain abnormalities [24]. Succinate dehydrogenase deficiency, a mitochondrial disorder, has been found to be associated with LVNC [64]. Mitochondrial DNA (mtDNA) mutations found in patients with LVNC include G3460A, which is also found in Leber's hereditary optic neuropathy, [65] and A3243G, a skeletal muscle heteroplasmic mutation in a patient with complete heart block, myopathy, and nail–patella syndrome [66, 67]. Additional reports include a man with ragged red fibers, complex partial seizures, limb wasting, and an A8381G mtDNA change in the MT-ATP8 gene [68, 69], and a patient with hearing impairment, ophthalmoplegia, central nervous system abnormalities, polyneuropathy, diabetes mellitus, and multiple mtDNA changes (A15662G, T3398C, T4216C, and G15812A) in the MT-ND1 (NADH dehydrogenase subunit 1) and MT-CYB genes [70].

The specific role of mitochondrial dysfunction in the etiology of noncompacted myocardium is not known. As the mitochondrion is essential for cardiac development and function, providing most of the energy for contraction and ion transport through mitochondrial oxidative phosphorylation, generating most of the endogenous reactive oxygen species as a toxic byproduct, and regulating programmed cell death [71], it follows that defects in mtDNA mutations, and/or other aspects of mitochondrial metabolism, would be likely to impact cardiac development, leading to noncompaction.

Other metabolic diseases described with LVNC include myoadenylate deaminase deficiency, an autosomal recessive, exercise-related myopathy, described in a man with myalgia, sinus bradycardia, who was found to have a mutation in the myoadenylate deaminase deficiency disease-causing locus AMPD1 [68, 69]. More recently, LVNC was described in a 2 year old girl with vitamin B12 (cobalamin) deficiency and a homozygous mutation in MMACHC specifically associated with combined methylmalonic aciduria and homocystinuria (cobalamin C type) [72].

Neuromuscular disorders are often associated with various types of cardiomyopathy. Duchene and Becker muscular dystrophy, and limb-girdle muscular dystrophy have been noted to be associated with cardiomyopathy and are classified as dystrophinopathies [66, 67, 73, 74]. These dystrophinopathies may also demonstrate features of LVNC [66, 67]. Other neuromuscular disorders described with LVNC include Charcot Marie Tooth disease and myotonic dystrophy [75, 76].

Many other genetic syndromes describe LVNC as one of their features [77]. There has been a recent spurt of publications and the ever expanding list includes Danon disease, Anderson-Fabry disease, Turner syndrome [77, 78], trisomy 13 [79], and 22q11.2 deletion syndrome [54], malformations syndromes—microphthalmia with linear skin defects [80], Roifman syndrome [81], Melnick Needles syndrome [82], nailpatella syndrome [66, 67] Noonan syndrome [83], and congenital contractural arachnodactyly (Beals syndrome) [84].

12.8 Epidemiology and Demographics

LVNC has been diagnosed in all age groups. In the original case series of isolated noncompaction by Chin et al, the median age at the time of diagnosis was 7 years (range:11 months-22 years) [1]. The true echocardiographic prevalence of LVNC is difficult to ascertain, mainly due to the referral bias to specialist centers and no standardized diagnostic criteria. In one echocardiographic series of patients with LVNC, the prevalence was 0.014% of patients referred to the echocardiography laboratory [19]. By contrast, another series of patients with ejection fraction <45% reported definite or probably LVNC in 3.7% [49]. Certainly there has been an increased incidence of LVNC with improved awareness by physicians and advances in cardiovascular imaging. Men appear to be affected more frequently than women, with males accounting for 56–82% of cases in the four largest reported series [1, 9, 19, 85].

12.9 Clinical Presentation

Noncompaction is identified incidentally or is found to be present in patients presenting with one or a combination of three major clinical manifestations [1, 9, 14].

1. Heart failure
2. Arrhythmias
3. Embolic events.

Clinical characteristics of patients from five study populations with noncompaction of the ventricular myocardium are presented in the Table 12.4.

A patient with noncompaction can present with findings that can range from asymptomatic LV dysfunction to severe disabling congestive heart failure. In the cohort with LVNC described in the initial report by Chin et al. depressed ventricular systolic function was noted in 63% of patients [1]. Over 70% of the patients in the largest series with LVNC had symptomatic heart failure [19]. In children with LVNC, the initial presentation may be as that of a restrictive cardiomyopathy [86, 88]. In a prospective case series of Japanese children with LVNC followed for up to 17 years, irrespective of the presence or absence of symptoms at the time of initial diagnosis, LV dysfunction developed in the majority [86].

Table 12.4 Clinical characteristics of patients from five study populations with left ventricular noncompaction

	Oechslin et al. [19]	Ritter et al. [9]	Ichida et al. [86]	Stollberger et al. [24]	Chin et al. [1]
Patient characteristics					
Patients	34	17	27	62	8
Females %	26	18	44	30	37
Age (years)	16–71	18–71	0–15	50 mean	0.9–22.5
Non-compacted segments %					
Apex	94	100	100	98	Most common
Inferior wall	84	100	70	8	–
Lateral wall	100		41	19	–
Mural thrombi %	9	6	0	–	25
Impaired left ventricular function %	82	76	60	58	63
Abnormal ECG %	94	88	88	92	88
Ventricular tachycardia %	41	47	0	18	38
Atrial fibrillation %	26	29	–	5	–
Systemic embolism %	21	24	0	–	38
Sudden death %	18	18	7	–	13

Source: Adapted from [87]

Diastolic dysfunction has been described in patients with ventricular noncompaction and is thought to be related to both abnormal relaxation and restrictive filling caused by the numerous prominent trabeculae [14].

Arrhythmias are not uncommon and can be a fatal mode of presentation for patients with ventricular noncompaction. Sudden cardiac death accounted for half of the deaths in the larger series of patients with LVNC [1, 9, 19, 20]. Although ventricular arrhythmias occurred in nearly 40% of patients in the initial description of LVNC by Chin et al. [1]; Ichida et al. described no cases of ventricular tachycardia or sudden death in the largest series of pediatric patients with LVNC [86]. Rhythm disturbances including paroxysmal supraventricular tachycardia and complete heart block have been reported in patients with LVNC [86]. Nonspecific findings on the resting electrocardiography (ECG) are found in the majority of patients with LVNC. ECG changes include LV hypertrophy, abnormal Q-waves, repolarization changes, T waves changes, ST segment abnormalities, axis shifts, intraventricular conduction abnormalities, and AV block [1, 9, 19, 86, 89] (Table 12.5). ECG findings consistent with Wolff-Parkinson-White syndrome have been described in up to 15% of pediatric patients [86, 90] but it was not observed in the two largest series of adults with isolated noncompaction [9, 19].

In three series of patients with LVNC, the occurrence of thromboembolic events, including cerebrovascular accidents, transient ischemic attacks, pulmonary embolism, and mesenteric infarction, ranged from 21% to 38% [1, 9, 19]. Embolic complications are possibly related to development of thrombi due to combination of

Table 12.5 Electrocardiographic abnormalities associated with left ventricular noncompaction

Axis shifts
Abnormal Q-waves
Intraventricular conduction abnormalities
AV block
Repolarization changes
LV hypertrophy
ST-segment abnormalities
T-wave changes
Atrial fibrillation
Paroxysmal supraventricular tachycardia
WPW-syndrome
Bigemini ventricular extrasystoles
Ventricular tachycardia
Ventricular fibrillation

Source: Adapted from [118]

factors that alter flow through the ventricle including an extensively trabeculated ventricle, depressed systolic function and development of atrial fibrillation [9, 14]. Of note, however, no systemic embolic events were reported in the largest pediatric series with LVNC [86].

An association between LVNC and facial dysmorphisms, including a prominent forehead, low-set ears, strabismus, high-arching palate, and micrognathia, was described by Chin et al. [1]. One third of children with LVNC in the series by Ichida et al. had similar dysmorphic facial features [86]. No associated dysmorphic facial features were observed in two adult populations with LVNC [9, 19]. An association between noncompaction and neuromuscular disorders has also been described with as many as 82% of patients having some form of neuromuscular disorder [24, 74].

More recently acquired and reversible LVNC has been described. This includes athletes, in whom the significance of this morphological finding is unclear and can cause confusion in otherwise healthy subjects [10, 11]. Other cases of acquired LVNC have been documented in sickle cell anaemia, pregnancy and chronic kidney disease [10, 11, 25, 91].

12.10 Diagnostic Criteria of Ventricular Noncompaction

The diagnosis is most commonly made morphologically by 2-dimensional echocardiography in combination with color Doppler technique (Figs. 12.1 and 12.2). The predominant feature demonstrated is a thickened left ventricular wall consisting of two layers, a thin compacted epicardial layer and a thickened endocardial layer with multiple prominent ventricular trabeculations with deep intertrabecular recesses. Color Doppler imaging is used to demonstrate the flow of blood through the deep recesses in continuity with the ventricular cavity [14].

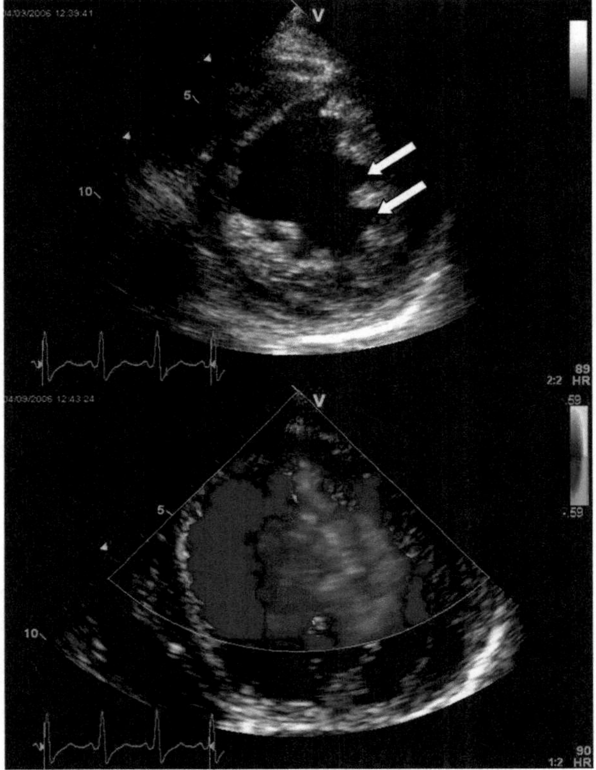

Fig. 12.1 Two-dimensional echocardiography

Echocardiographic studies have shown that noncompaction is found predominantly in the apical and inferior wall region [9]. RV apex has been described in over 40% of patients in one case series [9]. Noncompaction is often found in association with depressed ventricular systolic function [19] which may coexist with impaired diastolic function. Furthermore impaired function is not confined to segments of affected myocardium but may also affect what appears to be macroscopically 'normal' myocardium [19].

In an attempt to standardize the diagnosis, three echocardiographic criteria have been proposed to diagnose noncompaction. It must be noted that there is no universally accepted definition of LVNC [92]. Chin et al. were the first to describe a quantitative approach to diagnose noncompaction using a trabeculation trough (X) to peak (Y) ratio in end-diastole [1]. The parasternal long-axis view for the basal and mid-papillary levels, and the subcostal or apical 4-chamber view for the apical segments were used to measure the X:Y ratio. A progressive decrease in the X:Y ratio, and an increase in total LV posterior wall thickness from the base to the apex was reported in LVNC patients compared to controls in the study [1]. While the original paper did not provide a cut-off for the X:Y ratio to diagnose LVNC, the subsequent publications report an X:Y ratio of ≤ 0.5 in diastole

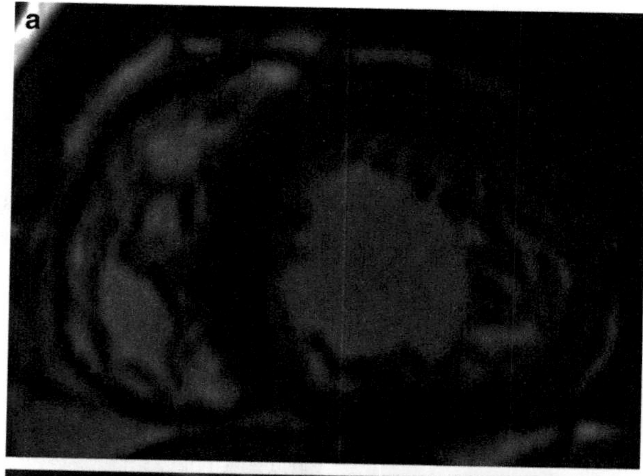

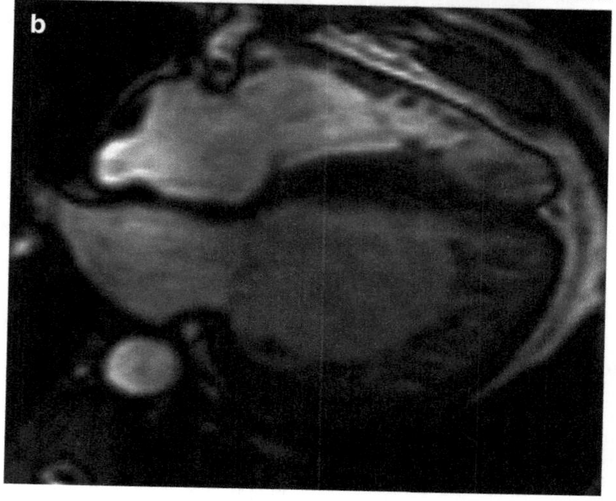

Fig. 12.2 Transthoracic echocardiography demonstrating prominent trabeculation (**a**) with color flow mapping demonstrating blood flow into the deep intertrabecular recesses in the left ventricle (**b**)

from short-axis view to diagnose LVNC [92]. However, this criteria has not been widely accepted into clinical practice [14, 20]. Later on, first Oechslin et al. and later Jenni et al. described the abnormally thickened myocardium as a two layered structure, with a normally compacted epicardial layer and a thickened endocardial layer [19, 21]. They proposed a quantitative evaluation for the diagnosis of LVNC by determining the ratio of maximal thickness of the noncompacted to compacted layers (measured at end systole in a parasternal short axis view), with a ratio >2 being diagnostic of LVNC. One advantage of this criteria is that it allows differentiation of the trabeculations of LVNC from that observed with DCM or hypertensive cardiomyopathy [21]. Stollberger et al. have proposed that LVNC is characterized by the presence of three or more coarse, prominent trabeculations apical to the papillary muscles, which have the same echogenicity as the myocardium, move synchronously with it, are not connected to the papillary muscles, and are surrounded by intertrabecular spaces, which are perfused from the ventricular cavity [24]. Similarities between Oechslin et al. and Stollberger et al. comprise the description of trabeculation and intertrabecular recesses communicating with and perfused from the ventricular cavity. Differences between these two definitions are the absence of an anatomic landmark to differentiate between trabeculations and papillary muscles in Oechslin's definition and the absence of the number of trabeculations as a criterium of LVNC [19]. Stollberger et al.'s definition on the contrary uses the anatomical landmark "apically to the papillary muscles" and requires the number of trabeculations [24]. A further difference between the two definitions includes the ratio of noncompacted to compacted layer at end-systole, which is a key criterium in Oechslin's definition and not included in Stollberger's definition. To unify the two definitions, in a recent review, Stollberger's et al have proposed that for future echocardiographic studies and clinical applications, it would be useful to differentiate between definite, probable, and possible LVNC [93]. Definite LVNC is said to present if both definitions are completely fulfilled. Probable LVNC is present if only either Oechslin's or Stollberger's criteria are fulfilled. Possible LVNC is present if the number of trabeculations is lower than four or if the ratio of noncompacted to compacted layer is less than two. There is limited concordance between different echocardiographic criteria. Transesophageal echocardiography and contrast echocardiography may be used when transthoracic studies cannot reliably exclude other processes [85, 94]. One report described the use of contrast echocardiography with sonicated albumin in a patient with LVNC [94].

Although echocardiography has been the diagnostic test of choice for noncompaction, other modalities have been used for the diagnosis, including contrast ventriculography [29, 94, 95] cardiac computed tomography [95, 96] and MRI [30, 32, 97].

MRI has shown a good correlation with echocardiography for localization and extent of noncompaction [30] (Fig. 12.3) and is particularly useful when echocardiography is inconclusive. Furthermore, It is proposed that the differences in MRI signal intensity in noncompacted myocardium can be used to identify substrate for potentially lethal arrhythmias [97]. It is now possible with MRI techniques such as gradient echo sequences to differentiate LVNC accurately from noncompacted areas of the LV as observed in healthy volunteers and, in patients with cardiomyopathies and concentric LV hypertrophy. The diagnostic criteria for LVNC on MRI include a diastolic ratio of noncompacted to compacted layer of greater than 2.3 [98], and an LV trabecular mass >20% of the total LV mass [99]. Cardiac Computed Tomography can be used in cases where MRI in contraindicated [100].

Tests such as invasive electrophysiological studies have not been widely used in patients with LVNC. Although, signal averaged electrocardiography in five children with LVNC showed late potentials in three and prolonged QT dispersion in one [30]. It is proposed that similar tests can be used to identify individuals at increased risk for ventricular arrhythmias and sudden death.

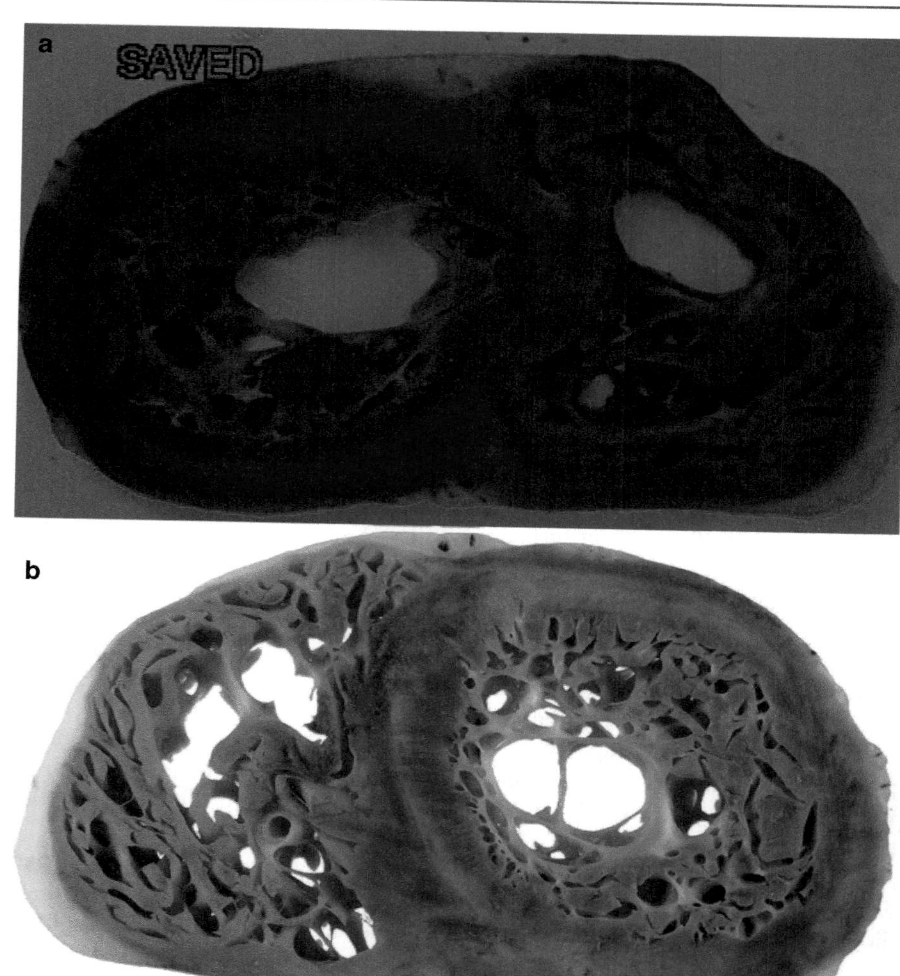

Fig. 12.3 MRI images demonstrating non-compacted fibres in short axis (**a**) and long axis views (**b**). Note noncompacting fibres are mainly confined to *posterior* and *lateral walls*

12.11 Differential Diagnosis

Any condition that results in prominent trabeculae with or without deep recesses may mimic LVNC. Apical HCM, DCM, arrhythmogenic right ventricular dysplasia, endocardial fibroelastosis, cardiac metastases, LV thrombus are some of the more common causes that should be borne in mind when considering the diagnosis of LVNC [14, 24, 28, 85]. It is recommended that one should be wary of making the diagnosis too readily, especially in the presence of impaired ventricular function [101].

Patients with LV hypertrophy secondary to pressure overload from systemic hypertension or congenital LV outflow tract obstruction are known to demonstrate excessive trabeculae [21, 54]. The existing trabeculae appear abnormally prominent with deep intertrabecular recesses as the myocardial hypertrophy involves the trabeculae as well as the outer compact layer. However this can be distinguished from LVNC by the preservation of the ratio of the noncompacted to compacted layer of myocardium [1, 21]. This is not to say that patients with LVNC cannot develop myocardial hypertrophy as a compensatory mechanism [9, 18, 22, 23, 87, 102, 103], however the ratio of non-compacted to compacted myocardium is not preserved. In addition, myocardial thickening in cases with primary noncompaction of the myocardium has been described to spare the regions of hypertrabeculation [104].

As previously noted, the absence of sinusoids (direct communications between the ventricular cavity and the coronary circulation) is another criterion that has frequently been cited for diagnosing primary myocardial noncompaction. These sinusoids develop as a means of decompression of the ventricular cavity in cases with semilunar valve atresia with an intact ventricular septum and are never present in otherwise structurally normal hearts [105–107]. They are mostly found in patients with pulmonary atresia and only rarely involve the LV [106, 107]. In these instances, excessive myocardial trabeculations, if present, are secondary to myocardial hypertrophy and not a form of primary myocardial disease.

12.12 Prognosis

The clinical course and prognosis of patients with noncompaction of the myocardium is highly variable. It can range from a prolonged asymptomatic course to rapidly progressive heart failure with resultant heart transplantation or death [20, 22, 23, 54, 86, 95, 108]. Transient recovery of ventricular function followed by later deterioration has been reported in infants [54], but the usual clinical course is one of rapid deterioration once symptoms develop [9, 88, 103]. In a group of children with myocardial noncompaction followed for up to 17 years, LV dysfunction developed in the vast majority, regardless of the presence of symptoms at initial diagnosis [88]. Ritter et al. followed 17 symptomatic adults for 6 years. Of which eight patients had died (47.1%) and two underwent heart transplantation [9]. In another series of 34 adults with myocardial noncompaction, 47% either died or underwent cardiac transplantation during the follow-up period of 44 ± 39 months [19].

The occurrences of ventricular arrhythmias, systemic emboli, and death was considerably lower in a large pediatric series from Japan [86] compared with those of adults. Increased age, higher LV end diastolic diameter at presentation, New York Heart Association class III or IV, permanent or persistent atrial fibrillation, bundle branch block, and the association with neuromuscular disease have been found to be predictors for increased mortality [19, 109]. Patients with these high-risk features are candidates for early and aggressive therapeutic interventions.

12.13 Management

Management of noncompaction of the ventricular myocardium centers on the management of the three major clinical manifestations: heart failure, arrhythmias, and systemic embolic events. Systolic and diastolic ventricular dysfunctions are treated with standard medical therapy [87]. Although, there are no large trials in patients with noncompaction, there is anecdotal evidence of the beneficial effects of the ß-blocker carvedilol on LV dysfunction, mass, and neurohormonal dysfunction [33]. Biventricular pacemakers may have a role to play in the treatment of patients with severely symptomatic heart failure, poor LV function, and prolonged intraventricular conduction [87]. Cardiac transplantation should be given consideration for those with refractory congestive heart failure [110, 111].

Due to the high incidence of arrhythmias in patients with LVNC, annual ambulatory ECG monitoring is prudent. Automated implantable cardioverter defibrillators (ICD) have an important role in the management of LVNC, although more work is required on stratifying patients according to risk of sudden cardiac death [87]. ICD use is currently not recommended as primary prophylaxis in LVNC alone, however maybe indicated in the setting of impaired systolic function based on current guidelines [112]. ICD is indicated for secondary prophylaxis after documented hemodynamically compromising sustained ventricular tachycardia or aborted sudden death [113]. Use of long term prophylactic anticoagulant therapy for all patients with ventricular noncompaction remains a controversial topic as the true prevalence of embolic phenomenon has not been established and hence the risk-benefit analysis cannot be done. However, the prevention of embolic complications remains an important issue. Whilst some authors recommend long-term prophylactic anticoagulation for all patients with ventricular noncompaction [9, 19] others advise anticoagulation only for patients with additional risk factors such as atrial fibrillation, evidence of thrombus or associated ventricular dysfunction [114, 115].

Clinical screening is recommended for asymptomatic first degree relatives of a patients with LVNC [116]. This should include a thorough genetic history, clinical

Table 12.6 Key points

1. LVNC is an uncommon cause of cardiomyopathy
2. It is widely thought to be related to arrested myocardial development
3. The genetic origin as well as the underlying pathogenesis remains unclear
4. It has a classical histopathological pattern and distinctive appearance on echocardiography and MRI which allows differentiation from other cardiomyopathies
5. LVNC is clinically characterized by a high prevalence of heart failure, thromboembolic complications and arrhythmias
6. Management of LVNC centers on these three major clinical manifestations
7. The clinical course and the prognosis of LVNC patients is highly variable
8. Increasing age, a dilated LV, symptoms of New York Heart Association class III or IV severity, atrial fibrillation, bundle branch block, and should lower the threshold for more aggressive management
9. The high incidence of familial occurrence warrants echocardiographic familial screening

history of possible symptoms, examination, electrocardiogram and echocardiogram. The role of genetic testing in asymptomatic subjects remains undefined. In asymptomatic relatives of a patient with an identified pathological mutation, targeted sequences may be of benefit [117]. Due to association of neuromuscular disorders and facial dysmorphism with noncompaction, their evaluation and treatment are required to complete the management [87, 118] (Table 12.6).

References

1. Chin TK, Perloff JK, Williams RG, et al. Isolated noncompaction of left ventricular myocardium. A study of eight cases. Circulation. 1990;82(2):507–13.
2. Dusek J, Ostadal B, Duskova M. Postnatal persistence of spongy myocardium with embryonic blood supply. Arch Pathol. 1975;99(6):312–7.
3. Maron BJ, Towbin JA, Thiene G, et al. Contemporary definitions and classification of the cardiomyopathies: an American Heart Association Scientific Statement from the Council on Clinical Cardiology, Heart Failure and Transplantation Committee; Quality of Care and Outcomes Research and Functional Genomics and Translational Biology Interdisciplinary Working Groups; and Council on Epidemiology and Prevention. Circulation. 2006;113(14):1807–16.
4. Jenni R, Goebel N, Tartini R, et al. Persisting myocardial sinusoids of both ventricles as an isolated anomaly: echocardiographic, angiographic, and pathologic anatomical findings. Cardiovasc Intervent Radiol. 1986;9(3):127–31.
5. Elliott P, Andersson B, Arbustini E, et al. Classification of the cardiomyopathies: a position statement from the european society of cardiology working group on myocardial and pericardial diseases. Eur Heart J. 2008;29(2):270–6.
6. Lauer RM, Fink HP, Petry EL, et al. Angiographic demonstration of intramyocardial sinusoids in pulmonary-valve atresia with intact ventricular septum and hypoplastic right ventricle. N Engl J Med. 1964;271:68–72.
7. Ozkutlu S, Ayabakan C, Celiker A, et al. Noncompaction of ventricular myocardium: a study of twelve patients. J Am Soc Echocardiogr. 2002;15(12):1523–8.
8. Biagini E, Ragni L, Ferlito M, et al. Different types of cardiomyipathy associated with isolated ventricular noncompaction. Am J Cardiol. 2006;98(6):821–4.
9. Ritter M, Oechslin E, Sutsch G, et al. Isolated noncompaction of the myocardium in adults. Mayo Clin Proc. 1997;72(1):26–31.
10. Gati S, Chandra N, Bennett RL, et al. Increased left ventricular trabeculation in highly trained athletes: do we need more stringent criteria for the diagnosis of left ventricular non-compaction in athletes? Heart. 2013;99(6):401–8.
11. Gati S, Papadakis M, Van Niekerk N, et al. Increased left ventricular trabeculation in individuals with sickle cell anaemia: physiology or pathology? Int J Cardiol. 2013;168(2):1658–60.
12. Harvey RP. Patterning the vertebrate heart. Nat Rev Genet. 2002;3(7):544–56.
13. Srivastava D, Olson EN. A genetic blueprint for cardiac development. Nature. 2000;407(6801):221–6.
14. Agmon Y, Connolly HM, Olson LJ, et al. Noncompaction of the ventricular myocardium. J Am Soc Echocardiogr. 1999;12(10):859–63.
15. Eisenberg LM, Markwald RR. Cellular recruitment and the development of the myocardium. Dev Biol. 2004;274(2):225–32.
16. Bernanke DH, Velkey JM. Development of the coronary blood supply: changing concepts and current ideas. Anat Rec. 2002;269(4):198–208.
17. Freedom RM, Yoo SJ, Perrin D, et al. The morphological spectrum of ventricular noncompaction. Cardiol Young. 2005;15(4):345–64.

18. Zambrano E, Marshalko SJ, Jaffe CC, et al. Isolated noncompaction of the ventricular myocardium: clinical and molecular aspects of a rare cardiomyopathy. Lab Investig. 2002;82(2):117–22.
19. Oechslin E, Attenhofer Jost CH, Rojas JR, et al. Long-term follow-up of 34 adults with isolated left ventricular noncompaction: a distinct cardiomyopathy with poor prognosis. J Am Coll Cardiol. 2000;36(2):493–500.
20. Rigopoulos A, Rizos IK, Aggeli C, et al. Isolated left ventricular noncompaction: an unclassified cardiomyopathy with severe prognosis in adults. Cardiology. 2002;98(1–2):25–32.
21. Jenni R, Oechslin E, Schneider J, et al. Echocardiographic and pathoanatomical characteristics of isolated left ventricular non-compaction: a step towards classification as a distinct cardiomyopathy. Heart. 2001;86(6):666–71.
22. Bleyl SB, Mumford BR, Brown-Harrison MC, et al. Xq28-linked noncompaction of the left ventricular myocardium: prenatal diagnosis and pathologic analysis of affected individuals. Am J Med Genet. 1997;72(3):257–65.
23. Bleyl SB, Mumford BR, Thompson V, et al. Neonatal, lethal noncompaction of the left ventricular myocardium is allelic with Barth syndrome. Am J Hum Genet. 1997;61(4):868–72.
24. Stollberger C, Finsterer J, Blazek G. Left ventricular hypertrabeculation/noncompaction and association with additional cardiac abnormalities and neuromuscular disorders. Am J Cardiol. 2002;90(8):899–902.
25. Markovic NS, Dimkovic N, Damjanovic T, et al. Isolated ventricular noncompaction in patients with chronic renal failure. Clin Nephrol. 2008;70(1):72–6.
26. Arbustini E, Favalli V, Narula N, et al. Left ventricular noncompaction. A distinct genetic cardiomyopathy? J Am Coll Cardiol. 2016;68(9):949–66.
27. Allenby PA, Gould NS, Schwartz MF, et al. Dysplastic cardiac development presenting as cardiomyopathy. Arch Pathol Lab Med. 1988;112(12):1255–8.
28. Boyd MT, Seward JB, Tajik AJ, et al. Frequency and location of prominent left ventricular trabeculations at autopsy in 474 normal human hearts: implications for evaluation of mural thrombi by two-dimensional echocardiography. J Am Coll Cardiol. 1987;9(2):323–6.
29. Engberding R, Bender F. Identification of a rare congenital anomaly of the myocardium by two-dimensional echocardiography: persistence of isolated myocardial sinusoids. Am J Cardiol. 1984;53(11):1733–4.
30. Junga G, Kneifel S, Von Smekal A, et al. Myocardial ischaemia in children with isolated ventricular non-compaction. Eur Heart J. 1999;20(12):910–6.
31. Jenni R, Oechslin EN, van der Loo B. Isolated ventricular non-compaction of the myocardium in adults. Heart. 2007;93(1):11–5.
32. Soler R, Rodriguez E, Monserrat L, et al. MRI of subendocardial perfusion deficits in isolated left ventricular noncompaction. J Comput Assist Tomogr. 2002;26(3):373–5.
33. Toyono M, Kondo C, Nakajima Y, et al. Effects of carvedilol on left ventricular function, mass, and scintigraphic findings in isolated left ventricular non-compaction. Heart. 2001;86(1):E4.
34. Hoedemaekers Y, Caliskan D, Majoor-Krakauer I, et al. Cardiac beta-myosin heavy chain defects in two families with non-compaction cardiomyopathy: linking non-compaction to hypertrophic, restrictive, and dilated cardiomyopathies. Eur Heart J. 2007;28(22):2732–7.
35. Klaassen S, Probst S, Oechslin E, et al. Mutations in sarcomere protein genes in left ventricular noncompaction. Circulation. 2008;117(22):2893–901.
36. Sasse-Klaassen S, Probst S, Gerull B, et al. Novel gene locus for autosomal dominant left ventricular noncompaction maps to chromosome 11p15. Circulation. 2004;109(22):2720–3.
37. Xing Y, Ichida F, Matsuoka T, et al. Genetic analysis in patients with left ventricular noncompaction and evidence for genetic heterogeneity. Mol Genet Metab. 2006;88(1):71–7.
38. Digilio MC, Marino B, Bevilacqua M, et al. Genetic heterogeneity of isolated noncompaction of the left ventricular myocardium. Am J Med Genet. 1999;85(1):90–1.
39. Aras D, Tufekcioglu O, Ergun K, et al. Clinical features of isolated ventricular noncompaction in adults long-term clinical course, echocardiographic properties, and predictors of left ventricular failure. J Card Fail. 2006;12(9):726–33.

40. Charron P, Arad M, Arbustini E, et al. Genetic counselling and testing in cardiomyopathies: a position statement of the European Society of Cardiology Working Group on Myocardial and Pericardial Diseases. Eur Heart J. 2010;31(22):2715–26.
41. Zaragoza MV, Arbustini E, Narula J. Noncompaction of the left ventricle: primary cardiomyopathy with an elusive genetic etiology. Curr Opin Pediatr. 2007;19(46):619–27.
42. Ichida F, Tsubata S, Bowles KR, et al. Novel gene mutations in patients with left ventricular noncompaction or Barth syndrome. Circulation. 2001;103(9):1256–63.
43. Marziliano N, Mannarino S, Nespoli L, et al. Barth syndrome associated with compound hemizygosity and heterozygosity of the TAZ and LDB3 genes. Am J Med Genet A. 2007;143(9):907–15.
44. Vatta M, Mohapatra B, Jimenez S, et al. Mutations in Cypher/ZASP in patients with dilated cardiomyopathy and left ventricular non-compaction. J Am Coll Cardiol. 2003;42(11):2014–27.
45. Luedde M, Ehlermann P, Weichenhan D, et al. Severe familial left ventricular noncompaction cardiomyopathy due to a novel troponin T (TNNT2) mutation. Cardiovasc Res. 2010;86(3):452–60.
46. Luxan G, Casanova J, Martinez-Poveda B, et al. Mutations in the NOTCH pathway regulator MIB1 cause left ventricular noncompaction cardiomyopathy. Nature Med. 2013;19(2):193–201.
47. Arndt A, Schafer S, Drenckhahn J, et al. Fine mapping of the 1p36 deletion syndrome identifies mutation of PRDM16 as a cause of cardiomyopathy. Am J Hum Genet. 2013;93(1):67–77.
48. Probst S, Oechslin E, Schuler P. Sarcomere gene mutations in isolated left ventricular noncompaction cardiomyopathy do not predict clinical phenotype. Circ Cardiovasc Genet. 2011;4(4):367–74.
49. Sandhu R, Finkelhor R, Gunawardena D, et al. Prevalence and characteristics of left ventricular noncompaction in a community hospital cohort of patients with systolic dysfunction. Echocardiography. 2008;25(1):8–12.
50. Hermida-Prieto M, Monserrat L, Castro-Beiras A, et al. Familial dilated cardiomyopathy and isolated left ventricular noncompaction associated with lamin A/C gene mutations. Am J Cardiol. 2004;94(1):50–4.
51. Bione S, D'Adamo P, Maestrini E, et al. A novel X-linked gene, G4.5 is responsible for Barth syndrome. Nat Genet. 1996;12(4):385–9.
52. Chen R, Tsuji T, Ichida F, Bowles KR, et al. Mutation analysis of the G4.5 gene in patients with isolated left ventricular noncompaction. Mol Genet Metab. 2002;77(4):319–25.
53. Kenton AB, Sanchez X, Coveler KJ, et al. Isolated left ventricular noncompaction is rarely caused by mutations in G4.5, alpha-dystrobrevin and FK binding protein-12. Mol Genet Metab. 2004;82(2):162–6.
54. Pignatelli RH, McMahon CJ, Dreyer WJ, et al. Clinical characterization of left ventricular noncompaction in children: a relatively common form of cardiomyopathy. Circulation. 2003;108(21):2672–8.
55. Thienpont B, Mertens L, Buyse G, et al. Left-ventricular non-compaction in a patient with monosomy 1p36. Eur J Med Genet. 2007;50(3):233–6.
56. Kanemoto N, Horigome H, Nakayama J, et al. Interstitial 1q43-q43 deletion with left ventricular noncompaction myocardium. Eur J Med Genet. 2006;49(3):247–53.
57. Benson DW, Silberbach GM, Kavanaugh-McHugh A, et al. Mutations in the cardiac transcription factor NKX2.5 affect diverse cardiac developmental pathways. J Clin Invest. 1999;104(11):1567–73.
58. Schott JJ, Benson DW, Basson CT, et al. Congenital heart disease caused by mutations in the transcription factor NKX2-5. Science. 1998;281(5373):108–11.
59. Pauli RM, Scheib-Wixted S, Cripe L, et al. Ventricular noncompaction and distal chromosome 5q deletion. Am J Med Genet. 1999;85(4):419–23.
60. Pashmforoush M, Lu JT, Chen H, et al. Nkx2-5 pathways and congenital heart disease; loss of ventricular myocyte lineage specification leads to progressive cardiomyopathy and complete heart block. Cell. 2004;117(3):373–86.

61. Schlame M, Ren M. Barth syndrome, a human disorder of cardiolipin metabolism. FEBS Lett. 2006;580(23):5450–5.
62. Scaglia F, Towbin JA, Craigen WJ, et al. Clinical spectrum, morbidity, and mortality in 113 pediatric patients with mitochondrial disease. Pediatrics. 2004;114(4):925–31.
63. Yaplito-Lee J, Weintraub R, Jamsen K, et al. Cardiac manifestations in oxidative phosphorylation disorders of childhood. J Pediatr. 2007;150(4):407–11.
64. Davili Z, Johar S, Hughes C, et al. Succinate dehydrogenase deficiency associated with dilated cardiomyopathy and ventricular noncompaction. Eur J Pediatr. 2007;166(8):867–70.
65. Finsterer J, Stollberger C, Kopsa W, et al. Wolff-Parkinson-White syndrome and isolated left ventricular abnormal trabeculation as a manifestation of Leber's hereditary optic neuropathy. Can J Cardiol. 2001;17(4):464–6.
66. Finsterer J, Stollberger C, Feichtinger H. Non-compaction on autopsy in Duchenne muscular dystrophy. Cardiology. 2007;108(3):161–3.
67. Finsterer J, Stollberger C, Steger C, et al. Complete heart block associated with noncompaction, nail-patella syndrome, and mitochondrial myopathy. J Electrocardiol. 2007;40(4): 352–4.
68. Finsterer J, Schoser B, Stollberger C. Myoadenylate-deaminase gene mutation associated with left ventricular hypertrabeculation/non-compaction. Acta Cardiol. 2004;59(4):453–6.
69. Finsterer J, Stollberger C, Schubert B. Acquired left ventricular hypertrabeculation/noncompaction in mitochondriopathy. Cardiology. 2004;102(4):228–30.
70. Finsterer J, Bittner R, Bodingbauer M, et al. Complex mitochondriopathy associated with 4 mtDNA transitions. Eur Neurol. 2000;44(1):37–41.
71. Wallace DC. Mitochondrial diseases in man and mouse. Science. 1999;283(5407):1482–8.
72. Tanpaiboon P, Callahan PF, Sloan J, et al. Noncompaction of the ventricular myocardium and hydrops fetalis in cobalamin C deficiency. Programme and abstracts of the American Society of Human Genetics Annual Meeting. 2006. Ref Type: Abstract.
73. Lofiego C, Biagini E, Pasquale F, et al. Wide spectrum of presentation and variable outcomes of isolated left ventricular non-compaction. Heart. 2007;93(1):65–71.
74. Stollberger C, Finsterer J, Blazek G, et al. Left ventricular non-compaction in a patient with Becker's muscular dystrophy. Heart. 1996;76(4):380.
75. Corrado G, Checcarelli N, Santarone M, et al. Left ventricular hypertrabeculation/noncompaction with PMP22 duplication-based Charcot-Marie-Tooth disease type 1A. Cardiology. 2006;105(3):142–5.
76. Finsterer J, Stolberger C, Kopsa W. Noncompaction in myotonic dystrophy type 1 on cardiac MRI. Cardiology. 2005;103(3):167–8.
77. OMIM Online Mendelian Inheritance in Man. 2017. Ref Type: Internet Communication.
78. Van Heerde M, Hruda J, Hazekamp MG. Severe pulmonary hypertension secondary to a parachute-like mitral valve, with the left superior caval vein draining into the coronary sinus, in a girl with Turner's syndrome. Cardiol Young. 2003;13(4):364–6.
79. McMahon CJ, Chang AC, Pignatelli RH, et al. Left ventricular noncompaction cardiomyopathy in association with trisomy 13. Pediatr Cardiol. 2005;26(4):477–9.
80. Kherbaoui-Redouani L, Eschard C, Bednarek N, et al. Cutaneous aplasia, noncompaction of the left ventricle and severe cardiac arrhythmia: a new case of MLS syndrome (microphtalmia with linear skin defects). Arch Pediatr. 2003;10(3):224–6.
81. Mandel K, Grunebaum E, Benson L. Noncompaction of the myocardium associated with Roifman syndrome. Cardiol Young. 2001;11(2):240–3.
82. Wong JA, Bofinger MK. Noncompaction of the ventricular myocardium in Melnick-Needles syndrome. Am J Med Genet. 1997;71(1):72–5.
83. Amann G, Sherman FS. Myocardial dysgenesis with persistent sinusoids in a neonate with Noonan's phenotype. Pediatr Pathol. 1992;12(1):83–92.
84. Matsumoto T, Watanabe A, Migita M, et al. Transient cardiomyopathy in a patient with congenital contractural arachnodactyly (Beals syndrome). J Nippon Med Sch. 2006;73(5):285–8.
85. Maltagliati A, Pepi M. Isolated noncompaction of the myocardium: multiplane transesophageal echocardiography diagnosis in an adult. J Am Soc Echocardiogr. 2000;13(11):1047–9.

86. Ichida F, Hamamichi Y, Miyawaki T, et al. Clinical features of isolated noncompaction of the ventricular myocardium: long-term clinical course, hemodynamic properties, and genetic background. J Am Coll Cardiol. 1999;34(1):233–40.
87. Weiford BC, Subbarao VD, Mulhern KM. Noncompaction of the ventricular myocardium. Circulation. 2004;109(24):2965–71.
88. Hook S, Ratliff NB, Rosenkranz E, et al. Isolated noncompaction of the ventricular myocardium. Pediatr Cardiol. 1996;17(1):43–5.
89. Reynen K, Bachmann K, Singer H. Spongy myocardium. Cardiology. 1997;88(6):601–2.
90. Yasukawa K, Terai M, Honda A, et al. Isolated noncompaction of ventricular myocardium associated with fatal ventricular fibrillation. Pediatr Cardiol. 2001;22(6):512–4.
91. Gati S, Papadakis M, Papamichael ND, et al. Reversible de novo left ventricular trabeculations in pregnant women: implications for the diagnosis of left ventricular noncompaction in low-risk populations. Circulation. 2014;130(6):475–83.
92. Oechslin E, Jenni R. Left ventricular noncompaction revisited: a distinct phenotype with genetic heterogeneity? Eur Heart J. 2011;32(12):1446–56.
93. Finsterer J, Stollberger C. Definite, probable, or possible left ventricular hypertrabeculation/noncompaction. Int J Cardiol. 2008;123(2):175–6.
94. Koo BK, Choi D, Ha JW, et al. Isolated noncompaction of the ventricular myocardium: contrast echocardiographic findings and review of the literature. Echocardiography. 2002;19(2):153–6.
95. Conces DJ, Ryan T, Tarver RD. Noncompaction of ventricular myocardium: CT appearance. AJR Am J Roentgenol. 1991;156(4):717–8.
96. Hamamichi Y, Ichida F, Hashimoto I, et al. Isolated noncompaction of the ventricular myocardium: ultrafast computed tomography and magnetic resonance imaging. Int J Cardiovasc Imaging. 2001;17(4):305–14.
97. Daimon Y, Watanabe S, Takeda S, et al. Two-layered appearance of noncompaction of the ventricular myocardium on magnetic resonance imaging. Circ J. 2002;66(6):619–21.
98. Petersen SE, Selvanayagam JB, Wiesmann F, et al. Left ventricular non-compaction: insights from cardiovascular magnetic resonance imaging. J Am Coll Cardiol. 2005;46(1):101–5.
99. Jacquier A, Thuny F, Jop B, et al. Measurement of trabeculated left ventricular mass using cardiac magnetic resonance imaging in the diagnosis of left ventricular non-compaction. Eur Heart J. 2010;31(9):1098–104.
100. Melendez-Ramirez G, Castillo-Castellon F, Espinola-Zavaleta N, et al. Left ventricular noncompaction: a proposal of new diagnostic criteria by multidetector computed tomography. J Cardiovasc Comput Tomogr. 2012;6(5):346–54.
101. Kohli SK, Pantazis AA, Shah JS, et al. Diagnosis of left-ventricular non-compaction in patients with left-ventricular systolic dysfunction: time for a reappraisal of diagnostic criteria? Eur Heart J 2008;29, 1:89-95.
102. Lengyel M. Isolated left ventricular noncompaction – first description in a Hungarian patient. Orv Hetil. 2002;143(27):1651–3.
103. Mizuno Y, Thompson TG, Guyon JR, et al. Desmuslin, an intermediate filament protein that interacts with alpha-dystrobrevin and desmin. Proc Natl Acad Sci U S A. 2001;98(11):6156–61.
104. Finsterer J, Stollberger C, Feichtinge H. Histological appearance of left ventricular hypertrabeculation/noncompaction. Cardiology. 2002;98(3):162–4.
105. Calder AL, Co EE, Sage MD. Coronary arterial abnormalities in pulmonary atresia with intact ventricular septum. Am J Cardiol. 1987;59(5):436–42.
106. Emmanouilides GC, Riemenschneider TA, Allen HD, et al. Hypoplastic left heart syndrome. In: Moss and Adams heart disease in infants, children and adolescents. Baltimore: Williams and Wilkins; 1995. p. 1133–53.
107. Emmanouilides GC, Riemenschneider TA, Allen HD, et al. Pulmonary atresia and intact ventricular septum. In: Moss and Adams heart disease in infants, children, and adolescents. Baltimore: Williams and Wilkins; 1995. p. 962–83.
108. Murphy RT, Thaman R, Gimeno Blanes J, et al. Natural history and familial characteristics of isolated left ventricular non-compaction. Eur Heart J. 2005;26(2):187–92.

109. Stollberger C, Winkler-Dworak M, Blazek G, et al. Prognosis of left ventricular hypertrabeculation/noncompaction is dependent on cardiac and neuromuscular comorbidity. Int J Cardiol. 2007;121(2):189–93.
110. Conraads V, Paelinck B, Vorlat A, et al. Isolated non-compaction of the left ventricle: a rare indication for transplantation. J Heart Lung Transplant. 2001;20(8):904–7.
111. Stamou SC, Lefrak EA, Athari FC, et al. Heart transplantation in a patient with isolated noncompaction of the left ventricular myocardium. Ann Thorac Surg. 2004;77(5):1806–8.
112. Hunt SA, Abraham WT, Chin MH, et al. 2009 focused update incorporated into the ACC/AHA 2005 Guidelines for the Diagnosis and Management of Heart Failure in Adults: a report of the American College of Cardiology Foundation/American Heart Association Task Force on Practice Guidelines: developed in collaboration with the International Society for Heart and Lung Transplantation. Circulation. 2009;119(14):e391–479.
113. Kobza R, Steffel J, Erne P, et al. Implantable cardioverter-defibrillator and cardiac resynchronization therapy in patients with left ventricular noncompaction. Heart Rhythm. 2010;7(11):1545–9.
114. Stollberger C, Finsterer J. Thrombi in left ventricular hypertrabeculation/noncompaction – review of the literature. Acta Cardiol. 2004;59(3):341–4.
115. Stollberger C, Finsterer J. Trabeculation and left ventricular hypertrabeculation/noncompaction. J Am Soc Echocardiogr. 2004;17(10):1120–1.
116. Hershberger RE, Lindenfeld J, Mestroni L, et al. Genetic evaluation of cardiomyopathy – a Heart Failure Society of America practice guideline. J Card Fail. 2009;15(2):83–97.
117. Towbin J, Lorts A, Jefferies J. Left ventricular non-compaction cardiomyopathy. Lancet. 2015;386(9995):813–25.
118. Finsterer J, Stollberger C, Blazek G. Neuromuscular implications in left ventricular hypertrabeculation/noncompaction. Int J Cardiol. 2006;110(3):288–300.

Inherited Arrhythmias: LQTS/SQTS/CPVT 13

Andrea Mazzanti and Silvia G. Priori

Abstract

"Inherited Arrhythmias" or "channelopathies" are familial disorders caused by mutations in genes coding for channel-proteins that control the electrical activity of the heart. These mutations predispose affected individuals to the development of life-threatening ventricular arrhythmias (polymorphic ventricular tachycardia/ventricular fibrillation) either by altering the fine-tuned equilibrium of ionic currents in the cardiac action potential, or by disrupting the electromechanical coupling in cardiomyocytes. Channelopathies are dangerous conditions, accounting for up to one third of sudden deaths in young individuals with a structurally "normal" heart. Every time an inherited arrhythmia syndrome is diagnosed in a patient, his/her family members may be predisposed to the same potentially lethal arrhythmias. If a timely diagnosis is reached, however, simple and efficacious preventive measures may be applied in most cases. Genetic information plays a pivotal role for the diagnosis of inherited arrhythmias and may help in the clinical management of patients and their relatives.

Keywords

Inherited arrhythmias • Long QT syndrome • Short QT syndrome • Sudden cardiac death • Genetics

A. Mazzanti
Istituti Clinici Scientifici Maugeri SpA SB, Pavia, Italy

S.G. Priori (✉)
Department of Cardiology, University of Pavia, Pavia, Italy

Salvatore Maugeri Foundation IRCCS, Pavia, Italy

Fondazione Salvatore Maugeri, University of Pavia, Pavia, Italy
e-mail: silvia.priori@fsm.it

D. Kumar, P. Elliott (eds.), *Cardiovascular Genetics and Genomics*,
https://doi.org/10.1007/978-3-319-66114-8_13

13.1 Introduction

The term "inherited arrhythmias" (or "channelopathies") defines a group of cardiac conditions caused by mutations in genes coding for channel-proteins that control the electrical activity of the heart. In the absence of macroscopic or microscopic structural heart defects, these mutations favor the development of ventricular tachycardia (VT) or ventricular fibrillation (VF) either by altering the ionic currents that regulate the duration of cardiac action potential (as in the case of Long QT syndrome, LQTS, and Short QT Syndrome, SQTS), or by disrupting the calcium cycle, which constitutes the basis for the electromechanical coupling in cardiomyocytes (e.g. Catecholaminergic Polymorphic VT, CPVT) [1, 2]. The clinical relevance of channelopathies lies in the fact that they are responsible for up to one third of sudden cardiac deaths (SCD) occurring in young patients with a structurally "normal" heart at post mortem investigations [2–5].

Taken as a group, channelopathies share some important features:

- They are rare disorders, with a prevalence ranging from 1 in 2000 for LQTS to less than 1 in 10,000 for SQTS and CPVT. Globally, however, they might affect up to 1 in 1000 unselected individuals from the general population.
- They are monogenic disorders that are most often transmitted in an autosomal dominant pattern, although they are typically characterized by incomplete penetrance and variable expressivity.
- They are clinically heterogeneous entities, with phenotypes ranging from asymptomatic, to palpitations, syncope, or SCD, which may occur as the first manifestation of the disease in apparently healthy individuals.
- They may be easily diagnosed with an electrocardiogram (ECG) recorded either at rest or during exercise, according to the specific condition.
- Genetic information allows for intervention at various stages in patient management, including diagnosis, risk stratification, and choice of therapy [3].

Once a channelopathy is diagnosed, simple prophylactic measures may be prescribed to reduce the arrhythmic risk of most patients. Therapeutic options include lifestyle changes (e.g. the avoidance of strenuous exercise in patients with LQTS or CPVT), antiarrhythmic drugs, or even the use of implantable cardioverter defibrillators (ICD) in selected cases [4, 5].

In the following sections we will outline the key features of three "inherited arrhythmias", beginning with the Long QT Syndrome, the first channelopathy described and therefore the most thoroughly understood with regard to risk stratification of patients and pharmacological treatment. We will then approach the mirror entity of LQTS, Short QT Syndrome, one of the rarest and most lethal channelopathies, described based on fewer than 200 patients in the literature. Finally, we will discuss Catecholaminergic Polymorphic Ventricular Tachycardia, highlighted because of the promising results of an innovative genetic therapy applied to animal models that aim to cure this disease.

Throughout this chapter we will make reference to the "Guidelines for the Management of Patients with Ventricular Arrhythmias and the Prevention of Sudden

Cardiac Death," published by the European Society of Cardiology in 2015 [5]. We will also reference two consensus documents released by major international heart rhythm societies for the diagnosis and management of "inherited primary arrhythmia syndromes" [4] and the appropriate use of genetic testing in these inheritable conditions [3].

13.2 Long QT Syndrome

13.2.1 Introduction

The definition of Long QT Syndrome (LQTS) includes a class of diseases characterized by the following traits: (1) prolonged ventricular repolarization reflected by the QT interval on surface ECG, (2) morphological abnormalities of the T waves, and (3) the susceptibility to develop a special form of polymorphic VT (termed *torsade de pointes*), especially during phases of adrenergic stimulation.

13.2.2 Clinical Case

DT, female, was born in 1981. At the age of 5 years, she experienced two syncopal episodes while playing in the courtyard. In both cases she lost her consciousness abruptly and recovered spontaneously after a few moments without urine loss or seizures. Neurological assessment was negative, while the electrocardiogram revealed the presence of a long QT interval (Fig. 13.1, panel a: RR 680 ms, QT 420 ms, QTc 509 ms). Beta-blocker therapy was started with propranolol 50 mg/day divided in

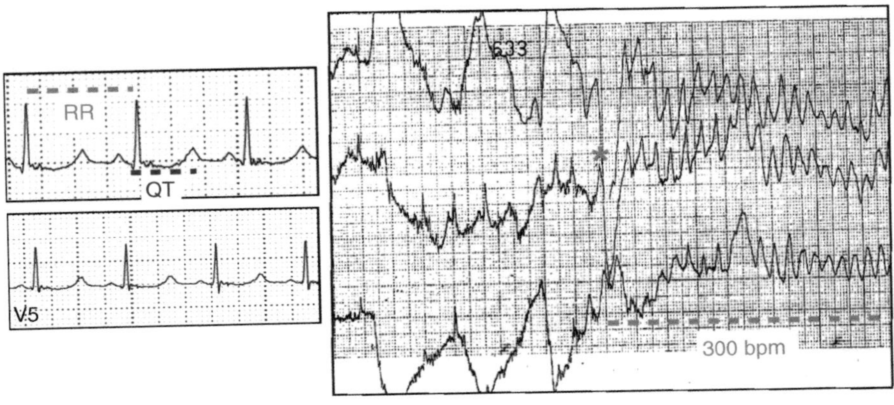

Fig. 13.1 Long QT syndrome. Panel (**a**) Baseline electrocardiogram shows the prolonged QT interval: RR 680 ms, QT 420 ms, QTc 509 ms. The broad-base morphology of the T wave is suggestive for type 1 Long QT Syndrome. The red dotted line identifies the RR interval; the blue dotted line identifies the QT interval. Panel (**b**) Exercise stress test with evidence of polymorphic VT with a heart rate of approximately 300 b.p.m. initiated by a premature ventricular contraction, indicated by the red asterisk

three doses (2.5 mg/kg/day) and experienced no arrhythmic episodes for the subsequent 3 years, undergoing annual controls with exercise stress test and ECG Holter.

At the age of 8, she experienced a sudden loss of consciousness while exercising on the treadmill (at the stage of 75 W with the Bruce protocol) during a routine medical control at our Center and an episode of polymorphic VT initiated by premature ventricular contractions in a short-long-short sequence was recorded (Fig. 13.1, panel b). The patient recovered spontaneously after 10 s. Since we considered that the dose of beta-blockers might have been too low for her body weight, we increased propranolol to 80 mg divided in three doses (3 mg/kg/day) per day and she repeated the exercise stress test after a week. She reached a higher stage of exercise (100 W) and no arrhythmias were documented. On this regard, it is vital to stress the importance of adapting the dose of beta-blockers to the increasing body weight during childhood and adolescence and to monitor their chronotropic control performing regular exercise stress tests on therapy.

At the age of 15, we changed therapy to increase the compliance of the patient and nadolol 80 mg twice a day was started (2.7 mg/kg/day) without further symptoms or ventricular arrhythmias documented. She has remained asymptomatic for the past 19 years, and during her first pregnancy at the age of 34 no arrhythmic episodes occurred. She continued her therapy without problems and she delivered the baby naturally without complications. The baby does not carry the pathogenic mutation and has a normal QT interval.

13.2.3 Familial and Genetic Study

The genetic testing performed in the patient revealed a point mutation in the intron region (c.1032+1 g>a) of the *KCNQ1* gene that originated a splice site error.

No history of sudden death or syncope was present in the family. Both parents had normal ECG. When they underwent genetic screening, neither the parents nor the brother and sister carried the *KCNQ1* variant identified in the proband. Therefore the *KCNQ1* was presumed to have arisen de novo.

13.2.4 Epidemiology

Patients with LQTS have been described in all ethnic groups. The prevalence of the autosomal dominant LQTS in Caucasians is estimated at 1:2000 [4], whereas the autosomal recessive form is far less frequent (1 in 200,000 according to epidemiological data from Northern Europe [6]).

13.2.5 Genetic Variants

Up to today 17 variants of congenital LQTS are known, caused mainly by mutations in genes encoding for subunits of potassium, sodium, or calcium voltage-dependent ion channels (Table 13.1).

Table 13.1 Clinical forms of long QT syndrome and related genes

Clinical LQTS Phenotype	LQTS Type	Frequency (%)	Gene symbol	Locus	Protein	Functional effect
Autosomal dominant LQTS without extracardiac manifestations (Romano-Ward Sdr)	LQT1	40–55	*KCNQ1*	11p15.5-p15.4	Potassium channel, voltage-gated, KQT-like subfamily, member 1	Loss of function; reduction of IKs current
	LQT2	30–45	*KCNH2*	7q36.1	Potassium channel, voltage-gated, subfamily H, member 2	Loss of function; reduction of IKr current
	LQT3	5	*SCN5A*	3p22.2	Sodium channel, voltage-gated, type V, alpha subunit	Gain of function; increase of sodium current
	LQT4	<1	*ANK2*	4q25-q26	Ankyrin 2	Loss of function (several target proteins)
	LQT5	<1	*KCNE1*	21q22.11-q22.12	Potassium channel, voltage-gated, ISK-related subfamily, member 1	Loss of function; reduction of IKs current
	LQT6	<1	*KCNE2*	21q22.11	Potassium channel, voltage-gated, ISK-related subfamily, member 2	Loss of function; reduction of IKr current
	LQT9	<1	*CAV3*	3p25.3	Caveolin 3	Secondary gain of function of sodium channel
	LQT10	<1	*SCN4B*	11q23.3	Sodium channel, voltage-gated, type IV, beta subunit	Secondary gain of function of sodium channel
	LQT11	<1	*AKAP9*	7q21.2	A-kinase anchor protein 9	Loss of function; reduction of IKs current
	LQT12	<1	*SNTA1*	20qll.21	Syntrophin, alpha-1	Secondary gain of function of sodium channel
	LQT13	<1	*KCNJ5*	11q24.3	Potassium channel, inwardly rectifying, subfamily J, member 5	Loss of function; reduction of IK-Ach current
	LQT14	<1	*CALM1*	14q32.11	Calmoduline 1	Loss of function, reduction in calcium-binding affinity
	LQT15	<1	*CALM2*	2p21	Calmoduline 2	Loss of function, reduction in calcium-binding affinity
	LQT16	<1	*CALM3*	19q13.2-q13.3	Calmoduline 3	Loss of function, reduction in calcium-binding affinity

(continued)

Table 13.1 (continued)

Clinical LQTS Phenotype	LQTS Type	Frequency (%)	Gene symbol	Locus	Protein	Functional effect
Autosomal dominant LQTS with extracar-diac manifesta-tions	LQT7 (ATS)	<1	*KCNJ2*	17q24.3	Potassium channel, inwardly rectifying, subfamily J, member 2	Loss of function; reduction of IK1 current
	LQT8 (TS)	<1	*CACNA1C*	12p13.33	Calcium channel, voltage-dependent, L type, alpha-lC subunit	Gain of function; increase of calcium current
Autosomal recessive LQTS with congenital deafness (Jervell and Lange-Nielsen Sdr)	JLN1	<1	*KCNQ1*	11p15.5-p15.4	Potassium channel, voltage-gated, KQT-like subfamily, member 1	Loss of function; reduction of IKs current
	JLN2	<1	*KCNE1*	21q22.11	Potassium channel, voltage-gated, ISK-related subfamily, member 1	Loss of function; reduction of IKs current
Autosomal recessive LQTS without extracar-diac manifesta-tions			*TRDN*	6q22.31	Triadine	Loss of function, loss of cardiac Ca2+ release units, impaired excitation-contraction coupling

ATS Andersen Tawil syndrome, *TS* Timothy syndrome, *JLN* Jervell and Lange-Nielsen syndrome

The first three subtypes, LQT1 to LQT3, account for 75% of LQTS cases [4]: 70% of all LQTS are secondary to loss-of-function mutations affecting either the Kv7.1 potassium channel (LQT1, gene *KCNQ1*) or the Kv11.1 potassium channel (LQT2, gene *KCNH2*), while about 5% are secondary to gain-of-function mutations in the Nav1.5 sodium channel (LQT3, gene *SCN5A*). The other "minor" LQTS genes are responsible for 5% of cases, while for the remaining 20% of patients the genetic background remains elusive [3], though new LQTS-related genes are continuously identified.

The two most recent forms of LQTS described are related to mutations in the genetic coding for the proteins triadin and calmodulin. Cardiac triadin (gene *TRDN*) is a transmembrane protein located on the sarcoplasmic reticulum (SR) and involved in the release of calcium ions from the SR that mediates the calcium homeostasis of the cardiomyocyte (see the section on CPVT within this chapter). In 2015 Altmann et al. found that 4 of 33 unrelated children with QT prolongation and severe exercise-induced arrhythmias carried either homozygous or compound heterozygous frameshift *TRDN* mutations [7].

Calmodulin (or CaM, an abbreviation for calcium-modulated protein) is a multifunctional intermediate calcium-binding messenger protein expressed in all eukaryotic cells, where it acts as part of a calcium signal transduction pathway by interacting with several target proteins such as kinases or phosphatases. CaM is encoded by three genes (*CALM1*, *CALM2*, and *CALM3*), all of which harbor pathogenic variants linked to LQTS with early and severe expressivity [8, 9].

The principal forms of LQTS may be grouped in the three following clinical categories:

1. Autosomal dominant LQTS (or Romano-Ward Syndrome), which includes LQT1-6 and LQT9-15 and is characterized by an isolated prolongation of the QT interval;
2. Autosomal dominant LQTS with extra-cardiac manifestation, which includes:
   - The Andersen-Tawil Syndrome (ATS), characterized by a prolonged QT interval, prominent U waves, facial dysmorphisms and hyper/hypokalemic periodic paralysis. Half of ATS cases are caused by mutations in the *KCNJ2*-encoded Kir2.1 potassium channel (LQT7).
   - The Timothy Syndrome (TS, or LQT8), which shows prolonged QT, syndactyly, cardiac malformations, autism spectrum disorders and facial dysmorphisms. LQT8 results from "gain-of-function" mutations in the *CACNA1C*-encoded L-type calcium channel alpha subunit.
3. Autosomal recessive LQTS, including:
   - Jervell and Lange-Nielsen Syndrome, which combines an extremely prolonged QT interval and congenital deafness and is caused by the same (homozygous) or different (compound heterozygous) *KCNQ1* or *KCNE1* mutations, received from both parents;
   - Triadin related LQTS, which represents an overlapping form of LQTS and CPVT.

13.2.6 Diagnosis

The diagnosis of LQTS relies primarily on the corrected measurement of the QT interval for heart rate (QTc) using Bazett's formula. From a technical standpoint, it is important to standardize the method of measuring the QT interval. The highest diagnostic accuracy in LQTS families has been observed for QTc measured in leads II and V5 of 12-lead ECGs. Thus, QT should be obtained in one of these leads [10]. Furthermore, when using the Bazett formula to correct heart rate, it is important to remember that the formula is linear for heart rates between 60 and 100 beats/min. Finally, considering the adaptation of the QT to changes in heart rate presents some delay (hysteresis), it is recommended to avoid QT measurement when the heart rate shows beat-to-beat instability. Whenever it is not possible to achieve a stable heart rate (such as in atrial fibrillation), it is reasonable to select the recording showing less variability of the RR interval [11].

Secondary causes of QT prolongation (drugs or electrolyte imbalance) need to be excluded when assessing the ECG of a patient with suspected LQTS.

According to the current definition [5], LQTS is diagnosed in patients with a cardiac arrest (CA) or syncope and a QTc >460 ms in repeated electrocardiograms, whereas in asymptomatic individuals without a family history of LQTS, a QTc >480 ms is required to establish the diagnosis [5].

Although a prolonged ventricular repolarization is the hallmark of LQTS, up to one third of carriers of a pathogenic mutation exhibit normal QTc values (incomplete penetrance). These "silent" mutation carriers are considered "affected" according to the current guidelines, having a higher risk of arrhythmias than the general population (10% from birth to 40 years [12]) and consequently need treatment [5]. In cases with less evident QT prolongation, a score (the so called "Schwartz Score") has been created that combines the age of the patient, clinical and family history, and the QTc duration, providing a probability of the diagnosis of LQTS [13].

Aside from the prolonged ventricular repolarization, patients with LQTS present with peculiar electro-morphological alterations. These alterations tend to be gene-specific, and may help in identifying the syndrome. Notches on the T-wave, for instance, are typical for LQT2 and indicate a higher risk for arrhythmic events. Long sinus pauses are common among LQT3 patients.

13.2.7 Clinical Manifestations

The clinical manifestations of LQTS are secondary to a distinctive form of polymorphic VT, termed *torsade de pointes*, characterized by fast bursts of ventricular complexes that twist 180° around the isoelectric line and lead to syncopal events. The precipitants for arrhythmias are often gene-specific, with most events occurring during physical or emotional stress in LQT1, sudden noises in LQT2 and during sleep in LQT3 patients [4].

The mean age of onset of symptoms is 14 years [14]; earlier manifestations predict a severe prognosis. Among untreated patients, the natural history is represented by the occurrence of several syncopal episodes, eventually leading to SCD (annual incidence of SCD between 0.3% and 1% from birth to 40 years [12]). In a non-negligible proportion of patients, however, SCD is the first manifestation of the syndrome, hence the rationale for treating asymptomatic patients.

Interestingly, LQTS patients are also at high risk for atrial arrhythmias, probably due to the prolonged atrial repolarization that may contribute to the initiation of atrial fibrillation. This might have prognostic relevance for both the risk of stroke and inappropriate shocks in patients with an ICD. Zellerhoff S. et al. assessed the occurrence of atrial arrhythmias in 21 LQTS patients and in 21 matched controls using ICD or pacemakers as monitors of atrial rhythm and found that 7 of 21 (33%) of the LQTS patients developed self-terminating atrial arrhythmias, versus only one control patient ($P < 0.05$) [15].

13.2.8 Risk Stratification

Clinical, electrocardiographic, genetic and demographic parameters should be integrated in the risk stratification of LQTS patients.

Patients with history of CA/arrhythmic syncope present a higher risk of SCD as compared to asymptomatic ones, especially if arrhythmias occur during the first year of life. Survivors of a CA have a high risk of recurrences, even while receiving beta-blockers (14% within 5 years [16]) and, in general, should receive an ICD as secondary prevention of SCD [5].

Similarly, the occurrence of syncope during therapy with adequate dosage of beta-blockers calls for aggressive treatment [5].

In asymptomatic individuals, the QT interval itself is the principal indicator of risk [12]: patients with QTc >500 ms (and especially >550 ms) are at high risk for SCD [12]. Further, ECG markers to consider in risk stratification are the presence of T wave *alternans* and long sinus pauses followed by T wave abnormalities that are signs of electrical instability [4].

Genetic information gives an important contribution to risk stratification and it is now possible to delineate a gene-specific profile for the risk of SCD: LQT1 patients are in the lowest risk category, as compared to LQT2 and LQT3 [12]. Additionally, mutations in specific regions of a protein have been correlated to the clinical severity: mutations in the cytoplasmic loops of LQT1 [17] and mutations in the pore region of LQT2 [18] are associated with a high risk of arrhythmias. More recently, mutation-specific risk stratification has been proposed and some highly malignant LQTS variants, such as the KCNQ1-A341V [19], have been recognized.

The highest malignancy is related to the autosomal recessive form of LQTS, the Jervell and Lange-Nielsen Syndrome, characterized by a very early onset and major QTc prolongation, and in which beta-blockers have limited efficacy [20].

One of the most appealing opportunities in risk stratification of LQTS patients derives from the opportunity to integrate genetic and clinical parameters to provide a truly personalized approach to patient management. Data from the International LQTS Registry have shown that male gender is associated with a 3-fold increase in the risk of life-threatening cardiac events during childhood [21] and this effect is especially evident in LQT1 families [21]. Interestingly, however, after puberty an opposite trend has been observed and females maintain a higher risk than males during adulthood. Sauer et al. [22] in an analysis of 812 positively genotyped LQTS patients found that women between the ages of 18–40 years old show a higher risk (2.7 fold) and higher cumulative probability (11% vs. 3%) of aborted CA and SCD as compared to men. Importantly, females (especially LQT2 women) show a peak of arrhythmic risk in the postpartum period [23].

After the age of 40, LQTS women still exhibit a significantly higher arrhythmic risk than men [22], and this appears to counterbalance the increased male risk due to acquired cardiovascular pathologies in the older age groups. Buber et al. [24] showed a genotype-specific association with the risk for cardiac events during the perimenopausal period, including a pronounced increase in the risk for arrhythmic events (mainly recurrent syncope) among LQT2 women and an opposite reduction in LQT1 women. A partial exception to this comes from LQT3, in which males exhibit an increased risk of SCD across their entire life-span [12].

Finally, it is noteworthy that up to 10% of genotyped LQTS patients may harbor a second pathogenic mutation in one of the LQTS-related genes and, according to data published by Westenskow et al., they are at increased risk of CA (OR, 3.5; 95% CI, 1.2–9.9) compared to patients with 1 or no identified mutation [25].

13.2.9 Management

Lifestyle modifications to limit the exposure to arrhythmic triggers should be applied to all LQTS patients. These include: avoidance of drugs prolonging QT interval (for a comprehensive list: www.crediblemeds.org), abstention from strenuous exercise (especially swimming) in LQT1 patients and reduction of exposure to abrupt loud noises in LQT2 patients.

Beta-blockers are the mainstay pharmacological therapy for LQTS [4]. They are indicated in all LQTS patients, including those with a genetic diagnosis and normal QTc, unless there is a contraindication. Long-acting non-selective beta-blockers (e.g. Nadolol 1–2 mg/kg/day or sustained-release Propranolol 3–5 mg/kg/day) are preferred due to improved compliance. Selective beta-blockers (e.g. metoprolol) may have a role in asthmatic patients [4].

In LQT3 patients refractory to beta-blockers, sodium channel blockers (especially mexiletine) have shown to be efficacious in reducing both QT interval and arrhythmic events. Our group demonstrated 20 years ago that mexiletine effectively shortened the QT interval in LQT3 patients [26]. Recently, we found that long-term treatment with mexiletine significantly reduced the occurrence of arrhythmic events in a cohort of 32 LQT3 patients treated for a median time of three years: the annual rate of LQTS-related syncope and CA dropped from 10.3% before treatment to 0.7% during therapy ($p = 0.0097$) [27].

In high-risk patients who are intolerant or refractory to beta-blockers, especially infants and children in whom ICD therapy may be relatively dangerous, Left Cardiac Sympathetic Denervation (LCSD) should be considered to reduce the probability for arrhythmias [4]. Olde Nordkamp et al. published a retrospective study on 11 symptomatic LQTS patients who underwent LCSD due to therapy-refractory cardiac events finding that the annual cardiac event rate decreased in 8/10 patients who survived LCSD, but after 2 years the probability of complete cardiac event-free survival was 59%, demonstrating that LCSD is a therapeutic option, but not a cure [28] for these patients.

ICD therapy is indicated in the few patients with a high arrhythmic risk despite therapy, such as survivors of a CA or those who experience a syncopal event while on beta-blockers [4]. Conversely, the use of an ICD in asymptomatic individuals who have never tried beta-blockers is generally not indicated [4]. According to current guidelines the prophylactic ICD therapy might be considered in addition to beta-blocker therapy in asymptomatic carriers of a pathogenic mutation in *KCNH2* or *SCN5A* when QTc exceeds 500 ms in repeated measures [5].

13.3 Short QT Syndrome

13.3.1 Introduction

The Short QT Syndrome (SQTS) is defined by an abbreviated duration of cardiac repolarization, which represents both its diagnostic hallmark on the surface ECG and the substrate for the development of VF. Since the 1990s, an association between a shorter than normal QT interval with an increased risk of sudden death was postulated, and in 2003 SQTS was identified as an autonomous cause of familial SCD [29] (Fig. 13.2).

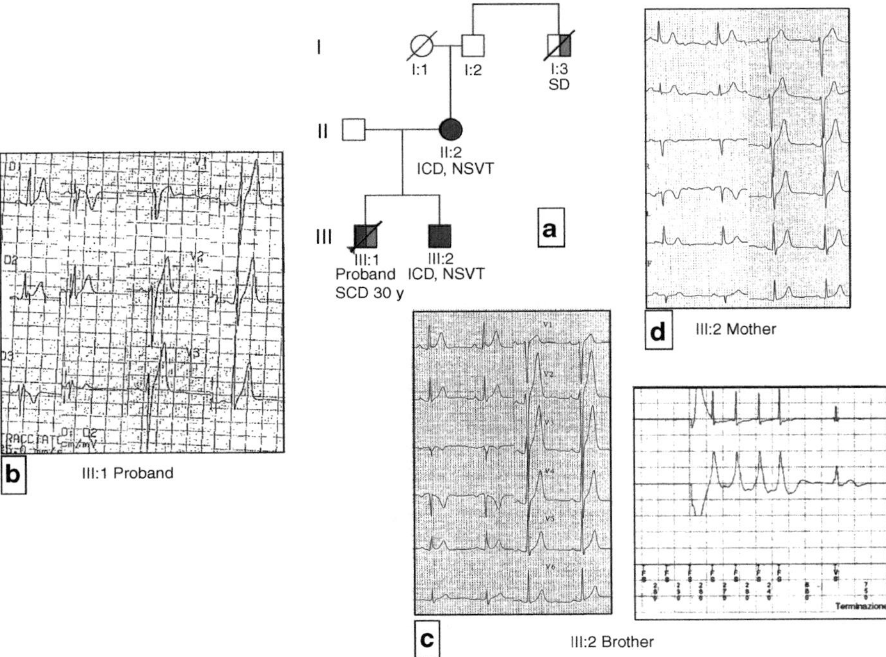

Fig. 13.2 Short QT syndrome. Panel (**a**) The three-generation pedigree shows a family with Short QT Syndrome and several cases of sudden death. Circles identify females, squares identify males. Blue identifies individuals who exhibited Short QT on electrocardiogram. The red identifies individuals who expired from sudden death (SD). *ICD* implantable cardioverter defibrillator, *NSVT* non-sustained ventricular tachycardia. Panel (**b**) The ECG of the proband exhibited RR 1100 ms, QT 290 ms, QTc 277 ms. The symmetrical and peaked T waves are typical of Short QT Syndrome. Panel (**c**) The brother of the proband exhibited a short QT interval: RR 880 ms, QT 300 ms, QTc 320 ms. His ICD recorded episodes of fast non-sustained ventricular tachycardia (maximum 8 beats with a minimum RR interval of 240 ms). Panel (**d**) The mother of the proband exhibited a short QT interval: RR 880 ms, QT 300 ms, QTc 320 ms

13.3.2 Clinical Case

FT, male, died suddenly while sleeping at the age of 30. He was previously asymptomatic. A 12 lead electrocardiogram (ECG) recorded before CA for routine medical examination revealed the presence of an extremely short QT interval (RR 1100 ms, QT 290 ms, QTc 277 ms, Fig. 13.3, panel b). Post-mortem examination revealed only minor abnormalities of the myocardium; no DNA was available for molecular autopsy.

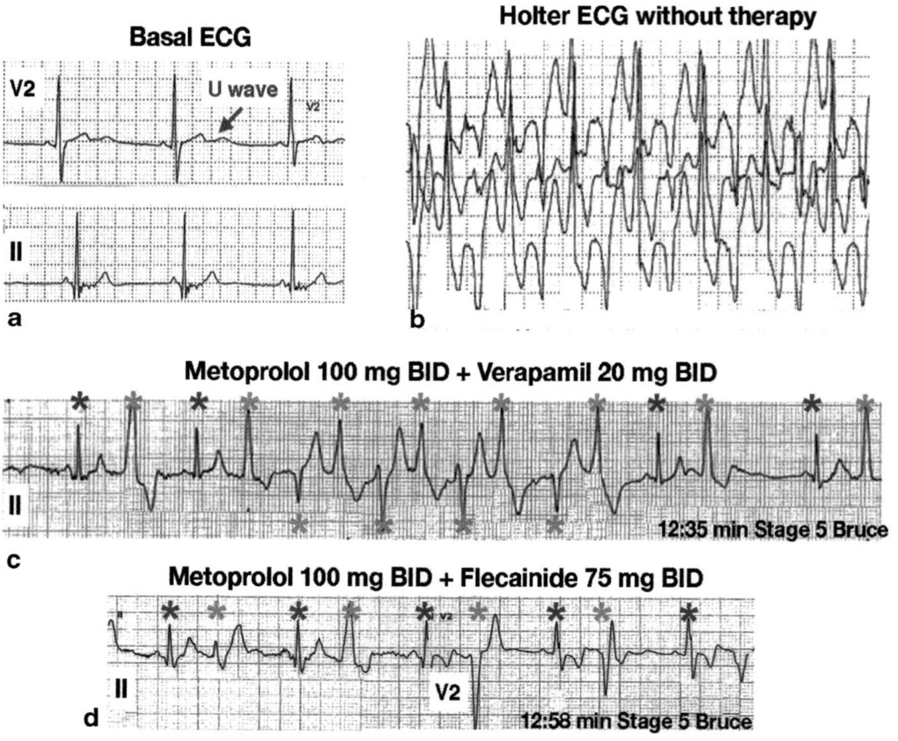

Fig. 13.3 Catecholaminergic polymorphic ventricular tachycardia. Panel (**a**) Baseline ECG of a patient affected by CPVT characterized by sinus bradycardia (heart rate 49 bpm), normal atrioventricular and intraventricular conduction and normal QT interval (QTc 416 ms). The arrow identifies the prominent U wave, typical of CPVT. Panel (**b**) Holter ECG recorded before initiating beta-blocker therapy, which shows an episode of bidirectional VT, typical of CPVT, characterized by a 180° beat-to-beat rotation of the ectopic QRS complexes on the frontal plane. This child was running at the moment of the recording. Panel (**c**) ECG recording from an exercise stress test performed while on therapy with metoprolol 100 mg BID and verapamil 20 mg BID shows a run of bidirectional VT arisen at the peak of the exercise. Panel (**d**) Verapamil was changed to flecainide 75 mg BID, which suppressed dramatically the complex arrhythmias. At the peak of the exercise (comparable with the previous test), the only arrhythmias were bigeminal ventricular polymorphic beats. Red asterisks identify premature ventricular contractions, blue asterisks identify sinus beats

The brother RT, who 5 years younger, was asymptomatic at the time of clinical observation. His ECG also revealed a short QT (RR 880 ms, QT 300 ms, QTc 320 ms, Fig. 13.3, panel c) interval and for this reason he was treated with hydroquinidine 500 mg BID, and his QTc increased to 400 ms. Due to severe gastric intolerance, however, he withdrew from the therapy. He therefore received an ICD, which recorded some episodes of fast non-sustained VT (maximum 8 beats, Fig. 13.3, panel c). No sustained arrhythmias or appropriate shocks have been recorded over 5 years of follow-up.

ECG of the mother of the two patients revealed a short QT interval (RR 880 ms, QT 300 ms, QTc 320 ms; Fig. 13.3, panel d), in the absence of clinical manifestations. She tried hydroquinidine 500 mg BID (QTc 385 ms), but refused to continue the therapy and preferred to have an ICD implanted. As in her son's case, some episodes of rapid non-sustained VT were recorded. No sustained arrhythmias or appropriate shocks have been recorded over 5 years of follow-up.

The genetic testing performed on the mother failed to identify any mutation in one of the principal genes related to the SQTS.

13.3.3 Epidemiology

Less than 200 SQTS patients have been reported in the literature [30, 31], reflecting the rarity of the disease (estimated prevalence <1:10,000).

13.3.4 Genetic Variants

SQTS is an autosomal dominant disease and it has been connected to five genes encoding for potassium (*KCNH2*, *KCNQ1*, *KCNJ2*) and calcium (*CACNA1C* and *CACNB2*) conducting channels. The yield of genetic screening is low, only 20% overall [31], because each gene accounts for less than 5% of index cases [3, 31]. Interestingly, three of these genes are also associated with variants of LQTS (LQT2, LQT1 and LQT7). This peculiarity, wherein mutations of the same genes result in both abnormally prolonged and abnormally shortened repolarization, has an obvious biophysical explanation. Mutations responsible for LQTS cause a reduction ("loss-of-function") in the potassium current conducted by the ion channels encoded by the *KCNQ1*, *KCNH2* and *KCNJ2* genes. Conversely, mutations responsible for SQTS cause an increase ("gain-of-function") in the current conducted by the same potassium channels, thus shortening repolarization. Loss-of-function mutations in the genes encoding alpha- and beta-subunits of the L-type cardiac calcium channel (*CACNA1C* and *CACNB2*) have been associated to a mixed phenotype of SQTS and Brugada Syndrome (BrS) [32].

Despite the reduced number of families with a positive genotype reported in the literature, some genotype-phenotype correlations have been attempted [30, 33]. Patients with *KCNH2*-related mutations (type 1 SQTS, or SQT1) constitute a subgroup with shorter QT intervals, higher prevalence of atrial fibrillation (AF) at a young age and a more constant response to quinidine in comparison to non-SQT1 ones [30]. As will be discussed, however, risk stratification according to genotype or phenotype is still being explored.

13.3.5 Diagnosis

As with all channelopathies, the diagnosis is based on the duration of the QT interval on a standard 12-lead ECG recorded at rest. QTc values ≤360 ms combined with a confirmed pathogenic mutation, symptoms or familial history of SCD at a young age are suggestive of the disease [5]. Individuals with QTc ≤340 ms are considered affected, even when they are asymptomatic [5, 31]. As for the LQTS, it is important that the QT interval is measured when the heart rate is close to 60 beats/min. This is especially important in young males, who tend to have low heart rates at rest: in the context of bradycardia, the Bazett's formula induces over-correction and this may cause the false diagnosis of SQTS. In uncertain cases the exercise stress test may be useful in recognizing SQTS patients, who show a reduced adaptation of the QT interval to the increase of heart rate. In a case-control study Giustetto et al. analyzed the behavior during exercise of 21 SQTS patients, demonstrating that the mean variation of the absolute QT interval from rest to peak effort was 48 ± 14 ms in SQTS patients vs. 120 ± 20 ms in age and gender matched controls ($P < 0.0001$) [34].

13.3.6 Clinical Manifestations

SQTS is highly lethal, and the probability of a CA by the age of 40 years exceeds 40% [31]. Unfortunately, a CA is the first manifestation of the disease in 40% of probands [31].

Symptoms may begin extremely early, even in the neonatal period [29, 31], and in fact, SQTS has been advocated as one of the possible causes for the Sudden Infant Death Syndrome [4].

In some patients, especially those with type 1 SQTS, the disease may manifest as early onset "lone" AF [29].

13.3.7 Risk Stratifications and Management

The clinical manifestations of SQTS are variable, even within the same family, and a risk stratification scheme for these patients is not yet available. In contrast with LQTS, a relation between the degree of QT interval shortening and an increased susceptibility to arrhythmias has not been demonstrated [31], nor has there been any data presented in support of the use of genotype to assess cardiac risk [31]. Importantly, no clinical predictors of risk have been identified in asymptomatic individuals [31].

SQTS patients who survived an episode of CA are candidates for an ICD, because the rate of recurrence reaches 10% per year [31]. Similarly, an ICD is recommended for patients who have documented spontaneous VT, with or without syncope [4]. On the contrary, there are no data to support the implantation of an ICD in asymptomatic SQTS patients and therefore risk stratification needs to be personalized.

Among pharmacological options to reduce the occurrence of life-threatening arrhythmias, quinidine (a class Ia antiarrhythmic drug) seems promising, because it may normalize the duration of the QT interval (especially in patients with *KCNH2* mutations) and it may also reduce ventricular vulnerability during programmed electrical stimulation, irrespective of the genotype [30, 35]. According to current recommendations, quinidine may be considered in asymptomatic patients with a diagnosis of SQTS and a family history of SCD or in patients who qualify for an ICD but present a contra-indication to the ICD or refuse it [5]. Data on the clinical efficacy of quinidine, however, is lacking so that more data from long-term follow-up of patients is needed.

13.4 Catecholaminergic Polymorphic Ventricular Tachycardia

13.4.1 Introduction

Catecholaminergic polymorphic ventricular tachycardia (CPVT) is a malignant arrhythmogenic syndrome characterized by adrenergic-mediated bidirectional and polymorphic VT that leads to syncope and CA during exercise or sudden emotions.

13.4.2 Clinical Case

CM, male, was born in 1987. At the age of 2 and 4 years he experienced two episodes of dizziness while playing.

The clinical evaluation performed at the emergency department was indifferent, the ECG was normal (Fig. 13.3, panel a) and a diagnosis of symptomatic hypoglycemia was suspected. Investigations proceeded, and at the age of 7 years a run of exercise-induced sustained bidirectional VT was recorded by a 24-h Holter ECG (Fig 13.3, panel b). Beta-blocker therapy was started with propranolol 3 mg/kg/day (divided in three doses) and verapamil 4 mg/kg/day (divided in three doses) was added shortly after because of the persistence of complex ventricular arrhythmias at the exercise stress test. He remained asymptomatic for the subsequent three years, undergoing annual controls with exercise stress test and ECG Holter monitoring until the age of 11 years, when he experienced syncope while playing football. At the moment of the event he was on therapy with propranolol 60 mg/day and verapamil 80 mg/day.

An ICD was implanted in that occasion; the beta-blocker was changed to nadolol and subsequently to metoprolol when the first was temporarily discontinued.

No further arrhythmic episodes were documented up to the age of 22, when the patient received an appropriate ICD shock, which interrupted a sustained VT triggered by a sudden emotion. In that occasion the patient had not been compliant with the therapy for some days. The exercise stress test performed during a follow-up visit 6 years later, showed the persistence of 8 beats of bidirectional VT arising at the peak of the effort (Fig. 13.3, panel c). Therefore the therapy was switched to metoprolol 200 mg/day (divided in two doses) and flecainide 150 mg/day (divided in two doses), which proved to be successful in suppressing complex ventricular arrhythmias (Fig. 13.3, panel d).

He has remained asymptomatic since then.

13.4.3 Familial and Genetic Study

No history of sudden death or syncope was present in the family.

Genetic screening identified a *RyR2* missense mutation (Ser2246Leu) through Sanger analysis. The genetic screening in the mother did not identify the variant found in the proband; moreover she had normal ECG and exercise stress test. No clinical or genetic information could have been acquired from the father, who refused to undergo clinical and genetic evaluation.

13.4.4 Epidemiology

CPVT is an extremely rare disease, with the most commonly quoted prevalence being 1:10,000. This is an approximate estimate, however, because CPVT patients have a normal resting ECG, and it is impossible to distinguish between low frequency of the disease and diagnostic underestimation.

13.4.5 Genetic Variants

Two principal CPVT genetic variants are known: an autosomal dominant form caused by mutations in the *RyR2* gene encoding for the cardiac ryanodine receptor, and an autosomal recessive form related to mutations in the *CASQ2* gene encoding for cardiac calsequestrin.

Both the autosomal dominant and the autosomal recessive variants lead to arrhythmias via a shared mechanism that alters the calcium homeostasis in cardiomyocytes [36]. In physiological conditions, RYR2 opens briefly during the early plateau phase of the action potential and mediates a massive release of calcium from the SR that initiates the contraction of the cardiomyocyte (i.e. the systolic phase of the cardiac cycle) [37]. After systole is completed, calcium ions are actively pumped back into the SR by the SR Ca-ATPase (SERCA2a) to allow for the relaxation of cardiac muscle (i.e. the diastolic phase), thereby completing this “calcium cycle”

[36]. Mutations in both *RyR2* and *CASQ2*, the gene that encodes the SR calcium-binding protein calsequestrin, cause spontaneous leakage of calcium ions from the SR in diastole, particularly during intense adrenergic activation, such as strenuous physical activity or emotions. The resultant calcium overload induces the development of delayed after-depolarizations that can trigger supraventricular and ventricular extrasystoles, which have the potential to degenerate into sustained hyperkinetic arrhythmias [38, 39].

Approximately 55% of CPVT index cases carry a mutation in the *RyR2* gene, while the prevalence of *CASQ2* mutations is estimated at 5%. As with LQTS, the recessive form is considered more malignant than the dominant variant. Because it is unclear whether *CASQ2* mutations may also cause autosomal dominant transmission of the phenotype, it appears reasonable to screen *CASQ2* in sporadic *RyR2*-negative index cases.

A partial phenotypic overlap exists between LQTS and CPVT: some carriers of LQT4 (gene *Ank2*), LQT7 (Andersen-Tawil Syndrome), or Triadin variants may exhibit bidirectional or stress induced ventricular arrhythmias in their ECG. It is currently debated whether these cases should be regarded as variants of LQTS that mimic CPVT or whether *KCNJ2*, *Ank2* and *TRDN* should be considered as new CPVT genes.

13.4.6 Diagnosis

CPVT patients show normal resting ECGs. Sinus bradycardia and large U waves have been reported in some patients, but neither finding is specific enough to allow a diagnosis. Typically, exercise stress testing or strong emotions elicit the appearance of ventricular premature beats that increase in complexity in parallel with the heart rate and culminate with the pathognomonic bi-directional or polymorphic VT. The term "bi-directional" VT refers to the 180° rotation on the frontal plane of the QRS complexes of the ectopic beats. Adrenergically induced supraventricular arrhythmias (premature atrial contractions, runs of supraventricular tachycardia and bursts of atrial fibrillation) are also common in CPVT.

13.4.7 Clinical Manifestations

Clinical manifestations of CPVT are stress-induced syncope and CA. The mean age of first symptoms is 8 years [40], but the onset of arrhythmias may also occur in adulthood. The clinical course is severe, as 30% of patients experience at least one syncope before age 10 and nearly 60% of affected individuals have symptomatic arrhythmias before age 40 [40].

Sudden CA can be the first manifestation of CPVT in up to 30% of cases [40]. Therefore, *RyR2* mutations may be regarded as a cause of adrenergically mediated idiopathic VF, which may justify genetic testing in such cases [5].

13.4.8 Risk Stratifications

There are few indicators of risk for adverse outcomes in CPVT. The occurrence of CA before diagnosis, but not of syncope, is associated with a higher risk of arrhythmic episodes at follow-up [41]. Similarly, diagnosis in childhood is a predictor of severe prognosis.

After diagnosis, the lack of beta-blocker therapy is an independent predictor for arrhythmic events [4].

Furthermore, the persistence of complex ventricular arrhythmias during exercise testing is a marker for a worse outcome [4].

Genetic information has not yet been able to contribute to risk stratification in CPVT patients, but genotype-phenotype correlations are emerging. Current data have shown that patients with a *RyR2* mutation in the C-terminal channel-forming domain showed an increased risk of non-sustained VT, compared to those with N-terminal domain mutations [4].

The autosomal recessive form of CPVT related to *CASQ2* mutations has been related to a more severe prognosis than that of *RyR2* mutations.

13.4.9 Management

According to current guidelines, patients with CPVT should restrict physical activity and reduce exposure to stressful stimuli [5, 39]. As a consequence of the adrenergic drive for arrhythmias in CPVT, the most effective pharmacological therapy is non-selective beta-blockers, titrated at the maximum tolerated dose in the absence of contraindications (e.g. asthma). Nadolol (1–2 mg/kg/day) is considered the most clinically effective choice [41, 42]; in countries where nadolol is not available, sustained-release Propranolol (3–5 mg/kg/day) can be used. Selective beta-blockers (e.g. metoprolol) may have a role in asthmatic patients [4].

Since SCD may occur also in silent carriers of a pathogenic mutation, these patients should receive beta-blockers even when they do not exhibit arrhythmias during the exercise stress test [5]. In the case series published by Hayashi et al. in 2012, 2 of 16 (13%) mutation carriers with negative exercise stress test had a CA during follow-up, in the absence of therapy [43].

It is important for patients to understand the need for compliance with therapy [5]. According to clinical experience, many patients who have had arrhythmic events while on therapy might have been non-compliant; the abrupt withdrawal of beta-blockade, in fact, may induce a rebound effect of catecholamines on the heart [44].

Remarkably, even with appropriate use of beta-blockers, up to one third of CPVT patients may experience recurrent arrhythmic events or show persistence of complex arrhythmias at exercise stress test [41]. Patients with arrhythmias refractory to beta-blockers should receive flecainide (a Class IC antiarrhythmic) at the dosage of 1.5–4.5 mg/kg/day as additional therapy [5]. This indication is based on the data published in 2009 by Watanabe et al., who reported that two CPVT patients refractory to beta-blockers had a complete suppression of adrenergic-induced arrhythmias with the use of flecainide [45]. The result was further confirmed by van der Werf et al., who demonstrated an acute suppression of exercise-induced ventricular arrhythmias in 76% of 33 CPVT patients with persistent arrhythmias despite beta-blocker therapy [46].

Patients who experience recurrent symptoms and/or ICD shocks despite optimal medical therapy may benefit from LCSD [5]. De Ferrari et al. observed a statistically significant reduction of arrhythmic events after LCSD in a cohort of 38 symptomatic CPVT patients over a follow-up period of 43 months [47]. The complexity of this procedure and the potential complications (e.g. pneumothorax) [48] require a specialized surgical center, therefore limiting the broad use of this technique, which has obtained a Class IIb recommendation in current guidelines for the prevention of SCD (it may be considered, but efficacy is less well established by evidence) [5].

Finally, in patients who are at particularly high risk of CA, an ICD is indicated. Candidates are patients who have survived a CA or those who have experienced syncope or sustained VT despite optimal medical therapy and LCSD [5]. To reduce the risk of inappropriate shocks that may have a pro-arrhythmic effect, it is important to concurrently administer beta-blockers and to program the ICD carefully (long delays before shock delivery and high cut-off rates).

The next therapeutic target for channelopathies is the search for a "cure" aimed at restoring a gene's normal function. Promising experimental approaches to "gene-therapy" are currently underway in CPVT, with encouraging results from animal models. Such studies achieved favorable results in the autosomal recessive form of CPVT related to the *CASQ2* gene. Our group demonstrated that infection of a viral vector carrying wild-type calsequestrin induces long-term expression of a properly functioning gene in a knockout murine model [49].

Conclusions

The seminal discovery of LQTS 50 years ago validated the concept that predisposition to SCD may be a heritable trait, prompting the characterization of a set of primary electrical cardiac disorders with a genetic basis, now known as "channelopathies".

From the collaborative efforts of cardiologists, geneticists and basic scientists, genetic information has entered into the arena of clinical practice as a vital and specialized branch of medicine: "molecular cardiology".

Genetic studies now play a key role in the diagnosis of channelopathies and may assist in the early detection of apparently unaffected individuals. The emergence of gene-based risk stratification algorithms and gene-specific treatments have led to the possibility for the implementation of preventive measures with the intention of reducing the potential lethality associated with these diseases.

The next step in the evolution of genetic studies is the search for an elusive cure, aimed at restoring a gene's normal function. With several promising experimental approaches to gene-therapy currently underway, the future, hopefully, is not so far away.

References

1. Mazzanti A, O'Rourke S, Ng K, Miceli C, Borio G, Curcio A, Esposito F, Napolitano C, Priori SG. The usual suspects in sudden cardiac death of the young: a focus on inherited arrhythmogenic diseases. Expert Rev Cardiovasc Ther. 2014;12:499–519.
2. Abriel H, Zaklyazminskaya EV. Cardiac channelopathies: genetic and molecular mechanisms. Gene. 2013;517:1–11.
3. Ackerman MJ, Priori SG, Willems S, Berul C, Brugada R, Calkins H, Camm AJ, Ellinor PT, Gollob M, Hamilton R, Hershberger RE, Judge DP, Le Marec H, McKenna WJ, Schulze-Bahr E, Semsarian C, Towbin JA, Watkins H, Wilde A, Wolpert C, Zipes DP. HRS/EHRA expert consensus statement on the state of genetic testing for the channelopathies and cardiomyopathies. Europace. 2011;13:1077–109.
4. Priori SG, Wilde AA, Horie M, Cho Y, Behr ER, Berul C, Blom N, Brugada J, Chiang CE, Huikuri H, Kannankeril P, Krahn A, Leenhardt A, Moss A, Schwartz PJ, Shimizu W, Tomaselli G, Tracy C. HRS/EHRA/APHRS expert consensus statement on the diagnosis and management of patients with inherited primary arrhythmia syndromes. Heart Rhythm. 2013;10:1932–63.
5. Priori SG, Blomstrom-Lundqvist C, Mazzanti A, Blom N, Borggrefe M, Camm JA, Elliott PM, Fitzsimons D, Hatala R, Hindricks G, Kirchhof P, Kjeldsen K, Kuck KH, Hernandez Madrid A, Nikolaou N, Norekval TM, Spaulding C, Van Veldhuisen DJ. 2015 ESC guidelines for the management of patients with ventricular arrhythmias and the prevention of sudden cardiac death. Eur Heart J. 2015;36:2793–867.
6. Tranebjaerg L, Bathen J, Tyson J, Bitner-Glindzicz M. Jervell and Lange-Nielsen syndrome: a Norwegian perspective. Am J Med Genet. 1999;89:137–46.
7. Altmann HM, Tester DJ, Will ML, Middha S, Evans JM, Eckloff BW, Ackerman MJ. Homozygous/compound heterozygous triadin mutations associated with autosomal-recessive long-QT syndrome and pediatric sudden cardiac arrest: elucidation of the triadin knockout syndrome. Circulation. 2015;131:2051–60.
8. Makita N, Yagihara N, Crotti L, Johnson CN, Beckmann BM, Roh MS, Shigemizu D, Lichtner P, Ishikawa T, Aiba T, Homfray T, Behr ER, Klug D, Denjoy I, Mastantuono E, Theisen D, Tsunoda T, Satake W, Toda T, Nakagawa H, Tsuji Y, Tsuchiya T, Yamamoto H, Miyamoto Y, Endo N, Kimura A, Ozaki K, Motomura H, Suda K, Tanaka T, Schwartz PJ, Meitinger T, Kaab S, Guicheney P, Shimizu W, Bhuiyan ZA, Watanabe H, Chazin WJ, George AL. Novel calmodulin (CALM2) mutations associated with congenital arrhythmia susceptibility. Circ Cardiovasc Genet. 2014;7:466–74.
9. Boczek NJ, Gomez-Hurtado N, Ye D, Calvert ML, Tester DJ, Kryshtal DO, Hwang HS, Johnson CN, Chazin WJ, Loporcaro CG, Shah M, Papez AL, Lau YR, Kanter R, Knollmann BC, Ackerman MJ. Spectrum and prevalence of CALM1-, CALM2-, and CALM3-encoded calmodulin variants in long QT syndrome and functional characterization of a novel long QT syndrome-associated calmodulin missense variant, E141G. Circ Cardiovasc Genet. 2016;9:136–46.
10. Monnig G, Eckardt L, Wedekind H, Haverkamp W, Gerss J, Milberg P, Wasmer K, Kirchhof P, Assmann G, Breithardt G, Schulze-Bahr E. Electrocardiographic risk stratification in families with congenital long QT syndrome. Eur Heart J. 2006;27:2074–80.
11. Lepeschkin E, Surawicz B. The measurement of the Q-T interval of the electrocardiogram. Circulation. 1952;6:378–88.
12. Priori SG, Schwartz PJ, Napolitano C, Bloise R, Ronchetti E, Grillo M, Vicentini A, Spazzolini C, Nastoli J, Bottelli G, Folli R, Cappelletti D. Risk stratification in the long-QT syndrome. N Engl J Med. 2003;348:1866–74.
13. Schwartz PJ, Crotti L. QTc behavior during exercise and genetic testing for the long-QT syndrome. Circulation. 2011;124:2181–4.
14. Moss AJ, Schwartz PJ, Crampton RS, Tzivoni D, Locati EH, MacCluer J, Hall WJ, Weitkamp L, Vincent GM, Garson A Jr, et al. The long QT syndrome. Prospective longitudinal study of 328 families. Circulation. 1991;84:1136–44.

15. Zellerhoff S, Pistulli R, Monnig G, Hinterseer M, Beckmann BM, Kobe J, Steinbeck G, Kaab S, Haverkamp W, Fabritz L, Gradaus R, Breithardt G, Schulze-Bahr E, Bocker D, Kirchhof P. Atrial arrhythmias in long-QT syndrome under daily life conditions: a nested case control study. J Cardiovasc Electrophysiol. 2009;20:401–7.
16. Moss AJ, Zareba W, Hall WJ, Schwartz PJ, Crampton RS, Benhorin J, Vincent GM, Locati EH, Priori SG, Napolitano C, Medina A, Zhang L, Robinson JL, Timothy K, Towbin JA, Andrews ML. Effectiveness and limitations of beta-blocker therapy in congenital long-QT syndrome. Circulation. 2000;101:616–23.
17. Barsheshet A, Goldenberg I, OU J, Moss AJ, Jons C, Shimizu W, Wilde AA, McNitt S, Peterson DR, Zareba W, Robinson JL, Ackerman MJ, Cypress M, Gray DA, Hofman N, Kanters JK, Kaufman ES, Platonov PG, Qi M, Towbin JA, Vincent GM, Lopes CM. Mutations in cytoplasmic loops of the KCNQ1 channel and the risk of life-threatening events: implications for mutation-specific response to beta-blocker therapy in type 1 long-QT syndrome. Circulation. 2012;125:1988–96.
18. Moss AJ, Zareba W, Kaufman ES, Gartman E, Peterson DR, Benhorin J, Towbin JA, Keating MT, Priori SG, Schwartz PJ, Vincent GM, Robinson JL, Andrews ML, Feng C, Hall WJ, Medina A, Zhang L, Wang Z. Increased risk of arrhythmic events in long-QT syndrome with mutations in the pore region of the human ether-a-go-go-related gene potassium channel. Circulation. 2002;105:794–9.
19. Brink PA, Crotti L, Corfield V, Goosen A, Durrheim G, Hedley P, Heradien M, Geldenhuys G, Vanoli E, Bacchini S, Spazzolini C, Lundquist AL, Roden DM, George AL Jr, Schwartz PJ. Phenotypic variability and unusual clinical severity of congenital long-QT syndrome in a founder population. Circulation. 2005;112:2602–10.
20. Schwartz PJ, Spazzolini C, Crotti L, Bathen J, Amlie JP, Timothy K, Shkolnikova M, Berul CI, Bitner-Glindzicz M, Toivonen L, Horie M, Schulze-Bahr E, Denjoy I. The Jervell and Lange-Nielsen syndrome: natural history, molecular basis, and clinical outcome. Circulation. 2006;113:783–90.
21. Goldenberg I, Moss AJ, Peterson DR, McNitt S, Zareba W, Andrews ML, Robinson JL, Locati EH, Ackerman MJ, Benhorin J, Kaufman ES, Napolitano C, Priori SG, Qi M, Schwartz PJ, Towbin JA, Vincent GM, Zhang L. Risk factors for aborted cardiac arrest and sudden cardiac death in children with the congenital long-QT syndrome. Circulation. 2008;117: 2184–91.
22. Sauer AJ, Moss AJ, McNitt S, Peterson DR, Zareba W, Robinson JL, Qi M, Goldenberg I, Hobbs JB, Ackerman MJ, Benhorin J, Hall WJ, Kaufman ES, Locati EH, Napolitano C, Priori SG, Schwartz PJ, Towbin JA, Vincent GM, Zhang L. Long QT syndrome in adults. J Am Coll Cardiol. 2007;49:329–37.
23. Seth R, Moss AJ, McNitt S, Zareba W, Andrews ML, Qi M, Robinson JL, Goldenberg I, Ackerman MJ, Benhorin J, Kaufman ES, Locati EH, Napolitano C, Priori SG, Schwartz PJ, Towbin JA, Vincent GM, Zhang L. Long QT syndrome and pregnancy. J Am Coll Cardiol. 2007;49:1092–8.
24. Buber J, Mathew J, Moss AJ, Hall WJ, Barsheshet A, McNitt S, Robinson JL, Zareba W, Ackerman MJ, Kaufman ES, Luria D, Eldar M, Towbin JA, Vincent M, Goldenberg I. Risk of recurrent cardiac events after onset of menopause in women with congenital long-QT syndrome types 1 and 2. Circulation. 2011;123:2784–91.
25. Westenskow P, Splawski I, Timothy KW, Keating MT, Sanguinetti MC. Compound mutations: a common cause of severe long-QT syndrome. Circulation. 2004;109:1834–41.
26. Ruan Y, Liu N, Bloise R, Napolitano C, Priori SG. Gating properties of SCN5A mutations and the response to mexiletine in long-QT syndrome type 3 patients. Circulation. 2007;116:1137–44.
27. Mazzanti A, Maragna R, Faragli A, Monteforte N, Bloise R, Memmi M, Novelli V, Baiardi P, Bagnardi V, Etheridge SP, Napolitano C, Priori SG. Gene-specific therapy with mexiletine reduces arrhythmic events in patients with long QT syndrome type 3. J Am Coll Cardiol. 2016;67:1053–8.

28. Olde Nordkamp LR, Driessen AH, Odero A, Blom NA, Koolbergen DR, Schwartz PJ, Wilde AA. Left cardiac sympathetic denervation in the Netherlands for the treatment of inherited arrhythmia syndromes. Neth Hear J. 2014;22:160–6.
29. Gaita F, Giustetto C, Bianchi F, Wolpert C, Schimpf R, Riccardi R, Grossi S, Richiardi E, Borggrefe M. Short QT syndrome: a familial cause of sudden death. Circulation. 2003;108:965–70.
30. Giustetto C, Schimpf R, Mazzanti A, Scrocco C, Maury P, Anttonen O, Probst V, Blanc JJ, Sbragia P, Dalmasso P, Borggrefe M, Gaita F. Long-term follow-up of patients with short QT syndrome. J Am Coll Cardiol. 2011;58:587–95.
31. Mazzanti A, Kanthan A, Monteforte N, Memmi M, Bloise R, Novelli V, Miceli C, O'Rourke S, Borio G, Zienciuk-Krajka A, Curcio A, Surducan AE, Colombo M, Napolitano C, Priori SG. Novel insight into the natural history of short QT syndrome. J Am Coll Cardiol. 2014;63:1300–8.
32. Antzelevitch C, Pollevick GD, Cordeiro JM, Casis O, Sanguinetti MC, Aizawa Y, Guerchicoff A, Pfeiffer R, Oliva A, Wollnik B, Gelber P, Bonaros EP Jr, Burashnikov E, Wu Y, Sargent JD, Schickel S, Oberheiden R, Bhatia A, Hsu LF, Haissaguerre M, Schimpf R, Borggrefe M, Wolpert C. Loss-of-function mutations in the cardiac calcium channel underlie a new clinical entity characterized by ST-segment elevation, short QT intervals, and sudden cardiac death. Circulation. 2007;115:442–9.
33. Harrell DT, Ashihara T, Ishikawa T, Tominaga I, Mazzanti A, Takahashi K, Oginosawa Y, Abe H, Maemura K, Sumitomo N, Uno K, Takano M, Priori SG, Makita N. Genotype-dependent differences in age of manifestation and arrhythmia complications in short QT syndrome. Int J Cardiol. 2015;190:393–402.
34. Giustetto C, Scrocco C, Schimpf R, Maury P, Mazzanti A, Levetto M, Anttonen O, Dalmasso P, Cerrato N, Gribaudo E, Wolpert C, Giachino D, Antzelevitch C, Borggrefe M, Gaita F. Usefulness of exercise test in the diagnosis of short QT syndrome. Europace. 2015;17:628–34.
35. Gaita F, Giustetto C, Bianchi F, Schimpf R, Haissaguerre M, Calo L, Brugada R, Antzelevitch C, Borggrefe M, Wolpert C. Short QT syndrome: pharmacological treatment. J Am Coll Cardiol. 2004;43:1494–9.
36. Fabiato A. Calcium-induced release of calcium from the cardiac sarcoplasmic reticulum. Am J Physiol. 1983;245:C1–14.
37. Bers DM. Sarcoplasmic reticulum Ca release in intact ventricular myocytes. Front Biosci. 2002;7:d1697–711.
38. Priori SG, Napolitano C. Intracellular calcium handling dysfunction and arrhythmogenesis: a new challenge for the electrophysiologist. Circ Res. 2005;97:1077–9.
39. Imberti JF, Underwood K, Mazzanti A, Priori SG. Clinical challenges in catecholaminergic polymorphic ventricular tachycardia. Heart Lung Circ. 2016;8:777–83.
40. Priori SG, Napolitano C, Memmi M, Colombi B, Drago F, Gasparini M, DeSimone L, Coltorti F, Bloise R, Keegan R, Cruz Filho FE, Vignati G, Benatar A, DeLogu A. Clinical and molecular characterization of patients with catecholaminergic polymorphic ventricular tachycardia. Circulation. 2002;106:69–74.
41. Hayashi M, Denjoy I, Extramiana F, Maltret A, Buisson NR, Lupoglazoff JM, Klug D, Hayashi M, Takatsuki S, Villain E, Kamblock J, Messali A, Guicheney P, Lunardi J, Leenhardt A. Incidence and risk factors of arrhythmic events in catecholaminergic polymorphic ventricular tachycardia. Circulation. 2009;119:2426–34.
42. Leren IS, Saberniak J, Majid E, Haland TF, Edvardsen T, Haugaa KH. Nadolol decreases the incidence and severity of ventricular arrhythmias during exercise stress testing compared with beta-selective beta-blockers in patients with catecholaminergic polymorphic ventricular tachycardia. Heart Rhythm. 2015;2:433–40.
43. Hayashi M, Denjoy I, Hayashi M, Extramiana F, Maltret A, Roux-Buisson N, Lupoglazoff JM, Klug D, Maury P, Messali A, Guicheney P, Leenhardt A. The role of stress test for predicting genetic mutations and future cardiac events in asymptomatic relatives of catecholaminergic polymorphic ventricular tachycardia probands. Europace. 2012;14:1344–51.

44. Leenhardt A, Lucet V, Denjoy I, Grau F, Ngoc DD, Coumel P. Catecholaminergic polymorphic ventricular tachycardia in children. A 7-year follow-up of 21 patients. Circulation. 1995;91:1512–9.
45. Watanabe H, Chopra N, Laver D, Hwang HS, Davies SS, Roach DE, Duff HJ, Roden DM, Wilde AA, Knollmann BC. Flecainide prevents catecholaminergic polymorphic ventricular tachycardia in mice and humans. Nat Med. 2009;15:380–3.
46. van der Werf C, Kannankeril PJ, Sacher F, Krahn AD, Viskin S, Leenhardt A, Shimizu W, Sumitomo N, Fish FA, Bhuiyan ZA, Willems AR, van der Veen MJ, Watanabe H, Laborderie J, Haissaguerre M, Knollmann BC, Wilde AA. Flecainide therapy reduces exercise-induced ventricular arrhythmias in patients with catecholaminergic polymorphic ventricular tachycardia. J Am Coll Cardiol. 2011;57:2244–54.
47. De Ferrari GM, Dusi V, Spazzolini C, Bos JM, Abrams DJ, Berul CI, Crotti L, Davis AM, Eldar M, Kharlap M, Khoury A, Krahn AD, Leenhardt A, Moir CR, Odero A, Olde Nordkamp L, Paul T, Roses INF, Shkolnikova M, Till J, Wilde AA, Ackerman MJ, Schwartz PJ. Clinical management of catecholaminergic polymorphic ventricular tachycardia: the role of left cardiac sympathetic denervation. Circulation. 2015;131:2185–93.
48. Odero A, Bozzani A, De Ferrari GM, Schwartz PJ. Left cardiac sympathetic denervation for the prevention of life-threatening arrhythmias: the surgical supraclavicular approach to cervicothoracic sympathectomy. Heart Rhythm. 2010;7:1161–5.
49. Denegri M, Bongianino R, Lodola F, Boncompagni S, De Giusti VC, Avelino-Cruz JE, Liu N, Persampieri S, Curcio A, Esposito F, Pietrangelo L, Marty I, Villani L, Moyaho A, Baiardi P, Auricchio A, Protasi F, Napolitano C, Priori SG. Single delivery of an adeno-associated viral construct to transfer the CASQ2 gene to knock-in mice affected by catecholaminergic polymorphic ventricular tachycardia is able to cure the disease from birth to advanced age. Circulation. 2014;129:2673–81.

Inherited Arrhythmias: Brugada Syndrome and Early Repolarisation Syndrome

14

Pieter G. Postema, Krystien V.V. Lieve, and Arthur A.M. Wilde

Abstract

In this chapter a detailed overview on Brugada syndrome and the early repolarisation syndrome is presented. These two disease entities are associated with malignant arrhythmias and sudden death in otherwise healthy young adults and even children. We discuss their history, clinical perspectives (including patient characteristics and epidemiology), the pathway to the diagnosis, pathophysiological mechanisms (including genetic associations) and review clinical risk stratification and treatment. With this chapter we aim to provide a thorough insight in the knowledge base that has developed in these entities in the past decades and we specifically included current debates and uncertainties that are relevant to daily practice and influence our judgements. Undoubtedly our understanding of these syndromes will continue to develop and influence the management of patients and their families in the coming years. Relevant topics for future research in these syndromes are likewise provided. We sincerely hope that this chapter is of practical use for al health care professionals and researchers in this field and that it will contribute to a better understanding and care for affected patients and their families.

P.G. Postema • K.V.V Lieve
Academic Medical Centre, Department of Clinical and Experimental Cardiology, New Amsterdam, The Netherlands

A.A.M Wilde (✉)
Academic Medical Centre, Department of Clinical and Experimental Cardiology, New Amsterdam, The Netherlands

Princess Al-Jawhara Al-Brahim Centre of Excellence in Research of Hereditary Disorders, Jeddah, Kingdom of Saudi Arabia
e-mail: a.a.wilde@amc.uva.nl

D. Kumar, P. Elliott (eds.), *Cardiovascular Genetics and Genomics*,
https://doi.org/10.1007/978-3-319-66114-8_14

Keywords
Brugada syndrome • Early repolarisation syndrome • Electrocardiography • Ventricular fibrillation • Sudden death, pathophysiology • Mutations • Clinical management

14.1 Introduction: Brugada Syndrome

The brothers Pedro and Josep Brugada described the Brugada syndrome as a distinct clinical entity in 1992. In their initial publication, they reported eight patients with a specific ECG pattern (Fig. 14.1) and repeated episodes of aborted sudden cardiac death [1]. The contemporary concept of Brugada syndrome is a disorder characterized by sudden cardiac death at relatively young age, with familial segregation, an apparent absence of gross structural abnormalities or ischemic heart disease, and specific electrocardiographic characteristics [2, 3]. Sudden cardiac death is caused by fast polymorphic ventricular tachycardia (VT) and ventricular fibrillation (VF) that typically occur in situations associated with an increased vagal tone. In some patients with Brugada syndrome, fever or drugs provoke the electrocardiographic characteristics and the life-threatening arrhythmias. Brugada syndrome is characterized on the electrocardiogram (ECG) by ST segment elevation directly followed by a negative T-wave in the right precordial leads and in leads positioned one or two intercostal space higher (Fig. 14.2), also referred to as a coved type Brugada ECG [4–6] or type 1 Brugada ECG [3]. This specific ECG hallmark typically fluctuates over time, and in some patients it may only be elicited after provocation with class 1A or class 1C antiarrhythmic drugs [7, 8].

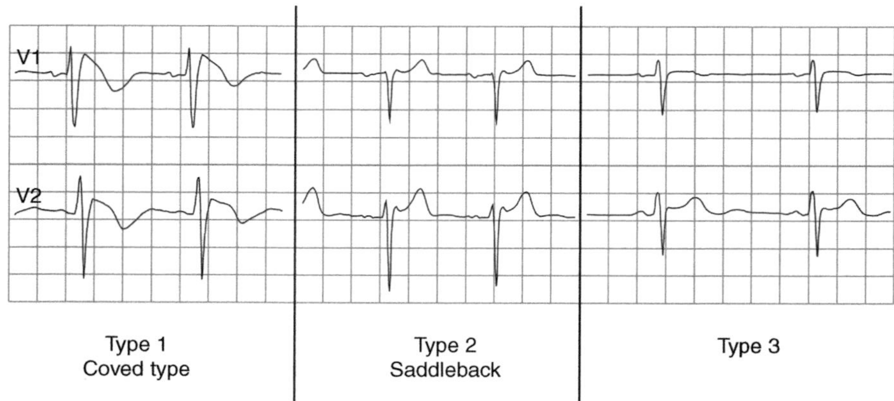

Fig. 14.1 ST segment morphologies recognized in Brugada syndrome: type 1, 2 and 3 (type 2 and 3 also recognized as type 2 only)

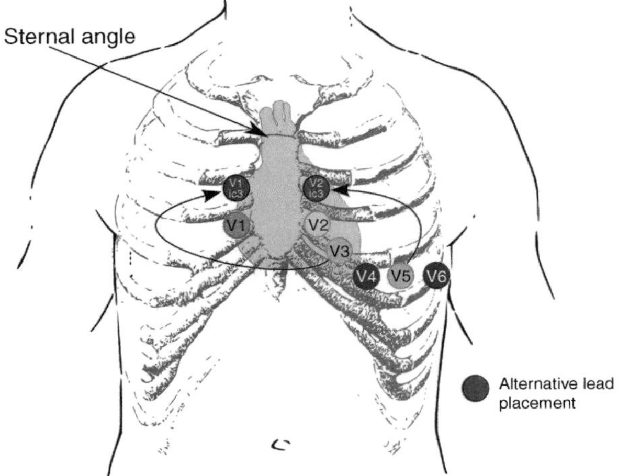

Fig. 14.2 Placement of the ECG leads in Brugada syndrome. For use in practice, V3 and V5 are often relocated from their original positions to V1 in the 3rd intercostal space (V1ic3) and in V2ic3. They may even be placed in the 2nd intercostal space (V1ic2, V2ic2)

In retrospect, the type 1 Brugada ECG was described as early as 1953 in three otherwise healthy patients who presented with atypical substernal discomfort or for routine medical testing [9]. One year later, ten more patients were described with ST elevation in the right precordial leads, including again clear-cut type 1 ECGs, without apparent heart disease and lack of events during follow-up [10]. Furthermore, 3 years before the publication of Brugada and Brugada in 1992, the characteristic Brugada ECG has been described in one out of six cases of VF without apparent heart disease [11].

In the late 1970s and 1980s in the United States, unexplained nocturnal death was reported in many refugees from East and Southeast Asia, mainly men [12]. This pattern of sudden death during sleep was already known for many centuries in Japan by the name Pokkuri (sudden unexpected death at night), and it was often prayed for as to end life without pain and suffering [13]. In the Philippines the same phenomenon is known as Bangungut (moaning and dying during sleep), in northeast Thailand as laitai (died during sleep), and in Laos as non-laitai (sleep death) [14, 15]. When studied, a considerable number of these patients displayed a Brugada-type ECG [14].

Different genes have been associated with Brugada syndrome since its description. First, in the late 1990s, cardiac sodium channel (*SCN5A*) mutations were documented in Brugada syndrome patients [16, 17]. Studies using heterologous expression in Xenopus oocytes demonstrated that these mutations resulted in loss-of-function of the cardiac sodium channels. Well over 300 *SCN5A* mutations associated with Brugada syndrome have been described [18], but *SCN5A* mutations are present in only 15%–30% of clinically diagnosed cases. Some Brugada-'mutations' have been found in control populations as well or were not proven to segregate with the phenotype, challenging their pathogenicity [19–23]. Second, the gene which encodes for the glycerol-3-phosphate dehydrogenase 1-like protein (*GPD1L*), was correlated with Brugada syndrome in a single large family [24, 25]. In their report,

London et al. report a reduction of sodium current in human embryonic kidney (HEK) cells expressing the mutated *GPD1L* gene versus wild-type controls, alike the *SCN5A* mutations linked with Brugada syndrome [26]. Third, loss-of-function missense mutations in the genes encoding for the L-type calcium channel (*CACNA1C*, *CACNB2* and *CACNA2D1*) were reported in Brugada syndrome patients [27, 28]. Additionally, in a subset of these patients carrying a calcium channel mutation, the heart rate corrected QT interval appeared to be shorter than normal. Finally, in rare cases mutations in *SCN1B*, *SCN2B*, *SCN3B*, *SCN10A*, *KCND3*, *KCNE3*, *KCNJ8*, *ABCC9*, *TRPM4*, *SLMAP*, *MOG1*, *PKP2*, FGF12, and *HCN4* have been associated with Brugada syndrome [29–43].

Notwithstanding the identification of as yet unknown genetic mutations and pathophysiologic mechanisms, clinical decision making in Brugada syndrome remains a daunting task. Implantation of an implantable cardioverter defibrillator (ICD) is the generally accepted therapy for the prevention of sudden death in patients affected by Brugada syndrome [44–48]. Oral therapy with quinidine may also prove valuable [49–55]. Importantly, risk stratification in asymptomatic patients is heavily debated, as it is still unclear how to correctly identify the large number of patients who will not develop life-threatening arrhythmias and how to prevent over-treating patients with ICD-therapy and its own associated morbidity and mortality [48, 56, 57].

14.2 Clinical Presentation

14.2.1 Epidemiology

The prevalence of the Brugada ECG is estimated at 1/2000 [58]. This is quite similar to long QT syndrome with an estimated prevalence of 1/2000 [59], but less than hypertrophic cardiomyopathy with a prevalence of 1/500 [60]. The exact prevalence of Brugada-like ECGs is difficult to estimate partly because the specific ECG pattern typically fluctuates over time and can be intermittently concealed [61, 62]. Furthermore, many patients with a spontaneous or inducible Brugada ECG are asymptomatic, and therefore will not come under medical attention and will remain without diagnosis. Also higher placed right precordial leads will often not be purposely used. The prevalence of the spontaneous Brugada syndrome ECG also seems to vary between different regions in the world (Fig. 14.3). Brugada syndrome would be most prevalent in East and Southeast Asia, particularly Japan, Thailand, and the Philippines, where it is part of the sudden unexplained (nocturnal) death syndrome (SUDS or SUNDS), which has been described as a major cause of death among young men [14, 92, 93]. In Europe, Brugada syndrome is also quite extensively described [20, 44, 94]. In the northern part of Europe [70] as well as in the United States [90] its prevalence seems to be lower. The worldwide prevalence of the spontaneous type 1 Brugada ECG from current prevalence studies (Fig. 14.3) is 0.05 ± 0.14% and of the type 2–3 ECG this is 0.17 ± 1.38% (n = 437,190).

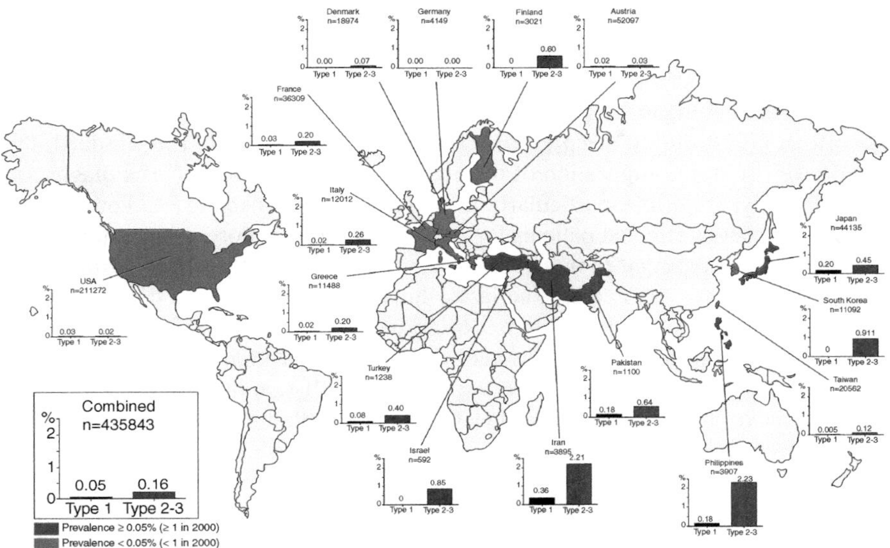

Fig. 14.3 Combined prevalence data of the spontaneous Brugada syndrome ECG in different parts of the world from 2000 to 2012. Bars represent mean prevalence in percentages. Only reports in English were considered. Prevalence studies in adolescents or children [63–65] were discarded for this figure. As the type 1 ECG was only recognized after the first consensus report [3], prevalence in two studies was acknowledged as type 1 only [66, 67], a coved type ECG was acknowledged as type 1, a saddleback or suspicious ECG as type 2–3. It should be noted that the populations studied and the methods used vary importantly. This figure is similar to [58]. Austria [68], Denmark [69], Finland [70], France [71, 72], Germany [73], Greece [74], Turkey [75], Israel [76], Iran [77], Italy [78], Japan [66, 79–83], Pakistan [84], Philippines [85], South Korea [86, 87], Taiwan [88], USA [67, 89–91]

14.2.2 The Patient

Malignant arrhythmic events can occur at all ages, from childhood to the elderly [1, 95, 96] with a peak around the fourth decade [2] of life. To our knowledge, the youngest patient clinically diagnosed with Brugada syndrome was 2 days old, [97] and the oldest 85 years old [98]. It has been estimated that Brugada syndrome is responsible for 4–12% of all sudden cardiac deaths and up to 20% of sudden cardiac deaths in patients without apparent structural heart disease [99]. However, these estimations have not been verified and may well be overestimating the true casualties due to Brugada syndrome. Still, Brugada syndrome may also be a cause of sudden infant death syndrome (SIDS) [95, 100]. Some patients present with palpitations or dizziness, but increasingly the clinical scenario is the detection of a Brugada ECG in an asymptomatic individual [72, 94, 101]. In a meta-analysis in 2007 of 1217 Brugada syndrome patients (defined by a spontaneous or inducible Brugada ECG and excluding case reports) the majority was asymptomatic (59%, range 0–80%) [102]. In a more recent meta-analysis of 1312 subjects the number of asymptomatic patients was even higher (67%) [103].

When sudden death occurs, it is most likely the result of fast polymorphic VT originating from the right ventricle/right ventricular outflow tract [104], which subsequently degenerates into VF leading to cardio-circulatory arrest. The onset of these life-threatening arrhythmias typically occurs in situations with an augmented vagal tone [105], during sleep [106], or after large meals [107, 108]. Indeed, the latter gave rise to the suggestion of the use of a "full stomach test" as a diagnostic tool [109]. Hyperthermia, particularly fever, may also provoke the ECG or arrhythmias in a subset of affected patients [55, 110–114]. Furthermore, a large number of drugs have been reported to induce Brugada syndrome, or Brugada syndrome-like ECG characteristics; for example antiarrhythmic drugs, anti-anginal drugs, psychotropic drugs, and also substances like cocaine and alcohol [2, 3, 115]. Some Brugada syndrome patients may experience agonal respiration at night, when arrhythmias are most prevalent [14, 106]. This is explained by self-terminating VT, which can provoke (recurrent) syncope [116–119]. Clinical presentation with sustained monomorphic ventricular tachyarrhythmia, although quite uncommon, has also been described [120–125].

In most patients, premature ventricular complexes are scarce during 24-hour Holter monitoring, but premature ventricular complexes can occur [116] and may increase before the spontaneous onset of VF [126]. The morphology of the preceding premature ventricular contractions appears to be identical to the first beat of VF. Repetitive episodes of VF may be initiated by premature ventricular contractions of similar morphology [126]. Most premature ventricular contractions have a left bundle branch block morphology, indicating an origin in the right ventricle. There seems to be a predilection site of origin in the right ventricular outflow tract, but also extra systoles from the right ventricular free wall, septum and apex contribute and are capable of initiating VF [104]. Further confirmation of the relationship between these right ventricular extra systoles and VF was derived from a study in three Brugada syndrome patients using endocardial catheter ablation of focal triggers of VF at different sites in the right ventricle [127]. This therapy resulted in the absence of further episodes of tachy-arrhythmias during short-term follow-up. Large studies using this strategy of endocardial ablation of VF-initiating extrasystoles with long-term follow-up are lacking, however. Moreover, epicardial ablation has now emerged as a more promising treatment [128].

Although the most impressive ECG characteristics in Brugada syndrome are the changes in the right precordial leads, other ECG abnormalities are frequently occurring. Supraventricular arrhythmias, mainly atrial fibrillation, are very common with a prevalence between 10 and 39% [129–132]. Supraventricular arrhythmias were found to be more prevalent in patients who had an indication for ICD for either symptoms or inducible VT/VF during electrophysiological study [133, 134]. Importantly, atrial arrhythmias may often lead to inappropriate ICD shocks [47, 48, 56, 57, 134, 135].

For a syndrome that inherits as an autosomal dominant trait with equal transmission to both genders, there is a striking male to female ratio of 4 to 1 [102, 103, 136]. Testosterone is probably a contributor to this gender disparity; surgical castration of two Brugada syndrome patients for prostate cancer normalized their ECGs [137], and testosterone levels in Brugada syndrome patients were found to be higher when compared to controls [138]. Sex hormones were suggested to modulate potassium and calcium currents during the repolarisation phase of the action potential [139]. Where testosterone may shorten the action potential duration [140], oestrogen may lengthen action potential duration [141]. Furthermore, a different distribution of certain ionic currents, particularly I_{to}, in males versus females may contribute [140]. Whether a difference in, for example, structural changes (fibrosis) may also play a role is uncertain.

14.3 Electrocardiography and Diagnosis

14.3.1 The Brugada ECG

Since its description in 1992, the signature sign of Brugada syndrome is its characteristic ECG [1, 44]. Patients with a spontaneous Brugada ECG and symptoms are considered to be at a high risk for sudden death secondary to VT/VF [44, 46, 94, 103, 136]. The electrocardiographic manifestation of Brugada syndrome is typically dynamic and may often be concealed. The latter has important consequences for risk stratification and follow-up of these patients, as patients with dynamic ECGs can still be at risk for future arrhythmic events [107, 142, 143]. Furthermore, the ECG may be influenced or elicited by hyperthermia and drugs.

The diagnosis of Brugada syndrome requires the demonstration of the "type 1" ECG pattern (Fig. 14.1) [2, 3, 144]. Since 2013, this type 1 Brugada ECG consists of ≥2 mm J point elevation in at least one of the right precordial leads (V1 and V2), in the standard 4th, or in the 3rd or 2nd intercostal space, gradually descending into a negative T-wave (also known as a "coved type" morphology of the ST-T segment). While between 2002 and 2013, V3 was also included but higher right precordial leads were not included in the consensus criteria (although they were increasingly used by many expert centres in the world). In some patients, the Brugada syndrome type 1 ECG is exclusively diagnosed in the leads positioned in the 3rd or 2nd intercostal space [5, 6, 145]. The reason why the characteristic Brugada ECG can be found in different intercostal spaces is most probable due to varying positions of the right ventricular outflow tract [146]. Importantly, with the higher placement of the V1 and V2 leads (Fig. 14.2), sensitivity increases and there do not seem to be false-positive test results [147]. Also the prognosis of patients with a spontaneous type 1 morphology exclusively in the leads positioned in the third intercostal seems to be similar to patients with a spontaneous type 1 morphology in V1 and V2 [148]. However, large prospective and long-term follow-up studies in the use of higher placed V1 and V2 are still lacking.

The type 1 ECG may be spontaneously present or provoked by drugs or hyperthermia. In the first and the second consensus report, the definite diagnosis of Brugada syndrome required, in addition to the type 1 ECG, either documented VT or VF, a family history of sudden cardiac death at <45 years old, coved-type ECGs in family members, syncope, inducibility of VT/VF with programmed electrical stimulation, or nocturnal agonal respiration [2, 3]. In the third consensus report in 2013, these additions were abandoned and only the ECG pattern, in the absence of an alternative diagnosis ('phenocopy'), was regarded sufficient for the diagnosis of Brugada syndrome.

Previously, there were two other ECG patterns recognized in Brugada syndrome, a type 2 and a type 3 ECG, although they are not considered to be specific and, importantly, not diagnostic (Fig. 14.1). Since 2013, these both ECG patterns have been renamed to type 2 patterns. This can be a "saddleback" appearance; consisting of ≥2 mm J elevation followed by a descending ST segment that does not reach the baseline and then giving rise to a positive or biphasic T-wave or a type 3 Brugada ECG with the morphology of a type 1 or saddleback ECG with ≥2 mm J elevation but characterized by a smaller magnitude of the ST elevation (≤1 mm) [144, 149]. Due to its typical dynamic nature, the type 1 ECG can change from and to a type 2 or normal ECG spontaneously or under influence of hyperthermia or drugs. Interestingly, the magnitude of ST elevation does not differ between Brugada syndrome patients with or without a *SCN5A* mutation [22]. As discussed earlier in this chapter, many drugs and substances are capable of inducing a type 1 ECG in patients with Brugada syndrome. For clinical purposes this knowledge is used as a diagnostic tool to evoke a type 1 ECG in patients suspected of Brugada syndrome who do not display a spontaneous type 1 ECG, for example, in case of symptoms (syncope, aborted sudden cardiac death) or as part of familial screening for Brugada syndrome. For this purpose, sodium channel blockers such as ajmaline, flecainide, pilsicainide, or procainamide are mostly used (Table 14.1) [2, 3]. The diagnostic accuracy of drug challenge in patients suspected of Brugada syndrome is higher with the use of ajmaline over flecainide, while equally safe [150]. Safety of drug challenges for Brugada syndrome is ensured when the test is performed using continuously 12-lead ECG monitoring, with cardioverter defibrillators and advanced cardiac life support close at hand and discontinuation of the test when a type 1 ECG is obtained, when ventricular extra systoles or VT develops or when the QRS duration increases more than 30% [3]. As a type 1 ECG is associated with ventricular arrhythmias, drugs or substances associated with a type 1 ECG need to be avoided in patients diagnosed with Brugada syndrome (Table 14.2). Particular attention should also be given to general anesthesia in Brugada syndrome patients [151–155].

Table 14.1 Drugs used for provocation of the Brugada ECG

Drug	Dosage (mg/kg)
Ajmaline	IV 1
Flecainide	IV 2
Procainamide	IV 10
Pilsicainide	IV 1

Notes: IV denotes intravenously. Ajmaline administration particularly differs between studies/centres (e.g., bolus every minute versus continuous administration, total dose in 5 min versus 10 mg/min up to maximal dose). Flecainide may be administered over 10 min or also as 10 mg/min. Flecainide is often maximized at 150 mg. Procainamide and pilsicainide are more routinely administered over 10 min

Table 14.2 Drugs known to induce Brugada or Brugada-like ECGs and arrhythmias

Anti-arrhythmic drugs	
1	To be avoided by Brugada syndrome patients
	Ajmaline, allapinine, ethacizine, flecainide, pilsicainide, procainamide, propafenone
2	Preferably avoided by Brugada syndrome patients
	Amiodarone, cibenzoline, disopyramide, lidocaine, propranolol, verapamil, vernakalant
Anesthetics	
1	To be avoided by Brugada syndrome patients
2	Bupivacaine, Procaine, Propofol Preferably avoided by Brugada syndrome patients Ketamine, Tramadol
Psychotropic drugs	
1	To be avoided by Brugada syndrome patients
	Amitriplyline, clomipramine, desipramine, lithium, loxapine, nortriptyline, oxcarbazepine, trifluoperazine
2	Preferably avoided by Brugada syndrome patients
	Bupropion, carbamazepine, clothiapine, cyamemazine, dosulepine, doxepine, fluoxetine, fluvoxamine, imipramine, lamotrigine, maprotiline, paroxetine, perphenazine, phenytoin, thioridazine
Other drugs and substances	
1	To be avoided by Brugada syndrome patients
2	Acetylcholine, alcohol (toxicity), cannabis, cocaine, ergonovine
	Preferably avoided by Brugada syndrome patients
	Demenhydrinate, diphenhydramine, edrophonium, indapamide, metoclopramide, terfenadine/fexofenadine

Source: Status of www.BrugadaDrugs.org in May 2016, adapted from [115], see www.BrugadaDrugs.org

The administration of isoprotenerol, a β-receptor agonist, and/or quinidine may effectively be used to treat repetitive ventricular arrhythmias or electrical storms [50, 105, 156–159].

As mentioned earlier, hyperthermia also evokes a type 1 ECG or ventricular arrhythmias in a (large) subset of Brugada syndrome patients. Several reports revealed the presence of a type 1 ECG or episodes of arrhythmias during febrile illness, often in children [55, 113, 114, 121, 160–163]. Elevation of the core body temperature e.g. during hot baths may have a similar effect [164] and in Russia hot baths are even discouraged for Brugada patients (www.BrugadaDrugs.org/patient-letter/). It also seems that patients with a fever induced Type-1 ECG have a slightly higher risk than patients with only a drug-induced Type-1 ECG [165]. Treating fever with antipyretic agents such as paracetamol (U.S.: Acetaminophen) and/or antibiotics may prove valuable in these cases. If hyperthermia persists and arrhythmias cannot be counteracted, cooling the patient by all means may be the ultimate rescue (personal communication Dr. Pedro Brugada, ESC congress 2006).

There is a wide differential diagnosis of clinical conditions accompanied by coved-like or elevated ST segments in the right precordial ECG leads, and these should be ruled out before a conclusive diagnosis of Brugada syndrome is made (Table 14.3) [3].

Table 14.3 Differential diagnosis for ST segment abnormalities in the right precordial ECG leads

Abnormalities
Right or left bundle branch block, left ventricular hypertrophy
Acute myocardial ischemia or infarction
Acute myocarditis
Right ventricular ischemia or infarction
Dissecting aortic aneurysm
Acute pulmonary thromboemboli
Various central and autonomic nervous system abnormalities
Heterocyclic antidepressant overdose
Duchenne muscular dystrophy
Friedreich's ataxia
Thiamine deficiency
Hypercalcemia
Hyperkalemia
Cocaine intoxication
Mediastinal tumor compressing right ventricular outflow tract
Arrhythmogenic right ventricular dysplasia/cardiomyopathy
Long QT syndrome type 3
Other conditions
Early repolarisation syndrome
Other normal variants (particularly in men)

Source: Adapted from [3]

When these conditions result in a type 1 or type 2 Brugada ECG these conditions have recently been named Brugada phenocopies [166, 167]. Relatively common causes include early repolarisation [168], myocardial infarction or ventricular aneurysms [72, 169], vasospastic angina [170, 171], electrolyte disturbances such as hyperkalemia or hypercalcemia [172–175], pericarditis or myocarditis [176–178]. The differentiation from Brugada syndrome can be made after resolution of the clinical condition (if possible), followed by performing a Brugada syndrome provocation test (e.g. using ajmaline) when the ECG turned non-diagnostic.

14.3.2 Other Electrocardiographic Characteristics

Other ECG characteristics associated with Brugada syndrome include conduction defects in the atria, conduction system, and ventricles. Frequently present are broad P-waves [145], long PQ interval [22], prolonged corrected sinus node recovery times, prolonged His-Ventricle intervals (HV), which may or may not be accompanied by prolonged Atrio-His (AH) intervals [130, 132, 134], sinus and AV node dysfunction [179], QRS axis deviation [1, 180], and broad QRS complexes [22, 145, 180]. Conduction interval prolongation is frequently associated with the presence of *SCN5A* mutations [22]. Furthermore, *SCN5A* mutations in Brugada syndrome patients may, as in Lev-Lenègres disease, worsen the phenotypic expression of the disease with ageing and may lead to the necessity of pacemaker implantation [132, 181, 182]. Although there is some variability of the heart rate corrected QT interval (QTc), it does not seem to prolong importantly when a type 1 Brugada ECG or VF develops [1, 126, 145, 180]. This clearly distinguishes Brugada syndrome from long QT syndrome where excessive QTc prolongation is the hallmark of the disease [183]. However, overlap syndromes between Brugada syndrome and long QT syndrome (type 3) exist, based on a multidysfunctional sodium channel caused by specific *SCN5A* mutations [184–188]. Interestingly, the phenotype of one of these mutations (*SCN5A* 1795insD) shares many similarities with mouse model carrying the murine equivalent mutation (*SCN5A* 1798insD) with bradycardia, right ventricular conduction slowing, an increased vulnerability for arrhythmias and QTc prolongation [189]. Conversely, shortened QTc intervals were noted in a subset of Brugada syndrome patients with calcium channel mutations [27]. However, data regarding the calcium channel mutation and/or shortened QTc intervals are limited.

Wide S-waves in the inferior and lateral leads are frequently observed before and after a type 1 ECG develops during drug challenge, which may mirror simultaneous slowing of right ventricular activation [145, 180, 190]. This is reflected in the possible prognostic value of wide and deep S-waves in lead I as a predictor of future VT/VF events [191, 192]. S-waves ≥80 ms in lead V1 appear to be a good predictor for a history of VF [193] but a possible prognostic value is not well studied.

Signal-averaged ECGs show more variation in filtered QRS duration and late potentials in symptomatic patients [105, 107, 194–197]. Late potentials are generally regarded as delayed and disorganized ventricular activation and are related to ventricular tachy-arrhythmias [198]. Particularly in Brugada syndrome, however, other mechanisms have also been proposed: late potentials might for example represent a delayed second upstroke of the epicardial action potential, a local phase 2 reentry [99]. These latter proposals have, however, not yet been validated as primary or cooperative pathophysiologic mechanisms of late potentials in Brugada syndrome (nor in other diseases).

Like late potentials, QRS fractionation or fragmentation is regarded as a sign of delayed and disorganized ventricular activation [199]. In Brugada syndrome, QRS fractionation might also have prognostic value regarding future arrhythmic events [200, 201].

In some reports of patients who presented with VF, ST elevation in the inferior and/or lateral leads has been described in the absence of electrolyte disturbances, hypothermia, or myocardial ischemia [202–207]. In a French family, different *SCN5A* mutation carrying family members displayed either inferior or right precordial coved-type ST segment elevation [208]. At present it still remains uncertain if these patients have the same characteristics as has been described in patients with solely right precordial coved-type ST segments.

14.4 Pathophysiology and Genetics

14.4.1 Arrhythmia Mechanisms

Ventricular arrhythmias in Brugada syndrome often originate from ventricular extra systoles in the right ventricle, which subsequently initiate polymorphic VT or VF. The exact pathophysiology behind Brugada syndrome is, however, still not clear and there might be different electrophysiological mechanisms involved. It seems that an increased vulnerability of the ventricles is present before the onset of VF. The coupling interval (i.e., the timing) of the premature ventricular complex, for example, may be important. In most electrophysiological studies, short coupled extra systoles (<200 ms) were necessary to induce VF while the coupling interval of the first premature ventricular complex of spontaneous VF is often (far) more than 300 ms [105, 126, 201]. There might also be a relation between the vulnerability of the ventricle and the preceding RR interval following for example an extra systole, which may augment ST elevation and eventually degenerate into VF [209]. Notwithstanding the associated risk for sudden cardiac death of a type 1 ECG, it is not necessary for arrhythmias in Brugada syndrome, as was shown in Holter and ICD recordings documentation suggesting that there might be distinct—albeit possibly related—electrophysiological mechanisms involved. Moreover, a substantial number of patients with spontaneous type 1 ECGs will never have any symptoms [9, 10, 210].

14.4.2 The Coved ST Segment

Ever since the first descriptions of Brugada syndrome, authors have been investigating possible mechanisms for this characteristic ECG feature [1, 8, 10, 211–214]. Currently, there are two theories explaining the pathophysiology underlying the Brugada syndrome: the repolarisation and the depolarization hypothesis [215]. Yan and Antzelevitch have developed the repolarisation hypothesis in canine right ventricular wedge preparations [216]. This hypothesis has attracted most support in the first 15 years after the description by the Brugada brothers in 1992. In this canine model, simultaneously measured epicardial and endocardial electrograms showed loss of action potential dome in the epicardium only when the wedge preparation was exposed to a potassium channel opener (pinacidil) or a combination of a sodium channel blocker (flecainide) and acetylcholine. This resulted in a transmural dispersion of repolarisation with different lengths of action potentials across different cardiac layers, ST segment elevation on the ECG and it created a vulnerable window for ('phase 2') re-entry to occur between these layers and degenerate into ventricular tachyarrhythmias. Isoprotenerol, 4-aminopyridine, and quinidine were able to restore this loss of action potential dome, normalize the ST segments, and prevent the ventricular arrhythmias. This model resolves around a heterogeneous expression of the transient outward potassium current I_{to}. This current seems to be expressed to a higher degree in the canine epicardium compared with the endocardium [217], in the right ventricle more than in the left ventricle [218], and in males more than in females [140], resulting in a higher susceptibility for I_{to} augmentation over other currents and a consequential higher risk for ventricular tachyarrhythmias. Relative augmentation of I_{to} would be enhanced by sodium current (I_{Na}) reduction, either by a loss-of-function sodium channel mutation or sodium channel blockade. Furthermore, reduction of the calcium current (I_{Ca}) and augmentation of the ATP-driven potassium current ($I_{K\text{-}ATP}$) would give similar effects [211].

The second hypothesis explaining the coved-type morphology resolves around a depolarization disorder [219] and is now regarded as the leading hypothesis. In this hypothesis, conduction slowing or conduction delay in the right ventricular outflow tract (RVOT) causes the type 1 morphology in the right precordial leads. Most evidence for this model is derived from clinical studies [105, 128, 180, 190, 195–197, 220–223]. The slowing of conduction originates in concert with subtle structural abnormalities (fibrosis, see below) [224]. Furthermore, conduction slowing in concordance with these structural abnormalities will create the vulnerability for re-entrant activation in the right ventricle and give rise to ventricular extra systoles and VT/VF (Fig. 14.4). The marked conduction slowing in atria and ventricles, which is seen during drug challenges with sodium channel blockers and in *SCN5A* mutation carriers particularly, further supports this model [145, 215, 227]. However, as with many diseases, it may be that Brugada syndrome is not explained by one single mechanism [219, 228]. The final common pathway of a spontaneous or inducible coved-type ECG and the vulnerability for ventricular arrhythmias may be started by distinct but cooperative mechanisms and may require tailored risk stratifications and treatment. Moreover, cooperative pathophysiological mechanisms such as structural myocardial abnormalities and gene–gene interactions are probably important modifiers or risk.

14.4.3 Structural Changes

The consensus criteria for Brugada syndrome recommend the exclusion of gross structural myocardial derangements in conjunction with the documentation of a type 1 ECG (see section Electrocardiography and Diagnosis) before a conclusive diagnosis of Brugada syndrome can be made [2, 144]. This reflects the initial hypothesis that Brugada syndrome is an electrical disease involving cardiac ion channel abnormalities and thus requires the absence of structural changes as opposed to, for example, hypertrophic cardiomyopathy. This issue has, however, been debated. Similarities between Brugada syndrome and arrhythmogenic (right) ventricular cardiomyopathy were early on suggested by many centres, even starting before the sentinel paper of the Brugada brothers in 1992 [11, 229, 230]. Biventricular endomyocardial biopsies in 18 Brugada syndrome patients showed myocarditis, cardiomyopathy-like changes, or fatty infiltration in the right ventricle of all patients (without a control group) [231]. Furthermore, in 8 out of these 18 patients (45%) there were similar findings in the left ventricle. Both magnetic resonance imaging (MRI) and echocardiography were negative in all patients. Interestingly, patients

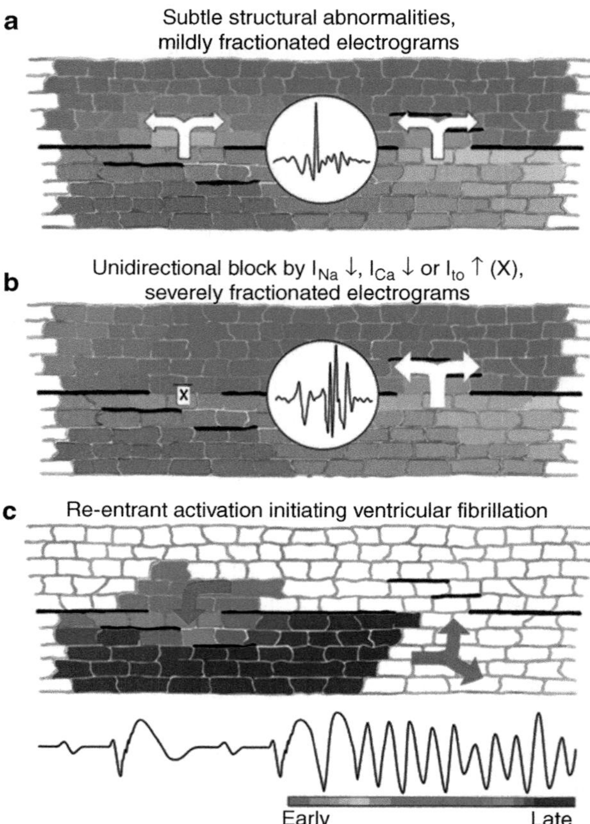

Fig. 14.4 This illustration (adjusted from the illustration of Hoogendijk et al.[225] with permission) shows the induction of re-entrant arrhythmia by current-to-load mismatch in myocardium containing two isthmuses due to subtle structural abnormalities (fibrosis). (**a**) During normal conditions, the redundancy in excitatory current makes conduction successful over both isthmuses and there is no re-entrant activation. Local electrograms will show mild fractionation. (**b**) Reduction of the cardiac sodium current (INa) or L-type calcium current (ICa) or an increase of the transient outward current (Ito) lowers the excitatory current and can cause unidirectional conduction block depending on the local geometry of the myocardium. Here, activation is blocked (X) at the left but not at the right isthmus. Local electrograms will show severe fractionation. (**c**) The asymmetrical distribution of the structural discontinuities at the left isthmus makes conduction in the opposite direction successful, and activation re-enters the proximal myocardium, causing re-entry, which in turn can initiate ventricular fibrillation. The coved type ECG, including fractionation, before the onset of the arrhythmia can be appreciated and is caused by excitation failure in adjacent myocardium in the right ventricular outflow tract [225, 226]. Ablation therapy [128] is targeted at the fractionated electrograms to close the gaps/isthmuses, and thereby resolving the excitation failure (coved type ST segments) and the substrate for re-entrant activation and ventricular fibrillation. Colours depict activation time; black indicates fibrous tissue between myocardial cells

with fatty infiltration and cardiomyopathy-like changes all had a *SCN5A* mutation. In another report, right ventricular fibrosis and epicardial fatty infiltration was documented in the explanted heart of a *SCN5A* mutation carrying Brugada syndrome patient who experienced intolerable numbers of ICD discharges (up to 129 appropriate shocks in 5 months) [232]. This patient also had no clinically detected cardiac structural abnormalities many years before transplant. In an elegant collaboration between different centres with detailed post-mortem and biopsy material analysis again fibrosis, connexion-43 and conduction abnormalities were found in concert [224]. In a study using endocardial mapping it was noted that Brugada syndrome patients showed increased (although still modest) electrogram fractionation and abnormal conduction velocity restitution, both also related to structural changes [190]. Finally, the sentinel report of Nademanee and co-workers on epicardial ablation of the substrate of Brugada syndrome showed complex fractionated electrograms at the RV outflow tract, with ablation terminating the substrate and ECG characteristics of Brugada syndrome [128]. The fractionated electrograms also appeared to coincide with areas of fibrosis [224]. These reports suggest that there are cooperative functional and subclinical structural derangements in Brugada syndrome, which may be enhanced by mutations in the sodium channel. In support of this hypothesis, mice and human data illustrate that *SCN5A* mutations may lead to impressive fibrosis accompanied by conduction disturbances, mainly in the right ventricle, which worsens with ageing [233–236]. Interestingly, a meta-analysis into risk stratification for ventricular tachyarrhythmias did not find an increased risk for patients carrying a *SCN5A* mutation [136]. The uncovering of *PKP2* mutations characteristic for arrhythmogenic (right) ventricular cardiomyopathy in patients with Brugada syndrome (and leading to decreased sodium current) further strengthened the association between structural abnormalities and Brugada syndrome [29, 237]. Fibrosis is probably underdetected in clinical practice as the clinical modalities to assess structural cardiac changes (echo, CT and MRI) are incapable of detecting mild or diffuse abnormalities although mild derangements have been noted [238–242].

14.4.4 Genetics of Brugada Syndrome

SCN5A mutations have been identified in about 15–30% of patients [20, 22]. Although efforts in screening 16 putatively associated genes identified another ion channel (the calcium channel), this still only resulted in a mutation diagnosis in 24% of patients [27]. When Brugada syndrome is present in children however, the amount of uncovered mutations, specifically *SCN5A* mutations, can be considerably higher [243].

The first mutation in Brugada syndrome patients was identified in a collaborative effort of clinics in Europe and the United States in 1998 [16]. A loss-of-function mutation in the *SCN5A* gene, encoding the pore-forming α-subunit of the human cardiac sodium channel protein (Nav1.5) was present in three out of six families with Brugada syndrome. Mutations leading to loss of sodium channel function can lead to a variety of disorders [244, 245]: Brugada syndrome (OMIM 601144), (progressive) cardiac conduction defects also known as Lev-Lenègres disease (OMIM 113900) [246], sick sinus syndrome (OMIM 608567) [247], Sudden infant death syndrome (OMIM 272120) [95, 100], and dilated cardiomyopathy associated with conduction defects and arrhythmias (OMIM 601154) [248]. In combination with other (atrial-specific modifier) genes, a loss-of-function defect may cause atrial standstill [249]. Mutations leading to a gain of function of the channel may cause long QT syndrome type 3 (OMIM 603830) [250] and also sudden infant death syndrome (OMIM 272120) [251, 252]. As mentioned earlier, certain mutations in the cardiac sodium channel gene may lead to combined phenotypes of loss-of-function and gain-of-function mutations, also referred to as an overlap syndrome [184–187]. *SCN5A* promoter polymorphisms in a haplotype variant may lead to variability in phenotypic expression as was shown in a study demonstrating slower cardiac conduction with a gene-dose effect in patients of Asian origin [253]. The same holds for common *SCN5A* polymorphisms or the combination of different *SCN5A* mutations that may modulate the expression of the mutant gene(s) and disease [254–257].

Loss-of-function cardiac calcium channel mutations have been demonstrated in Brugada syndrome patients [27]. These mutations involved the L-type calcium channel encoded by *CACNA1C* for the pore-forming Cav1.2 α1 subunit, and *CACNB2* for the Cavβ2b subunit involved in channel activation modulation of the α1 subunit. Mutations in the *GPD1L* gene have also been linked to Brugada syndrome in a single family [24, 25] and associates with reduced sodium current. This gene probably does not contribute more than 1% in Brugada syndrome [258, 259].

Exon mutations or duplications in the *SCN5A* gene and a large number of other candidate genes (Caveolin-3, Irx-3, Irx-4, Irx-5, Irx-6, Plakoglobin, Plakophilin-2, *SCN1B*, *SCN2B*, *SCN3B*, *SCN4B*, *KCNH2*, *KCNQ1*, *KCNJ2*, *KCNE1*, *KCNE2*, *KCNE3*, *KCND3*, *KCNIP2*, *KCNJ11*, and *CACNA2D1*) have been investigated in *SCN5A* mutation-negative Brugada syndrome patients with little success [27, 258]. Nevertheless, also mutations in several of these and other genes (*SCN1B*, *SCN2B*, *SCN3B*, *SCN10A*, *CACNA2D1*, *KCND3*, *KCNE3*, *KCNJ8*, *ABCC9*, *TRPM4*, *SLMAP*, *MOG1*, *PKP2*, FGF12, and *HCN4*) have finally been associated with Brugada syndrome [28–43]. It should, however, be acknowledged that in many of these reports segregation with the phenotype was not investigated or documented. In addition, variants in all these genes, except *SCN5A*, were also identified in equal numbers, in control patients or in existing next-generation sequencing data cohorts [40, 260]. This importantly challenges the pathogenicity and thus the association with Brugada syndrome of many of these rare genetic variants [23, 40, 260]. Recently it has actually been suggested that Brugada syndrome is not a monogenetic disease but an oligogenetic disease [261], where a (small) number of genetic hits together give rise to the clinical phenotype.

Interestingly, a study revealed common gene expression levels in Brugada syndrome patients irrespective of the culprit gene [262]. This expression pattern involved not only cardiac sodium channel and its subunits, but also potassium channels and calcium channels.

Typically for Brugada syndrome, and other Mendelian disorders, is an incomplete penetrance and variable expression of the disease [263]. Hence, not all mutation carriers are affected by the same degree and will thus not require the same treatment. Even so, the importance of diagnosing mutation carriers with little or no phenotypic expression of the disease is important because they still have a 50% chance of transmitting the genetic defect to their offspring, who in turn may be seriously symptomatic at young age. It is, however, not clear whether presymptomatic genetic testing in children of Brugada syndrome patients is to be advised [264]. As symptomatic Brugada syndrome is rare in children, risk stratification is imperfect, and treatment may do more harm than good (see also the section on Clinical Decision Making), the consequences of a positive test result of presymptomatic genetic testing should be carefully considered [243].

14.5 Clinical Decision Making

14.5.1 Risk Stratification

After diagnosing Brugada syndrome, risk stratification for future ventricular arrhythmias is mandatory. The prognosis and risk stratification of Brugada syndrome patients is, however, debated. Risk for future ventricular arrhythmias is generally accepted to be high in patients who are known to have already experienced life-threatening ventricular arrhythmias, that is, patients with a history of aborted sudden cardiac death. Syncope, dizziness or nocturnal agonal respiration can also be caused by ventricular arrhythmias and are thus often regarded as high-risk features. However, the assumption that these symptoms are indeed arhythmogenic in origin can be erroneous and other causes of these symptoms should also be sought.

A meta-analysis combined a history of sudden cardiac death and/or syncope as representative for a history of ventricular arrhythmias and found a relative risk (RR) of 3.34 [95% confidence interval (CI) 2.13–4.93] for the combined event of sudden cardiac death, syncope, or ICD shock during follow-up [136]. Also male gender, RR 3.47 (95% CI 1.58–7.63), and a spontaneous type 1 ECG versus a drug-induced type 1 ECG, RR 4.65 (95% CI 2.25–9.58), were positively associated with the occurrence of the combined events (sudden cardiac death and/or syncope) during follow-up. A family history of sudden cardiac death, *SCN5A* mutation, or inducible ventricular arrhythmias during electrophysiological study was not associated with events during follow-up in that meta-analysis. Importantly, these risk factors are probably not independent.

As the majority of Brugada patients are asymptomatic but can experience ventricular arrhythmias in the future, there is a dire need for reliable risk stratification in these patients. The role of the inducibility of ventricular arrhythmias during electrophysiological study in this matter has long been debated [2, 3, 46, 94, 265, 266]. A meta-analysis in 2007 to assess its prognostic role was not able to identify a significant role with regard to arrhythmic events during follow-up [102]. In a combined effort of 14 centres in France and Japan, it was shown that 45% of the 220 studied Brugada syndrome patients received an ICD following inducibility of ventricular arrhythmias during electrophysiological study whilst being asymptomatic [47]. In this study there was an 8% rate of appropriate shocks for ventricular arrhythmias during >3 years follow-up, and a relatively low (2 to 5 times lower) rate of appropriate shocks in asymptomatic patients compared to the patients with syncope or aborted sudden cardiac death. There were no other factors (like a spontaneous type 1 ECG) apart from a clinical history of syncope or aborted sudden cardiac death predicting appropriate shocks. Of importance, approximately 20% of patients in each group suffered from inappropriate shocks during follow-up. In a follow-up study in 2013 [48], the number of asymptomatic patients implanted with an ICD because of inducibility had grown to 87%, notably some in combination with other risk factors such as a spontaneous type 1 ECG. Interestingly, the number of patients who had already experienced a cardiac arrest and were inducible was lower (53%) than the number of patients who were asymptomatic and were inducible (87%). Again, inducibility could not be identified as a useful parameter to separate the patients who will and who will not progress to arrhythmias during follow-up. Importantly, ICD-complications, including fatal events, did occur in these patients with a primary prevention ICD. This notwithstanding, being asymptomatic at inclusion, still associated with about 1% of appropriate ICD interventions per year. Whether all these patients were indeed saved from a sudden death will never be known [267] but probably some of these events (if not a considerable number), would have been terminated spontaneously without sudden death. Importantly, programming longer detection intervals and higher cut-off rates for VF also seems to reduce inappropriate shock rates without compromising ICD safety [48, 268]. In 2016, another meta-analysis on inducibility was published, also including data from earlier studies [103]. In this paper, in contrast to earlier studies, additive value of inducibility to symptoms and presenting ECGs was found. Still it should be noted that 527 out of 1312 patients (40%) was inducible, while 65 patients (5%) experienced events (5 with sudden cardiac arrest and 60 with ICD shocks, 21 of whom being asymptomatic at presentation) during a median follow up of 38 months.

Non-invasive risk stratification has been attempted in relatively small cohorts of patients and yielded the strongest predictive value in spontaneous changes in the right precordial ST segments [107, 142, 143]. A standard cardiology workup including echocardiogram, 24-hour Holter, and an exercise test may be valuable to exclude differential diagnoses and to assess baseline conditions. There could be added value in 24-h 12-lead Holter monitoring as a number of patients with spontaneous type-1 ECGs will be uncovered [61, 62]. Thorough cardiac imaging using MRI or CT does not seem to add significant clinical value at present, unless arrhythmogenic right ventricular cardiomyopathy needs to be excluded.

A summary of the current literature on risk stratification in patients who did not yet experience a cardiac arrest, suggests that symptoms likely to be related to ventricular arrhythmias in combination with a spontaneous type-1 ECG identifies the patients at highest risk for future life-threatening arrhythmic events. Conversely, as asymptomatic patients without a spontaneous type-1 ECG have a (very) low risk of experiencing these arrhythmias, and the currently available treatment option (ICD implantation) may do more harm than good [56, 57], they should be identified as low risk. The combination of several characteristics to assess the risk profile is probably very worthwhile, and has been suggested [269, 270]. Undoubtedly, risk stratification should be re-evaluated in all patients during long-term follow-up using up-to-date consensus criteria.

14.5.2 Treatment

The most effective therapy to treat ventricular arrhythmias in Brugada syndrome is an ICD. Patients may, however, still experience intolerable numbers of ICD shocks, up to 150 a day [121], as an ICD does not lower the vulnerability of the heart for ventricular arrhythmias and ICDs are often programmed to quickly react—probably also treating VT/VF episodes that would have terminated spontaneously [267]. In some patients in earlier days, heart transplantation has been considered to be the only remaining option to diminish VT/VF events [271]. Cardiologists should carefully weigh possible benefits versus possible harm, quality of life, and costs of ICDs, as event rates are generally low and complications (in particular inappropriate shocks) are high in this population [47, 48, 57]. ICD implantation in the young specifically denotes several battery replacements, re-implantations over many decades, increased morbidity and even ICD-related mortality [48]. Still, in individual cases it might be considered to also implant an ICD in Brugada patients who are considered to have a low risk profile but who have an intolerable and uncontrollable anxiety that severely diminishes their quality of life and impairs their daily activities e.g. because they have lost a family member due to sudden cardiac death.

Acute lowering of the vulnerability of the heart for ventricular arrhythmias may be accomplished by treating hyperthermia (e.g., cooling, antipyretics, antibiotics), correcting electrolyte disturbances, and the administration of quinidine and/or isoproterenol [55, 110, 157, 160, 162]. Further chronic oral treatment with quinidine or several other agents may also prove valuable [50, 52, 272–279]. Excluding differential diagnoses in case of acute events is still mandatory as tachyarrhythmias not due to Brugada syndrome may display a devastating response on isoproterenol [280].

All patients with Brugada syndrome should receive a list of avoidable drugs and substances, including a number of antiarrhythmic drugs (particularly several class Ia & Ic drugs), psychotropic drugs (e.g. tricyclic antidepressants and lithium), anaesthetics (e.g. bupivacaine and propofol) and substances like cocaine, and excessive use of alcohol; see www.BrugadaDrugs.org [115]. Of note, some of these drugs, particularly propofol have been used frequently without untoward events. Still, the increased risk for arrhythmias should be recognized and be anticipated on. Furthermore, patients should be instructed to obtain an ECG in case of fever at least once (and if negative maybe every 5 years or so) to assess whether their form of Brugada syndrome is hyperthermia sensitive.

Special interest has emerged in the last years for ablation therapy to prevent (or even cure?) ventricular arrhythmias [127, 128, 281–283]. Especially the epicardial approach with ablation of late and fractionated electrograms of the right ventricular outflow tract seems to be very promising with abolition of inducibility, resolution of the characteristic ECG and a diminishing of recurrent episodes of VT/VF [128]. A randomized trial is currently prepared and should provide the first results around 2020 [284].

Long-term follow-up is mandatory in all Brugada syndrome patients. Symptomatic patients will have more frequent visits, but also asymptomatic patients should be seen with regular intervals for reassessment of the risk for arrhythmic events and genetic counselling in case of children. Genetic counselling should be advised for all adult patients.

14.6 Future Research

The knowledge and awareness of Brugada syndrome will continue to increase. In the first years after the description in 1992, many severely symptomatic patients were recognized, which led to the notion that Brugada syndrome is a malignant disease that is hard to manage [1, 44]. However, many asymptomatic patients have now been diagnosed and one of the great challenges for the future is to develop reliable risk stratification for arrhythmic events in this group of patients [144, 285]. Risk stratification and treatment in the paediatric population affected with Brugada syndrome, although limited in numbers, should also receive our continued attention. The pathophysiology of the ventricular arrhythmias and the coved-type ECG in the right precordial leads has been and will continue to be a major area of research. Although many animal and computer models are available, detailed descriptions of human data will continue to be important and will guide therapeutic interventions. Finally, further characterization of the (potentially complex) genetic origin of Brugada syndrome will help to identify those silent carriers, and their offspring, who might be at risk and may clarify the complicated genotype–phenotype relationship in Brugada syndrome patients.

14.7 Early Repolarisation Syndrome

14.7.1 Introduction

Already in 1936, in the era of the string galvanometer, common variations at the end of the QRS complex and the early ST segment were described. Shipley and Hallaran (Cleveland Ohio) noted in their study of 200 healthy men and women between the age of 20 and 35 (i.e. before the possible onset of significant coronary artery disease), and with a normal physical examination, in up to 44% percent of traces slurring or notching of the terminal QRS occurred [286]. In the same paper, ST-elevation was noted in up to 25% of males and up to 16% in females. In the years thereafter, also in 12-lead ECGs and in vectorcardiograms, ST-elevation, notching and slurring was found to be a frequent finding in apparently healthy individuals, particularly in young and athletic individuals and in those from African descent [287–291]. The term 'early repolarisation' to describe (common) inferolateral ST-elevation has been attributed to Grant, Estes and Doyle in their 1951 paper on the 12-lead ECG and vectorcardiogram [292, 293]. In later years, some authors even used the statement early repolarisation *syndrome* to describe this normal variant with ST-elevation, notching or slurring in the inferolateral leads [294, 295]. Currently we use early repolarisation *syndrome* only for those patients with an early repolarisation *pattern* in conjunction with a history of otherwise unexplained malignant ventricular arrhythmias [144].

Although considered a benign variation for decades [293, 294, 296], also because of its frequent occurrence in the young and healthy, since the 1990s several case reports of 'idiopathic' ventricular fibrillation with the presence of inferolateral ST elevation were published [202, 205, 297]. In 2008 the interest in early repolarisation, including notching and slurring, truly pivoted with the near simultaneous publication of two cohort studies investigating an association between the occurrence of malignant ventricular arrhythmias and an inferolateral early repolarisation pattern. Haïssaguerre and colleagues from 22 centres reviewed 206 case subjects who were resuscitated after cardiac arrest due to idiopathic ventricular fibrillation and compared these patients to 412 matched control subjects without obvious heart disease [298]. It appeared that an elevation of the QRS–ST junction of at least 0.1 mV from baseline in the inferior or lateral leads, manifested as QRS slurring or notching, was more frequent in case subjects (31 vs. 5%, $p < 0.001$). In a very comparable study, albeit with lower numbers, almost simultaneously published by Rosso and colleagues from three centres [299], 45 patients with idiopathic ventricular fibrillation were compared to 124 matched control subjects. Again, J-point elevation, particularly in the inferior and lateral extremity leads, was more common among cases (42 vs. 13%, $p = 0.001$). One year later, in 2009, a large community based study of 10,864 middle-aged subjects also noted an association between ST-elevation in the inferior leads and an increased risk of death due to cardiac causes [300]. Since then, many more papers have been published on the association between early repolarisation and an increased risk for cardiac events [301–304].

Still, in the AHA/ACC/HRS 2009 consensus statement on ECG interpretation, early repolarisation was continued to be described as 'a statement that is used frequently to characterise a normal QRS-T variant with J-point elevation' [305]. In 2011, two distinguished electrocardiographists even labelled the statement early repolarisation (and its accomplice 'J-wave') to be inappropriate and confusing [306]. In 2013, in the HRS/EHRA/APHRS consensus statement on the diagnosis and management of patients with inherited primary arrhythmia syndromes, the diagnosis of early repolarisation *syndrome* was reserved for those subjects who actually were resuscitated from otherwise unexplained ventricular fibrillation or polymorphic ventricular tachycardia in the presence of J-point elevation $\geq$0.1 mV in $\geq$2 contiguous inferior and/or lateral leads [144]. The early repolarisation *pattern* could be diagnosed with the same criteria but in the absence of (a strong suggestion of) malignant arrhythmias [144]. However, ongoing debate on nomenclature and definitions of early repolarisation led to the establishment of another consensus statement by many of the previous mentioned authors and specifically included terminal QRS notching or slurring *without* the need for ST-segment elevation [307].

A genetic basis for the early repolarisation syndrome is still under investigation and is currently suggested by anecdotal observations of an increased familial appearance of the early repolarisation pattern in concert with otherwise unexplained sudden deaths [308, 309]. In search for genetic variants in one severely affected patient, a *KCNJ8* gene variant was uncovered in a candidate gene approach including 21 genes [310]. However, in the same study an additional 156 early repolarisation syndrome patients were also tested for variants in *KCNJ8*, but this analysis failed to identify more proof of an association of early repolarisation syndrome with genetic variants in *KCNJ8*. In other candidate gene approach studies, variants in *KCNJ8* (the same variant), *CACNA1C*, *CACNB2*, (both unsuccessfully tested in the previous *KCNJ8* study) and *CACNA2D1* were documented as possible susceptibility genes for early repolarisation syndrome [28, 41]. However, in a subsequent study this specific *KCNJ8* variant (S422L) was found to be actually very common in Ashkenazi Jews, and not apparently associated with early repolarisation, not even in a homozygous boy [311]. In 2015 however, in the ESC guideline on ventricular arrhythmias, it was still claimed that no clear evidence of familial transmission of the early repolarisation syndrome exists [312]. This is mainly due to the relatively frequent occurrence of these variants in patients or cohorts without signs of early repolarisation syndrome.

The treatment of early repolarisation syndrome, in line with the 2013 consensus statement, is particularly aimed at preventing sudden death from recurrent malignant arrhythmia by a secondary prevention ICD implantation. During electrical storm isoproterenol can be useful in patients with a diagnosis of early repolarisation syndrome, while quinidine can be useful for secondary prevention of malignant arrhythmias in these patients [144, 313].

14.7.2 Clinical Presentation

14.7.2.1 Epidemiology

The prevalence of the early repolarisation pattern in the general population has been estimated at 1–13% but increases to 15–70% when studying cases of idiopathic ventricular fibrillation [298–301, 303, 314–317]. Differences in the prevalence of early repolarisation are mainly due to the type of population studied and the definition of early repolarisation that is used. Also, studies have shown that the early repolarisation pattern is intermittently present [315], which challenges the determination of its exact prevalence. Even though no clear regional differences in its prevalence have been observed, as for example have been seen in the Brugada syndrome, the early repolarisation pattern is more prevalent among blacks than in whites [318]. One study observed a higher prevalence of early repolarisation in aboriginal Australians compared to white Australians [319]. A rather high prevalence of the early repolarisation pattern has also been reported in a Japanese cohort of atomic-bomb survivors [301].

Early repolarisation is further predominantly found in the paediatric population, in males, young physically active individuals and in athletes [320]. In the athletes, case-control studies have estimated the prevalence of the early repolarisation pattern between 10 and 90% [321], and also here it is thought that the early repolarisation pattern is a most often a benign variant and associated with a low risk of arrhythmic events. It has been hypothesized that early repolarisation is influenced by hormonal factors since its prevalence is higher in the paediatric population. Furthermore, after puberty its prevalence increases (16–25%) in male subjects and decreases in female subjects (11–4%) [322, 323].

14.7.2.2 The Patient

Only an extremely small minority of the patients with the early repolarisation pattern will ever experience any symptoms of the early repolarisation *syndrome* (i.e. ventricular fibrillation), this is partly due to the high prevalence of the early repolarisation *pattern* in the young and healthy [321]. The early repolarisation pattern may be intermittently present and is can be modulated by vagal tone, heart rate and drugs [313, 316, 324, 325]. The Valsalva manoeuvre may unmask the early repolarisation pattern on the ECG. However, the sensitivity of the test is low (45%), and evidence relies predominantly upon one study [308]. Disappearance of the pattern may occur during exercise and infusion of isoproterenol [325].

Before the onset of VF, an increase in the amplitude of early repolarisation, can be seen as compared to baseline values [298, 326, 327]. For example, in the study of Haïssaguerre the J-point amplitude increased from 2.6 ± 1 to 4.1 ± 2 mm ($P < 0.001$) before the onset of VF [298]. This initial increase in the amplitude of the ERS may be subsequently followed by a ventricular ectopic beat with a short coupling interval that initiates ventricular fibrillation. It appears that this ectopy preceding VF most often arises from the left ventricle inferior wall [298]. In a follow-up study of IVF patients, patient with ERS had a higher risk for future cardiac events (41 vs. 23%) (HR 2.1; 95% confidence interval (CI), 1.2–3.5; $P = 0.008$) compared to those without ERS [298].

In the general population, the early repolarisation pattern has also been linked to an increased risk of cardiac events. A community based prospective study [300], analysed 10,864 Finnish subjects with a mean age of 44 ± 8 years old. In this study, patients with a J-wave amplitude of ≥0.1 mV in the inferior leads carried an increased risk of death from cardiac causes (adjusted relative risk (RR) 1.28, confidence interval (CI) 1.04–1.59) and this relative risk rose even further in patients with a J-wave amplitude of >0.2 mV in the inferior leads (adjusted RR 2.98; 95% CI 1.85–4.92) and from arrhythmia (adjusted RR 2.92; 95% CI 1.45–5.89). In another population-based prospective study including 1945 patients [303], the presence of an early repolarisation pattern was associated with cardiac and all-cause mortality, especially in those of younger age (35–54 years old) and male sex (hazard ratio 2.65; 95% CI 1.21–5.83). An inferior early repolarisation pattern further increased cardiac mortality (hazard ratio 3.15; 95% CI 1.58–6.28) for both sexes and particularly in male subjects between 35 and 54 years of age (hazard ratio 4.27; 95% CI 1.90–9.61). Important in this respect is that there seems to be a time dependent risk over very long follow-up (up to 20 years). Whether the early repolarisation pattern was still present before the event and what the association is with comorbidities like, e.g., ischaemic heart disease, is uncertain however.

Other studies have shown that the presence of the early repolarisation pattern may be a modulator of risk for sudden death in the setting of comorbidities. Tikkanen et al. studied the association between early repolarisation and risk of sudden death during an acute coronary event [328]. In this case-control study including 432 cases with a mean age 66 ± 11 years they found that the risk of sudden cardiac death was increased in patients with the early repolarisation pattern (odds ratio (OR), 1.85; 95% CI, 1.23–2.80). Specifically, in those patients with an early repolarisation pattern with a horizontal/descending ST segment predicted the occurrence of sudden cardiac death (OR, 2.04; 95% CI, 1.25–3.34). After multivariate adjustments the presence of the early repolarisation pattern with horizontal/descending ST segment remained as independent predictors of sudden cardiac death. A comparable association of increased risk of cardiac events in the setting of other pathologies has been observed in patients with inherited cardiac arrhythmia syndromes. For example, in a retrospective cohort study of catecholaminergic polymorphic ventricular tachycardia (CPVT) patients, those with an early repolarisation pattern were at increased risk for arrhythmic events when compared to CPVT patients without early repolarisation [329]. Such an association has also been found in the long QT syndrome type 1 and type 2 [330] and in Brugada syndrome [204].

14.7.3 Electrocardiography and Diagnosis

The diagnosis of early repolarisation syndrome is made *per exclusionem*. In survivors of a cardiac arrest due to ventricular fibrillation or polymorphic ventricular tachycardia, an extensive work-up in search of a diagnosis is recommended [312]. This will often include sequential ECGs and 24-h ECG-monitoring, coronary angiography and echo, while also exercise testing, detailed ECG analysis using signal averaging or brisk standing, magnetic resonance imaging (MRI), drug provocation with sodium channel blockers and endocardial biopsies should be considered. When all these tests turn negative while at the same time a clear early repolarisation pattern is evident, a diagnosis of early repolarisation syndrome can be made [144, 331, 332].

The criteria for the early repolarisation pattern have been susceptible for discussion and are not uniform across many papers (Fig. 14.5). One consensus statement on this topic specifically includes terminal QRS notching and slurring with or without concomitant ST-elevation as essential to the early repolarisation pattern [307]. Their definition incorporates terminal QRS notching or slurring with either elevation of the QRS–ST junction (also named J-termination or 'Jt') of at least 0.1 mV from baseline and/or elevation of the J-peak (in the case of a notch) of at least 0.1 mV from baseline in the inferior or lateral leads. Moreover, the consensus view of that group of authors was that in the absence of terminal QRS notching or slurring, ST- or Jt-elevation alone should *not* be reported as early repolarisation [307]. This last statement could clearly be in conflict with the HRS/EHRA/APHRS

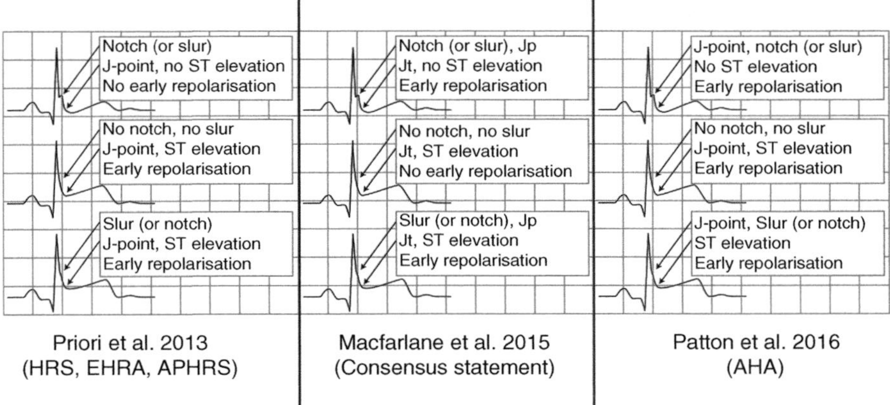

Fig. 14.5 Early repolarisation pattern examples and classification according to different statements [307, 333, 334]. Jp denotes J-peak, Jt denotes J-termination (a.k.a. QRS end or J-point). In the Patton paper the J-amplitude/ST elevation is measured at the peak of the notch or the start of the slur, instead of at the end of the QRS. In all statements, ST elevation, J-point or J-peak should be ≥0.1 mV and present in ≥2 contiguous inferior and/or lateral leads

2013 consensus statement which *only* mentions J-point elevation ≥0.1 mV in ≥2 contiguous inferior and/or lateral leads [144]. This is because the J-point is generally considered to be the QRS-ST junction or J-termination and when elevated this does not necessarily combine with a notched or slurred terminal QRS. In the 2016 AHA scientific statement yet another definition is suggested, [333] which also seems to be in conflict with the 2015 Macfarlane paper. In this 2016 AHA statement, early repolarisation includes ST- or Jt-elevation *with* or *without* notching or slurring (similar to the 2013 HRS/EHRA/APHRS statement). However, specific to this statement, the measurement of the J-elevation is performed on the peak of the notch or at the start of the slur, as opposed to the 2013 and 2015 statements.

Another important aspect of early repolarisation is the direction of the ST-segment; being either horizontal or down-sloping versus upsloping [335]. Tikkanen et al. in a follow-up paper of their earlier study, evaluated the ST-segment in athletes and in middle-aged subjects from the general population, and noted that only a horizontal or down-sloping ST-segment after terminal QRS-notching or slurring associated with an increased risk for arrhythmic death [300, 336]. Also a secondary analysis of the Rosso study showed that a horizontal or down-sloping ST-segment was more common in the subjects who suffered from idiopathic ventricular fibrillation than in the control subjects [335]. This has led to the suggestion to describe the early repolarisation pattern as either benign (upsloping) or malign (horizontal or down-sloping) [335]. This does not imply, however, that an upsloping ST-segment after a QRS notch or slur is always benign, as still about 30% of patients with early repolarisation syndrome will only show this 'benign' pattern [335, 337].

14.7.4 Pathophysiology

The pathophysiological mechanisms underlying early repolarisation syndrome are currently far from clear. The absence of a well-defined genetic substrate, the common occurrence of the early repolarisation pattern in the young and healthy, and the obligatory absence of any other known primary electrical disease or (signs of) cardiomyopathy, complicates this further. Although some authors have shared early repolarisation syndrome and Brugada syndrome under the common denominator 'J-wave syndromes' [338], others have opposed this practice [306, 339]. Whether the notching or slurring of the terminal QRS complex is actually a depolarisation or a repolarisation phenomenon is also still unclear [339–341]. Certainly there is a clear distinction between the mechanisms underlying Brugada syndrome and early repolarisation syndrome as is mirrored on the reverse reaction on different provocations and the inherent difference in the localisation of the aberrant ST-elevation. While in early repolarisation tachycardia, hyperthermia, isoproterenol and sodium blocker administration will decrease the ST-elevation, it will increase ST-elevation in Brugada syndrome [110, 180, 324, 325, 342–344]. Also, in Brugada syndrome there is evidence of conduction delay and of abnormal endocardial and particularly epicardial electrograms [22, 128, 190], while this is not the case in early repolarisation syndrome [337]. In contrast, in both Brugada syndrome and early repolarisation syndrome, an increased vagal tone is associated with ST-elevation [105, 109, 308, 337].

14.7.5 Genetics

For the comprehensive and authoritative Online Mendelian Inheritance in Man compendium, early repolarisation associated with ventricular fibrillation (OMIM 613601) still awaits confirmation of a genetic association [245]. The first study into the genetic underpinning of early repolarisation syndrome was published in 2009 by the group of Haïssaguerre et al. shortly after their pivotal 2008 paper [298, 310]. In this study, a severely affected 14-year-old female is described who suffered from >100 cardiac arrests due to ventricular fibrillation and displayed a prominent early repolarisation pattern (mostly prominent notching). Detailed genetic evaluation of many candidate genes (*KCNQ1*, *KCNE1*, *KCNH2*, *KCNE2*, *KCNJ2*, *KCNJ8*, *KCNJ11*, *ABCC9*, *KCNJ5*, *KCNJ3*, *KCND3*, *IRX3*, *IRX5*, *SCN5A*, *SCN1B*, *NCX1*, *CACNA1C*, *CACNB2*, *CALR*, *CASQ2* and *ANK2*) revealed a missense variant (p.S422L) in the *KCNJ8* gene encoding the Kir6.1 subunit of the K-ATP channel. This variant was absent in 764 control alleles from healthy controls, and, importantly, was also absent in a cohort of 156 additional early repolarisation syndrome patients. The mother of the patient did not have this same variant and the father denied testing, so no segregation analysis was available. In the year thereafter, an association with the *KCNJ8*-S422L variant was replicated by Medeiros-Domingo et al. [41]. In this study 101 unrelated patients with Brugada syndrome (n = 87) or early repolarisation syndrome (n = 14), were evaluated for *KCNJ8* variants, and in 1 Brugada patient and in 1 early repolarisation syndrome patient the same S422L variant was found (and absent in

1200 control alleles). Additional analyses showed that this variant was able to significantly increase the K-ATP current of Kir6.1, suggesting a gain-of-function mutation. However, in sharp contrast to these two studies suggestive of a pathogenic role for *KCNJ8*, and particularly for the S422L variant, in a subsequent study in Ashkenazi Jews this association was questioned [311]. The *KCNJ8*-S422L appeared to be rather prevalent in this population (4%) and was not apparently associated with an early repolarisation pattern nor syndrome, not even in a homozygous boy.

Further studies into the genetic underpinning of early repolarisation syndrome suggested a role for calcium channel mutations. Burashnikov et al. evaluated multiple candidate genes (*CACNA1C*, *CACNB2*, *CACNA2D1*, *KCNH2*, *KCNQ1*, *KCNJ8*, *KCNE1*, *KCNE2*, *KCNE3*, *KCNE4*, *SCN1B*, and *SCN3B*) in a cohort of unrelated probands with Brugada syndrome (n = 162), early repolarisation syndrome or pattern n = 24) and idiopathic ventricular fibrillation (n = 19). In their patients with early repolarisation syndrome or pattern, they found mutations in *CACNA1C*, *CACNB2* (both unsuccessfully tested in the 2009 *KCNJ8* study) and *CACNA2D1*. However, these variants were still only found in single cases among many tested subjects without proof of familial segregation.

There have also been reports of other possible associated genes, particularly *SCN5A*. One report suggested loss-of-function mutations in *SCN5A* to be associated with early repolarisation syndrome in the absence of a Brugada phenotype in 3 out of 50 early repolarisation syndrome patients [345]. However, in this report there was clear evidence of conduction slowing and abnormal right precordial ST segments in these three patients, while a Brugada syndrome was not definitely excluded in the absence of potent sodium channel blockade with ajmaline or higher placed right precordial leads. Again, familial segregation was not demonstrated. In another report the *ABCC9* gene was implicated to be associated with the early repolarisation syndrome [37]. In 4 out 150 probands with either the early repolarisation pattern of syndrome or Brugada syndrome, a variant in the *ABCC9* gene was found. One of the tested variants indeed caused a gain-of-function of the K-ATP channel Kir6.1. These authors also reported that the father of one of these patients also carried the same variant and also showed the early repolarisation pattern, now indeed suggesting familial segregation.

As mentioned earlier, in the 2015 ESC guideline on ventricular arrhythmias, it is stated that no clear evidence of familial transmission of the early repolarisation syndrome exists [312]. There are, however, reports on early repolarisation in families [308, 309]. In the Nunn et al. study, family members of probands diagnosed with the sudden arrhythmic death syndrome (SADS), were evaluated and were compared to matched controls. They found that inferolateral J-point elevation was more common in SADS-relatives as compared to controls (23 vs. 11%) and suggested that this inferolateral J-point elevation may indeed be a marker of pro-arrhythmic trait or even a marker of pro-arrhythmia. In the Gouraud et al. study, the relatives of four families affected by the early repolarisation syndrome were studied. They found that an early repolarisation pattern was indeed common among family members (33–61%), and suggestive of an autosomal dominant mode of inheritance.

An inherent problem in the genetic underpinning of early repolarisation syndrome remains that the alleles from a (phenotyped) control cohort can barely cover the extremely low incidence of the cases with a genetic variant. As long as there is no proof of genetic linkage with the phenotype a plausible genetic explanation for early repolarisation syndrome will remain a challenging issue. Illustrative to this point is that the largest study into the identification of genetic variants predisposing to the early repolarisation *pattern* did not provide supporting evidence for a genetic substrate [346]. In this study, a genome-wide association meta-analysis in 7482 subjects for the discovery stage, and in 7151 subjects for the replication stage (combined prevalence of the early repolarisation pattern 2.9–9.8%), no variants found in the discovery stage could be replicated. Combined meta-analysis results also failed to reach genome-wide significance.

14.7.6 Clinical Decision Making

14.7.6.1 Risk Stratification

Risk stratification in early repolarisation syndrome is not particularly difficult; as these patients have already experienced malignant ventricular arrhythmias resulting in cardiac arrest and resuscitation, these patients have a class I indication for secondary protection by an ICD [144]. However, the problem in risk stratification arises in those with an early repolarisation pattern. As mentioned earlier, an upsloping ST-segment is considered to be more probable benign, while a horizontal or downsloping ST-segment is considered to be more probable malignant [300, 335, 336]. This knowledge base underlies a class 2b recommendation to consider prophylactic ICD implantation in patients with a malignant early repolarisation pattern and/or in those with a previous syncope suggestive to be a tachyarrhythmia [144]. Importantly, there are currently no other parameters of risk in early repolarisation, including programmed stimulation [347]. In asymptomatic patients with an isolated early repolarisarion pattern, prophylactic ICD implantation is not recommend (class III recommendation) [144]. Whether patients with an overlap phenotype of Brugada syndrome and an early repolarisation pattern have a distinct risk profile is currently uncertain and it is advised to follow the regular risk stratification process for both.

14.7.6.2 Treatment

As mentioned earlier, secondary prevention for sudden death due to malignant arrhythmias can be established with ICD implantation. In a multi-centre study on drug therapy in early repolarisation syndrome it was documented that isoproterenol can be used to treat patients during electrical storm and that quinidine can be used to suppress recurrent arrhythmias on the long term [313]. Importantly, the other tested drugs in this cohort were ineffective to control arrhythmias and included mexiletine, verapamil, flecainide, propafenone, pilsicainide and also amiodarone (the latter seemed to be effective in 1 out of 6 patients during electrical storm though). There is currently no evidence that patients with early repolarisation syndrome should avoid specific drugs, in contrast to Brugada syndrome, Long QT syndrome and catecholaminergic polymorphic VT.

14.7.7 Future Research

Although the early repolarisation pattern has been known since the early years of electrocardiology (even before the recognition of the importance of a prolonged QT interval), the early repolarisation syndrome is a rather new entity. As mentioned earlier, we are also still struggling with the definition of the early repolarisation pattern, precluding uniformity in the research in this area. Another very important issue in the coming years will be to gain experience in the recognition of patients without symptoms but a high propensity for malignant arrhythmias in the future. These patients could be prophylactically treated with quinidine for example. However, as the early repolarisation pattern affects 5–60% and seldom up to 90% of investigated cohorts of presumably healthy individuals, and true early repolarisation syndrome is a particularly rare entity, this unmistakably is a daunting task. Lastly, although evidence for a monogenic substrate for early repolarisation syndrome is currently lacking, there will probably be genetic variants influencing the phenotype. This might possibly also have impact on screening and prophylactic treatment in the future.

References

1. Brugada P, Brugada J. Right bundle branch block, persistent ST segment elevation and sudden cardiac death: a distinct clinical and electrocardiographic syndrome. A multicenter report. J Am Coll Cardiol. 1992;20:1391–6.
2. Antzelevitch C, Brugada P, Borggrefe M, et al. Brugada syndrome: report of the second consensus conference. Heart Rhythm. 2005;2:429–40.
3. Wilde AA, Antzelevitch C, Borggrefe M, et al. Proposed diagnostic criteria for the Brugada syndrome: consensus report. Circulation. 2002;106:2514–9.
4. Brugada J, Brugada R, Brugada P. Right bundle-branch block and ST-segment elevation in leads V1 through V3: a marker for sudden death in patients without demonstrable structural heart disease. Circulation. 1998;97:457–60.
5. Sangwatanaroj S, Prechawat S, Sunsaneewitayakul B, et al. New electrocardiographic leads and the procainamide test for the detection of the Brugada sign in sudden unexplained death syndrome survivors and their relatives. Eur Heart J. 2001;22:2290–6.
6. Shimizu W, Matsuo K, Takagi M, et al. Body surface distribution and response to drugs of ST segment elevation in Brugada syndrome: clinical implication of eighty-seven-lead body surface potential mapping and its application to twelve-lead electrocardiograms. J Cardiovasc Electrophysiol. 2000;11:396–404.
7. Krishnan SC, Josephson ME. ST segment elevation induced by class IC antiarrhythmic agents: underlying electrophysiologic mechanisms and insights into drug-induced proarrhythmia. J Cardiovasc Electrophysiol. 1998;9:1167–72.
8. Miyazaki T, Mitamura H, Miyoshi S, et al. Autonomic and antiarrhythmic drug modulation of ST segment elevation in patients with Brugada syndrome. J Am Coll Cardiol. 1996;27:1061–70.
9. Osher HL, Wolff L. Electrocardiographic pattern simulating acute myocardial injury. Am J Med Sci. 1953;226:541–5.
10. Edeiken J. Elevation of the RS-T segment, apparent or real, in the right precordial leads as a probable normal variant. Am Heart J. 1954;48:331–9.
11. Martini B, Nava A, Thiene G, et al. Ventricular fibrillation without apparent heart disease: description of six cases. Am Heart J. 1989;118:1203–9.

12. Baron RC, Thacker SB, Gorelkin L, et al. Sudden death among Southeast Asian refugees. An unexplained nocturnal phenomenon. JAMA. 1983;250:2947–51.
13. Hattori K, McCubbin MA, Ishida DN. Concept analysis of good death in the Japanese community. J Nurs Scholarsh. 2006;38:165–70.
14. Nademanee K, Veerakul G, Nimmannit S, et al. Arrhythmogenic marker for the sudden unexplained death syndrome in Thai men. Circulation. 1997;96:2595–600.
15. Otto CM, Tauxe RV, Cobb LA, et al. Ventricular fibrillation causes sudden death in Southeast Asian immigrants. Ann Intern Med. 1984;101:45–7.
16. Chen Q, Kirsch GE, Zhang D, et al. Genetic basis and molecular mechanism for idiopathic ventricular fibrillation. Nature. 1998;392:293–6.
17. Rook MB, Bezzina Alshinawi C, Groenewegen WA, et al. Human SCN5A gene mutations alter cardiac sodium channel kinetics and are associated with the Brugada syndrome. Cardiovasc Res. 1999;44:507–17.
18. Napolitano C. Inherited arrhythmias database. In: Study Group Mol. Basis Arrhythm; 2007. http://www.fsm.it/cardmoc/.
19. Napolitano C. Just another Brugada syndrome mutation? Heart Rhythm. 2007;4:54–5.
20. Priori SG, Napolitano C, Gasparini M, et al. Clinical and genetic heterogeneity of right bundle branch block and ST-segment elevation syndrome: a prospective evaluation of 52 families. Circulation. 2000;102:2509–15.
21. Probst V, Wilde AA, Barc J, et al. SCN5A mutations and the role of genetic background in the pathophysiology of Brugada syndrome. Circ Cardiovasc Genet. 2009;2:552–7.
22. Smits JP, Eckardt L, Probst V, et al. Genotype-phenotype relationship in Brugada syndrome: electrocardiographic features differentiate SCN5A-related patients from non-SCN5A-related patients. J Am Coll Cardiol. 2002;40:350–6.
23. Wilde AA, Ackerman MJ. Exercise extreme caution when calling rare genetic variants novel arrhythmia syndrome susceptibility mutations. Heart Rhythm. 2010;7:1883–5.
24. London B, Michalec M, Mehdi H, et al. Mutation in glycerol-3-phosphate dehydrogenase 1 like gene (GPD1-L) decreases cardiac Na+ current and causes inherited arrhythmias. Circulation. 2007;116:2260–8.
25. Weiss R, Barmada MM, Nguyen T, et al. Clinical and molecular heterogeneity in the Brugada syndrome: a novel gene locus on chromosome 3. Circulation. 2002;105:707–13.
26. Tan HL, Bezzina CR, Smits JP, et al. Genetic control of sodium channel function. Cardiovasc Res. 2003;57:961–73.
27. Antzelevitch C, Pollevick GD, Cordeiro JM, et al. Loss-of-function mutations in the cardiac calcium channel underlie a new clinical entity characterized by ST-segment elevation, short QT intervals, and sudden cardiac death. Circulation. 2007;115:442–9.
28. Burashnikov E, Pfeiffer R, Barajas-Martinez H, et al. Mutations in the cardiac L-type calcium channel associated with inherited J wave syndromes and sudden cardiac death. Heart Rhythm. 2010;7:1872–82.
29. Cerrone M, Lin X, Zhang M, et al. Missense mutations in Plakophilin-2 cause sodium current deficit and associate with a Brugada syndrome phenotype. Circulation. 2014;129:1092–103.
30. Crotti L, Marcou CA, Tester DJ, et al. Spectrum and prevalence of mutations involving BrS1-through BrS12-susceptibility genes in a cohort of unrelated patients referred for Brugada syndrome genetic testing: implications for genetic testing. J Am Coll Cardiol. 2012;60:1410–08.
31. Delpon E, Cordeiro JM, Nunez L, et al. Functional effects of KCNE3 mutation and its role in the development of Brugada syndrome. Circ Arrhythm Electrophysiol. 2008;1:209–18.
32. Duthoit G, Fressart V, Hidden-Lucet F, et al. Brugada ECG pattern: a physiopathological prospective study based on clinical, electrophysiological, angiographic, and genetic findings. Front Physiol. 2012;3:474.
33. Giudicessi JR, Ye D, Tester DJ, et al. Transient outward current (I(to)) gain-of-function mutations in the KCND3-encoded Kv4.3 potassium channel and Brugada syndrome. Heart Rhythm. 2011;8:1024–32.
34. Hennessey JA, Marcou CA, Wang C, et al. FGF12 is a candidate Brugada syndrome locus. Heart Rhythm Off J Heart Rhythm Soc. 2013;10:1886–94.

35. Hu D, Barajas-Martinez H, Burashnikov E, et al. A mutation in the beta 3 subunit of the cardiac sodium channel associated with Brugada ECG phenotype. Circ Cardiovasc Genet. 2009;2:270–8.
36. Hu D, Barajas-Martínez H, Pfeiffer R, et al. Mutations in SCN10A are responsible for a large fraction of cases of Brugada syndrome. J Am Coll Cardiol. 2014;64:66–79.
37. Hu D, Barajas-Martínez H, Terzic A, et al. ABCC9 is a novel Brugada and early repolarization syndrome susceptibility gene. Int J Cardiol. 2014;171:431–42.
38. Ishikawa T, Sato A, Marcou CA, et al. A novel disease gene for Brugada syndrome: sarcolemmal membrane-associated protein gene mutations impair intracellular trafficking of hNav1.5. Circ Arrhythm Electrophysiol. 2012;5:1098–107.
39. Kattygnarath D, Maugenre S, Neyroud N, et al. MOG1: a new susceptibility gene for Brugada syndrome. Circ Cardiovasc Genet. 2011;4:261–8.
40. Le Scouarnec S, Karakachoff M, Gourraud J-B, et al. Testing the burden of rare variation in arrhythmia-susceptibility genes provides new insights into molecular diagnosis for Brugada syndrome. Hum Mol Genet. 2015;24:2757–63.
41. Medeiros-Domingo A, Tan B-H, Crotti L, et al. Gain-of-function mutation S422L in the KCNJ8-encoded cardiac K(ATP) channel Kir6.1 as a pathogenic substrate for J-wave syndromes. Heart Rhythm Off J Heart Rhythm Soc. 2010;7:1466–71.
42. Riuró H, Beltran-Alvarez P, Tarradas A, et al. A missense mutation in the sodium channel β2 subunit reveals SCN2B as a new candidate gene for Brugada syndrome. Hum Mutat. 2013;34:961–6.
43. Watanabe H, Koopmann TT, Le Scouarnec S, et al. Sodium channel beta1 subunit mutations associated with Brugada syndrome and cardiac conduction disease in humans. J Clin Invest. 2008;118:2260–8.
44. Brugada J, Brugada R, Antzelevitch C, et al. Long-term follow-up of individuals with the electrocardiographic pattern of right bundle-branch block and ST-segment elevation in precordial leads V1 to V3. Circulation. 2002;105:73–8.
45. Kusmirek SL, Gold MR. Sudden cardiac death: the role of risk stratification. Am Heart J. 2007;153:25–33.
46. Priori SG, Napolitano C, Gasparini M, et al. Natural history of Brugada syndrome: insights for risk stratification and management. Circulation. 2002;105:1342–7.
47. Sacher F, Probst V, Iesaka Y, et al. Outcome after implantation of a cardioverter-defibrillator in patients with Brugada syndrome. A multicenter study. Circulation. 2006;114:2317–24.
48. Sacher F, Probst V, Maury P, et al. Outcome after implantation of cardioverter-defibrillator in patients with Brugada syndrome: a multicenter study - part 2. Circulation. 2013;128:1739–47.
49. Alings M, Dekker L, Sadee A, Wilde A. Quinidine induced electrocardiographic normalization in two patients with Brugada syndrome. Pacing Clin Electrophysiol. 2001;24:1420–2.
50. Belhassen B, Glick A, Viskin S. Efficacy of quinidine in high-risk patients with Brugada syndrome. Circulation. 2004;110:1731–7.
51. Belhassen B, Glick A, Viskin S. Excellent long-term reproducibility of the electrophysiologic efficacy of quinidine in patients with idiopathic ventricular fibrillation and Brugada syndrome. Pacing Clin Electrophysiol. 2009;32:294–301.
52. Belhassen B, Rahkovich M, Michowitz Y, et al. Management of Brugada syndrome: a 33-year experience using electrophysiologically-guided therapy with class 1A antiarrhythmic drugs. Circ Arrhythm Electrophysiol. 2015;8:1393–402.
53. Hermida JS, Denjoy I, Clerc J, et al. Hydroquinidine therapy in Brugada syndrome. J Am Coll Cardiol. 2004;43:1853–60.
54. Mok NS, Chan NY, Chiu AC. Successful use of quinidine in treatment of electrical storm in Brugada syndrome. Pacing Clin Electrophysiol. 2004;27:821–3.
55. Probst V, Denjoy I, Meregalli PG, et al. Clinical aspects and prognosis of Brugada syndrome in children. Circulation. 2007;115:2042–8.
56. Olde Nordkamp LRA, Postema PG, Knops RE, et al. Implantable cardioverter-defibrillator harm in young patients with inherited arrhythmia syndromes: a systematic review and meta-analysis of inappropriate shocks and complications. Heart Rhythm. 2016;13:443–54.

57. Olde Nordkamp LRA, Wilde AAM, Tijssen JGP, et al. The ICD for primary prevention in patients with inherited cardiac diseases: indications, utilization and outcome. A comparison with secondary prevention. Circ Arrhythm Electrophysiol. 2013;6:91–100.
58. Postema PG. About Brugada syndrome and its prevalence. Europace. 2012;14:925–8.
59. Schwartz PJ, Stramba-Badiale M, Crotti L, et al. Prevalence of the congenital long-QT syndrome. Circulation. 2009;120:1761–7.
60. Maron BJ, Gardin JM, Flack JM, et al. Prevalence of hypertrophic cardiomyopathy in a general population of young adults. Echocardiographic analysis of 4111 subjects in the CARDIA Study. Coronary artery risk development in (young) adults. Circulation. 1995;92:785–9.
61. Cerrato N, Giustetto C, Gribaudo E, et al. Prevalence of type 1 brugada electrocardiographic pattern evaluated by twelve-lead twenty-four-hour holter monitoring. Am J Cardiol. 2015;115:52–6.
62. Richter S, Sarkozy A, Veltmann C, et al. Variability of the diagnostic ECG pattern in an ICD patient population with Brugada syndrome. J Cardiovasc. 2009;20:69–75.
63. Oe H, Takagi M, Tanaka A, et al. Prevalence and clinical course of the juveniles with Brugada-type ECG in Japanese population. Pacing Clin Electrophysiol. 2005;28:549–54.
64. Yamakawa Y, Ishikawa T, Uchino K, et al. Prevalence of right bundle-branch block and right precordial ST-segment elevation (Brugada-type electrocardiogram) in Japanese children. Circ J. 2004;68:275–9.
65. Yoshinaga M, Anan R, Nomura Y, et al. Prevalence and time of appearance of Brugada electrocardiographic pattern in young male adolescents from a three-year follow-up study. Am J Cardiol. 2004;94:1186–9.
66. Matsuo K, Akahoshi M, Nakashima E, et al. The prevalence, incidence and prognostic value of the Brugada-type electrocardiogram: a population-based study of four decades. J Am Coll Cardiol. 2001;38:765–70.
67. Monroe MH, Littmann L. Two-year case collection of the Brugada syndrome electrocardiogram pattern at a large teaching hospital. Clin Cardiol. 2000;23:849–51.
68. Schukro C, Berger T, Stix G, et al. Regional prevalence and clinical benefit of implantable cardioverter defibrillators in Brugada syndrome. Int J Cardiol. 2010;144:191–4.
69. Pecini R, Cedergreen P, Theilade S, et al. The prevalence and relevance of the Brugada-type electrocardiogram in the Danish general population: data from the Copenhagen City Heart Study. Europace. 2010;12:982–6.
70. Junttila MJ, Raatikainen MJ, Karjalainen J, et al. Prevalence and prognosis of subjects with Brugada-type ECG pattern in a young and middle-aged Finnish population. Eur Heart J. 2004; 25:874–8.
71. Blangy H, Sadoul N, Coutelour JM, et al. Prevalence of Brugada syndrome among 35,309 inhabitants of Lorraine screened at a preventive medicine centre. Arch Mal Coeur Vaiss. 2005;98:175–80.
72. Hermida JS, Lemoine JL, Aoun FB, et al. Prevalence of the brugada syndrome in an apparently healthy population. Am J Cardiol. 2000;86:91–4.
73. Sinner MF, Pfeufer A, Perz S, et al. Spontaneous Brugada electrocardiogram patterns are rare in the German general population: results from the KORA study. Europace. 2009;11:1338–44.
74. Letsas KP, Gavrielatos G, Efremidis M, et al. Prevalence of Brugada sign in a Greek tertiary hospital population. Europace. 2007;9:1077–80.
75. Bozkurt A, Yas D, Seydaoglu G, Acarturk E. Frequency of Brugada-type ECG pattern (Brugada sign) in Southern Turkey. Int Heart J. 2006;47:541–7.
76. Viskin S, Fish R, Eldar M, et al. Prevalence of the Brugada sign in idiopathic ventricular fibrillation and healthy controls. Heart. 2000;84:31–6.
77. Babaee Bigi MA, Aslani A, Shahrzad S. Prevalence of Brugada sign in patients presenting with palpitation in Southern Iran. Europace. 2007;9:252–5.
78. Gallagher MM, Forleo GB, Behr ER, et al. Prevalence and significance of Brugada-type ECG in 12,012 apparently healthy European subjects. Int J Cardiol. 2007;130:44–8.
79. Furuhashi M, Uno K, Tsuchihashi K, et al. Prevalence of asymptomatic ST segment elevation in right precordial leads with right bundle branch block (Brugada-type ST shift) among the general Japanese population. Heart. 2001;86:161–6.

80. Ito H, Yano K, Chen R, et al. The prevalence and prognosis of a Brugada-type electrocardiogram in a population of middle-aged Japanese-American men with follow-up of three decades. Am J Med Sci. 2006;331:25–9.
81. Miyasaka Y, Tsuji H, Yamada K, et al. Prevalence and mortality of the Brugada-type electrocardiogram in one city in Japan. J Am Coll Cardiol. 2001;38:771–4.
82. Sakabe M, Fujiki A, Tani M, et al. Proportion and prognosis of healthy people with coved or saddle-back type ST segment elevation in the right precordial leads during 10 years follow-up. Eur Heart J. 2003;24:1488–93.
83. Tsuji H, Sato T, Morisaki K, Iwasaka T. Prognosis of subjects with Brugada-type electrocardiogram in a population of middle-aged Japanese diagnosed during a health examination. Am J Cardiol. 2008;102:584–7.
84. Wajed A, Aslam Z, Abbas SF, et al. Frequency of Brugada-type ECG pattern (Brugada sign) in an apparently healthy young population. J Ayub Med Coll Abbottabad. 2008;20:121–4.
85. Gervacio-Domingo G, Isidro J, Tirona J, et al. The Brugada type 1 electrocardiographic pattern is common among Filipinos. J Clin Epidemiol. 2008;61:1067–72.
86. Shin SC, Ryu HM, Lee JH, et al. Prevalence of the Brugada-type ECG recorded from higher intercostal spaces in healthy Korean males. Circ J. 2005;69:1064–7.
87. Uhm JS, Hwang IU, YS O, et al. Prevalence of electrocardiographic findings suggestive of sudden cardiac death risk in 10,867 apparently healthy young Korean men. Pacing Clin Electrophysiol. 2011;34:717–23.
88. Juang JM, Phan WL, Chen PC, et al. Brugada-type electrocardiogram in the Taiwanese population-is it a risk factor for sudden death? J Formos Med Assoc. 2011;110:230–8.
89. Donohue D, Tehrani F, Jamehdor R, et al. The prevalence of Brugada ECG in adult patients in a large university hospital in the western United States. Am Heart Hosp J. 2008;6:48–50.
90. Greer RW, Glancy DL. Prevalence of the Brugada electrocardiographic pattern at the Medical Center of Louisiana in New Orleans. J La State Med Soc. 2003;155:242–6.
91. Patel SS, Anees SS, Ferrick KJ. Prevalence of a Brugada pattern electrocardiogram in an urban population in the United States. Pacing Clin Electrophysiol. 2009;32:704–8.
92. Gervacio-Domingo G, Punzalan FE, Amarillo ML, Dans A. Sudden unexplained death during sleep occurred commonly in the general population in the Philippines: a sub study of the National Nutrition and Health Survey. J Clin Epidemiol. 2007;60:567–71.
93. Vatta M, Dumaine R, Varghese G, et al. Genetic and biophysical basis of sudden unexplained nocturnal death syndrome (SUNDS), a disease allelic to Brugada syndrome. Hum Mol Genet. 2002;11:337–45.
94. Eckardt L, Probst V, Smits JP, et al. Long-term prognosis of individuals with right precordial ST-segment-elevation Brugada syndrome. Circulation. 2005;111:257–63.
95. Priori SG, Napolitano C, Giordano U, et al. Brugada syndrome and sudden cardiac death in children. Lancet. 2000;355:808–9.
96. Suzuki H, Torigoe K, Numata O, Yazaki S. Infant case with a malignant form of Brugada syndrome. J Cardiovasc. 2000;11:1277–80.
97. Sanatani S, Mahkseed N, Vallance H, Brugada R. The Brugada ECG pattern in a neonate. J Cardiovasc. 2005;16:342–4.
98. Huang MH, Marcus FI. Idiopathic Brugada-type electrocardiographic pattern in an octogenarian. J Electrocardiol. 2004;37:109–11.
99. Antzelevitch C. Late potentials and the Brugada syndrome. J Am Coll Cardiol. 2002;39:1996–9.
100. Skinner JR, Chung SK, Montgomery D, et al. Near-miss SIDS due to Brugada syndrome. Arch Dis Child. 2005;90:528–9.
101. Atarashi H, Ogawa S, Harumi K, et al. Three-year follow-up of patients with right bundle branch block and ST segment elevation in the right precordial leads: Japanese Registry of Brugada Syndrome. Idiopathic Ventricular Fibrillation Investigators. J Am Coll Cardiol. 2001;37:1916–20.
102. Paul M, Gerss J, Schulze-Bahr E, et al. Role of programmed ventricular stimulation in patients with Brugada syndrome: a meta-analysis of worldwide published data. Eur Heart J. 2007;28:2126–33.

103. Sroubek J, Probst V, Mazzanti A, et al. Programmed ventricular stimulation for risk stratification in the Brugada syndrome: a pooled analysis. Circulation. 2016;133:622–30.
104. Morita H, Fukushima-Kusano K, Nagase S, et al. Site-specific arrhythmogenesis in patients with Brugada syndrome. J Cardiovasc. 2003;14:373–9.
105. Kasanuki H, Ohnishi S, Ohtuka M, et al. Idiopathic ventricular fibrillation induced with vagal activity in patients without obvious heart disease. Circulation. 1997;95:2277–85.
106. Matsuo K, Kurita T, Inagaki M, et al. The circadian pattern of the development of ventricular fibrillation in patients with Brugada syndrome. Eur Heart J. 1999;20:465–70.
107. Ikeda T, Takami M, Sugi K, et al. Noninvasive risk stratification of subjects with a Brugada-type electrocardiogram and no history of cardiac arrest. Ann Noninvasive Electrocardiol. 2005;10:396–403.
108. Mizumaki K, Fujiki A, Nishida K, et al. Postprandial augmentation of bradycardia-dependent ST elevation in patients with Brugada syndrome. J Cardiovasc. 2007;18:839–44.
109. Ikeda T, Abe A, Yusu S, et al. The full stomach test as a novel diagnostic technique for identifying patients at risk of brugada syndrome. J Cardiovasc Electrophysiol. 2006;17:602–7.
110. Amin AS, Meregalli PG, Bardai A, et al. Fever increases the risk for cardiac arrest in the Brugada syndrome. Ann Intern Med. 2008;149:216–8.
111. Gonzalez Rebollo JM, Hernandez MA, Garcia A, et al. Recurrent ventricular fibrillation during a febrile illness in a patient with the Brugada syndrome. Rev Esp Cardiol. 2000;53:755–7.
112. Porres JM, Brugada J, Urbistondo V, et al. Fever unmasking the Brugada syndrome. Pacing Clin Electrophysiol. 2002;25:1646–8.
113. Skinner JR, Chung SK, Nel CA, et al. Brugada syndrome masquerading as febrile seizures. Pediatrics. 2007;119:e1206–11.
114. Tan HL, Meregalli PG. Lethal ECG changes hidden by therapeutic hypothermia. Lancet. 2007;369:78.
115. Postema PG, Wolpert C, Amin AS, et al. Drugs and Brugada syndrome patients: review of the literature, recommendations, and an up-to-date website (www.brugadadrugs.org). Heart Rhythm. 2009;6:1335–41.
116. Bjerregaard P, Gussak I, Kotar SL, et al. Recurrent syncope in a patient with prominent J wave. Am Heart J. 1994;127:1426–30.
117. Dubner SJ, Gimeno GM, Elencwajg B, et al. Ventricular fibrillation with spontaneous reversion on ambulatory ECG in the absence of heart disease. Am Heart J. 1983;105:691–3.
118. Kontny F, Dale J. Self-terminating idiopathic ventricular fibrillation presenting as syncope: a 40-year follow-up report. J Intern Med. 1990;227:211–3.
119. Patt MV, Podrid PJ, Friedman PL, Lown B. Spontaneous reversion of ventricular fibrillation. Am Heart J. 1988;115:919–23.
120. Boersma LV, Jaarsma W, Jessurun ER, et al. Brugada syndrome: a case report of monomorphic ventricular tachycardia. Pacing Clin Electrophysiol. 2001;24:112–5.
121. Dinckal MH, Davutoglu V, Akdemir I, et al. Incessant monomorphic ventricular tachycardia during febrile illness in a patient with Brugada syndrome: fatal electrical storm. Europace. 2003;5:257–61.
122. Mok NS, Chan NY. Brugada syndrome presenting with sustained monomorphic ventricular tachycardia. Int J Cardiol. 2004;97:307–9.
123. Ogawa M, Kumagai K, Saku K. Spontaneous right ventricular outflow tract tachycardia in a patient with Brugada syndrome. J Cardiovasc. 2001;12:838–40.
124. Rodríguez-Mañero M, Sacher F, de Asmundis C, et al. Monomorphic ventricular tachycardia in patients with Brugada syndrome: A multicenter retrospective study. Heart Rhythm Off J Heart Rhythm Soc. 2016;13:669–82.
125. Shimada M, Miyazaki T, Miyoshi S, et al. Sustained monomorphic ventricular tachycardia in a patient with Brugada syndrome. Jpn Circ J. 1996;60:364–70.
126. Kakishita M, Kurita T, Matsuo K, et al. Mode of onset of ventricular fibrillation in patients with Brugada syndrome detected by implantable cardioverter defibrillator therapy. J Am Coll Cardiol. 2000;36:1646–53.

127. Haissaguerre M, Extramiana F, Hocini M, et al. Mapping and ablation of ventricular fibrillation associated with long-QT and Brugada syndromes. Circulation. 2003;108:925–8.
128. Nademanee K, Veerakul G, Chandanamattha P, et al. Prevention of ventricular fibrillation episodes in Brugada syndrome by catheter ablation over the anterior right ventricular outflow tract epicardium. Circulation. 2011;123:1270–9.
129. Eckardt L, Kirchhof P, Loh P, et al. Brugada syndrome and supraventricular tachyarrhythmias: a novel association? J Cardiovasc Electrophysiol. 2001;12:680–5.
130. Morita H, Kusano-Fukushima K, Nagase S, et al. Atrial fibrillation and atrial vulnerability in patients with Brugada syndrome. J Am Coll Cardiol. 2002;40:1437–44.
131. Naccarelli GV, Antzelevitch C, Wolbrette DL, Luck JC. The Brugada syndrome. Curr Opin Cardiol. 2002;17:19–23.
132. Rossenbacker T, Carroll SJ, Liu H, et al. Novel pore mutation in SCN5A manifests as a spectrum of phenotypes ranging from atrial flutter, conduction disease, and Brugada syndrome to sudden cardiac death. Heart Rhythm. 2004;1:610–5.
133. Babai Bigi MA, Aslani A, Shahrzad S. Clinical predictors of atrial fibrillation in Brugada syndrome. Europace. 2007;9:947–50.
134. Bordachar P, Reuter S, Garrigue S, et al. Incidence, clinical implications and prognosis of atrial arrhythmias in Brugada syndrome. Eur Heart J. 2004;25:879–84.
135. Sarkozy A, Boussy T, Kourgiannides G, et al. Long-term follow-up of primary prophylactic implantable cardioverter-defibrillator therapy in Brugada syndrome. Eur Heart J. 2007;28:334–44.
136. Gehi AK, Duong TD, Metz LD, et al. Risk stratification of individuals with the Brugada electrocardiogram: a meta-analysis. J Cardiovasc Electrophysiol. 2006;17:577–83.
137. Matsuo K, Akahoshi M, Seto S, Yano K. Disappearance of the Brugada-type electrocardiogram after surgical castration: a role for testosterone and an explanation for the male preponderance. Pacing Clin Electrophysiol. 2003;26:1551–3.
138. Shimizu W, Matsuo K, Kokubo Y, et al. Sex hormone and gender difference–role of testosterone on male predominance in Brugada syndrome. J Cardiovasc. 2007;18:415–21.
139. Bidoggia H, Maciel JP, Capalozza N, et al. Sex differences on the electrocardiographic pattern of cardiac repolarization: possible role of testosterone. Am Heart J. 2000;140:678–83.
140. Di Diego JM, Cordeiro JM, Goodrow RJ, et al. Ionic and cellular basis for the predominance of the Brugada syndrome phenotype in males. Circulation. 2002;106:2004–11.
141. Pham TV, Robinson RB, Danilo P, Rosen MR. Effects of gonadal steroids on gender-related differences in transmural dispersion of L-type calcium current. Cardiovasc Res. 2002;53:752–62.
142. Tatsumi H, Takagi M, Nakagawa E, et al. Risk stratification in patients with Brugada syndrome: analysis of daily fluctuations in 12-lead electrocardiogram (ECG) and signal-averaged electrocardiogram (SAECG). J Cardiovasc Electrophysiol. 2006;17:705–11.
143. Veltmann C, Schimpf R, Echternach C, et al. A prospective study on spontaneous fluctuations between diagnostic and non-diagnostic ECGs in Brugada syndrome: implications for correct phenotyping and risk stratification. Eur Heart J. 2006;27:2544–54.
144. Priori SG, Wilde AA, Horie M, et al. Executive summary: HRS/EHRA/APHRS expert consensus statement on the diagnosis and management of patients with inherited primary arrhythmia syndromes. Heart Rhythm. 2013;10:1932–63.
145. Meregalli PG, Ruijter JM, Hofman N, et al. Diagnostic value of flecainide testing in unmasking SCN5A-related Brugada syndrome. J Cardiovasc Electrophysiol. 2006;17:857–64.
146. Veltmann C, Papavassiliu T, Konrad T, et al. Insights into the location of type I ECG in patients with Brugada syndrome: correlation of ECG and cardiovascular magnetic resonance imaging. Heart Rhythm Off J Heart Rhythm Soc. 2012;9:414–21.
147. Govindan M, Batchvarov VN, Raju H, et al. Utility of high and standard right precordial leads during ajmaline testing for the diagnosis of Brugada syndrome. Heart. 2010;96:1904–8.
148. Miyamoto K, Yokokawa M, Tanaka K, et al. Diagnostic and prognostic value of a type 1 Brugada electrocardiogram at higher (third or second) V(1) to V(2) recording in men with Brugada syndrome. Am J Cardiol. 2007;99:53–7.

149. Bayés de Luna A, Brugada J, Baranchuk A, et al. Current electrocardiographic criteria for diagnosis of Brugada pattern: a consensus report. J Electrocardiol. 2012;45:433–42.
150. Wolpert C, Echternach C, Veltmann C, et al. Intravenous drug challenge using flecainide and ajmaline in patients with Brugada syndrome. Heart Rhythm. 2005;2:254–60.
151. Cordery R, Lambiase P, Lowe M, Ashley E. Brugada syndrome and anesthetic management. J Cardiothorac Vasc Anesth. 2006;20:407–13.
152. Edge CJ, Blackman DJ, Gupta K, Sainsbury M. General anaesthesia in a patient with Brugada syndrome. Br J Anaesth. 2002;89:788–91.
153. Kim JS, Park SY, Min SK, et al. Anaesthesia in patients with Brugada syndrome. Acta Anaesthesiol Scand. 2004;48:1058–61.
154. Kloesel B, Ackerman MJ, Sprung J, et al. Anesthetic management of patients with Brugada syndrome: a case series and literature review. Can J Anaesth. 2011;58:824–36.
155. Santambrogio LG, Mencherini S, Fuardo M, et al. The surgical patient with Brugada syndrome: a four-case clinical experience. Anesth Analg. 2005;100:1263–6.
156. Jongman JK, Jepkes-Bruin N, Ramdat Misier AR, et al. Electrical storms in Brugada syndrome successfully treated with isoproterenol infusion and quinidine orally. Neth Hear J. 2007;15:151–4.
157. Ohgo T, Okamura H, Noda T, et al. Acute and chronic management in patients with Brugada syndrome associated with electrical storm of ventricular fibrillation. Heart Rhythm. 2007; 4:695–700.
158. Tanaka H, Kinoshita O, Uchikawa S, et al. Successful prevention of recurrent ventricular fibrillation by intravenous isoproterenol in a patient with Brugada syndrome. Pacing Clin Electrophysiol. 2001;24:1293–4.
159. Watanabe A, Kusano KF, Morita H, et al. Low-dose isoproterenol for repetitive ventricular arrhythmia in patients with Brugada syndrome. Eur Heart J. 2006;27:1579–83.
160. Chockalingam P, Rammeloo LA, Postema PG, et al. Fever-induced life-threatening arrhythmias in children harboring an SCN5A mutation. Pediatrics. 2011;127:e239–44.
161. Conte G, Dewals W, Sieira J, et al. Drug-induced brugada syndrome in children: clinical features, device-based management, and long-term follow-up. J Am Coll Cardiol. 2014;63:2272–9.
162. Saura D, Garcia-Alberola A, Carrillo P, et al. Brugada-like electrocardiographic pattern induced by fever. Pacing Clin Electrophysiol. 2002;25:856–9.
163. Todd SJ, Campbell MJ, Roden DM, Kannankeril PJ. Novel Brugada SCN5A mutation causing sudden death in children. Heart Rhythm. 2005;2:540–3.
164. Smith J, Hannah A, Birnie DH. Effect of temperature on the Brugada ECG. Heart. 2003;89:272.
165. Mizusawa Y, Morita H, Adler A, et al. Prognostic significance of fever-induced Brugada syndrome. Heart Rhythm. 2016;13(7):1515–20.
166. Baranchuk A, Nguyen T, Ryu MH, et al. Brugada phenocopy: new terminology and proposed classification. Ann Noninvasive Electrocardiol. 2012;17:299–314.
167. Gottschalk BH, Anselm DD, Brugada J, et al. Expert cardiologists cannot distinguish between Brugada phenocopy and Brugada syndrome electrocardiogram patterns. Europace. 2015;18(7):1095–100.
168. Gussak I, Antzelevitch C. Early repolarization syndrome: clinical characteristics and possible cellular and ionic mechanisms. J Electrocardiol. 2000;33:299–309.
169. Kataoka H. Electrocardiographic patterns of the Brugada syndrome in right ventricular infarction/ischemia. Am J Cardiol. 2000;86:1056.
170. Chinushi M, Kuroe Y, Ito E, et al. Vasospastic angina accompanied by Brugada-type electrocardiographic abnormalities. J Cardiovasc. 2001;12:108–11.
171. Sasaki T, Niwano S, Kitano Y, Izumi T. Two cases of Brugada syndrome associated with spontaneous clinical episodes of coronary vasospasm. Intern Med. 2006;45:77–80.
172. Douglas PS, Carmichael KA, Palevsky PM. Extreme hypercalcemia and electrocardiographic changes. Am J Cardiol. 1984;54:674–5.

173. Littmann L, Monroe MH, Taylor L, Brearley WD. The hyperkalemic Brugada sign. J Electrocardiol. 2007;40:53–9.
174. Postema PG, Vlaar AP, DeVries JH, Tan HL. Familial Brugada syndrome uncovered by hyperkalaemic diabetic ketoacidosis. Europace. 2011;13:1509–10.
175. Wu L-S, Wu C-T, Hsu LA, et al. Brugada-like electrocardiographic pattern and ventricular fibrillation in a patient with primary hyperparathyroidism. Europace. 2007;9(3):172–4. https://doi.org/10.1093/europace/eum002
176. Buob A, Siaplaouras S, Janzen I, et al. Focal parvovirus B19 myocarditis in a patient with Brugada syndrome. Cardiol Rev. 2003;11:45–9.
177. Hermida JS, Six I, Jarry G. Drug-induced pericarditis mimicking Brugada syndrome. Europace. 2007;9:66–8.
178. Kurisu S, Inoue I, Kawagoe T, et al. Acute pericarditis unmasks ST-segment elevation in asymptomatic Brugada syndrome. Pacing Clin Electrophysiol. 2006;29:201–3.
179. Morita H, Fukushima-Kusano K, Nagase S, et al. Sinus node function in patients with Brugada-type ECG. Circ J. 2004;68:473–6.
180. Postema PG, van Dessel PF, Kors JA, et al. Local depolarization abnormalities are the dominant pathophysiologic mechanism for the type-1 ECG in Brugada syndrome. A study of electrocardiograms, vectorcardiograms and body surface potential maps during ajmaline provocation. J Am Coll Cardiol. 2010;55:789–97.
181. Kyndt F, Probst V, Potet F, et al. Novel SCN5A mutation leading either to isolated cardiac conduction defect or Brugada syndrome in a large French family. Circulation. 2001;104:3081–6.
182. Probst V, Allouis M, Sacher F, et al. Progressive cardiac conduction defect is the prevailing phenotype in carriers of a Brugada syndrome SCN5A mutation. J Cardiovasc. 2006;17:270–5.
183. Schwartz PJ, Moss AJ, Vincent GM, Crampton RS. Diagnostic criteria for the long QT syndrome. An update. Circulation. 1993;88:782–4.
184. Bezzina C, Veldkamp MW, van den Berg MP, et al. A single Na(+) channel mutation causing both long-QT and Brugada syndromes. Circ Res. 1999;85:1206–13.
185. Grant AO, Carboni MP, Neplioueva V, et al. Long QT syndrome, Brugada syndrome, and conduction system disease are linked to a single sodium channel mutation. J Clin Invest. 2002;110:1201–9.
186. Makita N, Behr E, Shimizu W, et al. The E1784K mutation in SCN5A is associated with mixed clinical phenotype of type 3 long QT syndrome. J Clin Invest. 2008;118:2219–29.
187. Priori SG, Napolitano C, Schwartz PJ, et al. The elusive link between LQT3 and Brugada syndrome: the role of flecainide challenge. Circulation. 2000;102:945–7.
188. Veldkamp MW, Viswanathan PC, Bezzina C, et al. Two distinct congenital arrhythmias evoked by a multidysfunctional Na(+) channel. Circ Res. 2000;86:E91–7.
189. Remme CA, Verkerk AO, Nuyens D, et al. Overlap syndrome of cardiac sodium channel disease in mice carrying the equivalent mutation of human SCN5A-1795insD. Circulation. 2006;114:2584–94.
190. Postema PG, van Dessel PF, de Bakker JM, et al. Slow and discontinuous conduction conspire in Brugada syndrome: a right ventricular mapping and stimulation study. Circ Arrhythm Electrophysiol. 2008;1:379–86.
191. Calo L, Giustetto C, Martino A, et al. A new ECG marker of sudden death in Brugada syndrome: the S wave in lead I. J Am Coll Cardiol. 2016;67:1427–40.
192. Wilde AAM, Postema PG. Risk stratification in Brugada syndrome: the "impossible" made possible? J Am Coll Cardiol. 2016;67:1441–3.
193. Atarashi H, Ogawa S. New ECG criteria for high-risk Brugada syndrome. Circ J. 2003;67:8–10.
194. Eckardt L, Bruns HJ, Paul M, et al. Body surface area of ST elevation and the presence of late potentials correlate to the inducibility of ventricular tachyarrhythmias in Brugada syndrome. J Cardiovasc Electrophysiol. 2002;13:742–9.
195. Ikeda T, Sakurada H, Sakabe K, et al. Assessment of noninvasive markers in identifying patients at risk in the Brugada syndrome: insight into risk stratification. J Am Coll Cardiol. 2001;37:1628–34.

196. Kanda M, Shimizu W, Matsuo K, et al. Electrophysiologic characteristics and implications of induced ventricular fibrillation in symptomatic patients with Brugada syndrome. J Am Coll Cardiol. 2002;39:1799–805.
197. Nagase S, Kusano KF, Morita H, et al. Epicardial electrogram of the right ventricular outflow tract in patients with the Brugada syndrome: using the epicardial lead. J Am Coll Cardiol. 2002;39:1992–5.
198. Simson MB, Untereker WJ, Spielman SR, et al. Relation between late potentials on the body surface and directly recorded fragmented electrograms in patients with ventricular tachycardia. Am J Cardiol. 1983;51:105–12.
199. Das M, Suradi H, Maskoun W, et al. Fragmented wide QRS on a 12-Lead ECG: a sign of myocardial scar and poor prognosis. Circ Arrhythm Electrophysiol. 2008;1:258–68.
200. Morita H, Kusano KF, Miura D, et al. Fragmented QRS as a marker of conduction abnormality and a predictor of prognosis of Brugada syndrome. Circulation. 2008;118:1697–704.
201. Priori SG, Gasparini M, Napolitano C, et al. Risk stratification in Brugada syndrome results of the PRELUDE (PRogrammed ELectrical stimUlation preDictive valuE) registry. J Am Coll Cardiol. 2012;59:37–45.
202. Kalla H, Yan GX, Marinchak R. Ventricular fibrillation in a patient with prominent J (Osborn) waves and ST segment elevation in the inferior electrocardiographic leads: a Brugada syndrome variant? J Cardiovasc. 2000;11:95–8.
203. Ogawa M, Kumagai K, Yamanouchi Y, Saku K. Spontaneous onset of ventricular fibrillation in Brugada syndrome with J wave and ST-segment elevation in the inferior leads. Heart Rhythm. 2005;2:97–9.
204. Sarkozy A, Chierchia GB, Paparella G, et al. Inferior and lateral electrocardiographic repolarization abnormalities in Brugada syndrome. Circ Arrhythm Electrophysiol. 2009;2:154–61.
205. Takagi M, Aihara N, Takaki H, et al. Clinical characteristics of patients with spontaneous or inducible ventricular fibrillation without apparent heart disease presenting with J wave and ST segment elevation in inferior leads. J Cardiovasc. 2000;11:844–8.
206. Ueyama T, Shimizu A, Esato M, et al. A case of a concealed type of Brugada syndrome with a J wave and mild ST-segment elevation in the inferolateral leads. J Electrocardiol. 2007;40:39–42.
207. van den Berg MP, Wiesfeld AC. Brugada syndrome with ST-segment elevation in the lateral leads. J Cardiovasc Electrophysiol. 2006;17:1035.
208. Potet F, Mabo P, Le Coq G, et al. Novel brugada SCN5A mutation leading to ST segment elevation in the inferior or the right precordial leads. J Cardiovasc. 2003;14:200–3.
209. Matsuo K, Shimizu W, Kurita T, et al. Dynamic changes of 12-lead electrocardiograms in a patient with Brugada syndrome. J Cardiovasc. 1998;9:508–12.
210. Wilde A, Duren D. Sudden cardiac death, RBBB, and right precordial ST-segment elevation. Circulation. 1999;99:722–3.
211. Antzelevitch C. The Brugada syndrome: ionic basis and arrhythmia mechanisms. J Cardiovasc. 2001;12:268–72.
212. Brugada J, Brugada P. Further characterization of the syndrome of right bundle branch block, ST segment elevation, and sudden cardiac death. J Cardiovasc Electrophysiol. 1997;8:325–31.
213. Corrado D, Nava A, Buja G, et al. Familial cardiomyopathy underlies syndrome of right bundle branch block, ST segment elevation and sudden death. J Am Coll Cardiol. 1996;27:443–8.
214. Matsuo K, Shimizu W, Kurita T, et al. Increased dispersion of repolarization time determined by monophasic action potentials in two patients with familial idiopathic ventricular fibrillation. J Cardiovasc. 1998;9:74–83.
215. Wilde AA, Postema PG, Di Diego JM, et al. The pathophysiological mechanism underlying Brugada syndrome. Depolarization versus repolarization. J Mol Cell Cardiol. 2010;49:543–53.
216. Yan GX, Antzelevitch C. Cellular basis for the Brugada syndrome and other mechanisms of arrhythmogenesis associated with ST-segment elevation. Circulation. 1999;100:1660–6.
217. Litovsky SH, Antzelevitch C. Transient outward current prominent in canine ventricular epicardium but not endocardium. Circ Res. 1988;62:116–26.

218. Di Diego JM, Sun ZQ, Antzelevitch C. I(to) and action potential notch are smaller in left vs. right canine ventricular epicardium. Am J Phys. 1996;271:H548–61.
219. Meregalli PG, Wilde AA, Tan HL. Pathophysiological mechanisms of Brugada syndrome: depolarization disorder, repolarization disorder, or more? Cardiovasc Res. 2005;67:367–78.
220. Fujiki A, Usui M, Nagasawa H, et al. ST segment elevation in the right precordial leads induced with class IC antiarrhythmic drugs: insight into the mechanism of Brugada syndrome. J Cardiovasc Electrophysiol. 1999;10:214–8.
221. Izumida N, Asano Y, Doi S, et al. Changes in body surface potential distributions induced by isoproterenol and Na channel blockers in patients with the Brugada syndrome. Int J Cardiol. 2004;95:261–8.
222. Takami M, Ikeda T, Enjoji Y, Sugi K. Relationship between ST-segment morphology and conduction disturbances detected by signal-averaged electrocardiography in Brugada syndrome. Ann Noninvasive Electrocardiol. 2003;8:30–6.
223. Tukkie R, Sogaard P, Vleugels J, et al. Delay in right ventricular activation contributes to Brugada syndrome. Circulation. 2004;109:1272–7.
224. Nademanee K, Raju H, de Noronha SV, et al. Fibrosis, connexin-43, and conduction abnormalities in the Brugada syndrome. J Am Coll Cardiol. 2015;66:1976–86.
225. Hoogendijk MG, Potse M, Vinet A, et al. ST segment elevation by current-to-load mismatch: an experimental and computational study. Heart Rhythm. 2011;8:111–8.
226. Hoogendijk MG, Potse M, Linnenbank AC, et al. Mechanism of right precordial ST-segment elevation in structural heart disease: excitation failure by current-to-load mismatch. Heart Rhythm. 2010;7:238–48.
227. Veltmann C, Wolpert C, Sacher F, et al. Response to intravenous ajmaline: a retrospective analysis of 677 ajmaline challenges. Europace. 2009;11:1345–52.
228. Aiba T, Shimizu W, Hidaka I, et al. Cellular basis for trigger and maintenance of ventricular fibrillation in the Brugada syndrome model high-resolution optical mapping study. J Am Coll Cardiol. 2006;47:2074–85.
229. Martini B, Nava A. 1988-2003. Fifteen years after the first Italian description by Nava-Martini-Thiene and colleagues of a new syndrome (different from the Brugada syndrome?) in the Giornale Italiano di Cardiologia: do we really know everything on this entity? Ital Heart J. 2004;5:53–60.
230. Tada H, Aihara N, Ohe T, et al. Arrhythmogenic right ventricular cardiomyopathy underlies syndrome of right bundle branch block, ST-segment elevation, and sudden death. Am J Cardiol. 1998;81:519–22.
231. Frustaci A, Priori SG, Pieroni M, et al. Cardiac histological substrate in patients with clinical phenotype of Brugada syndrome. Circulation. 2005;112:3680–7.
232. Coronel R, Casini S, Koopmann TT, et al. Right ventricular fibrosis and conduction delay in a patient with clinical signs of Brugada syndrome: a combined electrophysiological, genetic, histopathologic, and computational study. Circulation. 2005;112:2769–77.
233. Bezzina CR, Rook MB, Groenewegen WA, et al. Compound heterozygosity for mutations (W156X and R225W) in SCN5A associated with severe cardiac conduction disturbances and degenerative changes in the conduction system. Circ Res. 2003;92:159–68.
234. Remme CA, Verkerk AO, Wilde AA, et al. Diversity in cardiac sodium channel disease phenotype in transgenic mice carrying a single SCN5A mutation. Neth Hear J. 2007;15: 235–8.
235. Royer A, van Veen TA, Le BS, et al. Mouse model of SCN5A-linked hereditary Lenegre's disease: age-related conduction slowing and myocardial fibrosis. Circulation. 2005;111:1738–46.
236. van Veen TA, Stein M, Royer A, et al. Impaired impulse propagation in Scn5a-knockout mice: combined contribution of excitability, connexin expression, and tissue architecture in relation to aging. Circulation. 2005;112:1927–35.
237. Forkmann M, Tomala J, Huo Y, et al. Epicardial ventricular tachycardia ablation in a patient with Brugada ECG pattern and mutation of PKP2 and DSP genes. Circ Arrhythm Electrophysiol. 2015;8:505–7.
238. Papavassiliu T, Wolpert C, Fluchter S, et al. Magnetic resonance imaging findings in patients with Brugada syndrome. J Cardiovasc. 2004;15:1133–8.

239. Rudic B, Schimpf R, Veltmann C, et al. Brugada syndrome: clinical presentation and genotype-correlation with magnetic resonance imaging parameters. Europace. 2015;18(9):1411–9.
240. Takagi M, Aihara N, Kuribayashi S, et al. Localized right ventricular morphological abnormalities detected by electron-beam computed tomography represent arrhythmogenic substrates in patients with the Brugada syndrome. Eur Heart J. 2001;22:1032–41.
241. Takagi M, Aihara N, Kuribayashi S, et al. Abnormal response to sodium channel blockers in patients with Brugada syndrome: augmented localised wall motion abnormalities in the right ventricular outflow tract region detected by electron beam computed tomography. Heart. 2003;89:169–74.
242. van Hoorn F, Campian ME, Spijkerboer A, et al. SCN5A mutations in Brugada syndrome are associated with increased cardiac dimensions and reduced contractility. PLoS One. 2012;7:e42037.
243. Andorin A, Behr ER, Denjoy I, et al. The impact of clinical and genetic findings on the management of young Brugada syndrome patients. Heart Rhythm Off J Heart Rhythm Soc. 2016;13:1274–82.
244. Koopmann TT, Bezzina CR, Wilde AA. Voltage-gated sodium channels: action players with many faces. Ann Med. 2006;38:472–82.
245. McKusick VA. OMIM - Online Mendelian Inheritance in Man. In: Natl. Cent. Biotechnol. Inf.; 2007. http://www.ncbi.nlm.nih.gov/sites/entrez?db=OMIM.
246. Schott JJ, Alshinawi C, Kyndt F, et al. Cardiac conduction defects associate with mutations in SCN5A. Nat Genet. 1999;23:20–1.
247. Benson DW, Wang DW, Dyment M, et al. Congenital sick sinus syndrome caused by recessive mutations in the cardiac sodium channel gene (SCN5A). J Clin Invest. 2003;112:1019–28.
248. McNair WP, Ku L, Taylor MR, et al. SCN5A mutation associated with dilated cardiomyopathy, conduction disorder, and arrhythmia. Circulation. 2004;110:2163–7.
249. Groenewegen WA, Firouzi M, Bezzina CR, et al. A cardiac sodium channel mutation cosegregates with a rare connexin40 genotype in familial atrial standstill. Circ Res. 2003;92:14–22.
250. Wang Q, Shen J, Li Z, et al. Cardiac sodium channel mutations in patients with long QT syndrome, an inherited cardiac arrhythmia. Hum Mol Genet. 1995;4:1603–7.
251. Ackerman MJ, Siu BL, Sturner WQ, et al. Postmortem molecular analysis of SCN5A defects in sudden infant death syndrome. JAMA. 2001;286:2264–9.
252. Wang DW, Desai RR, Crotti L, et al. Cardiac sodium channel dysfunction in sudden infant death syndrome. Circulation. 2007;115:368–76.
253. Bezzina CR, Shimizu W, Yang P, et al. Common sodium channel promoter haplotype in Asian subjects underlies variability in cardiac conduction. Circulation. 2006;113:338–44.
254. Baroudi G, Pouliot V, Denjoy I, et al. Novel mechanism for Brugada syndrome: defective surface localization of an SCN5A mutant (R1432G). Circ Res. 2001;88:E78–83.
255. Hong K, Guerchicoff A, Pollevick GD, et al. Cryptic 5' splice site activation in SCN5A associated with Brugada syndrome. J Mol Cell Cardiol. 2005;38:555–60.
256. Poelzing S, Forleo C, Samodell M, et al. SCN5A polymorphism restores trafficking of a Brugada syndrome mutation on a separate gene. Circulation. 2006;114:368–76.
257. Rossenbacker T, Schollen E, Kuiperi C, et al. Unconventional intronic splice site mutation in SCN5A associates with cardiac sodium channelopathy. J Med Genet. 2005;42:e29.
258. Koopmann TT, Beekman L, Alders M, et al. Exclusion of multiple candidate genes and large genomic rearrangements in SCN5A in a Dutch Brugada syndrome cohort. Heart Rhythm. 2007;4:752–5.
259. Rossenbacker T, Priori SG. The Brugada syndrome. Curr Opin Cardiol. 2007;22:163–70.
260. Kapplinger JD, Giudicessi JR, Ye D, et al. Enhanced classification of Brugada syndrome-associated and Long-QT syndrome-associated genetic variants in the SCN5A-encoded Na(v)1.5 cardiac sodium channel. Circ Cardiovasc Genet. 2015;8:582–95.
261. Bezzina CR, Barc J, Mizusawa Y, et al. Common variants at SCN5A-SCN10A and HEY2 are associated with Brugada syndrome, a rare disease with high risk of sudden cardiac death. Nat Genet. 2013;45:1409.

262. Gaborit N, Wichter T, Varro A, et al. Transcriptional profiling of ion channel genes in Brugada syndrome and other right ventricular arrhythmogenic diseases. Eur Heart J. 2009;30:487–96.
263. Wilde AA, Bezzina CR. Genetics of cardiac arrhythmias. Heart. 2005;91:1352–8.
264. Viskin S. Brugada syndrome in children: don't ask, don't tell? Circulation. 2007;115:1970–2.
265. Brugada J, Brugada R, Brugada P. Electrophysiologic testing predicts events in Brugada syndrome patients. Heart Rhythm. 2011;8:1595–7.
266. Wilde AA, Viskin S. EP testing does not predict cardiac events in Brugada syndrome. Heart Rhythm. 2011;8:1598–600.
267. Tung R, Zimetbaum P, Josephson ME. A critical appraisal of implantable cardioverter-defibrillator therapy for the prevention of sudden cardiac death. J Am Coll Cardiol. 2008;52:1111–21.
268. Moss AJ, Schuger C, Beck CA, et al. Reduction in inappropriate therapy and mortality through ICD programming. N Engl J Med. 2012;367:2275–83.
269. Delise P, Allocca G, Marras E, et al. Risk stratification in individuals with the Brugada type 1 ECG pattern without previous cardiac arrest: usefulness of a combined clinical and electrophysiologic approach. Eur Heart J. 2011;32:169–76.
270. Delise P, Allocca G, Sitta N, Di Stefano P. Event rates and risk factors in patients with Brugada syndrome and no prior cardiac arrest. A cumulative analysis of the largest available studies distinguishing ICD-recorded fast ventricular arrhythmias and sudden death. Heart Rhythm. 2014;11:252–8.
271. Ayerza MR, de Zutter M, Goethals M, et al. Heart transplantation as last resort against Brugada syndrome. J Cardiovasc. 2002;13:943–4.
272. Abud A, Bagattin D, Goyeneche R, Becker C. Failure of cilostazol in the prevention of ventricular fibrillation in a patient with Brugada syndrome. J Cardiovasc. 2006;17:210–2.
273. Chinushi M, Furushima H, Hosaka Y, et al. Ventricular fibrillation and ventricular tachycardia triggered by late-coupled ventricular extrasystoles in a Brugada syndrome patient. Pacing Clin Electrophysiol. 2011;34:e1–5.
274. Kaneko Y, Horie M, Niwano S, et al. Electrical storm in patients with Brugada syndrome is associated with early repolarization. Circ Arrhythm Electrophysiol. 2014;7:1122–8.
275. Marquez MF, Bonny A, Hernandez-Castillo E, et al. Long-term efficacy of low doses of quinidine on malignant arrhythmias in Brugada syndrome with an implantable cardioverter-defibrillator: a case series and literature review. Heart Rhythm. 2012;9:1995–2000.
276. Mizusawa Y, Sakurada H, Nishizaki M, Hiraoka M. Effects of low-dose quinidine on ventricular tachyarrhythmias in patients with Brugada syndrome: low-dose quinidine therapy as an adjunctive treatment. J Cardiovasc. 2006;47:359–64.
277. Murakami M, Nakamura K, Kusano KF, et al. Efficacy of low-dose bepridil for prevention of ventricular fibrillation in Brugada syndrome patients with and without SCN5A mutation. J Cardiovasc Pharmacol. 2010;56:389–95.
278. Sugao M, Fujiki A, Nishida K, et al. Repolarization dynamics in patients with idiopathic ventricular fibrillation: pharmacological therapy with bepridil and disopyramide. J Cardiovasc Pharmacol. 2005;45:545–9.
279. Tsuchiya T, Ashikaga K, Honda T, Arita M. Prevention of ventricular fibrillation by cilostazol, an oral phosphodiesterase inhibitor, in a patient with Brugada syndrome. J Cardiovasc. 2002;13:698–701.
280. Francis J, Sankar V, Nair VK, Priori SG. Catecholaminergic polymorphic ventricular tachycardia. Heart Rhythm. 2005;2:550–4.
281. Brugada J, Pappone C, Berruezo A, et al. Brugada syndrome phenotype elimination by epicardial substrate ablation. Circ Arrhythm Electrophysiol. 2015;8:1373–81.
282. Széplaki G, Ozcan EE, Osztheimer I, et al. Ablation of the epicardial substrate in the right ventricular outflow tract in a patient with brugada syndrome refusing implantable cardioverter defibrillator therapy. Can J Cardiol. 2014;30:1249.e9–1249.e11.
283. Talib AK, Yui Y, Kaneshiro T, et al. Alternative approach for management of an electrical storm in Brugada syndrome:Importance of primary ablation within a narrow time window. J Arrhythmia. 2016;32:220–2.

284. Wilde AAM, Nademanee K. Epicardial substrate ablation in Brugada syndrome: time for a randomized trial! Circ Arrhythm Electrophysiol. 2015;8:1306–8.
285. Zipes DP, Camm AJ, Borggrefe M, et al. ACC/AHA/ESC 2006 Guidelines for management of patients with ventricular arrhythmias and the prevention of sudden cardiac death: a report of the American College of Cardiology/American Heart Association Task Force and the European Society of Cardiology Committee for practice guidelines (writing committee to develop guidelines for management of patients with ventricular arrhythmias and the prevention of sudden cardiac death): developed in collaboration with the European Heart Rhythm Association and the Heart Rhythm Society. Circulation. 2006;114:e385–484.
286. Shipley RA, Hallaran WR. The four-lead electrocardiogram in two hundred normal men and women. Am Heart J. 1936;11:325–245.
287. Goldman MJ. RS-T segment elevation in mid- and left precordial leads as a normal variant. Am Heart J. 1953;46:817–20.
288. Goldman MJ. Normal variants in the electrocardiogram leading to cardiac invalidism. Am Heart J. 1960;59:71–7.
289. Hiss RG, Lamb LE, Allen MF. Electrocardiographic findings in 67,375 asymptomatic subjects. X. Normal values. Am J Cardiol. 1960;6:200–31.
290. Myers GB, Klein HA. Normal variations in multiple precordial leads. Am Heart J. 1947;34:785–808.
291. Seriki O, Smith AJ. The electrocardiogram of young Nigerians. Am Heart J. 1966;72:153–7.
292. Grant RP, Estes EH, Doyle JT. Spatial vector electrocardiography; the clinical characteristics of S-T and T vectors. Circulation. 1951;3:182–97.
293. Mehta M, Jain AC, Mehta A. Early repolarization. Clin Cardiol. 1999;22:59–65.
294. Kambara H, Phillips J. Long-term evaluation of early repolarization syndrome (normal variant RS-T segment elevation). Am J Cardiol. 1976;38:157–6.
295. Morace G, Padeletti L, Porciani MC, Fantini F. Effect of isoproterenol on the "early repolarization" syndrome. Am Heart J. 1979;97:343–7.
296. Surawicz B, Parikh SR. Prevalence of male and female patterns of early ventricular repolarization in the normal ECG of males and females from childhood to old age. J Am Coll Cardiol. 2002;40:1870–6.
297. Aizawa Y, Tamura M, Chinushi M, et al. Idiopathic ventricular fibrillation and bradycardia-dependent intraventricular block. Am Heart J. 1993;126:1473–4.
298. Haissaguerre M, Derval N, Sacher F, et al. Sudden cardiac arrest associated with early repolarization. N Engl J Med. 2008;358:2016–23.
299. Rosso R, Kogan E, Belhassen B, et al. J-point elevation in survivors of primary ventricular fibrillation and matched control subjects: incidence and clinical significance. J Am Coll Cardiol. 2008;52:1231–8.
300. Tikkanen JT, Anttonen O, Junttila MJ, et al. Long-term outcome associated with early repolarization on electrocardiography. N Engl J Med. 2009;361:2529–37.
301. Haruta D, Matsuo K, Tsuneto A, et al. Incidence and prognostic value of early repolarization pattern in the 12-lead electrocardiogram. Circulation. 2011;123:2931–7.
302. Rollin A, Maury P, Bongard V, et al. Prevalence, prognosis, and identification of the malignant form of early repolarization pattern in a population-based study. Am J Cardiol. 2012; 110:1302–8.
303. Sinner MF, Reinhard W, Müller M, et al. Association of early repolarization pattern on ECG with risk of cardiac and all-cause mortality: a population-based prospective cohort study (MONICA/KORA). PLoS Med. 2010;7:e1000314.
304. Wu S-H, Lin X-X, Cheng Y-J, et al. Early repolarization pattern and risk for arrhythmia death: a meta-analysis. J Am Coll Cardiol. 2013;61(6):645–50. https://doi.org/10.1016/j.jacc.2012.11.023
305. Rautaharju PM, Surawicz B, Gettes LS, et al. AHA/ACCF/HRS recommendations for the standardization and interpretation of the electrocardiogram: part IV: the ST segment, T and U waves, and the QT interval: a scientific statement from the American Heart Association Electrocardiography and Arrhythmias Committee, Council on Clinical Cardiology; the

American College of Cardiology Foundation; and the Heart Rhythm Society. Endorsed by the International Society for Computerized Electrocardiology. J Am Coll Cardiol. 2009;53:982–91.

306. Surawicz B, Macfarlane PW. Inappropriate and confusing electrocardiographic terms: J-wave syndromes and early repolarization. J Am Coll Cardiol. 2011;57:1584–6.
307. Macfarlane PW, Antzelevitch C, Haissaguerre M, et al. The early repolarization pattern: a consensus paper. J Am Coll Cardiol. 2015;66:470–7.
308. Gourraud J-B, Le Scouarnec S, Sacher F, et al. Identification of large families in early repolarization syndrome. J Am Coll Cardiol. 2013;61:164–72.
309. Nunn LM, Bhar-Amato J, Lowe MD, et al. Prevalence of J-point elevation in sudden arrhythmic death syndrome families. J Am Coll Cardiol. 2011;58:286–90.
310. Haissaguerre M, Chatel S, Sacher F, et al. Ventricular fibrillation with prominent early repolarization associated with a rare variant of KCNJ8/K channel. J Cardiovasc. 2009;20:93–8.
311. Veeramah KR, Karafet TM, Wolf D, et al. The KCNJ8-S422L variant previously associated with J-wave syndromes is found at an increased frequency in Ashkenazi Jews. Eur J Hum Genet. 2014;22:94–8.
312. Priori SG, Blomström-Lundqvist C, Mazzanti A, et al. 2015 ESC Guidelines for the management of patients with ventricular arrhythmias and the prevention of sudden cardiac death: The task force for the management of patients with ventricular arrhythmias and the prevention of sudden cardiac death of the European Society of Cardiology (ESC) endorsed by: Association for European Paediatric and Congenital Cardiology (AEPC). Europace. 2015;17:1601–87. https://doi.org/10.1093/europace/euv319.
313. Haissaguerre M, Sacher F, Nogami A, et al. Characteristics of recurrent ventricular fibrillation associated with inferolateral early repolarization role of drug therapy. J Am Coll Cardiol. 2009;53:612–9.
314. Abe A, Ikeda T, Tsukada T, et al. Circadian variation of late potentials in idiopathic ventricular fibrillation associated with J waves: insights into alternative pathophysiology and risk stratification. Heart Rhythm Off J Heart Rhythm Soc. 2010;7:675–82.
315. Derval N, Simpson CS, Birnie DH, et al. Prevalence and characteristics of early repolarization in the CASPER registry: cardiac arrest survivors with preserved ejection fraction registry. J Am Coll Cardiol. 2011;58:722–8.
316. Nam GB, Ko KH, Kim J, et al. Mode of onset of ventricular fibrillation in patients with early repolarization pattern vs. Brugada syndrome. Eur Heart J. 2010;31:330–9.
317. Rosso R, Adler A, Halkin A, Viskin S. Risk of sudden death among young individuals with J waves and early repolarization: putting the evidence into perspective. Heart Rhythm Off J Heart Rhythm Soc. 2011;8:923–9.
318. Muramoto D, Yong CM, Singh N, et al. Patterns and prognosis of all components of the J-wave pattern in multiethnic athletes and ambulatory patients. Am Heart J. 2014;167:259–66.
319. Brosnan MJ, Kumar S, LaGerche A, et al. Early repolarization patterns associated with increased arrhythmic risk are common in young non-Caucasian Australian males and not influenced by athletic status. Heart Rhythm Off J Heart Rhythm Soc. 2015;12:1576–83.
320. Junttila MJ, Sager SJ, Freiser M, et al. Inferolateral early repolarization in athletes. J Interv Card Electrophysiol Int J Arrhythm Pacing. 2011;31:33–8.
321. Aagaard P, Baranowski B, Aziz P, Phelan D. Early repolarization in athletes: a review. Circ Arrhythm Electrophysiol. 2016;9:e003577.
322. Noseworthy PA, Tikkanen JT, Porthan K, et al. The early repolarization pattern in the general population: clinical correlates and heritability. J Am Coll Cardiol. 2011;57:2284–9.
323. Sager SJ, Hoosien M, Junttila MJ, et al. Comparison of inferolateral early repolarization and its electrocardiographic phenotypes in pre- and postadolescent populations. Am J Cardiol. 2013;112:444–8.
324. Roten L, Derval N, Sacher F, et al. Ajmaline attenuates electrocardiogram characteristics of inferolateral early repolarization. Heart Rhythm. 2012;9:232–9.
325. Roten L, Derval N, Sacher F, et al. Heterogeneous response of J-wave syndromes to beta-adrenergic stimulation. Heart Rhythm Off J Heart Rhythm Soc. 2012;9:1970–6.

326. Nam GB, Kim YH, Antzelevitch C. Augmentation of J waves and electrical storms in patients with early repolarization. N Engl J Med. 2008;358:2078–9.
327. Shinohara T, Takahashi N, Saikawa T, Yoshimatsu H. Characterization of J wave in a patient with idiopathic ventricular fibrillation. Heart Rhythm Off J Heart Rhythm Soc. 2006;3:1082–4.
328. Tikkanen JT, Wichmann V, Junttila MJ, et al. Association of early repolarization and sudden cardiac death during an acute coronary event. Circ Arrhythm Electrophysiol. 2012;5:714–8.
329. Tülümen E, Schulze-Bahr E, Zumhagen S, et al. Early repolarization pattern: a marker of increased risk in patients with catecholaminergic polymorphic ventricular tachycardia. Europace. 2015;18:1587–92. https://doi.org/10.1093/europace/euv357.
330. Laksman ZWM, Gula LJ, Saklani P, et al. Early repolarization is associated with symptoms in patients with type 1 and type 2 long QT syndrome. Heart Rhythm Off J Heart Rhythm Soc. 2014;11:1632–8.
331. van der Werf C, van Langen IM, Wilde AA. Sudden death in the young: what do we know about it and how to prevent? Circ Arrhythm Electrophysiol. 2010;3:96–104.
332. Viskin S, Postema PG, Bhuiyan ZA, et al. The response of the QT-interval to the brief tachycardia provoked by standing. A bedside test for diagnosing Long-QT syndrome. J Am Coll Cardiol. 2010;55:1955–61.
333. Patton KK, Ellinor PT, Ezekowitz M, et al. Electrocardiographic early repolarization: a scientific statement from the American Heart Association. Circulation. 2016;133:1520–9.
334. Priori SG, Wilde AA, Horie M, et al. HRS/EHRA/APHRS expert consensus statement on the diagnosis and management of patients with inherited primary arrhythmia syndromes expert consensus statement on inherited primary arrhythmia syndromes. Heart Rhythm. 2013;10:e75–e106.
335. Adler A, Rosso R, Viskin D, et al. What do we know about the "malignant form" of early repolarization? J Am Coll Cardiol. 2013;62:863–8.
336. Tikkanen JT, Junttila MJ, Anttonen O, et al. Early repolarization: electrocardiographic phenotypes associated with favorable long-term outcome. Circulation. 2011;123:2666–73.
337. Sacher F, Lim HS, Haissaguerre M. Sudden cardiac death associated with J wave elevation in the inferolateral leads: insights from a multicenter registry. J Electrocardiol. 2013;46:456–60.
338. Antzelevitch C, Yan G-X, Viskin S. Rationale for the use of the terms J-wave syndromes and early repolarization. J Am Coll Cardiol. 2011;57:1587–90.
339. Postema PG, Wilde AAM. Do J waves constitute a syndrome? J Electrocardiol. 2013;46:461–5.
340. Hoogendijk MG, Potse M, Coronel R. Critical appraisal of the mechanism underlying J waves. J Electrocardiol. 2013;46:390–4.
341. Wellens HJ. Early repolarization revisited. N Engl J Med. 2008;358:2063–5.
342. Amin AS, de Groot EA, Ruijter JM, et al. Exercise-induced ECG changes in Brugada syndrome. Circ Arrhythm Electrophysiol. 2009;2:531–9.
343. Obeyesekere MN, Klein GJ, Nattel S, et al. A clinical approach to early repolarization. Circulation. 2013;127:1620–9.
344. Osborn JJ. Experimental hypothermia; respiratory and blood pH changes in relation to cardiac function. Am J Phys. 1953;175:389–98.
345. Watanabe H, Nogami A, Ohkubo K, et al. Electrocardiographic characteristics and SCN5A mutations in idiopathic ventricular fibrillation associated with early repolarization. Circ Arrhythm Electrophysiol. 2011;4:874–81.
346. Sinner MF, Porthan K, Noseworthy PA, et al. A meta-analysis of genome-wide association studies of the electrocardiographic early repolarization pattern. Heart Rhythm Off J Heart Rhythm Soc. 2012;9:1627–34.
347. Mahida S, Derval N, Sacher F, et al. Role of electrophysiological studies in predicting risk of ventricular arrhythmia in early repolarization syndrome. J Am Coll Cardiol. 2015;65:151–9.

Inherited Conduction Disease and Atrial Fibrillation

15

Claire Martin and Pier Lambiase

Abstract

Normal atrial contraction requires homogeneous electrical propagation through the myocardium. Disruption of the structural or ionic components of the sinus node, atrial myocytes or conduction system can result in sinus bradycardia, atrial fibrillation (AF) or premature atrioventicular block.

This chapter discusses the key molecular mechanisms determining the development of AF & conduction disorders. Both may exist as a monogenic disease, and research in these cases in animal models or human tissue focuses on investigating expression of specific genes coding ion channels, cytoskeletal complexes or transcription factors.

Alternatively, patients with AF/conduction disease may have a genetic background that predisposes to the disease without it necessarily segregating in a family. Research approaches examine genetic variants in the human population, through candidate single nucleotide polymorphism studies or genome wide association studies. Knowledge of potentially causative genes and association loci may lead to the development of targeted treatment strategies for these conditions utilising the underlying molecular pathway(s). This chapter will systematically explore these aspects.

C. Martin
Department of Cardiology, UCL, Barts Heart Centre, London, UK

P. Lambiase (✉)
Department of Cardiology, Barts Heart Centre, Institute of Cardiovascular Science, UCL, London, UK
e-mail: d.lambiase@ucl.ac.uk

D. Kumar, P. Elliott (eds.), *Cardiovascular Genetics and Genomics*,
https://doi.org/10.1007/978-3-319-66114-8_15

Keywords
Inherited conduction disease • Atrial fibrillation • Genomics • Mutations • Common genetic variants

15.1 Introduction

Normal atrial contraction requires an electromechanical impulse to propagate in an orderly way across myocardial cells. Any disruption in the structural and ionic components may result in chaotic electrical activity known as atrial fibrillation (AF). Similarly, a break down in the structural or electrical integrity of the sinus node or conduction system can result in conduction system disease.

This chapter will discuss the main molecular mechanisms known to underlie the development of AF and conduction system disorders, focusing on the genes and association loci that have been linked to these conditions and the possible ways in which treatment options for these conditions could be influenced by knowledge of the underlying genetic pathways.

Research efforts have focused on two approaches—examining genetic variants in the human population, and then investigating expression of specific genes in animal models or human tissue. Genetics in the human may involve analysis of AF/conduction disease as a monogenic disease in individuals with primary electrical disease, analysis of AF/conduction disease presenting in the setting of another familial disease, or the genetic background that might predispose to the disease without it necessarily segregating in a family. The first two pathways provide definitive insight into the aetiology and require analysis of families with the disease segregating across generations and following Mendelian inheritance in the context of a large effect size.

The third method involves investigating common variants. This can be performed through candidate single nucleotide polymorphism (SNP) studies, where a relatively small number of SNPs are examined in genes that are suspected to be associated with a disease, and uses known biology or associations to select the most relevant SNPs. Alternatively, genome wide association studies (GWAS) examine millions of SNPs throughout a large population sample for unsuspected associations and can identify new biological mechanisms. Non-related cases of AF/conduction disease matched to controls by age and gender are compared to identify differences in segregation of genetic backgrounds between both groups that may explain susceptibility to the disease. These methods examine common variants which have a small effect size, conferring susceptibility to AF along with a number of acquired factors or co-morbidities (Fig. 15.1).

Studies looking at alterations in gene expression of ion channels and regulatory subunits are usually performed in animal models of the disease, but can be undertaken on a more limited scale in humans. They provide information on molecular changes triggered by the disease, which may uncover the mechanisms leading to, for example, conduction disease or that allow paroxysmal AF to become

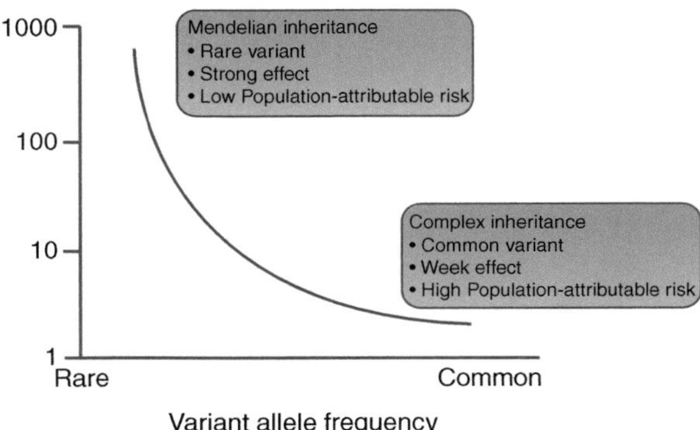

Fig. 15.1 Allele frequencies and risk in families and populations. Adapted from Darbar and Roden [251]

permanent. In AF for example, this may provide insight into whether changes in the atria form the aetiology of the disease, are a maladaptation or a compensatory mechanism [1–3].

15.2 Cardiac Conduction Disease

Conduction diseases encompass an important group of potentially life-threatening cardiac conditions accounting for approximately 50% of the one million permanent pacemakers implanted worldwide each year [4]. Morgagni was the first In 1761 to link recurrent fainting episodes with a slow pulse in a family, and similar observations were later made by Adams and Stokes. The development of the electrocardiogram at the end of the nineteenth century provided tighter definitions of related phenotypes, but it was not until 1964 that two independent researchers published reports on a form of progressive CCD combining clinical observations, ECG recordings and detailed post mortem studies of the heart [5, 6]. Their descriptions were subtly different, with Lev describing a diffuse fibrotic degeneration through the fibrous skeleton of the heart, whilst in Lenègre's description the fibrosis was limited to the conduction fibres. However, both involved progressive conduction slowing through the His-Purkinje system with left bundle branch block (LBBB) or right bundle branch block (RBBB) and widening of QRS complexes leading to complete AV block and sometimes causing syncope or sudden cardiac death (SCD). Lenègre-Lev Syndrome is now synonymous with 'Progressive Cardiac Conduction Disease' (PCCD).

Thus, conduction diseases comprise a heterogeneous group of conditions that may be either inherited or acquired, and either associated with structural abnormalities of the heart or manifest as 'primary electrical diseases' [7]. Cardiac activation is initiated in the sino-atrial node with the rate of depolarization dependent on the magnitude of the Na^+ (sodium) current involving Na^+ channel function and availability. The depolarizing current then spreads between cells through intercellular gap junctions. These each comprise hemi-channels, each containing 6 connexin protein subunits (Fig. 15.2) [8], which are low-resistance channels that provide

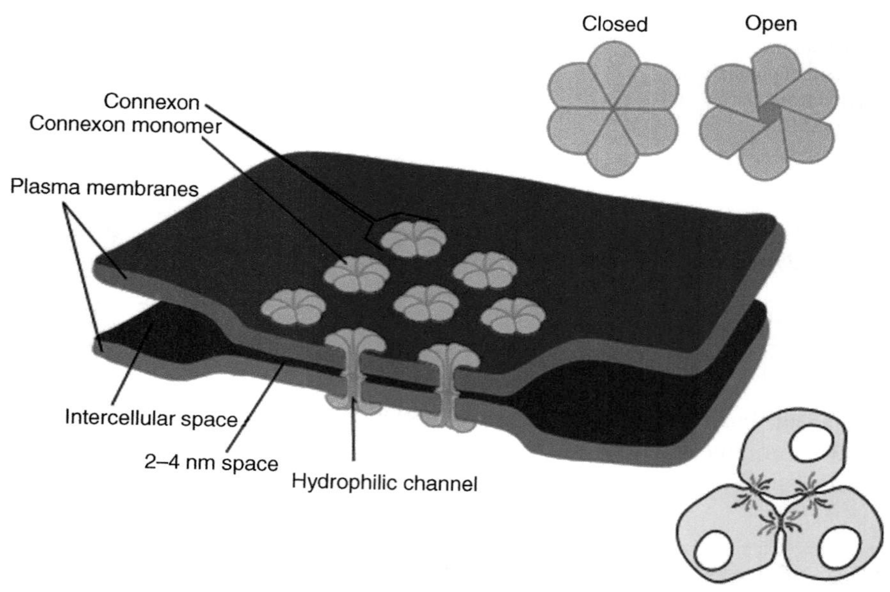

Fig. 15.2 Gap junction structure. From Mariana Ruiz

electrical coupling and intercellular electrical communication [9]. Thus conduction disease can result in abnormalities in any of the molecular components involved in electrophysiological activity, contractile function and cell–cell adhesion.

15.2.1 Sodium Channel Mutations Causing PCCD

15.2.1.1 SCN5A

The first gene to be associated with PCCD was *SCN5A*, which encodes the alpha subunit of the voltage gated Na^+ channel. Na^+ channels are essential for the transmission of the cardiac impulse through both the fast conducting system and the working myocardium [10], and it is therefore unsurprising that 'loss-of-function' mutations might result in conduction disease. In 1999, Schott's group [11] described a family with PCCD with various types of conduction disorder displayed in its members: RBBB, LBBB, left anterior or posterior hemi-block and long PR intervals. These defects were progressive over time (Fig. 15.3). Linkage analysis mapped the disease locus to chromosome 3 near *SCN5A*. Direct sequencing of affected members identified a splice donor site mutation in exon 22 of *SCN5A* (IVS.22+2T≥C) in 25 affected members. These observations suggest that PCCD associates *SCN5A* loss of function together with an additional permissive factor related to aging. Heterozygote Scn5a+/− mice demonstrate prolonged PR intervals, AV block and prolonged QRS intervals that worsen with age, associated with a pronounced myocardial rearrangement, including fibrosis and redistribution of connexin43 expression [12, 13].

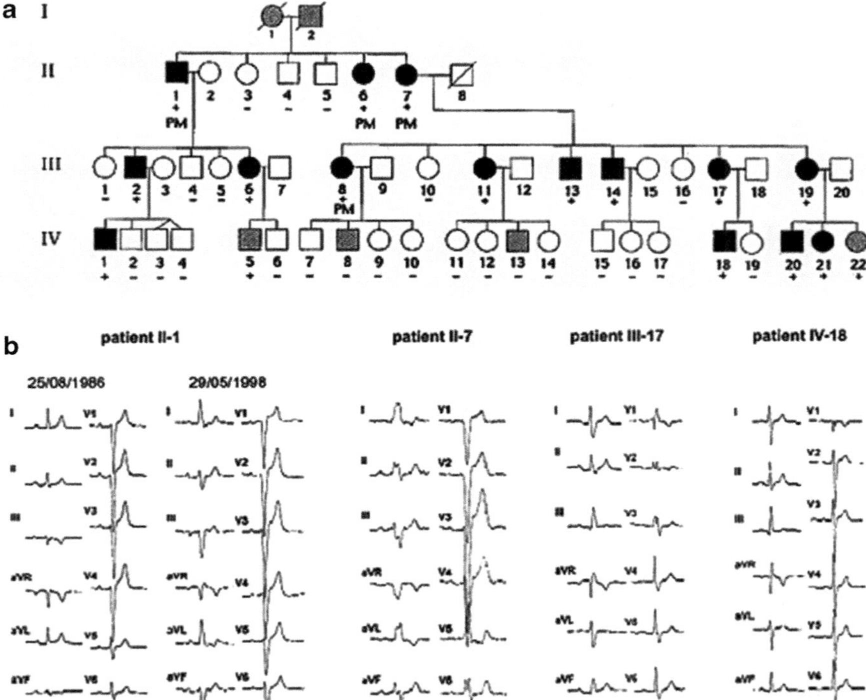

Fig. 15.3 (**a**) Pedigree of the French family identified by Schott et al. Patients with an unknown status (stippled) were not included in the linkage study. Individuals carrying the mutation are indicated (+), as are patients with a pacemaker (PM). (**b**). Representative ECGs from the French family. Patient II-1 had an unspecified conduction defect (QRS duration 120 ms) at age 60, but at age 72 had left anterior hemi-block with wide QRS complexes and a long PR interval (240 ms). ECGs from patients II-7, III-17 and IV-18 show complete LBBB, complete RBBB and left posterior hemi-block, respectively. Adapted with permission from Schott et al. [11]

There have subsequently been many reports identifying new *SCN5A* mutations causing PCCD or non-progressive CCD. Mutations have been found in various locations on *SCN5A* (Fig. 15.4), and have been postulated to give rise to loss of Na^+ channel function. Some mutations result in a non-functioning protein [14–16], whilst in others there is a defect in the trafficking mechanisms or in the channel gating behaviour once the protein is inserted into the membrane [17–21]. In the case of a Dutch family segregating a specific missense allele (G514C), the mutation causes unequal depolarizing shifts in the voltage-dependence of activation and inactivation such that a smaller number of channels are activated at typical threshold voltages [17]. Two *SCN5A* mutations causing isolated conduction disturbances (G298S and D1595N) are also predicted to reduce channel availability by enhancing the tendency of channels to undergo slow inactivation in combination with a complex mix of gain- and loss-of-function defects [22].

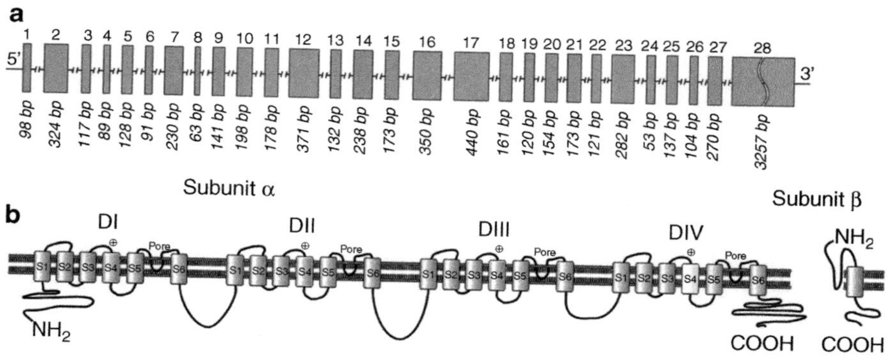

Fig. 15.4 Location of identified SCN5A mutations that result in conduction system disease. *common polymorphism. Adapted with permission from Moric et al. [255]. For complete updated list of SCN5A variants associated with PCCD see http://www.fsm.it/cardmoc/

There are also cases in which individuals with severe impairment in conduction have inherited mutations from both parents. Lupoglazoff et al. described a child homozygous for a missense *SCN5A* allele (V1777M) who exhibited rate-dependent atrio-ventricular (AV) conduction block [23]. In a separate report, probands from 3 families exhibited perinatal sinus bradycardia progressing to atrial standstill ('congenital sick sinus syndrome' (SSS)) and were found to have compound heterozygosity for mutations in *SCN5A* [24]. Compound heterozygosity in *SCN5A* has also been observed in 2 cases of neonatal wide complex tachycardia and a generalized cardiac conduction defect [18]. These unusually severe examples of *SCN5A*-linked cardiac conduction disorders illustrate the clinical consequence of near complete loss of Na^+ channel function.

Recently, mutations have been found which have a modulator effect on SCN5A. Niu et al. [25] described a W1421X mutation where four generations of a family demonstrated cardiac conduction abnormalities and several cases of SCD. However, one member with the mutation was unaffected, and was found to have a second mutation *SCN5A-R1193Q,* postulated to have a protective role in moderating the impact of the first mutation. Polymorphisms in connexin genes have also been found to have effects. Groenewegen et al. [26] identified *SCN5A-D1275N* co-segregating with two connexin40 genotypes in familial atrial standstill (AS). Whilst SCN5A-D1275N channels showed only a small depolarizing shift in activation compared with wild type the combined effect led to the severe conduction defects.

All the above variants result in purely functional conduction disorders; however, *SCN5A* mutations may also result in structural abnormalities along with CCD. In 2004, a large family with members suffering from sinus node dysfunction, arrhythmia and ventricular dysfunction, was found to harbour *SCN5A-D1275N* [27] demonstrating that genes encoding ion channels can also be associated with dilated structural phenotypes. Since then, other families with SCN5A mutations have been identified who display heart failure and atrial arrhythmias as well as conduction disorder [28–30]. Whilst it is possible that such structural abnormalities arise through tachycardia-induced cardiomyopathy, most evidence suggests that DCM may well be a primary manifestation of the *SCN5A* mutation [41]. This may result from interactions of the cardiac Na^+ channel with cytoskeletal components or through altered calcium homeostasis as a consequence of alterations in intracellular Na^+ concentrations ([Na]i).

15.2.1.2 SCN5A Overlap Syndrome

SCN5A mutations are associated not only with CCD but also Long QT (LQT3) and Brugada Syndromes (BrS). A gain-of-function mutation of the Na^+ channel is seen in LQT3 leading to a more prolonged depolarizing current, increasing the action potential duration (APD). BrS is associated with reduced Na^+ channel function and is characterized electrocardiographically by ST elevation in the right precordial leads and RBBB. Whilst isolated PCCD does not usually involve the ECG changes seen with BrS or LQT3, *SCN5A* mutations may also be associated with more complex phenotypes that appear to represent combinations of the characteristics of BrS, conduction system disease and LQT3 (Fig. 15.5). In one example, deletion of

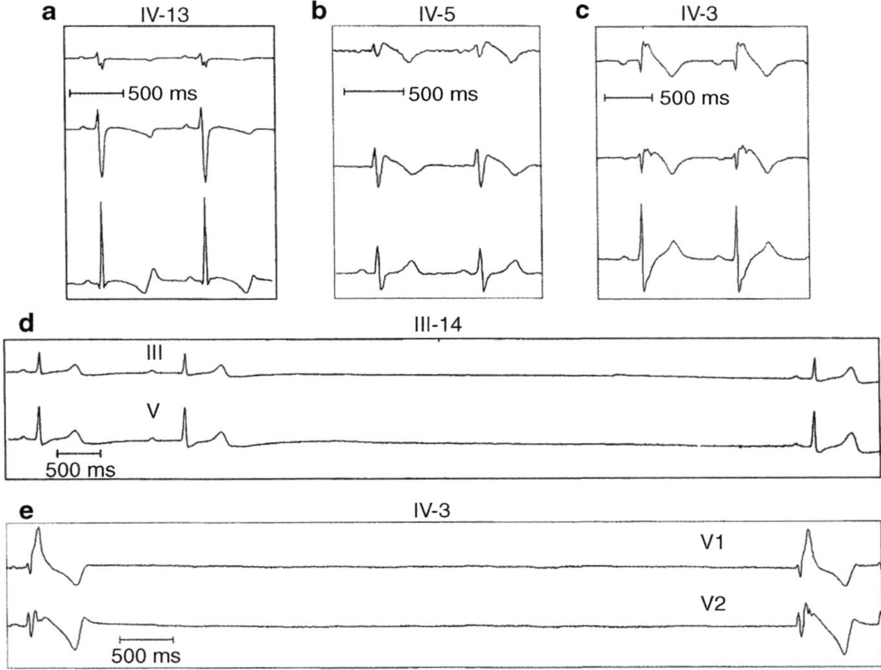

Fig. 15.5 ECG traces of mutation carriers showing leads V1, V2, and V5. (**a**) QT interval prolongation (**b**) ST segment elevation (patient IV-5 of the pedigree). (**c**) ST segment elevation and right bundle branch block (patient IV-3 of the pedigree). (**d**) First-degree AV block and E sinus arrest (patient III-14 of the pedigree). Reproduced with permission from Grant et al. [31]

lysine-1500 in *SCN5A* was associated with impaired inactivation, resulting in a persistent Na^+ current, but also reduction in Na_V channel availability by opposing shifts in voltage-dependence of inactivation and activation [31]. These complex relationships between genotype and phenotype may underlie clinical findings that individuals with BrS and an identifiable *SCN5A* mutation have longer PR intervals [32] and may experience more bradyarrhythmias [33] than BrS individuals with BrS who do not have an identifiable *SCN5A* mutation. However, Lenègre-Lev and Brugada Syndromes remain two distinct clinical entities, as only those individuals with a BrS phenotype display ST elevation and ventricular arrhythmias.

15.2.1.3 SCN1B

The cardiac Na^+ channel protein $Na_v1.5$ constitutes the pore-forming subunit of a multi-protein complex [34]. There are at least four beta subunits that modulate the expression and function of the Na^+ channel [35]. 3 pathogenic mutations have been found in the *SCN1B* gene, encoding the Na^+ channel β1 subunit, which decreased the $Na_v1.5$ mediated current in cellular expression system compared with controls [36].

15.2.1.4 SCN10A

Several large GWAS have demonstrated that loci within the SCN10A, encoding the Na^+ channel $Na_v1.8$, associate with AV conduction [37] and BrS [38]. A recent study has demonstrated cardiac expression of *SCN10A*, and identified an association of a non-synonymous SNP in the *SCN10A* with prolonged cardiac conduction. The PR interval is shorter in *Scn10a–/–* mice than in wild-type mice, suggesting that SCN10A in humans acts to lengthen cardiac conduction, and that this SNP in *SCN10A* is a gain-of-function variant [39]. Furthermore there is evidence that a cardiac enhancer in SCN10A interacts with and regulates the promoter of SCN5A, thus providing an explanation for how SCN10A genetic variants may affect conduction [40].

15.2.2 Other Genes Causing CCD in Structurally Normal Hearts

Mutations in genes encoding other relevant proteins have been identified in families with conduction disorders, although these do not usually exhibit the progression with age seen in Lenègre-Lev syndrome. Often mutations at the same site may result in either purely functional conduction defects or may also be associated with dilated or restrictive cardiomyopathy or other structural defects.

15.2.2.1 Connexins

There are four connexin isoforms in the human heart, which have a regional distribution. Cx40 are found in large, Cx43 in medium, Cx45 in small and Cx31.9 in ultra-small conductance gap junction channels respectively [41]. Mutations in connexins have been linked to abnormal cardiac activation and conduction disorders. A causal relationship between nucleotide substitutions in gene coding for Cx40 and progressive familial heart block has been demonstrated, with heterologous expression resulting in a reduction in junctional conductance and diffuse localization of Cx40 proteins at plasma membrane without formation of gap junctions [42].

15.2.2.2 TRPM4

There have been several descriptions of CCD in families in South Africa, with progressive RBBB and other conduction disturbances and a family history of SCD, which has been termed type I progressive familial heart block (PFHB) [43–45]. A distinct clinical entity, PFHB type II was also characterized, with complete heart block but narrow complexes. A similar disease was prevalent in Lebanon, with conduction defects, especially RBBB, progressive over time [46, 47]. A number of microsatellite markers in the South African and Lebanese families have been mapped to chromosome 19q13.2-13 [48, 49]. Subsequently, the genetic interval for the PFHBI disease locus has been defined, with a missense mutation in *TRPM4* isolated as the cause of blunted cardiac conduction in several branches of a large Afrikaner family [50]. *TRPM4* encodes a Ca^{2+}-activated channel (CAN) in in vitro expression systems [51] and has been suggested to contribute to the transient inward current (I_{ti}) initiated by Ca^{2+} waves. The *PFHBI*-associated mutation, which results in an amino acid sequence change in the TRPM4 N terminus, was found to lead to constitutive SUMOylation of TRPM4 and impaired TRPM4 endocytosis, resulting in a dominant gain of TRPM4 channel function (Fig. 15.6).

More recently, three more mutations in TRPM4 were reported in French and Lebanese families with PCCD [52]. Functional experiments expressing these three mutant variants of TRPM4 suggested a similar gain-of-function phenomenon

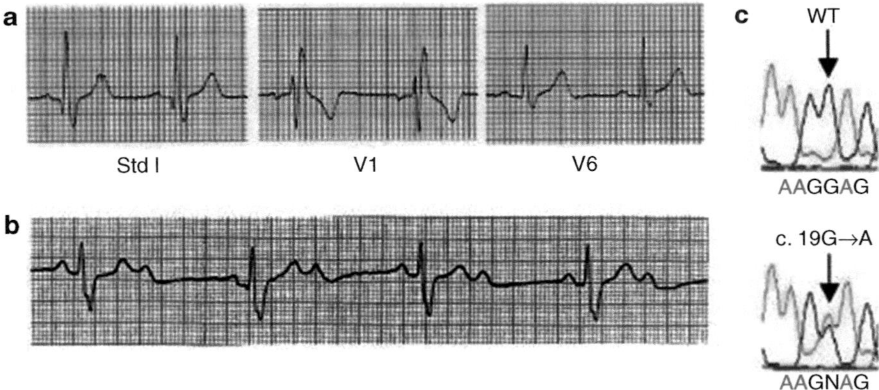

Fig. 15.6 (**a**, **b**) Cardiac phenotype of PFHBI patients. (**a**) Sinus rhythm with a RBBB in an 8-year-old asymptomatic boy on a standard 12-lead ECG, with leads Std I, V1, and V6 shown. (**b**) 2:1 atrioventricular node block (atrial rate, 76 bpm; ventricular rate, 38 bpm) with a broad QRS complex on Holter monitoring in a 54-year-old man who had recently become symptomatic. ECGs were recorded at a 25 mm/s paper speed and 10 mm/mV signal amplitude. (**c**) TRPM4 missense mutation in exon 1 associated with PFHBI. Electropherograms show TRPM4 WT sequence and the heterozygous sequence change c.19G→A in the DNA of PFHBI-affected individuals. Reproduced with permission from Kruse et al. [50]

related to altered deSUMOylation. In another recent study [53], an additional six TRPM4 mutations in patients with RBBB and AV block were identified, but electrophysiological or biochemical studies have yet to be carried out in order to elucidate the potential mechanisms involved. Altogether, these recent studies strongly suggest that TRPM4 plays a key role in the pathogenesis of genetically determined conduction disorders. It may be that gain-of-function mutant TRPM4 channels lead to cell membrane depolarization in the conduction system, thus reducing the number of available Na^+ channels and resulting in the observed conduction abnormalities.

15.2.2.3 KCNK17

In a PCCD patient with idiopathic VF, whole exome sequencing has identified a missense mutation in the KCNK17 gene [54], which encodes the potassium (K^+) channel TASK-4. A gain of function of TASK-4-mediated current may reduce the availability of Na^+ current by depolarizing the membrane of conduction system cells.

15.2.3 CCD Associated With Structural Cardiac Defects

Cardiac transcription factors are known to be critical in formation of the cardiac conduction system as well as cardiac septation and morphogenesis. It is thought that 10% of sporadic congenital heart disease involve de novo mutations which may affect cardiac conduction [55–57]. For example, the molecular pathway involving *TBX5*, *NKX2.5* and *Id2* genes controls specification of ventricular myoctyes into the ventricular conduction system lineage [58] as well as formation of the cardiac chambers and endocardial cushions, and modifies gene expression of ion channel proteins that contribute to properties of conduction system and contraction of myocardium [59]. Mutations have been linked to CCD associated with congenital heart disease [60].

15.2.3.1 NKX2.5

NKX2.5 (cardiac-specific homeobox) regulates proliferation of atrial working and conduction myocardium in coordination with the Notch pathway [61]. *NKX2.5* mutations have been identified in cases of CCD, and also Wenckebach conduction block, ventricular non-compaction and SCD. These cases are associated with septal defects [62] and a variety of other congenital heart defect phenotypes such as tetralogy of Fallot, truncus arteriosus, double outlet right ventricle, L-transposition of great arteries, interrupted aortic arch and hypoplastic left heart syndrome [63–65].

15.2.3.2 Tbx5

Mutations in the gene encoding the T-box transcription factor *Tbx5* have been found in 2 families with Holt-Oram syndrome [66]. This syndrome has an autosomal dominant transmission pattern and may include radial ray upper limb abnormalities, cardiac septation defect and coarctation [67, 68]. A range of conduction disorders may be seen, such as sinus bradycardia or AV block, even in the absence of overt structural heart disease. Mutations in the *TBX3* gene, which lies close to *TBX5* on chromosome 12q24, result in ulnar-mammary syndrome. A case of contiguous deletions of both *TBX5* and *TBX3* displaying clinical features of both, had rapidly progressive cardiac conduction disease [69].

15.2.3.3 Others

An intact cytoskeleton is required for proper myocyte structure and is involved in cell signalling processes. Mutations in genes encoding cytoskeletal proteins can lead to cardiomyopathy or muscular dystrophy, an example being the LMNA A/C gene, encoding laminin. However, often the first and most prominent disease manifestation is isolated CCD, without or before the development of detectable structural cardiac abnormalities. It appears that mutations in cytoskeletal proteins directly or indirectly alter ion channel function. This is supported by recent studies showing that alpha-syntrophin interacts with the alpha-subunit of the cardiac Na^+ channel, thereby regulating its membrane expression and gating behaviour [70]. Interactions of cytoskeletal proteins with mutant Na^+ channels may explain the exaggerated fibrosis seen in some cases of Lenègre-Lev syndrome [16, 18].

Mutations in *PRKAG2* encoding an AMP-activated protein kinase, have been found in cases of both isolated CCD [71] and conduction disease with cardiac hypertrophy [72]. These mutations may influence cardiac conduction by affecting the phosphorylation state of several cardiac ion channels; for example T172D that is known to affect the inactivation properties of the human cardiac Na^+ channel in heterologous cell expression [73].

Inborn errors of metabolism that affect normal transport and metabolism of fatty acids due to enzymatic defects may present as conduction disease and atrial arrhythmias without structural heart disease, although they can also be associated with cardiomyopathies. Usually, patients have defects in enzymes that regulate mitochondrial transport of long-chain fatty acids [74]. The accumulation of fatty acid metabolites downstream from the enzyme defect cannot only be myotoxic, but may also influence ion channels. They have been shown to reduce the inward rectifying K^+ and depolarizing Na^+ current, to activate Ca^{2+} channels, and to impair gap-junction hemi-channel interaction [75].

15.2.4 The Role of Common Genetic Variants

Several GWAS have identified variants in multiple loci that show evidence of association with heart rate [37, 76–78] (Fig. 15.7). Although none of the heart rate loci have shown association with the risk of AV block, SSS, pacemaker implantation or sudden cardiac death individually, a higher genome-wide polygenic score (GPS) was associated with reduced risk of SSS and pacemaker implantation. A range of approaches, including proteomics experiments and gene expression quantitative trait locus analysis, labelled 49 of the 234 genes located within the 21 loci as candidate genes for heart rate regulation [79]. Experiments in animal models supported a role in heart rate regulation for 20 of the 31 candidate genes tested, including ones

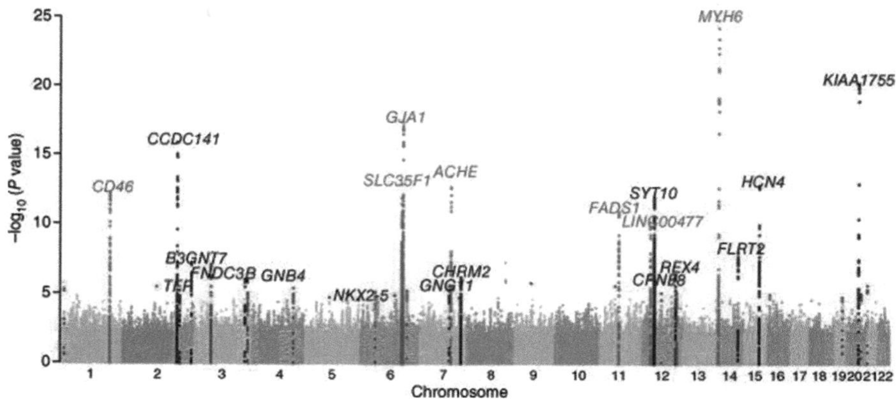

Fig. 15.7 Manhattan plot of SNPs associated with heart rate. The 7 loci that were previously identified are highlighted in light blue; the 14 newly associated loci are highlighted in dark blue. Loci that reached $P < 3 \times 10^{-5}$ after stage 1 but did not reach $P < 5 \times 10^{-8}$ after multi-stage meta-analysis are highlighted in red. Reproduced with permission from den Hoed et al. [79]

that have a role in embryonic development (*EPHB4*, *PLXNA2*, *PLD1* and *CALCRL*), as well as those with a role in the pathophysiology of dilated cardiomyopathy, congestive heart failure and/or SCD (*TTN*, *MFN1*, *CHRM2* and *PLD1*). These findings provide new insights into the mechanisms that regulate heart rate and may impact upon management strategies in future.

15.2.5 Management of Patients With Inherited PCCD

PCCD is diagnosed mainly in the presence of unexplained progressive conduction abnormalities in patients under 50. The index patient should have clinical data collected including history, family history, 12 lead ECG and an echo/MRI to investigate the presence of structural heart disease. Early onset PCCD in a structurally normal heart should trigger PCCD genetic testing [80].

There is currently no genotype based risk stratification strategy, but with genotype positive patients there should be a low threshold for investigating symptoms or ECG findings. Patients should avoid drugs with conduction slowing properties and there should be active treatment of fever in SCN5A mutation carriers to minimise the risk of ventricular arrhythmias. A recent HRS/EHRA/APHRS expert consensus statement concludes that pacemaker implantation should be recommended in PCCD patients with either intermittent or permanent third degree and high grade AV block, or symptomatic Mobitz I or II second degree AV block (class I recommendation). PPM can be useful in PCCD patients with bifascicular block with or without first degree AV block (class IIa recommendation) [81]. Targeted genetic screening of first degree relatives of a mutation positive PCCD patients is also recommended, to allow prospective follow up of asymptomatic mutation carriers.

15.2.6 Conclusions

There have been recent advances in the understanding of the development and pathophysiology of CCD, and in particular in the genetic backgrounds behind rare forms of familial PCCD. A large number of genes have been linked to cardiac conduction disorders. Genotype-phenotype correlations have demonstrated that PCCD is associated not only with aging, but also processes that lead to AV block and intraventricular block. Once more is known regarding the genetic pathways determining cardiac conduction, genetic analysis may become a routine part of management, with gene-mutation based risk stratification helping to determine optimal timing for pacemaker implantation. Mechanistically driven preventative strategies might also be employed to slow the development of the disease e.g. to modulate transcription or improve ion channel trafficking.

15.3 Atrial Fibrillation

AF is the most common cardiac arrhythmia, estimated to affect 1–2% of the UK population. Its prevalence is increasing and is estimated to have doubled by 2040 [82, 83]. The most serious chronic sequelae of AF include stroke, heart failure, and dementia with devastating effects on an individual's health and high socio-economic costs [84].

The increased incidence of AF is driven partly by ageing populations, but other factors are also implicated. Although hypertension remains the most well described risk marker, metabolic factors also play a part. Investigators of the Framingham Heart Study estimated that obesity was associated with a 50% increase in risk of AF [85]. A linear association has been reported between BMI and AF and short-term increases in body mass contributed substantially to risk of AF [86]. Although some of the effects of obesity might be haemodynamic (e.g., through impaired ventricular relaxation or atrial stretch), more direct metabolic effects seem likely [85, 86]. Diabetes is also independently associated with AF [87]. Epidemiological data for prevalence of AF in racial groups and various geographical locations provide evidence of intrinsic (presumably genetic) interactions. Black people have a higher prevalence of hypertension and metabolic disease but a lower incidence of AF than a comparable white population [88].

AF is a clinically and genetically heterogeneous condition, which can be thought of as representing the final common phenotype of multiple diverse pathways. Conditions that promote AF involve atrial structural, electrical and autonomic abnormalities and/or remodelling that lead to re-entry or triggered activity [89]. Slow conduction velocities and short effective refractory periods (ERP) allow the establishment and stabilization of multiple re-entrant circuits (Fig. 15.8). Delayed afterdepolarizations (DAD) emerge from abnormal Ca^{2+} release from the sarcoplasmic reticulum during diastole, acting as triggers for re-entry or, when sustained, as a focal source for AF [90, 91].

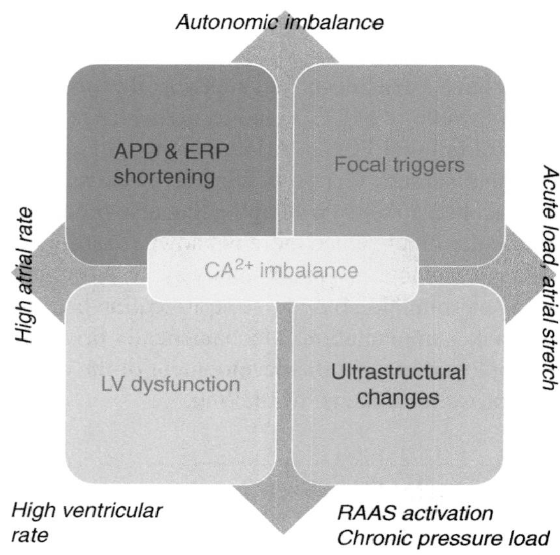

Fig. 15.8 The interaction between structural and functional anomalies promoting AF and Left ventricular dysfunction. Adapted from Kirchhof et al. [256]

15.4 AF as a Monogenic Disease

If AF occurs in the absence of any obvious predisposing factors it is known as 'lone AF' [92]. Lone AF can be thought of as a primary electrical disease caused by changes in ionic currents. It was in fact first reported in a family in 1943 [93], and it is estimated that 5% of pts with AF and up to 15% of individuals with lone AF may have a familial form [94]. There have been significant advances in the last 10 years in investigating the genetic elements of AF, with data from the Framingham study and Icelandic population showing that parental AF leads to a relative risk of AF in offspring of 4.7, if parents are affected before 60 years [95, 96]. The risk of developing lone AF at young age increases with the number affected of relatives with lone AF and decreasing age at onset in family members [97]. While this may of course reflect common exposure to environmental factors, it is likely that genetic susceptibility plays a significant role [94–96, 98, 99].

Various AF loci and genes with large effect sizes in AF kindreds have been identified in positional cloning and linkage analyses. The first AF locus was discovered in 1997 [100]; to date, mutations in over 25 genes have been associated with AF, including those encoding cardiac gap junctions, signalling molecules, ion channels and accessory subunits (Table 15.1). Gain or loss of function mutations in genes encoding proteins controlling cardiac depolarization or repolarization can increase susceptibility to AF (Fig. 15.9). Cardiac APD shortening has been shown to lead to re-entrant wavelets [101, 102], whilst prolonging the ERP enhances the likelihood of early afterdepolarsiations (EADs) [103, 104]. Interestingly, both gain and loss of function mutations in the same gene can cause AF.

Table 15.1 Atrial fibrillation genetic variants identified in families and individuals

Gene	Gene name	Function	References
ABCC9	ATP-binding cassette, subfamily C,member 9	I_{KATP} current	[213]
GATA4	Transcription factor GATA-4	Cardiac development	[116, 170, 182, 214]
GATA5	Transcription factor GATA-5	Cardiac development	[117, 182, 215]
GATA6	Transcription factor GATA-6	Cardiac development	[216–218]
GJA5	Connexin 40	Formation of atrial gap junctions	[119, 193, 219–222]
GREM2	Gremlin-2	BMP antagonist	[223]
HCN4	Hyperpolarization activated cyclic nucleotide-gated K^+ channel 4	I_f current	[224]
JPH2	Junctophilin-2	Ca^{2+} homeostasis	[225]
KCNA5	K^+ voltage-gated channel, shaker-related subfamily, member 5	I_{Kur} current	[125, 143, 145, 149]
KCND3	K^+ voltage-gated channel, Shal-related subfamily, member 3	I_{to1} current	[140]
KCNE1	K^+ voltage-gated channel, Isk-related family, member 1	K_v channel activity modulation	[139]
KCNE2	K^+ voltage-gated channel, Isk-related family, member 2	K_v channel activity modulation	[153]
KCNE3	K^+ voltage-gated channel, Isk-related family, member 3	K_v channel activity modulation	[226]
KCNE5	KCNE1-like	K_v channel activity modulation	[227]
KCNH2	K^+ voltage-gated channel, subfamily H (eag-related), member 2	I_{Kr} current	[80, 228]
KCNJ2	K^+ inwardly-rectifying channel, subfamily J, member 2	I_{K1} current	[141, 142]
KCNJ5	Potass K^+ ium inwardly-rectifying channel, subfamily J, member 5	I_{KACh} current	[229]
KCNJ8	K^+ inwardly-rectifying channel, subfamily J, member 8	I_{KATP} current	[230]
KCNQ1	K^+ voltage-gated channel, KQT-like subfamily, member 1	I_{Ks} current	[105, 107, 108, 231–234]
LMNA	Lamin A/B	Nuclear envelope structure	[202, 203]
NKX2.5	Homeobox protein Nkx2.5	Cardiac development	[113]
NPPA	Natriuretic Peptide Precursor A	Systemic sodium homeostasis	[197, 235]
NUP155	Nucleoporin 155	Nuclear pore formation	[236]
PITX2c	Paired-like homeodomain 2c	Great vein development, left right asymmetry	[114]
RYR2	Ryanodine Receptor 2	Ca^{2+} release from sarcoplasmic reticulum	[237]

(continued)

Table 15.1 (continued)

Gene	Gene name	Function	References
SCN1B	Na^+ channel, voltage-gated, type I, beta subunit	I_{Na} current modulation	[103, 238]
SCN2B	Na^+ channel, voltage-gated, type II, beta subunit	I_{Na} current modulation	[103]
SCN3B	Na^+ channel, voltage-gated, type III, beta subunit	I_{Na} current modulation	[120, 121]
SCN4B	Na^+ channel, voltage-gated, type IV, beta subunit	I_{Na} current modulation	[224]
SCN5A	Na^+ channel, voltage-gated, type V, alpha subunit	I_{Na} current	[148, 151, 152, 239–241]

Adapted from Tucker and Ellinor [212]

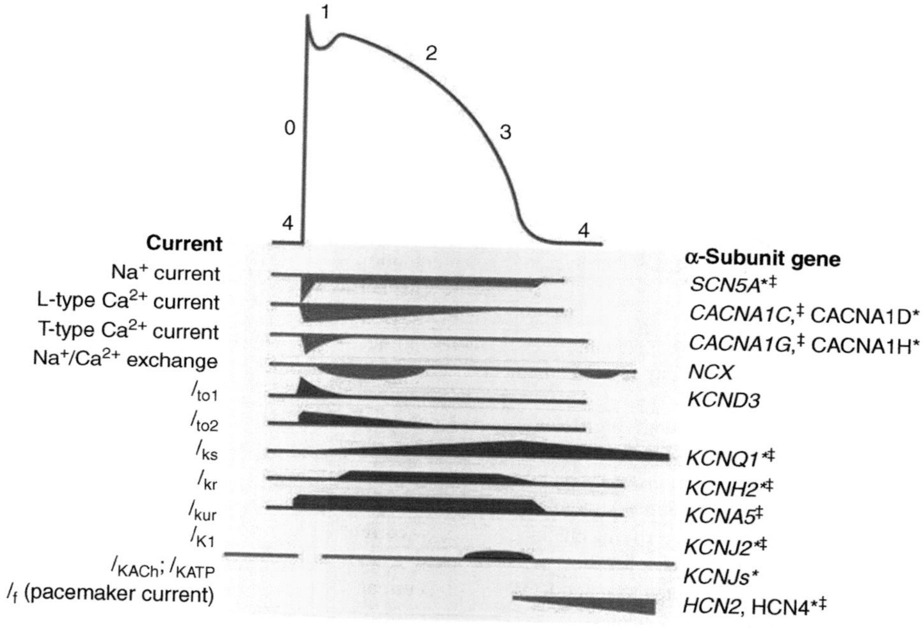

Fig. 15.9 The AP is initiated by a rapid influx of Na ions (phase 0), followed by early (phases 1 and 2) and late (phase 3) stages of repolarization, before returning to the resting membrane potential (phase 4). Repolarization is controlled by a balance between inward (red) and outward (blue) currents. The genes encoding the major currents of the atrial AP are shown. *Function-modifying subunit. #Mutation in this gene associated with atrial fibrillation. Reproduced with permission from Darbar and Roden [251]

15.4.1 Genes Associated With AF

15.4.1.1 Potassium Channel Mutations

One model proposed for AF pathogenesis describes reduced atrial ERP as a substrate for re-entrant arrhythmias [101]. This model is supported by reports of gain-of-function mutations in genes encoding subunits of cardiac ion channels responsible for generating repolarising K^+ currents; these mutations are predicted to decrease atrial APD and, therefore refractoriness. Familial AF has been associated with mutations in KCNQ1, which encodes the pore-forming alpha subunit of the cardiac K^+ channel Iks. In one mutation, functional studies have demonstrated an increase in current density, along with altered gating and kinetic properties, which results in shorter APD and ERP [105]. Other gain of function mutations have also been described [106, 107]. Another gain of function mutation in KCNQ1 has been identified with high penetrance in 5 different families with early onset AF, which also leads to an abnormal QTc, syncope and SCD [108].

KCNE1-5 encodes the regulator beta subunits of IKs, and mutations in these genes resulting in gain of function of IKs have been identified in families with AF (KCNE1: [109], KCNE2: [110], KCNE3: [111], KCNE4 [112], KCNE5: [113]). KCNH2 encodes the alpha subunit IKr; mutations in this gene resulting in increased IKr have been related to Short QT Syndrome (SQTS) and AF [112, 114, 115].

KCNJ2 encodes the inward rectifier channel Kir2.1 responsible for the IK1 current, which determines the late phase [3] of repolarisation and maintains the resting membrane potential (phase 4). Missense mutations causing gain of function have been identified in a Chinese family with AF [116]. KCNJ8 encodes the cardiac KATP channel Kir6.1, which controls a non-voltage-gated inwardly rectifying K^+ current, and leads to shortened APD under conditions of metabolic stress [117]. A missense mutation causing gain of function [118] has been identified in a cohort of lone AF patients [117].

The KCNA5 gene encodes the atria specific $K_v1.5$ channel which plays a role in the ultra-rapid delayed rectifier K^+ channel I_{Kur} involved in cardiac repolarization. *A* deletion in a kindred with early-onset lone familial AF [119] disrupts a proline-rich motif involved in tyrosine-kinase regulation of I_{Kur}, and renders the channel kinase-resistant. The precise mechanism for AF in this kindred is not certain, and might involve gain-of-function or loss-of-function of I_{Kur} but importantly, this study established the tyrosine-kinase signalling pathway as a potential therapeutic target in AF. A nonsense mutation causing loss of function has been identified in a familial case of AF [120], leading to APD prolongation and EADs. These data also predicted increased vulnerability to stress-induced triggered activity, and carriers of this *KCNA5* variant were prone to develop AF when challenged with isoproterenol [120]. This postulated mechanism for increased susceptibility to AF is supported by two studies in which investigators discovered loss-of-function mutations in *KCNA5* in patients with lone AF [103, 121]. Therefore, AF-associated mutations are likely to trigger AF by multiple mechanisms other than shortening of the atrial APD [122, 123]. The high prevalence of early-onset AF in patients with congenital long QT syndrome also supports a similar mechanism for AF in these patients [124].

Lastly, the ABCC9 gene encodes the SUR2A KATP channel subunit, which provides electrical stability under stress, including adrenergic challenge. A missense mutation causing loss of function has been identified in a case of early onset AF originating from triggers in the vein of Marshall [125].

15.4.1.2 Na+ Channel Mutations

As mentioned above, the SCN5A gene encodes the alpha subunit of the cardiac Na^+ channel which controls the I_{Na} current involved in cardiac depolarization. Rare variants in SCN5A have been identified in a familial form of AF, several of which cause overlapping phenotypes with cardiomyopathy [126]. 8 mutations in SCN5A have been seen in a cohort of lone AF patients, leading to decreased transient peak current and increased sustained current [127]. Both gain or loss of function alterations in cardiac Na^+ current can be involved in early onset AF.

SCN1B-4B encodes modifying beta subunits of the cardiac Na^+ channel. Loss of function mutations have been found in cohort of AF patients (SCN1B and SCN2B: [128], SCN3B: [129], as well as in patients with BrS [130]. SCN1Bb encodes the second beta1 transcript, Navbeta1B. A missense mutation has been found in patients with lone AF and with BrS [131], resulting in decreased peak Na^+ current and increased $K_v4.3$ transient outward current. [132].

15.4.1.3 Non-ion Channel Mutations

Table 15.1 also summarises known genes other than ion channels associated with AF. The NUP155 gene on chromosome 5q13 76 encodes nucleoporin, a component of the nuclear pore complex involved in nucleo-cytoplasmic transport. An AF locus has been mapped to chromosome 5q13 in a large AF family with autosomal recessive inheritance [133], which was then identified as NUP155 [134]. A homozygous mutation was seen in all affected family members, and heterozygous knock-out (KO) mice also demonstrated an AF phenotype.

NPPA encodes ANP, a circulating hormone produced in cardiac atria involved in BP regulation through natriuresis, diuresis and vasodilation [135]. In a family with an autosomal dominant pattern of AF, a heterozygous frameshift mutation in NPPA co-segregated with AF, and the mutant peptide shortened the atrial APD and ERP in a rat heart model [136]. A novel missense mutation in NPPA also co-segregates with early onset AF [137].

GATA4 and GATA6 genes encode cardiac transcription factors. They work synergistically with NKX2-5 in regulation of target gene expression, especially cardiogenesis [138]. A GATA4 mutation has been identified in lone AF [139]. Other studies have shown GATA4 mutations which co-segregate with AF, and lead to a decreased transcriptional effect [140–142]. Two heterozygous GATA6 mutations in 2 of 110 probands with familial AF co-segregated with AF in an autosomal dominant pattern, and were also associated with congenital cardiac defect in 3 AF patients [143]. Other studies have shown mutations in GATA6 which co-segregate with AF and lead to decreased transcriptional activity [144, 145].

The LMNA gene, mentioned above in conjunction with PCCD, encodes lamin A/C, an intermediate filament protein associated with inner nuclear membrane. A heterozygous missense mutation in LMNA have been seen in a family with AF as well as SVT, VE, muscle weakness and SCD [146]. Two further variants have been identified in two probands with AF, one with episodes of AV block, the other with reduced LV function, LBBB and a family history of heart disease [147].

The critical role of *PITX2* in the development of the pulmonary myocardium (see more below) has led investigators to examine other developmental genes important for atrial differentiation and cardiac development. A novel interaction was identified between AF and a rare variant (Q76E) within the coding region of gremlin-2 (*GREM2*; an antagonist of bone morphogenetic protein), which increases its inhibitory activity and cardiac development [148]. In a Zebra fish model GREM2 is required for cardiac laterality and atrial differentiation, and GREM2 over-activity results in slower cardiac contraction and lower contraction velocity. BMP is regulated by PITX2, and it is possible that GREM2 acts as an upstream regulator.

Another mechanism by which rare ion-channel and signalling-molecule variants might increase susceptibility to AF is through abnormal and heterogeneous disturbance of cell-to-cell impulse propagation. GJA1 and GJA5 genes encode connexin 43 and connexin 40. Four heterozygous missense mutations in GJA1 have been identified in families with AF [149]. A frameshift mutation in GJA5 leading to a protein–trafficking defect not present in lymphocyte DNA i.e. genetic mosaicism, causes failure of electric coupling between cells and has been associated with familial AF [150]. Germline mutations have also been identified in *GJA5* in patients with lone AF, and impairment of cell-to-cell communication has been confirmed in functional studies [151–153]. Furthermore, common polymorphisms in the promoter region of *GJA5* have been associated with AF, and functional studies showed that this promoter haplotype was associated with reduced luciferase activity, which is indicative of cardiac conduction heterogeneity [154] and decreased activity of two transcription factors: Sp1 and GATA-4 [155]. These data suggest that rare genetic variants in connexin-40 modulate expression of this gap-junction protein, with reduced expression causing impaired electrical cell-to-cell communication and creating conduction heterogeneity and a substrate for AF maintenance.

15.4.2 The role of Common Genetic Variants

The aim in the use of GWAS is to validate genetic markers for the population and assess how accurately these can differentiate patients from controls. Rare variants usually exhibit a large effect, result in early-onset AF and show Mendelian inheritance. Candidate SNP studies examine a small number of SNPs suspected to associate with the disease and use known biology. Genome wide association studies (GWAS) have shown that common SNPs have a role in the development of AF (Table 15.2). As of 2014, nine SNPs had been associated with AF and may allow elucidation of biological pathways and the genetic component of the more common forms of AF (Fig. 15.10). Huge sample sets are needed to establish deleterious or protective rare variants. By increasing sample size, the AFGen Consortium (www.afgen.org) have recently identified 12 more loci for AF. Further studies from large sample sizes are underway currently and the NHLB1 TOPMed program for Whole Genome Sequencing in early-inset AF is also in progress.

From these studies, functional groups can be seen, with variants in transcriptions factors, ion channels and related proteins and known myocyte proteins

Table 15.2 Genes associated with AF through GWAS studies

Transcription factors	Ion channels and related proteins	Known myocyte proteins	Others
PITX2	KCNN3	MYOZ1	C90RF3
PRRX1	HCN4	TTN	SYNE2
ZFHX3	CAV1/2	PLN	CAND2
TBX5	GJA1		NEURL
CUX2	KCNN2		METTL11B
WNT8A	SCN5A		ANXA4
	KCNJ5		CEP68
			THRB
			ASAH1
			HSF2/ SERINC
			SH3PXD2A

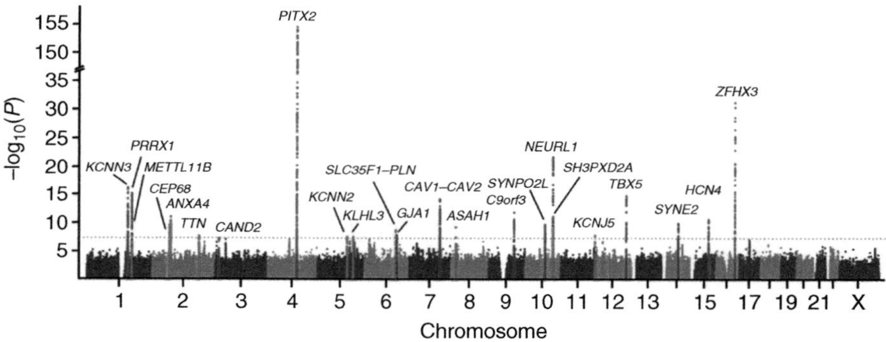

Fig. 15.10 Manhattan plot of meta-analysis results for genome-wide association with atrial fibrillation. The $-\log_{10}$ (P value) is plotted against the physical position of each SNP on each chromosome. The threshold for genome-wide significance, $P < 5 \times 10^{-8}$, is indicated by the dashed line. The previously reported loci for AF are indicated in blue, and the new loci that exceeded the genome-wide significance threshold are indicated in orange. Reproduced with permission from Christophersen et al. [257]

associating with AF. None of the GWAS hits are in amino-acid coding regions of genes. It would appear that they act instead as regulators of adjacent genes, possibly to alter the function of a promotor or enhancer, leading to up or down regulation of downstream processes. Work is needed to correlate GWAS hits with mRNA expression of genes located in the proximity of regions of SNPs. It should be remembered that the top hits from GWAS are not necessarily disease causing variants and GWAS hits may be in high linkage disequilibrium with low frequency variants [156].

15.4.2.1 4q25 Locus

The first SNP identified identified by GWAS was rs2200733, located in proximity of gene PITX2 on chromosome 4q25 and highly associated with AF [157]. The PITX2 gene encodes the paired-like transcription factor PITX2. In the human heart, PITX2c is the major isoform expressed [158] and is involved in the control of asymmetric cardiac morphogenesis [157]. A genetic variant on chromosome 4q25 has been associated with altered levels of PITX2 transcripts in left atrial (LA) tissue samples [159] and the role of PITX2 in the development of LA has been demonstrated in a KO mouse model [160]. It is thought to be required for the development of a sleeve of cardiomyocytes extending from the LA to the initial potion of the pulmonary veins [161]. This would fit with the known anatomical substrate for AF of ectopic foci from within PVs and posterior LA initiating and maintaining AF [162], and the basis of current strategy of pulmonary vein isolation as the cornerstone for ablation treatment [163].

Heterozygous KO PITXx +/− mice have normal cardiac morphology and function, but the expression of Ca^{2+} ion binding proteins, gap and tight junction and ion channels are altered, as well as showing differential expression of genes in Wnt signalling, a key fibrosis signalling pathway, with increased expression of collagen and extracellular matrix genes. Isolated mouse hearts go into AF during programmed pacing, showing shortened APDs and ERPs [164] (Fig. 15.11). Human studies have shown that PITX2c expression is decreased in patients with persistent AF [165]. There is much still to learn about PITx, including the mRNA levels in atrial tissue and target proteins.

15.4.2.2 Variants Modulating Cardiac Ion Channels

Several AF-susceptibility loci encoding cardiac ion channels have been identified. These include the K^+/Na^+ hyperpolarization-activated cyclic nucleotide-gated channel gene *HCN4* on chromosome 15q24, which encodes the cardiac pacemaker channel responsible for the funny current, and which as described above has been linked with sinus node dysfunction. The gene is expressed in most of the conduction system and is the predominant isoform of primary pacemaker in mouse hearts [166]. Rs13376333 is found on chromosome 1q21 in the KCNN3 gene, which encodes the small conductance Ca^{2+}-activated K^+ channel and is involved in atrial repolarization. Rabbit burst-pacing models which aim to mimic ectopic PV foci have shown that PV and atrial APDs are shortened, an effect inhibited by apamin which is known to block Ca^{2+}-activated K^+ channels [167].

Rs3807989 is found close to the caveolin-1 gene CAV-1 on chromosome 7q31, which encodes a cellular membrane protein selectively expressed in the atria and involved in signal transduction. This is expressed in atrial myoctyes, and is needed for the development of caveolae involved in electric signal transduction [168]. CAV1 KO mice have dilated cardiomyopathy and pulmonary hypertension [169]. Importantly, the caveolin-1 protein co-localises with, and negatively regulates the activity of, KCNH2 protein, a K^+ channel involved in cardiac repolarization, and *KCNH2* has been associated with AF in a candidate-gene association study [170].

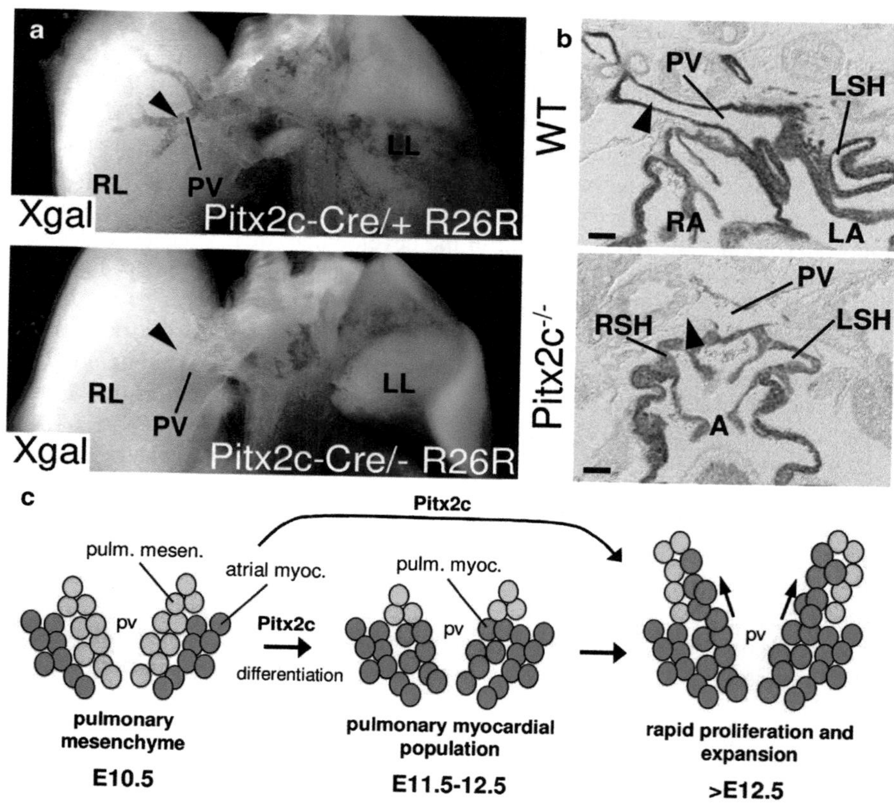

Fig. 15.11 The activity of β-galactosidase was detected in PITX2c-Cre/+R26R mice by using X-gal staining of embryos (**a**, upper panel). The absence of β -galactosidase activity in the Pitx2c-Cre/-R26R pulmonary vein indicates the deficiency of PITX2c myocardial cell (**a**, lower panel). Cardiac troponin I (cTnI) staining demonstrated differentiated myocardial cells in a wild-type heart (**b**, upper panel), but an absence of myocardial cells in the heart of a Pitx2c KO KO littermate (**b**, lower panel). The process of the development of pulmonary myocardium (pulm. myoc.) with either differentiation of pulmonary mesenchyme (pulm. mesen.) to myocardium or invasion of pulmonary vein by atrial myocardium requires presence of Pitx2c (**c**). *PV* indicates pulmonary vein, *LL* left lung, *RL* right lung, *RA* right atrium, *LSH* left sinus horn, *RSH* right sinus horn, *(R/L) A* right/left atrium. Reproduced with permission from Lubitz et al. [258]

15.4.2.3 GWAS Loci With Potential Links to Atrial Fibrosis

In 2009, two separate groups identified common risk alleles on chromosome 16q22 that associated with AF (OR 1.1–1.2). Both SNPs are close to the gene that encodes the zinc finger homeobox protein 3 (*ZFHX3*). Similarly to PITX2, ZFHX3 (also known as AT motif binding-factor 1) is a transcription factor that regulates skeletal muscle and neuronal development, with variable expression in many tissues, including the heart [171]. Interestingly, ZFHX3 regulates the transcription of the *POU1F1* gene (encoding POU class 1 homeobox 1), which not only facilitates DNA binding, but also modulates transcriptional activity of *PITX2* [172]. *ZFHX3* might also mediate its effect on the risk of

AF by modulating oxidative stress [173]. The gene associates with runt-related transcription factor 3 (RUNX3), which translocates in response to TGF-beta signalling and is an important fibrosis mediator [174, 175]. It might therefore increase susceptibility to AF by modulating pathways to increase inflammation and oxidative stress, which are important in pathogenesis of AF [176].

Rs3903239 is found on chromosome 1q24, 46kb upstream from PRRX1, which encodes a homeodomain transcription factor which is highly expressed in developing heart [177]. Studies in KO mice show that PRRX1 is needed for normal development of great vessels and lung vascularization, and is linked to pulmonary and liver fibrosis [37, 178].

SYNE2 encodes nesprin-2 that, with nesprin-1, forms a network in muscle linking the nucleoskeleton to nuclear membrane structures and the actin cytoskeleton [179]. α-Catenin interacts with nesprin-2 and emerin to regulate Wnt signalling-dependent transcription, a pathway implicated in fibrosis in the heart, kidney, and lung [180, 181]. Rs1152591 is found on chromosome 14q23 in the intron of gene SYNE2. Mutations are found in families with Emery-Dreifuss muscular dystrophy, who present with cardiomyopathy and cardiac conduction defects [177, 182]. Rs10821415 is in an open reading frame on chromosome 9, near to genes FBP1 and FBP2, which are involved in gluconeogenesis [177], although a further link has not yet been made. Rs10824026 is found on chromosome 10q22, 5 kb upstream of SYNPO2L [177], which encodes the cytoskeletal protein CHAP (cytoskeletal heart-enriched actin-associated protein). This is highly expressed in the Z-disc of cardiac and skeletal muscle and play an important role in skeletal and cardiac muscle development. Knock-down of this gene in zebrafish causes aberrant cardiac and skeletal muscle development and function [183]. It has been shown to be a susceptibility locus for AF in a family with autosomal dominant AF [100].

Taken together, there considerable evidence suggests that many common AF-susceptibility variants have the potential to modulate atrial fibrosis. Additionally, all these risk variants are likely to mediate their effect not only by regulating atrial conduction slowing, but also by modulating electrical remodelling processes that promote AF, such as shortening of the ERP.

15.4.2.4 Two Hit Hypothesis

Most patients with AF have one or more identifiable risk factors, such as hypertension or structural heart disease; however, many patients with these risk factors do not develop AF. Thus one might hypothesise that genetic determinants increase AF susceptibility in some individuals with other identifiable risk factors (genetic or acquired). In early GWAS, patients with non-familial AF were compared with controls and a small number of variants in candidate genes previously implicated in AF pathogenesis were tested. Subsequently, the GWAS paradigm of surveying the whole genome has been used successfully to identify new genomic loci contributing to AF susceptibility. For example, the risk of developing AF markedly increases (odds ratio [OR] 12–26) when a rare AF variant interacts with common AF risk alleles at the 4q25 locus [184]. Therefore, these data support the idea of a "two-hit" hypothesis—the combination of

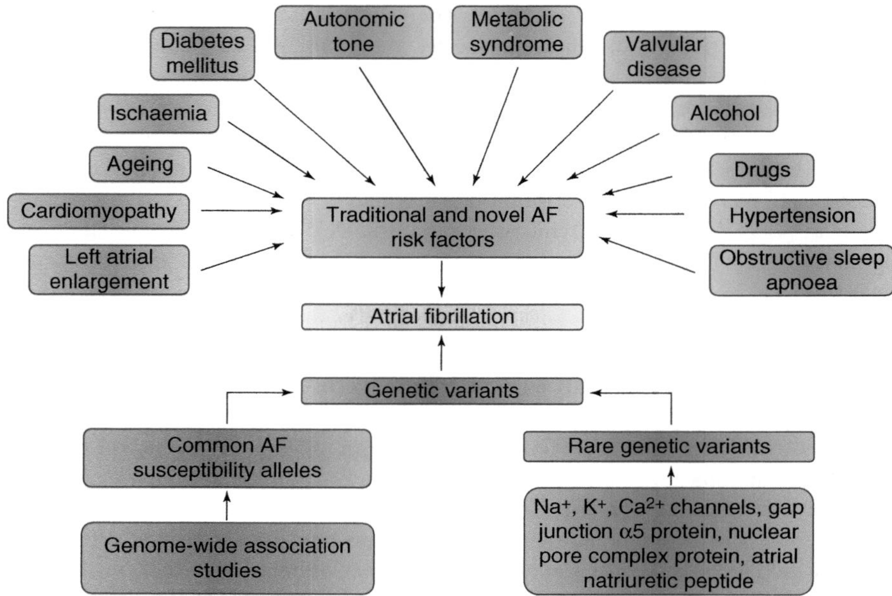

Fig. 15.12 Integration of environmental and genetic factors in AF pathogenesis. Adapted from Darbar and Roden [251]

a genetic variant with additional risk factors, such as left atrial dilatation or other genomic variants, is important in AF pathogenesis (Fig. 15.12) [185].

15.5 Bioinformatics

Exome data from NHLBI GO Exome Sequencing Project (ESP) (Seattle, WA, USA, URL. http://evs.gs.washington.edu/EVS/) reveals genetic variation in the general population. It uses next generation sequencing (NGS) of DNA from 6500 unrelated people recruited from different population studies, and is therefore representative of genetic variation in healthy subjects [127]. Rare variants associated with AF are mostly not present in the ESP population i.e. the variants are not random findings, but are disease-causing [186]. This is in contrast to studies showing that mutations previously thought to be disease causing in LQTS, sudden infant death syndrome (SIDS) and BrS show high prevalence in the ESP population and therefore may not in fact be disease causing [187–189].

15.6 Genetic Overlap With Other Cardiac Diseases

There is a large overlap between different genes involved in arrhythmic disease such as LQT, BrS, SQTS, SIDS, cardiomyopathy and AF. Indeed, most of the genes associated with AF are also associated with other arrhythmic diseases (Table 15.3).

Table 15.3 Genes implicated in overlap syndromes

	LQTS	BrS	SQTS	SIDS	Cardiomyopathy
KCNQ1	✓ [189]		✓ [189]	✓ [186]	
KCNE1	✓ [189, 242]			✓ [186]	
KCNE2	✓ [189, 242]			✓ [186]	
KCNE3	✓ [189, 242]	✓ [243]			
KCNE5		✓ [244]			
KCNJ8				✓ [186]	
KCNH2	✓ [189]	✓ [245]	✓ [189]	✓ [186]	
KCNJ2	✓ [189]		✓ [189]		
KCND3		✓ [246]			
SCN5A	✓ [189]	✓ [247]		✓ [186]	✓ [126]
SCN1Bb		✓ [131]		✓ [186]	
SCN3B		✓ [248]		✓ [186]	
ABCC9					✓ [249]
NPPA					✓ [250]
LMNA					✓ [187]
GJA1				✓ [186]	

Nine genes associated with AF have not been associated with other arrhythmic diseases (KCNE4, KCNA5, SCN2B, NUP155, GJA5, GATA4, GATA6, NKX2-5 and GREM2). These may be specific for AF, but another possibility is that these cohorts have simply not been examined yet. Patients with genetically proven SQTS or LQTS have a higher risk of early-onset AF [190, 191]. Early-onset AF occurs in 2% of patients with genetically proven LQTS as compared with a background prevalence of 0.1% [190]. In general, both shortened and prolonged QTc appear to be risk factors for AF, and especially lone AF [192].

15.7 Genetic Testing in AF

A recent HRS/EHRA expert consensus document has set out recommendations for genetic testing in channelopathies and cardiomyopathies [80]. Genetic testing is currently not indicated for AF as none of the known disease associated genes account for more than 5% of cases. Furthermore, there are no clear links between SNPs and clinical outcome.

A novel risk prediction model using data from 20,822 women without cardiovascular disease at baseline has been constructed [193]. This generates a genetic risk score using the 9 loci known to be common variants. Adding this genetic score to an AF risk algorithm improves the predictive accuracy, and may pave the way for the use of common variants for risk stratification. This may be a practical possibility with the advent of NGS, where the whole genome can be sequenced in a few days. This could lead to a personalized medicine approach, where specific variants could potentially predict whether the patient will elicit a response to a specific drug.

15.8 Role of Genomics in Therapy For AF

First line therapy for AF usually comprises anti-arrhythmic drugs, with a proportion of symptomatic patients selected for catheter ablation. Several factors contribute to the considerable variation in treatment options available—a lack of mechanism based and reliable effective treatments, together with adverse effects of both pharmacological and ablation therapy. Studies comparing rhythm and rate control have so far failed to show a survival benefit, and therefore there is an argument that there is no rationale in maintaining sinus rhythm if the patient has minimal symptoms [194]. However, maintaining sinus rhythm still has a role to play in the cases of symptomatic individuals, and large prospective studies now recruiting, may show a survival benefit including the prevention of progressive heart failure and stroke. Identifying genes responsible for AF will help understand its pathophysiology, especially in terms of heterogeneity of substrate and differences in disease mechanisms. Results from prospective, adequately powered, genotype directed clinical trials may allow us to then target therapy to the underlying molecular AF mechanisms in an individual patient, rather than relying on empiric approaches. Tailored therapy will lead to improved efficacy and reduced risk of adverse effects.

The response to drug therapy is highly variable between patients and there is currently little data to base selection of antiarrhythmic drugs in a particular individual. There is a lack of well-defined end points to measure efficacy of treatment. Often time to first symptom is used, but this correlates poorly with frequency of symptomatic episodes, and is unable to assess asymptomatic episodes. Limitations in continuous ambulatory monitoring technology has led to practical difficulties in assessing AF burden, but this is now easier with new miniaturised technology [195, 196].

Genetic factors have an important role in modulating drug responses. For rare ion-channel and other variants there are clear possible therapeutic implications. For example, in gain of function K^+ mutants, K^+ channel blockers such as sotolol might be employed. Equally, Na^+ channel blockers should be avoided if there is a loss-of-function variant in the Na^+ channel or its modifiers. However, although these mutations have a large effect size, they are rare and therefore the effects not widely applicable.

Common variants identified by GWAS have a greater aggregate effect, with combinations modulating AF risk. There have been few studies of genomic predictors of response to therapy, and they have been limited by being retrospective and of small sample size, meaning few results have been independently validated (Table 15.4). Reference 4q25 genotype has been independently associated with an improved response to class I or II antiarrhythmic drugs (OR 4.7). Beta1-adrenergic receptor polymorphisms (Arg389Gly) are significantly associated with inadequate ventricular rate control (OR 1.44) [197]. Loci with multiple SNPs associated with failure to response to 3 of more AV blocking drugs have been identified in 3 genes: MYO7A, SOX5, LANCL2. SOX5 codes for a transcription factor involved in the regulation of embryonic development and cell fate and is expressed in the heart. GWAS data have implicated SOX5 polymorphisms as PR modulators [37].

Table 15.4 Common genetic polymorphisms that modulate the response to therapies for AF

	Gene or SNP	Results	Replicated?	Reference
Rhythm control therapy	Angiotensin-converting enzyme I/D	D/D and I/D—increased AF recurrence after drugs	No	[252]
	Beta1-adrenergic receptor polymorphisms (G389R, S49G)	Arg389Arg—increased flecainide potency and increased HR during AF	Yes	[253]
	4q25: rs2200733, rs100334464; 16q22: rs7193343; 1q21: rs13376333	Re10033464—increased AF recurrence after drugs	Yes	[197]
	4q25: rs2200733, rs100334464	Any variant allele—increases early or late AF recurrence after ablation	Yes	[202, 254]
	4q25: rs2200733, rs100334464; 16q22: rs7193343; 1q21: rs13376333	Any common SNP increases AF recurrence after DCCV	No	[203]
Rate control therapy	Beta1-adrenergic receptor polymorphisms (G389R, S49G)	G389R—better rate control	Yes	[230]

Adapted from Darbar and Roden [251]

The NIH Pharmacogenomics Research Network [198] has recruited a large number of patients with well-characterized drug-response phenotypes. One project within the network is to establish a DNA repository for the large Catheter Ablation Versus Antiarrhythmic Drug Therapy for Atrial Fibrillation (CABANA) trial, in which two major approaches for the management of AF—ablation and drugs to maintain sinus rhythm—will be compared. Thus will hopefully allow investigators to address questions such as which patients are most likely to respond to, or develop complications with, ablation or drug therapy.

The Fire and Ice study [199] compared cryoballoon ablation and RF ablation. One clear point was that despite advances in technology and over 15 years' experience, recurrence rates have not dramatically fallen. The well-established parameters for determining ablation strategy include clinical presentation of AF, length of time in AF, LA diameter and presence of low voltage regions. However, genetic factors may help us better understand mechanisms for AF recurrence and therefore selection criteria for listing for ablation and allow a personalized approach in ablation strategy.

Using a candidate SNP approach, AF susceptibility alleles have been examined to identify which may potentially be associated with recurrence of AF after ablation. The main three loci which have been studied are 1q21/KCHN3, 4q25/PITX2 and 16q22/ZFHX3. No overall effect on recurrence has been found with 1q21/KCHN3 or 16q22/ZFHX3, with different effects seen depending on the cohort [200, 201]. 3 SNPs have been found at the 4q25/PITX2 locus—rs10033464, rs2200733, rs6843082. Of these, the rs2200733 has shown a significant association with AF recurrence in several European studies [201–203] but not in a Korean study [200].

There are several potential mechanisms for AF recurrence, including non-PV triggers, LA remodelling and PV sleeve reconnection. The current cornerstone for AF ablation is PVI, so those patients with non-PV triggers are likely to have worse outcomes as the procedure has not addressed the underlying mechanism for their arrhythmia. Mohanty et al. [204] tested 400 AF patients for an association between candidate panel of 16 SNPs and non-PV triggers. Two SNPs were associated with a lower risk of non-PV triggers, those at the SCN5A and 4q25/PITX2 loci, and two with a higher risk—4q25/PITx2 and ZFHx3. SNP 16q22 was associated with ectopic foci in the SVC in paroxysmal AF but not persistent AF, with a specificity of 97% in a single centre Japanese centre. PVI sleeve reconnection is a leading cause of recurrence of AF following ablation; however so far no studies have specifically examined genetic variants potentially associated with this. SNPs might also be independent predictors of AF recurrence after DCCV, with 4q25 SNPs showing higher recurrence of AF after DCCV.

The presence of LA fibrosis is also associated with poorer outcome following AF ablation [205], again because PVI does not address the issue of substrate in the rest of the LA. There have been several studies mostly in individual cohorts, with candidate genes involved in LA remodelling/fibrosis including ACEI/D [206, 207], CYP11B2 [207], AGT [208], IL6R [209], eNOS3 [210] and EPHX2 [211]. ACE I/D polymorphism may be the most promising, as it was found to be significant in both European and Asian cohorts.

Conclusion

Various rare, mostly 'private' genetic variants affecting only a single kindred that encode diverse ion-channel and signalling proteins have been found to increase the risk of developing AF through distinct genetic mechanisms. This diversity is likely to contribute to the genetic heterogeneity of AF and the differential response to therapies. The extent to which genetic variants, or combinations of genetic variants with variable penetrance determine susceptibility to AF is an area of active investigation.

Positional cloning and candidate-gene approaches have provided novel insights into the genetic mechanisms of AF, and since 2007 several GWAS have identified further genetic loci and genes implicated in AF. However, there is a disconnect between identifying genes and elucidating their mechanism. Indeed, some might argue that finding a GWAS is relatively straightforward, but determining function is not. The challenge now is to move from association to mechanism.

Current literature on genetic variation and AF ablation outcome is predominantly focused on common variants. Most studies have reported small or modest effect sizes and some contradictory findings. Previously reported associations need replication in larger cohorts of both European and non-European ancestries. Using additional genetic information could allow risk stratification based on pre-procedural characteristics to determine which patients are most likely to benefit, and tailoring ablation/drug/ablation-drug hybrid strategy for an individual patient. The development of genetic risk scores will likely be needed to clinically utilise common variant data. A large scale GWAS focused on AF recurrence after ablation may be useful to discover new genetic loci and determine the relative effect of SNPs on AF recurrence. From this, once we have a better understanding of the genetic basis of AF, we can translate this genetic knowledge to the care of patients. Critically, this should include assessment of how combinations of clinical and genetic factors predict development of AF and to what extent genomic variation adds to ordinary predictors such as hypertension or ischaemic heart disease.

References

1. Barth AS, Merk S, Arnoldi E, Zwermann L, Kloos P, Gebauer M, et al. Reprogramming of the human atrial transcriptome in permanent atrial fibrillation: expression of a ventricular-like genomic signature. Circ Res. 2005;96(9):1022–9.
2. Brugada R. Molecular biology of atrial fibrillation. Minerva Cardioangiol. 2004;52(2):65–72.
3. Barth AS, Hare JM. The potential for the transcriptome to serve as a clinical biomarker for cardiovascular diseases. Circ Res. 2006;98(12):1459–61.
4. Adán V, Crown LA. Diagnosis and treatment of sick sinus syndrome. Am Fam Physician. 2003;67(8):1725–32.
5. Lev M. The pathology of complete atrioventricular block. Prog Cardiovasc Dis. 1964;6:317–26.
6. Lenegre J. Etiology and pathology of bilateral bundle branch block in relation to complete heart block. Prog Cardiovasc Dis. 1964;6:409–44.
7. Martin CA, Huang CL-H, Grace AA. Progressive conduction diseases. Genet Card Arrhythm. 2010;2(4):509–19.
8. van Veen AA, van Rijen HV, Opthof T. Cardiac gap junction channels: modulation of expression and channel properties. Cardiovasc Res. 2001;51(2):217–29.
9. Kléber AG, Rudy Y. Basic mechanisms of cardiac impulse propagation and associated arrhythmias. Physiol Rev. 2004;84(2):431–88.
10. Herfst LJ, Rook MB, Jongsma HJ. Trafficking and functional expression of cardiac Na+ channels. J Mol Cell Cardiol. 2004;36(2):185–93.
11. Schott JJ, Alshinawi C, Kyndt F, Probst V, Hoorntje TM, Hulsbeek M, et al. Cardiac conduction defects associate with mutations in SCN5A. Nat Genet. 1999;23(1):20–1.
12. van Veen TAB, Stein M, Royer A, Le Quang K, Charpentier F, Colledge WH, et al. Impaired impulse propagation in Scn5a-knockout mice: combined contribution of excitability, connexin expression, and tissue architecture in relation to aging. Circulation. 2005;112(13):1927–35.
13. Martin CA, Zhang Y, Grace AA, Huang CL-H. In vivo studies of Scn5a+/− mice modeling Brugada syndrome demonstrate both conduction and repolarization abnormalities. J Electrocardiol. 2010;43(5):433–9.
14. Herfst LJ, Potet F, Bezzina CR, Groenewegen WA, Le Marec H, Hoorntje TM, et al. Na+ channel mutation leading to loss of function and non-progressive cardiac conduction defects. J Mol Cell Cardiol. 2003;35(5):549–57.
15. Kyndt F, Probst V, Potet F, Demolombe S, Chevallier JC, Baro I, et al. Novel SCN5A mutation leading either to isolated cardiac conduction defect or Brugada syndrome in a large French family. Circulation. 2001;104(25):3081–6.
16. Probst V, Kyndt F, Potet F, Trochu J-N, Mialet G, Demolombe S, et al. Haploinsufficiency in combination with aging causes SCN5A-linked hereditary Lenègre disease. J Am Coll Cardiol. 2003;41(4):643–52.
17. Tan HL, Bink-Boelkens MT, Bezzina CR, Viswanathan PC, Beaufort-Krol GC, van Tintelen PJ, et al. A sodium-channel mutation causes isolated cardiac conduction disease. Nature. 2001;409(6823):1043–7.

18. Bezzina CR, Rook MB, Groenewegen WA, Herfst LJ, van der Wal AC, Lam J, et al. Compound heterozygosity for mutations (W156X and R225W) in SCN5A associated with severe cardiac conduction disturbances and degenerative changes in the conduction system. Circ Res. 2003;92(2):159–68.
19. Valdivia CR, Ackerman MJ, Tester DJ, Wada T, McCormack J, Ye B, et al. A novel SCN5A arrhythmia mutation, M1766L, with expression defect rescued by mexiletine. Cardiovasc Res. 2002;55(2):279–89.
20. Viswanathan PC, Benson DW, Balser JR. A common SCN5A polymorphism modulates the biophysical effects of an SCN5A mutation. J Clin Invest. 2003;111(3):341–6.
21. Akai J, Makita N, Sakurada H, Shirai N, Ueda K, Kitabatake A, et al. A novel SCN5A mutation associated with idiopathic ventricular fibrillation without typical ECG findings of Brugada syndrome. FEBS Lett. 2000;479(1–2):29–34.
22. Wang DW, Viswanathan PC, Balser JR, George AL, Benson DW. Clinical, genetic, and biophysical characterization of SCN5A mutations associated with atrioventricular conduction block. Circulation. 2002;105(3):341–6.
23. Lupoglazoff JM, Cheav T, Baroudi G, Berthet M, Denjoy I, Cauchemez B, et al. Homozygous SCN5A mutation in long-QT syndrome with functional two-to-one atrioventricular block. Circ Res. 2001;89(2):E16–21.
24. Benson DW, Wang DW, Dyment M, Knilans TK, Fish FA, Strieper MJ, et al. Congenital sick sinus syndrome caused by recessive mutations in the cardiac sodium channel gene (SCN5A). J Clin Invest. 2003;112(7):1019–28.
25. Niu D-M, Hwang B, Hwang H-W, Wang NH, Wu J-Y, Lee P-C, et al. A common SCN5A polymorphism attenuates a severe cardiac phenotype caused by a nonsense SCN5A mutation in a Chinese family with an inherited cardiac conduction defect. J Med Genet. 2006;43(10):817–21.
26. Groenewegen WA, Firouzi M, Bezzina CR, Vliex S, van Langen IM, Sandkuijl L, et al. A cardiac sodium channel mutation cosegregates with a rare connexin40 genotype in familial atrial standstill. Circ Res. 2003;92(1):14–22.
27. McNair WP, Ku L, Taylor MRG, Fain PR, Dao D, Wolfel E, et al. SCN5A mutation associated with dilated cardiomyopathy, conduction disorder, and arrhythmia. Circulation. 2004;110(15):2163–7.
28. Olson TM, Michels VV, Ballew JD, Reyna SP, Karst ML, Herron KJ, et al. Sodium channel mutations and susceptibility to heart failure and atrial fibrillation. JAMA. 2005;293(4):447–54.
29. Laitinen-Forsblom PJ, Mäkynen P, Mäkynen H, Yli-Mäyry S, Virtanen V, Kontula K, et al. SCN5A mutation associated with cardiac conduction defect and atrial arrhythmias. J Cardiovasc Electrophysiol. 2006;17(5):480–5.
30. Ge J, Sun A, Paajanen V, Wang S, Su C, Yang Z, et al. Molecular and clinical characterization of a novel SCN5A mutation associated with atrioventricular block and dilated cardiomyopathy. Circ Arrhythm Electrophysiol. 2008;1(2):83–92.
31. Grant AO, Carboni MP, Neplioueva V, Starmer CF, Memmi M, Napolitano C, et al. Long QT syndrome, Brugada syndrome, and conduction system disease are linked to a single sodium channel mutation. J Clin Invest. 2002;110(8):1201–9.
32. Smits JPP, Eckardt L, Probst V, Bezzina CR, Schott JJ, Remme CA, et al. Genotype-phenotype relationship in Brugada syndrome: electrocardiographic features differentiate SCN5A-related patients from non-SCN5A-related patients. J Am Coll Cardiol. 2002;40(2):350–6.
33. Makiyama T, Akao M, Tsuji K, Doi T, Ohno S, Takenaka K, et al. High risk for bradyarrhythmic complications in patients with Brugada syndrome caused by SCN5A gene mutations. J Am Coll Cardiol. 2005;46(11):2100–6.
34. Shy D, Gillet L, Abriel H. Cardiac sodium channel NaV1.5 distribution in myocytes via interacting proteins: the multiple pool model. Biochim Biophys Acta. 2013;1833(4):886–94.
35. Brackenbury WJ, Isom LL. Na channel β subunits: overachievers of the ion channel family. Front Pharmacol. 2011;2:53.
36. Watanabe H, Koopmann TT, Le Scouarnec S, Yang T, Ingram CR, Schott J-J, et al. Sodium channel β1 subunit mutations associated with Brugada syndrome and cardiac conduction disease in humans. J Clin Invest. 2008;118(6):2260–8.

37. Pfeufer A, van Noord C, Marciante KD, Arking DE, Larson MG, Smith AV, et al. Genome-wide association study of PR interval. Nat Genet. 2010;42(2):153–9.
38. Bezzina CR, Barc J, Mizusawa Y, Remme CA, Gourraud J-B, Simonet F, et al. Common variants at SCN5A-SCN10A and HEY2 are associated with Brugada syndrome, a rare disease with high risk of sudden cardiac death. Nat Genet. 2013;45(9):1044–9.
39. Chambers JC, Zhao J, Terracciano CMN, Bezzina CR, Zhang W, Kaba R, et al. Genetic variation in SCN10A influences cardiac conduction. Nat Genet. 2010;42(2):149–52.
40. van den Boogaard M, Smemo S, Burnicka-Turek O, Arnolds DE, van de Werken HJG, Klous P, et al. A common genetic variant within SCN10A modulates cardiac SCN5A expression. J Clin Invest. 2014;124(4):1844–52.
41. Temple IP, Inada S, Dobrzynski H, Boyett MR. Connexins and the atrioventricular node. Heart Rhythm Off J Heart Rhythm Soc. 2013;10(2):297–304.
42. Makita N, Seki A, Sumitomo N, Chkourko H, Fukuhara S, Watanabe H, et al. A connexin40 mutation associated with a malignant variant of progressive familial heart block type I. Circ Arrhythm Electrophysiol. 2012;5(1):163–72.
43. Combrink JM, Davis WH, Snyman HW. Familial bundle branch block. Am Heart J. 1962;64:397–400.
44. Steenkamp WF. Familial trifascicular block. Am Heart J. 1972;84(6):758–60.
45. Van der Merwe PL, Weymar HW, Torrington M, Brink AJ. Progressive familial heart block (type I). A follow-up study after 10 years. South Afr Med J Suid-Afr Tydskr Vir Geneeskd. 1988;73(5):275–6.
46. Stéphan E, de Meeus A, Bouvagnet P. Hereditary bundle branch defect: right bundle branch blocks of different causes have different morphologic characteristics. Am Heart J. 1997;133(2):249–56.
47. Stephan E. Hereditary bundle branch system defect: survey of a family with four affected generations. Am Heart J. 1978;95(1):89–95.
48. Brink PA, Ferreira A, Moolman JC, Weymar HW, van der Merwe PL, Corfield VA. Gene for progressive familial heart block type I maps to chromosome 19q13. Circulation. 1995;91(6):1633–40.
49. de Meeus A, Stephan E, Debrus S, Jean MK, Loiselet J, Weissenbach J, et al. An isolated cardiac conduction disease maps to chromosome 19q. Circ Res. 1995;77(4):735–40.
50. Kruse M, Schulze-Bahr E, Corfield V, Beckmann A, Stallmeyer B, Kurtbay G, et al. Impaired endocytosis of the ion channel TRPM4 is associated with human progressive familial heart block type I. J Clin Invest. 2009;119(9):2737–44.
51. Launay P, Fleig A, Perraud AL, Scharenberg AM, Penner R, Kinet JP. TRPM4 is a Ca2+-activated nonselective cation channel mediating cell membrane depolarization. Cell. 2002;109(3):397–407.
52. Liu H, El Zein L, Kruse M, Guinamard R, Beckmann A, Bozio A, et al. Gain-of-function mutations in TRPM4 cause autosomal dominant isolated cardiac conduction disease. Circ Cardiovasc Genet. 2010;3(4):374–85.
53. Stallmeyer B, Zumhagen S, Denjoy I, Duthoit G, Hébert J-L, Ferrer X, et al. Mutational spectrum in the Ca(2+)--activated cation channel gene TRPM4 in patients with cardiac conductance disturbances. Hum Mutat. 2012;33(1):109–17.
54. Friedrich C, Rinné S, Zumhagen S, Kiper AK, Silbernagel N, Netter MF, et al. Gain-of-function mutation in TASK-4 channels and severe cardiac conduction disorder. EMBO Mol Med. 2014;6(7):937–51.
55. Bruneau BG. The developmental genetics of congenital heart disease. Nature. 2008;451(7181):943–8.
56. Bruneau BG, Srivastava D. Congenital heart disease: entering a new era of human genetics. Circ Res. 2014;114(4):598–9.
57. Zaidi S, Choi M, Wakimoto H, Ma L, Jiang J, Overton JD, et al. De novo mutations in histone-modifying genes in congenital heart disease. Nature. 2013;498(7453):220–3.
58. Moskowitz IPG, Kim JB, Moore ML, Wolf CM, Peterson MA, Shendure J, et al. A molecular pathway including Id2, Tbx5, and Nkx2-5 required for cardiac conduction system development. Cell. 2007;129(7):1365–76.

59. Sizarov A, Devalla HD, Anderson RH, Passier R, Christoffels VM, Moorman AFM. Molecular analysis of patterning of conduction tissues in the developing human heart. Circ Arrhythm Electrophysiol. 2011;4(4):532–42.
60. McCulley DJ, Black BL. Transcription factor pathways and congenital heart disease. Curr Top Dev Biol. 2012;100:253–77.
61. Nakashima Y, Yanez DA, Touma M, Nakano H, Jaroszewicz A, Jordan MC, et al. Nkx2-5 suppresses the proliferation of atrial myocytes and conduction system. Circ Res. 2014;114(7):1103–13.
62. Schott JJ, Benson DW, Basson CT, Pease W, Silberbach GM, Moak JP, et al. Congenital heart disease caused by mutations in the transcription factor NKX2-5. Science. 1998;281(5373):108–11.
63. Guntheroth W, Chun L, Patton KK, Matsushita MM, Page RL, Raskind WH. Wenckebach periodicity at rest that normalizes with tachycardia in a family with a NKX2.5 mutation. Am J Cardiol. 2012;110(11):1646–50.
64. Ouyang P, Saarel E, Bai Y, Luo C, Lv Q, Xu Y, et al. A de novo mutation in NKX2.5 associated with atrial septal defects, ventricular noncompaction, syncope and sudden death. Clin Chim Acta Int J Clin Chem. 2011;412(1–2):170–5.
65. McElhinney DB, Geiger E, Blinder J, Benson DW, Goldmuntz E. NKX2.5 mutations in patients with congenital heart disease. J Am Coll Cardiol. 2003;42(9):1650–5.
66. Basson CT, Huang T, Lin RC, Bachinsky DR, Weremowicz S, Vaglio A, et al. Different TBX5 interactions in heart and limb defined by Holt-Oram syndrome mutations. Proc Natl Acad Sci U S A. 1999;96(6):2919–24.
67. Baban A, Pitto L, Pulignani S, Cresci M, Mariani L, Gambacciani C, et al. Holt-Oram syndrome with intermediate atrioventricular canal defect, and aortic coarctation: functional characterization of a de novo TBX5 mutation. Am J Med Genet A. 2014;164A(6):1419–24.
68. Vaughan CJ, Basson CT. Molecular determinants of atrial and ventricular septal defects and patent ductus arteriosus. Am J Med Genet. 2000;97(4):304–9.
69. Bogarapu S, Bleyl SB, Calhoun A, Viskochil D, Saarel EV, Everitt MD, et al. Phenotype of a patient with contiguous deletion of TBX5 and TBX3: expanding the disease spectrum. Am J Med Genet A. 2014;164A(5):1304–9.
70. Ou Y, Strege P, Miller SM, Makielski J, Ackerman M, Gibbons SJ, et al. Syntrophin gamma 2 regulates SCN5A gating by a PDZ domain-mediated interaction. J Biol Chem. 2003;278(3):1915–23.
71. Gollob MH, Green MS, Tang AS, Gollob T, Karibe A, Ali Hassan AS, et al. Identification of a gene responsible for familial Wolff-Parkinson-White syndrome. N Engl J Med. 2001;344(24):1823–31.
72. Gollob MH, Seger JJ, Gollob TN, Tapscott T, Gonzales O, Bachinski L, et al. Novel PRKAG2 mutation responsible for the genetic syndrome of ventricular preexcitation and conduction system disease with childhood onset and absence of cardiac hypertrophy. Circulation. 2001;104(25):3030–3.
73. Light PE, Wallace CHR, Dyck JRB. Constitutively active adenosine monophosphate-activated protein kinase regulates voltage-gated sodium channels in ventricular myocytes. Circulation. 2003;107(15):1962–5.
74. Saudubray JM, Martin D, de Lonlay P, Touati G, Poggi-Travert F, Bonnet D, et al. Recognition and management of fatty acid oxidation defects: a series of 107 patients. J Inherit Metab Dis. 1999;22(4):488–502.
75. Bonnet D, Martin D, De Lonlay Null P, Villain E, Jouvet P, Rabier D, et al. Arrhythmias and conduction defects as presenting symptoms of fatty acid oxidation disorders in children. Circulation. 1999;100(22):2248–53.
76. Holm H, Gudbjartsson DF, Arnar DO, Thorleifsson G, Thorgeirsson G, Stefansdottir H, et al. Several common variants modulate heart rate, PR interval and QRS duration. Nat Genet. 2010;42(2):117–22.

77. Eijgelsheim M, Newton-Cheh C, Sotoodehnia N, de Bakker PIW, Müller M, Morrison AC, et al. Genome-wide association analysis identifies multiple loci related to resting heart rate. Hum Mol Genet. 2010;19(19):3885–94.
78. Cho YS, Go MJ, Kim YJ, Heo JY, Oh JH, Ban H-J, et al. A large-scale genome-wide association study of Asian populations uncovers genetic factors influencing eight quantitative traits. Nat Genet. 2009;41(5):527–34.
79. den Hoed M, Eijgelsheim M, Esko T, Brundel BJJM, Peal DS, Evans DM, et al. Identification of heart rate–associated loci and their effects on cardiac conduction and rhythm disorders. Nat Genet. 2013;45(6):621–31.
80. Ackerman MJ, Priori SG, Willems S, Berul C, Brugada R, Calkins H, et al. HRS/EHRA expert consensus statement on the state of genetic testing for the channelopathies and cardiomyopathies this document was developed as a partnership between the Heart Rhythm Society (HRS) and the European Heart Rhythm Association (EHRA). Heart Rhythm Off J Heart Rhythm Soc. 2011;8(8):1308–39.
81. Priori SG, Wilde AA, Horie M, Cho Y, Behr ER, Berul C, et al. HRS/EHRA/APHRS expert consensus statement on the diagnosis and management of patients with inherited primary arrhythmia syndromes. Heart Rhythm. 2013;10(12):1932–63.
82. Go AS, Hylek EM, Phillips KA, et al. Prevalence of diagnosed atrial fibrillation in adults: National implications for rhythm management and stroke prevention: the anticoagulation and risk factors in atrial fibrillation (atria) study. JAMA. 2001;285(18):2370–5.
83. Lloyd-Jones D, Adams RJ, Brown TM, Carnethon M, Dai S, De Simone G, et al. Executive summary: heart disease and stroke statistics–2010 update: a report from the American Heart Association. Circulation. 2010;121(7):948–54.
84. Grace AA, Roden DM. Systems biology and cardiac arrhythmias. Lancet Lond Engl. 2012;380(9852):1498–508.
85. Wang TJ, Parise H, Levy D, D'Agostino RB, Wolf PA, Vasan RS, et al. Obesity and the risk of new-onset atrial fibrillation. JAMA. 2004;292(20):2471–7.
86. Tedrow UB, Conen D, Ridker PM, Cook NR, Koplan BA, Manson JE, et al. The long- and short-term impact of elevated body mass index on the risk of new atrial fibrillation the WHS (women's health study). J Am Coll Cardiol. 2010;55(21):2319–27.
87. Nichols GA, Reinier K, Chugh SS. Independent contribution of diabetes to increased prevalence and incidence of atrial fibrillation. Diabetes Care. 2009;32(10):1851–6.
88. Magnani JW, Rienstra M, Lin H, Sinner MF, Lubitz SA, McManus DD, et al. Atrial fibrillation: current knowledge and future directions in epidemiology and genomics. Circulation. 2011;124(18):1982–93.
89. Cosio FG, Aliot E, Botto GL, Heidbüchel H, Geller CJ, Kirchhof P, et al. Delayed rhythm control of atrial fibrillation may be a cause of failure to prevent recurrences: reasons for change to active antiarrhythmic treatment at the time of the first detected episode. Europace. 2008;10(1):21–7.
90. Iwasaki Y, Nishida K, Kato T, Nattel S. Atrial fibrillation pathophysiology: implications for management. Circulation. 2011;124(20):2264–74.
91. Wakili R, Voigt N, Kääb S, Dobrev D, Nattel S. Recent advances in the molecular pathophysiology of atrial fibrillation. J Clin Invest. 2011;121(8):2955–68.
92. Fuster V, Rydén LE, Cannom DS, Crijns HJ, Curtis AB, Ellenbogen KA, et al. ACCF/AHA/HRS focused updates incorporated into the ACC/AHA/ESC 2006 guidelines for the management of patients with atrial fibrillation: a report of the American College of Cardiology Foundation/American Heart Association Task Force on practice guidelines developed in partnership with the European Society of Cardiology and in collaboration with the European Heart Rhythm Association and the Heart Rhythm Society. J Am Coll Cardiol. 2011;57(11):e101–98.
93. Wolff L. Familiar auricular fibrillation. New Engl J Med. 1943;229(396):7.
94. Darbar D, Herron KJ, Ballew JD, Jahangir A, Gersh BJ, Shen W-K, et al. Familial atrial fibrillation is a genetically heterogeneous disorder. J Am Coll Cardiol. 2003;41(12):2185–92.

95. Arnar DO, Thorvaldsson S, Manolio TA, Thorgeirsson G, Kristjansson K, Hakonarson H, et al. Familial aggregation of atrial fibrillation in Iceland. Eur Heart J. 2006;27(6):708–12.
96. Fox CS, Parise H, D'Agostino RB Sr, et al. Parental atrial fibrillation as a risk factor for atrial fibrillation in offspring. JAMA. 2004;291(23):2851–5.
97. Oyen N, Ranthe MF, Carstensen L, Boyd HA, Olesen MS, Olesen S-P, et al. Familial aggregation of lone atrial fibrillation in young persons. J Am Coll Cardiol. 2012;60(10):917–21.
98. Christophersen IE, Ravn LS, Budtz-Joergensen E, Skytthe A, Haunsoe S, Svendsen JH, et al. Familial Aggregation of Atrial Fibrillation A Study in Danish Twins. Circ Arrhythm Electrophysiol. 2009;2(4):378–83.
99. Ellinor PT, Yoerger DM, Ruskin JN, MacRae CA. Familial aggregation in lone atrial fibrillation. Hum Genet. 2005;118(2):179–84.
100. Brugada R, Tapscott T, Czernuszewicz GZ, Marian AJ, Iglesias A, Mont L, et al. Identification of a genetic locus for familial atrial fibrillation. N Engl J Med. 1997;336(13):905–11.
101. Nattel S. New ideas about atrial fibrillation 50 years on. Nature. 2002;415(6868):219–26.
102. Moe GK. Evidence for reentry as a mechanism of cardiac arrhythmias. Rev Physiol Biochem Pharmacol. 1975;72:55–81.
103. Yang Y, Li J, Lin X, Yang Y, Hong K, Wang L, et al. Novel KCNA5 loss-of-function mutations responsible for atrial fibrillation. J Hum Genet. 2009;54(5):277–83.
104. Shiroshita-Takeshita A, Brundel BJJM, Nattel S. Atrial fibrillation: basic mechanisms, remodeling and triggers. J Interv Card Electrophysiol Int J Arrhythm Pacing. 2005;13(3):181–93.
105. Chen Y-H, Xu S-J, Bendahhou S, Wang X-L, Wang Y, Xu W-Y, et al. KCNQ1 gain-of-function mutation in familial atrial fibrillation. Science. 2003;299(5604):251–4.
106. Hong K, Piper DR, Diaz-Valdecantos A, Brugada J, Oliva A, Burashnikov E, et al. De novo KCNQ1 mutation responsible for atrial fibrillation and short QT syndrome in utero. Cardiovasc Res. 2005;68(3):433–40.
107. Das S, Makino S, Melman YF, Shea MA, Goyal SB, Rosenzweig A, et al. Mutation in the S3 segment of KCNQ1 results in familial lone atrial fibrillation. Heart Rhythm Off J Heart Rhythm Soc. 2009;6(8):1146–53.
108. Bartos DC, Anderson JB, Bastiaenen R, Johnson JN, Gollob MH, Tester DJ, et al. A KCNQ1 mutation causes a high penetrance for familial atrial fibrillation. J Cardiovasc Electrophysiol. 2013;24(5):562–9.
109. Olesen MS, Bentzen BH, Nielsen JB, Steffensen AB, David J-P, Jabbari J, et al. Mutations in the potassium channel subunit KCNE1 are associated with early-onset familial atrial fibrillation. BMC Med Genet. 2012;13:24.
110. Yang Y, Xia M, Jin Q, Bendahhou S, Shi J, Chen Y, et al. Identification of a KCNE2 gain-of-function mutation in patients with familial atrial fibrillation. Am J Hum Genet. 2004;75(5):899–905.
111. Lundby A, Ravn LS, Svendsen JH, Haunsø S, Olesen S-P, Schmitt N. KCNE3 mutation V17M identified in a patient with lone atrial fibrillation. Cell Physiol Biochem. 2008;21(1–3):047–54.
112. Mann SA, Otway R, Guo G, Soka M, Karlsdotter L, Trivedi G, et al. Epistatic effects of potassium channel variation on cardiac repolarization and atrial fibrillation risk. J Am Coll Cardiol. 2012;59(11):1017–25.
113. Ravn LS, Aizawa Y, Pollevick GD, Hofman-Bang J, Cordeiro JM, Dixen U, et al. Gain of function in IKs secondary to a mutation in KCNE5 associated with atrial fibrillation. Heart Rhythm Off J Heart Rhythm Soc. 2008;5(3):427–35.
114. Hong K, Bjerregaard P, Gussak I, Brugada R. Short QT syndrome and atrial fibrillation caused by mutation in KCNH2. J Cardiovasc Electrophysiol. 2005;16(4):394–6.
115. Brugada R, Hong K, Dumaine R, Cordeiro J, Gaita F, Borggrefe M, et al. Sudden death associated with short-QT syndrome linked to mutations in HERG. Circulation. 2004;109(1):30–5.
116. Xia M, Jin Q, Bendahhou S, He Y, Larroque M-M, Chen Y, et al. A Kir2.1 gain-of-function mutation underlies familial atrial fibrillation. Biochem Biophys Res Commun. 2005;332(4):1012–9.

117. Delaney JT, Muhammad R, Blair MA, Kor K, Fish FA, Roden DM, et al. A KCNJ8 mutation associated with early repolarization and atrial fibrillation. Europace. 2012;14(10):1428–32.
118. Medeiros-Domingo A, Tan B-H, Crotti L, Tester DJ, Eckhardt L, Cuoretti A, et al. Gain-of-function mutation S422L in the KCNJ8-encoded cardiac K(ATP) channel Kir6.1 as a pathogenic substrate for J-wave syndromes. Heart Rhythm Off J Heart Rhythm Soc. 2010;7(10):1466–71.
119. Yang T, Yang P, Roden DM, Darbar D. A novel KCNA5 mutation implicates tyrosine kinase signaling in human atrial fibrillation. Heart Rhythm Off J Heart Rhythm Soc. 2010;7(9):1246–52.
120. Olson TM, Alekseev AE, Liu XK, Park S, Zingman LV, Bienengraeber M, et al. Kv1.5 channelopathy due to KCNA5 loss-of-function mutation causes human atrial fibrillation. Hum Mol Genet. 2006;15(14):2185–91.
121. Christophersen IE, Olesen MS, Liang B, Andersen MN, Larsen AP, Nielsen JB, et al. Genetic variation in KCNA5: impact on the atrial-specific potassium current IKur in patients with lone atrial fibrillation. Eur Heart J. 2013;34(20):1517–25.
122. Satoh T, Zipes DP. Cesium-induced atrial tachycardia degenerating into atrial fibrillation in dogs: atrial torsades de pointes? J Cardiovasc Electrophysiol. 1998;9(9):970–5.
123. Ehrlich JR, Zicha S, Coutu P, Hébert TE, Nattel S. Atrial fibrillation-associated minK38G/S polymorphism modulates delayed rectifier current and membrane localization. Cardiovasc Res. 2005;67(3):520–8.
124. Lemoine MD, Duverger JE, Naud P, Chartier D, Qi XY, Comtois P, et al. Arrhythmogenic left atrial cellular electrophysiology in a murine genetic long QT syndrome model. Cardiovasc Res. 2011;92(1):67–74.
125. Olson TM, Alekseev AE, Moreau C, Liu XK, Zingman LV, Miki T, et al. KATP channel mutation confers risk for vein of Marshall adrenergic atrial fibrillation. Nat Clin Pract Cardiovasc Med. 2007;4(2):110–6.
126. Darbar D, Kannankeril PJ, Donahue BS, Kucera G, Stubblefield T, Haines JL, et al. Cardiac sodium channel (SCN5A) variants associated with atrial fibrillation. Circulation. 2008;117(15):1927–35.
127. Olesen MS, Yuan L, Liang B, Holst AG, Nielsen N, Nielsen JB, et al. High prevalence of long QT syndrome-associated SCN5A variants in patients with early-onset lone atrial fibrillation. Circ Cardiovasc Genet. 2012;5(4):450–9.
128. Watanabe H, Darbar D, Kaiser DW, Jiramongkolchai K, Chopra S, Donahue BS, et al. Mutations in sodium channel β1- and β2-subunits associated with atrial fibrillation. Circ Arrhythm Electrophysiol. 2009;2(3):268–75.
129. Wang P, Yang Q, Wu X, Yang Y, Shi L, Wang C, et al. Functional dominant-negative mutation of sodium channel subunit gene SCN3B associated with atrial fibrillation in a Chinese GeneID population. Biochem Biophys Res Commun. 2010;398(1):98–104.
130. Hu D, Barajas-Martinez H, Burashnikov E, Springer M, Wu Y, Varro A, et al. A mutation in the beta 3 subunit of the cardiac sodium channel associated with Brugada ECG phenotype. Circ Cardiovasc Genet. 2009;2(3):270–8.
131. Olesen MS, Holst AG, Svendsen JH, Haunsø S, Tfelt-Hansen J. SCN1Bb R214Q found in 3 patients: 1 with Brugada syndrome and 2 with lone atrial fibrillation. Heart Rhythm Off J Heart Rhythm Soc. 2012;9(5):770–3.
132. Hu D, Barajas-Martínez H, Medeiros-Domingo A, Crotti L, Veltmann C, Schimpf R, et al. A novel rare variant in SCN1Bb linked to Brugada syndrome and SIDS by combined modulation of Na(v)1.5 and K(v)4.3 channel currents. Heart Rhythm Off J Heart Rhythm Soc. 2012;9(5):760–9.
133. Oberti C, Wang L, Li L, Dong J, Rao S, Du W, et al. Genome-wide linkage scan identifies a novel genetic locus on chromosome 5p13 for neonatal atrial fibrillation associated with sudden death and variable cardiomyopathy. Circulation. 2004;110(25):3753–9.
134. Zhang X, Chen S, Yoo S, Chakrabarti S, Zhang T, Ke T, et al. Mutation in nuclear pore component NUP155 leads to atrial fibrillation and early sudden cardiac death. Cell. 2008;135(6):1017–27.

135. Levin ER, Gardner DG, Samson WK. Natriuretic peptides. N Engl J Med. 1998;339(5):321–8.
136. Hodgson-Zingman DM, Karst ML, Zingman LV, Heublein DM, Darbar D, Herron KJ, et al. Atrial natriuretic peptide frameshift mutation in familial atrial fibrillation. N Engl J Med. 2008;359(2):158–65.
137. Abraham RL, Yang T, Blair M, Roden DM, Darbar D. Augmented potassium current is a shared phenotype for two genetic defects associated with familial atrial fibrillation. J Mol Cell Cardiol. 2010;48(1):181–90.
138. Zhang Y, Rath N, Hannenhalli S, Wang Z, Cappola T, Kimura S, et al. GATA and Nkx factors synergistically regulate tissue-specific gene expression and development in vivo. Dev Camb Engl. 2007;134(1):189–98.
139. Posch MG, Boldt L-H, Polotzki M, Richter S, Rolf S, Perrot A, et al. Mutations in the cardiac transcription factor GATA4 in patients with lone atrial fibrillation. Eur J Med Genet. 2010;53(4):201–3.
140. Yang Y-Q, Wang M-Y, Zhang X-L, Tan H-W, Shi H-F, Jiang W-F, et al. GATA4 loss-of-function mutations in familial atrial fibrillation. Clin Chim Acta Int J Clin Chem. 2011;412(19–20):1825–30.
141. Jiang J-Q, Shen F-F, Fang W-Y, Liu X, Yang Y-Q. Novel GATA4 mutations in lone atrial fibrillation. Int J Mol Med. 2011;28(6):1025–32.
142. Wang J, Sun Y-M, Yang Y-Q. Mutation spectrum of the GATA4 gene in patients with idiopathic atrial fibrillation. Mol Biol Rep. 2012;39(8):8127–35.
143. Yang Y-Q, Wang X-H, Tan H-W, Jiang W-F, Fang W-Y, Liu X. Prevalence and spectrum of GATA6 mutations associated with familial atrial fibrillation. Int J Cardiol. 2012;155(3):494–6.
144. Yang Y-Q, Li L, Wang J, Zhang X-L, Li R-G, Xu Y-J, et al. GATA6 loss-of-function mutation in atrial fibrillation. Eur J Med Genet. 2012;55(10):520–6.
145. Li J, Liu W-D, Yang Z-L, Yang Y-Q. Novel GATA6 loss-of-function mutation responsible for familial atrial fibrillation. Int J Mol Med. 2012;30(4):783–90.
146. Beckmann BM, Holinski-Feder E, Walter MC, Haserück N, Reithmann C, Hinterseer M, et al. Laminopathy presenting as familial atrial fibrillation. Int J Cardiol. 2010;145(2):394–6.
147. Saj M, Dabrowski R, Labib S, Jankowska A, Szperl M, Broda G, et al. Variants of the lamin A/C (LMNA) gene in non-valvular atrial fibrillation patients: a possible pathogenic role of the Thr528Met mutation. Mol Diagn Ther. 2012;16(2):99–107.
148. Müller II, Melville DB, Tanwar V, Rybski WM, Mukherjee A, Shoemaker MB, et al. Functional modeling in zebrafish demonstrates that the atrial-fibrillation-associated gene GREM2 regulates cardiac laterality, cardiomyocyte differentiation and atrial rhythm. Dis Model Mech. 2013;6(2):332–41.
149. Gollob MH, Jones DL, Krahn AD, Danis L, Gong X-Q, Shao Q, et al. Somatic mutations in the connexin 40 gene (GJA5) in atrial fibrillation. N Engl J Med. 2006;354(25):2677–88.
150. Thibodeau IL, Xu J, Li Q, Liu G, Lam K, Veinot JP, et al. Paradigm of genetic mosaicism and lone atrial fibrillation: physiological characterization of a connexin 43-deletion mutant identified from atrial tissue. Circulation. 2010;122(3):236–44.
151. Yang Y-Q, Liu X, Zhang X-L, Wang X-H, Tan H-W, Shi H-F, et al. Novel connexin40 missense mutations in patients with familial atrial fibrillation. Europace. 2010;12(10):1421–7.
152. Sun Y, Yang Y-Q, Gong X-Q, Wang X-H, Li R-G, Tan H-W, et al. Novel germline GJA5/connexin40 mutations associated with lone atrial fibrillation impair gap junctional intercellular communication. Hum Mutat. 2013;34(4):603–9.
153. Gu J-Y, Xu J-H, Yu H, Yang Y-Q. Novel GATA5 loss-of-function mutations underlie familial atrial fibrillation. Clin São Paulo Braz. 2012;67(12):1393–9.
154. Firouzi M, Ramanna H, Kok B, Jongsma HJ, Koeleman BPC, Doevendans PA, et al. Association of human connexin40 gene polymorphisms with atrial vulnerability as a risk factor for idiopathic atrial fibrillation. Circ Res. 2004;95(4):e29–33.
155. Firouzi M, Bierhuizen MFA, Kok B, Teunissen BEJ, Jansen AT, Jongsma HJ, et al. The human Cx40 promoter polymorphism -44G-->A differentially affects transcriptional regulation by Sp1 and GATA4. Biochim Biophys Acta. 2006;1759(10):491–6.

156. Holm H, Gudbjartsson DF, Sulem P, Masson G, Helgadottir HT, Zanon C, et al. A rare variant in MYH6 is associated with high risk of sick sinus syndrome. Nat Genet. 2011;43(4):316–20.
157. Gudbjartsson DF, Arnar DO, Helgadottir A, Gretarsdottir S, Holm H, Sigurdsson A, et al. Variants conferring risk of atrial fibrillation on chromosome 4q25. Nature. 2007;448(7151):353–7.
158. Franco D, Chinchilla A, Aránega AE. Transgenic insights linking pitx2 and atrial arrhythmias. Front Physiol. 2012;3:206.
159. Chung MK, Van Wagoner DR, Smith JD, Wirka RC, Topol EJ, Desai MY, et al. Abstract 4403: significant single nucleotide polymorphism associated with atrial fibrillation located on chromosome 4q25 in a whole genome association study and association with left atrial gene expression. Circulation. 2008;118(Suppl 18):S882.
160. Gage PJ, Suh H, Camper SA. Dosage requirement of Pitx2 for development of multiple organs. Dev Camb Engl. 1999;126(20):4643–51.
161. Mommersteeg MTM, Brown NA, Prall OWJ, de Gier-de Vries C, Harvey RP, AFM M, et al. Pitx2c and Nkx2-5 are required for the formation and identity of the pulmonary myocardium. Circ Res. 2007;101(9):902–9.
162. Mandapati R, Skanes A, Chen J, Berenfeld O, Jalife J. Stable microreentrant sources as a mechanism of atrial fibrillation in the isolated sheep heart. Circulation. 2000;101(2):194–9.
163. Haïssaguerre M, Jaïs P, Shah DC, Takahashi A, Hocini M, Quiniou G, et al. Spontaneous initiation of atrial fibrillation by ectopic beats originating in the pulmonary veins. N Engl J Med. 1998;339(10):659–66.
164. Kirchhof P, Kahr PC, Kaese S, Piccini I, Vokshi I, Scheld H-H, et al. PITX2c is expressed in the adult left atrium, and reducing Pitx2c expression promotes atrial fibrillation inducibility and complex changes in gene expression. Circ Cardiovasc Genet. 2011;4(2):123–33.
165. Chinchilla A, Daimi H, Lozano-Velasco E, Dominguez JN, Caballero R, Delpón E, et al. PITX2 insufficiency leads to atrial electrical and structural remodeling linked to arrhythmogenesis. Circ Cardiovasc Genet. 2011;4(3):269–79.
166. Herrmann S, Layh B, Ludwig A. Novel insights into the distribution of cardiac HCN channels: an expression study in the mouse heart. J Mol Cell Cardiol. 2011;51(6):997–1006.
167. Ozgen N, Dun W, Sosunov EA, Anyukhovsky EP, Hirose M, Duffy HS, et al. Early electrical remodeling in rabbit pulmonary vein results from trafficking of intracellular SK2 channels to membrane sites. Cardiovasc Res. 2007;75(4):758–69.
168. Gratton J-P, Bernatchez P, Sessa WC. Caveolae and caveolins in the cardiovascular system. Circ Res. 2004;94(11):1408–17.
169. Zhao Y-Y, Liu Y, Stan R-V, Fan L, Gu Y, Dalton N, et al. Defects in caveolin-1 cause dilated cardiomyopathy and pulmonary hypertension in knockout mice. Proc Natl Acad Sci U S A. 2002;99(17):11375–80.
170. Sinner MF, Pfeufer A, Akyol M, Beckmann B-M, Hinterseer M, Wacker A, et al. The non-synonymous coding IKr-channel variant KCNH2-K897T is associated with atrial fibrillation: results from a systematic candidate gene-based analysis of KCNH2 (HERG). Eur Heart J. 2008;29(7):907–14.
171. Sun X, Frierson HF, Chen C, Li C, Ran Q, Otto KB, et al. Frequent somatic mutations of the transcription factor ATBF1 in human prostate cancer. Nat Genet. 2005;37(4):407–12.
172. Qi Y, Ranish JA, Zhu X, Krones A, Zhang J, Aebersold R, et al. Atbf1 is required for the Pit1 gene early activation. Proc Natl Acad Sci U S A. 2008;105(7):2481–6.
173. Kim T-S, Kawaguchi M, Suzuki M, Jung C-G, Asai K, Shibamoto Y, et al. The ZFHX3 (ATBF1) transcription factor induces PDGFRB, which activates ATM in the cytoplasm to protect cerebellar neurons from oxidative stress. Dis Model Mech. 2010;3(11–12):752–62.
174. Verheule S, Sato T, Everett T, Engle SK, Otten D, Rubart-von der Lohe M, et al. Increased vulnerability to atrial fibrillation in transgenic mice with selective atrial fibrosis caused by overexpression of TGF-beta1. Circ Res. 2004;94(11):1458–65.
175. Mabuchi M, Kataoka H, Miura Y, Kim T-S, Kawaguchi M, Ebi M, et al. Tumor suppressor, AT motif binding factor 1 (ATBF1), translocates to the nucleus with runt domain transcrip-

tion factor 3 (RUNX3) in response to TGF-beta signal transduction. Biochem Biophys Res Commun. 2010;398(2):321–5.
176. Li J, Solus J, Chen Q, Rho YH, Milne G, Stein CM, et al. Role of inflammation and oxidative stress in atrial fibrillation. Heart Rhythm Off J Heart Rhythm Soc. 2010;7(4):438–44.
177. Ellinor PT, Lunetta KL, Albert CM, Glazer NL, Ritchie MD, Smith AV, et al. Meta-analysis identifies six new susceptibility loci for atrial fibrillation. Nat Genet. 2012;44(6):670–5.
178. Ihida-Stansbury K, McKean DM, Gebb SA, Martin JF, Stevens T, Nemenoff R, et al. Paired-related homeobox gene Prx1 is required for pulmonary vascular development. Circ Res. 2004;94(11):1507–14.
179. Mellad JA, Warren DT, Shanahan CM. Nesprins LINC the nucleus and cytoskeleton. Curr Opin Cell Biol. 2011;23(1):47–54.
180. He W, Dai C, Li Y, Zeng G, Monga SP, Liu Y. Wnt/beta-catenin signaling promotes renal interstitial fibrosis. J Am Soc Nephrol. 2009;20(4):765–76.
181. Homer RJ, Herzog EL. Recent advances in pulmonary fibrosis: implications for scleroderma. Curr Opin Rheumatol. 2010;22(6):683–9.
182. Zhang Q, Bethmann C, Worth NF, Davies JD, Wasner C, Feuer A, et al. Nesprin-1 and -2 are involved in the pathogenesis of Emery Dreifuss muscular dystrophy and are critical for nuclear envelope integrity. Hum Mol Genet. 2007;16(23):2816–33.
183. Beqqali A, Monshouwer-Kloots J, Monteiro R, Welling M, Bakkers J, Ehler E, et al. CHAP is a newly identified Z-disc protein essential for heart and skeletal muscle function. J Cell Sci. 2010;123(Pt 7):1141–50.
184. Ritchie MD, Rowan S, Kucera G, Stubblefield T, Blair M, Carter S, et al. Chromosome 4q25 variants are genetic modifiers of rare ion channel mutations associated with familial atrial fibrillation. J Am Coll Cardiol. 2012;60(13):1173–81.
185. Otway R, Vandenberg JI, Guo G, Varghese A, Castro ML, Liu J, et al. Stretch-sensitive KCNQ1 mutation A link between genetic and environmental factors in the pathogenesis of atrial fibrillation? J Am Coll Cardiol. 2007;49(5):578–86.
186. Andreasen C, Refsgaard L, Nielsen JB, Sajadieh A, Winkel BG, Tfelt-Hansen J, et al. Mutations in genes encoding cardiac ion channels previously associated with sudden infant death syndrome (SIDS) are present with high frequency in new exome data. Can J Cardiol. 2013;29(9):1104–9.
187. Andreasen C, Nielsen JB, Refsgaard L, Holst AG, Christensen AH, Andreasen L, et al. New population-based exome data are questioning the pathogenicity of previously cardiomyopathy-associated genetic variants. Eur J Hum Genet. 2013;21(9):918–28.
188. Risgaard B, Jabbari R, Refsgaard L, Holst AG, Haunsø S, Sadjadieh A, et al. High prevalence of genetic variants previously associated with Brugada syndrome in new exome data. Clin Genet. 2013;84(5):489–95.
189. Hedley PL, Jørgensen P, Schlamowitz S, Wangari R, Moolman-Smook J, Brink PA, et al. The genetic basis of long QT and short QT syndromes: a mutation update. Hum Mutat. 2009;30(11):1486–511.
190. Johnson JN, Tester DJ, Perry J, Salisbury BA, Reed CR, Ackerman MJ. Prevalence of early-onset atrial fibrillation in congenital long QT syndrome. Heart Rhythm Off J Heart Rhythm Soc. 2008;5(5):704–9.
191. Giustetto C, Schimpf R, Mazzanti A, Scrocco C, Maury P, Anttonen O, et al. Long-term follow-up of patients with short QT syndrome. J Am Coll Cardiol. 2011;58(6):587–95.
192. Nielsen JB, Graff C, Pietersen A, Lind B, Struijk JJ, Olesen MS, et al. J-shaped association between QTc interval duration and the risk of atrial fibrillation: results from the Copenhagen ECG study. J Am Coll Cardiol. 2013;61(25):2557–64.
193. Everett BM, Cook NR, Conen D, Chasman DI, Ridker PM, Albert CM. Novel genetic markers improve measures of atrial fibrillation risk prediction. Eur Heart J. 2013;34(29):2243–51.
194. Wyse DG, Waldo AL, DiMarco JP, Domanski MJ, Rosenberg Y, Schron EB, et al. A comparison of rate control and rhythm control in patients with atrial fibrillation. N Engl J Med. 2002;347(23):1825–33.

195. Israel CW, Grönefeld G, Ehrlich JR, Li Y-G, Hohnloser SH. Long-term risk of recurrent atrial fibrillation as documented by an implantable monitoring device: implications for optimal patient care. J Am Coll Cardiol. 2004;43(1):47–52.
196. Calkins H, Kuck KH, Cappato R, Brugada J, Camm AJ, Chen S-A, et al. HRS/EHRA/ECAS expert consensus statement on catheter and surgical ablation of atrial fibrillation: recommendations for patient selection, procedural techniques, patient management and follow-up, definitions, endpoints, and research trial design: a report of the Heart Rhythm Society (HRS) Task Force on Catheter and Surgical Ablation of Atrial Fibrillation. Developed in partnership with the European Heart Rhythm Association (EHRA), a registered branch of the European Society of Cardiology (ESC) and the European Cardiac Arrhythmia Society (ECAS); and in collaboration with the American College of Cardiology (ACC), American Heart Association (AHA), the Asia Pacific Heart Rhythm Society (APHRS), and the Society of Thoracic Surgeons (STS). Endorsed by the governing bodies of the American College of Cardiology Foundation, the American Heart Association, the European Cardiac Arrhythmia Society, the European Heart Rhythm Association, the Society of Thoracic Surgeons, the Asia Pacific Heart Rhythm Society, and the Heart Rhythm Society. Heart Rhythm Off J Heart Rhythm Soc. 2012;9(4):632–696.e21.
197. Parvez B, Vaglio J, Rowan S, Muhammad R, Kucera G, Stubblefield T, et al. Symptomatic response to antiarrhythmic drug therapy is modulated by a common single nucleotide polymorphism in atrial fibrillation. J Am Coll Cardiol. 2012;60(6):539–45.
198. Giacomini KM, Brett CM, Altman RB, Benowitz NL, Dolan ME, Flockhart DA, et al. The pharmacogenetics research network: from SNP discovery to clinical drug response. Clin Pharmacol Ther. 2007;81(3):328–45.
199. Kuck K-H, Brugada J, Fürnkranz A, Metzner A, Ouyang F, Chun KRJ, et al. Cryoballoon or radiofrequency ablation for paroxysmal atrial fibrillation. N Engl J Med. 2016;374(23):2235–45.
200. Choi E-K, Park JH, Lee J-Y, Nam CM, Hwang MK, Uhm J-S, et al. Korean atrial fibrillation (AF) network: genetic variants for AF do not predict ablation success. J Am Heart Assoc. 2015;4(8):e002046.
201. Shoemaker MB, Bollmann A, Lubitz SA, Ueberham L, Saini H, Montgomery J, et al. Common genetic variants and response to atrial fibrillation ablation. Circ Arrhythm Electrophysiol. 2015;8(2):296–302.
202. Husser D, Adams V, Piorkowski C, Hindricks G, Bollmann A. Chromosome 4q25 variants and atrial fibrillation recurrence after catheter ablation. J Am Coll Cardiol. 2010;55(8):747–53.
203. Benjamin Shoemaker M, Muhammad R, Parvez B, White BW, Streur M, Song Y, et al. Common atrial fibrillation risk alleles at 4q25 predict recurrence after catheter-based atrial fibrillation ablation. Heart Rhythm Off J Heart Rhythm Soc. 2013;10(3):394–400.
204. Mohanty S, Hall AW, Mohanty P, Prakash S, Trivedi C, Di Biase L, et al. Novel association of polymorphic genetic variants with predictors of outcome of catheter ablation in atrial fibrillation: new directions from a prospective study (DECAF). J Interv Card Electrophysiol Int J Arrhythm Pacing. 2016;45(1):7–17.
205. Akoum N, Daccarett M, McGann C, Segerson N, Vergara G, Kuppahally S, et al. Atrial fibrosis helps select the appropriate patient and strategy in catheter ablation of atrial fibrillation: a DE-MRI guided approach. J Cardiovasc Electrophysiol. 2011;22(1):16–22.
206. Ueberham L, Bollmann A, Shoemaker MB, Arya A, Adams V, Hindricks G, et al. Genetic ACE I/D polymorphism and recurrence of atrial fibrillation after catheter ablation. Circ Arrhythm Electrophysiol. 2013;6(4):732–7.
207. Zhang X-L, Wu L-Q, Liu X, Yang Y-Q, Tan H-W, Wang X-H, et al. Association of angiotensin-converting enzyme gene I/D and CYP11B2 gene -344T/C polymorphisms with lone atrial fibrillation and its recurrence after catheter ablation. Exp Ther Med. 2012;4(4):741–7.
208. Wang Q, Hu X, Li S, Wang X, Wang J, Zhang R, et al. Association of the angiotensinogen M235T polymorphism with recurrence after catheter ablation of acquired atrial fibrillation. J Renin-Angiotensin-Aldosterone Syst. 2015;16(4):888–97.

209. Wu G, Cheng M, Huang H, Yang B, Jiang H, Huang C. A variant of IL6R is associated with the recurrence of atrial fibrillation after catheter ablation in a Chinese Han population. PLoS One. 2014;9(6):e99623.
210. Shim J, Park JH, Lee J-Y, Uhm JS, Joung B, Lee M-H, et al. eNOS3 genetic polymorphism is related to post-ablation early recurrence of atrial fibrillation. Yonsei Med J. 2015;56(5):1244–50.
211. Wutzler A, Kestler C, Perrot A, Loehr L, Huemer M, Parwani AS, et al. Variations in the human soluble epoxide hydrolase gene and recurrence of atrial fibrillation after catheter ablation. Int J Cardiol. 2013;168(4):3647–51.
212. Tucker NR, Ellinor PT. Emerging directions in the genetics of atrial fibrillation. Circ Res. 2014;114(9):1469–82.
213. Lüke Y, Zaim H, Karakesisoglou I, Jaeger VM, Sellin L, Lu W, et al. Nesprin-2 giant (NUANCE) maintains nuclear envelope architecture and composition in skin. J Cell Sci. 2008;121(11):1887–98.
214. Deo M, Ruan Y, Pandit SV, Shah K, Berenfeld O, Blaufox A, et al. KCNJ2 mutation in short QT syndrome 3 results in atrial fibrillation and ventricular proarrhythmia. Proc Natl Acad Sci. 2013;110(11):4291–6.
215. Jabbari J, Olesen MS, Holst AG, Nielsen JB, Haunso S, Svendsen JH. Common polymorphisms in KCNJ5 [corrected] are associated with early-onset lone atrial fibrillation in Caucasians. Cardiology. 2011;118(2):116–20.
216. Lin H, Dolmatova EV, Morley MP, Lunetta KL, McManus DD, Magnani JW, et al. Gene expression and genetic variation in human atria. Heart Rhythm Off J Heart Rhythm Soc. 2014;11(2):266–71.
217. Takada F, Woude DLV, Tong H-Q, Thompson TG, Watkins SC, Kunkel LM, et al. Myozenin: an α-actinin- and γ-filamin-binding protein of skeletal muscle Z lines. Proc Natl Acad Sci. 2001;98(4):1595–600.
218. Brauch KM, Chen LY, Olson TM. Comprehensive mutation scanning of LMNA in 268 patients with lone atrial fibrillation. Am J Cardiol. 2009;103(10):1426–8.
219. Osio A, Tan L, Chen SN, Lombardi R, Nagueh SF, Shete S, et al. Myozenin 2 is a novel gene for human hypertrophic cardiomyopathy. Circ Res. 2007;100(6):766–8.
220. Frey N, Barrientos T, Shelton JM, Frank D, Rütten H, Gehring D, et al. Mice lacking calsarcin-1 are sensitized to calcineurin signaling and show accelerated cardiomyopathy in response to pathological biomechanical stress. Nat Med. 2004;10(12):1336–43.
221. Lubitz SA, Lunetta KL, Lin H, Arking DE, Trompet S, Li G, et al. Novel genetic markers associate with atrial fibrillation risk in Europeans and Japanese. J Am Coll Cardiol. 2014;63(12):1200–10.
222. Musunuru K, Strong A, Frank-Kamenetsky M, Lee NE, Ahfeldt T, Sachs KV, et al. From noncoding variant to phenotype via SORT1 at the 1p13 cholesterol locus. Nature. 2010;466(7307):714–9.
223. Petretto E, Sarwar R, Grieve I, Lu H, Kumaran MK, Muckett PJ, et al. Integrated genomic approaches implicate osteoglycin (Ogn) in the regulation of left ventricular mass. Nat Genet. 2008;40(5):546–52.
224. Duhme N, Schweizer PA, Thomas D, Becker R, Schröter J, Barends TRM, et al. Altered HCN4 channel C-linker interaction is associated with familial tachycardia–bradycardia syndrome and atrial fibrillation. Eur Heart J. 2013;34(35):2768–75.
225. Monti J, Fischer J, Paskas S, Heinig M, Schulz H, Gösele C, et al. Soluble epoxide hydrolase is a susceptibility factor for heart failure in a rat model of human disease. Nat Genet. 2008;40(5):529–37.
226. Yang Y-Q. A novel GATA5 loss-of-function mutation underlies lone atrial fibrillation. Int J Mol Med [Internet]. 2012 20 [cited 2016 Jul 24]. http://www.spandidos-publications.com/10.3892/ijmm.2012.1189.
227. Yang Y-Q, Wang J, Wang X-H, Wang Q, Tan H-W, Zhang M, et al. Mutational spectrum of the GATA5 gene associated with familial atrial fibrillation. Int J Cardiol. 2012;157(2):305–7.

228. GTEx Consortium. The genotype-tissue expression (GTEx) project. Nat Genet. 2013;45(6):580–5.
229. O'Roak BJ, Deriziotis P, Lee C, Vives L, Schwartz JJ, Girirajan S, et al. Exome sequencing in sporadic autism spectrum disorders identifies severe de novo mutations. Nat Genet. 2011;43(6):585–9.
230. Parvez B, Shoemaker MB, Muhammad R, Richardson R, Jiang L, Blair MA, et al. Common genetic polymorphism at 4q25 locus predicts atrial fibrillation recurrence after successful cardioversion. Heart Rhythm Off J Heart Rhythm Soc. 2013;10(6):849–55.
231. Hasegawa K, Ohno S, Ashihara T, Itoh H, Ding W-G, Toyoda F, et al. A novel KCNQ1 missense mutation identified in a patient with juvenile-onset atrial fibrillation causes constitutively open IKs channels. Heart Rhythm Off J Heart Rhythm Soc. 2014;11(1):67–75.
232. Ki C-S, Jung CL, Kim H, Baek K-H, Park SJ, On YK, et al. A KCNQ1 mutation causes age-dependant bradycardia and persistent atrial fibrillation. Pflugers Arch - Eur J Physiol. 2014;466(3):529–40.
233. Bartos DC, Duchatelet S, Burgess DE, Klug D, Denjoy I, Peat R, et al. R231C mutation in KCNQ1 causes long QT syndrome type 1 and familial atrial fibrillation. Heart Rhythm Off J Heart Rhythm Soc. 2011;8(1):48–55.
234. Lundby A, Ravn LS, Svendsen JH, Olesen S-P, Schmitt N. KCNQ1 mutation Q147R is associated with atrial fibrillation and prolonged QT interval. Heart Rhythm Off J Heart Rhythm Soc. 2007;4(12):1532–41.
235. Olesen MS, Refsgaard L, Holst AG, Larsen AP, Grubb S, Haunsø S, et al. A novel KCND3 gain-of-function mutation associated with early-onset of persistent lone atrial fibrillation. Cardiovasc Res. 2013;98(3):488–95.
236. Schnabel RB, Sullivan LM, Levy D, Pencina MJ, Massaro JM, D'Agostino RB, et al. Development of a risk score for atrial fibrillation (Framingham heart study): a community-based cohort study. Lancet Lond Engl. 2009;373(9665):739–45.
237. Patton KK, Ellinor PT, Heckbert SR, Christenson RH, DeFilippi C, Gottdiener JS, et al. N-terminal Pro-B-type natriuretic peptide is a major predictor of the development of atrial fibrillation. Circulation. 2009;120(18):1768–74.
238. Beavers DL, Wang W, Ather S, Voigt N, Garbino A, Dixit SS, et al. Mutation E169K in junctophilin-2 causes atrial fibrillation due to impaired RyR2 stabilization. J Am Coll Cardiol. 2013;62(21):2010–9.
239. Christophersen IE, Holmegard HN, Jabbari J, Sajadieh A, Haunsø S, Tveit A, et al. Rare variants in GJA5 are associated with early-onset lone atrial fibrillation. Can J Cardiol. 2013;29(1):111–6.
240. Shi H-F, Yang J-F, Wang Q, Li R-G, Xu Y-J, Qu X-K, et al. Prevalence and spectrum of GJA5 mutations associated with lone atrial fibrillation. Mol Med Rep. 2013;7(3):767–74.
241. Yang Y-Q, Zhang X-L, Wang X-H, Tan H-W, Shi H-F, Jiang W-F, et al. Connexin40 nonsense mutation in familial atrial fibrillation. Int J Mol Med. 2010;26(4):605–10.
242. Ohno S, Toyoda F, Zankov DP, Yoshida H, Makiyama T, Tsuji K, et al. Novel KCNE3 mutation reduces repolarizing potassium current and associated with long QT syndrome. Hum Mutat. 2009;30(4):557–63.
243. Delpón E, Cordeiro JM, Núñez L, Thomsen PEB, Guerchicoff A, Pollevick GD, et al. Functional effects of KCNE3 mutation and its role in the development of Brugada syndrome. Circ Arrhythm Electrophysiol. 2008;1(3):209–18.
244. Ohno S, Zankov DP, Ding W-G, Itoh H, Makiyama T, Doi T, et al. KCNE5 (KCNE1L) variants are novel modulators of Brugada syndrome and idiopathic ventricular fibrillation. Circ Arrhythm Electrophysiol. 2011;4(3):352–61.
245. Wilders R, Verkerk AO. Role of the R1135H KCNH2 mutation in Brugada syndrome. Int J Cardiol. 2010;144(1):149–51.
246. Giudicessi JR, Ye D, Tester DJ, Crotti L, Mugione A, Nesterenko VV, et al. Transient outward current (I(to)) gain-of-function mutations in the KCND3-encoded Kv4.3 potassium channel and Brugada syndrome. Heart Rhythm Off J Heart Rhythm Soc. 2011;8(7):1024–32.

247. Hedley PL, Jørgensen P, Schlamowitz S, Moolman-Smook J, Kanters JK, Corfield VA, et al. The genetic basis of Brugada syndrome: a mutation update. Hum Mutat. 2009;30(9):1256–66.
248. Ishikawa T, Takahashi N, Ohno S, Sakurada H, Nakamura K, On YK, et al. Novel SCN3B mutation associated with Brugada syndrome affects intracellular trafficking and function of Nav1.5. Circ J Off J Jpn Circ Soc. 2013;77(4):959–67.
249. Bienengraeber M, Olson TM, Selivanov VA, Kathmann EC, O'Cochlain F, Gao F, et al. ABCC9 mutations identified in human dilated cardiomyopathy disrupt catalytic KATP channel gating. Nat Genet. 2004;36(4):382–7.
250. Disertori M, Quintarelli S, Grasso M, Pilotto A, Narula N, Favalli V, et al. Autosomal recessive atrial dilated cardiomyopathy with standstill evolution associated with mutation of Natriuretic Peptide Precursor A. Circ Cardiovasc Genet. 2013;6(1):27–36.
251. Darbar D, Roden DM. Genetic mechanisms of atrial fibrillation: impact on response to treatment. Nat Rev Cardiol. 2013;10(6):317–29.
252. Darbar D, Motsinger AA, Ritchie MD, Gainer JV, Roden DM. ACE I/D polymorphism modulates symptomatic response to antiarrhythmic drug therapy in patients with lone atrial fibrillation. Heart Rhythm Off J Heart Rhythm Soc. 2007;4(6):743–9.
253. Nia AM, Caglayan E, Gassanov N, Zimmermann T, Aslan O, Hellmich M, et al. Beta1-Adrenoceptor polymorphism predicts flecainide action in patients with atrial fibrillation. PLoS ONE. 2010;5(7):e11421. http://www.ncbi.nlm.nih.gov/pmc/articles/PMC2896398/
254. Parvez B, Chopra N, Rowan S, Vaglio JC, Muhammad R, Roden DM, et al. A common β1-adrenergic receptor polymorphism predicts favorable response to rate control therapy in atrial fibrillation. J Am Coll Cardiol. 2012;59(1):49–56.
255. Moric E, Herbert E, Trusz-Gluza M, Filipecki A, Mazurek U, Wilczok T. The implications of genetic mutations in the sodium channel gene (SCN5A). Europace. 2003;5(4):325–34.
256. Kirchhof P, Bax J, Blomstrom-Lundquist C, Calkins H, Camm AJ, Cappato R, et al. Early and comprehensive management of atrial fibrillation: proceedings from the 2nd AFNET/EHRA consensus conference on atrial fibrillation entitled "research perspectives in atrial fibrillation". Europace. 2009;11(7):860–85.
257. Christophersen IE, Rienstra M, Roselli C, Yin X, Geelhoed B, Barnard J, et al. Large-scale analyses of common and rare variants identify 12 new loci associated with atrial fibrillation. Nat Genet. 2017;49(6):946–52.
258. Lubitz SA, Ozcan C, Magnani JW, Kääb S, Benjamin EJ, Ellinor PT. Genetics of atrial fibrillation implications for future research directions and personalized medicine. Circ Arrhythm Electrophysiol. 2010;3(3):291–9.

Cardiovascular Manifestations in Duchenne/Becker Muscular Dystrophy and Other Primary Myopathies

16

Douglas A. Stoller and Pradeep P.A. Mammen

Abstract

Patients with muscular dystrophy face a lifetime of physical challenges due to their neuromuscular disease. Physical challenges are faced on a daily basis, and as such this is the initial focus from a clinical perspective. Over the past decades, improvements in physical and respiratory therapy, coupled with advances in technology, have substantially improved quality of life for this patient group. Improvements in computer technology such as voice recognition have increased access to education and allowed greater independence for muscular dystrophy patients. Use of assisted cough techniques and ventilatory support, particularly non-invasive support, has significantly prolonged the lifespan of patients with neuromuscular disease, particularly Duchenne muscular dystrophy. As a result, cardiac disease is now thought to be the leading cause of death among those with Duchenne muscular dystrophy, and represents a new medical challenge for the current generation of patients.

Because skeletal and cardiac muscle share a common embryologic origin, the underlying genetic mutations generally impact both skeletal and cardiac muscle. Cardiac disease is common among patients with neuromuscular disease. Essentially all men with Duchenne muscular dystrophy will develop cardiomyopathy by age 18. In contrast, cardiac involvement in other muscular dystrophy patients depends on the specific subtype. For example, LGMD1B patients commonly have arrhythmias and cardiomyopathy while LGMD1C patients have isolated cases of hypertrophic cardiomyopathy. Patients with Becker muscular

D.A. Stoller
Division of Cardiovascular Medicine, University of Nebraska Medical Center, Omaha, NE, USA

P.P.A. Mammen (✉)
Internal Medicine and Integrative Biology, University of Texas Southwestern Medical Center, Dallas, TX, USA
e-mail: pradeep.mammen@utsouthwestern.edu

D. Kumar, P. Elliott (eds.), *Cardiovascular Genetics and Genomics*,
https://doi.org/10.1007/978-3-319-66114-8_16

dystrophy exhibit a broad range of cardiac phenotype—from patients with no cardiac involvement to those with severe cardiomyopathy requiring heart transplant.

Yet while cardiac disease is common, its scope and impact in neuromuscular patients is under recognized. Neurology clinics dedicated to muscular dystrophy are common, while only a handful of dedicated neuromuscular cardiomyopathy clinics exist (primarily at academic centers). Fewer still receive active treatment for cardiac disease.

In this chapter, we begin with a concise review of the basic assessment and workup of congestive heart failure in the general adult population. With this as a backdrop, the cardiac management of three common neuromuscular diseases—the dystrophinopathies, Limb-Girdle muscular dystrophy, and congenital muscular dystrophy.

Keywords
Adult cardiomyopathy • Becker muscular dystrophy • Duchenne muscular dystrophy • Limb-Girdle muscular dystrophy • Congenital muscular dystrophy

16.1 Introduction

Patients with muscular dystrophy face a lifetime of physical challenges due to their neuromuscular disease. Physical challenges are faced on a daily basis, and as such this is the initial focus from a clinical perspective. Over the past decades, improvements in physical and respiratory therapy, coupled with advances in technology, have substantially improved quality of life for this patient group [1]. Improvements in computer technology such as voice recognition have increased access to education and allowed greater independence for muscular dystrophy patients. Use of assisted cough techniques and ventilatory support, particularly non-invasive support, has significantly prolonged the lifespan of patients with neuromuscular disease, particularly Duchenne muscular dystrophy. As a result, cardiac disease is now thought to be the leading cause of death among those with Duchenne muscular dystrophy, and represents a new medical challenge for the current generation of patients.

Because skeletal and cardiac muscle share a common embryologic origin, the underlying genetic mutations generally impact both skeletal and cardiac muscle. Cardiac disease is common among patients with neuromuscular disease [2]. Essentially all men with Duchenne muscular dystrophy will develop cardiomyopathy by age 18. In contrast, cardiac involvement in other muscular dystrophy patients depends on the specific subtype. For example, LGMD1B patients commonly have arrhythmias and cardiomyopathy while LGMD1C patients have isolated cases of hypertrophic cardiomyopathy [3]. Patients with Becker muscular dystrophy exhibit a broad range of cardiac phenotype—from patients with no cardiac involvement to those with severe cardiomyopathy requiring heart transplant.

Yet while cardiac disease is common, its scope and impact in neuromuscular patients is under recognized. Neurology clinics dedicated to muscular dystrophy are common, while only a handful of dedicated neuromuscular cardiomyopathy clinics exist (primarily at academic centers). Fewer still receive active treatment for cardiac disease.

In this chapter, we begin with a concise review of the basic assessment and workup of congestive heart failure in the general adult population. With this as a backdrop, the cardiac management of three common neuromuscular diseases—the dystrophinopathies, Limb-Girdle muscular dystrophy, and congenital muscular dystrophy—will be reviewed and discussed.

16.2 General Management of Adult Cardiomyopathy

According to the most recent data available from the Centers of Disease Control and World Health organization, cardiac disease is the leading cause of death in the United State and the world at large. Heart failure, the clinical syndrome resulting from impaired cardiac flow due to abnormal filling or ejection, represents a major subset of all cardiac disease and is a common cardiac manifestation of neuromuscular disease. More than 5 million people in the United States have heart failure, with approximately 1 in 5 developing heart failure in one's adult lifetime [4].

All patients with known or suspected cardiac disease should undergo a thorough initial history and physical assessment [5]. A careful review of cardiac symptoms including chest pain, dyspnea, orthopnea, paroxysmal dyspnea, palpitations and syncope should be completed, especially in those with functional limitations. A three-generation family history is recommended in all patients with potential familial disease. The physical exam should include a thorough assessment of volume status via estimation of jugular venous pressure, perfusion of the distal extremities, and edema. Review of vital signs is particularly important in those with limited physical abilities, as tachycardia and narrow pulse pressure may be the only signs of impaired cardiac function.

In addition to a thorough history and physical exam, a thorough baseline laboratory assessment is useful for estimating risk and establishing a baseline for heart failure patients. The Seattle Heart Failure Model is a validated risk factor score which predicts 1, 2 and 5 year mortality based on a number of factors including age, ejection fraction, medications, and laboratory data. At a minimum, cardiac markers including troponin and B-type natriuretic peptide should be obtained at the initial assessment as both provide independent prognostic information. A baseline ECG should be obtained, and Holter monitoring is useful in patients with palpitations. Noninvasive cardiac imaging is likewise critical is assess for structural disease and systolic dysfunction. Cardiac MRI is preferred in suitable patients with cardiomyopathy to assess for delayed gadolinium enhancement, a prognostic marker of cardiac disease even in the absence of symptoms or systolic dysfunction.

Two important and complementary classification schemes are used in heart failure based on the initial assessment [5]. The American College of Cardiology

Foundation/American Heart Association (ACCF/AHA) classifies patients based on the risk and/or presence of cardiac disease. Stage A patients are at high risk for heart failure but currently have no detectable structural disease or symptoms; we would classify all muscular dystrophy patients would fall into this category. Stage B patients have evidence of structural heart disease (i.e. delayed gadolinium enhancement on cardiac MRI) but have no heart failure symptoms. Stage C patients have structural heart disease and symptoms, while Stage D patients require specialized interventions.

Secondly, the New York Heart Association (NYHA) functional classification groups patients by symptoms regardless of the underlying structural disease. NYHA class I patients have no symptoms with ordinary activity, while NYHA class II patients develop symptoms with exertion that mildly limit activity. NYHA class III patients remain asymptomatic at rest, but have marked physical limitation. Finally, NYHA class IV patients are symptomatic at rest or with any physical activity.

Therapy in heart failure is organized around the stage and symptom class for each patient. Heart failure management is based on numerous treatment trials resulting in a strong evidence base. The first line of heart failure treatment is medical therapy. Treatment of ACCF/AHA Stage A patients focuses on reducing the risk for subsequent heart failure. Aggressive treatment of hypertension and reducing the risk of ischemic heart disease by treating dyslipidemia and diabetes are common scenarios.

Stage B patients, asymptomatic by definition, are treated based on ejection fraction. Those with normal ejection fraction are treated essentially the same as Stage A patients. Stage B patients with systolic dysfunction (ejection fraction <50) should be treated with ACE inhibitors and beta blockers. Most of the experimental data in this subgroup is derived from patients with known CAD which accounts for a significant percentage of overall heart failure. That said, there is strong data supporting the use of ACE inhibitors in all patients with systolic function regardless of the etiology or presence of symptoms [6, 7]. Patients unable to tolerate an ACE inhibitor should be treated with angiotensin receptor blockers (ARBs) instead.

Stage C patients have structural heart disease and symptoms. All patients with systolic dysfunction should be treated with maximal doses of ACE inhibitors (ARBs if intolerant of ACE inhibitors) and beta blockers [5, 8]. ACE inhibitors have been shown to reduce mortality and hospitalizations regardless of symptom burden in those with and without the evidence of coronary disease. Data from multiple trials investigating ACE inhibitor therapy conclusively demonstrate reduced total mortality, heart failure related death, and heart failure hospitalization. Beta blockers are the second major class of medications shown to reduce mortality and hospitalization in heart failure. Similar to ACE inhibitor therapy, the benefits of beta blocker therapy are broad and include patients of all race, gender, and disease profile (with or without coronary disease, diabetes). Beta blocker therapy should be initiated once patients are clinically stable and not in decompensated heart failure.

It should be noted that specific beta blockers (metoprolol succinate, carvedilol, bisoprolol) are preferred in the management of heart failure [5, 9–12]. Unlike ACE inhibitors where all have shown consistent benefit, variation is present among beta blockers such that only those beta blockers with positive trial results are recommended (bisoprolol, carvedilol, or metoprolol succinate). While many cardiologists apply similar logic to ACE inhibitors (choosing enalopril or lisinopril), guidelines do not prefer one ACE inhibitor over another. Medical therapy with ACE inhibitors, beta blockers, and ARBs should be started at low doses and increased gradually to treatment targets established based on trial results (not response to therapy). Patients should undergo uptitration of medical therapy until target doses are met (lisinopril 20–40 mg daily, enalapril 10–20 mg twice daily, carvedilol 25 mg BID and metoprolol succinate 200 mg daily as examples) or they are unable to tolerate higher doses due to hypotension or worsening renal function. Dual therapy with low doses of beta blocker and ACE inhibitor is preferred over maximizing one at the expense of the other. Finally, lack of CHF symptoms should not delay initiation of medical therapy with ACE inhibitors or beta blockers. Both drugs have been shown to benefit asymptomatic patients and delay disease progression.

The third major class of medications for patients with Stage C heart failure are aldosterone receptor antagonists (ARBs) [5]. ARBs are typically added to medical regimens already including ACE inhibitors and beta blockers per treatment guidelines while these trials were conducted, although many believe ARBs are likely equally beneficial as ACE inhibitors and beta blockers. Mortality and hospitalization secondary to heart failure are reduced by ARB therapy. In randomized clinical trials, ARBs demonstrate a greater reduction in total mortality than either beta blockers or ACE inhibitors [13–15]. Benefit is seen for patients with a range of heart failure symptoms as well as patients after myocardial infarction. Care must be taken to avoid hyperkalemia or worsening renal function; therapy should only be started in patients with potassium less than 5 mEq/L and serum creatine less than 2.5 mg/dL. Both spironolactone and eplerenone should be started at low dose (12.5 mg daily and 25 mg daily, respectively) with close monitoring of bloodwork within 1 week of starting medication. In common use, nearly one quarter of patients will develop hyperkalemia. The dose of ARB should be reduced (or stopped) if potassium exceeds 5.5 mEq/L.

Several other classes of mediation for Stage C heart failure deserve mention [5, 8]. Combination hydralazine and isosorbide should be added to African American patients already on medical regimens including an ACE inhibitor and beta blocker based on the A-HeFT trial [16]. In the general heart failure population, ACE inhibitors have been shown to outperform vasodilator therapy but should be used in patients who cannot tolerate an ACE inhibitor or ARB (i.e. those with a history of angioedema or severe renal dysfunction). Diuretics are added in patients with evidence of volume overload on physical exam (elevated jugular venous pressure, peripheral edema or rales) as well as patients with elevated natriuretic peptides. Digoxin can be added to regimen for the goal of reducing hospitalizations, and importantly should not be discontinued in patients on stable regimens.

Medical therapy should be continued lifelong, even with complete reverse remodeling and the absence of symptoms.

Finally, appropriate Stage C patients should be considered for device therapy including an implantable cardioverter defibrillator (ICD) and cardiac resynchronization therapy (CRT) [5, 8]. Patients with severe systolic dysfunction are at increased risk for ventricular arrhythmias and sudden death. While medical therapy has been shown to reduce the risk of sudden death, further reduction of risk can be obtained with CRT and ICD therapy as primary prevention in appropriately selected patients [17–19]. Prior to implantation, patients should be first maximized on medical therapy (typically after 3–6 months), as cardiac remodeling will occur in a majority of patients. If severe systolic dysfunction (defined as an ejection fraction <35%) remains after medical therapy has been maximized, patients should be considered for an ICD. CRT therapy (pacing both right and left ventricles) should be considered in patients with severe systolic dysfunction and a wide QRS (>150 ms) with a left bundle branch pattern.

Stage D patients continue to have severe symptoms despite maximal therapy as described above [5]. Stage D patients have frequent hospitalizations, often exhibit declining renal function, and can be intolerant of guideline directed therapy such as ACE inhibitors and beta blockers. As a result, appropriately selected patients should be considered for chronic inotrope therapy, left ventricular assist devices (LVADs), and heart transplantation.

16.3 Dystrophinopathies

The dystrophin gene is the largest mammalian locus, and consists of 79 exons located at Xp21 [20]. First cloned by Louis Kunkel, dystrophin (~427 kDa) is a cytoskeletal scaffold protein that links actin to the dystrophin-sarcoglycan complex (Fig. 16.1). and is critical to membrane stability. Mutations in dystrophin result in membrane instability and increased susceptibility to damage from muscle contraction. Experimental evidence suggests that dystrophin is involved in signal transduction, and can interact with nitric oxide synthase [2]. Membrane instability also results in elevated serum levels of cardiac enzymes.

Mutations in dystrophin cause both Duchenne muscular dystrophy and the less-severe Becker muscular dystrophy [20]. Duchenne muscular dystrophy (incidence 1:3500) results from a complete lack of dystrophin. Symptoms present in early childhood, typically before the age of 5, and follow a predictable pattern (see below) [21]. Becker muscular dystrophy (incidence 1:19,000) results when overall dystrophin expression is reduced or the mutations result in protein truncation/alteration but not deletion. Unlike Duchenne, disease manifestations in Becker muscular dystrophy are variable in both onset and severity [1].

16.3.1 Duchenne Muscular Dystrophy

As noted, dystrophin is critical to membrane structure and stability. In its absence, the constant movement caused by myocardial contraction ultimately results in membrane damage. As a result, increases in intracellular calcium lead to proteolysis and ultimately destruction of cardiomyocytes. Regeneration of damaged and destroyed

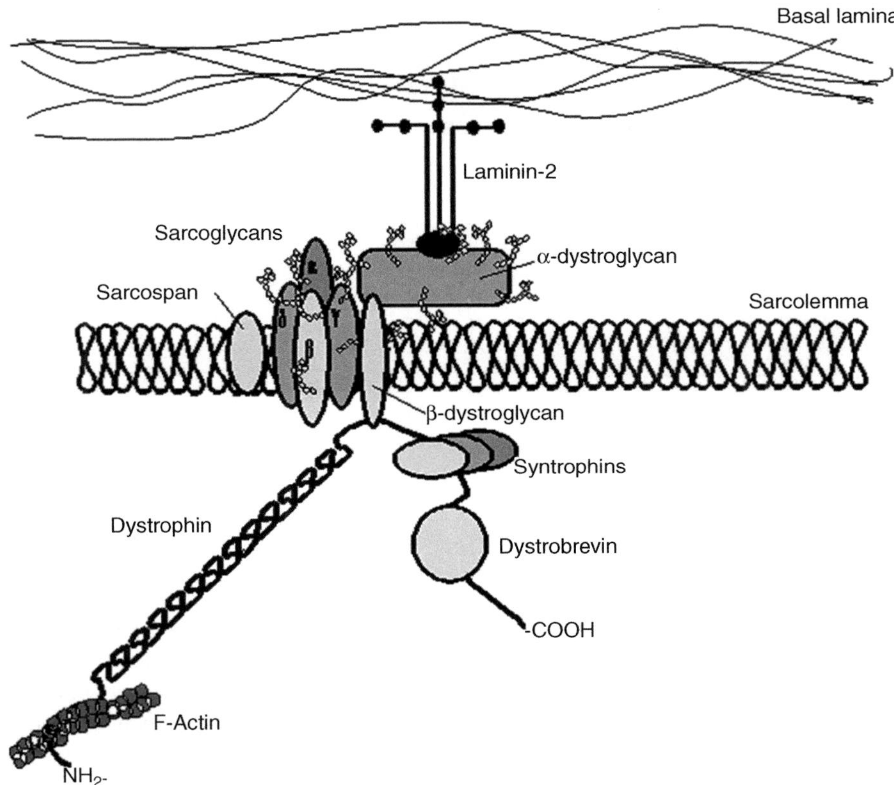

Fig. 16.1 Dystrophin-sarcoglycan membrane complex

cardiomyocytes is upregulated, but ultimately cardiomyocytes are replaced with fibrotic tissue when the repair process is overwhelmed.

Cardiac disease in Duchenne patients classically presents with abnormal ECG findings of an anterior QRS shift and tall R waves in precordial leads V1 and V2 due to characteristic scarring of the posterobasal wall [1, 22]. Fibrosis often extends to the lateral free wall including the posterior papillary muscle, and progresses from the base to apex of the heart. Necrosis is typically present at the junction between the myocardium and epicardial fat although at advanced stages transmural defects can develop. The coronary arteries can be involved although this is thought to be a secondary process (Fig. 16.2).

Because of the concomitant physical limitations, manifestations of cardiac disease in Duchenne patients are often vague. Symptoms may include fatigue, dyspnea, nausea from abdominal swelling, palpitations, and chest discomfort. Many patients will be asymptomatic until very advanced disease has developed. The cardiac physical exam can be similarly difficult. Tachycardia is common. Due to loss of dystrophin in vascular smooth muscle, patients often have low normal blood

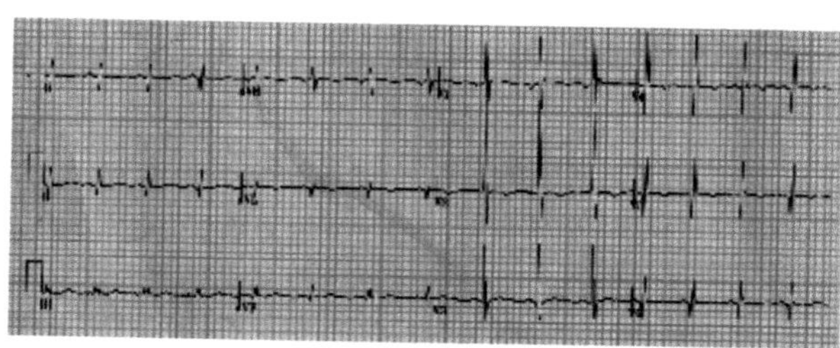

Fig. 16.2 ECG in DMD. Abnormal Q-waves in lateral (I & aVL), inferior (II, III, aVF) and apical (V5-6) leads. Abnormally tall R-waves in right precordial leads (V1-2). Widespread repolarization changes in chest leads

pressure and lukewarm extremities at baseline even though these signs are ominous in general heart failure patients. Assessment of jugular venous distention and the hepatojugular reflux are elevated in volume overload, but are uninformative in patients with ventilator support.

Given these challenges with history and physical exam, a workup via testing and imaging is vital for the care of Duchenne patients. On initial visits, we recommend a complete set of bloodwork including basic metabolic, endocrine and cardiac labs to allow calculation a Seattle Heart Failure Score. Baseline ECG and Holter monitoring are obtained to assess for arrhythmias. Cardiac MRI is strongly preferred to identify fibrosis and scarring via late gadolinium enhancement in addition to basic cardiac structure and function. In patients unable to complete a cardiac MRI, we recommend an echocardiogram with 3D assessment to allow more accurate measurement of chamber volumes. Strain imaging, a more sensitive measure of systolic function, can be informative but is not routinely completed by most echocardiography laboratories.

Essentially all patients with Duchenne muscular dystrophy will have cardiac manifestations by adulthood. Preclinical disease, typically an abnormal ECG, first presents before age 10 and then progresses [23]. Most common are right bundle branch block and repolarization abnormalities (50–60%), q waves (inferior and lateral) (~35%), wide QRS (~25%), and PR prolongation (~20%) [1, 24, 25]. Late gadolinium enhancement, typically involving the free wall of the left ventricle, precedes the development of systolic dysfunction, and is present in 60–70% of adults based on small patient series [26, 27]. Approximately 85% of patients with systolic dysfunction have +LGE. Dilated cardiomyopathy is most common (~3/4) with the remainder having hypertrophic cardiomyopathy [25]. Systolic dysfunction develops last and is present in approximately half of adults with DMD. Most patients will follow a continuum from ECG abnormalities only to hypertrophic cardiomyopathy and ultimately dilated cardiomyopathy [1].

Of note, the combination of systolic dysfunction and transmural fibrosis predicts adverse events in DMD/BMD. An impaired LV systolic function (LVEF $\leq$ 55%) and a "transmural" pattern of myocardial fibrosis independently predict the occurrence of adverse cardiac events in DMD/BMD patients. Even in DMD/BMD patients with relatively preserved LV-EF (55%), the simple and visually assessable parameter "transmural LGE" is of additive prognostic value [26].

Thousands of mutations causing Duchenne Muscular dystrophy have been identified. The vast majority, approximately 3/4, are exon deletions or duplications. The remaining quarter of mutations are point mutations [28]. Several studies have assessed whether genotype/phenotype relationships in Duchenne Muscular dystrophy with mixed conclusions. The first study published suggested that mutations in early (12, 14–17) and later (31–42) exons were associated with dilated cardiomyopathy (LV EF < 55 or LV dilation) [29]. A larger cohort analysis (n = 274 patients) from the same group was published 10 years later suggesting that patients with distal mutations were less likely to exhibit decreased ejection fraction or the presence of late gadolinium enhancement [30]. Other studies have not observed differences in mutation type or location and cardiac involvement. In one study of 205 patients from 184 families, dystrophin mutations were grouped by type (deletion, duplication, point mutation) and location (proximal or distal to exon 45). No correlation was present between mutation type or location and the age of onset for cardiac disease [31]. Ejection fraction was likewise not different based on mutation type. Similar data was observed in a third study where dystrophin mutations from 124 patients did not demonstrate that certain types or locations of mutations were associated with more severe cardiac phenotypes [32].

Current medical therapy for cardiomyopathy in Duchenne patients is derived from several small (in comparison to modern trials in adult cardiology) clinical trials coupled with established chronic heart failure regimens (See Table 16.1). Angiotensin-converting enzyme (ACEi) inhibitors are considered first line therapy based a multicenter double-blind, placebo controlled trial where approximately 60 children with normal baseline cardiac function were randomized to perindopril or placebo and treated for 3 years [33]. In the second phase of the trial, open label perindopril was given to all participants for an additional 24 months. The primary endpoints of the original trial were a drop in EF and the number of patients with LVEF < 45%. After 60 months, patients randomized to perindopril exhibited delayed onset to LV dysfunction (LVEF < 45%) although the mean EF was not different between treatment groups. More importantly, overall survival after 10 years was higher in those treated with perindopril compared to placebo (93% vs 66%, respectively) [34]. Further support of ACEi therapy was provided in a recently published trial which randomized patients with Duchenne or Becker muscular dystrophy with normal LVEF (>55%) and myocardial fibrosis on cardiac MRI to enalopril or placebo [35]. Treatment with enalopril slowed the progression of myocardial fibrosis, and fibrosis was associated with increased cardiovascular events.

Another promising therapy for Duchenne muscular therapy is aldosterone receptor blockade. Addition of ARB to medical therapy in chronic heart failure results in substantially reduced mortality and morbidity. A small randomized, double-blind, placebo-controlled multicenter trial of approximately 40 patients demonstrated benefit of ARB therapy added to ACEi [36]. Duchenne boys with normal EF and late gadolinium enhancement by cardiac MRI were randomized to eplerenone or placebo in addition to standard therapy with ACEi (or ARB). The primary outcome was change in left ventricular circumferential strain, a more sensitive marker of systolic function than ejection fraction, and EF. While systolic function declined in both

Table 16.1 Summary of clinical therapy studies in muscular dystrophy

Drug	Trial design	N	Result	Reference
Perindopril	Double blind, placebo controlled	N = 57 DMD Age 10–13 Normal EF ACEi vs placebo	Early treatment with ACEi delayed decline in LV systolic function and improved survival at 10 years	[33, 34]
Enalopril	Randomized, not blinded	N = 42 DMD or BMD Mean age 12 years EF > 50%, +fibrosis ACEi vs placebo	ACEi therapy slowed progression of myocardial fibrosis. Fibrosis was associated with CV events	[35]
Steroids	Cohort study	N = 86 DMD Mean age 9 years Mean EF 58% Steroids vs none	Steroid therapy was associated with reduced mortality and reduced onset of cardiomyopathy	[40, 41]
Eplerenone	Double blind, placebo controlled	N = 42 DMD Mean age 14.5 years EF > 45%, +fibrosis ACEi vs placebo	Eplerenone preserved LV systolic function as measured by LV strain	[36]
Carvedilol	Prospective, self-selected groups	N = 54 DMD Age 11–35 EF < 50, on ACEi Self-selected BB use	Use of BB resulted in improved survival, fewer arrhythmias, and less cardiac decline	[39]
Lisinopril and metoprolol	Cohort study	N = 42 DMD Mean age 14 years ACEi once EF < 55 BB once HR > 100	No difference in EF between group with ACEi vs ACEi + BB	[38]

treatment groups, treatment with epleronone resulted in significantly less systolic decline as measure by circumferential strain and EF.

Beta blocker therapy is recommended as outlined by chronic congestive heart failure guidelines although data supporting beta blocker therapy specifically in Duchenne muscular dystrophy remains is limited. No placebo controlled trials assessing beta blocker therapy in Duchenne muscular dystrophy exist. While small studies with patients treated with both ACE inhibitors and beta blockers demonstrate improved survival and remodeling, more recent work comparing patients on ACE inhibitors with and without beta blocker therapy did not demonstrate benefit from the addition of beta blockade [37, 38]. Improvement in EF was similar between groups treated with ACEi versus ACEi plus beta blocker (started once resting HR exceeded 100 beats per minute). One small open trial allowed Duchenne patients (n = 54 total) with depressed systolic function (EF < 50%) already on ACEi therapy were allowed to choose whether or not to receive carvedilol [39]. Patients treated with carvedilol exhibited significantly fewer cardiac events (death, severe arrhythmia or declining heart failure), although interpretation is limited by lack of randomization and blinding.

Corticosteroid therapy in childhood is supported based on restrospective analysis [40, 41]. Children treated with corticosteroids prior to onset of LV dysfunction exhibited less decline in LV systolic function than similar children not given steroids. Furthermore, a more recent cohort study comparing treatment of Duchenne patients with ACEi with or without steroids demonstrated higher overall survival in the steroid treatment cohort. In addition, steroid therapy added to ACEi significantly delayed the onset and development of cardiomyopathy. It should be noted that patients receiving steroid therapy were also started on ACEi therapy sooner than patients without steroids [41]. The mortality benefit from ACEi therapy alone is documented above [34]. How much of the observed mortality benefit in these observational studies is due to earlier initiation of ACEi therapy is not clear.

The cardiac implications of new experimental strategies including exon-skipping and nonsense mutation read-through therapies, enhanced utrophin expression, and phosphodiesterase 5 inhibitors are currently not known although trials in various phases are ongoing.

Current treatment guidelines for adults with Duchenne muscular dystrophy are basic, and as a result significant treatment variation exists between centers (See Table 16.2). Yearly assessments of systolic function are recommended after age 10. ACE inhibitors are considered first line therapy and should be initiated prior to the development of systolic dysfunction. Beta blockers and diuretics can be initiated based on general heart failure guidelines, while other medical therapies including aldosterone receptor blockade are not discussed. Symptoms consistent with arrhythmia such as palpitations should be assessed with Holter and/or event monitors.

We have established an algorithm to evaluate and treat patients with muscular dystrophy (See Table 16.3). A complete panel of labwork sufficient to calculate a Seattle Heart Failure score is obtained at the initiation visit and yearly thereafter. An ECG and Holter monitor is obtained to assess for arrhythmias. If normal, ECGs are obtained on an annual basis with additional Holter monitoring completed if and when new symptoms arise. Cardiac MRI is the preferred methodology of assessing cardiac structure and function given the added ability to assess for late gadolinium enhancement suggesting of scarring and fibrosis. Patients unable to complete a cardiac MRI undergo 3-D echocardiogram.

Based on the initial workup, an individualized treatment plan is developed. ACE inhibitors are initiated in all patients with Duchenne muscular dystrophy regardless of ejection fraction as long as blood pressure tolerates. Patients with evidence of late gadolinium enhancement on cardiac MRI are started on aldosterone antagonists. Beta blockade is reserved for patients with systolic dysfunction or sinus tachycardia. All medications are titrated to maximally tolerated doses consistent with chronic heart failure guidelines. ICD and CRT therapy is considered for patients meeting established criteria (EF $< 35\%$ for ICD therapy, QRS >150 ms with LBBB for CRT).

The likelihood of arrhythmic disease correlates with the severity of cardiomyopathy in most patients with Duchenne (and other dystrophin mutations). Requirement for permanent pacemaker placement is rare. ICD implantation is controversial, and when done should be in accordance with the patient's wishes and

Table 16.2 Summary of published recommendations for patients with muscular dystrophy [3, 5, 23, 51, 59, 60]

Duchenne muscular dystrophy
• Complete a baseline assessment of cardiac function (ECG, echocardiogram) at diagnosis or before age 6. Repeat cardiac assessments should be done at least yearly after age 10
• Signs or symptoms of arrhythmia should be investigated by Holter or event monitor.
• Early referral to cardiology for management
• Start ACE inhibitor therapy prior to evidence of cardiac dysfunction, preferably by age 10
• Beta blocker and mineralocorticoid receptor blockade therapy should be initiated per chronic heart failure guidelines
Becker muscular dystrophy
• Complete a baseline cardiac evaluation (ECG, echocardiogram) at diagnosis and every 2–5 years thereafter
• No specific recommendations regarding medical therapy beyond that recommended by chronic heart failure guidelines
Female carriers of dystrophin mutations
• Complete a baseline cardiac evaluation (ECG, echocardiogram) at diagnosis or in early adulthood (age 25–30) after the age of 16. Screen every 5 years thereafter
Limb-girdle muscular dystrophy
• For patients with variants known to have cardiac involvement, patients should undergo an ECG and echocardiogram or cardiac MRI
• Patients with an abnormality on cardiac testing (ECG, echocardiogram, or cardiac MRI) or symptoms of syncope, presyncope or palpitations should receive a Holter or event monitor to evaluate for arrhythmias
• Cardiology referral for patients with abnormal cardiac findings or symptoms suggestive of arrhythmia
• Permanent pacemaker may be considered for patients with any degree of atrioventricular block, regardless of symptoms
• Permanent pacemaker may be considered for patients with any degree of bifascicular block, regardless of symptoms
Congenital myopathy
• For patients with variants known to have cardiac involvement, patients should be closely followed for cardiac involvement
• An echocardiogram and ECG is recommended at diagnosis, prior to surgery, and when clinically indicated

established CHF guidelines (i.e. systolic dysfunction with LVEF <35% despite maximal medical therapy or after documentation of severe ventricular arrhythmias such as sustained ventricular tachycardia).

16.3.2 Becker Muscular Dystrophy

The presence of residual dystrophin expression distinguishes Becker Muscular dystrophy patients from those with Duchenne [1, 20, 42]. Available reports suggest that the distribution of genotypes in Becker Muscular dystrophy is similar to Duchenne although this may reflect mild selection bias. Nearly all studies assessing genotype

Table 16.3 Contemporary workup and management of muscular dystrophy

Initial assessment
1. Complete history and physical exam
2. Baseline blood work including complete blood count with differential, complete metabolic panel, pro-BNP, thyroid function studies, total CK, CK-MB, troponin, full lipid profile, uric acid level, hemoglobin A1c
3. Complete a 6 min walk test today to assess the submaximal exercise capacity
4. Baseline ECG and 24 h Holter monitor to assess for arrhythmias
5. Cardiac MRI with gadolinium to assess cardiac function & structure. 3D-echocardiograms are preferred in patients unable to undergo a cardiac MRI
6. Pursue genetic diagnosis for patients with variable cardiac involvement (LGMD, congenital myopathy)
Subsequent encounter(s) for potential medical therapy
• Initial choice of therapy is based on systolic function and presence of myocardial fibrosis on cardiac MRI
Normal EF → (−) myocardial fibrosis → start ACEi therapy
(+) myocardial fibrosis → start ACEi and aldosterone blockade therapy
Depressed EF → (−) myocardial fibrosis → start ACEi and BB therapy
(+) myocardial fibrosis → start ACEi, BB and aldosterone blockade therapy
• Uptitrate medical therapy to maximally tolerated doses
• Obtain an ECG and 6 min walk submaximal exercise test yearly. Holter and/or event monitors are obtained if new symptoms suggestive of arrhythmias arise.
• Repeat cardiac after imaging after patient is on maximal medical therapy or at least 1 year of therapy

are part of larger studies which include patients with Duchenne muscular dystrophy, and Becker patients with a more severe phenotype and therefore earlier presentation may have been included. Exon deletion and duplications are present in over 75% of patients, and deletion of exons 45–47 and 45–48 account for one third of Becker muscular dystrophy [28, 31]. Most important though is the impact on the mRNA reading frame. Patients with Becker muscular dystrophy are far more likely to have in-frame mutations thereby allowing at least some dystrophin expression. While frameshift and nonsense mutations are present in >75% of Duchenne patients, they account for approximately 50% of Becker patients.

Patients with Becker muscular dystrophy have a much broader range of phenotypes. Cardiomyopathy can develop at any point, and often does not correlate with skeletal muscle symptoms [1]. Genotype/phenotype correlation studies suggest that proximal mutations (proximal to exon 45), and specifically those in the *N*-terminal and rod domains, have a more severe cardiac phenotype [31]. Deletion mutations were also more severe than duplications.

The majority have patients with Becker muscular dystrophy will have an abnormal ECG (wide QRS, bundle branch block, or R > S in V1). Arrhythmias including supraventricular tachycardia and nonsustained ventricular tachycardia are present in ~20% and ~15%, respectively [43]. LV dysfunction or dilation occurs in 25–50%, usually in early adulthood (mean age 29) [31]. As with Duchenne, cardiac disease is progressive.

The treatment of cardiovascular disease in Becker muscular dystrophy has not been well studied in randomized trials, as treatment trials in muscular dystrophy patients have focused on patients with Duchenne muscular dystrophy. Because mutations in dystrophin result in both Duchenne and Becker muscular dystrophy, our approach is to treat Becker patients as we would Duchenne (See Table 16.3).

Albeit limited, advanced heart failure therapies have been utilized for the management of cardiomyopathy secondary to neuromuscular disease and Becker Muscular dystrophy specifically. A recent review of the Cardiac Transplant Research Database revealed 29 with muscular dystrophy patients (approximately half with Becker's Muscular Dystrophy) who received a heart transplant [44]. Overall survival at 1 and 5 years was similar compared to a matched cohort of heart transplant patients due to nonischemic cardiomyopathy. Left ventricular assist devices (LVAD) have been implanted in selected cases [45]. A review of Interagency Registry of Mechanical Circulatory Support (INTERMACS) found 10 cases of LVAD implantation including 7 patients with Becker muscular dystrophy [46]. While a very small cohort, overall survival and outcomes were similar to patients with dilated cardiomyopathy.

16.3.3 Female Carriers of Dystrophin Mutations

The clinical significance of dystrophin mutations in female carriers is underrecognized. The common understanding is that expression of dystrophin from the woman's normal copy is sufficient to prevent clinical symptoms, and in some cases this is true. Animal studies suggest 50% expression of dystrophin is enough to prevent cardiomyopathy [22]. However it is likewise true that a significant proportion of female carriers of dystrophin mutations will have cardiac manifestations [1, 47]. The underlying pathologic mechanism is thought to be skewed X-inactivation. To prevent overexpression, one of the X chromosomes in women is transcriptionally silenced, becoming the so called Barr body. Female carriers of dystrophin mutations thus have two distinct cell populations, one producing normal dystrophin and the other with mutated or absent dystrophin which in aggregate result in reduced dystrophin expression [48]. Skewing of X-inactivation thereby altering the amount of normal dystrophin expressed is thought to explain the observed clinical differences among this patient group [49].

The largest case series detailing cardiac manifestations in female carriers of dystrophin mutations includes approximately 200 women (~3/4 Duchenne and 1/4 Becker) between the ages of 5–69 years of which 164 were >16 years of age [47]. Patients were categorized as normal, preclinical (ECG abnormalities with normal or borderline systolic function), hypertrophic, arrhythmias, and dilated cardiomyopathy. Consistent with observations from men, cardiac disease progressed with age. By adulthood (age > 16 years), only 10% had no evidence of cardiac disease. The vast majority of women exhibited either preclinical (~45%) or hypertrophic (~30%) cardiac manifestations with no clear difference between Duchenne or Becker mutations. In a smaller case series of 25 Duchenne and 10 Becker carriers (median age 48 and 52 for Duchenne and Becker, respectively) utilizing cardiac

MRI, conclusions were slightly different [50]. While ECG abnormalities were only present in 6 of 25 Duchenne carriers, 18 of 25 exhibited delayed gadolinium enhancement and 10 of 25 had LV systolic dysfunction (average LVEF 45%). In contrast to the earlier case series, cardiac disease was less severe in Becker carriers. In the 10 Becker carriers, 2 exhibited ECG abnormalities, 5 delayed gadolinium enhancement and none had systolic dysfunction. The observation of increased cardiac involvement with age was again confirmed.

Limited direction regarding the management of female carriers of dystrophin mutations is available (See Table 16.2). The American Academy of Pediatrics recommends the carriers undergo an evaluation by a cardiologist with expertise in neuromuscular cardiomyopathy in early adulthood, with further cardiac screening every 5 years. Cardiac disease when present should be treated similarly to men with Duchenne or Becker muscular dystrophy [51].

16.4 Limb-Girdle Muscular Dystrophy

Limb-Girdle Muscular Dystrophy (LGMD) is a muscular dystrophy affecting the muscles of the shoulders and hips. LGMD can be inherited in both autosomal dominant (type 1) and autosomal recessive (type 2) patterns, and mutations in several genes result in the common phenotype of LGMD [3, 43, 52]. Mutations in myotilin (LGMD1A), lamin A/C (LGMD1B), caveolin-3 (LGMD1C), desmin (LGMD1E), the sarcoglycan protein family (LGMD2C-F), and titin (LGMD2J) are representative, and all result in the common muscular phenotype of LGMD.

Cardiac involvement in LGMD is gene specific and variable [52]. Some LGMD variants such as the sarcoglycan mutations can exhibit significant cardiac involvement while others have little reported clinical impact. LGMD variants with known cardiac involvement include LGMD1A (myotillin), LGMD1B (lamin), LGMD1D (DnaJ homolog subfamily B member 6), LGMD1E (desmin), and several LGMD2 variants (calpain-3, dysferlin, the sarcoglycans, telethonin, tripartite motif containing 32, titin, fukutin related protein, protein-O-mannosyl transferase 1, fukutin, protein-O-mannosyl transferase 2, protein O-linked mannose beta1,2-N-acetylglucosaminyl transferase, and dystroglycan). Of these, cardiac manifestations are typically most severe in patients with LGMD1B (lamin), LGMD2C-F (sarcoglycans), and LGMD2I (fukutin related protein) [3]. Of note, desmin (LGMD1E) mutations are a known cause of myofibrillar myopathy, often presenting with ventricular arrhythmias and cardiomyopathy.

Until the recent publication of the Italian LGMD registry experience (~400 patients), nearly all available data was from small case series and single centers [53]. Lamin mutations (LGMD1B) result in significant arrhythmias, with essentially all patients being affected. In the Italian registry experience, half required defibrillator placement with 3 of 13 ultimately undergoing heart transplant. Similar conclusions were made from a meta-analysis of lamin mutation carriers (both LGMD1B and Emery Dreyfus muscular dystrophy patients were included) [54]. Conduction disease precedes structural changes to the ventricle (usually dilation followed by systolic dysfunction) [55]. Pacemaker placement is common with 1/3 of patients undergoing placement, but importantly this did not alter the impact of sudden death. Death is sudden in nearly half of patients, and notably does not correlate with dilated cardiomyopathy or pacemaker placement, and pacemaker placement does not eliminate the risk of sudden death. Importantly, cardiac involvement preceded skeletal muscle symptoms in the majority.

Sarcoglycan mutations cause cardiac disease is comparable to that from dystrophin mutations (especially for LGMD2E) [43]. Cardiac disease typically presents in early adulthood, and will be present in approximately one third (Italian registry). In LGMD2E, most develop systolic dysfunction (~80% in one small series) while conduction disease seems to be less frequent (~25%).

Fukutin related protein mutations lead to cardiac disease in the majority of patients [53, 55]. A dilated cardiomoyopathy develops most frequently, and results in conduction disease (~30%) and systolic dysfunction (~40%) [43]. Cardiac and skeletal muscle involvement are not correlated.

Given the varied cardiac involvement and severity in LGMD, identifying the specific genetic mutation is important and provides significant prognostic information. We recommend an initial cardiac evaluation including ECG and cardiac MRI (or echocardiogram) at diagnosis or in early adulthood regardless of symptoms or genetic mutation. If the initial workup is normal and the mutation is known to be of low cardiac risk (LGMD1A, 1C, 2A, 2B, 2G, 2H, 2J) no further cardiac evaluation is needed unless cardiac symptoms manifest. In contrast, regular cardiac surveillance is indicated for patients with LGMD1B (lamin), 2C-2F (sarcoglycans), and 2I (fukutin related protine).

The treatment of cardiovascular disease in LGMD has not been studied in randomized trials. We follow a treatment algorithm similar to that described for dystrophin mutation carriers (See Table 16.3). LGMD1B patients in particular should be closely monitor for evidence of arrhythmias with regular ECGs and Holter/event monitoring, with consideration for PPM and/or ICD placement once conduction disease or ventricular dysrhythmias are documented. Advanced therapies including left ventricular assist devices and cardiac transplant is indicated in selected patients.

16.5 Congenital Muscular Dystrophy

Similar to LGMD, congenital muscular dystrophy (CMD) comprises a group of muscular dystrophies with the defining feature of presentation at birth [56]. Mutations in multiple genes result in CMD, some of which also cause LGMD (lamin, fukutin, and fukutin related protein). Cardiac involvement and severity in CMD is variable, like LGMD, and depends on the specific genetic mutation. What is known is based on small case series, and as CMD is a pediatric disease by definition much of the reporting is in children and not adults.

Mutations in the collagen VI (Ullrich and Bethlem CMD) and integrin seem to have little if any cardiac manifestations. Merosin-deficient CMD is the most common subtype with approximately one third of children exhibiting exhibit cardiac involvement and ECG abnormalities, dilated cardiomyopathy and systolic dysfunction have been reported [56, 57]. Cardiac involvement in CMD appears most common in patients with a dystroglycanopathy, and specifically those with fukutin mutations. Reduced systolic function is present in nearly all patients who reach adulthood, and heart failure has been identified as the cause of death in at least a fraction of patients. Dystroglycanopathy due to protein O-mannosyltransferase-2 (POMT2) mutations has also been reported have significant cardiac involvement with systolic dysfunction and dilated aortic root [58]. Mutations in lamin A/C can also cause a congenital form of LGMD1B, and are associated with arrhythmias similar to the adult-onset disease.

Given the heterogeneity of CMD, identifying the specific genetic mutation is again important and provides significant prognostic information. We recommend an initial cardiac evaluation including ECG, Holter and cardiac MRI (or echocardiogram) at diagnosis or in early adulthood regardless of symptoms or genetic mutation. Patients with CMD subtypes (specifically those mutations in merosin, fukutin, and lamin A/C) with known potential for cardiac involvement should undergo regular screening.

The treatment of cardiovascular disease in CMD has not been studied in randomized trials. We follow a treatment algorithm similar to that described for dystrophin mutation carriers (See Table 16.3).

16.6 Summary

Cardiac disease is common and often underappreciated in patients with muscular dystrophy. Advances in supportive therapies have led to improved outcomes such that cardiac disease is now a major cause of morbidity and mortality, especially in patients with dystrophin mutations. Mutations in dystrophin reduce protein expression and results in DMD (complete loss of dystrophin) and BMD (decreased expression of dystrophin). Cardiac disease is progressive, and early referral to cardiology facilitates risk stratification. Imaging with cardiac MRI is particularly useful, providing detailed structural assessment and identifying myocardial fibrosis which is often present prior to systolic dysfunction. ACEi therapy in particular should be started prior to the onset of cardiac dysfunction, and leads to improved survival in treated patients. Female carriers of dystrophin mutations are also at risk for cardiac disease, and should be screened and followed closely. In other muscular dystrophies including LGMD and CMD, cardiac involvement is variable and depends on the specific genetic mutation. As such, pursuit of a genetic diagnosis is recommended as this provides important prognostic information. Finally, advanced cardiac therapies including heart transplantation and left ventricular assist devices should be considered in carefully selected patients.

Acknowledgements None.

Funding Source

This textbook chapter was supported by grants awarded to Pradeep P. A. Mammen [National Institutes of Health Research Grants (R01-HL102478 and U54-AR068791)].

Disclosures

None.

References

1. Kamdar F, Garry DJ. Dystrophin-deficient cardiomyopathy. J Am Coll Cardiol. 2016; 67:2533–46.
2. McNally EM, MacLeod H. Therapy insight: cardiovascular complications associated with muscular dystrophies. Nat Clin Pract Cardiovasc Med. 2005;2:301–8.
3. Narayanaswami P, Weiss M, Selcen D, David W, Raynor E, Carter G, Wicklund M, Barohn RJ, Ensrud E, Griggs RC, Gronseth G, Amato AA, Guideline Development Subcommittee of the American Academy of Neurology, Practice Issues Review Panel of the American Association of Neuromuscular & Electrodiagnostic Medicine. Evidence-based guideline summary: diagnosis and treatment of limb-girdle and distal dystrophies: report of the guideline development subcommittee of the American Academy of Neurology and the practice issues review panel of the American Association of Neuromuscular & Electrodiagnostic Medicine. Neurology. 2014;83:1453–63.
4. Writing Group Members, Mozaffarian D, Benjamin EJ, Go AS, Arnett DK, Blaha MJ, Cushman M, Das SR, de Ferranti S, Despres JP, Fullerton HJ, Howard VJ, Huffman MD, Isasi CR, Jimenez MC, Judd SE, Kissela BM, Lichtman JH, Lisabeth LD, Liu S, Mackey RH, Magid DJ, McGuire DK, Mohler ER 3rd, Moy CS, Muntner P, Mussolino ME, Nasir K, Neumar RW, Nichol G, Palaniappan L, Pandey DK, Reeves MJ, Rodriguez CJ, Rosamond W, Sorlie PD, Stein J, Towfighi A, Turan TN, Virani SS, Woo D, Yeh RW, Turner MB, American Heart Association Statistics Committee, Stroke Statistics Subcommittee. Heart disease and stroke statistics-2016 update: a report from the American Heart Association. Circulation. 2016;133:e38–360.
5. Writing Committee Members, Yancy CW, Jessup M, Bozkurt B, Butler J, Casey DE Jr, Drazner MH, Fonarow GC, Geraci SA, Horwich T, Januzzi JL, Johnson MR, Kasper EK, Levy WC, Masoudi FA, McBride PE, McMurray JJ, Mitchell JE, Peterson PN, Riegel B, Sam F, Stevenson LW, Tang WH, Tsai EJ, Wilkoff BL, American College of Cardiology Foundation/American Heart Association Task Force on Practice Guidelines. 2013 ACCF/AHA guideline for the management of heart failure: a report of the American College of Cardiology Foundation/American Heart Association Task Force on practice guidelines. Circulation. 2013;128:e240–327.
6. The SOLVD Investigattors, Yusuf S, Pitt B, Davis CE, Hood WB Jr, Cohn JN. Effect of enalapril on mortality and the development of heart failure in asymptomatic patients with reduced left ventricular ejection fractions. N Engl J Med. 1992;327:685–91.
7. Jong P, Yusuf S, Rousseau MF, Ahn SA, Bangdiwala SI. Effect of enalapril on 12-year survival and life expectancy in patients with left ventricular systolic dysfunction: a follow-up study. Lancet. 2003;361:1843–8.
8. Heart Failure Society of America, Lindenfeld J, Albert NM, Boehmer JP, Collins SP, Ezekowitz JA, Givertz MM, Katz SD, Klapholz M, Moser DK, Rogers JG, Starling RC, Stevenson WG, Tang WH, Teerlink JR, Walsh MN. HFSA 2010 comprehensive heart failure practice guideline. J Card Fail. 2010;16:e1–194.
9. Effects of carvedilol, a vasodilator-beta-blocker, in patients with congestive heart failure due to ischemic heart disease. Australia-New Zealand Heart Failure Research Collaborative Group. Circulation. 1995;92:212-8.
10. Effect of metoprolol CR/XL in chronic heart failure: Metoprolol CR/XL randomised intervention trial in congestive heart failure (MERIT-HF). Lancet. 1999;353:2001-7.

11. Dargie HJ. Effect of carvedilol on outcome after myocardial infarction in patients with left-ventricular dysfunction: the CAPRICORN randomised trial. Lancet. 2001;357:1385–90.
12. The cardiac insufficiency bisoprolol study II (CIBIS-II): a randomised trial. Lancet. 1999;353:9–13.
13. Pitt B, Remme W, Zannad F, Neaton J, Martinez F, Roniker B, Bittman R, Hurley S, Kleiman J, Gatlin M, Eplerenone Post-Acute Myocardial Infarction Heart Failure Efficacy and Survival Study Investigators. Eplerenone, a selective aldosterone blocker, in patients with left ventricular dysfunction after myocardial infarction. N Engl J Med. 2003;348:1309–21.
14. Pitt B, Zannad F, Remme WJ, Cody R, Castaigne A, Perez A, Palensky J, Wittes J. The effect of spironolactone on morbidity and mortality in patients with severe heart failure. Randomized aldactone evaluation study investigators. N Engl J Med. 1999;341:709–17.
15. Zannad F, McMurray JJ, Krum H, van Veldhuisen DJ, Swedberg K, Shi H, Vincent J, Pocock SJ, Pitt B, Group E-HS. Eplerenone in patients with systolic heart failure and mild symptoms. N Engl J Med. 2011;364:11–21.
16. Taylor AL, Ziesche S, Yancy C, Carson P, D'Agostino R Jr, Ferdinand K, Taylor M, Adams K, Sabolinski M, Worcel M, Cohn JN, African-American Heart Failure Trial Investigators. Combination of isosorbide dinitrate and hydralazine in blacks with heart failure. N Engl J Med. 2004;351:2049–57.
17. Abraham WT, Fisher WG, Smith AL, Delurgio DB, Leon AR, Loh E, Kocovic DZ, Packer M, Clavell AL, Hayes DL, Ellestad M, Trupp RJ, Underwood J, Pickering F, Truex C, McAtee P, Messenger J, MIRACLE Study Group. Multicenter InSync Randomized Clinical Evaluation. Cardiac resynchronization in chronic heart failure. N Engl J Med. 2002;346:1845–53.
18. Bardy GH, Lee KL, Mark DB, Poole JE, Packer DL, Boineau R, Domanski M, Troutman C, Anderson J, Johnson G, McNulty SE, Clapp-Channing N, Davidson-Ray LD, Fraulo ES, Fishbein DP, Luceri RM, Ip JH, Sudden Cardiac Death in Heart Failure Trial Investigators. Amiodarone or an implantable cardioverter-defibrillator for congestive heart failure. N Engl J Med. 2005;352:225–37.
19. Moss AJ, Zareba W, Hall WJ, Klein H, Wilber DJ, Cannom DS, Daubert JP, Higgins SL, Brown MW, Andrews ML, Multicenter Automatic Defibrillator Implantation Trial II Investigators. Prophylactic implantation of a defibrillator in patients with myocardial infarction and reduced ejection fraction. N Engl J Med. 2002;346:877–83.
20. Flanigan KM. Duchenne and Becker muscular dystrophies. Neurol Clin. 2014;32:671–88. viii
21. Bushby K, Finkel R, Birnkrant DJ, Case LE, Clemens PR, Cripe L, Kaul A, Kinnett K, McDonald C, Pandya S, Poysky J, Shapiro F, Tomezsko J, Constantin C, Group DMDCCW. Diagnosis and management of Duchenne muscular dystrophy, part 1: diagnosis, and pharmacological and psychosocial management. Lancet Neurol. 2010;9:77–93.
22. Romfh A, McNally EM. Cardiac assessment in duchenne and becker muscular dystrophies. Curr Heart Fail Rep. 2010;7:212–8.
23. Bushby K, Finkel R, Birnkrant DJ, Case LE, Clemens PR, Cripe L, Kaul A, Kinnett K, McDonald C, Pandya S, Poysky J, Shapiro F, Tomezsko J, Constantin C, Group DMDCCW. Diagnosis and management of Duchenne muscular dystrophy, part 2: implementation of multidisciplinary care. Lancet Neurol. 2010;9:177–89.
24. Corrado G, Lissoni A, Beretta S, Terenghi L, Tadeo G, Foglia-Manzillo G, Tagliagambe LM, Spata M, Santarone M. Prognostic value of electrocardiograms, ventricular late potentials, ventricular arrhythmias, and left ventricular systolic dysfunction in patients with Duchenne muscular dystrophy. Am J Cardiol. 2002;89:838–41.
25. Nigro G, Comi LI, Politano L, Bain RJ. The incidence and evolution of cardiomyopathy in Duchenne muscular dystrophy. Int J Cardiol. 1990;26:271–7.
26. Hor KN, Taylor MD, Al-Khalidi HR, Cripe LH, Raman SV, Jefferies JL, O'Donnell R, Benson DW, Mazur W. Prevalence and distribution of late gadolinium enhancement in a large population of patients with Duchenne muscular dystrophy: effect of age and left ventricular systolic function. J Cardiovasc Magn Reson. 2013;15:107.

27. Silva MC, Meira ZM, Gurgel Giannetti J, da Silva MM, Campos AF, Barbosa Mde M, Starling Filho GM, Ferreira Rde A, Zatz M, Rochitte CE. Myocardial delayed enhancement by magnetic resonance imaging in patients with muscular dystrophy. J Am Coll Cardiol. 2007;49:1874–9.
28. Juan-Mateu J, Gonzalez-Quereda L, Rodriguez MJ, Baena M, Verdura E, Nascimento A, Ortez C, Baiget M, Gallano P. DMD mutations in 576 dystrophinopathy families: a step forward in genotype-phenotype correlations. PLoS One. 2015;10:e0135189.
29. Jefferies JL, Eidem BW, Belmont JW, Craigen WJ, Ware SM, Fernbach SD, Neish SR, Smith EO, Towbin JA. Genetic predictors and remodeling of dilated cardiomyopathy in muscular dystrophy. Circulation. 2005;112:2799–804.
30. Tandon A, Jefferies JL, Villa CR, Hor KN, Wong BL, Ware SM, Gao Z, Towbin JA, Mazur W, Fleck RJ, Sticka JJ, Benson DW, Taylor MD. Dystrophin genotype-cardiac phenotype correlations in Duchenne and Becker muscular dystrophies using cardiac magnetic resonance imaging. Am J Cardiol. 2015;115:967–71.
31. Magri F, Govoni A, D'Angelo MG, Del Bo R, Ghezzi S, Sandra G, Turconi AC, Sciacco M, Ciscato P, Bordoni A, Tedeschi S, Fortunato F, Lucchini V, Bonato S, Lamperti C, Coviello D, Torrente Y, Corti S, Moggio M, Bresolin N, Comi GP. Genotype and phenotype characterization in a large dystrophinopathic cohort with extended follow-up. J Neurol. 2011;258:1610–23.
32. Ashwath ML, Jacobs IB, Crowe CA, Ashwath RC, Super DM, Bahler RC. Left ventricular dysfunction in duchenne muscular dystrophy and genotype. Am J Cardiol. 2014;114:284–9.
33. Duboc D, Meune C, Lerebours G, Devaux JY, Vaksmann G, Becane HM. Effect of perindopril on the onset and progression of left ventricular dysfunction in Duchenne muscular dystrophy. J Am Coll Cardiol. 2005;45:855–7.
34. Duboc D, Meune C, Pierre B, Wahbi K, Eymard B, Toutain A, Berard C, Vaksmann G, Weber S, Becane HM. Perindopril preventive treatment on mortality in Duchenne muscular dystrophy: 10 years' follow-up. Am Heart J. 2007;154:596–602.
35. Silva MC, Magalhaes TA, Meira ZM, Rassi CH, Andrade AC, Gutierrez PS, Azevedo CF, Gurgel-Giannetti J, Vainzof M, Zatz M, Kalil-Filho R, Rochitte CE. Myocardial fibrosis progression in Duchenne and Becker muscular dystrophy: a randomized clinical trial. JAMA Cardiol. 2017;2:190.
36. Raman SV, Hor KN, Mazur W, Halnon NJ, Kissel JT, He X, Tran T, Smart S, McCarthy B, Taylor MD, Jefferies JL, Rafael-Fortney JA, Lowe J, Roble SL, Cripe LH. Eplerenone for early cardiomyopathy in Duchenne muscular dystrophy: a randomised, double-blind, placebo-controlled trial. Lancet Neurol. 2015;14:153–61.
37. Ogata H, Ishikawa Y, Ishikawa Y, Minami R. Beneficial effects of beta-blockers and angiotensin-converting enzyme inhibitors in Duchenne muscular dystrophy. J Cardiol. 2009;53:72–8.
38. Viollet L, Thrush PT, Flanigan KM, Mendell JR, Allen HD. Effects of angiotensin-converting enzyme inhibitors and/or beta blockers on the cardiomyopathy in Duchenne muscular dystrophy. Am J Cardiol. 2012;110:98–102.
39. Matsumura T, Tamura T, Kuru S, Kikuchi Y, Kawai M. Carvedilol can prevent cardiac events in Duchenne muscular dystrophy. Intern Med. 2010;49:1357–63.
40. Markham LW, Kinnett K, Wong BL, Woodrow Benson D, Cripe LH. Corticosteroid treatment retards development of ventricular dysfunction in Duchenne muscular dystrophy. Neuromuscul Disord. 2008;18:365–70.
41. Schram G, Fournier A, Leduc H, Dahdah N, Therien J, Vanasse M, Khairy P. All-cause mortality and cardiovascular outcomes with prophylactic steroid therapy in Duchenne muscular dystrophy. J Am Coll Cardiol. 2013;61:948–54.
42. Mavrogeni S, Markousis-Mavrogenis G, Papavasiliou A, Kolovou G. Cardiac involvement in Duchenne and Becker muscular dystrophy. World J Cardiol. 2015;7:410–4.
43. Petri H, Sveen ML, Thune JJ, Vissing C, Dahlqvist JR, Witting N, Bundgaard H, Kober L, Vissing J. Progression of cardiac involvement in patients with limb-girdle type 2 and Becker muscular dystrophies: a 9-year follow-up study. Int J Cardiol. 2015;182:403–11.
44. Wu RS, Gupta S, Brown RN, Yancy CW, Wald JW, Kaiser P, Kirklin NM, Patel PC, Markham DW, Drazner MH, Garry DJ, Mammen PP. Clinical outcomes after cardiac transplantation in muscular dystrophy patients. J Heart Lung Transplant. 2010;29:432–8.

45. Ryan TD, Jefferies JL, Sawnani H, Wong BL, Gardner A, Del Corral M, Lorts A, Morales DL. Implantation of the HeartMate II and HeartWare left ventricular assist devices in patients with duchenne muscular dystrophy: lessons learned from the first applications. ASAIO J. 2014;60:246–8.
46. Seguchi O, Kuroda K, Fujita T, Fukushima N, Nakatani T. Advanced heart failure secondary to muscular dystrophy: clinical outcomes after left ventricular assist device implantation. J Heart Lung Transplant. 2016;35:831–4.
47. Politano L, Nigro V, Nigro G, Petretta VR, Passamano L, Papparella S, Di Somma S, Comi LI. Development of cardiomyopathy in female carriers of Duchenne and Becker muscular dystrophies. JAMA. 1996;275:1335–8.
48. Deng X, Berletch JB, Nguyen DK, Disteche CM. X chromosome regulation: diverse patterns in development, tissues and disease. Nat Rev Genet. 2014;15:367–78.
49. Giliberto F, Radic CP, Luce L, Ferreiro V, de Brasi C, Szijan I. Symptomatic female carriers of Duchenne muscular dystrophy (DMD): genetic and clinical characterization. J Neurol Sci. 2014;336:36–41.
50. Mavrogeni S, Bratis K, Papavasiliou A, Skouteli E, Karanasios E, Georgakopoulos D, Kolovou G, Papadopoulos G. CMR detects subclinical cardiomyopathy in mother-carriers of Duchenne and Becker muscular dystrophy. JACC Cardiovasc Imaging. 2013;6:526–8.
51. American Academy of Pediatrics Section on Cardiology and Cardiac Surgery. Cardiovascular health supervision for individuals affected by Duchenne or Becker muscular dystrophy. Pediatrics. 2005;116:1569–73.
52. Murphy AP, Straub V. The classification, natural history and treatment of the limb girdle muscular dystrophies. J Neuromuscul Dis. 2015;2:S7–S19.
53. Magri F, Nigro V, Angelini C, Mongini T, Mora M, Moroni I, Toscano A, D'Angelo MG, Tomelleri G, Siciliano G, Ricci G, Bruno C, Corti S, Musumeci O, Tasca G, Ricci E, Monforte M, Sciacco M, Fiorillo C, Gandossini S, Minetti C, Morandi L, Savarese M, Fruscio GD, Semplicini C, Pegoraro E, Govoni A, Brusa R, Del Bo R, Ronchi D, Moggio M, Bresolin N, Comi GP. The italian limb girdle muscular dystrophy registry: relative frequency, clinical features, and differential diagnosis. Muscle Nerve. 2017;55:55–68.
54. van Berlo JH, de Voogt WG, van der Kooi AJ, van Tintelen JP, Bonne G, Yaou RB, Duboc D, Rossenbacker T, Heidbuchel H, de Visser M, Crijns HJ, Pinto YM. Meta-analysis of clinical characteristics of 299 carriers of LMNA gene mutations: do lamin A/C mutations portend a high risk of sudden death? J Mol Med. 2005;83:79–83.
55. Kostareva A, Sejersen T, Sjoberg G. Genetic spectrum of cardiomyopathies with neuromuscular phenotype. Front Biosci (Schol Ed). 2013;5:325–40.
56. Finsterer J, Ramaciotti C, Wang CH, Wahbi K, Rosenthal D, Duboc D, Melacini P. Cardiac findings in congenital muscular dystrophies. Pediatrics. 2010;126:538–45.
57. Jones KJ, Morgan G, Johnston H, Tobias V, Ouvrier RA, Wilkinson I, North KN. The expanding phenotype of laminin alpha2 chain (merosin) abnormalities: case series and review. J Med Genet. 2001;38:649–57.
58. Martinez HR, Craigen WJ, Ummat M, Adesina AM, Lotze TE, Jefferies JL. Novel cardiovascular findings in association with a POMT2 mutation: three siblings with alpha-dystroglycanopathy. Eur J Hum Genet. 2014;22:486–91.
59. Bushby K, Muntoni F, Bourke JP. 107th ENMC international workshop: the management of cardiac involvement in muscular dystrophy and myotonic dystrophy. 7th–9th June 2002, Naarden, the Netherlands. Neuromuscul Disord. 2003;13:166–72.
60. McNally EM, Kaltman JR, Benson DW, Canter CE, Cripe LH, Duan D, Finder JD, Groh WJ, Hoffman EP, Judge DP, Kertesz N, Kinnett K, Kirsch R, Metzger JM, Pearson GD, Rafael-Fortney JA, Raman SV, Spurney CF, Targum SL, Wagner KR, Markham LW, Working Group of the National Heart, Lung, and Blood Institute, Parent Project Muscular Dystrophy. Contemporary cardiac issues in Duchenne muscular dystrophy. Working Group of the National Heart, Lung, and Blood Institute in collaboration with Parent Project Muscular Dystrophy. Circulation. 2015;131:1590–8.

Familial Cardiac Amyloidoses

17

Claudio Rapezzi, Christian Gagliardi, Fabrizio Salvi,
Ilaria Bartolomei, Candida Cristina Quarta,
and Agnese Milandri

Abstract

Amyloid heart disease is one of the most frequent types of cardiomyopathy with restrictive pathophysiology. The familial amyloidoses constitute an extremely heterogeneous group of diseases. The form linked to transthyretin (TTR) mutations is by far the most common variety of familial amyloidosis. The clinical picture is non-specific with progressive chronic heart failure. A definitive diagnosis can readily be made from cardiac histopathology with evidence of amyloid deposits in other tissues. However, amyloid heart disease remains underdiagnosed. Advances in cardiac imaging have resulted in greater recognition of cardiac amyloidosis in everyday clinical practice, but the diagnosis continues to be made in patients with late-stage disease, suggesting that more needs to be done to improve awareness of its clinical manifestations and the potential of therapeutic intervention to improve prognosis. The electrocardiographic and echocardiographic findings are often misleading and indistinguishable from other cardiac conditions including hypertrophic cardiomyopathy and coronary artery disease. In most cases, since the clinical manifestations of systemic amyloidosis are manifold, patients may be referred to any one of a variety of specialists (especially hematologists, nephrologists and neurologists) without necessarily referred to the cardiologist. For patients with transthyretin amyloidosis, there are numerous disease modifying therapies that are currently in late-phase clinical trials.

C. Rapezzi (✉) • C. Gagliardi • C.C. Quarta • A. Milandri
Department of Experimental, Diagnostic and Specialty Medicine, Alma Mater Studiorum University of Bologna, Bologna, Italy
e-mail: claudio.rapezzi@unibo.it; christian.gagliardi@hotmail.it; ccquarta@gmail.com; agnesemilandri@hotmail.it

F. Salvi • I. Bartolomei
Department of Neuroscience, Bellaria Hospital, Bologna, Italy
e-mail: fabrizio.salvi@gmail.com; ilaria.bartolomei@gmail.com

D. Kumar, P. Elliott (eds.), *Cardiovascular Genetics and Genomics*,
https://doi.org/10.1007/978-3-319-66114-8_17

Keywords
Amyloidosis • Transthyretin • Prealbumin • Cardiomyopathies • Echocardiography
Heart failure • Magnetic resonance imaging • Radionuclide imaging

17.1 Introduction

Amyloid heart disease is one of the most frequent types of cardiomyopathy with restrictive pathophysiology. The clinical picture is non-specific with progressive chronic heart failure. A definitive diagnosis can readily be made from cardiac histopathology with evidence of amyloid deposits in other tissues. However, amyloid heart disease remains underdiagnosed. The electrocardiographic and echocardiographic findings are often misleading and indistinguishable from other cardiac conditions including hypertrophic cardiomyopathy and coronary artery disease. In most cases, since the clinical manifestations of systemic amyloidosis are manifold, patients may be referred to any one of a variety of specialists (especially hematologists, nephrologists and neurologists) without necessarily referred to the cardiologist.

The familial amyloidoses constitute an extremely heterogeneous group of diseases. The form linked to transthyretin (TTR) mutations (conventionally abbreviated as ATTR) is by far the most common variety of familial amyloidosis. This chapter provides an overview of current knowledge regarding the pathogenesis, diagnosis and treatment of familial amyloid heart disease in general, and of ATTR-related cardiomyopathy in particular. The cardiac involvement in ATTR is considered within the context of the broader spectrum of clinical manifestations of the disease. The section dedicated to therapy is addressed separately related to questions of general supportive care, liver transplantation (including combined heart-liver transplantation), and the current state of pharmacologic treatment. The chapter concludes with a brief summary on the clinical aspects of non-TTR related cardiac amyloidoses.

17.2 The Amyloidogenic Process

The term amyloidosis refers to a large group of disorders caused by the extracellular deposition of insoluble amyloid fibrils composed of abnormally folded proteins. These disorders can affect probably around 21 proteins [1, 2], but the fibrillary deposits share distinctive structural and tinctorial properties, particularly an amorphous eosinophilic appearance under light microscopy using routine histological stains; "apple-green" birefringence after Congo-red staining under a polarized light microscope (Fig. 17.1); presence of rigid non-branching fibrils 7.5–10 nm in diameter on electron microscopy; and a predominantly antiparallel β-sheet secondary structure visible under infrared and X-ray diffraction [1, 2].

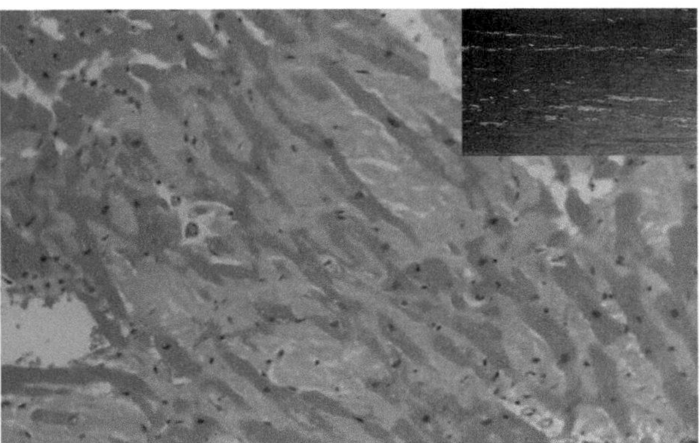

Fig. 17.1 Characteristic histological findings in the myocardium of a patient with amyloidotic cardiomyopathy. The amyloid deposits (pale pink with hematoxylin and eosinstaining) diffusely infiltrate the myocardial tissue, anatomically and functionally separating the cells from one another. The typical apple-green appearance (inset) can be seen at Congo red staining under polarized light. (photograph kindly provided by Dr. Ornella Leone)

The mechanisms by which different monomers with different biomechanical properties bind together to form regular amyloid fibrils is not understood, but three pathophysiologic steps in amyloid formation are recognised: (1) a peculiar short aminoacid sequence within the precursor protein; (2) an adequate supply of an amyloid precursor protein to allow deposition; (3) a slow but constant turnover of the resulting amyloid deposits [2–4]. The primary structure of fibril precursor proteins is undoubtedly a major determinant of their amyloidogenicity, but it is possible that any protein is intrinsically capable of producing amyloid fibrils in the presence of particular conditions [2–4]. There are several ways in which potentially pathogenic mis-folded proteins can form. The protein may have an intrinsic propensity to assume a pathologic conformation during ageing (e.g. transthyretin (TTR) in systemic senile amyloidosis) or at persistently high concentrations in serum (β_2 microglobulin in patients undergoing long-term hemodialysis). Another mechanism involves the replacement of a single amino acid in the protein, such as in hereditary amyloidosis. A third mechanism stems from proteolytic remodelling of the protein precursor, as in the case of β-amyloid precursor protein in Alzheimer's disease. These mechanisms can act independently or in conjunction with (and in addition to) the intrinsic amyloidogenic potential of the pathogenic protein. Other factors may act synergistically in amyloid deposition. For example, the protein precursor must reach a critical local concentration to trigger fibril formation, a process enhanced by local environmental factors and by interactions with extracellular matrices. Some peptides are highly fibrillogenic at high concentrations, while others are normally incorporated in larger protein precursors and become available for fibril formation only after proteolytic cleavage, such as the Aβ-peptide in Alzheimer's disease [3].

In the case of TTR protein, evidence suggests that under particular conditions (including pH, ionic strength, and protein concentration), its native structure can be destabilised by amyloidogenic mutations. Such protein mutations induce conformational changes leading to dissociation of the TTR tetramers into partially unfolded non-native monomers capable of forming high molecular-mass soluble aggregates and self-assembling into amyloid fibrils (Fig. 17.2) [4].

17.3 Mechanisms of Amyloid Induced Tissue Damage

Amyloid can cause organ and tissue damage in several ways. A major factor is the replacement of normal tissue by amyloid, leading to loss of the organ's mechanical function. However, infiltration cannot by itself completely explain the spectrum of clinical, instrumental and biological manifestations of amyloid diseases. For instance, it has been observed that similar or lesser amounts of cardiac amyloid deposits (as evaluated by echocardiography) have significantly worse functional and prognostic impact in patients with light chain amyloidosis than in patients with transthyretin amyloidosis [4, 5]. Furthermore, the amount of amyloid in an organ does not provide an accurate indicator of the clinical consequences of the disease. For example, patients with AL amyloidosis without hepatic failure may harbor

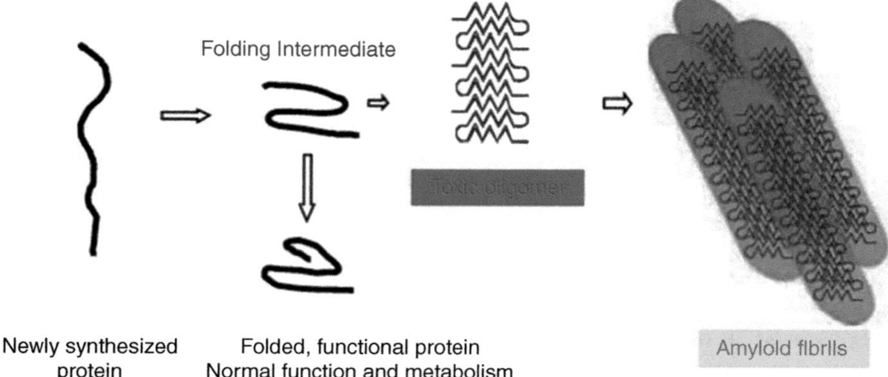

Fig. 17.2 Example of how an amyloid filament is thought to be formed. For many amyloid fibril proteins, the aggregation is believed to start from intermediates in the folding process, giving rise to a nucleus from which filament formation proceeds. There is strong evidence that oligomeric aggregates (also called protofibrils), which occur before mature fibrils are formed, exert toxic effects on cells whilst the full-blown fibrils are more inert. Amyloid fibrils usually consist of two or several thin filaments (indicated to the right in the figure) twisted around each other. The width of the definite amyloid fibril is around 10 nm. (Illustration based on data from Hou et al. [4])

abundant protein deposits in their livers. By contrast, in ATTR small amounts of amyloidotic infiltration of the peripheral nerves may be accompanied by severe neurologic impairment. In vitro, synthetic amyloidotic fibrils can exert lethal toxic effects on various cell types [6–8] always via induction of apoptosis [9]. Although the underlying mechanisms remain unclear, a variety of factors, including oxidative stress [10, 11], cell membrane destruction [12, 13], and formation of pathological ion channels [12, 14] have been implicated. It is now thought that cell toxicity largely occurs in the early stages of fibril formation. Experiments with several amyloid fibril proteins manufactured in vitro [13] suggest that smaller oligomeric aggregates (so-called protofibrils or intermediate-sized toxic amyloid particles) are probably toxic whereas the mature fibrils from the same peptides may not be [15].

17.4 Classification of Amyloidosis

The modern classification of amyloidosis, proposed by the World Health Organization nomenclature subcommittee (Table 17.1), is based on the precursor protein [16]. According to this classification, the amyloid protein is designated "protein A" followed by a suffix (e.g. ATTR), where A stands for amyloid and the suffix specifies the protein (this name is also used to identify the disease). The types of amyloidosis are subdivided into acquired or hereditary. Amyloid distribution may be focal, localized or systemic. The most common form of systemic amyloidosis is AL (where L stands for light-chain immunoglobulin), which was formerly known as "primary amyloidosis". The incidence of AL in Western countries is approximately 1 new case per 100,000 person-years [17]. Hereditary systemic amyloidoses are much less common; they are secondary to deposition of various proteins, including TTR, apolipoprotein A-I and A-II, lysozyme, gelsolin, cystatin C, and fibrinogen A α-chain. Senile systemic amyloidosis stems from deposition of amyloid derived from wild-type TTR (i.e. with a normal amino acid sequence). For reasons that remain unclear, wild-type TTR-related amyloidosis is almost exclusively a disorder of old men and mainly affects the heart.

17.5 TTR-Related Familial Amyloidosis

TTR-related familial amyloidosis (hereafter referred to as ATTR) is the most frequent form of hereditary systemic amyloidosis. TTR is a tetrameric plasma transport protein for the thyroid hormone and retinol-binding protein/vitamin A, which is synthesized in the liver (and in small amounts in the choroidal plexus and retinal epithelium). TTR is a single polypeptide chain of 127 amino acid residues encoded by a single gene on Chromosome 18 which spans approximately 7 kb and has four exons [3, 4].

Table 17.1 Nomenclature and classification of amyloidosis

Amyloidosis	Protein precursor	Systemic/Localized	Clinical syndrome/ Association
AL	Immunoglobulin light-chain (κ or λ)	S, L	• Primary • Myeloma-associated
AH	Immunoglobulin heavy-chain	S, L	• Primary • Myeloma-associated
AA	(Apo) serum AA	S	• Secondary • Reactive
ATTR	Transthyretin (TTR)	S L?	• Senile (TTR wild-type) • Familial (TTR mutated) • Tenosynovium
AApoAI	Apolipoprotein-AI	S	• Familial
		L	• Aortic
AApoAII	Apolipoprotein-AII	S	• Familial
AGel	Gelsolin	S	• Familial
ALys	Lysozyme	S	• Familial
AFib	Fibrinogen α-chain	S	• Familial
ACys	Cystatin C	S	• Familial
ABri	ABriPP	S L?	• Familial dementia (British)
Aβ	Aβ-protein precursor (AβPP)	L	• Alzheimer's disease • Ageing
APrP	Prion protein	L	• Spongioform encephalopathies
$A\beta_2M$	β_2-microglobulin	S	• Haemodialysis
		L?	• Joints
ACal	(Pro)calcitonin	L	• C-cell thyroid tumors
AIAPP	Islet amyloid polypeptide	L	• Islets of Langherans • Insulinomas
AANF	Atrial natriuretic factor	L	• Cardiac atria
APro	Prolactin	L	• Ageing pituitary • Prolactinomas
AIns	Insulin	L	• Iatrogenic
AMed	Lactadherin	L	• Senile aortic
Aker	Kerato-epithelin	L	• Familial cornea

ATTR is inherited in an autosomal dominant fashion with balanced sex distribution and variable penetrance. Over 80 different amyloidogenic mutations have been identified around the world, many of which have been found in single individuals or families ("private mutations") [3, 4, 18]. Most ATTR carriers are heterozygous for a pathogenic mutation and express both normal and variant TTR. The majority of TTR mutations derive from a single nucleotide substitution [4, 18]. An exception is the deletion of an entire 3-base codon (Val122Ile) [19, 20]. Development of the disease is probably the result of changes in primary structure of the protein, modulated by various genetic and possibly also environmental factors (although present in the blood from birth, variant TTR is does not start to produce amyloid until adulthood) [21].

A few of the TTR mutations are found in extended kindreds in particular locations around the world. The most common of these is the substitution of methionine for valine at position 30 (Val30Met), which leads to "type I familial amyloid polyneuropathy" (FAP) [22]. The Val30Met variety of ATTR amyloidosis has major geographical clusters in Portugal, Sweden and in Japan with smaller clusters in more than a dozen other countries [23] (Fig. 17.3). These three countries are geographically distant, and a consanguineous relationship between populations has not been identified. The issue of whether there is a common origin for a mutant allele has not been completely resolved. The hypothesis that the worldwide clusters of FAP (Val30Met) all originate from a mutant allele in the Portuguese kindred was based on historically documented commercial relations. Recently, Ohmori et al. compared haplotypes in several cohorts of patients with FAP and concluded that a common founder could conceivably link Portuguese and Japanese patients and Portuguese and Spanish patients, but could not account for Swedish and other patients [24].

The prevalence of Val30Met genotype is particularly high (about 1.5%) in northern Sweden, although the penetrance is only about 2% [23]. In Portugal the disease prevalence rate is estimated at 1 in 1000 [23]. In Japan, Val30Met families with early-onset neuropathy were initially identified in two limited areas (Arao district and Ogawa village), while a late-onset non-endemic type of Val30Met ATTR was reported in a wide distribution throughout the country [23]. In Sweden, in addition

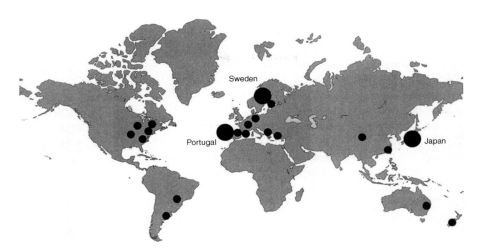

Fig. 17.3 Distribution of familial amyloidotic polyneuropathy (FAP) in the world. Locations of clusters of patients with FAP amyloidogenic mutated transthyretin Val30Met described in previous reports and obtained from personal communications are presented. The size of the circles is related to the number of patients at each location. (From Ando et al. [23] with permission)

to the endemic foci of Val30Met, Ala45Ser and Tyr69His mutations have been observed [25]. The Leu111Me mutation has been reported in Denmark, were it is the cause of so-called familial amyloidotic cardiomyopathy (FAC) [26, 27].

The Val30Met type is the most common cause of ATTR in the UK and Ireland [28]. In France, a large population of Portuguese Val30Met families coexists with families of French descent (in these families prevalence of Val30Met is no higher than 40%) [29–31]. High genotypic heterogeneity is also apparent in Italy, where at least 15 different TTR mutations have been identified (about 35% of affected families have Val30Met and Glu89Gln also appears to be relatively frequent [32]). Certain mutations are mainly observed in the USA [23, 30]. Leu58His (in families originating in Germany), Thr60Ala (in families of Irish descent), and Val122Ile, which is present in 4% of black people [19, 33]. The high prevalence of Val122Ile within the large Afro-American community probably makes this variety not only the most common familial amyloid cardiomyopathy, but perhaps also the most frequent form of amyloid heart disease (including AL) [19].

17.5.1 Clinical Profiles and Genotype-Phenotype Correlations

ATTR is characterized by a high degree of phenotypic as well as genotypic heterogeneity. Phenotypic heterogeneity is linked to at least three different factors: (1) the type of TTR mutation; (2) geographic distribution; (3) the type of aggregation (endemic or non-endemic).

In the "classic" endemic TTR Val30Met type of FAP, prevalent in Portugal and Japan, the disorder is inherited as an autosomal dominant trait with balanced sex distribution. Sensorimotor polyneuropathy is the prominent feature. The neuropathy usually starts at 30–35 years of age with small-fiber dysfunction in the lower limbs very similar to the neuropathy of diabetes mellitus, with lack of thermal appreciation is often an early feature [18, 23]. Dysesthesias may be prominent with or without varying degrees of pain. Motor function tends to be well maintained (sensory dissociation) until the sensory neuropathy has reached an advanced phase. Sensory loss in the lower extremities slowly progresses upwards from the feet and ankles to the knees and beyond, with similar symptoms eventually developing in the upper extremities. Autonomic neuropathy tends to occur relatively early and leads to severe orthostatic hypotension, disturbed bowel movement with constipation and diarrhoea, erectile dysfunction in men, bladder retention and urinary incontinence [18, 23]. In some men, sexual impotence is the initial clinical symptom. Nerve conduction studies can be a valuable tool for detecting peripheral nerve involvement.

Electrophysiological findings can help distinguish polyneuropathy from localized abnormalities, such as median neuropathy at the wrist (carpal tunnel syndrome). Serial studies can help follow the course of peripheral nerve abnormality [18, 23].

In the subgroup of Japanese and Portuguese patients with the non-endemic, "late-onset" Val30Met TTR mutation, autonomic dysfunction is milder, and sensory loss and cardiomyopathy are more common than in early-onset cases of FAP [18, 23]. The clinical profile of Swedish patients is different in that the average age at onset is the mid-1950s, penetrance at around 50%, and progression of the disease considerably slower than in Japanese and Portuguese patients [24, 25].

The carpal tunnel syndrome is a relatively frequent feature of ATTR irrespective of a particular mutation and occasionally may be the only clinical manifestation. Vocal hoarseness can occur due to recurrent laryngeal nerve palsy, and the "scalloped pupil" deformity, which is essentially pathognomonic for FAP, is due to amyloid deposition in ciliary nerves of the eye [18]. Vitreous opacities accompany about 20% of TTR mutations, and may be the first manifestation of FAP [34, 35]. TTR amyloid in the vitreous is probably the result of synthesis by the retinal pigment epithelium. Amyloid fibrils in the vitreous are predominantly (about 90–95%) composed of variant TTR, which is less prevalent (60–65%) in fibrils found in nerve and cardiac tissue [18].

In a characteristic, oculoleptomeningeal form of FAP, that can be induced by several TTR mutations, cerebral amyloid angiopathy and ocular amyloidosis are common [34]. Cerebral amyloid angiopathy is characterized by amyloid deposition in the cortex and leptomeninges [18, 34]. Typical clinical central nervous system manifestations include stroke, seizures, hydrocephalus, spastic paralysis, spinal cord infarction or, later, cerebral hemorrhage [18, 34]. Although amyloid deposits in the meningocerebrovascular system were thought to be the cause of central nervous system symptoms, the precise mechanism of amyloid formation remains to be elucidated. Renal involvement is generally not a feature of transthyretin-associated cardiac amyloidosis.

17.5.2 Amyloidotic Cardiac Involvement

Amyloid can infiltrate various cardiovascular structures, including the conduction system, the atrial and ventricular myocardium, valvular tissue, the coronary arteries and the large arteries [1, 2, 36–39]. The conduction system is commonly affected in cardiac amyloidosis, leading to sino-atrial node disease, atrial fibrillation, atrioventricular and bundle branch block, and ventricular tachycardia. Myocardial infiltration progressively increases the thickness of left and right ventricular walls and of the interatrial septum (Fig. 17.4). Involvement of cardiac valves leads to formation of nodules or diffuse thickening of the leaflets accompanied by a variable degree (generally mild) of valvular regurgitation. Deposition in the coronary arteries most frequently involves intramural arteries and may lead to myocardial ischemia in spite of angiographically normal epicardial vessels.

Cardiac amyloidosis (CA) is generally considered to be a myocardial disease with "hypertrophic phenotype" and restrictive physiology that leads to diastolic heart failure [40, 41]. However, any representative cohort of patients with amyloid heart disease will display a spectrum of diastolic filling abnormalities, with the restrictive pattern seen only in advanced stages of the disease. The left ventricular filling pattern generally

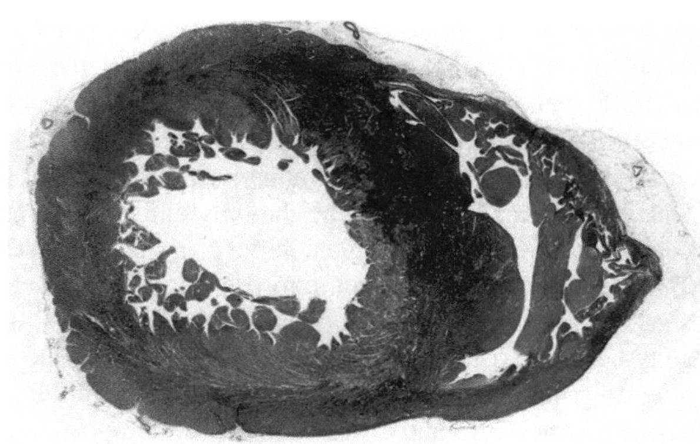

Fig. 17.4 Macrosopic cross-section at the mid-ventricular level of a heart explanted from an ATTR patient during combined heart-liver transplantation. The amyloid (pale pink with hematoxylin and eosin staining) has diffusely infiltrated the myocardium, and in many areas has completely replaced the normal myocardial tissue (photograph kindly provided by Dr. Ornella Leone)

evolves from an abnormal relaxation pattern, through a pseudonormal phase, to a restrictive pattern [36, 40]. Left ventricular systolic function can be impaired in patients with overt heart failure, although the left ventricular ejection fraction is often only mildly reduced (without left ventricular enlargement). Abnormalities in long axis function of both ventricles (detectable at tissue Doppler echocardiography) are frequent and appear earlier. [40–43]. Microvascular amyloidotic coronary infiltration can occur even in the absence of ventricular wall thickening, and may lead to systolic/diastolic "ischemic" dysfunction in the context of a dilated non-hypertrophic left ventricle. This presentation of amyloidosis is rare, probably being found in less than 1–2% of patients with cardiac involvement [36, 44].

17.5.3 Prevalence and Clinical Spectrum of Cardiac Involvement in ATTR

In ATTR, the frequency and type of cardiac involvement is related to the specific TTR mutation, geographic area (Portugal, Japan, Sweden, other countries), and endemic/non-endemic aggregation. Severity of cardiac involvement ranges widely from asymptomatic atrioventricular and bundle branch blocks to severe, rapidly progressive heart failure secondary to restrictive cardiomyopathy.

As a general rule, patients with the Val30Met mutation who come from endemic foci tend to have less severe heart involvement in comparison with individuals who carry the same mutation but come from a non-endemic area or have mutations other than Val30Met [23, 37, 38, 45]. In endemic areas of Portugal and Japan, conduction disturbances are the single most frequent form of cardiac involvement, whereas congestive heart failure due to amyloidotic cardiomyopathy is a rare, age-related manifestation. Patients in non-endemic areas of the same countries are more prone to develop severe cardiac amyloidosis [23, 37, 38]. Elsewhere, the likelihood and severity of cardiomyopathy varies with the type of mutation. TTR-CA may be due to specific mutations that have a predominant involvement of the heart (Val122Ile, Leu111Met, Ile68Leu) or ATTRwt. Ile68Leu and Leu111Met are mutations reported almost exclusively in Italy and Denmark, respectively, causing a severe cardiomyopathy at early age with a malignant course. In the US, ATTRwt followed by Val122Ile and Thr60Ala mutations are most common. In an Italian setting, a broad spectrum of cardiac abnormalities was observed (Fig. 17.5), with prevalence ranging from 24% for cardiomyopathies with restrictive physiology to 80% for any type of ECG abnormality [32]. Remarkably, cardiomyopathy of varying degrees of severity was found in the context of all but one of the TTR mutations encountered in this specialist center. Notably, in many non-Val30Met mutations, amyloidotic cardiomyopathy was the predominant or the exclusive clinical manifestation of ATTR (Table 17.2). In some of these mutations, neurological manifestations can be mild or absent with low penetrance, thereby simulating sporadic forms of non-ATTR amyloidotic cardiomyopathy, or even hypertrophic cardiomyopathy caused by sarcomeric protein gene mutations.

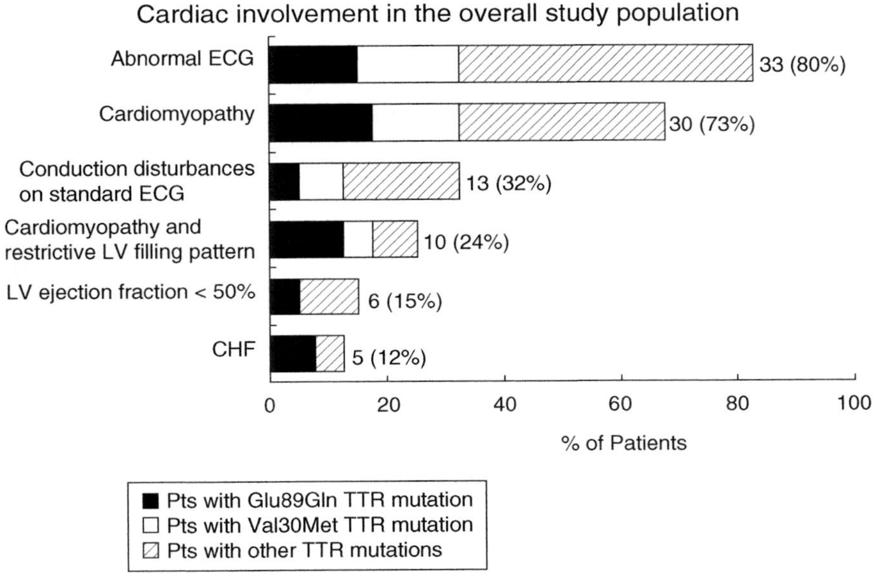

Fig. 17.5 Prevalence of different manifestations of cardiac involvement in a series of 41 ATTR patients referred to a specialised Italian tertiary centre. (From Rapezzi et al. [32])

Table 17.2 List of the main TTR mutations subdivided according to three prevalent clinical profiles

Prevalent polyneuropathy	Cys10Arg, Asp18Glu, Ala25Ser, Ala25Thr, Val28Met, Val30Ala, Val30Leu, Val30Met, Phe33Ile, Phe33Leu, Phe33Val, Arg34Thr, Lys35Asn, Ala36Pro, Asp38Ala, Phe44Ser, Ala45Asp, Gly47Arg, Gly47Val, Thr49Ala, Thr49Ile, Ser50Arg, Ser52Pro, Glu54Gly, Glu54Lys, Leu55Pro, Leu55Gln, Leu58Arg, Thr59Lys, Glu61Lys, Lys70Asn, Val71Ala, Ile73Val, Ser77Phe, Ile84Thr, Glu89Lys, Ala91Ser, Ser112Ile, Tyr114His, Tyr116Ser, Val122Ala
Prevalent myocardial involvement	Asp18Asn, Val20Ile, Ser23Asn, Pro24Ser, Phe33Cys, Glu42Asp, Glu42Gly, Ala45Ser, Ala45Thr, Gly47Ala, Thr49Pro, Ser50Ile, Glu51Gly, His56Arg, Leu58His, Thr60Ala, Phe64Leu, Ile68Leu, Tyr69Ile, Ser77Tyr, Ala81Thr, Ile84Asn, Ile84Ser, Glu89Gln, Gln92Lys, Ala97Gly, Arg103Ser, Ile107Val, Leu111Met, Ala120Ser, Val122Ile
Prevalent leptomeningeal involvement	Leu12Pro, Asp18Gly, Val30Gly, Gly53Glu, Phe64Ser, Ile84Ser, Tyr114Cys.

17.5.4 Diagnostic Examinations

17.5.4.1 Electrocardiography

The ECG is rarely normal in patients with cardiac amyloidosis [46–49]. About 10–15% of patients present with atrial fibrillation. The spectrum of QRS and repolarization alterations includes low ECG voltage (presence of QRS voltage amplitude ≤0.5 mV in all limb leads, or ≤1 mV in all precordial leads), pseudo-infarct patterns (anterior, inferior or lateral) (Fig. 17.6), left anterior hemiblock, right bundle branch block, and ischemic-type or non-specific T-wave abnormalities [46–49]. Low QRS voltage is considered the most typical ECG finding in cardiac amyloidosis, especially when coexistent with increased left ventricular wall thickness. In a series of patients with cardiomyopathy of suspected amyloidotic origin, the combination of low QRS voltage and interventricular septal thickness >1.98 cm provided a sensitivity of 72% and a specificity of 91% for a biopsy proven diagnosis of (mainly AL) cardiac amyloidosis [48]. Our experience [50] of patients affected by amyloidotic cardiomyopathy suggests that the prevalence of low QRS voltage at presentation may be significantly lower in ATTR than in AL (about 30 versus 50%). This observation underlines the importance of pursuing any clinical suspicion of ATTR amyloidotic cardiomyopathy, even in the absence of reduced QRS voltage.

17.5.4.2 Echocardiography

Echocardiography is the main non-invasive instrumental examination for detection of cardiac involvement, since it can reveal several features that are suggestive of cardiac amyloidosis (Fig. 17.7) [45, 51–57]. It has to be remembered, however, that such features commonly appear only in the later stages of disease [36, 39]. Thus, echocardiographic

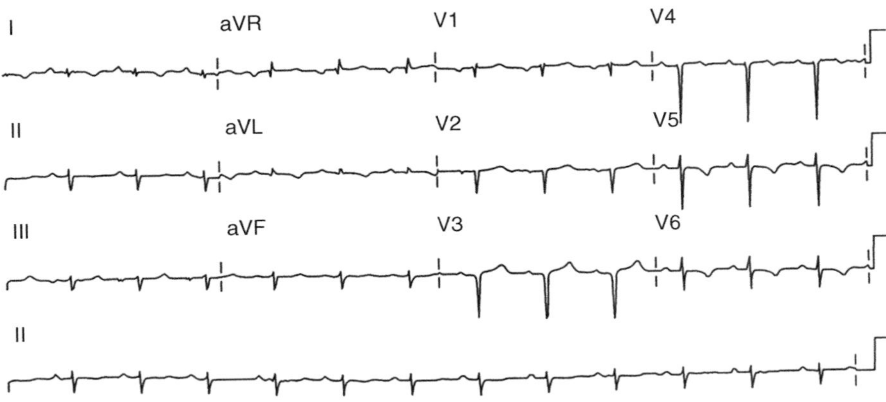

Fig. 17.6 Characteristic ECG from an ATTR patient with amyloidotic cardiomyopathy. The most striking features are low QRS voltage in the limb leads, anterior "pseudo-infarction" pattern, and diffuse "ischemic" T-wave abnormalities

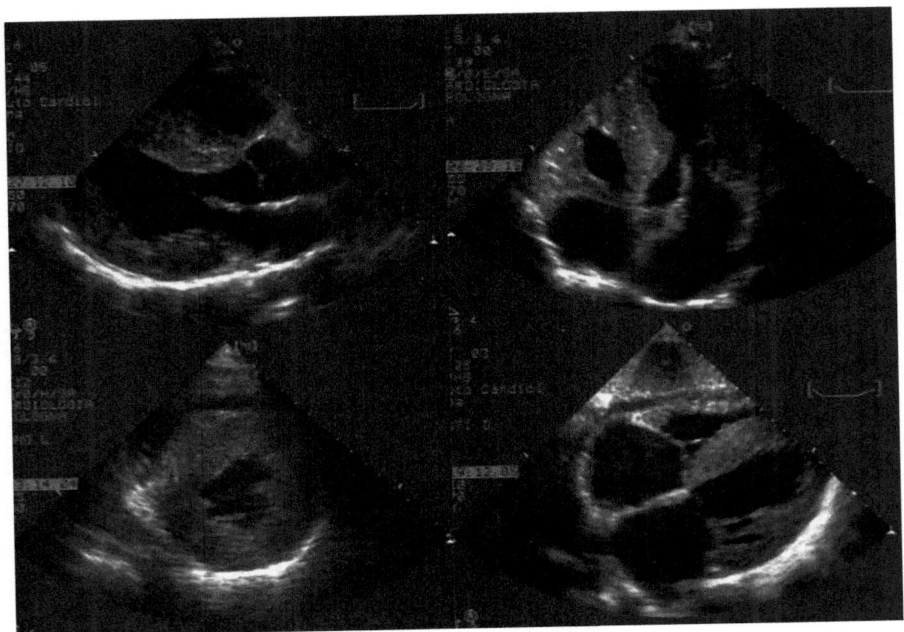

Fig. 17.7 Characteristic echocardiograms from four different ATTR patients affected by amyloidotic cardiomyopathy. The most striking shared feature is the increased thickness of the interventricular septum and free left ventricular wall. In the top right panel (4-chamber view), thickening of the mitral valve is also apparent. In the bottom right panel (subcostal view), thickening can also be seen in the free right ventricular wall and interatrial septum

images must be interpreted in the context of the clinical picture and other examinations, and they cannot be used in isolation for diagnostic confirmation. The most frequent echocardiographic finding is increased thickness of the interventricular septum and of the left ventricular free wall. This finding is often erroneously referred to as "hypertrophy", whereas in reality it corresponds to amyloidotic myocardial infiltration. Other characteristic echocardiographic findings include:

- increased right ventricular wall thickness;
- increased interatrial septal thickness;
- diffuse granular appearance of the myocardium;
- atrioventricular valve thickening;
- pericardial effusion.

Much stress has been laid on the diagnostic relevance of the granular or speckled appearance of the ventricular myocardium at echocardiography. However, recognition of a "granular pattern" remains subjective and current imaging technology may enhance myocardial echogenicity while at the same time attenuating granularity [39]. Nevertheless, the current definition of amyloidotic cardiomyopathy [56] is based on echocardiographic criteria: end-diastolic thickness of the interventricular septum >1.2 cm (in the absence of any other cause of ventricular hypertrophy) plus two or more of the following: (a) homogeneous atrioventricular valve thickening, (b) atrial septum thickening, and (c) sparkling/granular appearance of the ventricular septum.

The ventricles are usually not dilated in amyloidotic cardiomyopathy. The left ventricular ejection fraction tends to be normal or only slightly reduced, but the wall thickening velocity is frequently depressed. Similarly, the long-axis function of the left ventricle is often reduced even in the early phases of the disease when radial fractional shortening is still conserved, and this can be appreciated both by tissue Doppler imaging techniques and by 2-dimensional (2D) speckle-tracking imaging [36, 57]. In general, strain parameters in CA have been shown to be much more altered than in other causes of left ventricle hypertrophy. In particular, longitudinal strain (LS) in amyloidotic cardiomyopathy has an unusual pattern characterized by a severe impairment of strain at the base and a relative "apical sparing", that differentiates CA from other cardiomyopathies [58].

Echo-Doppler evaluation provides particularly relevant information regarding the diastolic phase of ventricular function. The frequency and types of diastolic abnormalities is related to the different phases of the disease. In particular, a true "restrictive filling pattern" is generally encountered only in advanced amyloidotic cardiomyopathy [40].

17.5.4.3 Magnetic Resonance Imaging

Magnetic resonance imaging (MRI) with delayed gadolinium enhancement is useful for detection of amyloidotic myocardial infiltration [59–62]. Gadolinium tends to accumulate within the interstitium infiltrated by amyloid (Fig. 17.8), leading to a late

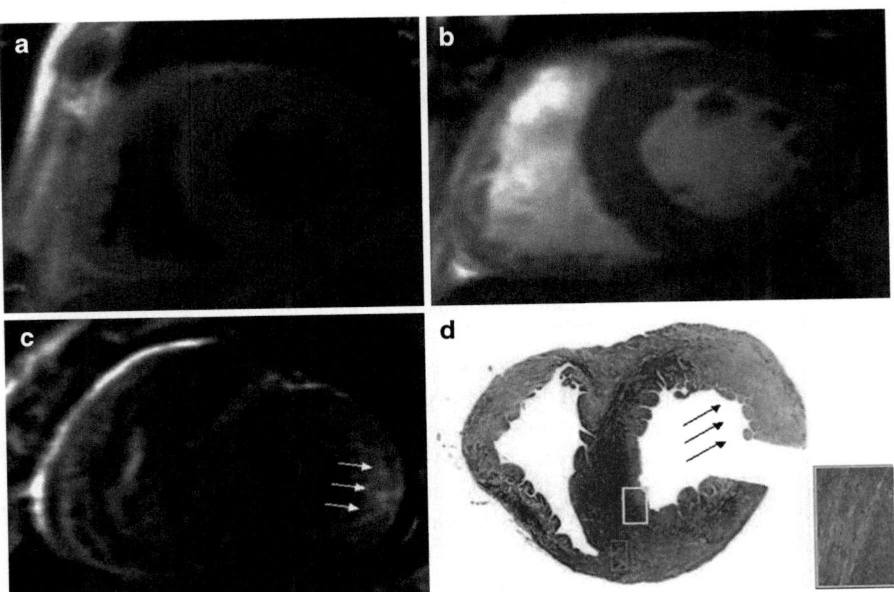

Fig. 17.8 In a 43 year old man with familial transthyretin related cardiac amyloidosis, conventional cardiac magnetic resonance (CMR) with (**a**) black blood fast spin echo and (**b**) bright blood fast gradient echo sequences shows increased left and right ventricular thicknesses. (**c**) Gadolinium inversion recovery fast gradient echo also shows a large transmural zone of strong, patchy hyperenhancement (arrows). (**d**) After combined heart and liver transplantation, myocardial histological analysis showed diffuse amyloid deposition with characteristic green birefringence on Congo red staining (inset) and an area of massive infiltration (arrows) corresponding to the strong, patchy enhancement seen on Gd-CMR. (From Perugini et al. [60]); with permission

enhancement effect, most often in the subendocardium [59], and less commonly in localized and transmural distributions [60, 63]. A unique feature of delayed-enhancement MRI in amyloidotic cardiomyopathy is the dark appearance of the blood pool, due to similar T1 values of the myocardium and blood (produced by high myocardial uptake and fast blood pool washout) [59]. Although MRI certainly provides relevant information in the diagnostic work up, its diagnostic accuracy and predictive value has not yet been studied in real-world situations where a variety of primary/secondary myocardial diseases have to be considered in the differential diagnosis.

T1 mapping is a new technique where a quantitative signal from the myocardium is measured, either before contrast (native T1) or after contrast administration [45, 64–66]. In CA native myocardial T1 is increased both in AL and ATTR patients. T1 values are higher in AL-CA compared with ATTR-CA, whilst the extracellular volume is higher in ATTR than in AL [67]. Native T1 is an early disease marker, being elevated before the onset of left ventricle hypertrophy, presence of late gadolinium enhancement or elevation in blood biomarkers and can be used in patients with renal impairement as it requires no contrast administration. Combined, native T1 mapping and measures of extracellular volume (ECV) post contrast can delineate three aspects of CA including amyloid burden or infiltration via measure of ECV, edema via measure of native T1 and myocyte response via measure of intracellular volume. This approach can provide a better understanding of the pathophysiological processes that may be used to monitor disease progression and response to therapy. Current limitations of the T1 imaging are the effect of confounding pathologies such as myocardial edema and platform dependent variation in normal ranges for T1.

17.5.4.4 Nuclear Scintigraphy

Scintigraphy is another important non-invasive examination for diagnosis and monitoring of amyloidosis [36, 39, 68, 69]. I^{123}-labeled serum amyloid P (SAP) specifically binds with all types of fibril (via a calcium-mediated mechanism). Its consequent accumulation in all amyloid deposits provides valuable information on the presence and topography of amyloid deposits in the body, making it possible to monitor progression and therapeutic response [68]. Unfortunately, SAP scanning is restricted to a very few centres and it cannot image the beating heart.

The 99mTc-phosphate derivatives, originally developed for bone imaging, were observed to accumulate in the early healing phase after acute myocardial infarction. In the early 1980s, 99mTc-PYP imaging was first described as a potential diagnostic test for CA following reports describing increased cardiac uptake in patients with amyloid heart disease [70–72]. More recently in Europe, studies have evaluated the diagnostic role of the tracer 99mTc-3,3-diphosphono-1,2-propanodicarboxylic (DPD) in cardiac amyloidosis [69, 73, 74] (Fig. 17.9). Altogether, the data show that ATTR-CA is avid for bone tracers, whereas uptake in AL-CA is either absent or only mild. The molecular bases for this differential uptake is unknown, but it has been suggested that the preferential binding to ATTR may be a result of higher calcium content. Since bone scintigraphy has a high diagnostic accuracy for imaging ATTR-CA, in selected patients with a moderate-intense myocardial radiotracer uptake and the absence of a detectable monoclonal protein in serum or urine, the diagnosis of ATTR CA is reliably without the need for histology [75]. Moreover, bone tracers seem to be useful for early identification of ATTR-CA and may more closely correlate with amyloid load than estimates from CMR [76]. Additionally, there is also uptake in skeletal muscle and soft tissues, which may appear to attenuate bone signal [77]. 18F-florbetapir is approved for imaging beta amyloid protein in the brain. Recent studies have shown that it is also taken up in the heart in patients with ATTR-CA and AL-CA. Similar findings have been reported for another beta amyloid imaging agent 11C-PiB [78]. These agents hold great promise for absolute quantification of amyloid burden.

17.5.4.5 Endomyocardial Biopsy

Endomyocardial biopsy (EMB) readily provides histological evidence of amyloid heart disease; false negatives are uncommon given the widespread myocardial

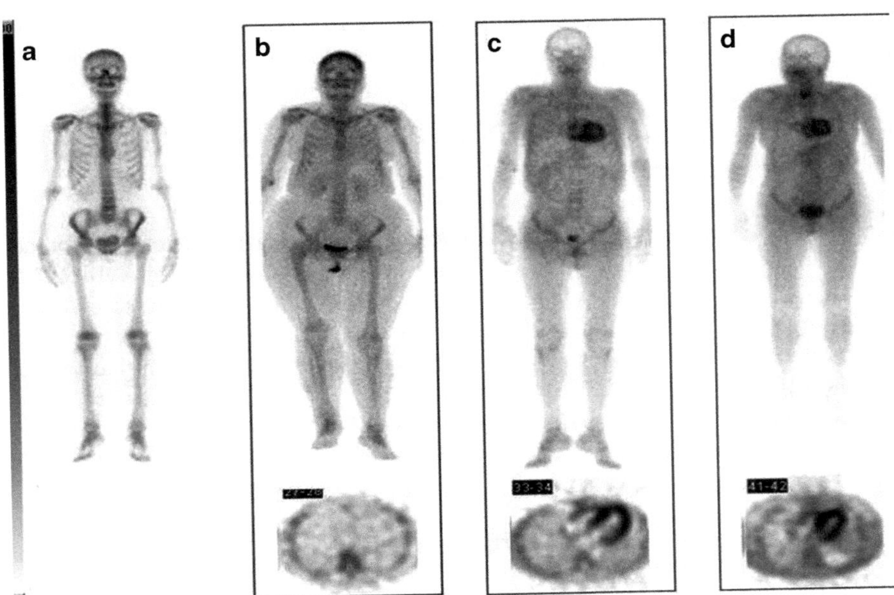

Fig. 17.9 Representative examples illustrating the spectrum of 99mTc-DPD uptake among patients with TTR-related or AL cardiac amyloidosis and unaffected controls (top row: whole-body scans, anterior view; bottom row: cross sectional views of cardiac SPECT in the same patients). (**a**) Unaffected control subject without visually detectable uptake. (**b**) Patient with AL amyloidosis and echocardiographic documentation of cardiac involvement without any visually detectable sign of myocardial 99mTc-DPD uptake; mild uptake of the tracer is visible only at soft tissue level. (**c**, **d**) Two patients with TTR-related amyloidosis and echocardiographic documentation of cardiac involvement, both showing strong myocardial 99mTc-DPD uptake (with absent bone uptake); in one of the patients (**d**), splanchnic uptake is also visible. (From Perugini et al. [69]); with permission

diffusion of amyloid deposits [79–81]. Since the ventricular walls are commonly thickened, biopsy carries a very low risk of cardiac perforation.

17.5.4.6 Cardiac Biomarkers

In AL cardiac amyloidosis, Troponin T and B-natriuretic peptide (BNP) plasma concentrations both tend to be elevated, even in the context of only limited ventricular dysfunction and mild or absent symptoms of congestive heart failure [82–86]. Both Troponin and BNP values can be useful to stratify the prognosis of AL patients and monitor their response to therapy [82–85]. Fewer biomarker data are available for ATTR [10, 86–88]. Taken together these studies show that NT-pro-BNP, BNP and troponin are frequently increased in ATTR as a consequence of both hemodynamic abnormalities and direct toxic effects of precursor proteins in some mutations. Recently, Grogan et al. have proposed a staging system with important prognostic implication for patients with wild-type TTR [88].

17.5.5 ATTR Amyloidosis Versus AL and Systemic Senile Amyloidosis

Hitherto, we have mainly considered amyloidotic cardiac involvement in the broad context of a systemic amyloidosis which infiltrates the heart. Although ATTR, AL and systemic senile cardiac amyloidosis share many features, there are some important differences (Table 17.3) [5, 89]. Compared to AL cardiac amyloidosis (the most common form), ATTR seems to be characterised by slightly greater ventricular wall thickness, less pronounced systolic and diastolic cardiac dysfunction with lower ventricular filling pressures, and lower prevalence of low QRS voltage. Furthermore, ATTR cardiac amyloidosis patients less often develop heart failure symptoms or die from cardiovascular complications.

17.5.5.1 Diagnosis of ATTR Cardiac Amyloidosis

Clinical Suspicion

From the cardiologist's standpoint, two main clinical scenarios can be distinguished in ATTR: (1) a clinical picture characterized by neurological impairment or a prexisting diagnosis of FAP; (2) heart muscle disease in the absence of a neurological diagnosis. If there is a strong suspicion or an existing diagnosis of FAP, the cardiologist's role is to look for signs of cardiac involvement. In such situations, ECG and echocardiography generally provide all the necessary diagnostic information. To recognise very early signs of myocardial involvement, careful observation of the longitudinal left ventricular function with tissue-Doppler echocardiography is particularly revealing.

Table 17.3 Comparison of the characteristics of the three main forms of systemic cardiac amyloidosis: summary of the literature (and the authors' experience)

	AL	Systemic senile amyloidosis	ATTR
Ventricular walls	Mild thickening	Greatly thickened	Moderate thickening
A-V valve involvement	Sometimes	Sometimes	Frequent
Diastolic dysfunction	Often moderate	Often mild	Sometimes
Systolic dysfunction	Sometimes	Frequent	Occasionally
Low QRS voltage	Frequent	Occasionally	Sometimes
Left bundle branch block	Sometimes	Occasionally	Sometimes
^{99}Tc-DPD myocardial uptake	Absent/weak	Strong	Strong
Severe heart failure	Very frequent	Frequent	Occasionally
Prognosis	Poor	Fair	Fair

The situation in which there is no neurological suspicion of FAP is much more challenging for cardiologists. Patients may be present with heart failure symptoms, arrhythmias, syncope, orthostatic hypertension, or ECG/echocardiographic abnormalities in the absence of symptoms. Differentiation from cardiomyopathies of other etiology can be difficult and not infrequently results in misdiagnosis of cardiac amyloidosis as familial hypertrophic cardiomyopathy. However, the particular echocardiographic signs described above should raise suspicion of amyloidotic etiology once "hypertrophic cardiomyopathy" has been recognized. Perhaps the single most useful sign is the presence of low or normal QRS voltage despite increased left ventricular wall thickness (Fig. 17.10). Unfortunately, this highly specific sign is not very sensitive and is more frequent in AL than in TTR-related amyloidosis.

Apart from evident neurological manifestations, other clinical pointers for a diagnosis of hereditary ATTR amyloidosis include:

- familial neurological disease (even in the absence of a precise diagnosis of FAP).
- a personal history of carpal tunnel syndrome.
- sensorimotor peripheral neuropathy.
- unexplained intense muscular pain in the leg and burning sensations;

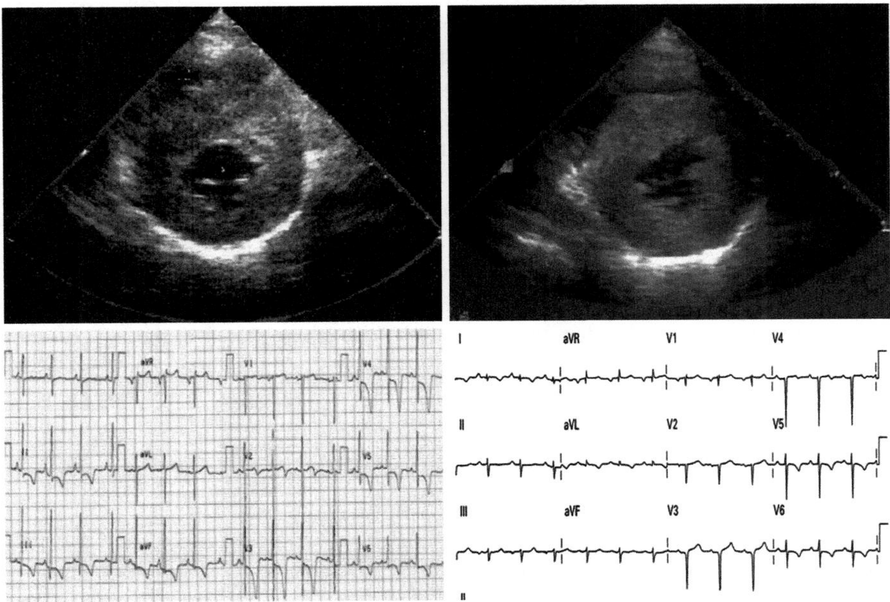

Fig. 17.10 Echocardiograms and ECG from a patient with sarcomeric hypertrophic cardiomyopathy (left) and amyloidotic cardiomyopathy (right). Despite similar degrees of left ventricular "hypertrophy"at echocardiography, the ECG are profoundly different (left ventricular hypertrophy and strain in the patient with sarcomeric hypertrophic cardiomyopathy versus low QRS voltage in the patient with amyloidotic cardiomyopathy)

– autonomic nervous system dysfunction (eg dyshydrosis, erectile dysfunction, diarrhoea alternating with constipation).
– vitreous opacity.

Since some of these signs can be very mild, and not necessarily self-reported by the patient, an active search is mandatory.

Tissue Diagnosis

Table 17.4 summarises the main features that can facilitate a differential etiological diagnosis between the tree main forms of systemic amyloidosis. Since AL amyloidosis is the most common form of the disease, a search for clonal plasma-cell dyscrasia is generally the first step. A detailed description of the sequence of diagnostic tests used for plasma cell dyscrasia can be found elsewhere [2, 36, 56]. Histological evidence of amyloid deposits is essential for a final diagnosis of amyloidosis. The diagnostic accuracy of an extra-cardiac biopsy depends on the type of amyloidosis and on the analyzed tissue [45]. In general, the yield of an extra-cardiac biopsy (lip, skin, salivary gland, or gastrointestinal tract) is higher in AL than in familial ATTR and, however, is very low in ATTR wild-type [90]. In ATTR, peri-umbilical fat biopsy, especially in patients with wild type ATTR has a sensitivity of <20% [90]. Thus, while a fat pad biopsy is a preferred initial site, expecially in AL, a negative result is insufficient to exclude the diagnosis and an EMB should be performed.

The final goal of a biopsy, following the documentation of amyloid infiltration, is to provide a definite etiologic classification. Immunohistochemistry remains the most widely available method for fibril typing [45]. Its diagnostic value is very high in AA amyloidosis and in most cases of ATTR amyloidosis, but the results are not always definitive in patients with AL amyloidosis. The most frequent pitfall is the coexistence of positivity for more than one type of antisera, typically those for TTR and lambda or kappa-chains, which are the result of the antibody binding to circulating proteins present in the pathological specimen. In a recent series, 8/15 patients with monoclonal gammopathy, showed strong TTR staining in the histological samples whereas mass spectrometry demonstrated light chain amyloid in 5 of these 8 patients

Table 17.4 Main features that facilitate a differential aetiological diagnosis between the three main forms of systemic amyloidosis

	AL	ATTR	Systemic senile amyloidosis
Suggestive clinical/instrumental signs	Present	Present	Present
Amyloid in biopsy from affected organ or abdominal fat	Positive	Positive	Positive (myocardium)
Plasma-cell dyscrasia	Present	Absent	Absent
Transthyretin mutation	Absent	Present	Absent
Immunohistochemistry	Positive for κ or λ light chains	Positive for TTR	Positive for TTR
Characteristic neurological signs	Sometimes	Yes	Sometimes
Echocardiographic findings suggestive of amyloidotic cardiomyopathy	Sometimes	Sometimes	Yes

[91]. Mass spectrometric analysis of amyloid is a technique recently introduced for fibril typing [92]. This method involves laser micro-dissection and laser capture of amyloid using a microscope followed by tryptic digestion and tandem mass spectrometry. Computer algorithms match the peptides to a reference database.

17.6 Therapy of Cardiac Amyloidoses

17.6.1 Disease Modifying Treatments (Liver Transplantation and New Drugs)

Current specific treatment for TTR-CA is focused on different steps in the TTR amyloid cascade including silencing of TTR production, TTR stabilization and amyloid clearance from tissues [45, 93–95].

Because 95% of TTR protein is produced by the liver, orthotropic liver transplantation (OLT) has been used in ATTRm to replace amyloidogenic mutant with wild-type TTR and theoretically arrest amyloid formation. According to the FAP World Transplant Registry, more than 2000 OLT procedures have been performed in a total of 12 different countries, most of all in patients with Val30Met mutation with a primary neuropathic phenotype [96]. OLT is considered a preventative measure to forestall the development of the sensorimotor neuropathy or multiple organ involvement. Survival after transplantation in Val30Met patients is >50% at 20 years [96]. Since the liver function of TTR liver transplant recipients is otherwise normal, their livers have been transplanted into high risk recipients ("domino liver transplant"), causing TTR amyloidosis in recipients several years late [97]. While survival is prolonged by liver transplantation [96], there is slowing but not arrest of disease progression. This is attributed to deposition of wild type TTR amyloid in the heart from the transplanted liver causing progressive cardiac dysfunction. Patients with fragmented ATTR fibrils (type A) developed HF after OLT while those who had intact ATTR fibrils (type B) did not deteriorate to the same degree [98]. The scarcity of organ availability, the need for lifelong immunosuppression, the relatively older age of affected subjects make transplantation an unsuitable option for facing TTR-CA.

Both RNA interference (RNAi) and antisense oligonucleotides (ASOs) have been used to inhibit hepatic expression of amyloidogenic TTR. These therapies capitalize on endogenous cellular mechanism for controlling gene expression in which siRNAs or ASOs, mediates the destruction of target messenger RNA (mRNA) essential for TTR production. These agents cause a robust and durable reduction in genetic expression (knockdown) of TTR and retinol binding protein [99–102]. Both methods of silencing have completed recruitment for phase III trials in TTR peripheral neuropathy with results expected in 2017 but a phase III trial in TTR cardiomyopathy was recently suspended.

TTR stabilizers have demonstrated efficacy in FAP [103, 104] but their efficacy in TTR-CA is unknown. Diflunisal, a nonsteroidal anti-inflammatory drug, binds and stabilizes common familial TTR variants against acid-mediated fibril formation in vitro and has been tested in human clinical trials [103]. Use of diflunisal is controversial given the known consequences of chronic inhibition of cyclooxygenase enzymes including gastrointestinal bleeding, renal dysfunction, fluid retention, and hypertension that may precipitate HF in vulnerable individuals. Tafamidis is a novel compound that binds to the thyroxine-binding sites of the TTR tetramer, inhibiting its dissociation into monomers [105] and blocking the rate-limiting step in the TTR amyloidogenesis cascade. A phase III clinical trial with tafamidis in TTR cardiac amyloidosis is ongoing and the results are expected in 2018.

Eepigallocatechin gallate (EGCG), the most abundant flavonoid in green tea, inhibits amyloid fibril formation in vitro, leading to open label trials in TTR-CA [106].

Doxycycline disrupts fibril formation [107] and when combined with bile salt, tauroursodeoxycholic acid demonstrated a synergistic effect on removal of tissue TTR deposits in an animal model, leading to ongoing open label trials in humans. Disruption/clearance of amyloid fibrils is a particularly relevant target. Various monoclonal antibodies are in developmental stages including NEOD001 and PRX004 (Prothena) targeted at AL and ATTR amyloid respectively, and an anti-SAP antibody (GSK) which target serum amyloid P component which decorates deposited amyloid fibrils.

17.6.2 Prevention and Treatment of Cardiovascular Complications

In the absence of widely available specific treatments for any of the etiologically distinct forms of cardiac amyloidosis, the main therapeutic aims are to relieve symptoms, treat congestive heart failure, and prevent arrhythmic and thromboembolic complications [36, 39]. Diuretics are essential for treatment of venous congestion. However, their use must be judicious, as pre-load reduction in patients with overt restrictive physiology may reduce ventricular filling pressures, leading to decreased cardiac output and hypotension. Large resistant pleural effusions (particularly frequent in AL) may indicate the presence of pleural amyloidotic involvement, [108] occasionally necessitating recurrent pleural taps or even pleurodesis. Digoxin must be used with caution, due to its high arrhythmogenicity in the amyloidotic substrate [1]. Indeed, the high propensity of this drug to bind with amyloid fibrils [109] can easily lead to clinical manifestations of digoxin toxicity, even in the presence of apparently "therapeutic" serum levels [36]. Maintenance of sinus rhythm is important, since development of atrial fibrillation worsens diastolic dysfunction, and a rapid ventricular response may further compromise the pumping function.

The decision whether or not to start antithrombotic therapy is complex, particularly in AL where risk of hemorrhage is high. In ATTR, hemorrhagic events appear to be less common. Anticoagulation with warfarin is mandatory for patients with paroxysmal or permanent atrial fibrillation and flutter. It has also been suggested that transesophageal echocardiography is useful to identify patients that have atrial dysfunction despite sinus rhythm (by revealing spontaneous echo contrast or atrial appendage Doppler velocities below 40 cm/s). In such cases, warfarin may be indicated in view of the risk of thrombus formation in the atrial appendage [40].

No controlled study is available regarding the effects of β-blocker used in amyloidosis, whether for rate control of atrial fibrillation or for treatment of heart failure, but rate reduction with β-blockers can cause a critical decrease in cardiac output without providing benefits in terms of reverse ventricular remodelling. Calcium channel blockers are contraindicated, since these drugs often exert relevant negative inotropic effects [110, 111].

In heart failure generally, ACE inhibitor or angiotensin receptor blockers are standard therapy. However, for patients with cardiac amyloidosis these drugs must be administered with extreme caution due to the elevated risk of inducing or exacerbating hypotension.

Although sudden death is frequent in amyloidosis [112, 113], very little is known about the underlying cause of most events. Sudden death has reportedly been caused by advanced atrioventricular block, ventricular tachycardia/fibrillation, and electromechanical dissociation. Implantable cardiac defibrillators have been used only in a small number of cases in the absence of any documented effect on survival. Although some centers use amiodarone to try to prevent arrhythmias and sudden death in patients with amyloidotic cardiomyopathy, studies of efficacy are lacking. If cardioversion is performed to treat atrial fibrillation, use of a temporary prophylactic pacemaker is advisable due to the risk that the abnormal sinus node may fail. When amyloidosis patients present with bradyarrhythmias, clinicians may feel justified to proceed to prophylactic pacemaker implantation earlier than they normally would with other patients. In the presence of restrictive physiology, dual-chamber devices should be preferred [112].

Neurogenic orthostatic hypotension is difficult to prevent and treat. General prophylactic non-pharmacologic measures and Midodrine, a peripheral, selective, direct α1-adrenoreceptor agonist, which is the only medication approved by the Food and Drug Administration for the treatment of orthostatic hypotension) are the only palliative treatments that can be offered to patients [114]. Phosphodiesterase inhibitors can be used to treat erectile dysfunction [115].

17.6.3 Combined 'Heart-Liver' Transplantation

Cardiac involvement can affect the success of OLT and the patient's postoperative outcome in at least two different ways. Patients with amyloidotic cardiomyopathy have an increased perioperative morbidity and mortality. Indeed, any cardiological complication which leads to low cardiac output or increased filling pressure in the perioperative phase can fatally damage the transplanted liver, thereby threatening the life of the recipient and wasting a precious life-saving organ. Cardiovascular complications account for about two-fifths of deaths after OLT (almost half of which of which occur within the first 3 months) [97]. The second major problem is progression of cardiomyopathy even after successful OLT. This phenomenon has been echocardiographically documented, especially (though not exclusively) in patients with mutations other than Val30Met. After OLT, some patients with the Leu30 variant of ATTR have shown an increased proportion of amyloid derived from wild-type

TTR in their myocardial tissue [38]. Furthermore, slow but progressive amyloidotic cardiomyopathy has been observed after OLT even in patients whose cardiac involvement was only mild up to the time of transplantation. It is currently thought that although wild-type TTR is only weakly amyloidogenic, its potential for myocardial deposition can increase dramatically in the presence of a pre-existing template of amyloid in the heart. These considerations provide the rationale for combined heart-liver transplantation in selected patients [116, 117]. The number of such interventions is currently limited (with no more than 30 reports available in the literature). Combined heart-liver transplantation is a technically challenging procedure which is necessarily the province of a few highly specialized centers. The degree of neurological impairment and the patient's nutritional status are thought to be the two major factors influencing long-term outcome [118]. Encouragingly, the cardiac grafts do not appear to be affected by amyloid during follow-up.

The main indication for combined heart-liver transplantation is presence of severe heart failure due to amyloidotic cardiomyopathy in a patient without advanced neurological involvement. Combined heart-liver transplantation has also been proposed as a therapeutic option for patients affected by mutations other than Val30Met who are candidates for OLT and who have an echocardiographic diagnosis of cardiomyopathy (even in the absence of major cardiovascular symptoms) [32].

17.7 Other Hereditary Amyloidoses

Other mutated genes which can induce systemic disease with variable patterns of organ involvement and clinical severity include apolipoprotein A-I (AApoAI), apolipoprotein A-II (AApoAII), lysozyme (ALys), gelsolin (AGel), fibrinogen Aa (AFib), and Cystatin C (ACys). Clinically relevant cardiac involvement mainly occurs in patients with apolipoprotein A-I mutation.

17.7.1 Apolipoprotein A-I Amyloidosis (AApoAI)

Apolipoprotein A-I is the main constituent of high-density lipoprotein particles (the ApoAI gene is located on chromosome 11). About half of apolipoprotein AI is synthesized in the liver and the other half in the small intestine [18, 119]. Twelve different ApoAI gene mutations (mostly single nucleotide substitutions) have been associated with deposition of apolipoprotein A-I amyloid [3, 120]. All forms of apolipoprotein A-I amyloidosis are inherited as autosomal dominant traits, but clinical onset varies from the third decade of life to advanced age and the penetrance is not known (although it is probably greater than 50%). Unlike ATTR, the kidney is the most frequently affected organ, and death is usually caused by renal failure. Other sites of involvement include liver, spleen, and occasionally the heart. In rare cases, cardiac involvement can lead to massive hypertrophy with very diminutive ventricular cavities [121]. In contrast to most cases of AL, in apolipoprotein A-I amyloidosis proteinuria is usually very limited.

17.7.2 Apolipoprotein A-II Amyloidosis (AApoAII)

Like apolipoprotein AI, apolipoprotein AII, is predominantly synthesized by the liver and the intestines. Apolipoprotein AII amyloidosis is the most recently discovered hereditary systemic form of the disease. It is an autosomal dominant amyloidosis caused by point mutations in the apoAII gene. Clinically, it characterized by early adult onset of progressive renal failure. Dialysis and renal transplantation are currently the only two therapeutic options, both of which are palliative [122]. After transplantation, recurrence of amyloid deposition in the graft is rare and progression of any other organ involvement tends to be very slow [122].

17.7.3 Lysozyme Amyloidosis (ALys)

Lysozyme is a ubiquitous bacteriolytic enzyme present in both external secretions and in leukocytes, macrophages, gastrointestinal cells and hepatocytes; its physiologic role is not clear. Lysozyme amyloidosis is an autosomal dominant "nonneuropathic" form of hereditary amyloidosis, associated with four different lysozyme gene mutations (Trp64Arg Ile56Thr, Asp67His, Phe57Ile) [123]. Gastrointestinal involvement has been seen in nearly all reported cases of lysozyme amyloidosis, varying from mild abdominal discomfort to severe malabsorption syndrome [123]. Megaloblastic anemia due to acid folic deficiency secondary to amyloid deposition in the small intestine [124] and bleeding of the gastrointestinal tract have also been described.

Renal manifestations are frequent in lysozyme amyloidosis [124, 125] Other clinical manifestations that have been described include "sicca syndrome" [126], bone marrow infiltration, [127] and heart involvement [128, 129].

17.7.4 Gelsolin (AGel)

Gelsolin amyloidosis is rather common in Finland [18, 130, 131] but very rare elsewhere. This type of amyloidosis stems from a mutation (Asp187Asn) in plasma gelsolin, an actin-modulating protein that takes part in the clearance of actin filaments [132, 133]. The main clinical manifestations are corneal lattice dystrophy, cranial neuropathy, and cutis laxa. Peripheral and autonomic neuropathy, and cardiac or renal involvement can also occur [134]. Lattice corneal dystrophy is pathognomonic, greatly facilitating diagnosis of the condition [135].

17.7.5 Fibrinogen Aa Amyloidosis (AFib)

Fibrinogen amyloidosis (AFib) is an autosomal dominant disease with low penetrance, caused by point mutations in the fibrinogen A alpha chain gene (about six amyloidogenic mutations in the fibrinogen Aα-chain have been identified, the most common being Glu526Val [136]. Kidneys are the main site of amyloid deposition. Cardiac involvement has yet to be reported.

17.7.6 Cystatin C Amyloidosis (ACys)

This disease, documented in a seven generation pedigree in northwest Iceland (hereditary cerebral haemorrhage with amyloidosis, Icelandic type, HCHWA-I) is a rare, fatal, autosomal dominant condition, directly linked to a Leu68Gln mutation in the cystatin C protein sequence, a cysteine protease inhibitor [137]. Mutant cystatin C forms amyloid in brain arteries and arterioles, and to a lesser degree in tissues outside the central nervous system such as the skin, lymph nodes, testis, spleen, submandibular salivary glands, and adrenal cortex.

17.8 Key Points

1. Systemic amyloidoses are complex entities, which are widely underdiagnosed.
2. ATTR (i.e. transthyretin-related familial amyloidosis) is the most frequent form of hereditary systemic amyloidosis. It is characterized by a high degree of genotypic (over 80 different amyloidogenic mutations) and phenotypic heterogeneity. The clinical spectrum of ATTR ranges from almost exclusive neurologic involvement (within a clearly familial context) to apparently sporadic cases with a strictly cardiological presentation.
3. Phenotypic heterogeneity is linked to at least three different factors: the type of TTR mutation, the geographic distribution, and the type of aggregation (endemic or non-endemic).
4. Cardiac amyloidosis is generally considered to be a myocardial disease with "hypertrophic phenotype" and restrictive physiology. However, any representative cohort of patients with amyloid heart disease will display a spectrum of diastolic filling abnormalities, with the restrictive pattern manifesting only in advanced stages of the disease.
5. The single most useful sign to arouse diagnostic suspicion of cardiac amyloidosis is the presence of low or normal QRS voltage at ECG despite increased left ventricular wall thickness at echocardiography.
6. Histologic evidence of amyloid deposits is essential for a final diagnosis of amyloidosis. However, in a patient with a genetically proven diagnosis of ATTR, echocardiographic identification of unexplained ventricular hypertrophy provides clinical evidence of the specific disease.
7. Since the liver is mainly responsible for TTR production, orthotopic liver transplantation can provide a "surgical gene therapy" for ATTR and must be considered as soon as possible for all patients with clinically evident, molecularly confirmed disease
8. The biologic process underlying TTR cardiac amyloidosis has led to the development of numerous therapies that are currently in late phase clinical trials.

9. Combined heart-liver transplantation can be offered to patients with severe heart failure due to amyloidotic cardiomyopathy, or to patients affected by mutations other than Val30Met who are candidates for OLT and who have an echocardiographic diagnosis of cardiomyopathy (even in the absence of major cardiovascular symptoms).

References

1. Falk RH, Comenzo RL, Skinner M. The systemic amyloidoses. N Engl J Med. 1997;337:898–909.
2. Merlini G, Bellotti V. Molecular mechanisms of amyloidosis. N Engl J Med. 2003;349:583–96.
3. Merlini G, Westermark P. The systemic amyloidoses: clearer understanding of the molecular mechanisms offers hope for more effective therapies. J Intern Med. 2004;255:159–78.
4. Hou X, Aguilar MI, Small DH. Transthyretin and familial amyloidotic polyneuropathy. Recent progress in understanding the molecular mechanism of neurodegeneration. FEBS J. 2007;274:1637–50.
5. Dubrey SW, Cha K, Skinner M, et al. Familial and primary (AL) cardiac amyloidosis: echocardiographically similar diseases with distinctly different clinical outcomes. Heart. 1997;78:74–82.
6. Yankner BA, Dawes LR, Fisher S, Villa-Komaroff L, Oster-Granite ML, Neve RL. Neurotoxicity of a fragment of the amyloid precursor associated with Alzheimer's disease. Science. 1989;245:417–20.
7. May PC, Boggs LN, Fuson KS. Neurotoxicity of human amylin in rat primary hippocampal cultures: similarity to Alzheimer's disease amyloid-b neurotoxicity. J Neurochem. 1993;61:2330–3.
8. Jordan J, Galindo MF, Miller RJ, Reardon CA, Getz GS, LaDu MJ. Isoform-specific effect of apolipoprotein E on cell survival and beta-amyloid-induced toxicity in rat hippocampal pyramidal neuronal cultures. J Neurosci. 1998;18:195–204.
9. Wang C-N, Chi C-W, Lin Y-L, Chen C-F, Shiao Y-J. The neuroprotective effects of phytoestrogens on amyloid b protein-induced toxicity are mediated by abrogating the activation of caspase cascade in rat cortical neurons. J Biol Chem. 2001;276:5287–95.
10. Schubert D, Behl C, Lesley R, et al. Amyloid peptides are toxic via a common oxidative mechanism. Proc Natl Acad Sci U S A. 1995;92:1989–93.
11. Goodman Y, Mattson MP. K+ channel openers protect hippocampal neurons against oxidative injury and amyloid b-peptide toxicity. Brain Res. 1996;706:328–32.
12. Engström I, Ronquist G, Pettersson L, Waldenström A. Alzheimer amyloid beta-peptides exhibit ionophore-like properties in human erythrocytes. Eur J Clin Investig. 1995;25:471–6.
13. Janson J, Ashley RH, Harrison D, McIntyre S, Butler PC. The mechanism of islet amyloid polypeptide toxicity is membrane disruption by intermediate-sized toxic amyloid particles. Diabetes. 1999;48:491–8.
14. Mirzabekov TA, Lin M, Kagan BL. Pore formation by the cytotoxic islet amyloid peptide amylin. J Biol Chem. 1996;271:1988–92.
15. Kayed R, Head E, Thompson JL, et al. Common structure of soluble amyloid oligomers implies common mechanism of pathogenesis. Science. 2003;300:486–9.
16. Sipe JD, Benson MD, Buxbaum JN, et al. Nomenclature 2014: amyloid fibril proteins and clinical classification of the amyloidosis. Amyloid. 2014;21(4):221–4.
17. Gertz MA, Lacy MQ, Dispenzieri A. Amyloidosis. Hematol Oncol Clin North Am. 1999;13:1211–33.
18. Benson MD, Kincaid JC. The molecular biology and clinical features of amyloid neuropathy. Muscle Nerve. 2007;36:411–23.

19. Jacobson DR, Pastore R, Pool S, et al. Revised transthyretin Ile 122 allele frequency in African-Americans. Hum Genet. 1996;98:236–8.
20. Uemichi T, Liepnieks JJ, Waits RP, Benson MD. A trinucleotide deletion in the transthyretin gene (V122) in a kindred with familial amyloidotic polyneuropathy. Neurology. 1997;48:1667–70.
21. Harats N, Worth RM, Benson MD. Hereditary amyloidosis: evidence against early amyloid deposition. Arthritis Rheum. 1989;32:1474–6.
22. Andrade C. A peculiar form of peripheral neuropathy. Familial atypical generalized amyloidosis with special involvement of the peripheral nerves. Brain. 1952;75:408–27.
23. Ando Y, Nakamura M, Araki S. Transthyretin-related familial amyloidotic polyneuropathy. Arch Neurol. 2005;62:1057–62.
24. Ohmori H, Ando Y, Makita Y, et al. Common origin of the Val30Met mutation responsible for the amyloidogenic transthyretin type of familial amyloidotic polyneuropathy. J Med Genet. 2004;41:51–5.
25. Suhr OB, Svendsen IH, Andersson R, Danielsson A, Holmgren G, Ranløv PJ. Hereditary transthyretin amyloidosis from a Scandinavian perspective. J Intern Med. 2003;254:225–35.
26. Ranløv I, Alves IL, Ranløv PJ, Husby G, Costa PP, Saraiva MJ. A Danish kindred with familial amyloid cardiomyopathy revisited: identification of a mutant transthyretin-methionine111 variant in serum from patients and carriers. Am J Med. 1992;93:3–8.
27. Svendsen IH, Steensgaard-Hansen F, Nordvåg BY. A clinical, echocardiographic and genetic characterization of a Danish kindred with familial amyloid transthyretin methionine 111 linked cardiomyopathy. Eur Heart J. 1998;19:782–9.
28. Reilly MM, Staunton H, Harding AE. Familial amyloid polyneuropathy (transthyretin Ala-60) in north west Ireland: a clinical, genetic, and epidemiological study. J Neurol Neurosurg Psychiatry. 1995;59:45–9.
29. Plante-Bordeneuve V, Carayol J, Ferreira A, et al. Genetic study of transthyretin amyloid neuropathies: carrier risks among French and Portuguese families. J Med Genet. 2003;40:e120.
30. Planté-Bordeneuve V, Ferreira A, Lalu T, Zaros C, Lacroix C, Adams D, Said G. Diagnostic pitfalls in sporadic transthyretin familial amyloid polyneuropathy (TTR-FAP). Neurology. 2007;69:693–8.
31. Adams D, Reilly M, Harding AE, Said G. Demonstration of genetic mutation in most of the amyloid neuropathies with sporadic occurrence. Rev Neurol (Paris). 1992;148:736–41.
32. Rapezzi C, Perugini E, Salvi F, et al. Phenotypic and genotypic heterogeneity in transthyretin-related cardiac amyloidosis: towards tailoring of therapeutic strategies? Amyloid. 2006;13:143–53.
33. Jacobson DR, Pastore RD, Yaghoubian R, et al. Variant-sequence transthyretin (isoleucine 122) in late-onset cardiac amyloidosis in black Americans. N Engl J Med. 1997;336:466–73.
34. Goren H, Steinberg MC, Farboody GH. Familial oculoleptomeningeal amyloidosis. Brain. 1980;103:473–95.
35. Yazaki M, Connors LH, Eagle RC Jr, Leff SR, Skinner M, Benson MD. Transthyretin amyloidosis associated with a novel variant (Trp41Leu) presenting with vitreous opacities. Amyloid. 2002;9:263–7.
36. Falk RH. Diagnosis and management of the cardiac amyloidoses. Circulation. 2005;112:2047–60.
37. Hattori T, Takei Y, Koyama J, Nakazato M, Ikeda S. Clinical and pathological studies of cardiac amyloidosis in transthyretin type familial amyloid polyneuropathy. Amyloid. 2003;10:229–39.
38. Ikeda S. Cardiac amyloidosis: heterogenous pathogenic backgrounds. Intern Med. 2004;43:1107–14.
39. Selvanayagam JB, Hawkins PN, Paul B, Myerson SG, Neubauer S. Evaluation and management of the cardiac amyloidosis. J Am Coll Cardiol. 2007;50:2101–10.
40. Klein AL, Hatle LK, Burstow DJ, et al. Doppler characterization of left ventricular diastolic function in cardiac amyloidosis. J Am Coll Cardiol. 1989;13:1017–26.

41. Elliott P, Andersson B, Arbustini E, et al. Classification of the cardiomyopathies: a position statement from the European Society of Cardiology working group on myocardial and pericardial diseases. Eur Heart J. 2008;29:270–6.
42. Koyama J, Ray-Sequin PA, Davidoff R, et al. Useful of pulsed tissue Doppler imaging for evaluating systolic and diastolic left ventricular function in patients with AL (primary) amyloidosis. Am J Cardiol. 2002;89:1067–71.
43. Palka P, Lange A, Donnelly E, et al. Doppler echocardiographic features of cardiac amyloidosis. J Am Soc Echocardiogr. 2002;15:1353–60.
44. Pasotti M, Agozzino M, Concardi M, Merlini G, Rapezzi C, Arbustini E. Obstructive intramural coronary amyloidosis: a distinct phenotype of cardiac amyloidosis that can cause acute heart failure. Eur Heart J. 2006;27:1810.
45. Maurer MS, Elliott P, Comenzo R, Semigran M, Rapezzi C. Addressing common questions encountered in the diagnosis and management of cardiac amyloidosis. Circulation. 2017;135:1357–77.
46. Carroll JD, Gaasch WH, McAdam KP. Amyloid cardiomyopathy: characterization by a distinctive voltage/mass relation. Am J Cardiol. 1982;49:9–13.
47. Hamer JP, Janssen S, van Rijswijk MH, et al. Amyloid cardiomyopathy in systemic non-hereditary amyloidosis. Clinical, echocardiographic and electrocardiographic findings in 30 patients with AA and 24 patients with AL amyloidosis. Eur Heart J. 1992;13:623–7.
48. Rahman JE, Helou EF, Gelzer-Bell R, et al. Noninvasive diagnosis of biopsy-proven cardiac amyloidosis. J Am Coll Cardiol. 2004;43:410–5.
49. Murtagh B, Hammill SC, Gertz MA, et al. Electrocardiographic findings in primary systemic amyloidosis and biopsy-proven cardiac involvement. Am J Cardiol. 2005;95:535–7.
50. González-López E, Gallego-Delgado M, Guzzo-Merello G, et al. Wild-type transthyretin amyloidosis as a cause of heart failure with preserved ejection fraction. Eur Heart J. 2015;36(38):2585–94.
51. Cueto-Garcia L, Tajik AJ, Kyle RA, et al. Serial echocardiographic observations in patients with primary systemic amyloidosis: an introduction to the concept of early (asymptomatic) amyloid infiltration of the heart. Mayo Clin Proc. 1984;59:589–97.
52. Klein AL, Hatle LK, Taliercio CP, et al. Prognostic significance of Doppler measures of diastolic function in cardiac amyloidosis. A Doppler echocardiography study. Circulation. 1991;83:808–16.
53. Simons M, Isner JM. Assessment of relative sensitivities of non-invasive tests for cardiac amyloidosis in documented cardiac amyloidosis. Am J Cardiol. 1992;69:425–7.
54. Trikas A, Rallidis L, Hawkins P, et al. Comparison of usefulness between exercise capacity and echocardiographic indexes of left ventricular function in cardiac amyloidosis. Am J Cardiol. 1999;84:1049–54.
55. Lachmann HJ, Booth DR, Booth SE, et al. Misdiagnosis of hereditary amyloidosis as AL (primary) amyloidosis. N Engl J Med. 2002;346:1786–91.
56. Gertz MA, Comenzo R, Falk RH, et al. Definition of organ involvement and treatment response in immunoglobulin light chain amyloidosis (AL): a consensus opinion from the 10th international symposium on amyloid and amyloidosis. Am J Hematol. 2005;79:319–28.
57. Demir M, Paydas S, Cayli M, et al. Tissue Doppler is a more reliable method in early detection of cardiac dysfunction in patients with AA amyloidosis. Ren Fail. 2005;27:415–20.
58. Quarta CC, Solomon SD, Uraizee I, et al. Left ventricular structure and function in transthyretin-related versus light-chain cardiac amyloidosis. Circulation. 2014;129(18):1840–9.
59. Maceira AM, Joshi J, Prasad SK, et al. Cardiovascular magnetic resonance in cardiac amyloidosis. Circulation. 2005;111:186–93.
60. Perugini E, Rapezzi C, Piva T, et al. Non-invasive evaluation of the myocardial substrate of cardiac amyloidosis by gadolinium cardiac magnetic resonance. Heart. 2006;92:343–9.
61. Thomson LE. Cardiovascular magnetic resonance in clinically suspected cardiac amyloidosis: diagnostic value of a typical pattern of late gadolinium enhancement. J Am Coll Cardiol. 2008;51:1031–2.

62. Vogelsberg H, Mahrholdt H, Deluigi CC, et al. Cardiovascular magnetic resonance in clinically suspected cardiac amyloidosis: noninvasive imaging compared to endomyocardial biopsy. J Am Coll Cardiol. 2008;51:1022–30.
63. Syed IS, Glockner JF, Feng D, et al. Role of cardiac magnetic resonance imaging in the detection of cardiac amyloidosis. JACC Cardiovasc Imaging. 2010;3:155–64.
64. Fontana M, Banypersad SM, Treibel TA, et al. Native T1 mapping in transthyretin amyloidosis. JACC Cardiovasc Imaging. 2014;7:157–65.
65. Fontana M, Chung R, Hawkins PN, Moon JC. Cardiovascular magnetic resonance for amyloidosis. Heart Fail Rev. 2015;20:133–44.
66. Karamitsos TD, Piechnik SK, Banypersad SM, et al. Noncontrast T1 mapping for the diagnosis of cardiac amyloidosis. JACC Cardiovasc Imaging. 2013;6:488–97.
67. Dungu JN, Valencia O, Pinney JH, et al. CMR-based differentiation of AL and ATTR cardiac amyloidosis. JACC Cardiovasc Imaging. 2014;7:133–42.
68. Hawkins PN. Serum amyloid P component scintigraphy for diagnosis and monitoring amyloidosis. Curr Opin Nephrol Hypertens. 2002;11:649–55.
69. Perugini E, Guidalotti PL, Salvi F, et al. Noninvasive etiologic diagnosis of cardiac amyloidosis using 99mTc-3,3-diphosphono-1,2-propanodicarboxylic acid scintigraphy. J Am Coll Cardiol. 2005;46:1076–84.
70. Wizenberg TA, Muz J, Sohn YH, et al. Value of positive myocardial technetium-99m-pyrophosphate scintigraphy in the noninvasive diagnosis of cardiac amyloidosis. Am Heart J. 1982;103:468–73.
71. Falk RH, Lee VW, Rubinow A, et al. Sensitivity of technetium-99m-pyrophosphate scintigraphy in diagnosing cardiac amyloidosis. Am J Cardiol. 1983;51:826–30.
72. Gertz MA, Brown ML, Hauser MF, Kyle RA. Utility of technetium Tc 99m pyrophosphate bone scanning in cardiac amyloidosis. Arch Intern Med. 1987;147:1039–44.
73. Rapezzi C, Guidalotti P, Salvi F, et al. Usefulness of 99mTc-DPD scintigraphy in cardiac amyloidosis. J Am Coll Cardiol. 2008;51:1509–10. author reply 1510.
74. Rapezzi C, Quarta CC, Guidalotti PL, et al. Usefulness and limitations of 99mTc-3,3-diphosphono-1,2-propanodicarboxylic acid scintigraphy in the aetiological diagnosis of amyloidotic cardiomyopathy. Eur J Nucl Med Mol Imaging. 2011;38:470–8.
75. Gillmore JD, Maurer MS, Falk RH, et al. Nonbiopsy diagnosis of cardiac transthyretin amyloidosis. Circulation. 2016;133(24):2404–12.
76. Hutt DF, Quigley AM, Page J, et al. Utility and limitations of 3,3-diphosphono-1,2-propanodicarboxylic acid scintigraphy in systemic amyloidosis. Eur Heart J Cardiovasc Imaging. 2014;15:1289–98.
77. Hutt DF, Fontana M, Burniston M, et al. Prognostic utility of the Perugini grading of 99mTc-DPD scintigraphy in transthyretin (ATTR) amyloidosis and its relationship with skeletal muscle and soft tissue amyloid. Eur Heart J Cardiovasc Imaging. 2017;18(12):1344–50, https://doi.org/10.1093/ehjci/jew325.
78. Park MA, Padera RF, Belanger A, et al. 18F-Florbetapir binds specifically to myocardial light chain and transthyretin amyloid deposits: autoradiography study. Circ Cardiovasc Imaging. 2015;8:e002954.
79. Crotty TB, Li C-Y, Edwards WD, et al. Amyloidosis and endomyocardial biopsy: correlation of extent and pattern of deposition with amyloid immunophenotype in 100 cases. Cardiovasc Pathol. 1995;4:39–42.
80. Gertz MA, Grogan M, Kyle RA, Tajik AJ. Endomyocardial biopsy proven light chain amyloidosis (AL) without echocardiographic features of infiltrative cardiomyopathy. Am J Cardiol. 1997;80:93–5.
81. Ardehali H, Qasim A, Cappola T, et al. Endomyocardial biopsy plays a role in diagnosing patients with unexplained cardiomyopathy. Am Heart J. 2004;147:919–23.
82. Palladini G, Campana C, Klersy C, et al. Serum N-terminal pro-brain natriuretic peptide is a sensitive marker of myocardial dysfunction in AL amyloidosis. Circulation. 2003;107:2440–5.

83. Dispenzieri A, Kyle RA, Gertz MA, et al. Survival in patients with primary systemic amyloidosis and raised serum cardiac troponins. Lancet. 2003;361:1787–9.
84. Dispenzieri A, Lacy MQ, Katzmann JA, et al. Absolute values of immunoglobulin free light chains are prognostic in patients with primary systemic amyloidosis undergoing peripheral blood stem cell transplantation. Blood. 2006;107:3378–83.
85. Palladini G, Lavatelli F, Russo P, et al. Circulating amyloidogenic free light chains and serum N-terminal natriuretic peptide type B decrease simultaneously in association with improvement of survival in AL. Blood. 2006;107:3854–8.
86. Suhr OB, Anan I, Backman C, et al. Do troponin and B-natriuretic peptide detect cardiomyopathy in transthyretin amyloidosis? J Intern Med. 2008;263:294–301.
87. Kristen AV, Maurer MS, Rapezzi C, THAOS Investigators, et al. Impact of genotype and phenotype on cardiac biomarkers in patients with transthyretin amyloidosis - report from the transthyretin amyloidosis outcome survey (THAOS). PLoS One. 2017;12(4):e0173086.
88. Grogan M, Scott C, Kyle RA, Zeldenrust SR, et al. Natural history of wild type transthyretin cardiac amyloidosis and risk stratification using a novel staging system. J Am Coll Cardiol. 2016;68:1014.
89. Ng B, Connors LH, Davidoff R, et al. Senile systemic amyloidosis presenting with heart failure: a comparison with light chain-associated amyloidosis. Arch Intern Med. 2005;165:1425–9.
90. Fine NM, Arruda-Olson AM, Dispenzieri A, Zeldenrust SR, Gertz MA, Kyle RA, Swiecicki PL, Scott CG, Grogan M. Yield of noncardiac biopsy for the diagnosis of transthyretin cardiac amyloidosis. Am J Cardiol. 2014;113:1723–7.
91. Satoskar AA, Efebera Y, Hasan A, et al. Strong transthyretin immunostaining: potential pitfall in cardiac amyloid typing. Am J Surg Pathol. 2011;35:1685–90.
92. Vrana JA, Gamez JD, Madden BJ, et al. Classification of amyloidosis by laser microdissection and mass spectrometry-based proteomic analysis in clinical biopsy specimens. Blood. 2009;114:4957–9.
93. Castano A, Drachman BM, Judge D, Maurer MS. Natural history and therapy of TTR-cardiac amyloidosis: emerging disease-modifying therapies from organ transplantation to stabilizer and silencer drugs. Heart Fail Rev. 2015;20:163–78.
94. Dubrey S, Ackermann E, Gillmore J. The transthyretin amyloidoses: advances in therapy. Postgrad Med J. 2015;91:439–48.
95. Hawkins PN, Ando Y, Dispenzeri A, et al. Evolving landscape in the management of transthyretin amyloidosis. Ann Med. 2015;47:625–38.
96. Ericzon BG, Wilczek HE, Larsson M, et al. Liver transplantation for hereditary transthyretin amyloidosis: after 20 years still the best therapeutic alternative? Transplantation. 2015;99:1847–54.
97. Stangou AJ, Heaton ND, Hawkins PN. Transmission of sistemic transthyretin amyloidosis by means of domino liver transplantation. N Engl J Med. 2005;352:2356.
98. Gustafsson S, Ihse E, Henein MY, et al. Amyloid fibril composition as a predictor of development of cardiomyopathy after liver transplantation for hereditary transthyretin amyloidosis. Transplantation. 2012;93:1017–23.
99. Coelho T, Adams D, Silva A, et al. Safety and efficacy of RNAi therapy for transthyretin amyloidosis. N Engl J Med. 2013a;369:819–29.
100. Coelho T, Maia LF, da Silva AM, et al. Long-term effects of tafamidis for the treatment of transthyretin familial amyloid polyneuropathy. J Neurol. 2013b;260:2802–14.
101. Niemietz C, Chandhok G, Schmidt H. Therapeutic oligonucleotides targeting liver disease: TTR amyloidosis. Molecules. 2015;20:17944–75.
102. Ackermann EJ, Guo S, Booten S, et al. Clinical development of an antisense therapy for the treatment of transthyretin-associated polyneuropathy. Amyloid. 2012;19(Suppl 1):43–4.
103. Berk JL, Suhr OB, Obici L, et al. Repurposing diflunisal for familial amyloid polyneuropathy: a randomized clinical trial. JAMA. 2013;310:2658–67.

104. Coelho T, Maia LF, Martins da Silva A, et al. Tafamidis for transthyretin familial amyloid polyneuropathy: a randomized, controlled trial. Neurology. 2012;79:785–92.
105. Bulawa CE, Connelly S, Devit M, et al. Tafamidis, a potent and selective transthyretin kinetic stabilizer that inhibits the amyloid cascade. Proc Natl Acad Sci U S A. 2012;109: 9629–34.
106. Kristen AV, Lehrke S, Buss S, et al. Green tea halts progression of cardiac transthyretin amyloidosis: an observational report. Clin Res Cardiol. 2012;101:805–13.
107. Ward JE, Ren R, Toraldo G, et al. Doxycycline reduces fibril formation in a transgenic mouse model of AL amyloidosis. Blood. 2011;118:6610–7.
108. Berk JL, Keane J, Seldin DC, et al. Persistent pleural effusions in primary systemic amyloidosis: etiology and prognosis. Chest. 2003;124:969–77.
109. Rubinow A, Skinner M, Cohen AS. Digoxin sensitivity in amyloid cardiomyopathy. Circulation. 1981;63:1285–8.
110. Gertz MA, Falk RH, Skinner M, Cohen AS, Kyle RA. Worsening of congestive heart failure in amyloid heart disease treated by calcium channel–blocking agents. Am J Cardiol. 1985;55:1645.
111. Pollak A, Falk RH. Left ventricular systolic dysfunction precipitated by verapamil in cardiac amyloidosis. Chest. 1993;104:618–20.
112. Falk RH, Rubinow A, Cohen AS. Cardiac arrhythmias in systemic amyloidosis: correlation with echocardiographic abnormalities. J Am Coll Cardiol. 1984;3:107–13.
113. Wright BL, Grace AA, Goodman HJ. Implantation of a cardioverterdefibrillator in a patient with cardiac amyloidosis. Nat Clin Pract Cardiovasc Med. 2006;3:110–4.
114. Freeman R. Neurogenic orthostatic hypotension. N Engl J Med. 2008;358:615–24.
115. Obayashi K, Ando Y, Terazaki H, et al. Effect of sildenafil citrate (Viagra) on erectile dysfunction in a patient with familial amyloidotic polyneuropathy ATTR Val30Met. J Auton Nerv Syst. 2000;12:89–92.
116. Ruygrok PN, Gane EJ, McCall JL, et al. Combined heart and liver transplantation for familial amyloidosis. Intern Med J. 2001;31:66–7.
117. Arpesella G, Chiappini B, Marinelli G, et al. Combined heart and liver transplantation for familial amyloidotic polyneuropathy. J Thorac Cardiovasc Surg. 2003;125:1165–6.
118. Herlenius G, Larsson M, Ericzon BG. FAP world transplant register and domino/sequential register update. Transplant Proc. 2001;33:1367.
119. Nichols WC, Gregg RE, Brewer HB, Benson MD. A mutation in apolipoprotein A-I in the Iowa type of familial amyloidotic polyneuropathy. Genomics. 1990;8:318–23.
120. Benson MD. The hereditary amyloidoses. Best Pract Res Clin Rheumatol. 2003;17:909–27.
121. Hamidi L, Liepnieks JJ, Hamidi K, et al. Hereditary amyloid cardiomyopathy caused by a variant apolipoprotein A1. Am J Pathol. 1999;154:221–7.
122. Magy N, Liepnieks J, Kluvebeckerman B. Renal transplantation for apolipoprotein AII amyloidosis. Amyloid. 2003;10:224–8.
123. Granel B, Valleix S, Serratrice J, et al. Lysozyme amyloidosis: report of 4 cases and a review of the literature. Medicine (Baltimore). 2006;85:66–73.
124. Yood RA, Skinner M, Rubinow A, Talarico L, Cohen AS. Bleeding manifestations in 100 patients with amyloidosis. JAMA. 1983;249:1322–4.
125. Simon BG, Moutsopoulos HM. Primary amyloidosis resembling sicca syndrome. Arthritis Rheum. 1979;22:932–4.
126. Valleix S, Drunat S, Philit JB, et al. Hereditary renal amyloidosis caused by a new variant lysozyme W64R in a French family. Kidney Int. 2002;61:907–12.
127. Granel B, Serratrice J, Valleix S, et al. A family with gastrointestinal amyloidosis associated with variant lysozyme. Gastroenterology. 2002;123:1346–9.
128. Gillmore JD, Booth DR, Madhoo S, Pepys MB, Hawkins PN. Hereditary renal amyloidosis associated with variant lysozyme in a large English family. Nephrol Dial Transplant. 1999;14:2639–44.
129. Booth DR, Pepys MB, Hawkins PN. A novel variant of human lysozyme (T70N) is common in the normal population. Hum Mutat. 2000;16:180.

130. Sack GH, Dumars KW, Gummerson KS, Law A, McKusick VA. Three forms of dominant amyloid neuropathy. Johns Hopkins Med J. 1981;149:239–47.
131. Sunada Y, Shimizu T, Nakase H, et al. Inherited amyloid polyneuropathy type IV (gelsolin variant) in a Japanese family. Ann Neurol. 1993;33:57–62.
132. Levy E, Haltia M, Fernandez-Madrid I, et al. Mutation in gel gene in Finnish hereditary amyloidosis. J Exp Med. 1990;172:1865–7.
133. Maury CPJ, Kere J, Tolvanen R, de la Chapelle A. Finnish hereditary amyloidosis is caused by a single nucleotide substitution in the gelsolin gene. FEBS Lett. 1990;276:75–7.
134. Chastan N, Baert-Desurmont S, Saugier-Veber P, et al. Cardiac conduction alterations in a French family with amyloidosis of the Finnish type with the p.Asp187Tyr mutation in the GSN gene. Muscle Nerve. 2006;33:113–9.
135. Meretoja J. Genetic aspects of familial amyloidosis with corneal lattice dystrophy and cranial neuropathy. Clin Genet. 1973;4:173–85.
136. Tennent GA, Brennan SO, Stangou AJ, O'Grady J, Hawkins PN, Pepys MB. Human plasma fibrinogen is synthesized in the liver. Blood. 2007;109:1971–4.
137. Olafsson I, Grubb A. Hereditary cystatin C amyloid angiopathy. Amyloid. 2000;7:70–9.

Cardiovascular Manifestations of Myotonic Dystrophy

18

Umesh Vivekananda, Michael Hanna, and Chris Turner

Abstract

The myotonic dystrophies type 1 and type 2 are the most frequently inherited neuromuscular diseases of adult life. They are progressive multisystem disorders and predominantly affect the conduction system of the heart. Tachy and bradyarrhythmias are the predominant cardiac manifestation and are associated with up to 30% of all cause mortality in DM. Routine cardiac screening is recommended in all patients with a minimum of a yearly ECG, ECHO and 24 h Holter monitoring. In our practice we recommend electrophysiological studies when there are any abnormalities on the ECG. Future work will aim to define criteria for implantation of pacemakers and implantable cardioverter defibrillators.

Keywords

Neuromuscular • Myotonia • Trinucleotide repeat • Arrhythmia • Electrophysiological studies

U. Vivekananda
MRC Centre for Neuromuscular Disease, National Hospital for Neurology and Neurosurgery, London, UK
e-mail: umie@ucl.ac.uk

M. Hanna
Department of Clinical Neurology, UCLH National Hospital for Neurology and Neurosurgery, London, UK
e-mail: m.hanna@ucl.ac.uk

C. Turner (✉)
Centre for Neuromuscular Diseases, National Hospital for Neurology and Neurosurgery, London, UK
e-mail: chris.turner@uclh.nhs.uk

D. Kumar, P. Elliott (eds.), *Cardiovascular Genetics and Genomics*,
https://doi.org/10.1007/978-3-319-66114-8_18

18.1 Introduction

Myotonic dystrophy is the most frequently inherited neuromuscular disease of adult life and is genetically divided into type 1 and type 2 (DM1 and DM2). Estimates of the prevalence of myotonic dystrophy type 1 range from approximately 1:100,000 in some areas of Japan to approximately 1:10,000 in Iceland, with a European prevalence of 3–15 per 100,000 [1]. DM2 is less common, affecting approximately 1 in 20,000, although our personal experience in London UK suggests that it is significantly less common than DM2. Both DM1 and DM2 are progressive multisystem disorders with clinical and genetic features in common. DM1 has a wide phenotypic spectrum and DM2 tends to cause a milder phenotype with later onset of symptoms.

18.2 Genetics of Myotonic Dystrophy Type 1 and 2

DM1 is caused by the expansion of an unstable trinucleotide (CTG) repeat sequence in an untranslated, but transcribed, portion of the 3′ region of the myotonic dystrophy protein kinase (DMPK) gene located on chromosome 19q13.3 [2]. Normal individuals have between 5 and 37 repeats. Patients with between 38 and 49 CTG repeats are asymptomatic but are at risk of having children with larger repeats caused by intergenerational repeat expansion due to anticipation. Patients with greater than 49 repeats will usually manifest clinical features of myotonic dystrophy.

There is a correlation between longer CTG repeat expansions and an earlier age of onset and more severe disease, especially below 400 CTG repeats [3]. One explanation for the limited correlation of phenotype with repeat size above 400 is that the DMPK CTG trinucleotide repeat length is unstable in individuals with DM1, which leads to somatic mosaicism for the size of the CTG expansion [4]. The repeat size is stable in some postnatal tissues, for example leucocytes, but not in others, for example skeletal and cardiac muscle. The estimated progenitor allele length and level of somatic instability have recently been described as major modifiers of age of onset and support the hypothesis that the variation in disease severity between organs, within an individual, may partly be related to the level of somatic mosaicism within each organ [5]. Myotonic dystrophy type 2 is caused by a quadruplet repeat expansion of a complex repeat motif (TG)n(TCTG)n(CCTG)n in the first intron of the CNBP (cellular nucleic acid-binding protein; previously 'ZNF 9', zinc finger protein 9) gene [6].

18.3 Clinical Features of Myotonic Dystrophy Type 1 and 2

Myotonic dystrophy can affect skeletal and smooth muscle. Skeletal muscle involvement in DM1 is characterized by myotonia or muscle stiffness, which predominantly affects limb muscles but can involve face, jaw, tongue and swallowing.

Skeletal muscle can also degenerate or become "dystrophic" which may cause muscle weakness on the face, swallowing, neck, finger flexors and ankle dorsiflexors. In contrast, the weakness in DM2 typically affects proximal muscles, including the neck, elbow extension and hip flexors [7]. DM2 patients commonly have prominent muscle pain in comparison with DM1. Respiratory failure caused by respiratory muscle weakness, especially the diaphragm, is common in myotonic dystrophy type 1 and is associated with early mortality. The gastrointestinal tract can also be involved usually causing symptoms similar to irritable bowel syndrome. Endocrine abnormalities commonly seen in DM1 include insulin resistance, as well as disturbances of the thyroid, hypothalamus and gonads.

18.4 Cardiac Involvement in Myotonic Dystrophy Type 1 and 2

The heart is one of the most significant organs to be involved in myotonic dystrophy, and clinically usually manifests with arrhythmias. In one 10-year follow-up study of DM1 patients [8], the mean age of death was 53 years. There was a positive correlation between age of onset and age at death with 30% of the deaths due to cardiac complications. The cardiac abnormalities included sudden unexpected death, presumed to be due to asystole after atrioventricular block or from a ventricular tachyarrhythmia. A comparison of the cardiac defects between DM1 and DM2 patients suggested that cardiac abnormalities were more frequent in DM1 but were still present in DM2 [9].

Conduction abnormalities are found in 30–75% of DM1 patients [10]. They are pathologically associated with myocyte hypertrophy, fibrosis, focal fatty infiltration, and also lymphocytic infiltration, which can occur anywhere along the conduction system, including the His-Purkinje system [11]. As a consequence, an arrhythmia can be generated at any point in the conduction system. There is conflicting evidence on the relationship between CTG repeat size and degree of cardiac involvement. Earlier studies found no correlation between ECG or electrophysiological abnormalities during invasive testing and DNA mutation size [12]. More recent studies have found a direct linear correlation between CTG length and all measured characteristics of cardiac conduction including PR and QRS intervals [13, 14]. A correlation between the length of tetranucleotide repeat and cardiac defects has also been described in DM2, however, no relationship between repeat expansion size and other phenotypic features has been described.

18.5 Bradyarrhythmias

Cardiac involvement initially manifests as asymptomatic electrocardiographic (ECG) abnormalities, which are usually prolongation of the PR interval and QRS duration and have been reported in 65% of DM1 patients [13]. Severe abnormalities on the ECG, such as a non sinus rhythm, PR interval of greater than 240 ms,

QRS duration of greater than 120 ms, or second and third degree atrioventricular block, are an independent predictor, with moderate sensitivity, of sudden death in patients with DM1 [10]. Age, degree of skeletal muscle impairment and male gender were correlated with PR prolongation. A prolonged PR interval also correlated with the distribution and extent of conduction-system lesions found at autopsy [12, 15]. Prolongation of the PR segment occurs in approximately 20–40% of DM2 patients [16].

18.6 Tachyarrhythmias

18.6.1 Atrial

Sinus-node dysfunction can manifest as supraventricular tachycardias such as atrial fibrillation, atrial flutter, and atrial tachycardia. Atrial tachyarrhythmias independently predict both sudden death and death from progressive neuromuscular respiratory failure. This likely reflects the presence of atrial fibrosis indicative of conduction involvement and an increased risk of sudden death [10, 17].

18.6.2 Ventricular

Although ventricular arrhythmias are probably less common in myotonic dystrophy, they are much more likely to become unstable and potentially life threatening. Ventricular arrhythmias include monomorphic ventricular tachycardia, polymorphic ventricular tachycardia, and ventricular fibrillation. There are several mechanisms that can lead to ventricular arrhythmias, including fibro-fatty degeneration of myocardium or the fascicles serving as a catalyst for re-entry within the ventricular wall or fascicular re-entry, respectively [16]. DM patients are predisposed to bundle branch re-entry ventricular tachycardia (BBRVT) because a diseased conduction system is essential to this mechanism [18]. This results from a macro re-entry between the left and right fascicles. Generally, BBRVT makes up only 6% of monomorphic ventricular tachycardias. If present however, morbidity is significant as 75% of patients that have inducible BBRVT will present with either with syncope or sudden cardiac death.

Late potentials, which are low amplitude signals usually greater than 36 ms seen at the end of the QRS complex, may also be evident in DM1. They are an expression of delayed myocardial activation of the His-Purkinje system and usually caused by an abnormal conduction system. Late potentials are considered predictors of ventricular arrhythmias [19].

18.6.3 Cardiomyopathy

Structural cardiomyopathy is present in both DM1 and DM2 [20]. However, symptoms of heart failure are infrequent because of the reduced mobility and difficulties in reporting symptoms caused by cognitive deficits. This is illustrated in one study of 400 DM patients that found some form of structural heart disease in 20% of patients, but only 2% of the patients had overt symptoms of heart failure [21]. The existence of a myocardial equivalent of skeletal muscle myotonia (myocardial myotonia) has been suggested by assessment of diastolic function by echo Doppler parameters [22], however myocardium does not express the skeletal muscle chloride channel whose mis-splicing is probably the cause of skeletal muscle myotonia in DM1. Microvascular dysfunction has also been described in DM1 patients suffering from chest pain, exhibiting a positive thallium scan and normal coronary arteries [23]. Regional wall abnormalities can be seen on echocardiogram but usually represents non-ischaemic fibrosis. Mitral valve prolapse has been reported in 25–40% of most DM1 series [24]. Hypertrophic cardiomyopathy has only been described in case reports.

18.6.4 Investigations

We recommend a yearly ECG and at least a five yearly echocardiogram are performed as a minimum in all patients with DM1 and 2 [25]. The frequency of ECHO has been debated especially since clinical manifestation of Cardiac failure is uncommon. Medications used to improve myotonia, such as mexiletine, and excessive daytime sleepiness, such as modafinil, may also increase the risk of arrhythmias and cardiac surveillance should be more frequent in these patients.

If an ECG abnormality is detected, such as marked prolongation of the PR interval (>240 ms), QRS complex (>120 ms), any form of conduction block, any tachyarrhythmia or if the patient develops cardiac symptoms, such as pre-syncope and palpitations, then cardiology referral is advised. More prolonged cardiac monitoring to detect arrhythmias may be required including non-invasive Holter monitoring or invasive monitoring, such as the Reveal or LINQ devices.

18.6.5 Electrophysiological Studies (EPS)

We would recommend that patients with any of the electrocardiographic or cardiac clinical features described above, should be considered for EPS. This "invasive" strategy has been found to be associated with a higher rate of 9-year survival than a 'non-invasive" strategy i.e. no EPS [26]. However the strategy did not lead to an improvement in overall mortality because of increased mortality from other disorders such as respiratory failure. Therefore, our opinion is that EPS studies in at risk patients is necessary but probably not sufficient. In our experience, infra-hisian conduction may be abnormal in the absence of ECG abnormalities and the role of EPS in the context of a normal ECG is still under debate. In favour of an invasive strategy is that patients usually undertake cardiac testing at rest, and it is the onset of significant exertion that may promote unstable arrhythmias. In one study, 18% of patients with a normal 24-h Holter monitor had inducible ventricular tachyarrhythmias on EPS [12].

18.7 Echocardiography and Cardiac MRI

Although death from heart failure due to cardiomyopathy is rare in DM, left ventricular dysfunction is associated with increased mortality and sudden death. Two-dimensional echocardiography has been the study of choice, both in the initial work-up of DM patients and surveillance patients with symptoms of heart failure. Cardiac MRI due to its greater sensitivity and reproducibility than echocardiography may be a more accurate method of monitoring in the future. DM1 patients show a number of cardiac MRI features including left ventricular systolic dysfunction, ventricular dilatation, myocardial hypertrophy and fibrosis. These MRI features are strongly correlated with ECG conduction abnormalities although one study suggested 16% of patients with normal ECGs, had cardiac MRI features of DM1 [27].

18.8 Management

We would recommend that all DM patients with prolonged PR (>240 ms) or QRS interval (>120 ms), first degree or Mobitz type 1 heart block should be considered for assessment by EPS because of the risk that these earlier manifestations of cardiac disease are likely to lead to the development of more significant clinical features.

If a prolonged His-Ventricle or HV interval is assessed at EPS (>70 ms), a decision may be taken for prophylactic insertion of a permanent pacemaker [25]. As with the general population, Mobitz type 2 or third degree atrioventricular heart block are indications for PPM placement.

Pharmacological therapy for atrial tachyarrhythmias should be used with caution, as AV block is also a feature in myotonic dystrophy. Beta blockers and amiodarone are likely to be safe in DM but flecainide, quinidine and disopyramide should be avoided [28]. Supraventricular and ventricular tachyarrhythmias may be successfully treated with radiofrequency ablation [29].

In DM1, abnormal late potentials are an expression of conduction disease, and represent an important non-invasive clue to the presence of a prolonged HV interval. QRS duration ≥100 ms and low amplitude signals in the last 40 ms of QRS complex ≥36 ms can predict a prolonged HV interval at EPS with good sensitivity and specificity (80% and 83.3%, respectively) [10]. A prolonged HV interval contributes to BBRVT, which is important to recognise as it may be successfully treated with radiofrequency ablation [16].

Biventricular failure caused by DM can be treated with cardiac resynchronisation therapy via biventricular pacing [30], although in clinical practice, symptomatic cardiac failure is uncommon. Figure 18.1 summarises our suggested management plan.

Conclusions

Myotonic dystrophy type 1 is the most common form of adult-onset muscular dystrophy. DM type 1 and 2 are multi-system disorders that often affect the heart and cardiac causes contribute approximately 30% of all case mortality. The pathological involvement of the His-Purkinje system is the commonest clinical

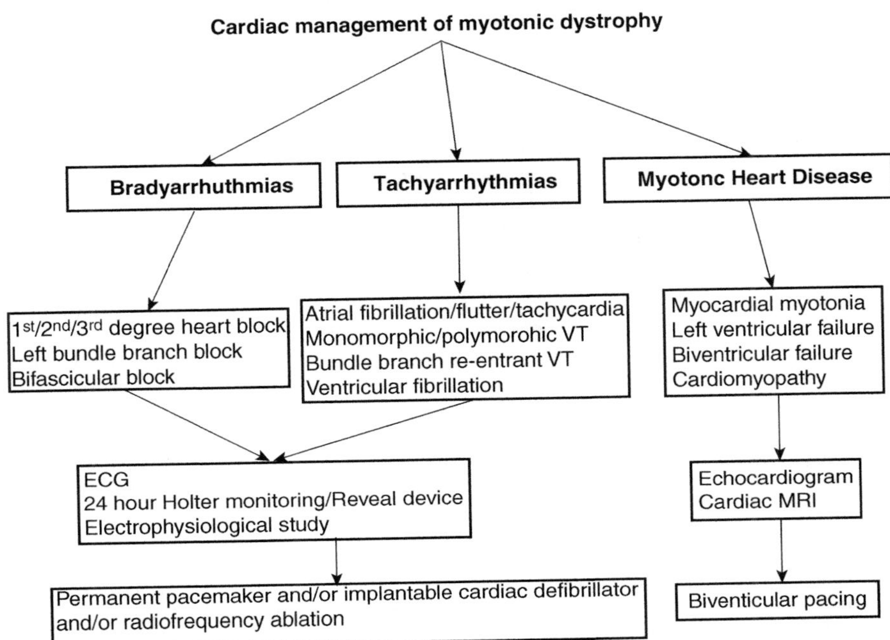

Fig. 18.1 Flow chart of the common cardiac manifestations of myotonic dystrophy, their investigation and management

manifestation of DM heart involvement and causes atrial and ventricular brady and tachyarrhythmias.

We recommend regular cardiac surveillance, even in asymptomatic patients, with at the least yearly ECG monitoring. Electrophysiological studies are an invasive tool in assessing the cardiac conduction system, which we would recommend in any patient with ECG or clinical evidence of His-Purkinje system involvement. Based on data derived from patients with ischaemic heart disease, there should be consideration of insertion of a permanent pacemaker if the patient has an HV interval of greater than 70 ms. Future studies need to clarify which patients groups are at most risk of significant life-threatening arrhythmia so that appropriate, but potentially invasive, surveillance and management can be targeted at the correct populations of patients.

References

1. Harper PS. Myotonic dystrophy. 3rd ed. Philadelphia: W.B. Saunders; 2001.
2. Brook JD, McCurrach ME, Harley HG, Buckler AJ, Church D, Aburatani H, Hunter K, Stanton VP, Thirion JP, Hudson T. Molecular basis of myotonic dystrophy: expansion of a trinucleotide (CTG) repeat at the 3′ end of a transcript encoding a protein kinase family member. Cell. 1992;69(2):385.

3. Hamshere MG, Harley H, Harper P, Brook JD, Brookfield JF. Myotonic dystrophy: the correlation of (CTG) repeat length in leucocytes with age at onset is significant only for patients with small expansions. J Med Genet. 1999;36(1):59–61.
4. Lavedan C, Hofmann-Radvanyi H, Shelbourne P, Rabes JP, Duros C, Savoy D, Dehaupas I, Luce S, Johnson K, Junien C. Myotonic dystrophy: size- and sex-dependent dynamics of CTG meiotic instability, and somatic mosaicism. Am J Hum Genet. 1993;52(5):875–83.
5. Morales F, Couto JM, Higham CF, Hogg G, Cuenca P, Braida C, Wilson RH, et al. Somatic instability of the expanded CTG triplet repeat in myotonic dystrophy type 1 is a heritable quantitative trait and modifier of disease severity. Hum Mol Genet. 2012;21(16):3558–67. https://doi.org/10.1093/hmg/dds185.
6. Liquori CL, Ricker K, Moseley ML, Jacobsen JF, Kress W, Naylor SL, Day JW, Ranum LP. Myotonic dystrophy type 2 caused by a CCTG expansion in intron 1 of ZNF9. Science. 2001;293(5531):864–7. https://doi.org/10.1126/science.1062125.
7. Day JW, Ricker K, Jacobsen JF, Rasmussen LJ, Dick KA, Kress W, Schneider C, et al. Myotonic dystrophy type 2: molecular, diagnostic and clinical spectrum. Neurology. 2003;60(4):657–64.
8. Mathieu J, Allard P, Potvin L, Prévost C, Bégin P. A 10-year study of mortality in a cohort of patients with myotonic dystrophy. Neurology. 1999;52(8):1658–62.
9. Wahbi K, Meune C, Bécane HM, Laforêt P, Bassez G, Lazarus A, Radvanyi-Hoffman H, Eymard B, Duboc D. Left ventricular dysfunction and cardiac arrhythmias are frequent in type 2 myotonic dystrophy: a case control study. Neuromuscul Disord. 2009;19(7):468–72. https://doi.org/10.1016/j.nmd.2009.04.012.
10. Groh WJ, Groh MR, Saha C, Kincaid JC, Simmons Z, Ciafaloni E, Pourmand R, et al. Electrocardiographic abnormalities and sudden death in myotonic dystrophy type 1. N Engl J Med. 2008;358(25):2688–97. https://doi.org/10.1056/NEJMoa062800.
11. Kennel AJ, Titus JL, Merideth J. Pathologic findings in the atrioventricular conduction system in myotonic dystrophy. Mayo Clin Proc. 1974;49(11):838–42.
12. Lazarus A, Varin J, Ounnoughene Z, Radvanyi H, Junien C, Coste J, Laforet P, et al. Relationships among electrophysiological findings and clinical status, heart function, and extent of DNA mutation in myotonic dystrophy. Circulation. 1999;99(8):1041–6.
13. Groh WJ, Lowe MR, Zipes DP. Severity of cardiac conduction involvement and arrhythmias in myotonic dystrophy type 1 correlates with age and CTG repeat length. J Cardiovasc Electrophysiol. 2002;13(5):444–8.
14. Melacini P, Villanova C, Menegazzo E, Novelli G, Danieli G, Rizzoli G, Fasoli G, Angelini C, Buja G, Miorelli M. Correlation between cardiac involvement and CTG trinucleotide repeat length in myotonic dystrophy. J Am Coll Cardiol. 1995;25(1):239–45.
15. Babuty D, Fauchier L, Tena-Carbi D, Poret P, Leche J, Raynaud M, Fauchier JP, Cosnay P. Is it possible to identify Infrahissian cardiac conduction abnormalities in myotonic dystrophy by non-invasive methods? Heart. 1999;82(5):634–7.
16. McNally EM, Sparano D. Mechanisms and management of the heart in myotonic dystrophy. Heart. 2011;97(13):1094–100. https://doi.org/10.1136/hrt.2010.214197.
17. Nguyen HH, Wolfe JT, Holmes DR, Edwards WD. Pathology of the cardiac conduction system in myotonic dystrophy: a study of 12 cases. J Am Coll Cardiol. 1988;11(3):662–71.
18. Merino JL, Carmona JR, Fernández-Lozano I, Peinado R, Basterra N, Sobrino JA. Mechanisms of sustained ventricular tachycardia in myotonic dystrophy: implications for catheter ablation. Circulation. 1998;98(6):541–6.
19. Pelargonio G, Dello Russo A, Sanna T, De Martino G, Bellocci F. Myotonic dystrophy and the heart. Heart. 2002;88(6):665–70.
20. Bhakta D, Lowe MR, Groh WJ. Prevalence of structural cardiac abnormalities in patients with myotonic dystrophy type I. Am Heart J. 2004;147(2):224–7. https://doi.org/10.1016/j.ahj.2003.08.008.
21. Bhakta D, Groh MR, Shen C, Pascuzzi RM, Groh WJ. Increased mortality with left ventricular systolic dysfunction and heart failure in adults with myotonic dystrophy type 1. Am Heart J. 2010;160(6):1137–1141., 1141.e1. https://doi.org/10.1016/j.ahj.2010.07.032.

22. Fragola PV, Caló L, Luzi M, Mammarella A, Antonini G. Doppler echocardiographic assessment of left ventricular diastolic function in myotonic dystrophy. Cardiology. 1997;88(6):498–502.
23. Itoh H, Shimizu M, Horita Y, Ino H, Taguchi T, Kajinami K, Yagi K, Chujo D, Mabuchi H. Microvascular ischemia in patients with myotonic dystrophy. Jpn Circ J. 2000;64(9):720–2.
24. Phillips MF, Harper PS. Cardiac disease in myotonic dystrophy. Cardiovasc Res. 1997;33(1):13–22.
25. Sovari AA, Bodine CK, Farokhi F. Cardiovascular manifestations of myotonic dystrophy-1. Cardiol Rev. 2007;15(4):191–4. https://doi.org/10.1097/CRD.0b013e318070d1a7.
26. Wahbi K, Meune C, Porcher R, Bécane HM, Lazarus A, Laforêt P, Stojkovic T, et al. Electrophysiological study with prophylactic pacing and survival in adults with myotonic dystrophy and conduction system disease. JAMA. 2012;307(12):1292–301. https://doi.org/10.1001/jama.2012.346.
27. Hermans MCE, Faber CG, Bekkers SCAM, de Die-Smulders CEM, Gerrits MM, Merkies ISJ, Snoep G, Pinto YM, Schalla S. Structural and functional cardiac changes in myotonic dystrophy type 1: a cardiovascular magnetic resonance study. J Cardiovasc Magn Reson. 2012;14:48. https://doi.org/10.1186/1532-429X-14-48.
28. Bassez G, Lazarus A, Desguerre I, Varin J, Laforêt P, Bécane HM, Meune C, et al. Severe cardiac arrhythmias in young patients with myotonic dystrophy type 1. Neurology. 2004;63(10):1939–41.
29. Muraoka H, Negoro N, Terasaki F, Nakakoji T, Kojima S, Hoshiga M, Sugino M, Hosokawa T, Ishihara T, Hanafusa T. Re-entry circuit in ventricular tachycardia due to focal fatty-fibrosis in a patient with myotonic dystrophy. Intern Med. 2005;44(2):129–35.
30. Kilic T, Vural A, Ural D, Sahin T, Agacdiken A, Ertas G, Yildiz Y, Komsuoglu B. Cardiac resynchronization therapy in a case of myotonic dystrophy (Steinert's disease) and dilated cardiomyopathy. Pacing Clin Electrophysiol. 2007;30(7):916–20. https://doi.org/10.1111/j.1540-8159.2007.00782.x.

Marfan Syndrome and Related Disorders

19

John C.S. Dean and Bart Loeys

Abstract

Marfan syndrome is the best known of the hereditary aortopathies, but its clinical variability and multisystem involvement often make diagnosis and management challenging. The skeletal and ocular findings overlap with other conditions, but FBN1 genetic testing and clinical assessment using the Ghent nosology is recommended. Loeys Dietz Syndrome is a related aortopathy, associated with changes in other genes in the same pathway (TGFBR1, TGFBR2, SMAD3, TGFB2, TGFB3 and SMAD2). Features such as cleft palate, bifid uvula, hypertelorism, craniosynostosis and osteoarthritis and the absence of ectopia lentis suggest Loeys Dietz. Trial evidence suggests that beta-blockers and angiotensin 2 receptor blockers delay dilatation of the Marfan aorta. Regular imaging is required to determine the timing of prophylactic aortic root surgery. Management of Loeys Dietz Syndrome follows similar principles, except that drug therapy has not been proven in trials, and more widespread imaging of the arterial tree and earlier surgery is recommended.

Keywords

Marfan • Ghent nosology • Loeys dietz • Aortopathy

J.C.S. Dean (✉)
North of Scotland Regional Genetics Service, Aberdeen Royal Infirmary, Aberdeen, Scotland
e-mail: john.dean@nhs.net

B. Loeys
Department of Clinical Genetics, Center for Medical Genetics, Antwerp University Hospital, Antwerp, Belgium
e-mail: bart.loeys@uantwerpen.be

D. Kumar, P. Elliott (eds.), *Cardiovascular Genetics and Genomics*,
https://doi.org/10.1007/978-3-319-66114-8_19

19.1 Introduction

Concern about a diagnosis of Marfan syndrome is usually raised in one of three clinical scenarios: the tall thin patient with arachnodactyly, joint hypermobility, pectus deformity or scoliosis, the patient with ectopia lentis, and the patient presenting with ascending thoracic aortic aneurysm with or without aortic, mitral or other valve disease. These clinical scenarios often overlap, and this clinical variability is a hallmark of Marfan syndrome, an autosomal dominant connective tissue disorder which can also have effects on the lungs, the skin and the dura mater. The various features are described in the Ghent nosology, which is commonly used to diagnose the condition. The overwhelming majority of cases are associated with mutation in the *FBN1* gene on chromosome 15, but there are pathogenic links between the fibrillin-1 protein and other proteins such as the transforming growth factor beta receptors (*TGFBR*) *1* and *2*. Some Marfan-like cases without lens involvement have been reported to have mutations in one of these genes rather than *FBN1*. To complicate the picture further, some rare *FBN1* mutations appear to have a mild effect and are found in patients who have some features of Marfan syndrome but do not fulfil the accepted diagnostic criteria. Such patients have been described as having a fibrillinopathy, because they do not fulfil the Marfan syndrome diagnostic criteria. Mutations in genes encoding components of the TGFbeta signalling cascade (*TGFB2/3, TGFBR1/2* and *SMAD2/3)* cause the related condition, Loeys-Dietz syndrome and these and other genes have recently been associated with a range of disorders from syndromic to isolated familial thoracic aortic aneurysm. In this chapter, we will discuss the diagnosis and management of Marfan syndrome, the evolving knowledge of genetic causes of thoracic aortic aneurysm and the implications of knowledge about Marfan management for these disorders.

19.2 Historical Background

Marfan syndrome is named after Antoine Bernard-Jean Marfan, a French paediatrician, who described a 5 year old girl (Gabrielle P) with long thin limbs, particularly noticeable in the fingers and toes, in an article published in Paris in 1896 [1]. He named this combination of skeletal findings dolichostenomelia. Gabrielle also had joint contractures and scoliosis. In 1902, Achard described an older patient with some similar features which were familial, and in 1912 and 1914 respectively, cardiac and ocular findings were added to the syndrome [2]. It is no longer certain whether Marfan's original patient had the condition which bears his name—it is now believed that she suffered from a Marfan-related condition, called Beals syndrome or congenital contractural arachnodactly. In 1955, McKusick described Marfan syndrome as a heritable disorder of connective tissue, and noted its variability [3], laying the foundations for later clinical and molecular descriptions of the condition. Histochemical studies and a positional cloning approach led to the identification of mutation in the fibrillin-1 gene as the usual cause of Marfan syndrome in 1991 [4]. In 1993, a large French family with a Marfan-like disorder was described where the condition showed linkage to chromosome 3 rather than fibrillin-1 [5, 6], but the issue of whether Marfan syndrome displays locus heterogeneity remained controversial. In 2005, coinciding with the discovery of *TGFBR2* mutations in the related Loeys-Dietz syndrome [7], mutation in *TGFBR2* on chromosome 3 was also found to underlie the so-called "non-ocular" form of Marfan syndrome, sometimes designated Marfan syndrome type 2 [8].

19.3 Defining Marfan Syndrome

Marfan syndrome (MIM 154700) as currently defined is a variable, autosomal dominant disorder of connective tissue whose cardinal features affect the cardiovascular system, eyes, and skeleton. The minimal birth incidence is around 1 in 9800 [9], and the prevalence may be around 1/5000 [10]. Progressive aortic dilatation, typically maximal at the sinus of Valsalva, associated with aortic valve incompetence leads to aortic dissection or rupture and is the principal cause of mortality in many cases, but mitral valve prolapse with incompetence may be significant, and lens dislocation, myopia, and arthralgia associated with chronic joint laxity can cause substantial morbidity. The most common clinical presentations are personal or family history of lens subluxation, personal or family history of aortic dissection or rupture, or in a young person with a tall, thin body habitus, long limbs, arachnodactyly, pectus deformities and sometimes scoliosis (Figs. 19.1 and 19.2). In each case, other findings in the clinical picture such as a high arched palate with dental crowding, skin striae distensae, recurrent hernia or recurrent pneumothorax may increase suspicion. Family history may be helpful, but around 27% of cases arise from new mutation [11]. Between 66 and 91% of bona fide Marfan syndrome patients have an identifiable *FBN1* mutation [12, 13], but *FBN1* mutations also cause some Marfan-like disorders or fibrillinopathies with a better prognosis, such as MASS phenotype, (MIM 604308, Mitral valve prolapse, mild non-progressive Aortic dilatation, Skin and Skeletal features), or isolated Ectopia Lentis, (MIM 129600) [10]. In addition, mutations in the TGF beta receptor 2 (*TGFBR2*) gene on chromosome 3 and in the *TGFBR1* gene on chromosome 9 cause Loeys Dietz Syndrome (OMIM 609192 and 610168) [7, 14] which can closely resemble Marfan syndrome, but without ectopia lentis [8, 15–17]. More recently mutations in *TGFB2*, *TGFB3*, *SMAD2* and *SMAD3* were also associated with Marfan/Loeys-Dietz like clinical presentations, often with familial aortic aneurysm and variable syndromic features (including for example, cleft palate, bifid uvula, hypertelorism, craniosynostosis, and for *SMAD3*, osteoarthritis) [18]. *TGFBR2* mutations at the R460 codon have also been described in families with non-syndromic familial thoracic ascending aortic aneurysm [19, 20] (FTAA3, OMIM 608967). Careful clinical assessment of patients with suspected Marfan syndrome is therefore essential to achieve an accurate clinical diagnosis, interpret genetic testing results correctly in a patient and their family, provide prognostic information and decide management options. To this end, the various features were codified in 1988 into the so-called Berlin criteria, revised as the Ghent nosology in 1996 [21] and revised again in 2010 [22]. Patients who can be

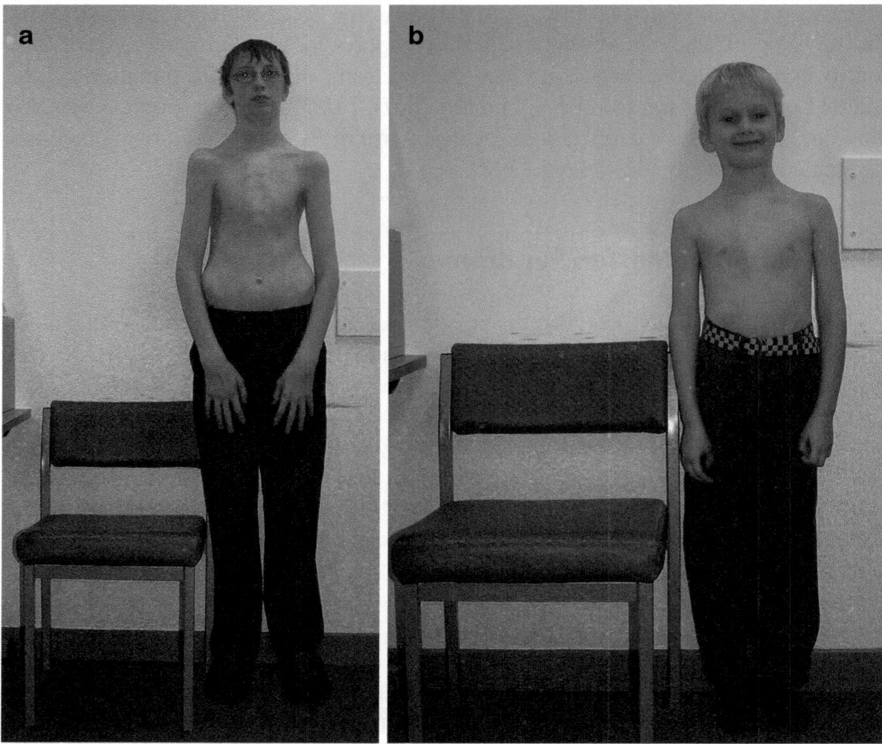

Fig. 19.1 (**a**) 13 year old boy with lens subluxation, skeletal system involvement and mild aortic root dilatation. He therefore fulfils the Ghent criteria on clinical findings alone. (**b**) 6 year old boy with skeletal system involvement and mild aortic root dilatation. His father died from an aortic dissection, but had never been evaluated using the Ghent nosology. A nonsense mutation in exon 54 of fibrillin 1 was detected in the boy allowing a diagnosis of Marfan syndrome to be confirmed, and appropriate follow-up and management to be arranged

diagnosed as affected using this nosology are likely to be at greater risk of cardiovascular complications, and need regular follow-up with prophylactic medical and surgical treatment, and lifestyle advice. The 2010 nosology can provide pointers to alternative genetic aetiologies. As the nosology is complex, it may be helpful to use an integrated care pathway in the clinic [23].

19.3.1 Diagnosis of Marfan Syndrome Using the Revised (2010) Ghent Nosology

There are five essential elements to the assessment of a patient for possible Marfan syndrome in the revised Ghent nosology [24]. These are family history, ectopia lentis, aortic dilatation or dissection, a so-called systemic score made up from the other features of Marfan syndrome, and the genetic test findings. In an adult, a diagnosis of Marfan

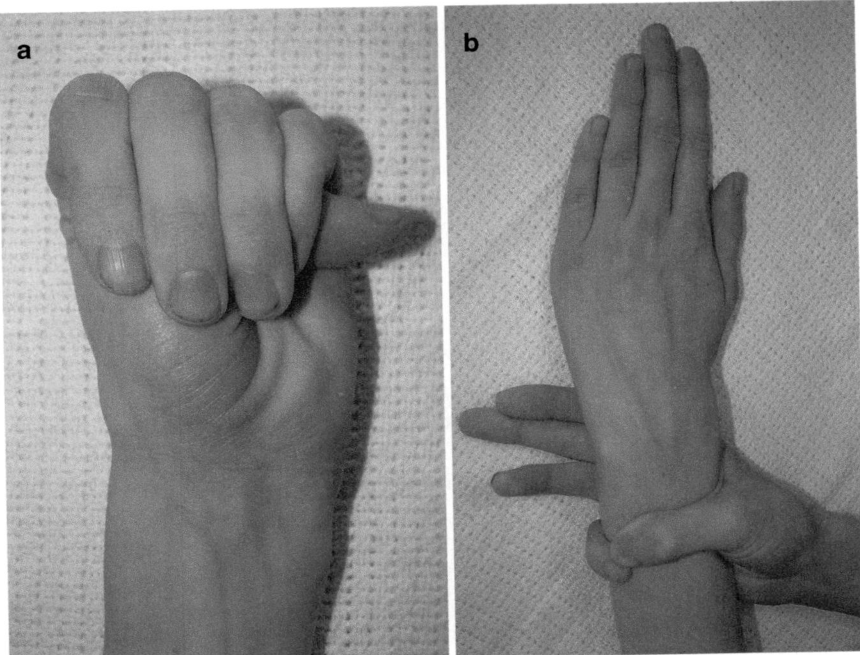

Fig. 19.2 Arachnodactyly. (**a**) Positive Steinberg thumb sign: entire thumb nail protrudes beyond ulnar border of hand. (**b**) Positive Walker-Murdoch wrist sign: thumb and fifth finger overlap when encircling the wrist. Both signs must be present to diagnose arachnodactyly

syndrome can be made if two elements of the assessment are positive in various combinations [Table 19.1], and the nosology also provides for the diagnosis of some other disorders when different criteria are met. Not all eventualities are covered in the published nosology, but the algorithms in Fig. 19.3 try to fill these gaps. In younger people, the algorithm is slightly simpler, to take account of the age dependent penetrance of some features (Fig. 19.4) [26, 27]. As Marfan syndrome cannot be excluded with confidence in many younger people, repeat evaluations should be offered (for example, at least at ages 5, 10 and 15 years) until age 20. The cardiovascular assessment requires measurement of the aortic diameter at the Sinuses of Valsalva, usually by transthoracic echocardiography (Fig. 19.4), and comparison with normal values based on age, gender, and body surface area, calculated from height and weight (Fig. 19.5) [21, 28–31]. The deviation from the normal range is usually expressed as a z-score [32]. Other imaging techniques such as transoesophageal echocardiography, or MRI scanning (Fig. 19.6) may be helpful in some cases [33], including those with severe pectus deformity. A pelvic X-ray to detect protrusio acetabulae [34], and lumbar MRI scan for dural ectasia should be carried out only if a positive finding would affect the diagnosis (i.e. result in the systemic score reaching 7 or higher). Ocular evaluation for myopia (due to increased globe length, measured by ultrasound), corneal flattening (measured by keratometry), hypoplastic iris or iris muscle and lens subluxation requires ophthalmology assessment.

Table 19.1 The Ghent 2010 nosology—diagnosis of Marfan requires 2 positive elements

Element	Finding
Cardiovascular	Aortic dilatation/dissection
Eyes	Ectopia lentis
Systemic score ≥7	Score of 14 additional clinical features (Table 19.2) Skeletal, skin, respiratory, dural ectasia, myopia, mitral valve prolapse
Family history	Unequivocally affected relative
Genetic testing	*FBN1* mutation known to cause Marfan

The differential diagnosis of a tall young person with Marfan-like skeletal features includes homocystinuria (MIM 236300), Beals syndrome or congenital contractural arachnodactyly (MIM 121050), Marshall-Stickler syndrome (MIM 108300, 604841, 184840), Ehlers-Danlos syndrome (MIM 130050), and MASS phenotype (MIM 604308). Where there is a family history of aortic aneurysm, Familial Thoracic Aortic Aneurysm (FTAA) should be considered (MIM 607086, other features of Marfan syndrome—mainly skeletal —may or may not be present). Additional clinical findings may suggest other disorders—bicuspid aortic valve and FTAA type 1 (MIM 607086), craniosynostosis, intellectual impairment and Shprintzen-Goldberg syndrome (MIM 182212), arterial tortuosity or widespread aneurysms, hypertelorism, bifid uvula/cleft palate, craniosynostosis, visceral rupture, joint hypermobility, thin skin with atrophic scarring, and Loeys-Dietz syndrome [14] or intellectual impairment, velopharyngeal insufficiency and Lujan-Fryns syndrome (MIM 309520). The initial evaluation of patients with possible Marfan syndrome requires a multi-disciplinary approach including clinical genetics, cardiology, ophthalmology and radiology. Deciding when to refer a patient for such an assessment may be facilitated by using the "seven-signs" score (Table 19.2), which is much simpler to administer in a busy clinic [35]. Referral for further evaluation should be considered for anyone in the moderate or high risk groups.

19.3.2 Using the Ghent Criteria in the Clinic

Assessment of a patient using the Ghent 2010 nosology is simpler than using the 1996 nosology, which required assessment of 30 features. In Ghent 2010, a diagnosis of Marfan can be achieved in the presence of only two findings: aortic dilatation and ectopia lentis or aortic dilatation and an *FBN1* mutation. A comparison of the two nosologies in the same group of 1009 patients suggested that slightly fewer are diagnosed by the Ghent 2010 nosology, which the authors attributed to diagnosis of some cases as Isolated Ectopia Lentis, and MASS phenotype in Ghent 2010, who would have been diagnosed as Marfan in Ghent 1996 [36]. In addition, some patients can be diagnosed as Marfan under the 2010 criteria, who would not have been so diagnosed under 1996, because they had fewer extra cardiac or ocular features. Neither nosology correlates completely with the likelihood of finding an *FBN1* mutation: for example, a study of patients reported to the Fibrillin-1 Universal Marfan Database [37] demonstrated that *FBN1* mutations are sometimes found in

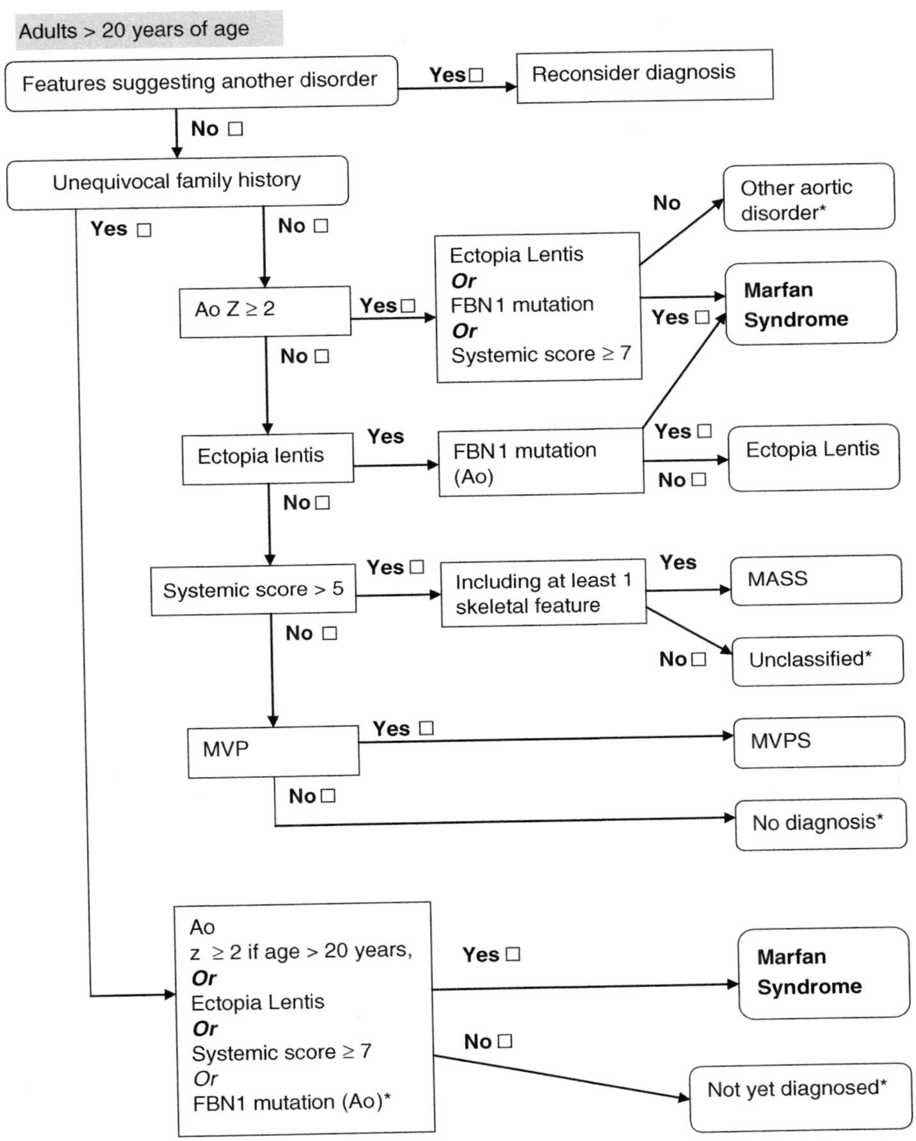

Fig. 19.3 Algorithms for applying the Ghent 2010 nosology in the clinic. (a) adults. Note: Ao z ≥ 2 means Aortic Sinus Diameter Cornell z score > 2 or Aortic dissection/aneurysm. FBN1 mutation (Ao) means Fibrillin 1 mutation known to be associated with aortic dilatation. *Outcome/feature not part of 2010 Ghent Nosology as published. (**b**) young people under the age of 20 years. Note: Young people (<20 years) with no family history, systemic score <7, aortic root z < 3 and no FBN1 mutation may be diagnosed "non-specific connective tissue disorder" and followed up until adult. Young people (<20 years) with an FBN1 mutation but aortic root z < 3 may be diagnosed "potential Marfan syndrome". Young people (<20 years) with a positive family history, but who fall into the "Not yet diagnosed" category should be followed up and periodically re-evaluated at least until age 20

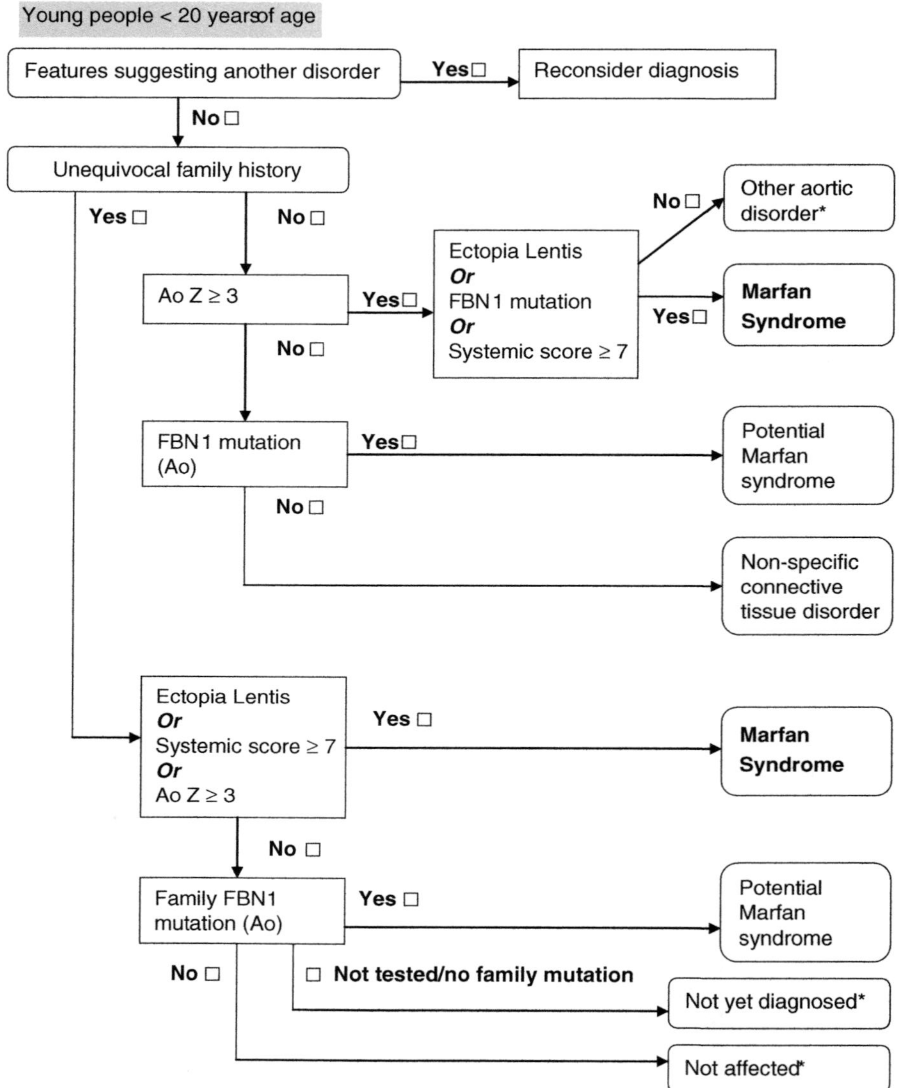

Fig. 19.3 (continued)

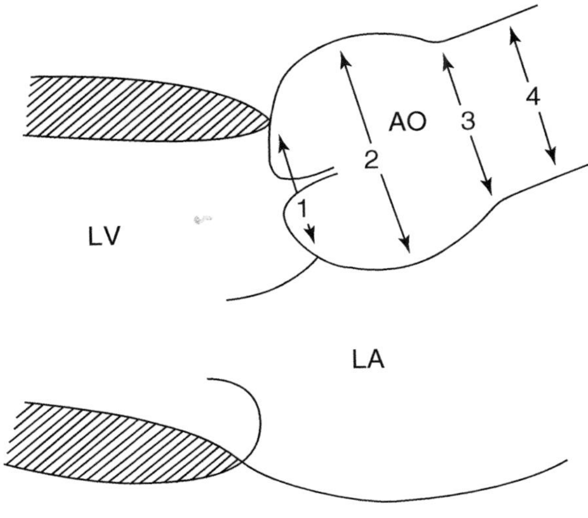

Fig. 19.4 Diagram of the aortic root as seen at echocardiography. The aortic diameter should be measured at the aortic annulus (1), the sinuses of Valsalva (2), the supra-aortic ridge (3), and the proximal ascending aorta (4). In Marfan syndrome, dilatation usually starts at the sinuses of Valsalva, so this measurement is critical in monitoring the early evolution of the condition. Diameters must be related to normal values for age and body surface area. After Roman et al. [25] with permission

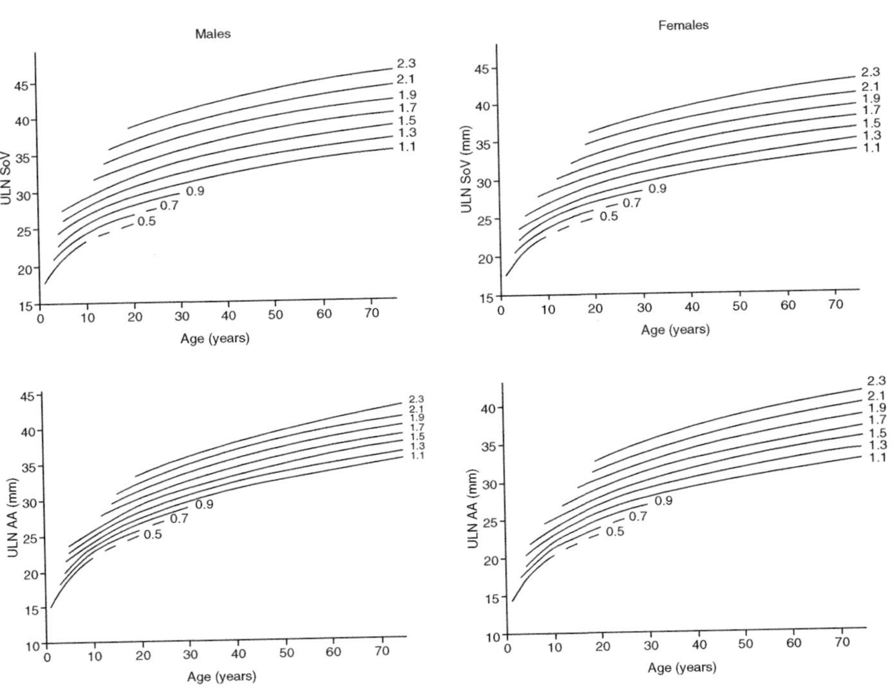

Fig. 19.5 Nomograms displaying the upper limit of normal for the Sinuses of Valsalva and Ascending Aortic diameters as a function of Body Surface Area, age and gender. [28] Body surface area (BSA) is calculated using the Du Bois and Du Bois formula: BSA (m^2) = BSA = (Weight (kg) 0.425 × Height (cm) 0.725) × 0.007184 [29]

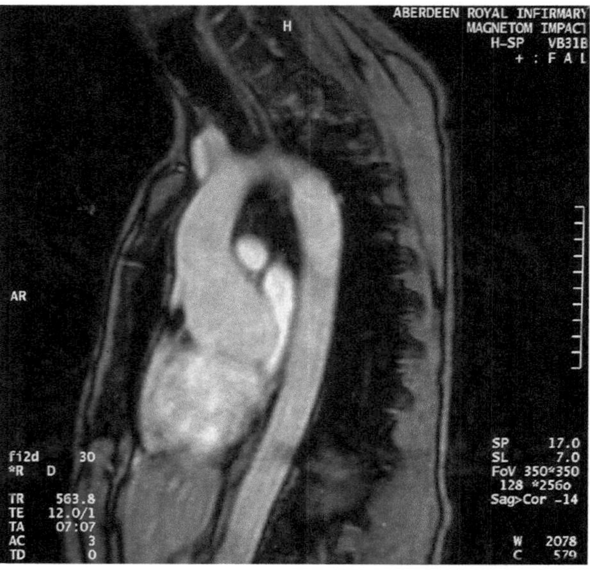

Fig. 19.6 Parasagittal cine magnetic resonance angiogram (MRA) showing dilated aortic root but with normal upper ascending, arch and descending aorta in a young adult

Table 19.2 The Ghent 2010 nosology—systemic score

Feature		Score
Wrist and thumb signs	Both present	3
	One present only	1
Pectus carinatum		2
Pectus excavatum/chest asymmetry		1
Hindfoot deformity	Hindfoot valgus and pes planus	2
	Pes planus alone	1
Protrusio acetabuli		2
Reduced ULSR* AND span/height ratio >1.05 (but no severe scoliosis)		1
Scoliosis or thoracolumbar kyphosis		1
Reduced elbow extension		1
3 or more facial features (dolichocephaly, enopthalmos, downslanting palpebral fissures, malar hypoplaisa, retrognathia)		1
Skin striae		1
Pneumothorax		2
Dural ectasia		2
Myopia >3 diopters		1
Mitral valve prolapse		1

Key: **ULSR* upper to lower segment ratio <0.85 in white adults, <0.78 in black adults; in children aged 0–5 years <1, 6–7 years <0.95, 8-9 years <0.9, 10 years and over, <0.85

patients who do not apparently fulfil the 1996 nosology. However, the clinical information available for the cases reported is incomplete—some may have fulfilled the nosology with more extensive clinical investigation, and the risk of aortic dilatation

Table 19.3 "Seven signs" of Marfan

Feature	Score
Family history of Marfan syndrome	2
Previous thoracic aortic surgery	1
Pectus excavatum	1
Wrist and thumb signs	1
History of pneumothorax	1
Skin striae	1
Ectopia lentis	4

Probability of Marfan syndrome: ≤1 point, low: 2 or 3 points, medium: ≥4 points, high

Table 19.4 Key issues in the assessment of Marfan syndrome

• Diagnosis or exclusion of Marfan syndrome in an individual should be based on the Ghent diagnostic nosology
• The initial assessment should include a personal history, detailed family history, and clinical examination including ophthalmology examination and transthoracic echocardiogram
• The aortic diameter at the Sinus of Valsalva should be related to normal values based on age and body surface area
• The development of scoliosis and protrusio acetabulae is age dependent, commonly occurring following periods of rapid growth. X-ray for these features, depending on age, if a positive finding would make the diagnosis of Marfan syndrome
• A pelvic MRI scan to detect dural ectasia is indicated if a positive finding would make the diagnosis of Marfan syndrome
• The Ghent nosology cannot exclude Marfan syndrome in children, because of the age dependent penetrance of many features
• Younger patients with a positive family history but unsuccessful DNA testing and insufficient clinical features to fulfil the diagnostic criteria, and younger patients with no family history who miss fulfilling the diagnostic criteria by one element only, should be offered further clinical evaluations at least until age 20, or until a diagnosis can be made
• Family history of aortic aneurysm may represent a disorder such as Familial Thoracic Aortic Aneurysm, where the use of the Ghent nosology to assess risk in relatives is inappropriate

in these "Ghent negative" cases with *FBN1* mutations is uncertain. Some *FBN1* variants are of uncertain clinical significance—only variants where there is evidence that they cause aortic dilatation should be used to make a diagnosis in the Ghent nosology [35]. The Scottish care pathway and clinical guideline were devised to make the use of the 1996 nosology more practical in the clinic—any degree of scoliosis is accepted, as is any degree of myopia, and X-ray for protrusio acetabulae, MRI for dural ectasia, and *FBN1* gene testing are each required only if a positive result would ensure a diagnosis of Marfan syndrome through the nosology [38]. These principles can also be applied in Ghent 2010, and the algorithms shown in Fig. 19.3 can be used as part of a diagnostic care pathway for adults and children using this nosology. The algorithms fill some gaps in the outcomes of the original description, and suggest that when there is a family history of Marfan syndrome, the presence of the causative *FBN1* mutation in a relative is sufficient to make the diagnosis. *FBN1* gene testing in the index case may therefore be offered to enable testing of relatives as well as to support the original diagnosis (Tables 19.3 and 19.4).

19.4 Molecular Pathology of Marfan Syndrome and Related Disorders

Classical Marfan syndrome is associated with mutation in *FBN1*, which encodes fibrillin-1, an important component of the elastic microfibril. Fibrillin-1 is a 350 kD glycoprotein, synthesized as a 375 kD precursor which is processed and secreted into the extra-cellular matrix (ECM). It polymerises to form microfibrils and helps to stabilise latent transforming growth factor β binding proteins (LTBPs) in the ECM [39]. LTBPs hold transforming growth factor β (TGF-β) in an inactive state [15]. A failure of the interaction between fibrillin-1 and LTBPs may result in excess TGF-β signalling [40]. Most fibrillin-1 mutations are missense, suggesting a dominant negative effect on microfibrillar assembly. Ectopia lentis tends to be associated with missense mutations causing cysteine substitutions within the epidermal growth factor (EGF)—like domains of the protein, but nonsense and frameshift mutations are seen in other cases, suggesting that while cysteine residues are important to the function of the suspensory ligament of the eye, either abnormal fibrillin-1 or reduced amounts of fibrillin-1 (haploinsufficiency) may cause other aspects of the Marfan phenotype [41]. In keeping with this hypothesis, protein truncating mutations tend to be associated with more severe skeletal and skin involvement, but are less common in cases with ectopia lentis [42]. Marked variability in severity has been documented—different mutations in the same codon can cause either severe neonatal Marfan syndrome, or classical adult Marfan syndrome. Similarly, mutations in the central region of the gene (exons 24–32), sometimes called the "neonatal region", may be associated with phenotypes ranging from severe neonatal Marfan syndrome to isolated ectopia lentis [10, 13, 15], although in general mutations in this region are associated with more severe disease [42]. Although it was thought that abnormalities of microfibril structure might play an architectural role in causing the Marfan phenotype, it is now clear that the role of fibrillin-1 in regulation of TGF-β signalling may be more pertinent. The discovery of *TGFBR1* and *TGFBR2* mutations in Loeys-Dietz syndrome, a Marfan related condition supports this, as does evidence from mouse models [15, 43]. *TGFBR1 or 2* mutations in humans are also associated with loss of elastin fibres, and fibre disarray. Although the *TGFBR1* and *2* mutations described so far are loss of function mutations, increased TGFβ signalling was found in patient tissues and Marfan mouse models, and TGFβ blockade by neutralising antibodies or angiotensin 2 type 1 (AT1) receptor blockers rescues the model phenotypes [7, 15, 44]. The pathogenic process must involve a complex disruption of TGFβ signalling yet to be fully elucidated.

19.5 Aspects of Clinical Management in Marfan Syndrome

Although clinical management of many genetic disorders is not backed by extensive trials and case series [23], there are a large number of published studies of Marfan syndrome, which were reviewed in the development of the

Scottish Marfan guideline. Some of the key studies will now be discussed, to provide a flavour of the evidence and dilemmas that influence Marfan management today.

19.5.1 Cardiovascular System in Marfan Syndrome

Cardiovascular complications of Marfan syndrome include mitral valve prolapse and regurgitation, left ventricular dilatation and cardiac failure, pulmonary artery dilatation, but aortic root dilatation is the most common cause of morbidity and mortality. Aortic valve incompetence usually arises in the context of a dilated aortic root, and the risk of aortic dissection (Fig. 19.6) increases when the diameter at the sinus of Valsalva exceeds 5 cm [31, 45], when the aortic dilatation is more extensive, when the rate of dilatation exceeds 1.5 mm per year, and where there is a family history of aortic dissection [45–48]. Myocardial infarction may occur if an aortic root dissection occludes the coronary ostia. Marfan syndrome mortality from aortic complications has decreased (70% in 1972, 48% in 1995) and life expectancy has increased (mean age at death 32 ± 16 years in 1972 versus 45 ± 17 years in 1998) [11] associated with increased medical and surgical intervention (Table 19.5).

The Marfan aorta is characterised by elastic fibre fragmentation and disarray, paucity of smooth muscle cells, and deposition of collagen and mucopolysaccharide between the cells of the media. These appearances are sometimes described as "cystic medial degeneration" although there are no true cysts present. This finding is not specific for Marfan syndrome and can also be found in other conditions such as LDS, FTAA and BAV with FTAA. Mucopolysaccharide deposition in the valves may cause valve leaflet thickening. Elastic fibre degeneration in the aorta is associated with reduced distensibility in response to the pulse pressure wave. This abnormal aortic compliance can be detected at any age by echocardiography [49] or gated MRI scanning [50], although it is less marked in children. Reduction of the systolic

Table 19.5 Key issues in cardiovascular management

• Beta blocker therapy should be considered at any age if the aorta is dilated, but prophylactic treatment may be more effective in those with an aortic diameter of less than 4 cm. Angiotensin receptor blockade is an alternative
• Risk factors for aortic dissection include aortic diameter greater than 5 cm, aortic dilatation extending beyond the sinus of Valsalva, rapid rate of dilatation (>5% per year, or 1.5 mm/year in adults), and family history of aortic dissection
• At least annual evaluation should be offered, comprising clinical history, examination and echocardiography. In children, serial echocardiography at 6–12 month intervals is recommended, the frequency depending on the aortic diameter (in relation to body surface area) and the rate of increase
• Prophylactic aortic root surgery should be considered when the aortic diameter at the Sinus of Valsalva exceeds 5 cm
• In pregnancy, there is an increased risk of aortic dissection if the aortic diameter exceeds 4 cm. Frequent cardiovascular monitoring throughout pregnancy and into the puerperium is advised

ejection impulse by beta-blockers might be expected to reduce the risk of aortic dissection in Marfan syndrome [48]. Studies in turkeys prone to aortic dissection showed improved survival with propranolol and two trials in Marfan patients (a randomised trial of propranolol therapy and a retrospective historically controlled trial of propranolol or atenolol therapy) demonstrated a reduced rate of aortic dilatation and fewer aortic complications in the treatment group [48, 51]. Some patients respond better than others, responders tending to be younger and showing improved aortic distensibility, reduced pulse wave velocity, smaller pre-treatment aortic diameters (less than 4 cm in one study) [46, 48, 49, 51–53]. Poor response may be associated with more extensive elastic fibre degeneration, either due to a more severe mutation, or more advanced disease. Beta-blockade should therefore be considered in all Marfan patients, including children. Some patients may not tolerate beta-blockers, and alternative drugs which reduce the ejection impulse such as calcium antagonists [54], and angiotensin-converting enzyme (ACE) inhibitors have been considered. ACE inhibitors also reduce vascular smooth muscle cell apoptosis in vitro through an angiotensin II type 2 (AT2) receptor dependent mechanism (apoptosis is implicated in the cystic medial degeneration seen in the Marfan aorta [55]). This theoretical benefit may be in addition to any haemodynamic effects. Enalapril improved aortic distensibility and reduced the rate of aortic dilatation compared with beta-blockers in one small clinical trial in children and adolescents [56]. In a mouse model, the angiotensin II type 1 (AT1) receptor antagonist losartan reduced aortic growth rate, and prevented elastic fibre degeneration, presumably through effects on TGFβ signalling as well as haemodynamic effects, although angiotensin II also stimulates Smad-2 dependent signalling in vascular smooth muscle cells and vessel wall fibrosis by an AT1 receptor dependent but TGFβ independent mechanism [44]. Furthermore, recent studies in another mouse model suggest that while losartan protects the aorta at any stage, neuralisation of TGFβ signalling using a monoclonal antibody exacerbates arterial disease if given early on, before the aneurysm has developed, but is protective when given later [57]. The authors of this study suggested that TGFβ signalling may be physiological early on, but pathological once the arterial damage has started to occur. A number of human trials of angiotensin receptor blockers (mainly Losartan) suggests that Losartan therapy does reduce the rate of aortic growth [58–61] although one study showed no effect [62]. This issue is important as a large aortic diameter is a predictor of dissection or rupture [63, 64]. Trials comparing Losartan with Atenolol suggested no difference between these drugs in reducing aortic growth [60, 65, 66]. No effect on clinical outcomes (dissection, elective aortic surgery, cardiovascular death) was seen but the trials were of short duration and the dose of atenolol was high and that of losartan normal [60]. Increasing aortic stiffness is another predictor of aortic dilatation and dissection in Marfan syndrome, and appears to be reduced by both Losartan and Atenolol although it is suggested that Losartan may do this by TGFbeta neutralisation and affecting smooth muscle relaxation while atenolol principally reduces pulse wave velocity [52, 67, 68] (Fig. 19.7).

Other drugs may also have prophylactic potential in Marfan syndrome: ACE inhibitors reduce angiotensin 2 production, and act on both AT1 and AT2 dependent

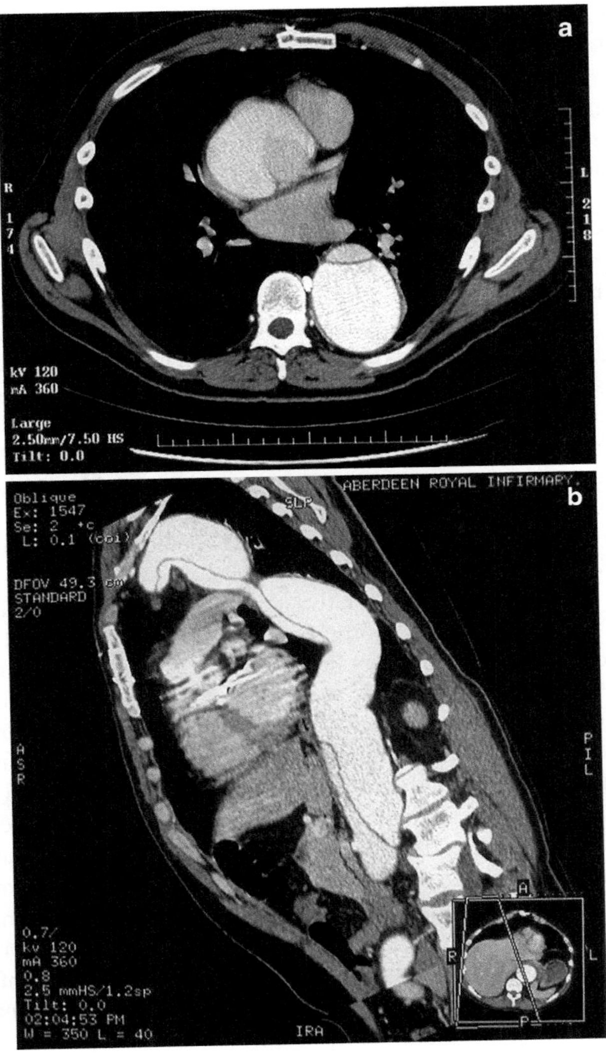

Fig. 19.7 (**a**) Axial CT scan at T7 of a Marfan patient showing dilated ascending and descending aorta with dissection flap anteriorly in the descending aorta and previous surgery to the ascending aorta. (**b**) Parasagittal reformatted CT of chest and abdomen in the same patient with contrast showing dilatation of the whole of the aorta with a spiral dissection from the arch through to the lower abdominal aorta. MR and CT images courtesy of Professor J Weir, Department of Radiology, Aberdeen Royal Infirmary

pathways—the benefit or otherwise of inhibiting both pathways is unknown. Matrix metalloproteinases (MMPs) are large endopeptidases which degrade matrix proteins including elastin. They may therefore contribute to the elastic fibre degeneration of Marfan syndrome. Their expression is closely regulated at several levels, but increased expression of MMP 2 and MMP 9 has been found in the Marfan aorta. In a mouse model, doxycyline, a nonspecific inhibitor of MMP 2 and 9 prevented thoracic aortic aneurysm, and suppressed upregulation of TGFβ expression [69]—no human data has yet been reported. Enalapril is known to decrease MMP-9 activity in non-Marfan patients [70]. In another study, abnormal flow mediated vasodilation of the brachial artery was demonstrated in Marfan patients, although agonist mediated vasodilation was normal [71]. This was attributed to abnormal endothelial cell mechanotransduction associated with abnormal fibrillin. Although the use of losartan and beta-blockers has the greatest evidence base at the moment, there may be other molecular targets for future pharmacological intervention.

If medical treatment fails, and the aortic root dilates to 5 cm or more, then prophylactic surgery should be considered [21, 45, 72]. One study suggests the threshold diameter should be 0.5 cm lower in affected women [47]. Other factors such as the rate of aortic growth, and family history of dissection should be taken into account. Numerous studies have shown better survival rates for prophylactic compared with emergency aortic surgery [45, 73], and improved longevity for Marfan patients who undergo prophylactic surgery compared with their untreated relatives [74]. Alternative procedures include the Bentall composite graft repair, in which both the aortic root and the aortic valve are replaced, or a valve conserving technique such as re-implantation of the native aortic valve in a Dacron tube (described by David) or remodelling of the aortic root (described by Yacoub) [75, 76]. The Bentall procedure has a low mortality in experienced hands with long term survival of around 80% at 5 years and 60% at 10 years [77], but requires lifelong anticoagulation post-operatively, whereas valve conserving techniques may avoid the need for anticoagulation. Use of a valve sparing procedure has been controversial as it is suggested that further deterioration of the aortic valve leaflets will require later valve replacement surgery. Recent case series have suggested that in expert hands, and in selected cases such as those where the aortic valve appears structurally normal (incompetence being due to annular dilatation) the medium term outcome is as good as the Bentall procedure, without the hazards of anticoagulation [78, 79]. In longer term follow-up (8 years), one series suggested a better outcome for valve conserving surgery, although this was attributed to preferential use of the Bentall procedure in higher risk patients. Thromboembolism was more common after the Bentall procedure (9% compared with 1% at 8 years) but re-operation was more common in patients who had undergone valve conserving surgery (6% compared with 2% at 8 years) [80]. There is certainly a case for considering a valve sparing procedure for children, women of childbearing age, and those in whom anticoagulation may be hazardous. As Marfan patients survive longer, re-operation for new aneurysms developing elsewhere in the arterial tree are becoming common—in one series, 70% developed second aneurysms requiring surgery [74]. Continuation of long-term medical prophylaxis after surgery is therefore strongly recommended [77] along with follow-up imaging of the descending and abdominal aorta [76]. Other cardiac valves may also be involved—mitral valve surgery is required in up to 10% of those requiring aortic root surgery [74].

19.5.2 Ocular System

Ocular features of Marfan syndrome include bilateral ectopia lentis (40–56%), myopia (28%) and retinal detachment (0.78%) [12, 81]. Lens dislocation into the anterior chamber may occur. Subluxation usually develops in early childhood, but may first present in the second decade [82]. Myopia is associated with an increased length of the globe and an increased risk of retinal detachment [83]. Early detection and correction of refractive errors prevents amblyopia—correction after the age of 12 years is less likely to restore visual acuity. Anisotropia (unequal refraction between the two eyes) and the possible anterior chamber abnormalities are further important considerations for management [83]. Ophthalmology assessment is important, and regular orthoptic review is recommended, particularly in childhood. Vitreolensectomy with laser prophylaxis to prevent retinal detachment can be effective in improving visual acuity in some patients [84].

19.5.3 Musculo-Skeletal System

Skeletal abnormalities develop and may progress during childhood. Scoliosis affects around 60% of Marfan patients and may progress rapidly during growth spurts, leading to marked deformity, pain and restricted ventilatory deficit. In adults, back pain (associated with scoliosis) is three times more frequent than in the general population [85]. Occasionally scoliosis may progress in adult life especially if the angle of curvature is >40°. Back pain is said to be more common in patients with dural ectasia but the evidence for this is problematic. Dural ectasia is present in 69% of Marfan patients by CT scan, and 95% by MRI imaging [86, 87]. In a study of 32 patients, dural ectasia was present in 76% of those with back pain, and 41% of those without [88]. Treatment of dural ectasia to manage back pain remains speculative [86]. Similarly, bone mineral density appears to be reduced at the spine and hip in Marfan syndrome [89, 90], but no associated increase in fracture rate has been observed.

Joint hypermobility is common, affecting 85% of children under 18, and 56% of adults with many patients suffering arthralgia, myalgia or ligamentous injury [91]. A Marfan-related myopathy with abnormal muscle fibrillin was described in one family [92] causing skeletal and respiratory muscle weakness. The significance of this for musculoskeletal symptoms in the wider Marfan patient group awaits further study.

19.5.4 Respiratory System

Pectus excavatum occurs in approximately two thirds of patients with Marfan syndrome, and when severe, can be associated with a restrictive ventilatory defect [93, 94]. It can cause difficulty with cardiac surgical procedures but correction is most often requested for cosmetic reasons. Patients with Marfan syndrome are more likely to have delayed wound healing following repair of pectus excavatum [95, 96]. Surgical correction in children should be avoided, as recurrence is common in this age group [95].

Spontaneous pneumothorax occurs in 4–11% of patients and may be associated with apical bullae [97, 98]. Recurrence is common, and there should be a low threshold for surgical intervention. Mechanical ventilation can exacerbate respiratory difficulties in Marfan neonates because of susceptibility to pneumothorax, bullae and emphysema.

Adult patients with Marfan syndrome have an increased tendency to upper airway collapse during sleep, causing obstructive sleep apnoea. This is associated with abnormalities of craniofacial structure. It may contribute to daytime somnolence, sometimes attributed to beta-blocker therapy [99].

19.5.5 Central Nervous System

Dural ectasia may reduce the effectiveness of epidural anaesthesia [100], and has been associated with intracranial hypotension-associated headache in some case reports [101]. Anterior sacral meningocele has been described rarely as a complication of Marfan syndrome, and may lead to diagnostic confusion when presenting as a pelvic or abdominal mass [102]. Cerebral haemorrhage and other neurovascular disorders are uncommon in Marfan patients [103], but intracranial aneurysms may be more common in the Loeys-Dietz syndrome [14].

19.6 Pregnancy in Marfan Syndrome

The risk of aortic dissection during pregnancy is increased, although women with Marfan syndrome who have had children have a similar lifetime risk of aortic dissection to those who have remained childless [104], despite the fact that the rate of aortic dilatation after childbirth may be higher in women who started pregnancy with an aortic root exceeding 4.5 cm in diameter [105]. It has been suggested that pregnancy acts as a "revealer" of those women likely to have dissections. Recently, also a possible link of aortic dissection to breast feeding has been suggested. Inhibition of collagen and elastin deposition in the aorta by oestrogen, the hyperdynamic hypervolaemic circulatory state of pregnancy [106] and conditions such as gestational hypertension and pre-eclampsia may be additional factors [107], although these last two conditions are less common in women on beta-blockers [105]. Aortic dissection occurs in around 4.5% of pregnancies in women with Marfan syndrome [107] and the risk is greater if the aortic root exceeds 4 cm at the start of pregnancy, or if it dilates rapidly [108]. More frequent monitoring of aortic diameter in pregnancy is advisable. If the aortic root dilates to 5 cm during the pregnancy, consideration should be given to immediate aortic replacement, early delivery or termination of pregnancy. There may be an increased risk of spontaneous preterm labour [105], but the frequencies of spontaneous miscarriage or postpartum haemorrhage are similar to those seen in the general population. The risk of aortic complications including Type B aortic dissection extends into the postpartum period [109, 110] and growth in aortic root diameter of >1 mm during pregnancy is a predictor of risk.

In about one third of the Marfan patients the *FBN1* mutation occurs de novo, but in two thirds the mutation is inherited from an affected parent. As Marfan syndrome is autosomal dominant, there is a 1 in 2 (50%) chance that the child of an affected person will inherit the disorder. Marfan patients seldom ask for prenatal diagnosis, although pre-implantation genetic diagnosis has been undertaken for families with prior molecular work up in the genetic clinic [111]. Ultrasound diagnosis is unreliable. Marfan patients should be offered genetic counselling before planning a family.

It is often difficult to diagnose Marfan syndrome in a newborn baby, but offspring of Marfan patients should be assessed early in life, with gene testing where possible, so that appropriate follow-up can be organised.

19.7 Marfan Syndrome and Sports

Although there have been no trials to investigate the effectiveness of sports limitation to avoid joint damage, common sense suggests that activities likely to stress the joints should be avoided. Heart rate, systolic blood pressure and cardiac output increase during both dynamic exercise (e.g. running) and static exercise (e.g. weight lifting). Peripheral vascular resistance and diastolic blood pressure tend to fall during dynamic exercise, but increase during static exercise [112]. Marfan patients should therefore avoid high intensity static exercise, but can be encouraged to participate in lower intensity dynamic exercise [113]. Contact sports are not advised, to protect the aorta and the lens of the eye, and scuba diving should be avoided because of the increased risk of pneumothorax.

19.8 Other Inherited Aortopathies

19.8.1 Loeys-Dietz Syndrome

In 2005, a novel autosomal dominant aortic aneurysm syndrome was identified and this entity is characterized by the triad of hypertelorism, bifid uvula/cleft palate, and arterial tortuosity with ascending aortic aneurysm/dissection. This disorder was firstly delineated in 10 families and designated Loeys-Dietz syndrome (LDS—MIM 60919) [7] showing multiple additional findings including craniosynostosis, Arnold Chiari type I malformation, dural ectasia, pectus deformity, scoliosis, arachnodactyly, club feet, patent ductus arteriosus, atrial septal defect, and bicuspid semilunar valves, but most importantly aneurysms/dissections throughout the arterial tree. Evaluation of a larger series of patients proved that the previously reported triad remains the most specific finding for this diagnosis [14], but also indicated the increased incidence of additional findings including congenital hip dislocation, dural ectasia, spondylolisthesis, cervical spine dislocation or instability, submandibular branchial cysts, osteoporosis with multiple fractures at a young age and defective tooth enamel. LDS patients may share several manifestations of the Marfan syndrome, but do not display ectopia lentis or significant dolichostenomelia, findings that are typical in Marfan syndrome.

Based on the central role of TGFβ signaling in cardiovascular, skeletal and craniofacial development, the genes encoding the TGFβ receptors (*TGFBR1* and *TGFBR2*) were considered as candidate genes. Also, a prior report had suggested that heterozygous loss-of-function mutations can cause a *TGFBR2* phenocopy of Marfan syndrome [8], a phenotype significantly overlapping with LDS. In the initial analysis of 10 patients with the classic, severe presentation of LDS (including typical craniofacial features; LDS-I) 6 mutations in *TGFBR2* and 4 in *TGFBR1* were identified [7]. While this observation intuitively corroborated the essential role of the TGFβ pathway in the pathogenesis of aortic aneurysm, it was not clear how a loss of function of the receptor for TFGβ could lead to upregulation of TGFβ activity, as had been previously observed in mouse models for Marfan syndrome. The study of fibroblasts derived from heterozygous patients with LDS failed to reveal any defect in the acute phase response to administered ligand and showed an apparent increase in TGFβ signaling after 24 h of ligand deprivation and a slower decline in the TGFβ signal after restoration of ligand. An even more informative result was the observation of increased expression of TGFβ-dependent gene products such as collagen and CTGF (connective tissue growth factor) and increased nuclear accumulation of pSmad2 in the aortic wall of patients with LDS, as well as in patients with Marfan syndrome.

Following the initial identification of *TGFBR* mutations in the first 10 patients with LDS, a more in-depth clinical and molecular study of 52 affected families, of which 40 had probands with typical clinical manifestations of LDS was published [14]. Mutations in *TGFBR1* or *TGFBR2* were found in all probands with typical LDS. As there is a clear phenotypic overlap between LDS and the vascular Ehlers-Danlos syndrome (EDS type IV), a cohort of 40 patients who presented with a vascular EDS-like syndrome, but did not bear the characteristic type III collagen abnormalities was investigated [14]. *TGFBR1* or *TGFBR2* mutations were identified in 12 probands presenting with this condition, which was initially referred to as LDS type II. The phenotype of these patients was characterised by velvety, translucent skin, easy bruising, atrophic scars, uterine rupture and arterial aneurysms/dissections within the cerebral, thoracic and abdominal circulations. Since the original discovery of *TGFBR1* and *TGFBR2* mutations in LDS, four additional genes coding for components of the TGFbeta signalling pathway have been associated with LDS like phenotypes. The LDS subtypes are now numbered according to the corresponding genes: LDS-type 1 (*TGFBR1*), type 2 (*TGFBR2*), type 3 (*SMAD3*), type 4 (*TGFB2*), type 5 (*TGFB3*). First, loss-of- function mutations in *SMAD3*, the first downstream effector, were shown to cause Aneurysms-Osteoarthritis syndrome (AOS) [114]. Since the original description of AOS, many families without osteoarthritis but with LDS-like features, such as hypertelorism, bifid uvula, and craniosynostosis, have been described, all features consistent with LDS. Moreover, *SMAD3*-mutation-positive patients seem to have the same severe cardiovascular outcome, putting this entity clearly within the LDS spectrum. Subsequently, *TGFB2* was the first TGFbeta ligand involved in aortic disease. Heterozygous loss-of-function mutations, were originally discovered in a total of 10 families and in two sporadic thoracic aortic aneurysm cases [115]. *TGFB2*-mutation-positive patients also present with a variable clinical phenotype overlapping with LDS. These features include hypertelorism, arterial tortuosity, bicuspid aortic valve, bifid uvula, clubfeet, and easy bruising. The cardiovascular findings in *TGFB2*-mutant patients initially seem to be less severe compared to those of other LDS types, but the full spectrum is still emerging; for example, intracranial aneurysms and subarachnoid hemorrhages have also recently been described in young adults with a *TGFB2* mutation. Most recently, another TGFbeta ligand, *TGFB3*, was also shown to play a role in syndromic aortic aneurysms and dissections [116]. In addition to LDS systemic features, typical cardiovascular features present in *TGFB3*-mutant patients include aneurysms and dissections, both occurring in the descending aorta and abdominal aorta, and mitral valve abnormalities, ranging from mild mitral valve prolapse to severe regurgitation with chordae rupture. In line with the findings regarding *TGFB2*, it was hypothesized that *TGFB3* mutations would lead to loss of function of TGFB3 but cause a paradoxical increase in TGFbeta signaling. Indeed, this hypothesis was confirmed by the demonstration of increased canonical and non-canonical TGFbeta signaling in the aortic wall of affected patients. Finally, a couple of patients with *SMAD2* mutations have reported with mild syndromic presentations of TAA [117]. The initially described natural history of LDS was characterised by aggressive arterial aneurysms (mean age at death, 26 years) and a high incidence of pregnancy-related complications. Obviously, the natural history of disease in LDS patients is far more aggressive than that of Marfan syndrome or vascular EDS, including aortic dissection in young childhood and/or at much lower aortic dimensions than in other connective tissue disorders. Patients with more severe outward systemic features had a poorer prognosis towards cardiovascular surgery and life expectancy. Importantly however, aneurysms in LDS appeared to be well-amenable to early and aggressive surgical intervention, in contrast to what is observed in vascular EDS, in which intra-operative mortality is very high due to the extreme fragility of the vessel walls. More recently, a wide spectrum of clinical phenotypes has been associated with *TGFBR1* and *2* mutations, ranging from isolated (familial) thoracic aortic aneurysm to severe syndromic LDS presentation with important outward features. So far, there are no apparent differences between the mutations found in patients with LDS versus those described as causing Marfan syndrome type 2 [8] or familial thoracic aortic aneurysm and dissection (FTAA) [118]. Indeed, identical mutations described as causing Marfan syndrome type 2 or FTAA have been identified in patients with typical LDS. Preliminary observations suggest that the aneurysmal phenotype is most severe in patients with *TGFBR1/2* and *SMAD3* and milder in patients with *TGFB2/3* and *SMAD2* mutations.

All this suggests that comprehensive clinical evaluation is critical for making the diagnostic distinction between the Marfan syndrome, LDS and the vascular EDS, and that in addition to molecular studies of *FBN1* (fibrillin-1) or *COL3A1* (collagen type III), genotyping of TGFbeta related genes can also be useful in the diagnostic work-up and further management of patients presenting with aortic aneurysms.

The management principles are largely based on previous experience with Marfan and vascular Ehlers-Danlos syndrome but are also guided by the differences between these diseases and Loeys-Dietz syndrome. Two important management differences distinguish patients with *FBN-1/COL3A1* mutations from TGFbeta-related gene positive patients. In the latter, more extensive imaging of the arterial tree (from head to pelvis) is indicated and earlier surgery at smaller aortic root dimensions is justifiable. Beta-adrenergic blockers or other medications are used to reduce hemodynamic stress. Angiotensin receptor blockers have been used in LDS but no randomized trials exist to proof their benefit. Aneurysms in LDS are amenable to early and aggressive surgical intervention (in contrast to vascular EDS, in which surgery is used as a last resort because of the extremely high rate of intraoperative complications and death). Many individuals can receive a valve-sparing procedure that precludes the need for chronic anticoagulation. Given the safety and the increasing availability of the valve-sparing procedure, this method is preferred. For young children with severe systemic findings of LDS, surgical repair of the ascending aorta should be considered once the maximal dimension exceeds the ninty-ninth percentile and the aortic annulus exceeds 1.8 cm, allowing the placement of a graft of sufficient size to accommodate growth.

For adolescents and adults, surgical repair of the ascending aorta should be considered once the maximal dimension approaches 4.0–4.5 cm. This recommendation is based on both numerous examples of documented aortic dissection in adults with aortic root dimensions at or below 4.0 cm and the excellent response to prophylactic surgery. An extensive family history of larger aortic dimension without dissection could alter this practice for individual patients. This practice may not eliminate risk of dissection and death, and earlier intervention based on family history or the patient's personal assessment of risk versus benefit may be indicated.

Conclusion

The Ghent nosology remains the most effective way of diagnosing or excluding Marfan syndrome, providing its limitations with respect to children are not forgotten. It can help to identify families with aortic dissection who do not have Marfan syndrome, but it should not be used to assess risk in such families. Despite the morbidity and mortality associated with Marfan syndrome and related disorders, appropriate medical and surgical management can improve and extend the lives of many patients, and advancing research holds the promise of further improvements in the future.

Acknowledgements The Scottish Marfan Guideline was developed in conjunction with colleagues from many disciplines as part of a project funded by the Clinical Resources and Audit Group of the Scottish Executive Department of Health. Bart Loeys is a senior clinical investigator of the Fund for Scientific Research Flanders.

References

1. Marfan AB-J. Un cas de déformation congénitgale des quatres membres, plus prononcée aux extremités, caractérisée par l'allongement des os avec un certain degré d'amincissiment. Bull Mem Soc Med Hop Paris. 1896;13:220–8.
2. Parish JG. Skeletal syndromes associated with arachnodactyly. Proc R Soc Med. 1960;53:515–8.
3. McKusick VA. Heritable disorders of connective tissue. III. The Marfan syndrome. J Chronic Dis. 1955;2:609–44.
4. Dietz HC, Cutting GR, Pyeritz RE, et al. Marfan syndrome caused by a recurrent de novo missense mutation in the fibrillin gene. Nature. 1991;352:337–9.
5. Boileau C, Jondeau G, Babron MC, et al. Autosomal dominant Marfan-like connective-tissue disorder with aortic dilation and skeletal anomalies not linked to the fibrillin genes. Am J Hum Genet. 1993;53:46–54.
6. Collod G, Babron MC, Jondeau G, et al. A second locus for Marfan syndrome maps to chromosome 3p24.2-p25. Nat Genet. 1994;8:264–8.
7. Loeys BL, Chen J, Neptune ER, et al. A syndrome of altered cardiovascular, craniofacial, neurocognitive and skeletal development caused by mutations in TGFBR1 or TGFBR2. Nat Genet. 2005;37:275–81.
8. Mizuguchi T, Collod-Beroud G, Akiyama T, et al. Heterozygous TGFBR2 mutations in Marfan syndrome. Nat Genet. 2004;36:855–60.
9. Gray JR, Bridges AB, Faed MJ, et al. Ascertainment and severity of Marfan syndrome in a Scottish population. J Med Genet. 1994;31:51–4.
10. Dietz HC, Pyeritz RE. Mutations in the human gene for fibrillin-1 (FBN1) in the Marfan syndrome and related disorders. Hum Mol Genet. 1995;4:1799–809.
11. Gray JR, Bridges AB, West RR, et al. Life expectancy in British Marfan syndrome populations. Clin Genet. 1998;54:124–8.
12. Loeys B, De BJ, Van AP, et al. Comprehensive molecular screening of the FBN1 gene favors locus homogeneity of classical Marfan syndrome. Hum Mutat. 2004;24:140–6.
13. Loeys B, Nuytinck L, Delvaux I, et al. Genotype and phenotype analysis of 171 patients referred for molecular study of the fibrillin-1 gene FBN1 because of suspected Marfan syndrome. Arch Intern Med. 2001;161:2447–54.
14. Loeys BL, Schwarze U, Holm T, et al. Aneurysm syndromes caused by mutations in the TGF-beta receptor. N Engl J Med. 2006;355:788–98.
15. Mizuguchi T, Matsumoto N. Recent progress in genetics of Marfan syndrome and Marfan-associated disorders. J Hum Genet. 2007;52:1–12.
16. Sakai H, Visser R, Ikegawa S, et al. Comprehensive genetic analysis of relevant four genes in 49 patients with Marfan syndrome or Marfan-related phenotypes. Am J Med Genet A. 2006;140:1719–25.
17. Singh KK, Rommel K, Mishra A, et al. TGFBR1 and TGFBR2 mutations in patients with features of Marfan syndrome and Loeys-Dietz syndrome. Hum Mutat. 2006;27:770–7.
18. Verstraeten A, Alaerts M, Van Laer L, Loeys B. Marfan syndrome and related disorders: 25 years of gene discovery. Hum Mutat. 2016;37(6):524–31.
19. Law C, Bunyan D, Castle B, et al. Clinical features in a family with an R460H mutation in transforming growth factor beta receptor 2 gene. J Med Genet. 2006;43:908–16.
20. Pannu H, Fadulu VT, Chang J, et al. Mutations in transforming growth factor-beta receptor type II cause familial thoracic aortic aneurysms and dissections. Circulation. 2005;112:513–20.
21. de Paepe AM, Devereux RB, Dietz HC, et al. Revised diagnostic criteria for the Marfan syndrome. Am J Med Genet. 1996;62:417–26.
22. Loeys BL, Dietz HC, Braverman AC, Callewaert BL, De Backer J, Devereux RB, Hilhorst-Hofstee Y, Jondeau G, Faivre L, Milewicz DM, Pyeritz RE, Sponseller PD, Wordsworth P, De Paepe AM. The revised Ghent nosology for the Marfan syndrome. J Med Genet. 2010;47:476–85.

23. Campbell H, Bradshaw N, Davidson R, et al. Evidence based medicine in practice: lessons from a Scottish clinical genetics project. J Med Genet. 2000;37:684–91.
24. Loeys BL, Dietz HC, Braverman AC, et al. The revised Ghent nosology for the Marfan syndrome. J Med Genet. 2010;47(7):476–85. https://doi.org/10.1136/jmg.2009.072785.
25. Roman MJ, Devereux RB, Kramer-Fox R, et al. Two-dimensional echocardiographic aortic root dimensions in normal children and adults. Am J Cardiol. 1989;64:507–12.
26. Joseph KN, Kane HA, Milner RS, et al. Orthopedic aspects of the Marfan phenotype. Clin Orthop Relat Res. 1992;277:251–61.
27. Lipscomb KJ, Clayton-Smith J, Harris R. Evolving phenotype of Marfan's syndrome. Arch Dis Child. 1997;76:41–6.
28. Campens L, Demulier L, De Groote K, et al. Reference values for echocardiographic assessment of the diameter of the aortic root and ascending aorta spanning all age categories. Am J Cardiol. 2014;114:914–20.
29. Du Bois D, Du Bois EF. A formula to estimate the approximate surface area if height and weight be known. Arch Intern Med. 1916;17:863–71.
30. Mosteller RD. Simplified calculation of body-surface area. N Engl J Med. 1987;317:1098.
31. Roman MJ, Rosen SE, Kramer-Fox R, et al. Prognostic significance of the pattern of aortic root dilation in the Marfan syndrome. J Am Coll Cardiol. 1993;22:1470–6.
32. Curtis AE, Smith TA, Ziganshin BA, Elefteriades JA. The mystery of the Z-score. Aorta. 2016;4:124–30.
33. Meijboom LJ, Groenink M, Van Der Wall EE, et al. Aortic root asymmetry in Marfan patients; evaluation by magnetic resonance imaging and comparison with standard echocardiography. Int J Card Imaging. 2000;16:161–8.
34. Yule SR, Hobson EE, Dean JC, et al. Protrusio acetabuli in Marfan's syndrome. Clin Radiol. 1999;54:95–7.
35. Von Kodolitsch Y, De Backer J, Shuler H, et al. Perspectives on the revised Ghent criteria for the diagnosis of Marfan syndrome. Appl Clin Genet. 2015;8(1):37–155.
36. Faivre L, Collod-Beroud G, Ades L, et al. The new Ghent criteria for Marfan syndrome: what do they change? Clin Genet. 2012;81:433–42.
37. Faivre L, Collod-Beroud G, Child A, et al. Contribution of molecular analyses in diagnosing Marfan syndrome and type I fibrillinopathies: an international study of 1009 probands. J Med Genet. 2008;45:384–90.
38. Dean JC. Marfan syndrome: clinical diagnosis and management. Eur J Hum Genet. 2007;15:724–33.
39. Robinson PN, Arteaga-Solis E, Baldock C, et al. The molecular genetics of Marfan syndrome and related disorders. J Med Genet. 2006;43:769–87.
40. Gelb BD. Marfan's syndrome and related disorders--more tightly connected than we thought. N Engl J Med. 2006;355:841–4.
41. Judge DP, Biery NJ, Keene DR, et al. Evidence for a critical contribution of haploinsufficiency in the complex pathogenesis of Marfan syndrome. J Clin Invest. 2004;114:172–81.
42. Faivre L, Collod-Beroud G, Loeys BL, et al. Effect of mutation type and location on clinical outcome in 1,013 probands with Marfan syndrome or related phenotypes and FBN1 mutations: an international study. Am J Hum Genet. 2007;81:454–66.
43. Dietz HC, Loeys B, Carta L, et al. Recent progress towards a molecular understanding of Marfan syndrome. Am J Med Genet C Semin Med Genet. 2005;139C:4–9.
44. Habashi JP, Judge DP, Holm TM, et al. Losartan, an AT1 antagonist, prevents aortic aneurysm in a mouse model of Marfan syndrome. Science. 2006;312:117–21.
45. Groenink M, Lohuis TA, Tijssen JG, et al. Survival and complication free survival in Marfan's syndrome: implications of current guidelines. Heart. 1999;82:499–504.
46. Legget ME, Unger TA, O'Sullivan CK, et al. Aortic root complications in Marfan's syndrome: identification of a lower risk group. Heart. 1996;75:389–95.
47. Meijboom LJ, Timmermans J, Zwinderman AH, et al. Aortic root growth in men and women with the Marfan's syndrome. Am J Cardiol. 2005a;96:1441–4.
48. Shores J, Berger KR, Murphy EA, et al. Progression of aortic dilatation and the benefit of long-term beta-adrenergic blockade in Marfan's syndrome. N Engl J Med. 1994;330:1335–41.

49. Rios AS, Silber EN, Bavishi N, et al. Effect of long-term beta-blockade on aortic root compliance in patients with Marfan syndrome. Am Heart J. 1999;137:1057–61.
50. Adams JN, Brooks M, Redpath TW, et al. Aortic distensibility and stiffness index measured by magnetic resonance imaging in patients with Marfan's syndrome. Br Heart J. 1995;73:265–9.
51. Salim MA, Alpert BS, Ward JC, et al. Effect of beta-adrenergic blockade on aortic root rate of dilation in the Marfan syndrome. Am J Cardiol. 1994;74:629–33.
52. Groenink M, de RA, Mulder BJ, et al. Changes in aortic distensibility and pulse wave velocity assessed with magnetic resonance imaging following beta-blocker therapy in the Marfan syndrome. Am J Cardiol. 1998;82:203–8.
53. Haouzi A, Berglund H, Pelikan PC, et al. Heterogeneous aortic response to acute beta-adrenergic blockade in Marfan syndrome. Am Heart J. 1997;133:60–3.
54. Rossi-Foulkes R, Roman MJ, Rosen SE, et al. Phenotypic features and impact of beta blocker or calcium antagonist therapy on aortic lumen size in the Marfan syndrome. Am J Cardiol. 1999;83:1364–8.
55. Nagashima H, Sakomura Y, Aoka Y, et al. Angiotensin II type 2 receptor mediates vascular smooth muscle cell apoptosis in cystic medial degeneration associated with Marfan's syndrome. Circulation. 2001;104:I282–7.
56. Yetman AT, Bornemeier RA, McCrindle BW. Usefulness of enalapril versus propranolol or atenolol for prevention of aortic dilation in patients with the Marfan syndrome. Am J Cardiol. 2005;95:1125–7.
57. Cook JR, Clayton NP, Carta L, et al. Dimorphic effects of transforming growth factor-β signaling during aortic aneurysm progression in mice suggest a combinatorial therapy for Marfan syndrome. Arterioscler Thromb Vasc Biol. 2015;35:911–17. https://doi.org/10.1161/ATVBAHA.114.305150.
58. Brooke BS, Habashi JP, Judge DP, et al. Angiotensin II blockade and aortic-root dilation in Marfan's syndrome. N Engl J Med. 2008;358:2787–95.
59. Groenink M, den Hartog AW, Franken R, et al. Losartan reduces aortic dilatation rate in adults with Marfan syndrome: a randomized controlled trial. Eur Heart J. 2013;34:3491–500.
60. Lacro RV, Dietz HC, Sleeper LA, et al. Atenolol versus losartan in children and young adults with Marfan's syndrome. N Engl J Med. 2014;371:2061–71.
61. Pees C, Laccone F, Hagl M, et al. Usefulness of losartan on the size of the ascending aorta in an unselected cohort of children, adolescents, and young adults with Marfan syndrome. Am J Cardiol. 2013;112:1477–83.
62. Milleron O, Arnoult F, Ropers J, et al. Marfan Sartan: a randomized, double blind, placebo-controlled trial. Eur Heart J. 2015;36:2160–6.
63. Elefteriades JA. Natural history of thoracic aortic aneurysms: indications for surgery, and surgical versus nonsurgical risks. Ann Thorac Surg. 2002;74:S1877–80.
64. Kuzmik GA, Sang AX, Elefteriades JA. Natural history of thoracic aortic aneurysms. J Vasc Surg. 2013;56:565–71.
65. Forteza A, Evangelista A, Sanchez V, et al. Efficacy of losartan vs. atenolol for the prevention of aortic dilation in Marfan syndrome: a randomized clinical trial. Eur Heart J. 2016;37:978–85.
66. Lacro RV, Dietz HC, Wruck LM, et al. Rationale and design of a randomized clinical trial of beta-blocker therapy (atenolol) versus angiotensin II receptor blocker therapy (losartan) in individuals with Marfan syndrome. Am Heart J. 2007;154:624–31.
67. Bhatt AB, Buck JS, Zuflacht JP, et al. Distinct effects of losartan and atenolol on vascular stiffness in Marfan syndrome. Vasc Med. 2015;20:317–25.
68. Kröner ES, Scholte AJ, de Koning PJ, et al. MRI-assessed regional pulse wave velocity for predicting absence of regional aorta luminal growth in Marfan syndrome. Int J Cardiol. 2013;167:2977–82.
69. Chung AW, Yang HH, Radomski MW, et al. Long-term doxycycline is more effective than atenolol to prevent thoracic aortic aneurysm in Marfan syndrome through the inhibition of matrix metalloproteinase-2 and -9. Circ Res. 2008;102:e73–85.
70. Williams A, Davies S, Stuart AG, et al. Medical treatment of Marfan syndrome: a time for change. Heart. 2008;94:414–21.

71. Wilson DG, Bellamy MF, Ramsey MW, et al. Endothelial function in Marfan syndrome: selective impairment of flow-mediated vasodilation. Circulation. 1999;99:909–15.
72. Meijboom LJ, Nollen GJ, Mulder BJM. Prevention of cardiovascular complications in Marfan syndrome. Vasc Dis Prev. 2004;1:79–86.
73. Gott VL, Cameron DE, Alejo DE, et al. Aortic root replacement in 271 Marfan patients: a 24-year experience. Ann Thorac Surg. 2002;73:438–43.
74. Finkbohner R, Johnston D, Crawford ES, et al. Marfan syndrome. Long-term survival and complications after aortic aneurysm repair. Circulation. 1995;91:728–33.
75. de Oliveira NC, David TE, Ivanov J, et al. Results of surgery for aortic root aneurysm in patients with Marfan syndrome. J Thorac Cardiovasc Surg. 2003;125:789–96.
76. Nataf P, Lansac E. Dilation of the thoracic aorta: medical and surgical management. Heart. 2006;92:1345–52.
77. Treasure T. Elective replacement of the aortic root in Marfan's syndrome. Br Heart J. 1993;69:101–3.
78. Bassano C, De Matteis GM, Nardi P, et al. Mid-term follow-up of aortic root remodelling compared to Bentall operation. Eur J Cardiothorac Surg. 2001;19:601–5.
79. Kallenbach K, Karck M, Pak D, et al. Decade of aortic valve sparing reimplantation: are we pushing the limits too far? Circulation. 2005;112:1253–9.
80. Patel ND, Weiss ES, Alejo DE, et al. Aortic root operations for Marfan syndrome: a comparison of the Bentall and valve-sparing procedures. Ann Thorac Surg. 2008;85:2003–10.
81. van den Berg JS, Limburg M, Hennekam RC. Is Marfan syndrome associated with symptomatic intracranial aneurysms? Stroke. 1996;27:10–2.
82. Maumenee IH. The eye in the Marfan syndrome. Trans Am Ophthalmol Soc. 1981;79:684–733.
83. Pyeritz RE, McKusick VA. The Marfan syndrome: diagnosis and management. N Engl J Med. 1979;300:772–7.
84. Hubbard AD, Charteris DG, Cooling RJ. Vitreolensectomy in Marfan's syndrome. Eye. 1998;12(Pt 3a):412–6.
85. Pyeritz RE, Francke U. The second international symposium on the Marfan syndrome. Am J Med Genet. 1993;47:127–35.
86. Fattori R, Nienaber CA, Descovich B, et al. Importance of dural ectasia in phenotypic assessment of Marfan's syndrome. Lancet. 1999;354:910–3.
87. Oosterhof T, Groenink M, Hulsmans FJ, et al. Quantitative assessment of dural ectasia as a marker for Marfan syndrome. Radiology. 2001;220:514–8.
88. Ahn NU, Sponseller PD, Ahn UM, et al. Dural ectasia is associated with back pain in Marfan syndrome. Spine. 2000;25:1562–8.
89. Giampietro PF, Peterson M, Schneider R, et al. Assessment of bone mineral density in adults and children with Marfan syndrome. Osteoporos Int. 2003;14:559–63.
90. Le Parc JM, Molcard S, Tubach F. Bone mineral density in Marfan syndrome. Rheumatology. 2001;40:358–9.
91. Grahame R, Pyeritz RE. The Marfan syndrome: joint and skin manifestations are prevalent and correlated. Br J Rheumatol. 1995;34:126–31.
92. Behan WM, Longman C, Petty RK, et al. Muscle fibrillin deficiency in Marfan's syndrome myopathy. J Neurol Neurosurg Psychiatry. 2003;74:633–8.
93. Scherer LR, Arn PH, Dressel DA, et al. Surgical management of children and young adults with Marfan syndrome and pectus excavatum. J Pediatr Surg. 1988;23:1169–72.
94. Streeten EA, Murphy EA, Pyeritz RE. Pulmonary function in the Marfan syndrome. Chest. 1987;91:408–12.
95. Arn PH, Scherer LR, Haller JA Jr, et al. Outcome of pectus excavatum in patients with Marfan syndrome and in the general population. J Pediatr. 1989;115:954–8.
96. Golladay ES, Char F, Mollitt DL. Children with Marfan's syndrome and pectus excavatum. South Med J. 1985;78:1319–23.
97. Hall JR, Pyeritz RE, Dudgeon DL, et al. Pneumothorax in the Marfan syndrome: prevalence and therapy. Ann Thorac Surg. 1984;37:500–4.

98. Wood JR, Bellamy D, Child AH, et al. Pulmonary disease in patients with Marfan syndrome. Thorax. 1984;39:780–4.
99. Cistulli PA, Gotsopoulos H, Sullivan CE. Relationship between craniofacial abnormalities and sleep-disordered breathing in Marfan's syndrome. Chest. 2001;120:1455–60.
100. Lacassie HJ, Millar S, Leithe LG, et al. Dural ectasia: a likely cause of inadequate spinal anaesthesia in two parturients with Marfan's syndrome. Br J Anaesth. 2005;94:500–4.
101. Rosser T, Finkel J, Vezina G, et al. Postural headache in a child with Marfan syndrome: case report and review of the literature. J Child Neurol. 2005;20:153–5.
102. Voyvodic F, Scroop R, Sanders RR. Anterior sacral meningocele as a pelvic complication of Marfan syndrome. Aust N Z J Obstet Gynaecol. 1999;39:262–5.
103. Wityk RJ, Zanferrari C, Oppenheimer S. Neurovascular complications of Marfan syndrome: a retrospective, hospital-based study. Stroke. 2002;33:680–4.
104. Pacini L, Digne F, Boumendil A, et al. Maternal complication of pregnancy in Marfan syndrome. Int J Cardiol. 2008;136:156.
105. Meijboom LJ, Drenthen W, Pieper PG, et al. Obstetric complications in Marfan syndrome. Int J Cardiol. 2006;110:53–9.
106. Immer FF, Bansi AG, Immer-Bansi AS, et al. Aortic dissection in pregnancy: analysis of risk factors and outcome. Ann Thorac Surg. 2003;76:309–14.
107. Chow SL. Acute aortic dissection in a patient with Marfan's syndrome complicated by gestational hypertension. Med J Aust. 1993;159:760–2.
108. Lind J, Wallenburg HC. The Marfan syndrome and pregnancy: a retrospective study in a Dutch population. Eur J Obstet Gynecol Reprod Biol. 2001;98:28–35.
109. Kuperstein R, Cahan T, Yoeli-Ullman R, et al. Risk of aortic dissection in pregnant patients with the Marfan syndrome. Am J Cardiol. 2017;119:132–7.
110. Roman MJ, Pugh NL, Hendershot TP, Devereux RB, Dietz H, Holmes K, Eagle KA, LeMaire SA, Milewicz DM, Morris SA, Pyeritz RE, Ravekes WJ, Shohet RV, Silberbach M, GenTAC Investigators. Aortic complications associated with pregnancy in Marfan syndrome: the NHLBI National Registry of Genetically Triggered Thoracic Aortic Aneurysms and Cardiovascular Conditions (GenTAC). J Am Heart Assoc. 2016;5:e004052. https://doi.org/10.1161/JAHA.116.004052.
111. Loeys B, Nuytinck L, Van AP, et al. Strategies for prenatal and preimplantation genetic diagnosis in Marfan syndrome (MFS). Prenat Diagn. 2002;22:22–8.
112. Salim MA, Alpert BS. Sports and Marfan syndrome - awareness and early diagnosis can prevent sudden death. Phys Sportsmed. 2001;29:80–93.
113. Maron BJ, Chaitman BR, Ackerman MJ, et al. Recommendations for physical activity and recreational sports participation for young patients with genetic cardiovascular diseases. Circulation. 2004;109:2807–16.
114. van de Laar IM, Oldenburg RA, Pals G, et al. Mutations in SMAD3 cause a syndromic form of aortic aneurysms and dissections with early-onset osteoarthritis. Nat Genet. 2011;43:121–6.
115. Lindsay ME, Schepers D, Bolar NA. Loss-of-function mutations in TGFB2 cause a syndromic presentation of thoracic aortic aneurysm. Nat Genet. 2012;44:922–7.
116. Bertoli-Avella AM, Gillis E, Morisaki H, et al. Mutations in a TGF-beta ligand, TGFB3, cause syndromic aortic aneurysms and dissections. J Am Coll Cardiol. 2015;65:1324–36.
117. Micha D, Guo DC, Hilhorst-Hofstee Y, et al. SMAD2 mutations are associated with arterial aneurysms and dissections. Hum Mutat. 2015;36:1145–9.
118. Pannu H, Avidan N, Tran-Fadulu V, et al. Genetic basis of thoracic aortic aneurysms and dissections: potential relevance to abdominal aortic aneurysms. Ann N Y Acad Sci. 2006;1085:242–55.

Cardiovascular Manifestations in Inherited Connective Tissue Disorders

20

Julie de Backer and Anne de Paepe

Abstract
Heritable connective tissue disorders comprise a heterogeneous group of entities with widespread manifestations in most of them. Increased understanding of the structure and function of the connective tissue had led to the identification of many additional diseases over the last decade. The spectrum of disorders affecting the cardiovascular system has broadened significantly and also includes disorders with no- or very limited-systemic manifestations. Important clinical and genetic overlap between these different entities exists. In this chapter, we provide an overview of the most common cardiovascular manifestations occurring in the setting of HCTD and discuss the most relevant disease entities in this context.

Keywords
Marfan syndrome • Connective tissue disorder • Aortic aneurysm • Aortic dissection • Aorta • Mitral valve prolapse

20.1 Heritable Connective Tissue Disorders

Heritable connective tissue disorders (HCTD) are Mendelian disorders that affect the normal development, maintenance and function of the hard (bone, cartilage) and/or soft (skin, blood vessels, cardiac valves, tendon and ligaments, ocular structures) connective tissues.

J. de Backer (✉) • A. de Paepe
Department of Cardiology and Medical Genetics, Ghent University Hospital, Ghent, Belgium
e-mail: Julie.debacker@ugent.be; Anne.depaepe@ugent.be

D. Kumar, P. Elliott (eds.), *Cardiovascular Genetics and Genomics*,
https://doi.org/10.1007/978-3-319-66114-8_20

The connective tissue is composed of sparsely distributed cells surrounded by an extracellular matrix. The extracellular matrix forms a complex three-dimensional network, composed of a wide variety of macromolecules, generally classified as fibrous proteins (elastin and collagen) and ground substance (a mixture of glycoproteins and glycosaminglycans) [1]. The components of the extracellular matrix are secreted and maintained by tissue specific cells. Variations in the composition of the extracellular matrix, determines the properties of the connective tissue. While its major function was initially thought to be mainly structural, it has now become clear that the connective tissue plays crucial roles in signal transmission and tissue homeostasis. Homeostasis requires not only an intact extracellular matrix but also intact cellular components. Indeed, bi-directional cross-talk between the matrix and the cells is very important. In the vascular structures, Smooth muscle cells (VSMC) also play an important role in this interaction. Alterations in the VSMC contractile function may therefor also lead to connective tissue disorders.

Defects due to genetic alterations in any of the genes encoding components of the connective tissue and its main interaction partners may lead to disease. With increasing knowledge of the composition and function of the connective tissue, the spectrum of CTD has expanded tremendously over the last decade and connective tissue diseases with cardiovascular involvement can now be classified into:

- Diseases caused by defects in structural components such as collagen and elastic fibers, e.g. FBN1, COL3A1
- Diseases caused by mutations in components of the VSMC contractile apparatus, e.g. ACTA2, MYH11
- Diseases caused by components in signaling pathways such as the TGFβ signaling cascade, e.g. TGFBR2, SMAD3

Many of these genetic conditions will give rise to syndromic entities, with manifestations in several organ systems. From a cardiovascular point of view however it is important to acknowledge that mutations in most of the genes related to these syndromic entities can also be encountered in patients presenting nonsyndromic (or isolated) aortic disease. These patients constitute a particular group as no outward features triggering the diagnosis are present and aortic aneurysms grow without symptoms in most cases and may evolve to life-threatening aortic dissections. With the expanding availability and efficiency of high throughput (next generation) genetic sequencing techniques, the threshold for genetic testing in patients with aortic disease has—and should—come down since this will allow timely detection of patients at risk for life-threatening complications.

In this chapter, we will first describe and define the main cardiovascular abnormalities encountered in HCTD after which we will provide an overview of the most relevant HCTD.

20.2 Description of the Main Cardiovascular Manifestations in HCTD

20.2.1 Aortic Aneurysms and Dissections

Aortic dilatation is defined as a diameter of the aorta exceeding ≥1.96 standard deviations of the normal expected diameter (i.e. the upper limit of the 95% confidence interval of the distribution in a large reference population) [2]. A commonly used method to quantify dilatation is to use z-scores. The z-score value of the aortic root at the level of the sinus of plays a crucial role in the diagnosis of MFS in the revised Ghent nosology, where an aortic root z-score >2 in adults and >3 in children is required for the diagnosis (see below). In other HCTD, z-score calculation is equally important since it allows correct identification of patients with aortic disease. Calculating z-scores in a correct way is extremely important and requires adequate normal values obtained in the right reference population using the same technique as applied in the individual patient. Differences in measuring techniques between pediatric cardiologists and adult cardiologists render comparison of values hazardous and one should be very careful to use the correct calculation method. Pediatric cardiologists will usually measure the aortic root diameters in systole, according to the inner-to-inner edge technique [3] whereas most adult cardiologists will measure at end diastole using the leading-to-leading edge technique [4] (Fig. 20.1). A recent study comparing pediatric and adult techniques showed that the pediatric method revealed a systematically lower diameter than the adult method of measuring; the correlation between both techniques was good [5]. Reference values for the pediatric methods are published by Gautier [6]—adult reference values have been provided by Devereux and Roman [2, 7]. Comparing various reference values in a cohort of adult MFS patients revealed that the more recently published calculation method by Devereux is more reliable than the initial publication by their group, mainly because the reference group was larger and because there was a continuous distribution of age. Correcting for height instead of for BSA may be more reliable, especially with the increasing amount of obese subjects [8].

In addition to its value in a diagnostic setting, aortic root diameters play an important role in determining the outcome in patients with aortic disease—a direct (but not absolute!) correlation between the diameter and risk for dissection has clearly been documented and the aortic diameter still is the most important factor in risk prediction and in defining the threshold for prophylactic surgery [9, 10].

An *aortic aneurysm* is defined as a local dilatation of the vessel exceeding 50% of the normal size at that location for that specific individual. In HCTD, aneurysms may develop in any part of the aorta as well as in its branching vessels in several entities.

Aortic dissection refers to splitting of the vessel wall as a result of an intimal tear, allowing blood to enter the aortic media layer and creating a false and true lumen in the vessel. Aortic dissection is followed either by an aortic rupture in the case of

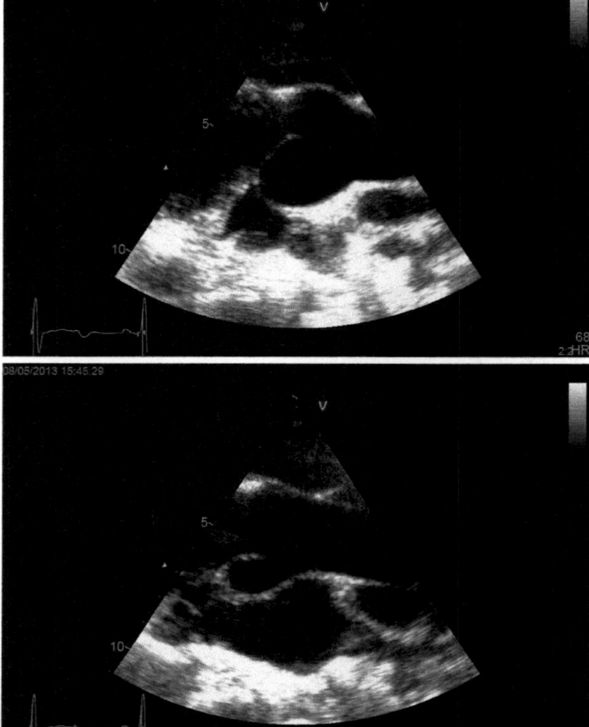

Fig. 20.1 Aortic root measurement with transthoracic echocardiography in the PSLAX view in a 14-year-old Marfan boy. On the left, measurement at end diastole, with the leading-to-leading edge principle, used in adult cardiology. On the right, measurement at end systole, with the inner-to-inner edge principle, used in pediatric cardiology. Note the 2 mm difference

adventitial disruption or by a re-entering into the aortic lumen through a second intimal tear.

Several classification systems have been used to describe aortic dissections with DeBakey and Stanford being the most common ones (Fig. 20.2). The DeBakey classification categorizes the dissection based on the location of the intimal tear and extent of the dissection, whereas the Stanford classification is based on whether or not the ascending aorta is involved. In this chapter, we will us the Stanford classification, unless stated otherwise. Stanford type A dissections originate proximal to the left subclavian artery and type B distal to the left subclavian artery. Both types are quite different with regards to outcome in the acute and long term setting as well as in treatment. Patients with type A aortic dissections suffer double the mortality from patients with type B dissections (25% versus 12%) [10–12]. The only life-saving treatment in acute type A dissection is urgent surgical intervention, leading to a decrease in mortality from 56.6% to 26.9% in the International Registry of Aortic Dissections (IRAD registry) [11, 13]. Conventionally, patients presenting with a type B dissection are treated medically with aggressive blood pressure lowering. Indications for surgery include any sign of organ ischemia (kidney, chordal spine, intestinal, leg) or rapidly growing aneurysms in the dissected areas [10].

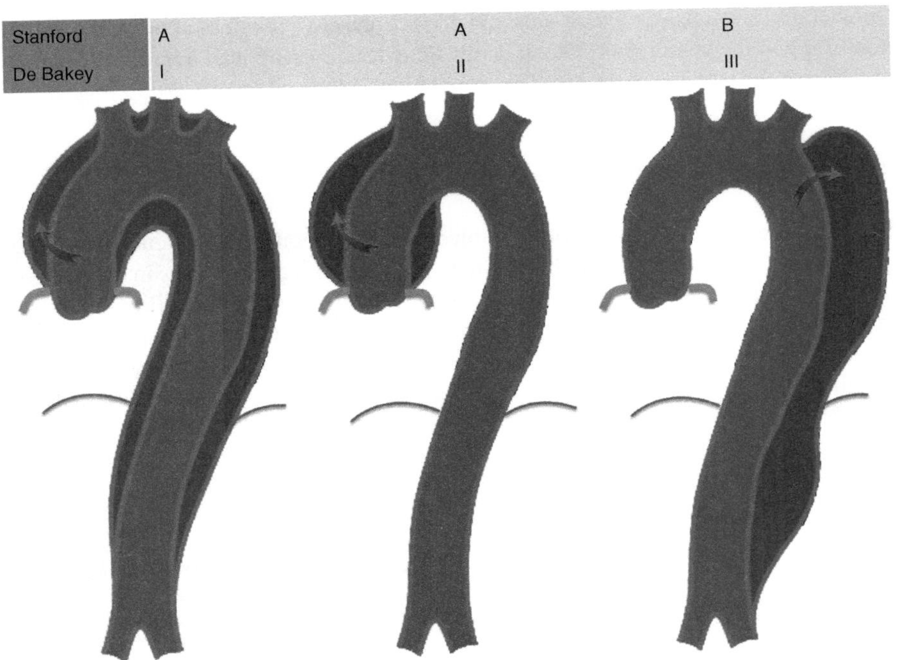

Fig. 20.2 Classification of aortic dissections according to Stanford and De Bakey

Endovascular procedures, commonly used for the treatment of aortic dissections in the general population are formally contra-indicated in patients with CTD due to a significant risk for stent displacement or rupture.

20.3 Pathophysiology of Aneurysms and Dissections in Connective Tissue Disorders: Current Concept

While initially, aortic aneurysms and dissections in connective tissue disorders were thought to result essentially form structural weakness, it has now clearly been established that the process is more complex and that the mutated components of the connective tissue also have important functional roles in signal transmission and maintaining tissue homeostasis. This current concept is known as mechanobiology of the vessel wall and is nicely reviewed in [14, 15]. Homeostasis implicates correct sensing by the cells in the vessel wall of their chemomechanical environment in order establish, maintain, remodel and—if necessary—repair the extracellular matrix to provide compliance as well as strength. Correct sensing of the signals in turn necessitates intact receptors that connect the ECM to intracellular actomyosin filaments as well as intact signaling molecules that transmit the information to the nucleus. Indeed, the clinical manifestation of aortic aneurysms and dissections at the macro (tissue) level are a reflection of important alterations on the micro (molecular) level. Aortic aneurysms and dissections are a result of abnormal mechanobiology in the vessel wall, which is related to the intrinsic wall abnormalities due to the underlying genetic defect. This concept is illustrated in Fig. 20.3

20.3.1 Arterial/Aortic Tortuosity

Reporting vessel tortuosity is often subjective and operator dependent, indicating the need for more objective methods. Such methods with applications in connective tissue disorders have been published recently, showing easy applicability and interesting correlations with the extent of the disease. The vertebral artery tortuosity index (VTI) based on distance factor is calculated by dividing the actual measured length of the vessel over the straight distance (both in cm) (Distance factor = [actual/straight length-1] × 100. An illustration is given in Fig. 20.4. VTI's exceeding 50 were associated with worse outcome [16].

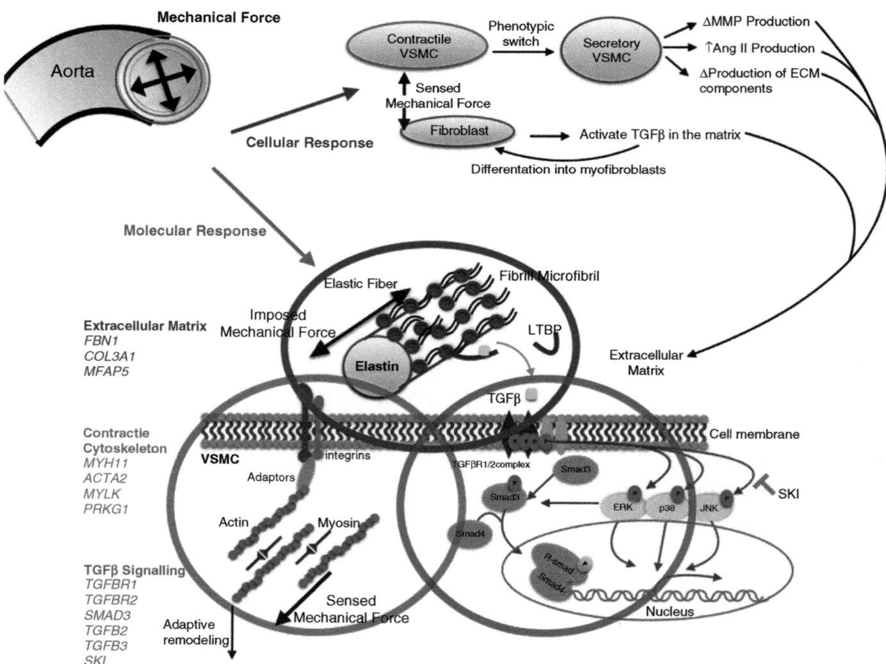

Fig. 20.3 Concept of mechanobiology underlying homeostasis in the thoracic aorta. Alterations, either due to higher imposed forces (hypertension) or due to (genetic) alterations in the various components required for proper sensing and/or transduction of the signal may lead to aneurysms/dissections. Mutations in the various components may affect the mechanical properties of the microfibrils or the signaling pathways, leading to an altered mechanotransduction signal and initiation of cellular response mechanisms including increased TGFβ signalling

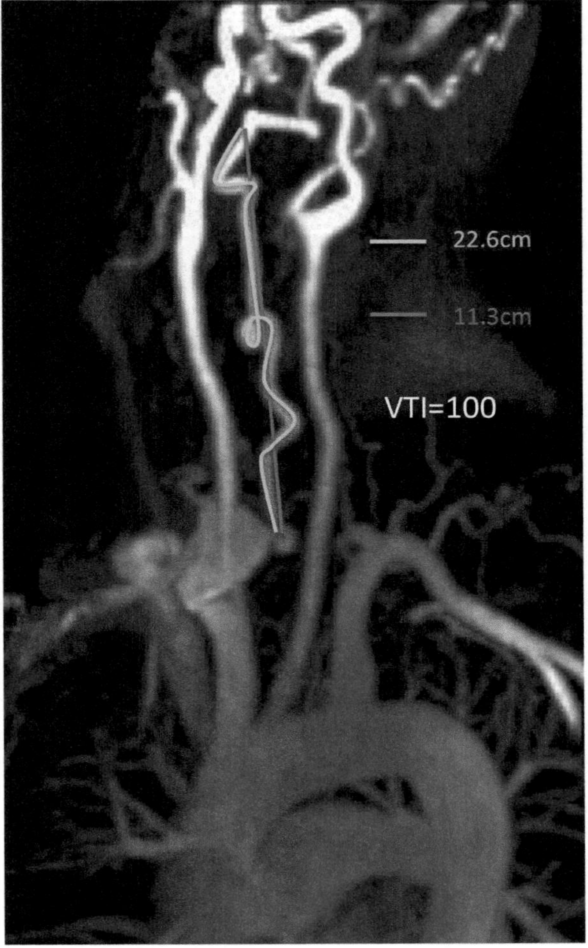

Fig. 20.4 Vertebral Tortuosity Index calculation in a patient with Loeys Dietz syndrome. Distance Factor = [actual(yellow)/straight(red) length-1] × 100

Similar methods and results have been obtained calculating the aortic tortuosity index in Marfan patients [17].

20.3.2 Mitral Valve Prolapse

Mitral valve prolapse is characterized by the displacement of an abnormally thickened mitral valve leaflet into the left atrium during systole in the long axis view on echocardiography [18]. By definition, the displacement from the mitral valve annular plane needs to exceed 2 mm. The presence of valve thickening which was used to discriminate between classic and non-classic prolapse [19] is no longer taken into account in more recent criteria.

Figure 20.5 gives an overview of cardiovascular manifestations in HCTD.

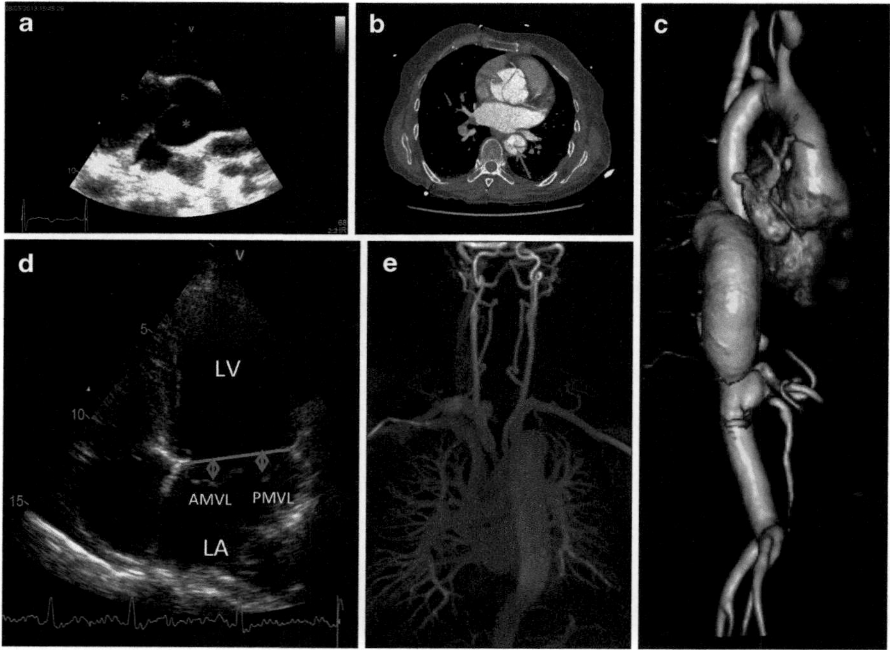

Fig. 20.5 Cardiovascular manifestations in HCTD. (**a**) Transthoracic echocardiogram (PSLAX) of an aortic root aneurysm (red asterisk) in a Marfan patient. (**b**) CT image of type A aortic dissection extending into the descending thoracic aorta in a Marfan patient. (**c**) MRI image of an aortic root aneurysm and an aneurysm of the descending thoracic aorta (after open surgery 14 years prior to this control). (**d**) Transthoracic echocardiogram (AP4CV) of Mitral Valve Prolapse—note the excursion of the Anterior and Posterior Mitral Valve Leaflets (AMVL and PMVL) into the left atrium (LA). *LV* left ventricle. (**e**) MRI image of the proximal aorta and head and neck vessels in a patient with Loeys-Dietz syndrome—note the marked arterial tortuosity

20.4 Heritable Connective Tissue Disorders with Cardiovascular Manifestations

20.4.1 Marfan Syndrome

20.4.1.1 Diagnosis

Marfan syndrome (MFS) is caused by mutations in the Fibrillin-1 gene (*FBN1*), encoding the fibrillin1 protein [20, 21]. Fibrillin1 is a glycoprotein and important component of the microfibrils displaying important structural and functional roles. Fibrillin1 is essential for elastic fiber formation and these fibers are in turn important for structural integrity of the aorta.

MFS is an eminent example of a pleiotropic disorder with manifestations in different organ systems including the ocular, cardiovascular and skeletal system. The diagnosis of MFS is based on the identification of clinical manifestations, as defined in the revised Ghent nosology [22]. Aortic root dilatation and lens luxation play a

Table 20.1 Diagnostic criteria for Marfan syndrome

In the absence of family history: MFS if
1. AoRD (Z ≥ 2) + EL
2. AoRD (Z ≥ 2) + *FBN1*
3. AoRD (Z ≥ 2) + Syst (≥7 pts)
4. EL + *FBN1* with known Aortic involvement
In the presence of family history (FH): MFS if
1. EL + FH of MFS (as defined above) = MFS
2. Syst (≥7 pts) + FH of MFS (as defined above) = MFS
3. Ao (Z ≥ 2 in adults, Z ≥ 3 in children) + FH of MFS (as defined above) = MFS

Adopted from [22]

cardinal role. A systemic score to assess additional features in various organ systems has been provided as an addition to the diagnostic clues and more importance has been assigned to the identification of an underlying FBN1 mutation (Table 20.1).

Cardiovascular manifestations in MFS are the major determinants of life expectancy in affected patients. Aortic root aneurysm ensuing a risk for fatal type A aortic dissection is the most threatening manifestation and definitely was the most important reason for early demise in MFS patients before the era of structured cardiovascular management in these patients including prophylactic aortic root surgery, medical treatment, life style advice and regular imaging [23, 24]. With better treatment options for aortic root aneurysms, the spectrum of cardiovascular disease in MFS has widened and now also includes heart failure, arrhythmias and distal aortic disease.

20.4.1.2 Aortic Aneurysms and Dissections in Marfan Syndrome

One out four Marfan patients will be diagnosed only after presenting with an aortic aneurysm or—dissection, emphasizing the crucial role of cardiology/cardiovascular surgery in the diagnostic setting of many patients [25].

Children with MFS may have normal aortic root dimensions in the early stages of the disease: at the age of 5 years, only 20% has an enlarged aortic root but by the age of 10 years, this will increase to 50% and by the age of 18 >80% will have developed aortic root dilatation [26]. Aortic root growth rate in MFS patients varies between 0.3 and 0.9 mm/year [27, 28], which is definitely higher when compared to the growth rate in the general population, estimated at 1 mm/decade [29].

Knowledge of the diagnosis is the most important factor to prevent aortic events, although a recent study from the large Dutch CONCOR cohort indicated that after a follow-up period of 8.3 years, 12.8% of the patients known with MFS had developed aortic dissection [30]. Furthermore, a recently reported surgical series indicated that 36% of MFS patients requiring aortic surgery presented with dissections [31]. These data clearly indicate that there still is a dare need to better diagnose and identify MFS patients at risk for dissection.

Despite the knowledge that dissections in MFS may occur at lower diameters [32], and after numerous attempts to refine the threshold at which aortic dissections may occur, the aortic root diameter continues to be the most important parameter used in daily clinical practice. According to the ESC guidelines on aortic disease, MFS patients need to be referred for prophylactic aortic root surgery when the aortic root reaches 50 mm, unless other risk factors including rapid growth (>3 mm/year), a positive family history for dissection, severe mitral or aortic valve disease or a desire for pregnancy are present, in which case the threshold is lowered to 45 mm [10]. The American (AHA/ACC) guidelines add a threshold of an indexed aortic root area (divided by the patient's height in meters) >10 which is considered a class IIa indication for surgery in the AHA guidelines (level of evidence C) [33, 34]. As pointed out above, a significant proportion of MFS patients will develop aortic dissection even when strictly applying the guidelines.

Options for risk better stratification have been explored and include functional imaging techniques and biomarkers. Aortic stiffness parameters have been explored and showed an added value in the abdominal aorta [35]. Arterial and aortic tortuosity indices are additional imaging characteristics that seem to have a prognostic value in MFS patients (Morris, Franken). Numerous biomarkers have been explored, including markers of inflammation such as MMP's, blood TGFβ levels or extracellular matrix protein metabolism products such as elastin or fibrillin fragments [36, 37] and miRNA's [38]. None of these markers are currently ready for use in clinical practice [39].

With better outcome of surgery and improved survival of MFS patients, repeat complications and interventions, often in more distal parts of the aorta tend to occur more frequently and indicate the need for careful follow-up, including regular imaging of the distal aorta. Determinants for repeat vascular surgeries include the presence of acute or chronic dissection at the time of the first surgery, hypertension after the first surgery and a history of smoking [31, 40].

20.4.1.3 Pulmonary Artery Dilatation

The pulmonary artery root has the same embryologic origin as the aortic root and the vessel wall characteristics are very similar with higher elastin content when compared to the more distal parts of the vessels. It is therefore not surprising that pulmonary root dilatation is a common feature in MFS patients, though it's clinical consequences are much milder as can be expected in this lower pressure vascular bed. Pulmonary artery dilatation was listed as a minor criterion in the initial Ghent diagnostic criteria for MFS but is no longer listed in the revised version. A cut-off value of 23 mm with ultrasound and of 30 mm with MRI has been suggested to define dilatation [41, 42].

20.4.1.4 Mitral Valve Prolapse

Mitral valve prolapse (MVP) is a very common feature in MFS patients, occurring in 30–50% of children and in 60–80% of adults (as compared to 1–2% in the general population) [42–45]. Not only does it occur more frequently, the outcome in MFS patients is also significantly worse with increased numbers of patients requiring surgery, developing heart failure or endocarditis (28% vs 13% in idiopathic MVP). The age at which events occur is also significantly lower in MFS patients when compared to idiopathic forms of MVP (35 vs 65 years) [43, 46]. 5–12% of MFS patients require primary MV surgery and 20% of patients undergoing aortic root surgery will undergo concomitant MV surgery. The outcome of repair techniques seems more favorable on the long term than replacement and is similar to the outcome in non-MFS patients [47, 48].

In pediatric series, MVP seems related to the degree of aortic root dilatation.

Severe MVP with significant regurgitation in association with severe tricuspid valve prolapse is a characteristic feature of neonatal Marfan syndrome, a very severe form of the disease presenting in neonatal life and leading to fatal demise due to heart failure and severe AV valve dysfunction in the first year of life in most cases [49].

20.4.1.5 Tricuspid Valve Prolapse

TVP has not led to any clinically relevant problems in MFS patients so far but should be recognized as a common feature and may therefore be helpful in a diagnostic setting. The presence of TVP seems to influence the outcome of MVP.

20.4.1.6 Cardiomyopathy

Several reports as well as a recent retrospective study have indicated that heart failure and sudden arrhythmic cardiac death are important causes of death in MFS patients and thus clearly deserve more attention [50]. Significant LV dilatation and dysfunction leading to heart failure sometimes even necessitating heart transplantation has been described in a few cases and seems to be a very rare complication in MFS [51, 52]

Subclinical intrinsic myocardial dysfunction on the other hand, has been reported in larger subsets of MFS patients of various ages by several independent research groups [53–59] and mildly increased LV dimensions have been demonstrated in a subset of patients with MFS [60]. The clinical evolution of MFS related CMP appears to be mild as we have recently demonstrated (campens).

Initially, valvular dysfunction and aortic stiffness in MFS were considered as the main factors underlying LV dysfunction. The current view is that the observed cardiac phenotype is caused by dysfunctional microfibrils [61]. This hypothesis is supported by the observation that microfibrils contribute to the mechanical stability and elasticity of several tissues. Additional evidence for intrinsic myocardial dysfunction was provided by recent insights obtained in mice with cardiomyocyte-specific Fbn1 hypomorphism ($Fbn1^{\alpha MHC-/-}$ mouse model), which demonstrates myocardial dysfunction in the absence of aortic disease [62]. These findings have led to the hypothesis that mutations in fibrillin-1 may underlie ventricular dysfunction by interfering with the structural properties of the myocardial tissue and/or with the process of mechanosignaling and mechanotransduction. Preliminary studies in different MFS mouse models support these hypotheses. Several mechanisms including alterations in integrin function and their interaction with AT1R have been studied and need further confirmation in humans.

20.4.1.7 Arrhythmias

A feature that is closely related to ventricular dysfunction in MFS is an increased risk for adverse arrhythmogenic events [63–65]. Ventricular arrhythmias have been documented in pediatric as well as in adult series. An association with increased NT-ProBNP levels, age, increased left ventricular size, ventricular ectopia and mitral valve prolapse has been evidenced [63–65]. The risk for sudden arrhythmic cardiac death in MFS appeared to be increased by 7 fold when compared to the risk in the general population in a recent study [65]. Specific Holter ECG based tools such as Heart Rate Turbulence and Deceleration Capacity have been proposed as predictive factors and deserve further exploration in larger studies [66].

20.4.1.8 Estimating Cardiovascular Outcome in MFS

It is beyond any doubt that aortic root aneurysm with its ensuing risk for life-threatening type A aortic dissection is the main determinant of outcome in MFS. Prior to the introduction of prophylactic aortic root surgery, a retrospective analysis indicated that MFS patients died in their 4th or 5th decade of life [67]. The introduction of the Bentall procedure, which went along with the start of the use of beta blockers in the 1970s has resulted in a 30 years increase in life expectancy [23, 24]—an achievement that has never been paralleled in cardiovascular disease.

Reported predictors of a worse outcome include

- Family History of cardiovascular events (defined as a history of aortic dissection, aortic surgery or non ischemic cardiovascular death in a first degree relative) [68]
- Smoking & Hypertension were the only determinants of the need for recurrent surgery in a large retrospective series of MFS patients [40]—this was not confirmed however in a more recent study [31]
- Male gender was associated with an increased aortic growth rate [27] and increased incidence of aortic surgery at baseline (38.0% vs. 19.4%) and during follow-up (24.0% vs. 15.1%), in the Dutch Concor registry [30] but was not associated with a risk for recurrent interventions in the surgical series[31, 40]
- Genotype: numerous studies addressing genotype/phenotype correlations in MFS have been performed but so far, very few have been reproducible. The only solid correlation is between mutations in the middle portion of the gene (exons 24–32) and neonatal Marfan syndrome, a specific entity at the severe end of the disease spectrum [69]. A potentially interesting finding related to cardiovascular disease is that nonsense or splicing mutations occurred more frequently in patients with an aortic event in a large cohort (N = 179) [70]. A similar observation was made in the Dutch Concor study where patients harboring a mutation predicting to lead to happloinsufficiency were at increased risk for cardiovascular death and aortic dissection when compared to patients with mutations leading to a dominant negative effect [30].
- Whether pregnancy as such is a trigger for aortic dissection in MFS is not fully elucidated yet—interpretation of reports on the association are often case reports or retrospective series, with an inherent ascertainment bias. Both hemodynamic and hormonal factors associated with pregnancy may have an adverse effect on the already fragile aorta in MFS patients. Many—if not most of the reported dissections have occurred in women unaware of the diagnosis or not receiving proper counselling or follow-up. In addition to its immediate effects, pregnancy

also influences long term outcome with an increased growth rate in Marfan women with an aortic root diameter above 40 mm (0.36 mm/year vs 0.14 mm/year in the childless Marfan women) [71] and increased rates of elective aortic surgery an aortic dissection in pregnant versus non-pregnant women [72].

20.4.1.9 Management of Cardiovascular Manifestations in MFS Patients

The mainstay of cardiovascular management in MFS constitutes of the avoidance of aortic dissection. This involves life-style adjustment including avoidance of strenuous exercise, blood pressure control and refraining from smoking and use of cocaine and amphetamines.

As already mentioned above, timely prophylactic aortic root surgery is life-saving in MFS. The operative mortality in emergency procedures is significantly higher when compared to elective procedures (1.5 vs 11.7%) [73]. Thresholds have been discussed above. The current preferred surgical techniques in MFS are the so-called valve sparing procedures as these do not require subsequent lifelong treatment with anticoagulants as does the classic Bentall procedure. Long-term outcome is good as has been evidenced in several large series. Surgery in the distal aorta in Marfan syndrome and other HCTD is more challenging. Endovascular procedures are conventionally not recommended, although recent reports show that carefully prepared hybrid procedures may be offered in selected cases [74]. In Marfan patients with aortic dissection, the use of endovascular stenting should only be considered in life-threatening emergencies, as a bridge to definite open procedures, since these aortas dilate progressively, resulting in high endoleak rates, a 12% mortality rate and a 14–18% need of a new surgical procedure [75, 76].

Medical treatment to slow down aortic root growth has been used since the seventies, when beta-blockers were introduced. The effect of these drugs is thought to be through lowering of wall shear stress (dp/dt). The only randomized study in MFS patient, published in 1994 showed a beneficial effect, although the study was underpowered to assess hard endpoints [77]. Promising perspectives for medical treatment arose with the identification of involvement of the TGFβ pathway in the pathophysiology of MFS. It was postulated that TGFβ inhibition with losartan (an angiotensin receptor blocker) would be beneficial in MFS, as was indicated by a study in a mouse model [78]. Several large-scale trials in humans have unfortunately not been able to recapitulate these findings in humans and currently; losartan is considered as a valid alternative in those patients intolerant for beta-blockers [79–83].

Women with MFS contemplating pregnancy require proper pre-pregnancy counselling covering both the genetic and cardiovascular aspects related to the disease. Women with an aortic root diameter above 45 mm are strongly discouraged to become pregnant without pre-emptive surgical repair. An aortic root diameter below 40 mm is generally considered as low-risk, although a completely safe diameter does not exist. In women with an aortic root diameter between 40 and 45 mm, recent aortic growth rate and a family history of aortic events are important factors to take into account in the counselling. Women with previous aortic root surgery remain at increased risk for complications including worsening aortic valve regurgitation or type B aortic dissection [84, 85].

20.4.2 Loeys-Dietz Syndrome

In 2005 a clinically distinct entity associated with aggressive aortic disease and caused by mutations in the TGFBR1 and two genes was described. The disease is characterized by aortic root aneurysms with a propensity to dissect at low diameters, involvement of the distal aorta and branching arteries and marked arterial tortuosity. Dysmorphic features including hypertelorism and cleft palate/bifid uvula are also encountered in these patients and the disease has been named after the senior authors initially describing the disease, Loeys and Dietz [86, 87]. Since the initial publication, mutations in other genes have been identified in patients displaying very similar phenotypic features, leading to the suggestion of different types of LDS, according to the underlying gene defect. LDS type 3 in this classification is caused by mutations in the Smad3 gene. As many patients with Smad3 mutations also exhibit osteoarthritis, this disease entity is also known as Aneurysm Ostearthritis syndrome [88, 89]. Visceral and iliac arteries appear to be more frequently involved in patients with SMAD3 mutations with more than half of the reported aneurysms being encountered in the abdomen in one study [90, 91]. Other genes in the TGFβ pathway that give rise to LDS like phenotypes include the TGFB2 and TGFB3 genes (see for more details Chapter 19).

The severity of the cardiovascular manifestations in patients with mutations in the TGFβ related genes is highly variable and subsets of patients have been reported with outcomes comparable to those observed in MFS cohorts [92, 93]. Patients with very little syndromic features have been reported by several groups and may be better categorized in the nonsyndromic H-TAD category (see below). A link between the severity of craniofacial abnormalities and the extent of cardiovascular manifestations has been suggested [87].

The extent- and aggressive course of vascular involvement in LDS patients justifies more extended vascular imaging (preferably with MRI) at regular intervals, at least in the early stages of the diagnosis until a stable status has been evidenced.

Mitral valve prolapse occurs less frequently in LDS when compared to MFS (20–30%) but can be seen in all types and even appeared to be a discriminating factor in patients harboring mutations in the TGFB2 gene [94]. Structural congenital heart defects are more prevalent in LDS than in the general population and include atrial septal defect (ASD), patent ductus arteriosus (PDA), and bicuspid aortic valve (BAV). In patients with Smad3 mutations, atrial fibrillation (24%) and left ventricular hypertrophy (18%) have been reported [95]. Impaired left ventricular systolic function has been reported in LDS type 1 [96]

No evidence in support of drug treatment in LDS patients has been published so far and management is largely extrapolated from the knowledge obtained in MFS.

Surgical outcome is good, at least for those procedures performed in planned elective circumstances [97]. A surgical series looking at the outcome in LDS patients who had been managed primarily as having Marfan syndrome showed similar risks for re-intervention in both groups [98]. The threshold at which to refer LDS patients for prophylactic surgery may be lowered to 45 mm [99] (Jondeau Circulation CV Genetics in press)

20.4.3 Vascular Ehlers Danlos Syndrome

Vascular Ehlers Danlos Syndrome (vEDS, formerly known is EDS type IV) is caused by mutations in the COL3A1 gene, encoding collagen type 3. Clinical features in vEDS patients are marked by pronounced and generalized tissue fragility. Vessels (both arterial and venous) are extremely friable and prone to dissection or rupture, often without preceding dilatation, rendering management particularly challenging. The gastro-intestinal tract and uterus are other organs at risk for rupture [100, 101].

Patients with vEDS suffer major clinical events at a young age with a documented mean age at a first event of 29 years in a recent comprehensive cohort of patients from France with confirmed COL3A1 mutations [102]. First major events in this cohort were predominantly arterial dissection/rupture (63%), followed by digestive complications (26%). Arterial complications were predominantly local dissections and aneurysms at the iliac, renal and carotid arteries—80% presented complications at multiple locations. These data are comparable to those from large series from the US [103, 104] (Pepin). The US series indicated an increased risk for events in males, which was not confirmed in the French cohort. In many vEDS patients, the diagnosis is often only made after the occurrence of a catastrophic vascular complication or at postmortem examination. As is the case for most of the connective tissue disorders reported in this chapter, mortality rates and fatal outcome of emergency procedures occur more frequently in patients who are unaware of the diagnosis. Multiple locations (synchronous) or recurring ruptures or dissections in different anatomical regions in medium sized arteries in individuals under the age 40 should raise this diagnostic consideration. The proximal and distal branches of the aortic arch, the descending thoracic aorta and abdominal aorta are often affected, as well as vertebral and carotid arteries. In a recent literature review, Berqvist et al. reported arterial rupture without underlying aneurysm in 33% of patients with a serious hemorrhagic complication [105]. Aneurysm and arterial-venous fistula in the cavernous portion of the carotid (often referred to as a carotid-cavernous sinus fistula, CCSF) is a rare condition with a higher than expected prevalence in people with vEDS.

Mitral valve prolapse has been reported in several older case reports of vEDS [106, 107] but subsequent larger studies could not confirm this finding [108] indicating that mitral valve prolapse is probably an aspecific finding in vEDS.

The unpredictability of the events renders management of patients with vascular Ehlers-Danlos syndrome particularly challenging. Blood pressure control and avoidance of activities involving strenuous exercise is essential. Because of significant risks of arterial pathology and fragility, any sudden onset of unusual pain needs prompt and meticulous investigation, by both clinical examination and appropriate non-invasive imaging.

In general, the management of a vascular dissection or rupture should be conservative, whenever possible. Special surgical preventive measures need to be taken into account and surgery is more likely to be successful if the surgeon is well-informed about the condition [109]. More recently developed techniques for endovascular repair have been used successfully in the right hands in small series [110]. The outcome of surgical management in such highly specialized centers is better than the average natural evolution but remains associated with high morbidity as demonstrated by complication in 46% in a series of 31 patients from the Mayo clinic and in 33% in 9 patients from the Johns Hopkins hospital [109, 110].

The pros and cons of serial vascular imaging, are elusive, but are probably at least potentially beneficial. One should balance the risk of causing anxiety against the potential benefits of detecting previously unknown aneurysms or progressive dilatations that are potentially treatable and potentially life-saving [109]. So far, the reduction of mortality or morbidity by serial imaging capable of predicting potential early signs of arterial wall weakness has not been systematically explored in vEDS.

The only drug with a proven beneficial effect in vEDS is the selective B1 receptor blocker with B2 mimetic properties, celiprolol. A multicenter randomized open label controlled trial with celiprolol in 53 patients was ended prematurely due to treatment benefit with a 36% reduction in vascular events in the treated group as compared to the untreated group [111]. It needs to be acknowledged though that the occurrence rate of vascular events remained high at 20% in the treated patient group.

20.4.4 Other Syndromic Heritable Connective Tissue Disorders

20.4.4.1 Multisystemic Smooth Muscle Cell Dysfunction Syndrome

The de novo R179H mutation in the ACTA2 gene causes a specific syndrome caused by generalized smooth muscle cell dysfunction [112]. Abnormal α-actin filaments lead to alterations in cellular contractile function. Clinical manifestations include hemodynamically significant patent ductus arteriosus necessitating intervention in neonatal life and early onset thoracic aortic aneurysms often requiring surgery in childhood. Additional cardiovascular features include dilatation of the pulmonary arteries, the aortic arch, suprarenal abdominal aorta and head and neck vessels. Aortic coarctation and aortopulmonary window have also been reported [113].

All patients also show cerebrovascular abnormalities on imaging studies with fusiform dilatation of the internal carotids and stenoses at the more terminal portions of these same vessels, reminiscent but not entirely similar to what is seen in Moya Moya disease [114, 115]. Other organ system manifestations include bilateral periventricular white matter hyperintensities suggesting concurrent angiographically occult small vessel disease [114], congenital mydriasis or fixed dilated pupils hypotonic bladder and malrotation, and hyperperistalsis of the gasto intestinal tract.

Pulmonary manifestations include asthma, cystic lung disease in infancy and primary pulmonary hypertension necessitating bilateral lung transplantation at the age 18 months in one case [112, 116, 117]. Other ACTA2 mutations lead to milder forms of nonsyndromic H-TAD (see below).

20.4.4.2 Shprintzen Goldberg Syndrome

Shprintzen Goldberg syndrome is a rare craniosynostosis syndrome characterized by dysmorphic features including a marfanoid habitus, exopthalmos, hypertelorism, downslanting palpebral fissures and developmental delay. Cardiovascular manifestations include aortic root dilatation/aneurysm and mitral valve prolapse. So far, no aortic dissection has been reported. The underlying gene defect has been identified as heterozygous mutations in exon 1 of the *SKI* gene [118, 119].

20.4.4.3 Arterial Tortuosity Syndrome

The hallmark of Arterial Tortuosity Syndrome (ATS) is marked tortuosity of the aorta and branching vessels. Arterial stenosis and aneurysms in the pulmonary and systemic vascular beds also occur frequently [120].

This autosomal recessive disorder is caused by mutations in a glucose transporter gene (*GLUT10*) [121].

20.4.4.4 Congenital Contractural Arachnodactylia

Congenital contractural arachnodactyly is a condition primarily affecting the skeleton with contractures of digits, elbows, and knees evident at birth, elongated long bones and kyphoscoliosis. In addition, the pinna of the ear is typically crumpled. Mitral valve prolapse and aortic root dilatation have been reported, with unknown frequency and generally in a milder degree than in MFS. Mutations in the *FBN2* gene account for about half of cases [122, 123].

20.4.5 Nonsyndromic Heritable Thoracic Aortic Disorders

Nonsyndromic H-TAD (NS H-TAD) is diagnosed in the presence of familial dilatation and/or dissection of the thoracic aorta, in the absence of MFS, LDS, vEDS or other syndromic features, and in the absence of other predisposing factors for aortic disease such as smoking or hypertension. NS H-TAD is inherited as an autosomal dominant trait with decreased penetrance and variable expression [124].

Even with the use of advanced next generation sequencing techniques, mutations in NS-HTAD patients are identified in less than 20% of cases [125, 126]. Multiple genes are involved and, as can be appreciated from Table 20.2, mutations in nearly all genes reported in the setting of syndromic H-TAD entities may give rise to NS H-TAD.

Currently known causal genes that have been identified so far in H-TAD can be grouped into those affecting structure (i.e. genes encoding extracellular matrix

(ECM) components (*FBN1, COL3A1, MFAP5, ELN, FBLN4*)) and those that affect the ability to modify structure in response to changes in mechanical load imposed on the aortic wall. The latter group can be divided into genes encoding various proteins involved in TGFβ signaling (*TGFBR1, TGFBR2, TGFB2, TGFB3, SMAD3*) and genes encoding proteins involved in vascular smooth muscle cell contractility (*ACTA2, MYH11*, MYLK, *PRKG1, FLNA*).

By definition, affected individuals with H-TAD present progressive aortic dilatation of the sinuses of Valsalva and/or ascending aorta and/or ascending aortic dissection. In the majority of cases, enlargement of the aorta precedes dissection [127]. In NS H-TAD, the onset and rate of progression of aortic dilatation is highly variable, with some individuals developing dilatation in childhood while others reach high age without aneurysms. A higher growth rate was observed in one study comparing familial to sporadic cases of TAD [128]. Individuals with familial H-TAD have a younger mean age at presentation than individuals with non-familial thoracic aortic aneurysms, but are older than individuals with Marfan syndrome [129]). Aortic dissection in childhood is rare.

An overview of main cardiovascular features of the syndromes described above and of NS H-TAD is provided in Table 20.2.

In 2007, 14 mutations in the ACTA2 gene were identified in 97 TAAD families, indicating this gene as a common underlying factor in TAD [130]. A recent study describing aortic features in a large series of patients with *ACTA2* mutations indicated that aortic events occurred in 48% of individuals, with the vast majority presenting with thoracic aortic dissections (88%) associated with 25% mortality. Type A dissections were more common than type B dissections (54% versus 21%), but the median age of onset of type B dissections was significantly younger than type A dissections (27 years versus 36 years). In this extensive series, the lifetime risk for an aortic event was 76%, suggesting that additional environmental or genetic factors play a role in the expression of aortic disease in individuals with *ACTA2* mutations [131]. Mitral valve prolapse in *ACTA2* mutation patients is reported in only 3% of cases which is in contrast to Marfan syndrome and Loeys Dietz syndrome and approaches the prevalence in the general population. Patients harbouring specific *ACTA2* mutations also show an increased risk for early onset stroke or coronary artery disease [131]

Patients with *MFAP5* mutations present with aortic root dilatation, mostly occurring at middle-age and associated with various and very mild syndromic features in some individuals (pectus deformities, mitral valve prolapse). Interestingly several patients also presented lone atrial fibrillation [132].

63% of the 31 patients reported with mutations in the *PRKG1* gene presented with aortic dissection, commonly at a young age (mean 31 years) [133] Patients with *MAT2A* mutations have a predisposition for thoracic aortic aneurysms/dissections. Bicuspid aortic valves are seen more frequently [134].

The majority of patients with a mutation in the *MYH11* gene also present a patent ductus arteriosus [135–138]. Aortic stiffness in mutation carriers is increased even in those without significant aortic dilatation [138].

Table 20.2 Overview of the main syndromic and nonsyndromic connective tissue disorders associated with cardiovascular disease and their main features

Disorder	Gene(s)	Main cardiovascular features
Syndromic heritable connective tissue disorders		
Marfan	*FBN1* [21], *TGFBR1&2* [125, 139], *SMAD3* [125], *TGFB2* [140]	Sinus of valsalva aneurysm, aortic dissection, mitral valve prolapse, main pulmonary artery dilatation, left ventricular dysfunction
Loeys-Dietz	*TGFBR1&2* [86, 87], *SMAD3*, *TGFB2* [141], *TGFB3* [99]	Sinus of valsalva aneurysm, aortic dissection, arterial aneurysms and dissections, arterial tortuosity, patent ductus arteriosus, atrial septal defect, bicuspid aortic valve
Vascular Ehlers-Danlos	*COL3A1*	Arterial rupture and dissection without preceding dilatation/aneurysm
Multisystemic smooth muscle dysfunction syndrome	*ACTA2* [112]	Ascending aortic aneurysm, aortic dissection, patent ductus arteriosus, aortic coarctation, aortopulmonary window, pulmonary arterial hypertension
Shprintzen-Goldberg syndrome	*SKI* [118, 119]	Mild aortic root dilatation, mitral valve prolapse
Arterial Tortuosity syndrome	*SLC2A10* [121]	Arterial tortuosity, arterial stenoses and aneurysms, mild aortic root dilatation
Congenital contractual arachnodactylia	*FBN2*	Mild aortic root dilatation
Nonsyndromic heritable thoracic aortic disorders	*ACTA2 (10–21%)*	Thoracic aortic aneurysm/dissection, cerebrovascular disease, coronary artery disease
	TGFBR1/2 (3–5%)	Thoracic aortic aneurysm/dissection
	FBN1 (3%)	Sinus valsalva aneurysms
	MYLK	Thoracic aortic aneurysm/dissections often at low aortic diameters
	SMAD3 (2%)	Intracranial and other arterial aneurysms
	TGFβ2	Mitral valve prolapse
	MYH11	Patent ductus arteriosus
	PRKG1	Aortic dissection at young age
	MAT2A	Bicuspid aortic valve
	MFAP5	Lone atrial fibrillation

References

1. Engel J, Chiquet M. An overview of extracellular matrix strcture and function. In: Mecham R, editor. The extracellular matrix: an overview. Biology of extracellular matrix. Berlin: Springer; 2011.
2. Devereux RB, de Simone G, Arnett DK, Best LG, Boerwinkle E, Howard BV, Kitzman D, Lee ET, Mosley TH, Weder A, Roman MJ. Normal limits in relation to age, body size and gender of two-dimensional echocardiographic aortic root dimensions in persons ≥15 years of age. Am J Cardiol. 2012;110:1189–94. https://doi.org/10.1016/j.amjcard.2012.05.063.

3. Lopez L, Colan SD, Frommelt PC, Ensing GJ, Kendall K, Younoszai AK, Lai WW, Geva T. Recommendations for quantification methods during the performance of a pediatric echocardiogram: a report from the Pediatric Measurements Writing Group of the American Society of Echocardiography Pediatric and Congenital Heart Disease Council. J Am Soc Echocardiogr. 2010;23:465–495. quiz 576–7. https://doi.org/10.1016/j.echo.2010.03.019.
4. Lang RM, Badano LP, Mor-Avi V, Afilalo J, Armstrong A, Ernande L, Flachskampf FA, Foster E, Goldstein SA, Kuznetsova T, Lancellotti P, Muraru D, Picard MH, Rietzschel ER, Rudski L, Spencer KT, Tsang W, Voigt J-U. Recommendations for cardiac chamber quantification by echocardiography in adults: an update from the American Society of Echocardiography and the European Association of Cardiovascular Imaging. J Am Soc Echocardiogr. 2015;28:1–39. e14. https://doi.org/10.1016/j.echo.2014.10.003.
5. Bossone E, Yuriditsky E, Desale S, Ferrara F, Vriz O, Asch FM. Normal values and differences in ascending aortic diameter in a healthy population of adults as Measured by the Pediatric versus Adult American Society of Echocardiography Guidelines. J Am Soc Echocardiogr. 2015. https://doi.org/10.1016/j.echo.2015.09.010.
6. Gautier M, Detaint D, Fermanian C, Aegerter P, Delorme G, Arnoult F, Milleron O, Raoux F, Stheneur C, Boileau C, Vahanian A, Jondeau G. Nomograms for aortic root diameters in children using two-dimensional echocardiography. Am J Cardiol. 2010;105:888–94. https://doi.org/10.1016/j.amjcard.2009.11.040.
7. Roman MJ, Devereux RB, Kramer-Fox R, O'Loughlin J. Two-dimensional echocardiographic aortic root dimensions in normal children and adults. AJC. 1989;64:507–12.
8. van Kimmenade RRJ, Kempers M, de Boer M-J, Loeys BL, Timmermans J. A clinical appraisal of different Z-score equations for aortic root assessment in the diagnostic evaluation of Marfan syndrome. Genet Med. 2013. https://doi.org/10.1038/gim.2012.172.
9. Elefteriades JA, Farkas EA. Thoracic aortic aneurysm clinically pertinent controversies and uncertainties. J Am College Cardiol. 2010;55:841–57. https://doi.org/10.1016/j.jacc.2009.08.084.
10. Erbel R, Aboyans V, Boileau C, Bossone E, Bartolomeo RD, Eggebrecht H, Evangelista A, Falk V, Frank H, Gaemperli O, Grabenwöger M, Haverich A, Iung B, Manolis AJ, Meijboom F, Nienaber CA, Roffi M, Rousseau H, Sechtem U, Sirnes PA, RSV A, CJM V, ESC Committee for Practice Guidelines. 2014 ESC Guidelines on the diagnosis and treatment of aortic diseases: document covering acute and chronic aortic diseases of the thoracic and abdominal aorta of the adult. The Task Force for the Diagnosis and Treatment of Aortic Diseases of the European Society of Cardiology (ESC). Eur Heart J. 2014;35:2873–926. https://doi.org/10.1093/eurheartj/ehu281.
11. Tsai TT, Evangelista A, Nienaber CA, Trimarchi S, Sechtem U, Fattori R, Myrmel T, Pape L, Cooper JV, Smith DE, Fang J, Isselbacher E, Eagle KA, International Registry of Acute Aortic Dissection (IRAD). Long-term survival in patients presenting with type A acute aortic dissection: insights from the International Registry of Acute Aortic Dissection (IRAD). Circulation. 2006;114:I350–6. https://doi.org/10.1161/CIRCULATIONAHA.105.000497.
12. Tsai TT, Fattori R, Trimarchi S, Isselbacher E, Myrmel T, Evangelista A, Hutchison S, Sechtem U, Cooper JV, Smith DE, Pape L, Froehlich J, Raghupathy A, Januzzi JL, Eagle KA, Nienaber CA, International Registry of Acute Aortic Dissection. Long-term survival in patients presenting with type B acute aortic dissection: insights from the International Registry of Acute Aortic Dissection. Circulation. 2006;114:2226–31. https://doi.org/10.1161/CIRCULATIONAHA.106.622340.
13. Mehta RH, Suzuki T, Hagan PG, Bossone E, Gilon D, Llovet A, Maroto LC, Cooper JV, Smith DE, Armstrong WF, Nienaber CA, Eagle KA, International Registry of Acute Aortic Dissection (IRAD) Investigators. Predicting death in patients with acute type a aortic dissection. Circulation. 2002;105:200–6.
14. Humphrey JD, Milewicz DM, Tellides G, Schwartz MA. Cell biology. Dysfunctional mechanosensing in aneurysms. Science. 2014;344:477–9. https://doi.org/10.1126/science.1253026.

15. Humphrey JD, Schwartz MA, Tellides G, Milewicz DM. Role of mechanotransduction in vascular biology: focus on thoracic aortic aneurysms and dissections. Circ Res. 2015;116:1448–61. https://doi.org/10.1161/CIRCRESAHA.114.304936.
16. Morris SA, Orbach DB, GEVA T, Singh MN, Gauvreau K, Lacro RV. Increased vertebral artery tortuosity index is associated with adverse outcomes in children and young adults with connective tissue disorders. Circulation. 2011;124:388–96. https://doi.org/10.1161/CIRCULATIONAHA.110.990549.
17. Franken R, Morabit el A, de Waard V, Timmermans J, Scholte AJ, van den Berg MP, Marquering H, Planken NRN, Zwinderman AH, Mulder BJM, Groenink M. Increased aortic tortuosity indicates a more severe aortic phenotype in adults with Marfan syndrome. Int J Cardiol. 2015;194:7–12. https://doi.org/10.1016/j.ijcard.2015.05.072.
18. Hayek E, Gring CN, Griffin BP. Mitral valve prolapse. Lancet. 2005;365:507–18. https://doi.org/10.1016/S0140-6736(05)17869-6.
19. Freed LA, Levy D, Levine RA, Larson MG, Evans JC, Fuller DL, Lehman B, Benjamin EJ. Prevalence and clinical outcome of mitral-valve prolapse. N Engl J Med. 1999;341:1–7. https://doi.org/10.1056/NEJM199907013410101.
20. Judge DP, Dietz HC. Marfan's syndrome. Lancet. 2005;366:1965–76. https://doi.org/10.1016/S0140-6736(05)67789-6.
21. Dietz HC, Cutting GR, Pyeritz RE, Maslen CL, Sakai LY, Corson GM, Puffenberger EG, Hamosh A, Nanthakumar EJ, Curristin SM. Marfan syndrome caused by a recurrent de novo missense mutation in the fibrillin gene. Nature. 1991;352:337–9. https://doi.org/10.1038/352337a0.
22. Loeys BL, Dietz HC, Braverman AC, Callewaert BL, De Backer J, Devereux RB, Hilhorst-Hofstee Y, Jondeau G, Faivre L, Milewicz DM, Pyeritz RE, Sponseller PD, Wordsworth P, de Paepe AM. The revised Ghent nosology for the Marfan syndrome. J Med Genet. 2010;47:476–85. https://doi.org/10.1136/jmg.2009.072785.
23. Silverman DI, Burton KJ, Gray J, Bosner MS, Kouchoukos NT, Roman MJ, Boxer M, Devereux RB, Tsipouras P. Life expectancy in the Marfan syndrome. AJC. 1995;75:157–60.
24. Pyeritz RE. Marfan syndrome: 30 years of research equals 30 years of additional life expectancy. Heart. 2008;95:173–5. https://doi.org/10.1136/hrt.2008.160515.
25. Sheikhzadeh S, Kusch ML, Rybczynski M, Kade C, Keyser B, Bernhardt AM, Hillebrand M, Mir TS, Fuisting B, Robinson PN, Berger J, Lorenzen V, Schmidtke J, Blankenberg S, Kodolitsch v Y. A simple clinical model to estimate the probability of Marfan syndrome. QJM. 2012;105:527–35. https://doi.org/10.1093/qjmed/hcs008.
26. Mueller GC, Stark V, Steiner K, Kodolitsch v Y, Rybczynski M, Weil J, Mir TS. Impact of age and gender on cardiac pathology in children and adolescents with Marfan syndrome. Pediatr Cardiol. 2012;34:991–8. https://doi.org/10.1007/s00246-012-0593-0.
27. Meijboom LJ, Timmermans J, Zwinderman AH, Engelfriet PM, Mulder BJM. Aortic root growth in men and women with the Marfan's syndrome. AJC. 2005;96:1441–4. https://doi.org/10.1016/j.amjcard.2005.06.094.
28. Roman MJ, Rosen SE, Kramer-Fox R, Devereux RB. Prognostic significance of the pattern of aortic root dilation in the Marfan syndrome. JAC. 1993;22:1470–6.
29. Campens L, Demulier L, De Groote K, Vandekerckhove K, De Wolf D, Roman MJ, Devereux RB, de Paepe A, De Backer J. Reference values for echocardiographic assessment of the diameter of the aortic root and ascending aorta spanning all age categories. Am J Cardiol. 2014;114:914–20. https://doi.org/10.1016/j.amjcard.2014.06.024.
30. Franken R, Groenink M, de Waard V, Feenstra HMA, Scholte AJ, van den Berg MP, Pals G, Zwinderman AH, Timmermans J, Mulder BJM. Genotype impacts survival in Marfan syndrome. Eur Heart J. 2016. https://doi.org/10.1093/eurheartj/ehv739.
31. Schoenhoff FS, Jungi S, Czerny M, Roost E, Reineke D, Mátyás G, Steinmann B, Schmidli J, Kadner A, Carrel T. Acute aortic dissection determines the fate of initially untreated aortic segments in Marfan syndrome. Circulation. 2013;127:1569–75. https://doi.org/10.1161/CIRCULATIONAHA.113.001457.

32. Pape LA, Tsai TT, Isselbacher EM, Oh JK, O'gara PT, Evangelista A, Fattori R, Meinhardt G, Trimarchi S, Bossone E, Suzuki T, Cooper JV, Froehlich JB, Nienaber CA, Eagle KA, on behalf of the International Registry of Acute Aortic Dissection (IRAD) Investigators. Aortic diameter >=5.5 cm is not a good predictor of type a aortic dissection: observations from the international registry of acute aortic dissection (IRAD). Circulation. 2007;116:1120–7. https://doi.org/10.1161/CIRCULATIONAHA.107.702720.
33. Svensson LG, Khitin L. Aortic cross-sectional area/height ratio timing of aortic surgery in asymptomatic patients with Marfan syndrome. J Thorac Cardiovasc Surg. 2002;123:360–1. https://doi.org/10.1067/mtc.2002.118497.
34. Hiratzka LF, Bakris GL, Beckman JA, Bersin RM, Carr VF, Casey DE, Eagle KA, Hermann LK, Isselbacher EM, Kazerooni EA, Kouchoukos NT, Lytle BW, Milewicz DM, Reich DL, Sen S, Shinn JA, Svensson LG, Williams DM, American College of Cardiology Foundation/American Heart Association Task Force on Practice Guidelines, American Association for Thoracic surgery, American College of Radiology, American Stroke Association, Society of Cardiovascular Anesthesiologists, Society for Cardiovascular Angiography and Interventions, Society of Interventional Radiology, Society of Thoracic Surgeons, Society for Vascular Medicine. 2010 ACCF/AHA/AATS/ACR/ASA/SCA/SCAI/SIR/STS/SVM guidelines for the diagnosis and management of patients with Thoracic Aortic Disease: a report of the American College of Cardiology Foundation/American Heart Association Task Force on Practice Guidelines, American Association for Thoracic Surgery, American College of Radiology, American Stroke Association, Society of Cardiovascular Anesthesiologists, Society for Cardiovascular Angiography and Interventions, Society of Interventional Radiology, Society of Thoracic Surgeons, and Society for Vascular Medicine. Circulation. 2010;121:e266–369. doi: https://doi.org/10.1161/CIR.0b013e3181d4739e
35. Nollen GJ, Groenink M, Tijssen JGP, Van Der Wall EE, Mulder BJM. Aortic stiffness and diameter predict progressive aortic dilatation in patients with Marfan syndrome. Eur Heart J. 2004;25:1146–52. https://doi.org/10.1016/j.ehj.2004.04.033.
36. Marshall LM, Carlson EJ, O'Malley J, Snyder CK, Charbonneau NL, Hayflick SJ, Coselli JS, Lemaire SA, Sakai LY. Thoracic aortic aneurysm frequency and dissection are associated with fibrillin-1 fragment concentrations in circulation. Circ Res. 2013;113:1159–68. https://doi.org/10.1161/CIRCRESAHA.113.301498.
37. Matt P, Schoenhoff F, Habashi J, Holm T, van Erp C, Loch D, Carlson OD, Griswold BF, Fu Q, De Backer J, Loeys B, Huso DL, NB MD, van Eyk JE, Dietz HC, GenTAC Consortium. Circulating transforming growth factor-beta in Marfan syndrome. Circulation. 2009;120:526–32. https://doi.org/10.1161/CIRCULATIONAHA.108.841981.
38. Jones JA, Stroud RE, O'Quinn EC, Black LE, Barth JL, Elefteriades JA, Bavaria JE, Gorman JH, Gorman RC, Spinale FG, Ikonomidis JS. Selective microRNA suppression in human thoracic aneurysms: relationship of miR-29a to aortic size and proteolytic induction. Circ Cardiovasc Genet. 2011;4:605–13. https://doi.org/10.1161/CIRCGENETICS.111.960419.
39. van Bogerijen GHW, Tolenaar JL, Grassi V, Lomazzi C, Segreti S, Rampoldi V, Elefteriades JA, Trimarchi S. Biomarkers in TAA-the Holy Grail. Prog Cardiovasc Dis. 2013;56:109–15. https://doi.org/10.1016/j.pcad.2013.05.004.
40. Finkbohner R, Johnston D, Crawford ES, Coselli J, Milewicz DM. Marfan syndrome. Long-term survival and complications after aortic aneurysm repair. Circulation. 1995;91:728–33.
41. Lundby R, Rand-Hendriksen S, Hald JK, Pripp AH, Smith H-J. The pulmonary artery in patients with Marfan syndrome: a cross-sectional study. Genet Med. 2012. https://doi.org/10.1038/gim.2012.82.
42. De Backer J, Loeys B, Devos D, Dietz H, de Sutter J, de Paepe A. A critical analysis of minor cardiovascular criteria in the diagnostic evaluation of patients with Marfan syndrome. Genet Med. 2006;8:401–8. https://doi.org/10.1097/01.gim.0000223550.41849.e3.
43. Pyeritz RE, Wappel MA. Mitral valve dysfunction in the Marfan syndrome. Clinical and echocardiographic study of prevalence and natural history. Am J Med. 1983;74:797–807.
44. Rybczynski M, Mir TS, Sheikhzadeh S, Bernhardt AMJ, Schad C, Treede H, Veldhoen S, Groene EF, Kühne K, Koschyk D, Robinson PN, Berger J, Reichenspurner H, Meinertz T,

von Kodolitsch Y. Frequency and age-related course of mitral valve dysfunction in the Marfan syndrome. Am J Cardiol. 2010;106:1048–53. https://doi.org/10.1016/j.amjcard.2010.05.038.
45. Lacro RV, Guey LT, Dietz HC, Pearson GD, Yetman AT, Gelb BD, Loeys BL, Benson DW, Bradley TJ, De Backer J, Forbus GA, Klein GL, Lai WW, Levine JC, Lewin MB, Markham LW, Paridon SM, Pierpont ME, Radojewski E, Selamet Tierney ES, Sharkey AM, Wechsler SB, Mahony L, Investigators PHN. Characteristics of children and young adults with Marfan syndrome and aortic root dilation in a randomized trial comparing atenolol and losartan therapy. Am Heart J. 2013;165:828–35. https://doi.org/10.1016/j.ahj.2013.02.019.
46. Rybczynski M, Treede H, Sheikhzadeh S, Groene EF, Bernhardt AMJ, Hillebrand M, Mir TS, Kühne K, Koschyk D, Robinson PN, Berger J, Reichenspurner H, Meinertz T, Kodolitsch v Y. Predictors of outcome of mitral valve prolapse in patients with the Marfan syndrome. Am J Cardiol. 2011;107:268–74. https://doi.org/10.1016/j.amjcard.2010.08.070.
47. Helder MRK, Schaff HV, Dearani JA, Li Z, Stulak JM, Suri RM, Connolly HM. Management of mitral regurgitation in Marfan syndrome: outcomes of valve repair versus replacement and comparison with myxomatous mitral valve disease. J Thorac Cardiovasc Surg. 2014;148:1020–4. https://doi.org/10.1016/j.jtcvs.2014.06.046.
48. Kunkala MR, Schaff HV, Li Z, Volguina I, Dietz HC, Lemaire SA, Coselli JS, Connolly H. Mitral valve disease in patients with marfan syndrome undergoing aortic root replacement. Circulation. 2013;128:S243–7. https://doi.org/10.1161/CIRCULATIONAHA.112.000113.
49. Buchhorn R, Kertess-Szlaninka T, Dippacher S, Hulpke-Wette M. Neonatal Marfan syndrome: improving the bad prognosis with a strict conservative treatment with carvedilol? OJTS. 2014;4:44–7. https://doi.org/10.4236/ojts.2014.42010.
50. Cameron DE, et al. Aortic Root Replacement in 372 Marfan Patients: Evolution of Operative Repair Over 30 Years. Ann Thorac Surg. 2009;87(5):1344–50
51. Knosalla C, Weng Y-G, Hammerschmidt R, Pasic M, Schmitt-Knosalla I, Grauhan O, Dandel M, Lehmkuhl HB, Hetzer R. Orthotopic heart transplantation in patients with Marfan syndrome. Ann Thorac Surg. 2007;83:1691–5. https://doi.org/10.1016/j.athoracsur.2007.01.018.
52. Audenaert T, de Pauw M, François K, de Backer J. Type B aortic dissection triggered by heart transplantation in a patient with Marfan syndrome. BMJ Case Rep. 2015. https://doi.org/10.1136/bcr-2015-211138.
53. Nollen GJ, Groenink M, Tijssen JGP, van der Wall EE, Mulder BJM. Aortic stiffness and diameter predict progressive aortic dilatation in patients with Marfan syndrome. Eur Heart J. 2004;25(13):1146–52. https://doi.org/10.1016/j.ehj.2004.04.033
54. de Backer JF, Devos D, Segers P, Matthys D, François K, Gillebert TC, de Paepe AM, de Sutter J. Primary impairment of left ventricular function in Marfan syndrome. Int J Cardiol. 2006;112:353–8. https://doi.org/10.1016/j.ijcard.2005.10.010.
55. Kiotsekoglou A, Moggridge JC, Bijnens BH, Kapetanakis V, Alpendurada F, Mullen MJ, Saha S, Nassiri DK, Camm J, Sutherland GR, Child AH. Biventricular and atrial diastolic function assessment using conventional echocardiography and tissue-Doppler imaging in adults with Marfan syndrome. Eur J Echocardiogr. 2009;10:947–55. https://doi.org/10.1093/ejechocard/jep110.
56. Kiotsekoglou A, Bajpai A, Bijnens BH, Kapetanakis V, Athanassopoulos G, Moggridge JC, Mullen MJ, Nassiri DK, Camm J, Sutherland GR, Child AH. Early impairment of left ventricular long-axis systolic function demonstrated by reduced atrioventricular plane displacement in patients with Marfan syndrome. Eur J Echocardiogr. 2008;9:605–13. https://doi.org/10.1093/ejechocard/jen003.
57. Kiotsekoglou A, Sutherland GR, Moggridge JC, Kapetanakis V, Bajpai A, Bunce N, Mullen MJ, Louridas G, Nassiri DK, Camm J, Child AH. Impaired right ventricular systolic function demonstrated by reduced atrioventricular plane displacement in adults with Marfan syndrome. Eur J Echocardiogr. 2008;10:295–302. https://doi.org/10.1093/ejechocard/jen239.
58. Rybczynski M, Koschyk DH, Aydin MA, Robinson PN, Brinken T, Franzen O, Berger J, Hofmann T, Meinertz T, Kodolitsch v Y. Tissue Doppler imaging identifies myocardial

dysfunction in adults with Marfan syndrome. Clin Cardiol. 2007;30:19–24. https://doi.org/10.1002/clc.3.
59. Alpendurada F, Wong J, Kiotsekoglou A, Banya W, Child A, Prasad SK, Pennell DJ, Mohiaddin RH. Evidence for Marfan cardiomyopathy. Eur J Heart Fail. 2010;12:1085–91. https://doi.org/10.1093/eurjhf/hfq127.
60. Meijboom LJ, Timmermans J, van Tintelen JP, Nollen GJ, De Backer J, van den Berg MP, Boers GH, Mulder BJM. Evaluation of left ventricular dimensions and function in Marfan's syndrome without significant valvular regurgitation. Am J Cardiol. 2005;95:795–7. https://doi.org/10.1016/j.amjcard.2004.11.042.
61. Campens L, Renard M, Trachet B, Segers P, Muiño Mosquera L, de Sutter J, Sakai L, de Paepe A, De Backer J. Intrinsic cardiomyopathy in Marfan syndrome: results from in-vivo and ex-vivo studies of the Fbn1(C1039G/+) model and longitudinal findings in humans. Pediatr Res. 2015;78:256–63. https://doi.org/10.1038/pr.2015.110.
62. Cook JR, Carta L, Bénard L, Chemaly ER, Chiu E, Rao SK, Hampton TG, Yurchenco P, Costa KD, Hajjar RJ, Ramirez F. Abnormal muscle mechanosignaling triggers cardiomyopathy in mice with Marfan syndrome. J Clin Invest. 2014. https://doi.org/10.1172/JCI71059DS1.
63. Chen S, Fagan LF, Nouri S, Donahoe JL. Ventricular dysrhythmias in children with Marfan's syndrome. Am J Dis Child. 1985;139:273–6.
64. Yetman AT, Bornemeier RA, McCrindle BW. Long-term outcome in patients with Marfan syndrome: is aortic dissection the only cause of sudden death? JAC. 2003;41:329–32.
65. Hoffmann BA, Rybczynski M, Rostock T, Servatius H, Drewitz I, Steven D, Aydin A, Sheikhzadeh S, Darko V, Kodolitsch v Y, Willems S. Prospective risk stratification of sudden cardiac death in Marfan's syndrome. Int J Cardiol. 2012:1–7. https://doi.org/10.1016/j.ijcard.2012.06.036.
66. Schaeffer BN, Rybczynski M, Sheikhzadeh S, Akbulak RO, Moser J, Jularic M, Schreiber D, Daubmann A, Willems S, Kodolitsch v Y, Hoffmann BA. Heart rate turbulence and deceleration capacity for risk prediction of serious arrhythmic events in Marfan syndrome. Clin Res Cardiol. 2015;104:1054–63. https://doi.org/10.1007/s00392-015-0873-9.
67. Murdoch JL, Walker BA, Halpern BL, Kuzma JW, McKusick VA. Life expectancy and causes of death in the Marfan syndrome. N Engl J Med. 1972;286:804–8. https://doi.org/10.1056/NEJM197204132861502.
68. Silverman DI, Gray J, Roman MJ, Bridges A, Burton K, Boxer M, Devereux RB, Tsipouras P. Family history of severe cardiovascular disease in Marfan syndrome is associated with increased aortic diameter and decreased survival. JAC. 1995;26:1062–7. https://doi.org/10.1016/0735-1097(95)00258-0.
69. Faivre L, Masurel-Paulet A, Collod-Beroud G, Callewaert BL, Child AH, Stheneur C, Binquet C, Gautier E, Chevallier B, Huet F, Loeys BL, Arbustini E, Mayer K, Arslan-Kirchner M, Kiotsekoglou A, Comeglio P, Grasso M, Halliday DJ, Béroud C, Bonithon-Kopp C, Claustres M, Robinson PN, Adès L, De Backer J, Coucke P, Francke U, de Paepe A, Boileau C, Jondeau G. Clinical and molecular study of 320 children with Marfan syndrome and related type I fibrillinopathies in a series of 1009 probands with pathogenic FBN1 mutations. Pediatrics. 2009;123:391–8. https://doi.org/10.1542/peds.2008-0703.
70. Baudhuin LM, Kotzer KE, Lagerstedt SA. Increased frequency of FBN1 truncating and splicing variants in Marfan syndrome patients with aortic events. Genet Med. 2015;17:177–87. https://doi.org/10.1038/gim.2014.91.
71. Meijboom LJ. Pregnancy and aortic root growth in the Marfan syndrome: a prospective study. Eur Heart J. 2005;26:914–20. https://doi.org/10.1093/eurheartj/ehi103.
72. Donnelly RT, Pinto NM, Kocolas I, Yetman AT. The immediate and long-term impactof pregnancy on aortic growth rate and mortality in women with Marfan syndrome. JAC. 2012;60:224–9. https://doi.org/10.1016/j.jacc.2012.03.051.
73. Gott VL, Greene PS, Alejo DE, Cameron DE, Naftel DC, Miller DC, Gillinov AM, Laschinger JC, Pyeritz RE. Replacement of the aortic root in patients with Marfan's syndrome. N Engl J Med. 1999;340:1307–13. https://doi.org/10.1056/NEJM199904293401702.

74. EER MD, JJI MD, AML MS, KM MD, EGSM MPH, DRJ MD, VK MD, EHB MD, JFSI MD, BWL MD, PhD LGSM. Beyond the aortic root: staged open and endovascular repair of arch and descending aorta in patients with connective tissue disorders. Ann Thorac Surg. 2016;101:906–12. https://doi.org/10.1016/j.athoracsur.2015.08.011.
75. Pacini D, Parolari A, Berretta P, Di Bartolomeo R, Alamanni F, Bavaria J. Endovascular treatment for type B dissection in Marfan syndrome: is it worthwhile? Ann Thorac Surg. 2013;95:737–49. https://doi.org/10.1016/j.athoracsur.2012.09.059.
76. Nordon IM, Hinchliffe RJ, Holt PJ, Morgan R, Jahangiri M, Loftus IM, Thompson MM. Endovascular management of chronic aortic dissection in patients with Marfan syndrome. J Vasc Surg. 2009;50:987–91. https://doi.org/10.1016/j.jvs.2009.05.056.
77. Shores J, Berger KR, Murphy EA, Pyeritz RE. Progression of aortic dilatation and the benefit of long-term beta-adrenergic blockade in Marfan's syndrome. N Engl J Med. 1994;330:1335–41. https://doi.org/10.1056/NEJM199405123301902.
78. Habashi JP, Judge DP, Holm TM, Cohn RD, Loeys BL, Cooper TK, Myers L, Klein EC, Liu G, Calvi C, Podowski M, Neptune ER, Halushka MK, Bedja D, Gabrielson K, Rifkin DB, Carta L, Ramirez F, Huso DL, Dietz HC. Losartan, an AT1 antagonist, prevents aortic aneurysm in a mouse model of Marfan syndrome. Science. 2006;312:117–21. https://doi.org/10.1126/science.1124287.
79. Lacro RV, Dietz HC, Sleeper LA, Yetman AT, Bradley TJ, Colan SD, Pearson GD, Selamet Tierney ES, Levine JC, Atz AM, Benson DW, Braverman AC, Chen S, De Backer J, Gelb BD, Grossfeld PD, Klein GL, Lai WW, Liou A, Loeys BL, Markham LW, Olson AK, Paridon SM, Pemberton VL, Pierpont ME, Pyeritz RE, Radojewski E, Roman MJ, Sharkey AM, Stylianou MP, Wechsler SB, Young LT, Mahony L, Investigators PHN. Atenolol versus losartan in children and young adults with Marfan's syndrome. N Engl J Med. 2014;371:2061–71. https://doi.org/10.1056/NEJMoa1404731.
80. Milleron O, Arnoult F, Ropers J, Aegerter P, Detaint D, Delorme G, Attias D, Tubach F, Dupuis-Girod S, Plauchu H, Barthelet M, Sassolas F, Pangaud N, Naudion S, Thomas-Chabaneix J, Dulac Y, Edouard T, Wolf J-E, Faivre L, Odent S, Basquin A, Habib G, Collignon P, Boileau C, Jondeau G. Marfan Sartan: a randomized, double-blind, placebo-controlled trial. Eur Heart J. 2015;36:2160–6. https://doi.org/10.1093/eurheartj/ehv151.
81. Groenink M, Hartog den AW, Franken R, Radonic T, de Waard V, Timmermans J, Scholte AJ, van den Berg MP, Spijkerboer AM, Marquering HA, Zwinderman AH, Mulder BJM. Losartan reduces aortic dilatation rate in adults with Marfan syndrome: a randomized controlled trial. Eur Heart J. 2013. https://doi.org/10.1093/eurheartj/eht334.
82. Forteza A, Evangelista A, Sánchez V, Teixido-Tura G, Sanz P, Gutiérrez L, Gracia T, Centeno J, Rodríguez-Palomares J, Rufilanchas JJ, Cortina J, Ferreira-Gonzalez I, García-Dorado D. Efficacy of losartan vs. atenolol for the prevention of aortic dilation in Marfan syndrome: a randomized clinical trial. Eur Heart J. 2015. https://doi.org/10.1093/eurheartj/ehv575.
83. Bowen J, Connolly H. Of Marfan's syndrome, mice, and medications. N Engl J Med. 2014. https://doi.org/10.1056/NEJMoa1404731.
84. Wanga S, Silversides C, Dore A, de Waard V, Mulder B. Pregnancy and thoracic aortic disease: managing the risks. Can J Cardiol. 2016;32:78–85. https://doi.org/10.1016/j.cjca.2015.09.003.
85. European Society of Gynecology (ESG), Association for European Paediatric Cardiology (AEPC), German Society for Gender Medicine (DGesGM), Regitz-Zagrosek V, Blomstrom Lundqvist C, Borghi C, Cifkova R, Ferreira R, Foidart J-M, JSR G, Gohlke-Baerwolf C, Gorenek B, Iung B, Kirby M, AHEM M, Morais J, Nihoyannopoulos P, Pieper PG, Presbitero P, Roos-Hesselink JW, Schaufelberger M, Seeland U, Torracca L, ESC Committee for Practice Guidelines. ESC guidelines on the management of cardiovascular diseases during pregnancy: the Task Force on the Management of Cardiovascular Diseases during Pregnancy of the European Society of Cardiology (ESC). Eur Heart J. 2011;32:3147–97. https://doi.org/10.1093/eurheartj/ehr218.
86. Loeys BL, Chen J, Neptune ER, Judge DP, Podowski M, Holm T, Meyers J, Leitch CC, Katsanis N, Sharifi N, FL X, Myers LA, Spevak PJ, Cameron DE, De Backer J, Hellemans J, Chen Y,

Davis EC, Webb CL, Kress W, Coucke P, Rifkin DB, de Paepe AM, Dietz HC. A syndrome of altered cardiovascular, craniofacial, neurocognitive and skeletal development caused by mutations in TGFBR1 or TGFBR2. Nat Genet. 2005;37:275–81. https://doi.org/10.1038/ng1511.

87. Loeys BL, Schwarze U, Holm T, Callewaert BL, Thomas GH, Pannu H, de Backer JF, Oswald GL, Symoens S, Manouvrier S, Roberts AE, Faravelli F, Greco MA, Pyeritz RE, Milewicz DM, Coucke PJ, Cameron DE, Braverman AC, Byers PH, de Paepe AM, Dietz HC. Aneurysm syndromes caused by mutations in the TGF-beta receptor. N Engl J Med. 2006;355:788–98. https://doi.org/10.1056/NEJMoa055695.
88. van de Laar IMBH, Oldenburg RA, Pals G, Roos-Hesselink JW, de Graaf BM, Verhagen JMA, Hoedemaekers YM, Willemsen R, Severijnen L-A, Venselaar H, Vriend G, Pattynama PM, Collée M, Majoor-Krakauer D, Poldermans D, Frohn-Mulder IME, Micha D, Timmermans J, Hilhorst-Hofstee Y, Bierma-Zeinstra SM, Willems PJ, Kros JM, Oei EHG, Oostra BA, Wessels MW, Bertoli-Avella AM. Mutations in SMAD3 cause a syndromic form of aortic aneurysms and dissections with early-onset osteoarthritis. Nat Genet. 2011;43:121–6. https://doi.org/10.1038/ng.744.
89. van de Laar IMBH, van der Linde D, Oei EHG, Bos PK, Bessems JH, Bierma-Zeinstra SM, van Meer BL, Pals G, Oldenburg RA, Bekkers JA, Moelker A, de Graaf BM, Mátyás G, Frohn-Mulder IME, Timmermans J, Hilhorst-Hofstee Y, Cobben JM, Bruggenwirth HT, Van Laer L, Loeys B, De Backer J, Coucke PJ, Dietz HC, Willems PJ, Oostra BA, de Paepe A, Roos-Hesselink JW, Bertoli-Avella AM, Wessels MW. Phenotypic spectrum of the SMAD3-related aneurysms-osteoarthritis syndrome. J Med Genet. 2011;49:47–57. https://doi.org/10.1136/jmedgenet-2011-100382.
90. van der Linde D, Verhagen HJM, Moelker A, van de Laar IMBH, Van Herzeele I, De Backer J, Dietz HC, Roos-Hesselink JW. Aneurysm-osteoarthritis syndrome with visceral and iliac artery aneurysms. YMVA. 2012;57:96–102. doi: https://doi.org/10.1016/j.jvs.2012.06.107
91. Martens T, Van Herzeele I, De Ryck F, Renard M, de Paepe A, François K, Vermassen F, De Backer J. Multiple aneurysms in a patient with aneurysms-osteoarthritis syndrome. Ann Thorac Surg. 2013;95:332–5. https://doi.org/10.1016/j.athoracsur.2012.05.085.
92. Attias D, Stheneur C, Roy C, Collod-Beroud G, Detaint D, Faivre L, Delrue M-A, Cohen L, Francannet C, Béroud C, Claustres M, Iserin F, Khau Van Kien P, Lacombe D, Le Merrer M, Lyonnet S, Odent S, Plauchu H, Rio M, Rossi A, Sidi D, Steg PG, Ravaud P, Boileau C, Jondeau G. Comparison of clinical presentations and outcomes between patients with TGFBR2 and FBN1 mutations in Marfan syndrome and related disorders. Circulation. 2009;120:2541–9. https://doi.org/10.1161/CIRCULATIONAHA.109.887042.
93. Teixido-Tura G, Franken R, Galuppo V, Gutiérrez García-Moreno L, Borregan M, Mulder BJM, García-Dorado D, Evangelista A. Heterogeneity of aortic disease severity in patients with Loeys-Dietz syndrome. Heart. 2016. https://doi.org/10.1136/heartjnl-2015-308535.
94. Renard M, Callewaert B, Malfait F, Campens L, Sharif S, Del Campo M, Valenzuela I, McWilliam C, Coucke P, de Paepe A, De Backer J. Thoracic aortic-aneurysm and dissection in association with significant mitral valve disease caused by mutations in TGFB2. Int J Cardiol. 2012;165:584–7. https://doi.org/10.1016/j.ijcard.2012.09.029.
95. van der Linde D, van de Laar IMBH, Bertoli-Avella AM, Oldenburg RA, Bekkers JA, Mattace-Raso FUS, van den Meiracker AH, Moelker A, van Kooten F, Frohn-Mulder IME, Timmermans J, Moltzer E, Cobben JM, Van Laer L, Loeys B, De Backer J, Coucke PJ, de Paepe A, Hilhorst-Hofstee Y, Wessels MW, Roos-Hesselink JW. Aggressive cardiovascular phenotype of aneurysms-osteoarthritis syndrome caused by pathogenic SMAD3 variants. JAC. 2012;60:397–403. https://doi.org/10.1016/j.jacc.2011.12.052.
96. Eckman PM, Hsich E, Rodriguez ER, Gonzalez-Stawinski GV, Moran R, Taylor DO. Impaired systolic function in Loeys-Dietz syndrome: a novel cardiomyopathy? Circ Heart Fail. 2009;2:707–8. https://doi.org/10.1161/CIRCHEARTFAILURE.109.888636.
97. Williams JA, Hanna JM, Shah AA, Andersen ND, McDonald MT, Jiang Y-H, Wechsler SB, Zomorodi A, McCann RL, Hughes GC. Adult surgical experience with Loeys-Dietz syndrome. Ann Thorac Surg. 2015;99:1275–81. https://doi.org/10.1016/j.athoracsur.2014.11.021.

98. Schoenhoff FS, Mueller C, Czerny M, Mátyás G, Kadner A, Schmidli J, Carrel T. Outcome of aortic surgery in patients with Loeys-Dietz syndrome primarily treated as having Marfan syndrome. Eur J Cardiothorac Surg. 2014. https://doi.org/10.1093/ejcts/ezu002.
99. MacCarrick G, Black JH, Bowdin S, El-Hamamsy I, Frischmeyer-Guerrerio PA, Guerrerio AL, Sponseller PD, Loeys B, Dietz HC. Loeys-Dietz syndrome: a primer for diagnosis and management. Genet Med. 2014. https://doi.org/10.1038/gim.2014.11.
100. Pepin MG, Murray ML, Byers PH. Vascular Ehlers-Danlos syndrome. In: Pagon RA, Adam MP, Ardinger HH, editors. Gene reviews. Seattle: University of Washington; 1999. www.ncbi.nlm.nih.gov-books-NBK1494.
101. Pagon RA, Adam MP, Ardinger HH, Bird TD, Dolan CR, Fong C-T, Smith RJ, Stephens K, Pepin MG, Byers PH. Ehlers-Danlos syndrome type IV. Seattle: University of Washington; 1993.
102. Frank M, Albuisson J, Ranque B, Golmard L, Mazzella J-M, Bal-Theoleyre L, Fauret A-L, Mirault T, Denarié N, Mousseaux E, Boutouyrie P, Fiessinger J-N, Emmerich J, Messas E, Jeunemaitre X. The type of variants at the COL3A1 gene associates with the phenotype and severity of vascular Ehlers-Danlos syndrome. Eur J Hum Genet. 2015. https://doi.org/10.1038/ejhg.2015.32.
103. Pepin MG, Schwarze U, Rice KM, Liu M, Leistritz D, Byers PH. Survival is affected by mutation type and molecular mechanism in vascular Ehlers-Danlos syndrome (EDS type IV). Genet Med. 2014;16:881–8. https://doi.org/10.1038/gim.2014.72.
104. Pepin M, Schwarze U, Superti-Furga A, Byers PH. Clinical and genetic features of Ehlers-Danlos syndrome type IV, the vascular type. N Engl J Med. 2000;342:673–80. https://doi.org/10.1056/NEJM200003093421001.
105. Bergqvist D, Björck M, Wanhainen A. Treatment of vascular Ehlers-Danlos syndrome: a systematic review. Ann Surg. 2013;258:257–61. https://doi.org/10.1097/SLA.0b013e31829c7a59.
106. Watanabe S, Ishimitsu T, Inoue K, Tomizawa T, Noguchi Y, Sugishita Y, Ito I. Type IV Ehlers-Danlos syndrome associated with mitral valve prolapse: a case report. J Cardiol Suppl. 1988;18:97–105. discussion 106
107. Jaffe AS, Geltman EM, Rodey GE, Uitto J. Mitral valve prolapse: a consistent manifestation of type IV Ehlers-Danlos syndrome. The pathogenetic role of the abnormal production of type III collagen. Circulation. 1981;64:121–5.
108. Dolan AL, Mishra MB, Chambers JB, Grahame R. Clinical and echocardiographic survey of the Ehlers-Danlos syndrome. Br J Rheumatol. 1997;36:459–62.
109. Oderich GS, Panneton JM, Bower TC, Lindor NM, Cherry KJ, Noel AA, Kalra M, Sullivan T, Gloviczki P. The spectrum, management and clinical outcome of Ehlers-Danlos syndrome type IV: a 30-year experience. YMVA. 2005;42:98–106. https://doi.org/10.1016/j.jvs.2005.03.053.
110. Brooke BS, Arnaoutakis G, McDonnell NB, Black JH. Contemporary management of vascular complications associated with Ehlers-Danlos syndrome. YMVA. 2010;51:131–9. https://doi.org/10.1016/j.jvs.2009.08.019.
111. Ong K-T, Perdu J, De Backer J, Bozec E, Collignon P, Emmerich J, Fauret A-L, Fiessinger J-N, Germain DP, Georgesco G, Hulot J-S, de Paepe A, Plauchu H, Jeunemaitre X, Laurent S, Boutouyrie P. Effect of celiprolol on prevention of cardiovascular events in vascular Ehlers-Danlos syndrome: a prospective randomised, open, blinded-endpoints trial. Lancet. 2010;376:1476–84. https://doi.org/10.1016/S0140-6736(10)60960-9.
112. Milewicz DM, Ostergaard JR, Ala-Kokko LM, Khan N, Grange DK, Mendoza-Londono R, Bradley TJ, Olney AH, Adès L, Maher JF, Guo D, Buja LM, Kim D, Hyland JC, Regalado ES. De novo ACTA2 mutation causes a novel syndrome of multisystemic smooth muscle dysfunction. Am J Med Genet A. 2010;152A:2437–43. https://doi.org/10.1002/ajmg.a.33657.
113. Yetman AT, Starr LJ, Bleyl SB, Meyers L, Delaney JW. Progressive aortic dilation associated with ACTA2 mutations presenting in infancy. Pediatrics. 2015;136:e262–6. https://doi.org/10.1542/peds.2014-3032.

114. Munot P, Saunders DE, Milewicz DM, Regalado ES, Ostergaard JR, Braun KP, Kerr T, Lichtenbelt KD, Philip S, Rittey C, Jacques TS, Cox TC, Ganesan V. A novel distinctive cerebrovascular phenotype is associated with heterozygous Arg179 ACTA2 mutations. Brain. 2012;135:2506–14. https://doi.org/10.1093/brain/aws172.
115. Khan N, Schinzel A, Shuknecht B, Baumann F, Ostergaard JR, Yonekawa Y. Moyamoya angiopathy with dolichoectatic internal carotid arteries, patent ductus arteriosus and pupillary dysfunction: a new genetic syndrome? Eur Neurol. 2004;51:72–7.
116. Meuwissen MEC, Lequin MH, Bindels-de Heus K, Bruggenwirth HT, Knapen MFCM, Dalinghaus M, de Coo R, van Bever Y, Winkelman BHJ, Mancini GMS. ACTA2 mutation with childhood cardiovascular, autonomic and brain anomalies and severe outcome. Am J Med Genet A. 2013;161A:1376–80. https://doi.org/10.1002/ajmg.a.35858.
117. Lemire BD, Buncic JR, Kennedy SJ, Dyack SJ, Teebi AS. Congenital mydriasis, patent ductus arteriosus, and congenital cystic lung disease: new syndromic spectrum? Am J Med Genet A. 2004;131:318–9. https://doi.org/10.1002/ajmg.a.30341.
118. Doyle AJ, Doyle JJ, Bessling SL, Maragh S, Lindsay ME, Schepers D, Gillis E, Mortier G, Homfray T, Sauls K, Norris RA, Huso ND, Leahy D, Mohr DW, Caulfield MJ, Scott AF, Destrée A, Hennekam RC, Arn PH, Curry CJ, Van Laer L, McCallion AS, Loeys BL, Dietz HC. Mutations in the TGF-β repressor SKI cause Shprintzen-Goldberg syndrome with aortic aneurysm. Nat Genet. 2012;44:1249–54. https://doi.org/10.1038/ng.2421.
119. Carmignac V, Thevenon J, Adès L, Callewaert B, Julia S, Thauvin-Robinet C, Gueneau L, Courcet J-B, Lopez E, Holman K, Renard M, Plauchu H, Plessis G, De Backer J, Child A, Arno G, Duplomb L, Callier P, Aral B, Vabres P, Gigot N, Arbustini E, Grasso M, Robinson PN, Goizet C, Baumann C, Di Rocco M, Del Pozo JS, Huet F, Jondeau G, Collod-Beroud G, Béroud C, Amiel J, Cormier-Daire V, Riviere J-B, Boileau C, de Paepe A, Faivre L. In-frame mutations in exon 1 of SKI cause dominant Shprintzen-Goldberg syndrome. Am J Hum Genet. 2012;91:950–7. https://doi.org/10.1016/j.ajhg.2012.10.002.
120. Wessels MW, Catsman-Berrevoets CE, Mancini GMS, Breuning MH, Hoogeboom JJM, Stroink H, Frohn-Mulder I, Coucke PJ, Paepe AD, Niermeijer MF, Willems PJ. Three new families with arterial tortuosity syndrome. Am J Med Genet A. 2004;131:134–43. https://doi.org/10.1002/ajmg.a.30272.
121. Coucke PJ, Willaert A, Wessels MW, Callewaert B, Zoppi N, De Backer J, Fox JE, Mancini GMS, Kambouris M, Gardella R, Facchetti F, Willems PJ, Forsyth R, Dietz HC, Barlati S, Colombi M, Loeys B, de Paepe A. Mutations in the facilitative glucose transporter GLUT10 alter angiogenesis and cause arterial tortuosity syndrome. Nat Genet. 2006;38:452–7. https://doi.org/10.1038/ng1764.
122. Gupta PA, Wallis DD, Chin TO, Northrup H, Tran-Fadulu VT, Towbin JA, Milewicz DM. FBN2 mutation associated with manifestations of Marfan syndrome and congenital contractural arachnodactyly. J Med Genet. 2004;41:e56.
123. Nishimura A, Sakai H, Ikegawa S, Kitoh H, Haga N, Ishikiriyama S, Nagai T, Takada F, Ohata T, Tanaka F, Kamasaki H, Saitsu H, Mizuguchi T, Matsumoto N. FBN2, FBN1, TGFBR1, and TGFBR2 analyses in congenital contractural arachnodactyly. Am J Med Genet A. 2007;143A:694–8. https://doi.org/10.1002/ajmg.a.31639.
124. Pyeritz RE. Heritable thoracic aortic disorders. Curr Opin Cardiol. 2014;29:97–102. https://doi.org/10.1097/HCO.0000000000000023.
125. Campens L, Callewaert B, Muiño Mosquera L, Renard M, Symoens S, de Paepe A, Coucke P, De Backer J. Gene panel sequencing in heritable thoracic aortic disorders and related entities – results of comprehensive testing in a cohort of 264 patients. Orphanet J Rare Dis. 2015;10:9. https://doi.org/10.1186/s13023-014-0221-6.
126. Wooderchak-Donahue W, VanSant-Webb C, Tvrdik T, Plant P, Lewis T, Stocks J, Raney JA, Meyers L, Berg A, Rope AF, Yetman AT, Bleyl SB, Mesley R, Bull DA, Collins RT, Ojeda MM, Roberts A, Lacro R, Woerner A, Stoler J, Bayrak-Toydemir P. Clinical utility of a next generation sequencing panel assay for Marfan and Marfan-like syndromes featuring aortopathy. Am J Med Genet A. 2015. https://doi.org/10.1002/ajmg.a.37085.

127. Milewicz DM, Chen H, Park ES, Petty EM, Zaghi H, Shashidhar G, Willing M, Patel V. Reduced penetrance and variable expressivity of familial thoracic aortic aneurysms/dissections. AJC. 1998;82:474–9.
128. Albornoz G, Coady M, Roberts M, Davies R, Tranquilli M, Rizzo J, Elefteriades J. Familial thoracic aortic aneurysms and dissections—incidence, modes of inheritance, and phenotypic patterns. Ann Thorac Surg. 2006;82:1400–5. https://doi.org/10.1016/j.athoracsur.2006.04.098.
129. Coady MA, Rizzo JA, Goldstein LJ, Elefteriades JA. Natural history, pathogenesis, and etiology of thoracic aortic aneurysms and dissections. Cardiol Clin. 1999;17:615–35.
130. Guo D-C, Pannu H, Tran-Fadulu V, Papke CL, Yu RK, Avidan N, Bourgeois S, Estrera AL, Safi HJ, Sparks E, Amor D, Adès L, McConnell V, Willoughby CE, Abuelo D, Willing M, Lewis RA, Kim DH, Scherer S, Tung PP, Ahn C, Buja LM, Raman CS, Shete SS, Milewicz DM. Mutations in smooth muscle α-actin (ACTA2) lead to thoracic aortic aneurysms and dissections. Nat Genet. 2007;39:1488–93. https://doi.org/10.1038/ng.2007.6.
131. Regalado ES, Guo D, Prakash S, Bensend TA, Flynn K, Estrera A, Safi H, Liang D, Hyland J, Child A, Arno G, Boileau C, Jondeau G, Braverman A, Moran R, Morisaki T, Morisaki H, Consortium MA, Pyeritz R, Coselli J, LeMaire S, Milewicz DM. Aortic disease presentation and outcome associated with ACTA2 mutations. Circ Cardiovasc Genet. 2015. https://doi.org/10.1161/CIRCGENETICS.114.000943.
132. Barbier M, Gross M-S, Aubart M, Hanna N, Kessler K, Guo D-C, Tosolini L, Ho-Tin-Noe B, Regalado E, Varret M, Abifadel M, Milleron O, Odent S, Dupuis-Girod S, Faivre L, Edouard T, Dulac Y, Busa T, Gouya L, Milewicz DM, Jondeau G, Boileau C. MFAP5 loss-of-function mutations underscore the involvement of matrix alteration in the pathogenesis of familial thoracic aortic aneurysms and dissections. Am J Hum Genet. 2014;95:736–43. https://doi.org/10.1016/j.ajhg.2014.10.018.
133. Guo D-C, Regalado E, Casteel DE, Santos-Cortez RL, Gong L, Kim JJ, Dyack S, Horne SG, Chang G, Jondeau G, Boileau C, Coselli JS, Li Z, Leal SM, Shendure J, Rieder MJ, Bamshad MJ, Nickerson DA, Kim C, Milewicz DM, GenTAC Registry Consortium, National Heart, Lung, and Blood Institute Grand Opportunity Exome Sequencing Project. Recurrent gain-of-function mutation in PRKG1 causes thoracic aortic aneurysms and acute aortic dissections. Am J Hum Genet. 2013;93:398–404. https://doi.org/10.1016/j.ajhg.2013.06.019.
134. Guo D-C, Gong L, Regalado ES, Santos-Cortez RL, Zhao R, Cai B, Veeraraghavan S, Prakash SK, Johnson RJ, Muilenburg A, Willing M, Jondeau G, Boileau C, Pannu H, Moran R, de Backer J, Bamshad MJ, Shendure J, Nickerson DA, Leal SM, Raman CS, Swindell EC, Milewicz DM, GenTAC Investigators, National Heart, Lung, and Blood Institute Go Exome Sequencing Project, Montalcino Aortic Consortium. MAT2A mutations predispose individuals to thoracic aortic aneurysms. Am J Hum Genet. 2015;96:170–7. https://doi.org/10.1016/j.ajhg.2014.11.015.
135. Zhu L, Vranckx R, van Kien PK, Lalande A, Boisset N, Mathieu F, Wegman M, Glancy L, Gasc J-M, Brunotte F, Bruneval P, Wolf J-E, Michel J-B, Jeunemaitre X. Mutations in myosin heavy chain 11 cause a syndrome associating thoracic aortic aneurysm/aortic dissection and patent ductus arteriosus. Nat Genet. 2006;38:343–9. https://doi.org/10.1038/ng1721.
136. Renard M, Callewaert B, Baetens M, Campens L, Macdermot K, Fryns J-P, Bonduelle M, Dietz HC, Gaspar IM, Cavaco D, Stattin E-L, Schrander-Stumpel C, Coucke P, Loeys B, de Paepe A, De Backer J. Novel MYH11 and ACTA2 mutations reveal a role for enhanced TGFbeta signaling in FTAAD. Int J Cardiol. 2011;165:314–21. https://doi.org/10.1016/j.ijcard.2011.08.079.
137. Pannu H, Tran-Fadulu V, Papke CL, Scherer S, Liu Y, Presley C, Guo D, Estrera AL, Safi HJ, Brasier AR, Vick GW, Marian AJ, Raman CS, Buja LM, Milewicz DM. MYH11 mutations result in a distinct vascular pathology driven by insulin-like growth factor 1 and angiotensin II. Human Molecular Genetics. 2007;16:2453–62. https://doi.org/10.1093/hmg/ddm201.
138. van Kien PK. Mapping of familial thoracic aortic aneurysm/dissection with patent ductus arteriosus to 16p12.2-p13.13. Circulation. 2005;112:200–6. https://doi.org/10.1161/CIRCULATIONAHA.104.506345.

139. Mizuguchi T, Collod-Beroud G, Akiyama T, Abifadel M, Harada N, Morisaki T, Allard D, Varret M, Claustres M, Morisaki H, Ihara M, Kinoshita A, Yoshiura K-I, Junien C, Kajii T, Jondeau G, Ohta T, Kishino T, Furukawa Y, Nakamura Y, Niikawa N, Boileau C, Matsumoto N. Heterozygous TGFBR2 mutations in Marfan syndrome. Nat Genet. 2004;36:855–60. https://doi.org/10.1038/ng1392.
140. Guo D-C, Hanna N, Regalado ES, Detaint D, Gong L, Varret M, Prakash SK, Li AH, d'Indy H, Braverman AC, Grandchamp B, Kwartler CS, Gouya L, Santos-Cortez RLP, Abifadel M, Leal SM, Muti C, Shendure J, Gross M-S, Rieder MJ, Vahanian A, Nickerson DA, Michel J-B, Jondeau G, Boileau C, Milewicz DM. TGFB2 mutations cause familial thoracic aortic aneurysms and dissections associated with mild systemic features of Marfan syndrome. Nat Genet. 2012;44:916–21. https://doi.org/10.1038/ng.2348.
141. Lindsay ME, Schepers D, Bolar NA, Doyle JJ, Gallo E, Fert-Bober J, Kempers MJE, Fishman EK, Chen Y, Myers L, Bjeda D, Oswald G, Elias AF, Levy HP, Anderlid B-M, Yang MH, Bongers EMHF, Timmermans J, Braverman AC, Canham N, Mortier GR, Brunner HG, Byers PH, Van Eyk J, Van Laer L, Dietz HC, Loeys BL. Loss-of-function mutations in TGFB2 cause a syndromic presentation of thoracic aortic aneurysm. Nat Genet. 2012;44:922–7. https://doi.org/10.1038/ng.2349.

Thoracic Aortic Dilatation, Aneurysm and Dissection

21

Michael Ibrahim and Nimesh D. Desai

Abstract

The thoracic aorta is an extremely sophisticated structure which allows for the smooth conversion of pulsatile ventricular output to continuous arterial perfusion. Its sophistication is determined by an increasingly well described network of interacting genes. When these genetic pathways are abnormal, the aorta is pre-disposed to dilation, aneurysm formation and associated risk of dissection. We here review the major genetic pathways involved through discussion of key clinical cases, and highlight areas of uncertainty where rapid advances are being made.

Keywords

Aortic sydromes • Genetic aortopathy • Aneurysm

21.1 Introduction

The thoracic aorta is a sophisticated and dynamic structure consisting of multiple cell types arranged in intimal, medial and adventitial layers [1]. It is ordinarily capable of transmitting the entire cardiac output approximately seventy times a minute for an entire lifetime and transforming intermittent cardiac ejection into continuous tissue perfusion, while withstanding the systemic blood pressure. This remarkable feat is achieved with little energy expenditure. It is also highly responsive to neurohormonal as well as biophysical signals and adapts to changes such as exercise and

M. Ibrahim • N.D. Desai (✉)
Division of Cardiovascular Surgery, Hospital of the University of Pennsylvania, Philadelphia, PA, USA
e-mail: Michael.Ibrahim@uphs.upenn.edu; nimesh.desai@uphs.upenn.edu

D. Kumar, P. Elliott (eds.), *Cardiovascular Genetics and Genomics*,
https://doi.org/10.1007/978-3-319-66114-8_21

pregnancy. The aorta's embryological formation and homeostasis depends on a large number of genes acting in concert.

Macroscopically, the normal thoracic aorta consists of a number of elements beginning at the aortic root (itself consisting of the aortic valve annulus, cusps, and sinuses of Valsalva), the ascending aorta (from the tubular portion of the aorta originating at the sinotubular junction to the innominate artery), the arch, and the descending aorta (Fig. 21.1). Aneurysmal dilation may affect any part of this system and is defined as permanent localized dilation of over 50% of the expected diameter. Ectasia describes dilation not reaching this cut-off. Arteriomegaly is defined as permanent, diffuse dilation of multiple arterial segments of at least 50%. The most feared sequela of aneurysmal dilation is aortic dissection, defined as disruption of the media layer with bleeding within and along the aortic wall.

Genetic influence upon these conditions may be thought of as (Table 21.1) [2]:

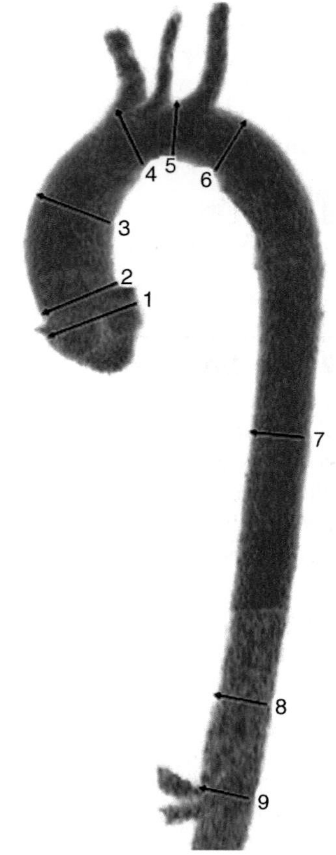

Fig. 21.1 Normal anatomy of the thoracoabdominal aorta with standard anatomic landmarks for reporting aortic diameter as illustrated on a volume-rendered CT image of the thoracic aorta. (1) Aortic sinuses of Valsalva; (2) Sinotubular junction; (3) Mid ascending aorta (midpoint in length between Nos. 2 and 4); (4) Proximal aortic arch (aorta at the origin of the innominate artery); (5) Mid aortic arch (between left common carotid and subclavian arteries); (6) Proximal descending thoracic aorta (begins at the isthmus, approximately 2 cm distal to left subclavian artery); (7) Mid descending aorta (midpoint in length between Nos. 6 and 8); (8) Aorta at diaphragm (2 cm above the celiac axis origin); (9) Abdominal aorta at the celiac axis origin

Table 21.1 Major categories of gene alterations driving inherited aortopathy

TGF-β Aortopathy (Syndromic)	Smooth Muscle Contraction Aortopathy (Non-syndromic)
MS	Familial Aortopathies
LDS	BAV
Multi-system involvement	Cardiovascular involvement
FBN1, TGFBR1, TGFBR2, TGFB2, TGFB3, SMAD2, SMAD3 and SKI	ACTA2, MYH11, MYLK, and PRKG1

1. Syndromic: multi-organ phenotype from heritable genetic defects centered on the transforming growth factor-β (TGF-β pathway). This includes the Marfan syndrome, Loeys-Dietz Syndrome and others.
2. Non-syndromic: these aortopathies are either familial with diverse genetic aeitologies (largely centered around the contractile apparatus) or are non-syndromic and are driven by conventional vascular risk factors including hypertension, age, smoking, diabetes and hypercholesterolemia.

Our improving genetic understanding is becoming more important to the management of thoracic aortic disease including risk stratification, operative planning and refined pharmacologic approaches.

21.2 Syndromic Aortopathies

21.2.1 Case 1

A 24 year old lady who has always been taller than her peers presents to your clinic for routine follow up of an aortic root aneurysm and mitral valve prolapse. Her clinical history includes recurrent inguinal hernias and shortsightedness. Her father reportedly had heart surgery. A transthoracic echocardiogram reveals a 4.2 cm ascending aortic aneurysm without valvular regurgitation. A CT angiogram shows 1.1 cm growth in the transverse diameter of the aneurysm since a year ago.

This case is prototypic of syndromic aortopathy: an inherited pleiotropic genetic disorder affecting the cardiovascular and other systems. In this case, a young lady presents with the classic features of the Marfan syndrome (MS). The commonest cardiovascular manifestations of MS include aortic root aneurysm and mitral valve prolapse. Its other systemic manifestations include overgrowth of long bones, reduced muscular mass, osteopenia and adiposity as well as craniofacial anomalies and ocular defects including ectopia lentis [3].

MS is rare autosomal dominant disease affecting 1 in 5000. A very few cases of autosomal recessive inheritance have been reported. The diagnosis of MS is not always straightforward. Clinical suspicion, especially in the absence of a clear family history, may be lowered by the variability in the phenotype. The diagnosis of MS is based on the revised Ghent nosology, a range of features agreed upon by expert consensus to be diagnostic [4]. In these criteria, the presence of ectopia lentis and aortic aneurysm are the cardinal features and are diagnostic even in the absence of a family history. If either of these two are absent, a defect in the fibrillin 1 gene with a number of associated systemic defects is required to be diagnostic, based on a scoring system. Fibrillin 1 mutations also underlie other genetic syndromes including mild aortic dilatation, skeleton and skin (MASS) syndrome and others [5].

In 1896, Antoine Marfan first described patients with the systemic features now recognized as pathognomonic for MS. The cardiac manifestations of this syndrome became apparent later in 1912. McKusick described the first series in the 1950s, characterized the cardiovascular defects in more detail and suggested MS represented a monogenetic inherited disorder [6]. Histological analysis of the Marfan aorta suggested what appeared to be pronounced medial degeneration, and defective tropoelastin deposition and collagen cross linking in early postnatal life. This led investigators to search for a genetic defect driving a structural weakness centered on impaired elastin formation, presumably driving aortic aneurysm formation. However, microdeletions in the only elastin gene in the human genome leads to Williams syndrome, characterized by supravalvular aortic stenosis and not dilation or aneurysm formation [7]. The same was true of point mutations in the elastin gene [8]. To complicate matters, some mutations in genes involved in elastogenesis do cause aneurysm formation, aortic tortuosity as well as stenosis, namely FBLN4 [9]. This demonstrates that similar genetic defects can result in markedly different phenotypes. These findings challenged the concept of a gene defect causing a simplistic structural weakness.

The fibrillin 1 gene was discovered to be the causative genetic defect in 1991 [10]. This defect is inherited in an autosomal dominant fashion. This very large gene located at 15q21.1 has structural homology with TGF-β binding proteins and contributes to the final structure of a microfibril. Indeed, the fibrillin gene interacts with the TGF-β signaling pathway to fine tune it. An important breakthrough in our understanding of this disease process came from the analysis of an animal model of fibrillin-1 gene defective mice who develop emphysema [11]. While their genetic defect is in the fibrillin-1 gene, they show significant TGF-β dysregulation characterized by TGF-β sequestration, with persistent activation driving marked apoptosis. The fact that the administration of TGF-β neutralizing antibodies could eliminate many of these phenotypic features is consistent with an excess of TGF-β being a key feature driving pathogenesis. A large number of studies now provide conclusive evidence that excessive TGF-β activation is a causal and initiating event in several manifestations of MS including mitral valve disease, aortic dilatation and skeletal myopathy. In a seminal paper, Habashi et al. showed that in a mouse model of MS, aortic dilation was caused by excessive TGF-β activation, and could be prevented with either neutralizing antibodies or angiotensin receptor blockade [12].

The spectrum of aortopathy in MS is wide. It may range from abnormal aortic stiffness to aortic dissection. The cardinal histologic features are elastic llamelae fragmentation, excessive collagen and mucopolysaccharide deposition and a paucity of vascular smooth muscle cells. At a macroscopic level, aneurysm formation principally affects the proximal thoracic aorta, especially the aortic root (in up to 80% of MS patients [13]) with severe aortoannular ectasia and dilated aortic sinuses and annulus.

The standardized clinical follow up of MS patients includes precautions (exercise limitations), beta blockade and serial imaging. The imaging modality of choice depends on the extent of the disease, but EKG gated computerized tomography (CT) provides rapid, detailed imaging. Cardiovascular magnetic resonance can also provide detailed imaging of the aorta. As noted above, in animal models of MS, angiotensin blockade appears to ameliorate aortic dilatation. Milleron et al., in a randomized clinical trial, showed that losartan reduced the blood pressure but did not limit aortic dilatation over a three year follow up period in MS patients [14], reaffirming the primacy of beta blockade. This conflicts with other data, for example from the COMPARE trial, showing that losartan can reduce aortic dilation in MS patients [15]. How can this conflicting data be reconciled? It appears that the specific MS genotype may influence the sensitivity to specific pharmacologic therapies as well as survival [16]. Franken et al. showed that losartan was effective in reducing the rate of aortic dilatation only in MS patients with FBN1 mutations causing haploinsufficiency, which (compared to patients with a dominant negative mutation) is associated with a 1.6X risk of any aortic complication and a 2.5X risk of cardiovascular death [17]. This may be because in haploinsufficiency the aortic wall is thinner, and more prone to damage, resulting in increased activation of angiotensin and TGF-β. Losartan is able to prevent this augmented TGF-β production, reducing blood pressure, proinflammatory and myofibroblast responses, and production of reactive oxygen species. Overall these data show that MS is not a single clinical entity and that improved understanding of the gene-phenotype interaction will lead to more tailored therapies.

By the age of 60, 100% of MS patients have aortic root dilatation of some degree and 75% have had aortic root replacement due to excessive dilatation, aortic dissection or aortic insufficiency [5]. In degenerative aortic aneurysm disease, a transverse dimension of 5.5 cm is generally used as the trigger for surgical evaluation of repair [18]. However, in patients with inherited aortopathy a smaller dimension of between 4 and 5 cm is suggested. This is a problematic area however, as repair too early exposes what is already a young patient population to the risks of complications unnecessarily. On the other hand, a significant number of patients experience a devastating progression of their disease at dimensions significantly smaller than those which would trigger repair under current guidelines. Is there a better way of evaluating risk in these patients? Franken et al. showed that circulating TGF-β levels could act as a risk marker as elevated levels correlated with larger aortic dimensions, a faster rate of growth and earlier aortic surgery [19]. MS patients with FBN1 mutations have low risk for dissection at diameters below 5.5 cm [20]. Small variations in the FBN1 gene called single nucleotide polymorphisms (SNPs) amongst people without MS, increases risk of aortic dilatation and dissection [21]. This may also be relevant to risk of dissection within MS populations, and studies are currently underway to assess this.

21.2.2 Case 2

A 22 male with a background of patent ductus arteriosus, and with multiple systemic features including hypertelorism and cleft palate with bifid uvula presents to your aortopathy clinic. CT angiogram reveals widespread tortuosity of the arterial tree and a 4.3 cm ascending aortic aneurysm.

There are a number of genetic aortopathy syndromes similar to MS including Loeys-Dietz syndrome (as in Case 2), aneurysm osteoarthritis syndrome, Ehlers-Danlos syndrome and others which all share aortic dilatation and aneurysm formation but additionally include multi-system involvement [22]. Loeys and Dietz described their syndrome in a series of patients who showed mutations in the TGF-β receptors 1 and 2 (genes TGFBR1 and TGFBR2). These patients have marfanoid features with hypertelorism, craniofacial anomalies, club feet, easy bruising and dystrophic scars. Their aortopathy is more variable than MS and can affect the entire vascular tree. Their propensity for aortic dilation and dissection is more pronounced, and they tend to dilate at younger ages and dissect at smaller transverse diameters than MS patients [23, 24]. As for MS, TGF-β signaling appears to play a major role.

The TGF-β pathway is a regulatory cytokine pathway which is responsible for directing embryogenesis and maintaining tissue homeostasis (reviewed in detail in [25]). Its expression is tightly regulated. TGF-β is activated by proteases, allowing TGF-β binding sites to bond with TGF-β ligands. This results in downstream signaling which occur in the canonical and non-canonical pathways.

In the canonical pathway, TGF-β ligand binding events trigger its receptor kinase, leading to the phosphorylation of regulatory molecules termed SMADs. Further signal transduction events lead to the formation of a complex with co-SMADs which is imported into the nucleus and regulates gene transcription. This signal transduction pathway is substantially antagonized by the proto-oncogene SKI which acts by repressing SMAD3 and inhibiting TGF-β signaling. Mutations in all the elements described in the canonical pathway are associated with syndromic aortopathy including LDS at the level of the TGF-β receptor (TGFB1, TGFBR2, TGFB2, TGFB3); aneurysm-osteoarthritis syndrome (SMAD3) and Shprintzen-Goldberg Syndrome (SKI1), which is a rare disease with many similarities to MS including craniofacial anomalies and aortopathy.

TGF-β signaling can also occurs through an alternative, SMAD independent pathways termed the non-canonical pathway. This involves a number of molecular players including RAS-MAPK, c-Jun and the Ras homolog gene family, member a which is a regulator of the serine/threonine kinase ROCK1 which influences many aspects of smooth muscle cell contraction [26]. Histologic analysis shows that overexpression of TGF-β is a hallmark in syndromic and non-syndromic aortopathy (below). Animal models suggest that mutations in canonical TGF-β signalling as described above in syndromic TAD, drive upregulation of the non-canonical pathway and an overall activation of TGF-β [27]. This likely occurs due to loss of inhibitory feedback from canonical pathways and resultant over-activation of non-canonical pathways. This is termed the TGF-β paradox and drives epithelial to mesenchymal cell fate transformation influencing fibrosis, wound repair and valve development.

In a similar fashion to that already discussed for MS, genetic factors may help to risk stratify and therefore inform management decisions in LDS. In LDS patients, who have TGFBR1 and TGFBR2 mutations, aortic dissection occurs at diameters less than 5.0 cm [23, 24]. In addition, these patients show aneurysms of other arteries. The TGFBR2 mutation appears to increase risk more than TGFBR1, especially in men [24]. These findings have led to the recommendation that these patients undergo operative management at 4.2 cm [18].

21.2.3 Case 3

A 37 year old female presents for surgical evaluation following a screening echocardiogram triggered due to her brother having known bicuspid aortic valve disease. She has no symptoms. An echocardiogram reveals a bicuspid aortic valve and 4.7 cm proximal ascending aorta without regurgitation.

Bicuspid aortic valve (BAV) is the commonest congenital heart defect and represents a complex familial syndrome. In first-degree relatives, there is a prevalence of 9% [28]. The connection between BAV and TAD was identified by Abbott in 1928. Initially thought of a simple mechanical consequence of post-stenotic blood flow, the aortic dilation of BAV is now properly understood to be a primary aortopathy. Unlike the other syndromes discussed above, which have a far lower incidence, the risk of dissection is diminutive; for example the incidence of MS is 0.02% with a risk of dissection of 40%, whereas BAV has an incidence of 1–2% and a risk of dissection of approximately 5% [29]. It is clear that a number of different gene mutations may give rise to BAV. For example, BAV is found in mice with mutations in Nkx2.5, Gata5, Nos3, Matr3, Adamts5, Brg1 and HoxA1 (reviewed in [22]). NOTCH1 mutations have been reliably and consistently associated with BAV syndrome in humans [30]. The aorta in BAV shows many features of primary aortopathy with increased elastic fibre damage, a relative deficiency in fibrillin 1 and augmented levels of matrix metallic proteinases and smooth muscle cell apoptosis [31–33]. The aortopathy in BAV occurs in distinct patterns affecting the aortic root alone in 10%, the ascending aorta alone in 10%, the ascending aorta and transverse arch in 28%, and the aortic root, ascending aorta and proximal transverse arch in 45% [34]. This suggests that our understanding of BAV disease as a single entity is likely overly simplistic.

No clear genetic basis nor pathophysiologic mechanism has been elucidated for BAV aortopathy. This is in part due to low penetrance and possible multi-genetic aetiology [35, 36]. While it is now thought that BAV is a type of aortopathy syndrome, it is not reasonable to extrapolate the cut-offs for management of syndromic TAD to BAV patients as this exposes this cohort to unacceptable surgical risk without a clear benefit [37].

21.3 Non-Syndromic Tad

21.3.1 Case 4

A 45 year old male presents with a 5.5 cm ascending aortic aneurysm following a screening chest CT. He is asymptomatic. He reports that his grandfather died of aortic dissection in his 1940s. He does not have diabetes, hypertension, hypercholesterolemia and is a lifelong non smoker.

Non-syndromic TAD can be subdivided into non-familial and familial varieties. Non familial non-syndromic TAD represents degenerative aortic dilatation and aneurysm formation as a consequence of conventional vascular risk factors including hypertension, hypercholesterolemia, smoking and diabetes. Familial non-syndromic TAD is a complex disorder affecting at least two family members. Aortic disease in these patients presents earlier in life, progress more rapidly and is not driven by classical vascular risk factors. It's genetics are more complex than the syndromic TADs and mutations appear to be centered on the contractile apparatus of vascular smooth muscle cells. The genes implicated include MYH11, MYLK, PRKG1 [38–40]. MFAP5 regulates the interaction between microfibrils and elastic fibres and has been found to be mutated in some forms of familial TAD [41]. MAT2a, a gene encoding a adenyltransferase highly expressed in aortic smooth muscle cells, is also found in some families with familial TAD [42]. The most common mutation accounting for familial TAD is ACTA2 which encodes for actin in vascular smooth muscle cells, and accounts for up to 14% of familial TAD [43]. Patients with ACTA2 mutations show variable penetrance, with some mildly or largely unaffected. On the other hand, some ACTA2 mutations portend a significant risk of dissection, at small dimensions typically below 5.0 cm [44]. These patients also typically have livedo reticularis, iris floccule, patent ductus arteriosus and BAV.

21.3.1.1 Clinical Management of Genetic TAD

The aim of the management of the patient cohorts described above is to avoid aortic dissection. To do this requires optimal medical management, surveillance of the thoracic aorta radiologically, risk stratification based on a combination of genetics, imaging and conventional risk factors in order to make sound recommendations on the timing (and nature) of operative management and thereby avoid the potentially devastating consequences of acute aortic dissection or rupture, while delaying the risks of surgery until necessary.

A number of imaging modalities can be used to assess these patients. Transthoracic echocardiography is a painless, noninvasive, rapid and non-radiating modality which is widely available. Measurements should be taken of internal diameters, perpendicular to blood flow. EKG-gated CT and MRI are also useful modalities with the advantage of imaging the entire thoracic aorta and beyond. In these modalities, external diameters perpendicular to blood flow should be recorded. These modalities are less prone to user variability, although standardization in recording is important. Use of the same modality and same reader over serial examinations is useful.

Current generation multi-detector helical CT has sensitivity and specificity approaching 100% for aortic dissection [45]. In an acute setting, CT is probably the single best imaging modality (unless the patient is unstable or very high risk, when transesophageal echocardiography should be performed). These generally include a non-contrast image to detect intramural haematoma, followed by a contrast phase to define dissection, reveal malperfusion and exclude rupture. The vascular tree should be imaged from the thoracic inlet to the pelvis including the iliac and femoral arteries.

The imaging modality of choice and frequency of screening is different for the different syndromes. For any aortopathy, the advent of interval symptoms should prompt immediate re-imaging, probably by EKG gated CT. In initial presentation of Marfan syndrome, a transthoracic echo to assess the extent of aortic root dilation and the presence of aortic regurgitation should be performed. This should be repeated at 6 months to assess for rapid progression. Once stability has been documented, it is recommended to image these patients annually, unless the aortic dimension exceeds 4.5 cm or there is rapid growth, or the patient is pregnant, when more frequent monitoring may be warranted. Conversely in a LDS patient or in a patient with a high risk mutation (including ACTA2, TGFBR1/TGFBR2 FBN1, and MYH11), it is important to assess the entire aorta in detail. In LDS specifically, owing to the propensity for dispersed aneurysms throughout the arterial tree, an MRI may be best for detecting such aneurysms and should be performed from the brain to the pelvis [46]. In addition, in Turner syndrome patients, it is important to image the heart and aorta to exclude BAV, coarctation and aortic dilatation; if initial imaging is reassuring, interval imaging every 5–10 years is appropriate, otherwise, annual screening is advised.

In addition, it is advisable that first degree relatives of those with thoracic aortic dilatation or high risk mutations undergo assessment to include genetic testing and imaging. If a first degree relative is identified with a mutation and proven to have aortic dilation, then assessment of second degree relatives is recommended also.

A risk reduction program to reduce the rate of progression of aortic dilation and avoid dissection is essential. Risk reduction consists of general measures including patient education and aggressive vascular risk factors modification: cessation of smoking, tight diabetes control, blood pressure control and treatment for hypercholesterolemia. Blood pressure goals for aortic dilation are less than 140/90 or less than 130/80 in those with diabetes or renal disease. It is uncontroversial that beta blockade is a first line agent, with the addition of ACE inhibitors or angiotensin receptor blockers in adition [47–49].

The normal aorta is highly adaptive and changes in the short and long term when faced with different environmental stressors. These pose a challenge in managing risk in patients with genetic TAD. Pregnancy accentuates the risk of rapid aortic dilation and dissection in syndromic TAD and if aortic dimensions exceed 4.0 cm in a MS patient contemplating pregnancy, she should be considered for preemptive surgical repair prior to pregnancy [50]. In any case, pregnancy in a patient with known aortopathy should trigger closer monitoring by serial imaging using non-radiating modalities. These patients should be counselled specifically about the risk of aortic dissection and the heritable nature of the disease. Exercise is another potential stress on the aorta. There is currently no outcomes research to support any specific recommendation. Most clinicians would advise against high exertion exercise which may increase aortic wall stress [51].

21.3.1.2 Operative Management

Having appropriately followed and risk stratified these patients, the key decision is timing and extent of surgery. Case 1 describes a young lady with MS who presents with an aortic root aneurysm and mitral valve disease. At 4.2 cm, the size of her aneurysm alone would make her a surgical candidate since the recommendation is to operate somewhere between 4.0 and 5.0 cm [18, 52]. In addition, she demonstrates rapid growth in excess of 0.5 cm/year, meeting an additional criteria for consideration for surgery. Further, she is a young female and may undergo the stress of pregnancy in the next decade. All in all, these features suggest operative management may be appropriate. The patient in this scenario also has mitral valve disease, which could be repaired concomitantly if it were causing moderate or severe regurgitation. Case 2 describes a patient with LDS and a 4.3 cm aortic aneurysm. Again this patient would meet the criteria for operative management based on an aortic diameter of greater than 4.2 cm in the setting of LDS [18]. Case 3 describes a lady with BAV and significant aortic aneurysm with a maximum diameter of 4.7 cm. BAV is classified as a genetic aortopathy and current guidelines recommend considering operative management for all these patients between 4.0 and 5.0 cm [18]. In addition, were she to require surgery for aortic valve disease (even if she did not have congenital BAV), it would be reasonable to consider repair at a dimension of greater than 4.5 cm. Case 4 describes a patient with familial, non-syndromic aortic aneurysm. These patients are considered for surgery in the same manner as syndromic patients described above. Details of the operative management of these patients is beyond the scope of this chapter. However, a brief overview of the thought process underlying these operations is given.

In patients with syndromic and familial TAD, aggressive resection of the aortic sinuses, ascending aorta and proximal arch is favored due to the risk of late reoperation when more conservative approaches are adopted [53]. This involves resection to the level of the innominate artery on the greater curvature and to the level of the subclavian on the lesser curvature. This so called aggressive hemi-arch approach provides good protection against future arch aneurysms. If the aneurysm extends well into the arch and descending thoracic aorta, full arch replacement is performed usually with the elephant trunk procedure [54]. Briefly, this is a staged procedure which involves replacement of the ascending aorta and arch with a Dacron graft, the distal end of which is sutured beyond the subclavian artery with the free end of the graft lying within the descending aneurysm. A Dacron cuff provides a distal attachment zone for an endovascular stent graft which is deployed in a second stage procedure, and whose proximal landing zone is the free elephant trunk in the descending aneurysm. Another consideration is treatment of the aortic valve. Often these patients do not require valve replacement. When valve replacement is required, the normal considerations apply in weighing biological and mechanical prostheses. In genetic TAD, including BAV, the pulmonary autograft root is not favored due to the potential for intrinsic disease.

Aortic dissection is a devastating sequela of TAD, and the management and risk stratification described above is designed to prevent it. Patients presenting with high risk features for aortic dissection, such as tearing retrosternal chest pain of sudden onset, evidence of malperfusion of abdominal viscera or extremity malperfusion/ blood pressure differential, known aortic valve disease, known genetic aortopathy, recent aortic manipulation or a new murmur of aortic regurgitation should have an emergent cardiac surgical evaluation. Initial management consists of EKG (coronary dissection is rare, meaning that ST changes make ischaemic cardiac pain more likely than aortic dissection, and management should be initially directed toward that unless the patient is high risk for aortic dissection). Urgent aortic imaging should be obtained. In a high risk patient with convincing features this may be performed via transesophageal imaging in the operating theatre. Otherwise, a stat CT should be obtained to investigate the extent of dissection and identify an intimal tear. There are five classes of intimal tear. Type I is classic false lumen formation with a septum and intimal tear. The lumens communicate, often in the descending aorta. Type II represents intramural haematoma, often without an obvious intimal tear which is found intraoperatively. Type III consists of intimal tear without haematoma an eccentric aortic bulge, and are difficult to detect; MS patients are prone to this. These may result in rupture. Type IV represents a penetrating atherosclerotic ulcer with localized haematoma. These often progress to Type I. Type V represent iatrogenic, often catheter induced or traumatic dissection. In addition, it is essential to define the extent of dissection, which is described by the Debakey or Stanford classifications.

Initial therapy focuses on heart rate and blood pressure reduction with intravenous beta blockade titrated to a heart rate of 60. If beta blockade is contraindicated, intravenous nondihydropyridine calcium channel blockers are used. If, following adequate heart rate reduction, the systolic BP remains over 120 then intravenous ACE inhibitors are used. For all dissections involving the ascending aorta, urgent operative management is mandatory unless contraindicated (normally due to devastating neurological injury or comorbidities). Evidence of ischaemia, especially combined generalized and localized branch artery ischaemia is highly predictive of mortality [55]. Medical management of descending dissections is appropriate in the absence of a complication such as malperfusion necessitating urgent operative intervention. In general, all aneurysmal aorta and the proximal dissection should be excised and replaced. Partial dissection of the root can be managed with valve resuspension, while extensive root dissection should be treated with full root replacement with a composite graft or valve sparing root replacement [56].

Conclusions

The thoracic aorta is an elegant and tightly regulated structure, normally able to withstand the systemic blood pressure and respond to physiologic stressors. Its embryogenesis and tissue homeostasis is choreographed by a wide array of genes. Mutations, mostly inherited, can make the aorta susceptible to dilation, aneurysm formation and dissection. There has been tremendous progress in understanding the genetic basis of inherited aortopathy, and in some cases this provides important clinical indicators of risk and responsiveness to various therapies. The full details of how this occurs, specific genotype/phenotype relationships and how our expanding knowledge of the genetics underlying these diseases ought to influence clinical management remains uncertain.

References

1. El-Hamamsy I, Yacoub MH. Cellular and molecular mechanisms of thoracic aortic aneurysms. Nat Rev. Cardiol. 2009;6(12):771–86.
2. Isselbacher EM, Lino Cardenas CL, Lindsay ME. Hereditary influence in thoracic aortic aneurysm and dissection. Circulation. 2016;133(24):2516–28.
3. Pepe G, et al. Marfan syndrome: current perspectives. Appl Clin Genet. 2016;9:55–65.
4. Loeys BL, et al. The revised Ghent nosology for the Marfan syndrome. J Med Genet. 2010;47(7):476–85.
5. Detaint D, et al. Cardiovascular manifestations in men and women carrying a FBN1 mutation. Eur Heart J. 2010;31(18):2223–9.
6. Mc KV. The cardiovascular aspects of Marfan's syndrome: a heritable disorder of connective tissue. Circulation. 1955;11(3):321–42.
7. Ewart AK, et al. Supravalvular aortic stenosis associated with a deletion disrupting the elastin gene. J Clin Invest. 1994;93(3):1071–7.
8. Li DY, et al. Elastin point mutations cause an obstructive vascular disease, supravalvular aortic stenosis. Hum Mol Genet. 1997;6(7):1021–8.
9. Renard M, et al. Altered TGFbeta signaling and cardiovascular manifestations in patients with autosomal recessive cutis laxa type I caused by fibulin-4 deficiency. Eur J Hum Genet. 2010;18(8):895–901.
10. Dietz HC, et al. Marfan syndrome caused by a recurrent de novo missense mutation in the fibrillin gene. Nature. 1991;352(6333):337–9.
11. Neptune ER, et al. Dysregulation of TGF-beta activation contributes to pathogenesis in Marfan syndrome. Nat Genet. 2003;33(3):407–11.
12. Habashi JP, et al. Losartan, an AT1 antagonist, prevents aortic aneurysm in a mouse model of Marfan syndrome. Science. 2006;312(5770):117–21.
13. Marsalese DL, et al. Marfan's syndrome: natural history and long-term follow-up of cardiovascular involvement. J Am Coll Cardiol. 1989;14(2):422–8. discussion 429-31
14. Milleron O, et al. Marfan Sartan: a randomized, double-blind, placebo-controlled trial. Eur Heart J. 2015;36(32):2160–6.
15. Groenink M, et al. Losartan reduces aortic dilatation rate in adults with Marfan syndrome: a randomized controlled trial. Eur Heart J. 2013;34(45):3491–500.
16. Franken R, et al. Genotype impacts survival in Marfan syndrome. Eur Heart J. 2016;37(43):3285–90.
17. Franken R, et al. Beneficial outcome of losartan therapy depends on type of FBN1 mutation in Marfan syndrome. Circ Cardiovasc Genet. 2015;8(2):383–8.
18. Hiratzka LF, et al. ACCF/AHA/AATS/ACR/ASA/SCA/SCAI/SIR/STS/SVM guidelines for the diagnosis and management of patients with thoracic aortic disease: executive summary. A report of the American College of Cardiology Foundation/American Heart Association Task Force on Practice Guidelines, American Association for Thoracic Surgery, American College of Radiology, American Stroke Association, Society of Cardiovascular Anesthesiologists, Society for Cardiovascular Angiography and Interventions, Society of Interventional Radiology, Society of Thoracic Surgeons, and Society for Vascular Medicine. Catheter Cardiovasc Interv. 2010;76(2):E43–86.

19. Franken R, et al. Circulating transforming growth factor-beta as a prognostic biomarker in Marfan syndrome. Int J Cardiol. 2013;168(3):2441–6.
20. Milewicz DM, Dietz HC, Miller DC. Treatment of aortic disease in patients with Marfan syndrome. Circulation. 2005;111(11):e150–7.
21. LeMaire SA, et al. Genome-wide association study identifies a susceptibility locus for thoracic aortic aneurysms and aortic dissections spanning FBN1 at 15q21.1. Nat Genet. 2011;43(10):996–1000.
22. Andelfinger G, Loeys B, Dietz H. A decade of discovery in the genetic understanding of thoracic aortic disease. Can J Cardiol. 2016;32(1):13–25.
23. Loeys BL, et al. Aneurysm syndromes caused by mutations in the TGF-beta receptor. N Engl J Med. 2006;355(8):788–98.
24. Tran-Fadulu V, et al. Analysis of multigenerational families with thoracic aortic aneurysms and dissections due to TGFBR1 or TGFBR2 mutations. J Med Genet. 2009;46(9):607–13.
25. Shi Y, Massague J. Mechanisms of TGF-beta signaling from cell membrane to the nucleus. Cell. 2003;113(6):685–700.
26. Shimizu Y, et al. ROCK-I regulates closure of the eyelids and ventral body wall by inducing assembly of actomyosin bundles. J Cell Biol. 2005;168(6):941–53.
27. Holm TM, et al. Noncanonical TGFbeta signaling contributes to aortic aneurysm progression in Marfan syndrome mice. Science. 2011;332(6027):358–61.
28. Guntheroth WG, Spiers PS. Does aortic root dilatation with bicuspid aortic valves occur as a primary tissue abnormality or as a relatively benign poststenotic phenomenon? Am J Cardiol. 2005;95(6):820.
29. Erbel R, Eggebrecht H. Aortic dimensions and the risk of dissection. Heart. 2006;92(1):137–42.
30. Garg V, et al. Mutations in NOTCH1 cause aortic valve disease. Nature. 2005;437(7056):270–4.
31. Bonderman D, et al. Mechanisms underlying aortic dilatation in congenital aortic valve malformation. Circulation. 1999;99(16):2138–43.
32. Nataatmadja M, et al. Abnormal extracellular matrix protein transport associated with increased apoptosis of vascular smooth muscle cells in marfan syndrome and bicuspid aortic valve thoracic aortic aneurysm. Circulation. 2003;108(Suppl 1):II329–34.
33. Fedak PW, et al. Vascular matrix remodeling in patients with bicuspid aortic valve malformations: implications for aortic dilatation. J Thorac Cardiovasc Surg. 2003;126(3):797–806.
34. Fazel SS, et al. The aortopathy of bicuspid aortic valve disease has distinctive patterns and usually involves the transverse aortic arch. J Thorac Cardiovasc Surg. 2008;135(4):901–7.
35. Cripe L, et al. Bicuspid aortic valve is heritable. J Am Coll Cardiol. 2004;44(1):138–43.
36. Martin LJ, et al. Whole exome sequencing for familial bicuspid aortic valve identifies putative variants. Circ Cardiovasc Genet. 2014;7(5):677–83.
37. Itagaki S, et al. Long-term risk for aortic complications after aortic valve replacement in patients with bicuspid aortic valve versus Marfan syndrome. J Am Coll Cardiol. 2015;65(22):2363–9.
38. Guo DC, et al. Recurrent gain-of-function mutation in PRKG1 causes thoracic aortic aneurysms and acute aortic dissections. Am J Hum Genet. 2013;93(2):398–404.
39. Wang L, et al. Mutations in myosin light chain kinase cause familial aortic dissections. Am J Hum Genet. 2010;87(5):701–7.
40. Zhu L, et al. Mutations in myosin heavy chain 11 cause a syndrome associating thoracic aortic aneurysm/aortic dissection and patent ductus arteriosus. Nat Genet. 2006;38(3):343–9.
41. Barbier M, et al. MFAP5 loss-of-function mutations underscore the involvement of matrix alteration in the pathogenesis of familial thoracic aortic aneurysms and dissections. Am J Hum Genet. 2014;95(6):736–43.
42. Guo DC, et al. MAT2A mutations predispose individuals to thoracic aortic aneurysms. Am J Hum Genet. 2015;96(1):170–7.
43. Guo DC, et al. Mutations in smooth muscle alpha-actin (ACTA2) lead to thoracic aortic aneurysms and dissections. Nat Genet. 2007;39(12):1488–93.
44. Regalado ES, et al. Aortic Disease Presentation and Outcome Associated With ACTA2 Mutations. Circ Cardiovasc Genet. 2015;8(3):457–64.

45. Yoshida S, et al. Thoracic involvement of type A aortic dissection and intramural hematoma: diagnostic accuracy--comparison of emergency helical CT and surgical findings. Radiology. 2003;228(2):430–5.
46. Sommer T, et al. Aortic dissection: a comparative study of diagnosis with spiral CT, multiplanar transesophageal echocardiography, and MR imaging. Radiology. 1996;199(2):347–52.
47. Shores J, et al. Progression of aortic dilatation and the benefit of long-term beta-adrenergic blockade in Marfan's syndrome. N Engl J Med. 1994;330(19):1335–41.
48. Brooke BS, et al. Angiotensin II blockade and aortic-root dilation in Marfan's syndrome. N Engl J Med. 2008;358(26):2787–95.
49. Mochizuki S, et al. Valsartan in a Japanese population with hypertension and other cardiovascular disease (Jikei Heart Study): a randomised, open-label, blinded endpoint morbidity-mortality study. Lancet. 2007;369(9571):1431–9.
50. Pearson GD, et al. Report of the National Heart, Lung, and Blood Institute and National Marfan Foundation Working Group on research in Marfan syndrome and related disorders. Circulation. 2008;118(7):785–91.
51. Cheng A, Owens D. Marfan syndrome, inherited aortopathies and exercise: what is the right answer? Heart. 2015;101(10):752–7.
52. Elefteriades JA. Natural history of thoracic aortic aneurysms: indications for surgery, and surgical versus nonsurgical risks. Ann Thorac Surg. 2002;74(5):S1877–80. discussion S1892–8
53. Donaldson RM, Ross DN. Composite graft replacement for the treatment of aneurysms of the ascending aorta associated with aortic valvular disease. Circulation. 1982;66(2 Pt 2):I116–21.
54. Greenberg RK, et al. Hybrid approaches to thoracic aortic aneurysms: the role of endovascular elephant trunk completion. Circulation. 2005;112(17):2619–26.
55. Augoustides JG, et al. Observational study of mortality risk stratification by ischemic presentation in patients with acute type A aortic dissection: the Penn classification. Nat Clin Pract Cardiovasc Med. 2009;6(2):140–6.
56. El-Hamamsy I, et al. State-of-the-art surgical management of acute type A aortic dissection. Can J Cardiol. 2016;32(1):100–9.

Genetics and Genomics of Coronary Artery Disease

22

Yoshiji Yamada and Yoshiki Yasukochi

Abstract

Coronary artery disease (CAD) is an important clinical problem because of its large contribution to mortality. Disease prevention is an important strategy for reducing the overall burden of CAD, with the identification of markers for disease risk being key both for risk prediction and for potential intervention to lower the chance of future cardiovascular events. Recent genome-wide association studies (GWAS) demonstrated that single nucleotide polymorphisms at chromosome 9p21.3 or other loci were associated with CAD. In this review, we summarize genetics of CAD and susceptibility loci and genes for this condition identified by GWASs. We also review in more detail studies that have revealed the association with CAD of genetic variants at chromosome 9p21.3 identified by GWASs. Such studies may provide insight into the function of implicated genes as well as into the role of genetic factors in the development of CAD.

Keywords

Coronary artery disease • Myocardial infarction • Genetics • Genomics Polymorphism • Genetic variant • Genome-wide association study

Y. Yamada (✉)
Department of Human Functional Genomics, Advanced Science Research Promotion Center, Mie University, Tsu, Mie, Japan

Department of Medical Genomics and Proteomics, Institute of Basic Sciences, Mie University Graduate School of Medicine, Tsu, Mie, Japan

Research Center for Genomic Medicine, Mie University, Tsu, Mie, Japan
e-mail: yamada@gene.mie-u.ac.jp

Y. Yasukochi
Department of Human Functional Genomics, Advanced Science Research Promotion Center, Mie University, Tsu, Mie, Japan
e-mail: hyasukou@proof.ocn.ne.jp, yasukouchi@gene.mie-u.ac.jp

D. Kumar, P. Elliott (eds.), *Cardiovascular Genetics and Genomics*,
https://doi.org/10.1007/978-3-319-66114-8_22

22.1 Introduction

Recent progress in human genetics and genomics research, highlighted by completion of the nucleotide sequences of the human genome by the Human Genome Project [1], has provided substantial benefits to clinical medicine, including facilitation of the characterization of disease pathogenesis at the molecular level and the development of panels of genetic markers for assessment of disease risk. In particular, determination of single nucleotide polymorphisms (SNPs) and haplotype blocks and the specification of tag SNPs in each haplotype block for diverse ethnic groups by the International HapMap Project [2] have led to increasingly effective approaches to the identification of genetic variation associated with various multifactorial diseases, providing new insight into the pathogenesis of these conditions. Furthermore, technological developments such as microarrays analyzing gene expression, genotypes of SNPs, or DNA methylation that provide huge amounts of genetic information have made possible the detection of genetic differences among individuals at the whole-genome level.

Selection of the most appropriate strategies for disease prevention or therapy on the basis of genetic information for a given individual is referred to as personalized or precision medicine. In conventional medicine, medications are prescribed on the basis of the diagnosis and severity of the disease. However, the efficacy of drugs and the incidence of side effects vary among individuals. The goal of treatment based on genetic or genomic information is to be able to predict therapeutic outcome or side effects in an individual, thereby increasing the effectiveness and safety of therapy. In addition, the clarification of disease etiologies at the molecular level and the identification of genetic variants that confer disease susceptibility are likely to contribute both to disease prevention and to the development of new medicines.

Coronary artery disease (CAD) is a serious clinical problem because of its large contribution to mortality. In the United States, the total numbers of individuals affected by CAD or myocardial infarction (MI) in 2012 were 15.5 million and 7.6 million, respectively. The annual incidence of new or recurrent MI or ultimately fatal CAD was 965,000, with an annual mortality of 370,213 from these conditions, in 2013 [3]. Despite recent advances in therapy, such as drug-eluting stents [4] for acute coronary syndrome, CAD remains the leading cause of death in the United States [3]. Disease prevention is an important strategy for reducing the overall burden of CAD, and the identification of biomarkers for disease risk is key both for risk prediction and for potential intervention to reduce the chance of future coronary events.

The main causal and treatable risk factors for CAD include hypertension, diabetes mellitus, dyslipidemia, chronic kidney disease, obesity, and smoking. In addition to these risk factors, recent studies have highlighted the importance of genetic factors and of interactions between multiple genes and environmental factors in this condition [5, 6]. The heritability of CAD was estimated to be 40–50% on the basis of family and twin studies [7]. The common forms of CAD are thus thought to be multifactorial and to be determined by many genes, each with a relatively small effect, working alone or in combination with modifier genes or environmental factors (or both). The "common disease, common variants hypothesis" proposes that genetic variants present in many normal individuals contribute to overall CAD risk. In addition, susceptibility to CAD may be conferred, in part, by rarer variants [8].

22.2 Familial Aggregation of CAD

Twin and family studies have established that CAD aggregates in families, with a family history of early-onset CAD having long been considered a risk factor for the disease [9]. The familial clustering of CAD might be explained in part by heritable quantitative variation in known CAD risk factors. However, evidence suggests that family history contributes to an increased risk of CAD independently of the known risk factors [10, 11]. High-risk families account for a substantial proportion of early-onset CAD cases in the general population [12]. A history of early-onset CAD in a first-degree relative approximately doubles a person's risk of CAD, although the reported relative risk ranges from 1.3 to 11.3 [11, 13–15]. The highest relative hazard of CAD-related death is seen in monozygotic twins, when one twin dies of early-onset CAD [11]. Furthermore, sibling history of MI seems to be a greater risk factor than parental history of early-onset CAD [16]. A family risk score for CAD has been proposed to evaluate the ratio of observed CAD events to expected events in an individual's first-degree relatives, with adjustment for age and sex at the onset of the first event [17]. A higher family risk score is associated with greater CAD risk [18].

22.3 CAD and MI Associated with Mendelian Disorders

Genes responsible for familial hypercholesterolemia and Tangier disease are the prototypical examples of causal genes for CAD and MI associated with Mendelian disorders. Familial hypercholesterolemia is an autosomal dominant disorder characterized by pronounced increases in the serum concentrations of total cholesterol and low density lipoprotein (LDL)–cholesterol. Cholesterol deposition accounts for the associated findings, which include tendon xanthomas and markedly increase the risk for CAD and MI. One of the underlying causes of familial hypercholesterolemia is a defect in the LDL receptor, which is responsible for the uptake of most circulating LDL-cholesterol by the liver. Familial hypercholesterolemia is an uncommon disorder, and homozygosity for an associated mutation results in exceptionally high LDL-cholesterol levels that lead to progressive CAD and MI in the first decade of life. In addition to mutations of the LDL receptor gene (*LDLR*), familial hypercholesterolemia can be caused by mutations in the apolipoprotein B100 gene (*APOB*), proprotein convertase subtilisin/kexin type 9 gene (*PCSK9*), cytochrome P450, family 7, subfamily A, polypeptide 1 gene (*CYP7A1*), and LDL receptor adaptor protein 1 gene (*ARH*). Studies of the molecular basis of familial hypercholesterolemia led to identification of the pathways of LDL-cholesterol metabolism and the subsequent development of HMG-CoA reductase inhibitors, statins [8, 18–22].

Rare allelic variants of genes thought to influence high density lipoprotein (HDL)–cholesterol metabolism, including those for ATP-binding cassette, subfamily A, member 1 (*ABCA1*), apolipoprotein A-I (*APOA1*), and lecithin-cholesterol acyltransferase (*LCAT*), are associated with syndromes characterized by a low plasma concentration of HDL-cholesterol but are also found in individuals from the general population with low HDL-cholesterol levels [23, 24]. Tangier disease is a rare autosomal recessive disorder characterized by diffuse deposition of cholesterol esters throughout the reticuloendothelial system and by the classic manifestation of enlarged yellow tonsils. Affected individuals have low plasma HDL-cholesterol levels as a result of loss-of-function mutations in *ABCA1* [25–27]. In families affected by Tangier disease, the onset of CAD occurs substantially earlier in mutation carriers than in noncarriers [28, 29]. The increased incidence of early-onset CAD in *ABCA1* mutation carriers is likely attributable to the accumulation of lipid-laden macrophage foam cells in the vascular wall and the consequent development and progression of atherosclerosis [30].

The genes for familial hypercholesterolemia and Tangier disease were identified by linkage analysis, given that each condition segregates in a Mendelian pattern with a clear marker for the presence of the mutant gene. Clinical genetic testing is available for both of these disorders. The efficacy of testing is limited, however, to confirmation of the clinical diagnosis in an individual with an abnormal lipid profile or to prenatal diagnosis. The real power of genetic testing is to identify at-risk individuals who cannot otherwise be identified because they lack other clinical or laboratory markers [20]. Several Mendelian disorders of lipid metabolism associated with increased CAD risk have yielded new insight into the mechanisms of CAD. The examination of disease pathogenesis and gene function in such Mendelian disorders may increase our understanding of the etiology of complex traits [31]. In addition, common variation in genes implicated in Mendelian disorders might be used to determine disease susceptibility in the general population [18].

22.4 Strategies for Genetic Analysis of CAD

There are two basic strategies for identifying genes that influence the predisposition to CAD: linkage analyses and association studies (Fig. 22.1). Linkage analysis involves the proposition of a model to account for the pattern of inheritance of a phenotype observed in a pedigree. It determines whether the phenotypic locus is transmitted together with genetic markers of known chromosomal position [32]. Linkage analysis is an effective means to identify highly penetrant genetic variants responsible for the disease in large multigenerational families that include many affected individuals with a Mendelian or Mendelian-like mode of inheritance. The power of linkage analysis, however, is limited in detection of genetic variants with low to moderate effects for multigene disorders with a low family penetrance. Association studies determine whether a certain allele occurs at a frequency higher than that expected by chance in individuals with a particular phenotype. Such an association is thus suggested by a statistically significant difference in the

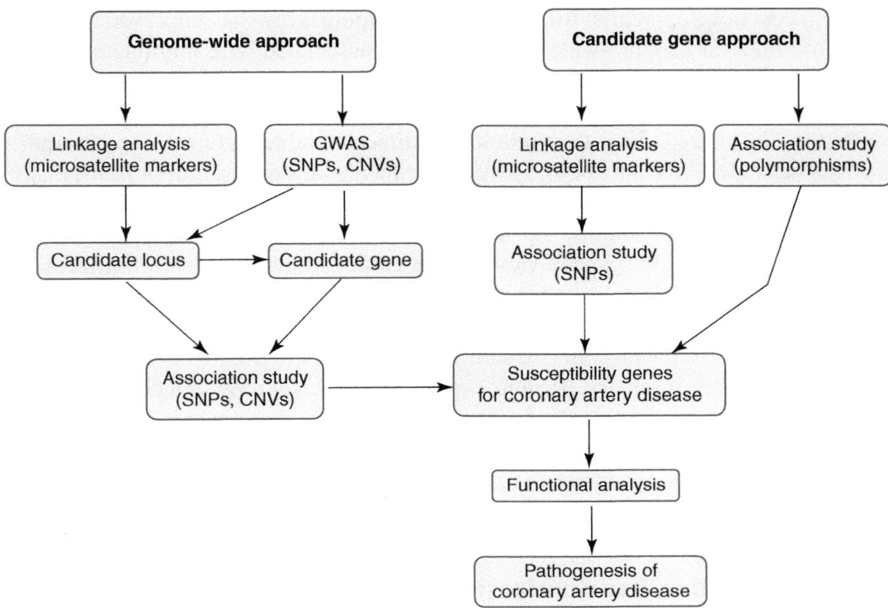

Fig. 22.1 Strategies for identifying susceptibility genes for coronary artery disease. There are two basic strategies for identifying genes that influence coronary artery disease or myocardial infarction, the genome-wide approach and the candidate gene approach, both of which rely on linkage analyses and association studies. In the genome-wide association study (GWAS), single nucleotide polymorphisms (SNPs) or copy number variations (CNVs) distributed throughout the entire genome are used to identify genomic regions that harbor genes that influence the trait of interest with a detectable effect size. The candidate gene approach involves the direct examination of whether an individual gene or genes might contribute to the trait of interest

prevalence of alleles with respect to the phenotype [33]. Association studies consisted of two strategies: the candidate gene approach and the genome-wide approach [34]. The candidate gene approach involves the direct examination of whether an individual gene or genes might contribute to the trait of interest. This strategy has been widely applied to analysis of the possible association between genetic variants and disease outcome, with genes selected on the basis of a priori hypotheses regarding their potential etiologic role. It is characterized as a hypothesis-testing approach because of the biological observation supporting the proposed candidate gene. The candidate gene approach is not able, however, to identify disease-associated polymorphisms in unknown genes. Numerous candidate genes and SNPs have been implicated, but those that show reproducible associations between risk allele and CAD or MI in replication studies are few. In the genome-wide approach, single nucleotide polymorphisms (SNPs) or copy number variations (CNVs) distributed throughout the entire genome are used to identify genomic regions that harbor genes that influence the trait of interest with a detectable effect size. This is a hypothesis-generating approach, allowing the detection of previously unknown potential trait loci.

The recent development of high-density genotyping arrays has improved the resolution of unbiased genome-wide scans for SNPs associated with multifactorial diseases [35]. Currently, the genome-wide association study (GWAS) makes use of high-throughput genotyping technologies that include up to 4.5 million markers for SNPs and CNVs to examine their relation to clinical conditions or measurable traits. GWASs have identified a lot of SNPs associated with various diseases or traits, many in genes not previously suspected of having a role in the condition studied, and some in genomic regions containing no known genes. GWASs represent a substantial advance in the search for genetic variants that confer susceptibility to multifactorial polygenic diseases. GWASs, however, had disadvantages that previously available marker sets were designed to identify common alleles [minor allele frequency (MAF) of ≥5%] and were not well suited to study the effects of low-frequency and rare variants within a gene of interest. Recent exome or whole genome sequencing studies have successfully uncovered a lot of low-frequency and rare variants and have systematically evaluated their associations with complex traits [36, 37]. A more cost-effective genotyping exome array including common, low-frequency, and rare variants were also used to perform exome-wide association studies [38].

22.5 Mendelian Randomization

Mendelian randomization analysis is a relatively recent development in genetic epidemiology based on Mendel's second law, which states that the inheritance of one trait is independent of that of other traits [39, 40]. It relies on common genetic polymorphisms that are known to influence exposure patterns (such as the propensity to drink alcohol) or to have effects equivalent to those produced by modifiable exposures (such as an increased serum cholesterol concentration). Associations between genetic variants and outcomes are not generally confounded by behavioral or environmental exposures, with the result that observational studies of genetic variants have similar properties to intention to treat analyses in randomized controlled trials. The simplest way of appreciating the potential of Mendelian randomization analysis is to consider applications of the underlying principles. The inferences that can be drawn from Mendelian randomization studies depend on the different ways in which genetic variants can serve as a proxy for environmentally modifiable exposures [41].

Key Points

- Twin and family studies have established that CAD aggregates in families, with a family history of early-onset CAD being considered a risk factor for the disease.
- Genes responsible for familial hypercholesterolemia and Tangier disease are the prototypical examples of causal genes for CAD and MI associated with Mendelian disorders.
- Genome-wide association studies have identified genetic variations that confer susceptibility to many common complex diseases.
- Mendelian randomization analysis is based on Mendel's second law, which states that the inheritance of one trait is independent of that of other traits.

22.6 GWAS of CAD or MI

Recent GWASs in European ancestry populations [42–49], African Americans [50], or Han Chinese [51, 52] have identified various genes and loci that confer susceptibility to CAD or MI. A meta-analysis of GWASs for CAD in European ancestry populations identified 46 loci with a genome-wide significance level and 104 variants at a false discovery rate of <5% [53]. These genetic variants typically have a MAF of ≥5% and a small individual effect size, and they collectively account for only ~10.6% of the heritability of CAD [53]. A more recent meta-analysis for CAD among European ancestry populations that included low-frequency (0.5% ≤ MAF < 5%) variants identified 58 loci with a genome-wide significance level and 202 independent variants at a false discovery rate of <5% [54]. These genetic variants together account for ~28% of the heritability of CAD, showing that genetic susceptibility to this condition is largely determined by common variants with small effect sizes [54, 55]. The GWASs and meta-analyses of GWASs have implicated chromosome 9p21.3 as well as various other loci and genes in predisposition to CAD or MI mainly in Caucasian populations. The published results of GWASs for CAD or MI [53, 54] are summarized in Table 22.1. In the following sections, the CDKN2B antisense RNA 1 gene (*CDKN2B-AS1*) located at chromosome 9p21.3 that was identified by GWASs and the proprotein convertase subtilisin/kexin type 9 gene (*PCSK9*) that was of particular interest in the genetics of CAD are reviewed.

Table 22.1 Chromosomal loci, genes, and SNPs shown to be associated with coronary artery disease or myocardial infarction by meta-analyses of genome-wide association studies [53, 54]

Chromosomal locus	Gene	SNP	Nucleotide (aminoacid) substitution
1p32.2	*PLPP3*	rs17114036	G→A
1p32		rs11206510	C→T
1p24		rs515135	G→A
1p21	*CELSR2*	rs646776	A→G
1q21	*IL6R*	rs4845625	C→T
1q42	*TAF1A*	rs17464857	T→G
2p24		rs16986953	G→A
2p21	*ABCG8*	rs6544713	C→T
2p11.2	*VAMP5*	rs1561198	A→G
2q22.3	*TEX41*	rs2252641	G→A
2q33.2	*WDR12*	rs6725887	C→T
3q22.3	*MRAS*	rs9818870	T→C
4q12	*NOA1*	rs17087335	G→T
4q31.2		rs1878406	C→T
4q32.1	*GUCY1A3*	rs7692387	G→A
5q31.1	*SLC22A4*	rs273909	T→C
6p24.1	*PHACTR1*	rs12526453	C→G
6p24.1	*ADTRP*	rs6903956	A→G
6p21.31	*ANKS1A*	rs17609940	G→C

(continued)

Table 22.1 (continued)

Chromosomal locus	Gene	SNP	Nucleotide (aminoacid) substitution
6p21	*KCNK5*	rs10947789	T→C
6q23.2	*TCF21*	rs12190287	C→G
6q25.3	*SLC22A3*	rs2048327	A→G
6q26	*PLG*	rs4252120	T→C
7p21.1	*HDAC9*	rs2023938	A→G
7q22.3	*BCAP29*	rs10953541	C→T
7q32.2	*ZC3HC1*	rs11556924	C→T (Arg→His)
7q36	*NOS3*	rs3918226	C→T
8p22	*LPL*	rs264	G→A
8q24.1		rs2954029	A→T
9p21	*CDKN2B*	rs3217992	G→A
9q34.2		rs579459	C→T
10p11.23	*KIAA1462*	rs2505083	T→C
10q11.21		rs2047009	A→C
10q23.2-q23.3	*LIPA*	rs11203042	C→T
10q24.32	*CNNM2*	rs12413409	G→A
11p15	*SWAP70*	rs10840293	G→A
11q22.3		rs974819	A→G
11q23.3	*ZPR1*	rs964184	C→G
12q21.3	*ATP2B1*	rs7136259	T→C
12q24	*SH2B3*	rs3184504	C→T (Arg→Trp)
12q24.22-q24.23	*KSR2*	rs11830157	T→G
13q12	*FLT1*	rs9319428	G→A
13q34	*COL4A1*	rs4773144	G→A
14q32	*HHIPL1*	rs2895811	T→C
15q22.33	*SMAD3*	rs56062135	C→T
15q25		rs7173743	C→T
15q26.1		rs8042271	G→A
15q26.1	*FURIN*	rs17514846	A→C
17p13.3	*SMG6*	rs216172	C→G
17p11.2		rs12936587	A→G
17q21.32	*UBE2Z*	rs46522	C→T
17q23	*BCAS3*	rs7212798	C→T
18q21.3		rs663129	C→T
19q13	*TOMM40*	rs2075650	G→A
19q13.11	*LOC400684*	rs12976411	A→T
19p13.2	*SMARCA4*	rs1122608	G→T
21q22.1		rs9982601	C→T
22q11.22	*POM121L9P*	rs180803	C→A

22.6.1 Chromosome 9p21.3 (*CDKN2B-AS1*)

Independent GWASs based on the use of SNP microarrays identified five SNPs on chromosome 9p21.3 that were associated with CAD or MI in several white cohorts [44, 45, 47, 49]. McPherson et al. [45] identified two susceptibility SNPs (rs10757274, rs2383206) that were located within 20 kbp of each other on chromosome 9p21.3 and were associated with CAD in a Canadian population and five other white cohorts. Helgadottir et al. [44] described an association between MI and two SNPs (rs2383207, rs10757278) located in the same 9p21.3 region in an Icelandic population, and they replicated the finding in four white cohorts. The same genetic locus (rs1333049) was also identified by a GWAS performed with 1926 CAD cases and 3000 controls from a British population [49], and the finding (rs1333049) was replicated in a German population [47]. This locus was then shown to be associated with ischemic stroke [56, 57]. Interestingly, the independent population-based case-control studies also identified several SNPs at 9p21.3 that were significantly associated with type 2 diabetes mellitus in white populations in England [58], Finland [59], and Sweden [60]. In addition to MI, a SNP rs10757278 at this locus was found to be associated with abdominal aortic aneurysm and intracranial aneurysm [61]. Schunkert et al. [62] genotyped rs1333049 (C→G) representing the 9p21.3 locus in seven case-control studies including a total of 4645 subjects with MI or CAD and 5177 controls. The risk allele (*C*) of this SNP was uniformly associated with MI or CAD in each study, with pooled analysis revealing the odds ratio per copy of the risk allele to be 1.29. Meta-analysis of rs1333049 in 12,004 cases and 28,949 controls provided further evidence for association of this SNP with MI or CAD, yielding an odds ratio of 1.24 per risk allele.

Although this broad replication of the association with chromosome 9p21.3 provides important new information on the molecular genetics of CAD and MI, the underlying mechanism is as yet elusive. The region is defined by two flanking recombination hot spots and contains the coding sequences of genes for two cyclin-dependent kinase inhibitors, *CDKN2A* and *CDKN2B* (Fig. 22.2). These genes play an important role in regulation of the cell cycle and belong to a family of genes that have been implicated in the pathogenesis of atherosclerosis as a result of their contribution to inhibition of cell growth by transforming growth factor, beta 1. However, the SNPs associated most strongly with MI or CAD lie considerably upstream of these genes, with the nearest being located 10 kbp upstream of *CDKN2B*. Therefore, other explanations for the association of the 9p21.3 region with MI or CAD was required to be considered [62].

The high-risk CAD haplotype at 9p21.3 [T (rs10116277)–T (rs6475606)–G (rs10738607)–T (rs10757272)–G (rs10757274)–G (rs4977574)–G (rs2891168)–G (rs1333042)–G (rs2383206)–G (rs2383207)–C (rs1333045)–G (rs10757278)–C (rs1333048)–C (rs1333049)] overlapped with CDKN2B antisense RNA 1 (*CDKN2B-AS1*), a large antisense non-protein coding RNA that was identified by

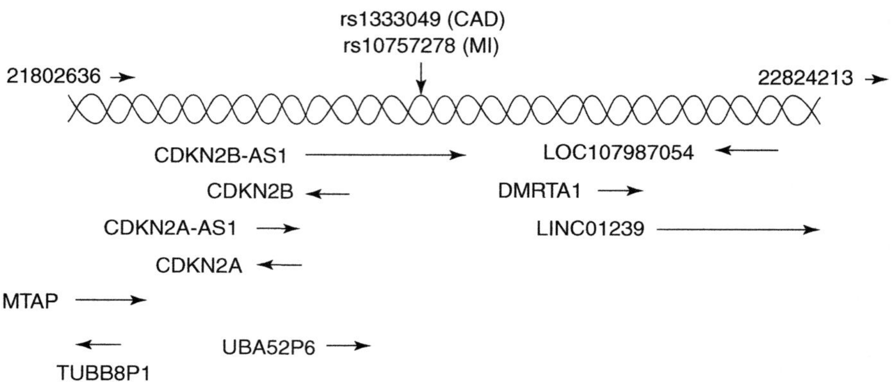

Fig. 22.2 Genomic region at chromosome 9p21.3. The SNPs at 9p21.3 associated with CAD or MI overlap with CDKN2B antisense RNA 1 (*CDKN2B-AS1*), a large antisense non-protein coding RNA

deletion analysis of an extended French family with hereditary melanoma–neural system tumors [63]. Reverse transcription and polymerase chain reaction analysis showed that *CDKN2B-AS1* is expressed in atheromatous human vessels (specimens of abdominal aortic aneurysm or carotid endarterectomy), which manifest a cell type profile similar to that of atherosclerotic coronary arteries. *CDKN2B-AS1* was found to be expressed in vascular endothelial cells, monocyte-derived macrophages, and coronary smooth muscle cells, all of which contribute to atherosclerosis [64].

Conserved noncoding sequence derived from the 9p21.3 risk allele exhibited significantly higher levels of enhancer activity compared to the reference conserved noncoding sequence. The observed difference in the regulatory activity of conserved noncoding sequence is attributable to rs1333045 (C→T) that is in strong linkage disequilibrium with representative SNPs of the previously defined 9p21.3 risk region. These findings indicate that the 9p21.3 risk allele alters activity of regulatory sequence which in turn may lead to changes in expression levels of *CDKN2B-AS1* or other genes relevant to atherosclerosis [65]. Furthermore, SNPs at the 9p21.3 may act as a molecular switch resulting in reciprocal changes in expression levels of the short and long *CDKN2B-AS1* transcripts. The risk allele may modify expression of cell cycle regulatory genes by reducing expression of the long *CDKN2B-AS1* transcript or by increasing expression of the short *CDKN2B-AS1* transcripts, thereby promoting a proliferative phenotype in arterial smooth muscle cells or other cell types relevant to atherosclerosis [65]. *CDKN2B-AS1* also interacts with polycomb repressive complex-1 and -2, leading to epigenetic silencing of other genes in this cluster and to alteration of expression of several genes related to cellular proliferation [65]. These observations suggest that a conserved noncoding sequence at the 9p21.3 locus has enhancer activity and that the risk allele of rs1333045 within conserved noncoding sequence increases transcriptional activity in vascular smooth muscle cells. The allelic variants at the 9p21.3 locus may thus mediate the increased predisposition to CAD or MI by altering expression levels of short and long *CDKN2B-AS1* transcripts, which in turn may affect cellular proliferation pathways [65].

Expression analysis in peripheral blood mononuclear cells revealed that transcripts *EU741058* and *NR_003529* of *CDKN2B-AS1* were increased in carriers of the risk haplotype. In contrast, transcript *DQ485454* remained unaffected, suggesting differential expression of *CDKN2B-AS1* transcripts at 9p21.3. Results were replicated in whole blood and atherosclerotic plaque tissue. Moreover, expression of *CDKN2B-AS1* transcripts (*EU741058*, *NR_003529*) was directly correlated with severity of atherosclerosis. These observations may provide evidence for an association of *CDKN2B-AS1*, but not *CDKN2A*, *CDKN2B*, *C9orf53*, or *MTAP*, with atherosclerosis and 9p21.3 genotype [66].

The 9p21.3 locus has also been associated with platelet reactivity and the increased platelet reactivity may explain the association with MI and ischemic stroke [67]. Visel et al. [68] examined mice deficient of the whole 70 kbp region at 9p21 and observed excessive proliferation of smooth muscle cells and also several neoplasms. These studies confirm that the 9p21 region is a regulator of the cyclin-dependent kinase inhibitors in mice as in humans [68, 69]. Harismendy et al. [70] observed a SNP in a STAT1-binding site located in the 58 kbp DNA region of 9p21. Given that interferon mediates its effect on inflammation, in part through the STAT1 sequence, interferon-γ may mediate the risk of 9p21 for CAD [70]. However, the effects of interferon-γ on CDKN2A/B are independent of the 9p21 risk variant [71]. Furthermore, the effects of type 1 interferon, including interferon-α-21, are not associated with the 9p21 risk variant [69, 72]. Although chromosome 9p21.3 region (*CDKN2B-AS1*) was confirmed to be a susceptibility locus for CAD or MI, the functional mechanisms by which SNPs at this locus confer susceptibility to these conditions have not been determined definitively.

22.6.2 PCSK9

The PCSK9 story is one of successful examples of how human genetic research identify a new therapeutic target and facilitate drug development. Abifadel et al. [73] discovered gain-of-function mutations (Ser127Arg, Phe216Leu) in *PCSK9*, which were associated with hypercholesterolemia and the increased prevalence of CAD. This was followed by a discovery of loss-of-function mutations (Tyr142X, Cys679X) in 2.6% of African-American individuals, which was associated with a 28% reduction in the mean plasma LDL-cholesterol concentration and an 88% reduction in the risk of CAD [74]. This observation demonstrated that a lifelong exposure to a relatively small reduction in plasma LDL-cholesterol levels protect individuals against CAD. PCSK9 increases plasma LDL-cholesterol by binding to the LDL receptor, leading to its degradation. Normally, LDL receptor binds to LDL-cholesterol, then internalizes and transfers LDL-cholesterol for degradation and recycles to the surface, which is prevented by PCSK9. Inhibition of PCSK9 represents a novel approach to lowering the plasma concentrations of LDL-cholesterol, and the most successful agent is a monoclonal antibody against PCSK9 [75, 76]. Inhibition of PCSK9 increases the removal of LDL-cholesterol from the plasma and is complementary to the effect of statin therapy that decreases its production. Thus, inhibition of PCSK9 provides a novel therapy for hyper-LDL-cholesterolemia that is required in the prevention of CAD [69].

Key Points

- Independent GWASs based on the use of SNP microarrays have identified five SNPs on chromosome 9p21.3 that were associated with CAD or MI in several white cohorts. Meta-analysis of rs1333049 provided further evidence for association of this SNP with MI or CAD, yielding an odds ratio of 1.24 per risk allele.
- Although broad replication of the association with chromosome 9p21.3 provides important new information on the molecular genetics of CAD and MI, the underlying mechanism is as yet elusive. Clarification of the functional relevance of SNPs at 9p21.3 to CAD and MI may provide insight into the pathogenesis of these conditions as well as into the role of genetic factors in their development.
- PCSK9 increases plasma LDL-cholesterol levels by binding to the LDL receptor, leading to its degradation. Gain-of-function mutations in PCSK9 were associated with hypercholesterolemia and the increased prevalence of CAD, whereas loss-of-function mutations in this gene were associated with decreases in plasma LDL cholesterol and risk of CAD.

22.7 Exome or Whole-Genome Sequencing Studies for CAD

Previous GWASs and meta-analyses of GWASs have implicated various loci and genes in predisposition to CAD or MI. Most of the genetic variants identified in these studies have a MAF of ≥5% and a small individual effect size. Given that these common variants explain only a fraction of the heritability of CAD and MI, low-frequency (0.5% ≤ MAF < 5%) or rare (MAF < 0.5%) variants with larger effect sizes likely contribute to the genetic architecture of this condition [77]. Technological development of next-generation sequencing have made possible the detection of low-frequency and rare variants in individuals at the whole-exome or -genome level.

Exome sequencing related to CAD has identified low-frequency or rare variants previously established genes involved in lipoprotein metabolism. These genes include those affecting plasma LDL cholesterol concentrations (*PSCK9*, *LDLR*, and *NPC1L1*) or plasma triglyceride levels (*APOA5*, *APOC3*, *LPL*, and *ANGPTL4*) [78–82]. A low-frequency variant in *SVEP1* was associated with CAD through a mechanism of action involves effects on systolic and diastolic blood pressure [79].

Whole-genome sequencing has identified rare loss-of function variants (12-bp deletion in intron 4, Trp158X) in *ASGR1* that are associated with decreases in plasma concentrations of LDL cholesterol and triglycerides and a reduced risk of CAD. These variants disrupt the function of ASGR1 and represent a link between the sialylation pathway and atherosclerotic diseases [83]. Whole-genome sequencing offers the additional benefit of identifying the low-frequency and rare variants in noncoding regulatory regions of an individual's genome. The effects sizes for such noncoding variants are not likely to be greater than those observed for causal variants within exons or common noncoding variants discovered by GWASs [84]. The discovery of loci not previously implicated by GWAS may be particularly challenging [85].

Key Points

- Technological development of next-generation sequencing has made possible the detection of low-frequency and rare variants in individuals at the whole-exome or -genome level.
- Exome sequencing has identified low-frequency or rare variants previously established genes affecting plasma LDL cholesterol concentrations (*PSCK9*, *LDLR*, and *NPC1L1*) or plasma triglyceride levels (*APOA5*, *APOC3*, *LPL*, and *ANGPTL4*).
- Whole-genome sequencing has identified rare loss-of function variants in *ASGR1* that are associated with decreases in plasma concentrations of LDL cholesterol and triglycerides and a reduced risk of CAD.

22.8 Clinical Implication

The increasing body of information garnered from studies on the genetics of CAD has resulted in the emergence of a greater understanding of the etiology of this disease. Such knowledge may have clinical implications for the prevention, diagnosis, prognosis, and treatment of CAD. The genes responsible for the pathogenesis of CAD as well as their encoded proteins are potentially important therapeutic targets in the design of new treatments for the disease. Genetic markers are potential diagnostic tools for assessment of individuals at risk of developing the disease. Genetic markers of the disease together with examination with laboratory or radiological examinations might also form the basis for promotion of preventive therapies in individuals at risk of CAD. It should remember, however, that gene-gene and gene-environment interactions make interpretation of information based on genetic markers of CAD more complex than is that of information based on markers for monogenic disorders. Another use of genetic markers might be to distinguish treatment responders from nonresponders and to identify patients who are at risk of developing unfavorable side effects. It is likely that the use of gene polymorphisms to predict the response to and adverse effects of therapies for CAD will increase in the future and will give rise to major advances in patient care. Genetic analysis of CAD is thus likely to have important direct clinical applications.

Conclusion

In this chapter, CAD and MI associated with single-gene disorders and the susceptibility loci and genes for common forms of these diseases are summarized. There has been a growing effort to find genetic variants that confer risk for CAD and MI as a means to understand the underlying biological events. Clarification of the functional relevance of SNPs at various loci to CAD and MI may provide insight into the pathogenesis of these conditions as well as into the role of genetic factors in their development. Such studies may ultimately lead to the personalized prevention of these conditions. In the future, we may have the ability to use specific agents particularized for certain genetic susceptibility factors, thereby increasing efficacy and limiting side effects of treatment. Identification of susceptibility genes for CAD and MI and clarification of the functional relevance of genetic variants to these conditions will thus contribute to the precision medicine of CAD and MI.

References

1. International Human Genome Sequencing Consortium. Finishing the euchromatic sequence of the human genome. Nature. 2004;431:931–45.
2. International HapMap 3 Consortium, Altshuler DM, Gibbs RA, Peltonen L, Altshuler DM, Gibbs RA, Peltonen L, et al. Integrating common and rare genetic variation in diverse human populations. Nature. 2010;467:52–8.
3. Mozaffarian D, Benjamin EJ, Go AS, Arnett DK, Blaha MJ, Cushman M, American Heart Association Statistics Committee, Stroke Statistics Subcommittee, et al. Heart disease and stroke statistics–2016 update: a report from the American heart association. Circulation. 2016;133:e38–e360.
4. Stefanini GG, Holmes DR Jr. Drug-eluting coronary-artery stents. N Engl J Med. 2013;368:254–65.
5. Topol EJ, Smith J, Plow EF, Wang QK. Genetic susceptibility to myocardial infarction and coronary artery disease. Hum Mol Genet. 2006;15:R117–23.
6. Yamada Y, Ichihara S, Nishida T. Molecular genetics of myocardial infarction. Genome Med. 2008;2:7–22.
7. Peden JF, Farrall M. Thirty-five common variants for coronary artery disease: the fruits of much collaborative labour. Hum Mol Genet. 2011;20:R198–205.
8. Arnett DK, Baird AE, Barkley RA, Basson CT, Boerwinkle E, Ganesh SK, American Heart Association Council on Epidemiology and Prevention, American Heart Association Stroke Council, Functional Genomics and Translational Biology Interdisciplinary Working Group, et al. Relevance of genetics and genomics for prevention and treatment of cardiovascular disease: a scientific statement from the American Heart Association Council on Epidemiology and Prevention, the Stroke Council, and the Functional Genomics and Translational Biology Interdisciplinary Working Group. Circulation. 2007;115:2878–901.
9. Scheuner MT. Genetic evaluation for coronary artery disease. Genet Med. 2003;5:269–85.
10. Murabito JM, Pencina MJ, Nam BH, D'Agostino RB Sr, Wang TJ, Lloyd-Jones D, Wilson PW, O'Donnell CJ. Sibling cardiovascular disease as a risk factor for cardiovascular disease in middle-aged adults. JAMA. 2005;294:3117–23.
11. Yusuf S, Hawken S, Ounpuu S, Dans T, Avezum A, Lanas F, INTERHEART Study Investigators, et al. Effect of potentially modifiable risk factors associated with myocardial infarction in 52 countries (the INTERHEART study): case-control study. Lancet. 2004;364:937–52.

12. Williams RR, Hunt SC, Heiss G, Province MA, Bensen JT, Higgins M, Chamberlain RM, Ware J, Hopkins PN. Usefulness of cardiovascular family history data for population-based preventive medicine and medical research (the Health Family Tree Study and the NHLBI Family Heart Study). Am J Cardiol. 2001;87:129–35.
13. Friedlander Y, Siscovick DS, Weinmann S, Austin MA, Psaty BM, Lemaitre RN, Arbogast P, Raghunathan TE, Cobb LA. Family history as a risk factor for primary cardiac arrest. Circulation. 1998;97:155–60.
14. Kaikkonen KS, Kortelainen ML, Linna E, Huikuri HV. Family history and the risk of sudden cardiac death as a manifestation of an acute coronary event. Circulation. 2006;114:1462–7.
15. Lloyd-Jones DM, Nam BH, D'Agostino RB Sr, Levy D, Murabito JM, Wang TJ, Wilson PW, O'Donnell CJ. Parental cardiovascular disease as a risk factor for cardiovascular disease in middle-aged adults: a prospective study of parents and offspring. JAMA. 2004;291:2204–11.
16. Nasir K, Michos ED, Rumberger JA, Braunstein JB, Post WS, Budoff MJ, Blumenthal RS. Coronary artery calcification and family history of premature coronary heart disease: sibling history is more strongly associated than parental history. Circulation. 2004;110:2150–6.
17. Li R, Bensen JT, Hutchinson RG, Province MA, Hertz-Picciotto I, Sprafka JM, Tyroler HA. Family risk score of coronary heart disease (CHD) as a predictor of CHD: the Atherosclerosis Risk in Communities (ARIC) study and the NHLBI family heart study. Genet Epidemiol. 2000;18:236–50.
18. Kullo IJ, Ding K. Mechanisms of disease: the genetic basis of coronary heart disease. Nat Clin Pract Cardiovasc Med. 2007;4:558–69.
19. Rader DJ, Cohen J, Hobbs HH. Monogenic hypercholesterolemia: new insights in pathogenesis and treatment. J Clin Invest. 2003;111:1795–803.
20. Robin NH, Tabereaux PB, Benza R, Korf BR. Genetic testing in cardiovascular disease. J Am Coll Cardiol. 2007;50:727–37.
21. Soutar AK, Naoumova RP. Mechanism of disease: genetic causes of familial hypercholesterolemia. Nat Clin Pract Cardiovasc Med. 2007;4:214–25.
22. Goldstein JL, Brown MS. Familial Hypercholesterolemia: Identification of a Defect in the Regulation of 3-Hydroxy-3-Methylglutaryl Coenzyme A Reductase Activity Associated with Overproduction of Cholesterol. PNAS 70(10):2804–8.
23. Cohen JC, Kiss RS, Pertsemlidis A, Marcel YL, McPherson R, Hobbs HH. Multiple rare alleles contribute to low plasma levels of HDL cholesterol. Science. 2004;305:869–72.
24. Frikke-Schmidt R, Nordestgaard BG, Jensen GB, Tybjaerg-Hansen A. Genetic variation in ABC transporter A1 contributes to HDL cholesterol in the general population. J Clin Invest. 2004;114:1343–53.
25. Bodzioch M, Orso E, Klucken J, Langmann T, Böttcher A, Diederich W, et al. The gene encoding ATP-binding cassette transporter 1 is mutated in Tangier disease. Nat Genet. 1999;22:347–51.
26. Brooks-Wilson A, Marcil M, Clee SM, Zhang LH, Roomp K, van Dam M, et al. Mutations in ABC1 in Tangier disease and familial high-density lipoprotein deficiency. Nat Genet. 1999;22:336–45.
27. Rust S, Rosier M, Funke H, Real J, Amoura Z, Piette JC, Deleuze JF, et al. Tangier disease is caused by mutations in the gene encoding ATP-binding cassette transporter 1. Nat Genet. 1999;22:352–5.
28. Clee SM, Kastelein JJ, van Dam M, Marcil M, Roomp K, Zwarts KY, et al. Age and residual cholesterol efflux affect HDL cholesterol levels and coronary artery disease in ABCA1 heterozygotes. J Clin Invest. 2000;106:1263–70.
29. van Dam MJ, de Groot GE, Clee SM, Hovingh GK, Roelants R, Brooks-Wilson A, et al. Association between increased arterial-wall thickness and impairment in ABCA1-driven cholesterol efflux: an observational study. Lancet. 2002;359:37–42.
30. Oram JF, Heinecke JW. ATP-binding cassette transporter A1: a cell cholesterol exporter that protects against cardiovascular disease. Physiol Rev. 2005;85:1343–72.
31. Antonarakis SE, Beckmann JS. Mendelian disorders deserve more attention. Nat Rev. Genet. 2006;7:277–82.

32. Ott J, Wang J, Leal SM. Genetic linkage analysis in the age of whole-genome sequencing. Nat Rev. Genet. 2015;16:275–84.
33. Cordell HJ, Clayton DG. Genetic association studies. Lancet. 2005;366:1121–31.
34. Lunetta KL. Genetic association studies. Circulation. 2008;118:96–101.
35. Hirschhorn JN, Daly MJ. Genome-wide association studies for common diseases and complex traits. Nat Rev. Genet. 2005;6:95–108.
36. Helgadottir A, Gretarsdottir S, Thorleifsson G, Hjartarson E, Sigurdsson A, Magnusdottir A, et al. Variants with large effects on blood lipids and the role of cholesterol and triglycerides in coronary disease. Nat Genet. 2016;48:634–9.
37. Lek M, Karczewski KJ, Minikel EV, Samocha KE, Banks E, Fennell T, Exome Aggregation Consortium, et al. Analysis of protein-coding genetic variation in 60,706 humans. Nature. 2016;536:285–91.
38. Yamada Y, Sakuma J, Takeuchi I, Yasukochi Y, Kato K, Oguri M, et al. Identification of STXBP2 as a novel susceptibility locus for myocardial infarction in Japanese individuals by an exome-wide association study. Oncotarget. 2017;8:33527–35.
39. Davey Smith G, Ebrahim S. "Mendelian randomization": Can genetic epidemiology contribute to understanding environmental causes of disease? Int J Epidemiol. 2003;32:1–22.
40. Keavney B. Genetic epidemiological studies of coronary heart disease. Int J Epidemiol. 2002;31:730–6.
41. Davey Smith G, Ebrahim S. What can mendelian randomization tell us about modifiable behavioural and environmental exposures? Br Med J. 2005;330:1076–9.
42. Coronary Artery Disease (C4D) Genetics Consortium, Steering and Writing Committee, Peden JF, Hopewell JC, Saleheen D, Chambers JC, Hager J, Soranzo N, Statistical Genetics and Bioinformatics, Goel A, Ongen H, Strawbridge RJ, Heath S, Mälarstig A, Helgadottir A, The MuTHER consortium, Eriksson P, Discovery cohorts, Offer A, Bowman L, Sleight P, Armitage J, Peto R, Abecasis G, Ahmed N, Replication cohorts, Spector T, Peltonen L, Nieminen MS, Sinisalo J, Salomaa V, Ripatti S, Bennett D, Leander K, et al. A genome-wide association study in Europeans and South Asians identifies five new loci for coronary artery disease. Nat Genet. 2011;43:339–44.
43. Erdmann J, Willenborg C, Nahrstaedt J, Preuss M, König IR, Baumert J, et al. Genome-wide association study identifies a new locus for coronary artery disease on chromosome 10p11.23. Eur Heart J. 2011;32:158–68.
44. Helgadottir A, Thorleifsson G, Manolescu A, Gretarsdottir S, Blondal T, Jonasdottir A, et al. A common variant on chromosome 9p21 affects the risk of myocardial infarction. Science. 2007;316:1491–3.
45. McPherson R, Pertsemlidis A, Kavaslar N, Stewart A, Roberts R, Cox DR, et al. A common allele on chromosome 9 associated with coronary heart disease. Science. 2007;316: 1488–91.
46. Reilly MP, Li M, He J, Ferguson JF, Stylianou IM, Mehta NN, et al. Identification of ADAMTS7 as a novel locus for coronary atherosclerosis and association of ABO with myocardial infarction in the presence of coronary atherosclerosis: two genome-wide association studies. Lancet. 2011;377:383–92.
47. Samani NJ, Erdmann J, Hall AS, Hengstenberg C, Mangino M, Mayer B, WTCCC and the Cardiogenics Consortium, et al. Genomewide association analysis of coronary artery disease. N Engl J Med. 2007;357:443–53.
48. Schunkert H, König IR, Kathiresan S, Reilly MP, Assimes TL, Holm H, CARDIoGRAM Consortium, Samani NJ, et al. Large-scale association analysis identifies 13 new susceptibility loci for coronary artery disease. Nat Genet. 2011;43:333–8.
49. Wellcome Trust Case Control Consortium. Genome-wide association study of 14,000 cases of seven common diseases and 3,000 shared controls. Nature. 2007;447:661–78.
50. Lettre G, Palmer CD, Young T, Ejebe KG, Allayee H, et al. Genome-wide association study of coronary heart disease and its risk factors in 8,090 African Americans: the NHLBI CARe Project. PLoS Genet. 2011;7:e1001300.
51. Lu X, Wang L, Chen S, He L, Yang X, Shi Y, Cheng J, Coronary ARtery DIsease Genome-Wide Replication And Meta-Analysis (CARDIoGRAM) Consortium, Peng X, Wu X, Liu D,

Yang Y, Chen R, Qiang B, Gu D. Genome-wide association study in Han Chinese identifies four new susceptibility loci for coronary artery disease. Nat Genet. 2012;44:890–4.

52. Wang F, CQ X, He Q, Cai JP, Li XC, Wang D, et al. Genome-wide association identifies a susceptibility locus for coronary artery disease in the Chinese Han population. Nat Genet. 2011;43:345–9.
53. CARDIoGRAMplusC4D Consortium, Deloukas P, Kanoni S, Willenborg C, Farrall M, Assimes TL, Thompson JR, DIAGRAM Consortium, CARDIOGENICS Consortium, MuTHER Consortium, Nikus K, Peden JF, Rayner NW, Rasheed A, Rosinger S, Rubin D, et al. Large-scale association analysis identifies new risk loci for coronary artery disease. Nat Genet. 2013;45:25–33.
54. Nikpay M, Goel A, Won HH, Hall LM, Willenborg C, Kanoni S, CARDIoGRAMplusC4D Consortium, et al. A comprehensive 1000 Genomes-based genome-wide association meta-analysis of coronary artery disease. Nat Genet. 2015;47:1121–30.
55. McPherson R, Tybjaerg-Hansen A. Genetics of coronary artery disease. Circ Res. 2016;118:564–78.
56. Gschwendtner A, Bevan S, Cole JW, Plourde A, Matarin M, Ross-Adams H, International Stroke Genetics Consortium, et al. Sequence variants on chromosome 9p21.3 confer risk for atherosclerotic stroke. Ann Neurol. 2009;65:531–9.
57. Matarin M, Brown WM, Singleton A, Hardy JA, Meschia JF, ISGS investigators. Whole genome analyses suggest ischemic stroke and heart disease share an association with polymorphisms on chromosome 9p21. Stroke. 2008;39:1586–9.
58. Zeggini E, Weedon MN, Lindgren CM, Frayling TM, Elliott KS, Lango H, Wellcome Trust Case-Control Consortium (WTCCC), McCarthy MI, Hattersley AT, et al. Replication of genome-wide association signals in UK samples reveals risk loci for type 2 diabetes. Science. 2007;316:1336–41.
59. Scott LJ, Mohlke KL, Bonnycastle LL, Willer CJ, Li Y, Duren WL, Erdos MR, et al. A genome-wide association study of type 2 diabetes in Finns detects multiple susceptibility variants. Science. 2007;316:1341–5.
60. Saxena R, Voight BF, Lyssenko V, Burtt NP, de Bakker PI, Chen H, et al. Genome-wide association analysis identifies loci for type 2 diabetes and triglyceride levels. Science. 2007;316:1331–6.
61. Helgadottir A, Thorleifsson G, Magnusson KP, Grétarsdottir S, Steinthorsdottir V, Manolescu A, et al. The same sequence variant on 9p21 associates with myocardial infarction, abdominal aortic aneurysm and intracranial aneurysm. Nat Genet. 2008;40:217–24.
62. Schunkert H, Götz A, Braund P, McGinnis R, Tregouet DA, Mangino M, Cardiogenics Consortium, et al. Repeated replication and a prospective meta-analysis of the association between chromosome 9p21.3 and coronary artery disease. Circulation. 2008;117:1675–84.
63. Pasmant E, Laurendeau I, Heron D, Vidaud M, Vidaud D, Bieche I. Characterization of a germ-line deletion, including the entire INK4/ARF locus, in a melanoma-neural system tumor family: identification of ANRIL, an antisense noncoding RNA whose expression coclusters with ARF. Cancer Res. 2007;67:3963–9.
64. Broadbent HM, Peden JF, Lorkowski S, Goel A, Ongen H, Green F, PROCARDIS consortium, et al. Susceptibility to coronary artery disease and diabetes is encoded by distinct, tightly linked SNPs in the ANRIL locus on chromosome 9p. Hum Mol Genet. 2008;17:806–14.
65. Jarinova O, Stewart AF, Roberts R, Wells G, Lau P, Naing T, et al. Functional analysis of the chromosome 9p21.3 coronary artery disease risk locus. Arterioscler Thromb Vasc Biol. 2009;29:1671–7.
66. Holdt LM, Beutner F, Scholz M, Gielen S, Gäbel G, Bergert H, et al. ANRIL expression is associated with atherosclerosis risk at chromosome 9p21. Arterioscler Thromb Vasc Biol. 2010;30:620–7.
67. Musunuru K, Post WS, Herzog W, Shen H, O'Connell JR, McArdle PF, et al. Association of single nucleotide polymorphisms on chromosome 9p21.3 with platelet reactivity: a potential mechanism for increased vascular disease. Circ Cardiovasc Genet. 2010;3:445–53.
68. Visel A, Zhu Y, May D, Afzal V, Gong E, Attanasio C, Blow MJ, Cohen JC, Rubin EM, Pennacchio LA. Targeted deletion of the 9p21 non-coding coronary artery disease risk interval in mice. Nature. 2010;464:409–12.

69. Roberts R. Genetics of coronary artery disease. Circ Res. 2014;114:1890–903.
70. Harismendy O, Notani D, Song X, Rahim NG, Tanasa B, Heintzman N, et al. 9p21 DNA variants associated with coronary artery disease impair interferon-γ signalling response. Nature. 2011;470:264–8.
71. Almontashiri NA, Fan M, Cheng BL, Chen HH, Roberts R, Stewart AF. Interferon-γ activates expression of p15 and p16 regardless of 9p21.3 coronary artery disease risk genotype. J Am Coll Cardiol. 2013;61:143–7.
72. Erridge C, Gracey J, Braund PS, Samani NJ. The 9p21 locus does not affect risk of coronary artery disease through induction of type 1 interferons. J Am Coll Cardiol. 2013;62:1376–81.
73. Abifadel M, Varret M, Rabès JP, Allard D, Ouguerram K, Devillers M, et al. Mutations in PCSK9 cause autosomal dominant hypercholesterolemia. Nat Genet. 2003;34:154–6.
74. Cohen JC, Boerwinkle E, Mosley TH Jr, Hobbs HH. Sequence variations in PCSK9, low LDL, and protection against coronary heart disease. N Engl J Med. 2006;354:1264–72.
75. Kastelein JJ, Nissen SE, Rader DJ, Hovingh GK, Wang MD, Shen T, Krueger KA. Safety and efficacy of LY3015014, a monoclonal antibody to proprotein convertase subtilisin/kexin type 9 (PCSK9): a randomized, placebo-controlled Phase 2 study. Eur Heart J. 2016;37:1360–9.
76. Ni YG, Di Marco S, Condra JH, Peterson LB, Wang W, Wang F, et al. A PCSK9-binding antibody that structurally mimics the EGF(A) domain of LDL-receptor reduces LDL cholesterol in vivo. J Lipid Res. 2011;52:78–86.
77. Manolio TA, Collins FS, Cox NJ, Goldstein DB, Hindorff LA, Hunter DJ, et al. Finding the missing heritability of complex diseases. Nature. 2009;461:747–53.
78. Do R, Stitziel NO, Won HH, Jørgensen AB, Duga S, Angelica Merlini P, NHLBI Exome Sequencing Project, Girelli D, Martinelli N, Farlow DN, MA DP, Roberts R, Stewart AF, et al. Exome sequencing identifies rare LDLR and APOA5 alleles conferring risk for myocardial infarction. Nature. 2015;518:102–6.
79. Myocardial Infarction Genetics and CARDIoGRAM Exome Consortia Investigators, Stitziel NO, Stirrups KE, Masca NG, Erdmann J, Ferrario PG, König IR, et al. Coding variation in ANGPTL4, LPL, and SVEP1 and the risk of coronary disease. N Engl J Med. 2016;374:1134–44.
80. Myocardial Infarction Genetics Consortium Investigators, Stitziel NO, Won HH, Morrison AC, Peloso GM, Do R, Lange LA, Fontanillas P, et al. Inactivating mutations in NPC1L1 and protection from coronary heart disease. N Engl J Med. 2014;371:2072–82.
81. TG and HDL Working Group of the Exome Sequencing Project, National Heart, Lung, and Blood Institute, Crosby J, Peloso GM, Auer PL, Crosslin DR, Stitziel NO, et al. Loss-of-function mutations in APOC3, triglycerides, and coronary disease. N Engl J Med. 2014;371:22–31.
82. Dewey FE, Gusarova V, O'Dushlaine C, Gottesman O, Trejos J, Hunt C, et al. Inactivating variants in ANGPTL4 and risk of coronary artery disease. N Engl J Med. 2016;374:1123–33.
83. Nioi P, Sigurdsson A, Thorleifsson G, Helgason H, Agustsdottir AB, Norddahl GL, et al. Variant ASGR1 Associated with a Reduced Risk of Coronary Artery Disease. N Engl J Med. 2016;374:2131–41.
84. Fuchsberger C, Flannick J, Teslovich TM, Mahajan A, Agarwala V, Gaulton KJ, et al. Familial hypercholesterolemia: identification of a defect in the regulation of 3-hydroxy-3-methylglutaryl coenzyme A reductase activity associated with overproduction of cholesterol. Proc Natl Acad Sci U S A. 1973;70:2804–8.
85. Assimes TL, Roberts R. Genetics: implications for prevention and management of coronary artery disease. J Am Coll Cardiol. 2016;68:2797–818.

Cardiovascular Manifestations of Immune-Mediated Inflammatory Disorders

23

Anna Abou-Raya and Suzan Abou-Raya

Abstract

Chronic immune-mediated inflammatory diseases (IMIDs) are characterized by a high prevalence of cardiovascular disease (CVD) which constitutes the leading cause of morbidity and mortality among such patients. The increase in CV events is attributed mainly to accelerated atherosclerosis and endothelial dysfunction with inflammation providing the pivotal link. The association of IMID with atherosclerosis suggests a common pathogenic mechanism. Genomic and proteomic studies performed on atherosclerotic plaques have confirmed the presence of gene and protein profile similar to that observed in autoimmune diseases with cardiovascular risks. Traditional risk assessment usually underestimates CVD risk in IMID. In IMID inflammation and autoimmunity further promote atherosclerosis. Evidence is accumulating indicating heterogeneity in the vascular involvement underlying different autoimmune rheumatic diseases. Recent research provides evidence that genes explain the higher prevalence of CVD in patients with chronic IMID. Epigenetic mechanisms seem to influence inflammation and CVD associated with IMID. Genomic and proteomic studies will aid to identify novel patterns of biomarkers, while together with the traditional risk factors, the novel non-taditional risk factors might help target better screening.

Keywords

Immune-mediated inflammatory diseases • Atherosclerosis, Cardiovascular disease • Inflammation • Traditional and non- traditional risk factors

A. Abou-Raya (✉) • S. Abou-Raya
Department of Internal Medicine, University of Alexandria Hospital, Alexandria, Egypt
e-mail: annaaraya@yahoo.com; suzanraya@yahoo.com

D. Kumar, P. Elliott (eds.), *Cardiovascular Genetics and Genomics*,
https://doi.org/10.1007/978-3-319-66114-8_23

23.1 Introduction

Chronic immune-mediated inflammatory diseases (IMID) such as Rheumatoid arthritis (RA), Systemic lupus erythematosus (SLE), Anti-phospholipid syndrome (APS), Sjögren's syndrome (SS), Systemic sclerosis (SSc), Psoriatic arthritis (PsA), Sarcoidosis and Vasculitis are characterized by a high prevalence of cardiovascular disease (CVD) which constitutes the leading cause of morbidity and mortality among such patients [1].

The spectrum of cardiovascular manifestations with chronic IMID is wide affecting the myocardium, endocardium including cardiac valves, pericardium and vasculature [1, 2].

An array of clinical studies have shown that chronic IMID have a higher prevalence of cardiovascular events compared to the general population. The increase in CV events is attributed mainly to accelerated atherosclerosis and endothelial dysfunction with inflammation providing the pivotal link [2–4].

Chronic IMID are linked to accelerated premature atherosclerosis. Cardiovascular diseases are chronic diseases associated with an inflammatory component and inflammation is a risk factor for coronary artery disease [5, 6].

Atherosclerosis is now recognized as an autoimmune-inflammatory disease. Both humoral and cellular immune mechanisms have been implicated to participate in the onset and progress of atheromatous lesions [6–9].

Recent genomic and transcriptomic studies have implicated certain cytokines, surface receptors, signalling pathways and cell types in the pathogenesis of inflammatory rheumatic diseases [9, 10]. The association of IMID with atherosclerosis suggests a common pathogenic mechanism. Genomic and proteomic studies performed on atherosclerotic plaques have confirmed the presence of gene and protein profile similar to that observed in autoimmune diseases with cardiovascular risks [11]. Traditional risk assessment usually underestimates CVD risk in IMID. In IMID inflammation and autoimmunity further promote atherosclerosis. Evidence is accumulating indicating heterogeneity in the vascular involvement underlying different autoimmune rheumatic diseases (Fig. 23.1). Epigenetic mechanisms seem to influence inflammation and CVD associated with IMID [12, 13]. The increased understanding of the mechanisms promoting damage has led to a focus on pro-inflammatory pathways. Some of the mechanisms that drive atherosclerotic plaque formation are shared with several autoimmune diseases although each disease may have particular immunologic abberrations.The application of genomic technologies have aided in explaining the common pathophysiological mechanism linking atherosclerosis and CVD in IMID such as RA and SLE [10–14].

Recent research provides evidence that genes explain the higher prevalence of CVD in patients with chronic IMID. The use of genetic profiling, has shown that specific genetic loci that have been linked with CVD risk in the general population have been found to be significantly increased in association with CVD risk among chronic IMID patients, for example the RA risk gene CFLAR-CASP8.These findings represent an important step towards characterising the genetic basis of CVD risk in chronic IMID [14–18].

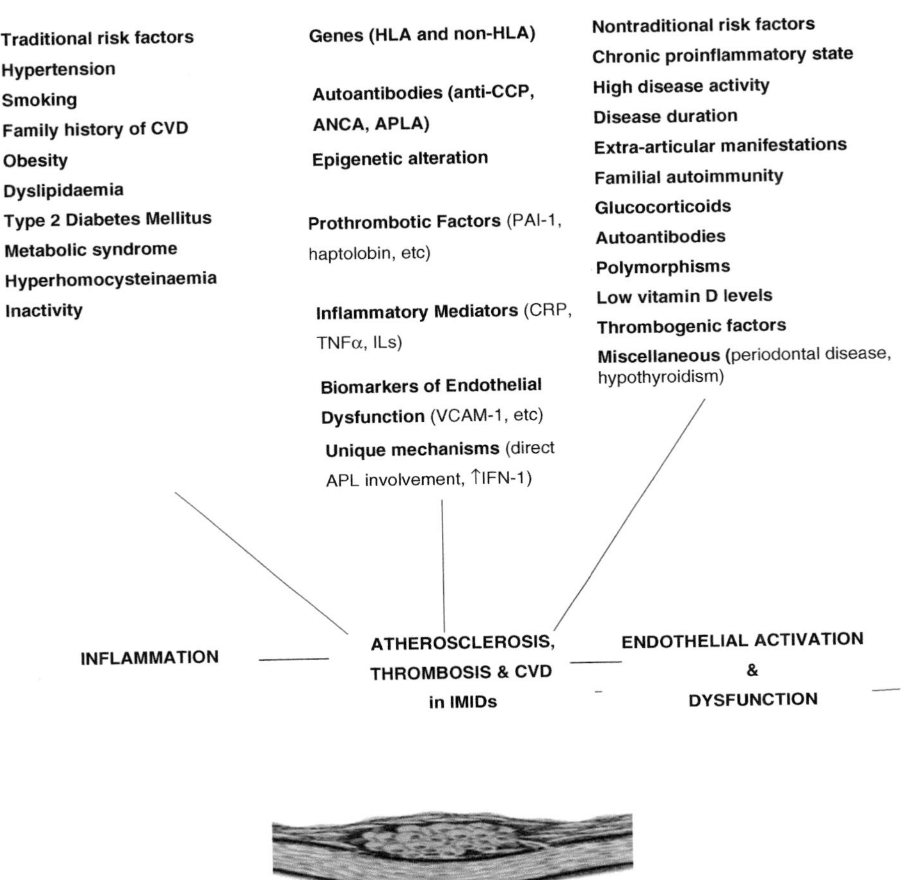

Fig. 23.1 Evidence is accumulating indicating heterogeneity in the vascular involvement underlying different autoimmune rheumatic diseases

23.2 Rheumatoid Arthritis

Cardiovascular disease is the leading cause of death in RA [1]. Ischemic heart disease secondary to atherosclerosis is the most prevalent cause of death associated with CVD in RA [19]. Cardiac involvement in RA also includes pericarditis and commonly coexistent pericardial effusion which can evolve into constrictive pericarditis, increased incidence of congestive heart failure, mitral and aortic valve involvement, rarely heart block and pulmonary hypertension secondary to lung fibrosis [20]. Systemic inflammation is the cornerstone of both RA and atherosclerosis.

Observational studies in RA cohorts with different characteristics report an increased incidence rate for CVD morbidity and mortality. Several studies indicate a double risk compared to the general population which is comparable to the cardiovascular risk in diabetes mellitus [21–23]. Traditional risk factors are incriminated, however traditional risk factors alone do not explain the higher cardiovascular risk in RA.

Cardiovascular risk is increased even before the clinical onset of RA. Studies have demonstrated that the first signs of atherosclerosis exist even before the onset of RA. Furthermore, early signs of atherosclerosis have been found to correlate with systemic inflammatory and disease severity markers [24, 25].

Rheumatoid arthritis and atherosclerosis are both regarded as inflammatory-driven diseases [24]. Epidemiological, clinical and laboratory studies have implicated chronic inflammation and immune dysregulation in RA and atherosclerosis [26, 27].

Yet, another factor that links atherosclerosis to RA is a common genetic background [19]. Several recent investigations report gene polymorphisms that are associated with a higher risk of CVD in RA. HLA-DRB1and CFLAR-CASP8 are examples of genes linked to increased cardiovascular risk in RA [19].

A wide array of subphenotypes and mortality due to CVD occur in RA including coronary artery disease, myocardial infarction (MI), peripheral vascular disease, hypertension, thrombosis and left ventricular diastolic dysfunction; the general prevalence reaching up to 50% [28].

In addition to the traditional risk factors (advanced age, male gender, smoking, obesity, sedentary lifestyle, family history of CVD, obesity, type 2 diabetes mellitus, metabolic syndrome, hypertension, dyslipidaemia and hyperhomocysteinaemia) [29, 30] several nontraditional risk factors are also associated with CVD and RA. HLA-DRB1 shared epitope (SE)- HLA-DRB1 alleles are related to chronic inflammation, high disease activity, endothelial dysfunction, increase in cardiovascular events, atherosclerotic plaques and premature mortality [29–33]. Being a carrier of a single copy of HLA-DRB1 SE is associated with increased risk of atherosclerotic plaques in RA [33].

Non-HLA genetic factors including polymorphisms in tumour necrosis factor alpha, interleukin 6 *(IL-6)*, endothelin-1, nuclear factor of kappa light polypeptide gene enhancer in B-cells 1(NF-kβ1), vascular endothelial growth factor-A(VEGFA), methylene tetrahydrofolate reductase(MTH-FR), TNF receptor-associated factor 1(TRAF1/C5), signal transducer and activator of transcription 4(STAT4), plasminogen activator inhibitor type-1(PAI-1), tumor necrosis factor receptor II(TNFR-II), acid 5 phosphatase locus (ACP1), factor XIIIA, lymphotoxin-A (LT-A), transforming growth factor beta (TGF-β), glutathione S-transferase (GSTT1) and galectin-2 (LGALS2) genes are associated with CVD risk and predisposition to cardiovacular complications in RA patients [34, 35].

RA-associated autoantibodies such as anti-cyclic citrullinated peptide antibodies (anti-CCP) and rheumatoid factor immunoglobulin M (RF-IgM) have been shown to be related related to impaired endothelial function and are independently associated with impaired left ventricular relaxation and development of IHD. Immune complexes from RF can be deposited in the endothelium leading to endothelial dysfunction and atherosclerosis through inflammatory reactions. RF titers are also independently predictive of endothelial dysfunction and increased mortality in RA [5, 9, 36–38].

Anti-oxidized low-density lipoprotein antibodies (anti-ox-LDL), antiphospholipid antibodies (APLA), anticardiolipins antibodies (ACLA), APLA, anti-apolipoprotein A-1(anti-ApoA-1), antiphosphorylcholine antibodies (anti-PC), anti-HSP: anti-heat shock proteins antibodies (anti-HSP 60/65) and anti- malondialdehyde modified LDL (anti-MDA-LDL) antibodies are associated with inflammation, atherosclerosis and increased risk for CVD [36–39].

Other non-traditional risk factors for CVD in RA patients include: extra-articular manifestations which increase CVD risk 3-fold;long duration of disease, prolonged RA with chronic inflammation have more extensive atherosclerosis; glucocorticoid use, patients receiving more than 7.5 mg per day have twice the risk of CVD; high disease activity (disease activity scores DAS-28) and the chronic proinflammatory state (high markers of inflammation-C-reactive protein (CRP), erythrocyte sedimentation rate (ESR), TNF-α), IL-6, interleukin-17 (IL-17), hepcidin, serum pentraxin-3 (sPTX-3) and haptoglobin are associated with increased risk of CVD and cardiovascular adverse events. Additional nontraditional risk factors that have been shown to increase the risk of CVD in RA patients are hypothyroidism which increases CVD risk 4-fold and periodontal disease [39–44].

23.3 Systemic Lupus Erythematosus and Antiphospholipid Syndrome

Systemic lupus erythematosus (SLE) and antiphospholipid syndrome (APS) are two highly related IMID associated with an increased risk of developing CVD [45]. Despite the great progresses made in understanding the pathological mechanisms leading to CVD in those pathologies, there is still the unmet need to improve long term prognosis [46–49]. Cardiovascular diseases in SLE and APS is thought to happen as the result of a complex interaction between traditional CVD risk factors, immune deregulation and disease activity [50, 51], including the synergic effect of cytokines, chemokines, adipokines, proteases, autoantibodies, adhesion receptors, oxidative stress and a plethora of intracellular signalling molecules. Genomic and epigenomic analyses have further allowed the identification of specific signatures explaining the proathero-thrombotic profiles of APS and SLE patients [52].

Patients with SLE are 5–6 times more likely to have a significant coronary event than people in the general population. Apart from the established risk factors mentioned above, a number of nontraditional novel risk factors are associated with CVD and SLE [53].

Cardiac involvement in SLE includes: pericarditis which is clinically significant in 25% of the cases although autopsy series have shown 60%–80% involvement, pericardial effusion (which may occur as a complication of renal failure), coronary atherosclerosis, acute coronary syndrome and valvular disease in the form of sterile vegetations (Libman-Sacks endocarditis) and mitral valve involvement [54, 55].

In SLE, the pathogenesis of CVD is multi-factorial and complex, involving an interaction between inflammation-induced and autoantibody-mediated vascular injury and thrombosis from the underlying disorder and traditional CVS risk factors. SLE-related factors seem to be involved in all stages of atherosclerosis [56].

Though the exact pathogenesis of atherosclerosis in systemic lupus remains elusive, an imbalance between endothelial damage and atheroprotection seems to be a central event [57]. Insults leading to endothelial damage in lupus include oxidized low density lipoprotein (oxLDL), autoantibodies against endothelial cells and phospholipids, type I interferons (IFN) and neutrophil extracellular traps (NETs) directly or through activation of type I IFN pathway [58–60]. Increased oxidative stress, reduced levels of the normally antioxidant high density lipoprotein (HDL), increased levels of proinflammatory HDL (piHDL) and reduced paraoxonase activity have been related to increased oxLDL levels [58–60].

Processes integral to the pathogenesis of SLE, including immune complex formation and complement activation are involved in endothelial injury and local inflammation. The upregulated CD40–CD40–ligand interactions in SLE may influence many processes, ranging from promoting inflammatory processes to contributing to thrombus formation. The CD40–CD40–ligand is another immune-mediated interaction, common to both SLE and atherosclerosis that leads to upregulation of adhesion molecules on endothelial cells [61]. Furthermore, several risk factors closely related to inflammation and autoimmunity (several auto antibodies and their respective autoantigens) have been identified as possible factors in development and progress of atherosclerosis namely; oxidized low density lipoprotein (LDL) and anti-oxidized LDL, beta 2-glycoprotein 1 [β2GP1 and anti-β2GP1], lupus anticoagulant, ACLA, APLA, heat shock(hsp) protein and anti-hsp autoantibody systems; activation of endothelial MMP-2 by MMP-9 contained in netosis bodies (NETs) as an important player in endothelial dysfunction and MMP-9 as a novel self-antigen in SLE [62–66].

A considerable genetic component for CVD is with interferon regulatory factor 8 (IRF8) as a strong susceptibility locus and tumour necrosis factor receptor-associated factors (TRAF3IP2) associated with the the occurrence of pericarditis [62, 67].

As with RA, longer disease duration, higher disease activity and increased levels of inflammatory markers (CRP, ESR), use of glucocorticoids (>10 mg/day), vasculopathy, menopausal status and use of hormone replacement therapy are associated with increased CVD risk in SLE patients. Recently, a number of studies have demonstrated that lower baseline levels of 25-hydroxy vitamin D are associated with more active SLE and increased risk for CVD [68–70].

23.3.1 Anti-Phospholipid Syndrome (APS)

The APS is a prothrombotic state that affects both the venous and arterial circulations. Cardiac involvement in APS includes: valve abnormalities (thickening of leaflets, valve dysfunction and sterile vegetations), thrombotic and atherosclerotic coronary occlusion, intracardiac thrombus, pulmonary hypertension, ventricular hypertrophy and dysfunction. Thrombotic events are the clinical hallmark of APS expressed as carotid disease, coronary artery disease, valvular thickening due to deposition of immune complexes and PVD, all of which are significant risk factors for stroke [71–75].

23.4 HLA-B27-Associated Spondyloarthropathies (SpA)

Spondyloarthropathies are chronic IMID associated with accelerated atherosclerosis and with a higher CVD risk than the general population [1]. Subclinical atherosclerosis manifested by endothelial dysfunction, carotid intima thickness and carotid plaques has been observed in ankylosing spondylitis and psoriatic arthritis [1].

Cardiovascular involvement in spondyloarthropathies includes frequent aortic root disease (dilatation and aortic valve regurgitation), venous thromboembolism (VTE), IHD, conduction disease in up to one third of cases which is generally progressive and rarely pericarditis [76]. Patients with AS, PsA and uSpA are at increased risk for acute coronary syndromes and stroke events, which emphasizes the importance of identification of and intervention against cardiovascular risk factors in SpA patients [77, 78].

The accumulation of CCR7 (chemokine receptor 7) positive cells in the vessel wall may be involved in endothelial dysfunction and subsequent accelerated atherogenesis. CCR7 plays a crucial role in T cell and monocyte migration/homing and in priming of naive T lymphocytes in non-lymphoid tissues in IMID. In AS, miRNA-16 and miRNA-221 are aberrantly expressed in T cells [79–81].

23.4.1 Psoriasis/Psoriatic Arthritis

Psoriasis/psoriatic arthritis (PsA) are common chronic, inflammatory, immune-mediated skin/arthritic diseases with a high incidence of atherosclerosis and cardiovascular disease [82–85].

Several studies have shown that patients with psoriasis, especially younger patients and those with more severe forms of psoriasis or with psoriatic arthritis, have a higher prevalence of risk factors and metabolic syndrome, as well as an increased risk of major cardiovascular events such as myocardial infarction, cerebrovascular disease, and peripheral arterial disease [86, 87].

Increased prevalence of subclinical atherosclerosis in PsA patients is caused by several traditional and non traditional risk factors. Risk factors associated with PsA include smoking, obesity, insulin resistance and metabolic syndrome. High disease activity and greater degrees of inflammation (as detected by disease activity indices and high levels of CRP, ESR) as well as longer disease duration are also associated with increased CVD risk [84–87].

There is a strong familial component to psoriatic disease as well as a complex array of genetic, immunologic, and environmental factors. The dominant genetic effect is located on chromosome 6p21.3 within the major histocompatibility complex region, accounting for one-third of genetic contribution. Genome-wide association studies (GWAS) identified additional genes, including skin barrier function, innate immune response, and adaptive immune response genes [88]. To date, 36 genes have reached genome-wide significance, accounting for approximately 22% of psoriasis (Ps) heritability. Prominent genes identified via GWAS include HLA-Cw6, IL12B, IL23R, IL23A, TNIP1, TNFAIP3, LCE3B-LCE3C, TRAF3IP2, NFkBIA, FBXL19, TYK2, IFIH1, REL, and ERAP1. Genes identified in psoriatic arthritis (PsA) has largely echoed those in Ps and include HLA-B/C, HLA-B, IL-12B, IL-23R, TNIP1, TRAF3IP2, FBXL19, and REL [88, 89]. The candidate genes identified in PsV/PsA have highlighted pathways of critical importance to psoriatic disease including distinct signaling pathways comprised of barrier integrity, innate immune response and adaptive immune response, mediated primarily by Th-17 and Th-1 signalling [88–90].

23.5 Sjögren's Syndrome

Sjögren's Syndrome (SS) is an epithelitis affecting the exocrine glands. The clinical spectrum of SS extends from autoimmune exocrinopathy to systemic involvement with vasculitis and extraglandular manifestations including CVD allbeit with a lower prevalence than the IMID mentioned above due primarily to the milder chronic inflammation present in SS. The CVD risk in SS patients is however rising primarily due to the population affected, namely postmenopausal women. Studies have demonstrated a high rate of subclinical atherosclerosis particularly in the carotid artery, suggesting endothelium dysfunction as a consequence of combined immunological and chronic inflammatory factors [91].

Risk factors for CVD in SS include the conventional CVD risk factors of diabetes mellitus and dyslipidaemia and the non traditional risk factors including: long duration of disease, chonic inflammatory state with elevated CRP, glucocorticoid use, presence of autoantibodies (anti-Ro/SS-A; anti-La/SS-B), haematological alterations (hypogammaglobulinaemia, thrombocytopaenia and soluble vascular adhesion molecules [s-VCAM-1]) and systemic involvement (articular, renal, *liver* central nervous system) all of which are associated with increased risk of stroke and IHD [91–93].

23.6 Systemic Sclerosis (SSc)

Systemic sclerosis (SSc), a complex disorder with a strong genetic predisposition, is characterized by fibrosis and widespread vascular pathology. Raynaud's phenomenon and digital ulceration are prominent manifestations of vascular involvement in SSc. Disease presentation is due to primarily microvascular but also macrovascular involvement. The vasculopathy typically affects capillaries and small arteries in the form of microvascular occlusive disease with vasospasm and intimal proliferation. Macrovascular involvement due to fibrosis, thickening, chronic intimal layer proliferation as well as increased atherosclerosis [94].

Cardiovascular involvement in *SSc* includes: pulmonary hypertension, pericarditis, pericardial effusion, coronary vasospasm, coronary microvascular disease, arrhythmias, conduction disturbances, hypertension and left ventricular dysfunction [95].

The traditional risk factors associated with CVD and *SSc* include diabetes mellitus, dyslipidaemia, hypertension, smoking and hyperhomocysteinaemia [94]. The nontraditional CVD risk factors in *SSc* include chronic inflammation (increased levels of CRP) and autoantibodies (anti-oxidized low-density lipoprotein/β2 glycoprotein I antibodies (anti-oxLDL/β2GPI) complex, anti-ox-LDL, anti-lipoprotein lipase antibodies (anti-LPL), anti-endothelial cell antibodies (AECA), anti-centromere, anti-HSP65/60, APLA, interferon regulatory factor 5 (IRF5), signal transducer and activator of transcription 4 (Stat4), protein tyrosine phosphatase, non-receptor type 22 (PTPN22) and B cell scaffold protein with ankyrin repeats 1 (BANK1), connective tissue growth factor (CTGF), T-box transcription factor (TBX21), Corf13-BLK, interleukin 10 receptor (IL-10R), interleukin 23 receptor (IL-23R), and tumour necrosis factor superfamily -TNFSF4 [96].

23.7 Sarcoidosis

Sarcoidosis is an idiopathic disease characterized by the presence of non-caseating granulomas in the involved organs. Sarcoid-mediated myocardial inflammation is associated with a regional impairment of coronary circulatory function [97].

Cardiac involvement is common and significantly alters the patient's prognosis. Manifestations of cardiac sarcoidosis include fibrotic cardiomyopathy, congestive heart failure, conduction abnormalities, atrial and ventricular arrhythmias, and sudden death. Cardiac complications are the second leading cause of sarcoidosis-related death, after respiratory complication. Studies have shown that the association between immune-suppressive treatment-related alterations in myocardial inflammation and changes in coronary vasodilator capacity suggests direct adverse effect of inflammation on coronary circulatory function in cardiac sarcoidosis [98].

Cardiac involvement in sarcoidosis occurs in the form of granulomatous infiltration of the heart in 25% of the cases of which 95% are asymptomatic and diagnosed using cardiac magnetic resonance imaging, the conerstone for diagnosing cardiac sarcoidosis rather than endomyocardial biopsy which may miss patchy infiltrates; and clinically heterogenous effects including dilated cardiomyopathy, congestive heart failure with an incidence of 10–30%, pericarditis, pulmonary *artery* hypertension due to lung fibrosis, ventricular tachycardia 2–42%, supraventricular tachycardia 0–15%, bundle branch block 12–61%, AV block 26–62% and sudden cardiac death 12–65% [97, 98].

23.8 Vasculitis

Premature atherosclerosis and increased cardiovascular morbidity and mortality has been documented in large, medium and small vessel systemic vasculitides [99]. Both humoral and cellular immune mechanisms are incriminated and are thought to contribute to accelerated atherosclerosis [100].

23.8.1 Giant Cell Arteritis

Giant cell arteritis (GCA) is a systemic IMID primarily affecting the elderly. It is characterized by inflammation of the adventitial layer of large and medium-sized arteries. Studies have demonstrated that initially there is a high concentration of proinflammatory cytokines (CRP, IL-1, IL-6, TNFα, interferon-gamma), autoantibodies particularly anti-neutrophil cytoplasmic antibody ANCA and T cells in the vessel wall. Later stages demonstrate growth factors promoting intimal growth and stenosis. Cardiac involvement involves mainly the aorta (15% of cases) and subclavian artery [101, 102].

Conclusions

A broad spectrum of cardiovascular phenotypes exists in IMID. Chronic immune-mediated inflammatory diseases have variable cardiac sequelae. A complex interaction between traditional and disease-specific traits exists. Additionally, interactions between environmental, immunological, epigenetic and genetic factors that result in downstream perturbations of complex and interactive biological networks all play a role in the development of atherosclerosis and CVD in autoimmune diseases. Identification of novel epigenetic targets and a better identification and understanding of epigenetic mechanisms involved in CVD, may provide novel therapeutic approaches in chronic IMID.

Further studies are needed to elucidate the different pathogenic mechanisms contributing to the development of atherothrombosis in IMID.

Genomic and proteomic studies will aid to identify novel patterns of biomarkers, while together with the traditional risk factors, the novel nontaditional risk factors might help target better screening. As regards the treatment targeted at underlying IMID as well as cardiac issues there are no definite guidelines, however until further research and disease specific predictor tools are available, evidence supports controlling disease activity aggressively, strict screening and management of modifiable traditional risk factors. Cardiovascular assessment should include various non-invasive imaging modalities including rest/stress ECG, echocardiography, nuclear technology, positron emission tomography and cardiac magnetic resonance (CMR) which detect ischaemia or inflammatory disease in IMID.

References

1. Durante A, Bronzato S. The increased cardiovascular risk in patients affected by autoimmune diseases: Review of the various manifestations. J Clin Med Res. 2015;7(6):379–84.
2. Roman MJ, Salmon JE. Cardiovascular manifestations of rheumatologic diseases. Circulation. 2007;116:2346–55.
3. Abou-Raya S, Abou-Raya A, Naim A, Abuelkheir H. Chronic inflammatory autoimmune disorders and atherosclerosis. Ann N Y Acad Sci. 2007;1107:56–67.
4. Sherer Y, Shoenfeld Y. Mechanisms of disease: atherosclerosis in autoimmune diseases. Nat Clin Pract Rheumatol. 2006;2(2):99–106.
5. Kahlenberg JM, Kaplan MJ. Mechanisms of premature atherosclerosis in rheumatoid arthritis and lupus. Annu Rev. Med. 2013;64:249–63.
6. Au K, Singh MK, Bodukam V, Bae S, Maranian P, Ogawa R, Spiegel B, et al. Atherosclerosis in systemic sclerosis: a systematic review and meta-analysis. Arthritis Rheum. 2011; 63(7):2078–90.

7. Frostegard J. Atherosclerosis in patients with autoimmune disorders. Arterioscler Thromb Vasc Biol. 2005;25(9):1776–85.
8. Hansson GK. Inflammation, atherosclerosis, and coronary artery disease. N Engl J Med. 2005;352(16):1685–95.
9. Bartoloni E, Shoenfeld Y, Gerli R. Inflammatory and autoimmune mechanisms in the induction of atherosclerotic damage in systemic rheumatic diseases: two faces of the same coin. Arthritis Care Res. 2011;63:178–83.
10. López-Pedrera C, Barbarroja N, Aguirre MA, Torres LA, Velasco F, Cuadrado MJ. Genomics and proteomics: a new approach for assessing thrombotic risk in autoimmune diseases. Lupus. 2008;17:904–15.
11. López-Pedrera C, Sanchez CP, Aguirre MA, Ramos-Casals M, Gonzalez MS, Rodriguez-Ariza A, Cuadrado MJ. Cardiovascular risk in systemic autoimmune diseases: Epigenetic mechanisms of immune regulatory functions. Clin Dev Immunol. 2012;2012:1–10.
12. Brooks WH, Le Dantec C, Pers JO, Youinou P, Renaudineau Y. Epigenetics and autoimmunity. J Autoimmun. 2010;34(3):J207–19.
13. Jungel A, Ospelt C, Gay S. What can we learn from epigenetics in the year 2009? Curr Opin Rheumatol. 2010;22(3):284–92.
14. Pascual V, Chaussabel D, Banchereau J. A genomic approach to human autoimmune diseases. Annu Rev. Immunol. 2010;28:535–71.
15. Eyre S, Bowes J, Diogo D, et al. High-density genetic mapping identifies new susceptibility loci for rheumatoid arthritis. Nat Genet. 2012;44:1336–40.
16. Stahl EA, Raychaudhuri S, Remmers EF, et al. Genomewide association study meta-analysis identifies seven new rheumatoid arthritis risk loci. Nat Genet. 2010;42:508–14.
17. Teague H, Mehta NN. The link between inflammatory disorders and coronary heart disease: a look at recent studies and novel drugs in development. Curr Atheroscler Rep. 2016;18:3.
18. Abou-Raya A, Abou-Raya S. Inflammation: a pivotal link between autoimmune diseases and atherosclerosis. Autoimmun Rev. 2006;5(5):331–7.
19. Symmons DP, Gabriel SE. Epidemiology of CVD in rheumatic disease, with a focus on RA and SLE. Nat Rev. Rheumatol. 2011;7:399–408.
20. Kitas GD, Gabriel SE. Cardiovascular disease in rheumatoid arthritis: state of the art and future perspectives. Ann Rheum Dis. 2011;63:1211–20.
21. Peters MJ, van Halm VP, Voskuyl AE, Smulders YM, Boers M, Lems WF, Visser M, et al. Does rheumatoid arthritis equal diabetes mellitus as an independent risk factor for cardiovascular disease? A prospective study. Arthritis Rheum. 2009;61(11):1571–9.
22. del Rincon ID, Williams K, Stern MP, Freeman GL, Escalante A. High incidence of cardiovascular events in a rheumatoid arthritis cohort not explained by traditional cardiac risk factors. Arthritis Rheum. 2001;44(12):2737–45.
23. Avina-Zubieta JA, Thomas J, Sadatsafavi M, Lehman AJ, Lacaille D. Risk of incident cardiovascular events in patients with rheumatoid arthritis: a meta-analysis of observational studies. Ann Rheum Dis. 2012;71(9):1524.
24. Montecucco F, Mach F. Common inflammatory mediators orchestrate pathophysiological processes in rheumatoid arthritis and atherosclerosis. Rheumatology. 2009;11–22(16):48.
25. Gonzalez A, Maradit Kremers H, Crowson CS, et al. The widening mortality gap between rheumatoid arthritis patients and the general population. Arthritis Rheum. 2007;56:3583–7.
26. Wick G, Knoflach M, Xu Q. Autoimmune and inflammatory mechanisms in atherosclerosis. Annu Rev. Immunol. 2004;22:361–403.
27. Matsuura E. Atherosclerosis and autoimmunity. Clin Rev. Allergy Immunol. 2009;37(1):1–3, 2009.
28. Goodson N, Marks J, Lunt M, Symmons D. Cardiovascular admissions and mortality in an inception cohort of patients with rheumatoid arthritis with onset in the 1980s and 1990s. Ann Rheum Dis. 2005;64(11):1595–601.
29. Gonzalez-Juanatey C, Llorca J, Gonzalez-Gay MA. Correlation between endothelial function and carotid atherosclerosis in rheumatoid arthritis patients with long-standing disease. Arthr Res Ther. 2011;13(3):R101.

30. Chung CP, Giles JT, Petri M, Szklo M, Post W, Blumenthal RS, Gelber AC, et al. Prevalence of traditional modifiable cardiovascular risk factors in patients with rheumatoid arthritis: comparison with control subjects from the multi-ethnic study of atherosclerosis. Semin Arthritis Rheum. 2012;41(4):535–44.
31. Farragher TM, Goodson NJ, Naseem H, Silman AJ, Thomson W, Symmons D, Barton A. Association of the HLA-DRB1 gene with premature death, particularly from cardiovascular disease, in patients with rheumatoid arthritis and inflammatory polyarthritis. Arthritis Rheum. 2008;58(2):359–69.
32. Gonzalez-Juanatey C, Testa A, Garcia-Castelo A, et al. HLADRB1 status affects endothelial function in treated patients with rheumatoid arthritis. Am J Med. 2003;114(8):647–52.
33. Mattey DL, Thomson W, Ollier WER, et al. Association of DRB1 shared epitope genotypes with early mortality in rheumatoid arthritis: results of eighteen years of follow up from the early rheumatoid arthritis study. Arthritis Rheum. 2007;56(5):1408–16.
34. Palomino-Morales R, Gonzalez-Juanatey C, VazquezRodriguez TR, et al. A1298C polymorphism in the MTHFR gene predisposes to cardiovascular risk in rheumatoid arthritis. Arthritis Res Ther. 2010;12(2):R71.
35. Lopez-Mejıas R, Garcıa-Bermudez M, Gonzalez-Juanatey C, et al. NFKB1-94ATTG ins/del polymorphism (rs28362491) is associated with cardiovascular disease in patients with rheumatoid arthritis. Atherosclerosis. 2012;224:426–9.
36. Toms TE, Panoulas VF, Smith JP, et al. Rheumatoid arthritis susceptibility genes associate with lipid levels in patients with rheumatoid arthritis. Ann Rheum Dis. 2011;70(6):1025–32.
37. Wang J, Hu B, Meng Y, Zhang C, Li K, Hui C. The level of malondialdehyde-modified LDL and LDL immune complexes in patients with rheumatoid arthritis. Clin Biochem. 2009;42(13–14):1352–7.
38. Hjeltnes G, Hollan I, Førre Ø, Wiik A, Mikkelsen K, Agewall S. Anti-CCP and RF IgM: predictors of impaired endothelial function in rheumatoid arthritis patients. Scand J Rheumatol. 2011;40(6):422–7.
39. Amaya-Amaya J, Sarmiento-Monroy JC, Mantilla R, Pineda-Tamayo R, Rojas-Villarraga A, Anaya JM. Novel risk factors for cardiovascular disease in rheumatoid arthritis. Immunol Res. 2013;56:267–86.
40. Dessein PH, Joffe BI, Veller MG, et al. Traditional and nontraditional cardiovascular risk factors are associated with atherosclerosis in rheumatoid arthritis. J Rheumatol. 2005;32(3):435–42.
41. Book C, Saxne T, Jacobsson LTH. Prediction of mortality in rheumatoid arthritis based on disease activity markers. J Rheumatol. 2005;32(3):430–4.
42. McCoy SS, Crowson CS, Gabriel SE, Matteson EL. Hypothyroidism as a risk factor for development of cardiovascular disease in patients with rheumatoid arthritis. J Rheumatol. 2012;39(5):954–8.
43. Abou-Raya A, Abou-Raya S, Abu-Elkheir H. Periodontal diease and 18 rheumatoid arthritis: is there a link? Scand J Rheumatol. 2005;34(5):408–10.
44. Turesson C, McClelland RL, Christianson TJH, Matteson EL. Severe extra-articular disease manifestations are associated with an increased risk of first ever cardiovascular events in patients with rheumatoid arthritis. Ann Rheum Dis. 2007;66(1):70–5.
45. Schoenfeld SR, Kasturi S, Costenbader KH. The epidemiology of atherosclerotic cardiovascular disease among patients with SLE: a systematic review. Semin Arthritis Rheum. 2013;43(1):77–95.
46. Petri MA, Kiani AN, Post W, Christopher-Stine L, Magder LS. Lupus atherosclerosis prevention study (LAPS). Ann Rheum Dis. 2011;70(5):760–5.
47. Magder LS, Petri M. Incidence of and risk factors for adverse cardiovascular events among patients with systemic lupus erythematosus. Am J Epidemiol. 2012;176(8):708–19.
48. Esdaile JM, Abrahamowicz M, Grodzicky T, et al. Traditional Framingham risk factors fail to fully account for accelerated atherosclerosis in systemic lupus erythematosus. Arthritis Rheum. 2001;44:2331–7.

49. Roman MJ, et al. Prevalence and correlates of accelerated atherosclerosis in systemic lupus erythematosus. N Engl J Med. 2003;349:2399–406.
50. Svenungsson E, Jensen-Urstad K, Heimburger M, Silveira A, Hamsten A, de Faire U, Witztum JL, et al. Risk factors for cardiovascular disease in systemic lupus erythematosus. Circulation. 2001;104(16):1887–93.
51. Petri M, Perez-Gutthann S, Spence D, Hochberg MC. Risk factors for coronary artery disease in patients with systemic lupus erythematosus. Am J Med. 1992;93:513–9.
52. Silva GL, Junta CM, Mello SS, et al. Profiling meta-analysis reveals primarily gene coexpression concordance between systemic lupus erythematosus and rheumatoid arthritis. Ann N Y Acad Sci. 2007;1110:33–46.
53. Knight JS, Kaplan MJ. Cardiovascular disease in lupus: insights and updates. Curr Opin Rheumatol. 2013;25:597–605.
54. Kay SD, Poulsen MK, Diederichsen AC, Voss A. Coronary, carotid, and lower-extremity atherosclerosis and their interrelationship in Danish patients with systemic lupus erythematosus. J Rheumatol. 2016;43:315–22.
55. Wu GC, Liu HR, Leng RX, et al. Subclinical atherosclerosis in patients with systemic lupus erythematosus: a systemic review and meta-analysis. Autoimmun Rev. 2016;15:22–37.
56. Skaggs BJ, Hahn BH, McMahon M. Accelerated atherosclerosis in patients with SLE—mechanisms and management. Nat Rev. Rheumatol. 2012;8:214–23.
57. Rajagopalan S, Somers EC, Brook RD, Kehrer C, Pfenninger D, Lewis E, Chakrabarti A, Richardson BC, Shelden E, McCune WJ, Kaplan MJ. Endothelial cell apoptosis in systemic lupus erythematosus: a common pathway for abnormal vascular function and thrombosis propensity. Blood. 2004;103:3677–83.
58. Sacre K, Criswell LA, McCune JM. Hydroxychloroquine is associated with impaired interferon-alpha and tumor necrosis factor-alpha production by plasmacytoid dendritic cells in systemic lupus erythematosus. Arthritis Res Ther. 2012;14:R155.
59. Telles R, Lanna CCD, Ferreira GA, Ribeiro A. Metabolic syndrome in patients with systemic lupus erythematosus: association with traditional risk factors for coronary heart disease and lupus characteristics. Lupus. 2010;19(7):803–9.
60. Yassin LM, Londono J, Montoya G, et al. Atherosclerosis development in SLE patients is not determined by monocytes ability to bind/endocytose Ox LDL. Autoimmunity. 2011;44(3): 201–10.
61. Kim KJ, Baek IW, Yoon CH, Kim WU, Cho CS. Elevated levels of soluble CD40 ligand are associated with antiphospholipid antibodies in patients with systemic lupus erythematosus. Clin Exp Rheumatol. 2017;35(5):823–30.
62. Absher DM, Li X, Waite LL, et al. Genome-wide DNA methylation analysis 20 of systemic lupus erythematosus reveals persistent hypomethylation of interferon genes and compositional changes to CD4+ T-cell populations. PLoS Genet. 2013;9(8):article e1003678.
63. Gomez-Pacheco L, Villa AR, Drenkard C, Cabiedes J, Cabral AR, Alarcon-Segovia D. Serum anti-β2-glycoproteinI and anticardiolipin antibodies during thrombosis in systemic lupus erythematosus patients. Am J Med. 1999;106(4):417–23.
64. Rho YH, Chung CP, Oeser A, et al. Novel cardiovascular risk factors in premature coronary atherosclerosis associated with systemic lupus erythematosus. J Rheumatol. 2008;35(9): 1789–94.
65. ShinzatoMM,BuenoC,VianaVST,BorbaEF,GoncalvesCR,BonfaE.Complement-fixingactivity of anti-cardiolipin antibodies in patients with and without thrombosis. Lupus. 2005;14(12): 953–8.
66. Carmona-Rivera C, Zhao W, Yalavarthi S, Kaplan MJ. Neutrophil extracellular traps induce endothelial dysfunction in systemic lupus erythematosus through the activation of matrix metalloproteinase-2. Ann Rheum Dis. 2015;74(7):1417–24.
67. Perricone C, Ciccacci C, Ceccarelli F, et al. TRAF3IP2 gene and systemic lupus erythematosus: association with disease susceptibility and pericarditis development. Immunogenetics. 2013;65:703–9.

68. Lertratanakul A, Wu P, Dyer A, et al. 25-Hydroxyvitamin D and cardiovascular disease in patients with systemic lupus erythematosus: Data from a large international inception cohort. Arthritis Care Res. 2014;66(80):1167–76.
69. Reynolds JA, Haque S, Berry JL, et al. 25-hydroxyvitamin D deficiency is associated with increased aortic stiffness in patients with systemic lupus erythematosus. Rheumatology. 2012;51(3):544–51.
70. Mok CC, Birmingham DJ, Leung HW, Hebert LA, Song H, Rovin BH. Vitamin D levels in Chinese patients with systemic lupus erythematosus: relationship with disease activity, vascular risk factors and atherosclerosis. Rheumatology. 2012;51(4):644–52.
71. Medina G, Gutierrez-Moreno AL, Vera-Lastra O, Saavedra MA, Jara LJ. Prevalence of metabolic syndrome in primary antiphospholipid syndrome patients. Autoimmun Rev. 2011;10(4):214–7.
72. Lopez LR, Simpson DF, Hurley BL, Matsuura E. OxLDL/beta2GPI complexes and autoantibodies in patients with systemic lupus erythematosus, systemic sclerosis, and antiphospholipid syndrome: pathogenic implications for vascular involvement. Ann N Y Acad Sci. 2005;1051:313–22.
73. Gurlek A, Ozdol C, Pamir G, Dincer I, Tutkak H, Oral D. Association between anticardiolipin antibodies and recurrent cardiac events in patients with acute coronary syndrome. Int Heart J. 2005;46:631–8.
74. Ribeiro AR, Carvalho JF. Traditional risk factors for cardiovascular disease in primary antiphospholipid syndrome (APS) when compared with secondary APS: a study with 96 patients. Acta Reumatol Port. 2010;35(1):36–41.
75. Tenedios F, Erkan D, Lockshin MD. Cardiac manifestations in the antiphospholipid syndrome. Rheum Dis Clin N Am. 2006;32(3):491–507.
76. Roldan CA, Chavez J, Wiest PW, Qualls CR, Crawford MH. Aortic root disease and valve disease associated with ankylosing spondylitis. J Am Coll Cardiol. 1998;32:1397–404.
77. Szabo SM, Levy AR, Rao SR, et al. Increased risk of cardiovascular and cerebrovascular diseases in individuals with ankylosing spondylitis: a population-based study. Arthritis Rheum. 2011;63(11):3294–304.
78. Peters MJ, van der Horst-Bruinsma IE, Dijkmans BA, Nurmohamed MT. Cardiovascular risk profile of patients with spondylarthropathies, particularly ankylosing spondylitis and psoriatic arthritis. Semin Arthritis Rheum. 2004;34(3):585–92.
79. Sulicka J, Surdacki A, Korkosz M, Mikołajczyk T, Strach M, Klimek E, Guzik T, Grodzicki T. Endothelial dysfunction is independent of inflammation and 22 altered CCR7 T cell expression in patients with ankylosing spondylitis. Clin Exp Rheumatol. 2017;35(5):844–9.
80. Lai NS, Yu HC, Chen HC, Yu CL, Huang HB, Lu MC. Aberrant expression of microRNAs in T cells from patients with ankylosing spondylitis contributes to the immunopathogenesis. Clin Exp Immunol. 2013;173(1):47–57.
81. Lai NS, Chou JL, Chen GCW, Liu SQ, Lu MC, Chan MWY. Association between cytokines and methylation of SOCS-1 in serum of patients with ankylosing spondylitis. Mol Biol Rep. 2014;41(6):3773–80.
82. Tam LS, Shang Q, Li EK, Tomlinson B, Chu TT, Li M, et al. Subclinical carotid atherosclerosis in patients with psoriatic arthritis. Arthritis Rheum. 2008;59:1322–3.
83. Kimhi O, Caspi D, Bornstein NM, Maharshak N, Gur A, Arbel Y, et al. Prevalence and risk factors of atherosclerosis in patients with psoriatic arthritis. Semin Arthritis Rheum. 2007;36:203–9.
84. Jamnitski A, Symmons D, Peters MJ, Sattar N, McInnes I, Nurmohamed MT. Cardiovascular comorbidities in patients with psoriatic arthritis: a systematic review. Ann Rheum Dis. 2013;72:211–6.
85. Raychaudhuri SK, Chatterjee S, Nguyen C, Kaur M, Jialal I, Raychaudhuri SP. Increased prevalance of the metabolic syndrome in patients with psoriatic arthritis. Metab Syndr Relat Disord. 2010;8(4):331.
86. Mehta NN, Azfar RS, Shin DB, Neimann AL, Troxel AB, Gelfand JM. Patients with severe psoriasis are at increased risk of cardiovascular mortality: cohort study using the General Practice Research Database. Eur Heart J. 2010;31:1000–6.

87. Tam LS, Tomlinson B, Chu TT, Li M, Leung YY, Kwok LW, et al. Cardiovascular risk profile of patients with psoriatic arthritis compared to controls - the role of inflammation. Rheumatology. 2008;47:718–23.
88. Gonzalez-Juanatey Llorca CJ, Miranda-Filloy JA, et al. Endothelial dysfunction 23 in psoriatic arthritis patients without clinically evident cardiovascular disease or classic atherosclerosis risk factors. Arthritis Care Res. 2007;57(2):287–93.
89. Zhang Z, Yuan J, Tian Z, Xu J, Lu Z. Investigation of 36 non-HLA (human leucocyte antigen) psoriasis susceptibility loci in a psoriatic arthritis cohort. Arch Dermatol Res. 2017; 309(2):71–7.
90. O'Rielly DD, Rahman P. Genetic, epigenetic and pharmacogenetic aspects of psoriasis and psoriatic arthritis. Rheum Dis Clin N Am. 2015;41(4):623–42.
91. Perez-De-Lis M, Akasbi M, Siso A, et al. Cardiovascular risk factors in primary Sjogren's syndrome: a case-control study in 624 patients. Lupus. 2010;19(8):941.
92. Gerli R, Vaudo G, Bocci EB, et al. Functional impairment of the arterial wall in primary Sjogren's syndrome: combined action of immunologic and inflammatory factors. Arthritis Care Res. 2010;62(5):712–8.
93. Kang J, Lin H. Comorbidities in patients with primary Sjogren's syndrome: a registry-based case-control study. J Rheumatol. 2010;37(6):1188–94.
94. Guiducci S, Distler O, Distler JH, Matucci-Cerinic M. Mechanisms of vascular damage in SSc—implications for vascular treatment strategies. Rheumatology. 2008;47(supplement 5):v18–20.
95. Chung L, Distler O, Hummers L, Krishnan E, Steen V. Vascular disease in systemic sclerosis. Int J Rheumatol. 2010;3(1):8.
96. Nussinovitch U, Shoenfeld Y. Atherosclerosis and macrovascular involvement in systemic sclerosis: myth or reality. Autoimmun Rev. 2011;10(5):259–66.
97. Chapelon-Abric C, Sene D, Saadoun D, Cluzel P, Vignaux O, Costedoat-Chalumeau N, Piette JC, Cacoub P. Cardiac sarcoidosis: diagnosis, therapeutic management and prognostic factors. Arch Cardiovasc Dis. 2017;110(8–9):456–65.
98. Kim JJS, Judson MA, Donnino R, Gold M, et al. Cardiac Sarcoidosis. Am Heart J. 2009;157(1):9–21.
99. Tervaert JW. Cardiovascular disease due to accelerated atherosclerosis in systemic vasculitides. Best Pract Res Clin Rheumatol. 2013;27:33–44.
100. Libby P. Pathophysiology of vasculitis. In: Creager MA, Beckman JA, editors. Vascular medicine: a companion to Braunwald's heart disease. 2nd ed; 2012. p. 126–32.
101. Mackie SL, Dasgula B. Vasculitis syndromes dealing with increased vascular risk and mortality in giant cell arteritis. Nat Rev. Rheumatol. 2014;10:264–5.
102. Amiri N, de Vera M, Choi HK, Sayre EC, Avina-Zubieta JA. Increased risk of cardiovascular disease in giant cell arteritis: a general population-based study. Rheumatology. 2016;55(1):33–40.

Genetics and Genomics of Stroke

24

Rhea Y.Y. Tan and Hugh S. Markus

Abstract

Stroke is defined as the acute onset of focal neurological disturbance arising due to a cerebrovascular cause, confirmed histopathologically or on imaging, where other causes have been excluded. Strokes may either be ischaemic (approximately 80% of cases) or haemorrhagic (20%). Although often thought of as a single disease, stroke represents the end stage of many different pathologies, each of which can result in cerebral ischaemia and/or haemorrhage. Therefore when investigating a stroke patient, investigations are performed to identify the underlying cause. Most cases of ischaemic stroke are caused by one of three pathologies: large vessel atherosclerotic disease (LVD), cerebral small vessel disease (SVD) or cardioembolism, although there are multiple rarer causes including cervical artery dissection. However, even with detailed investigation an underlying cause cannot be found in approximately a quarter of all ischaemic strokes. Haemorrhagic strokes are categorized according to the brain region they arise from; lobar or cortical haemorrhages are commonly caused by cerebral amyloid angiopathy, or an underlying structural lesion for example an arteriovenous malformation. Subcortical haemorrhages are usually associated with hypertension and believed to be often a manifestation of SVD.

This chapter will briefly outline the genetic basis of strokes in general, and highlight key examples of familial forms of stroke.

Keywords

Stroke • Genetics • Genomics • Cerebrovascular • CADASIL • CARASIL COL4A1 • NOTCH3 • HTRA1 • COL4A1 • COL4A2

R.Y.Y. Tan • H.S. Markus (✉)
Stroke Research Group, Department of Clinical Neurosciences, Cambridge Biomedical Campus, Cambridge, UK
e-mail: yyrt2@medschl.cam.ac.uk; hsm32@medschl.cam.ac.uk

D. Kumar, P. Elliott (eds.), *Cardiovascular Genetics and Genomics*,
https://doi.org/10.1007/978-3-319-66114-8_24

24.1 Introduction

Stroke is defined as the acute onset of focal neurological disturbance arising due to a cerebrovascular cause, confirmed histopathologically or on imaging, where other causes have been excluded [1]. Strokes may either be ischaemic (approximately 80% of cases) or haemorrhagic (20%) [2]. Although often thought of as a single disease, stroke represents the end stage of many different pathologies, each of which can result in cerebral ischaemia and/or haemorrhage. Therefore when investigating a stroke patient, investigations are performed to identify the underlying cause. Most cases of ischaemic stroke are caused by one of three pathologies: large vessel atherosclerotic disease (LVD), cerebral small vessel disease (SVD) or cardioembolism, although there are multiple rarer causes including cervical artery dissection [3]. However, even with detailed investigation an underlying cause cannot be found in approximately a quarter of all ischaemic strokes. Haemorrhagic strokes are categorized according to the brain region they arise from; lobar or cortical haemorrhages are commonly caused by cerebral amyloid angiopathy, or an underlying structural lesion for example an arteriovenous malformation. Subcortical haemorrhages are usually associated with hypertension and believed to be often a manifestation of SVD.

This chapter will briefly outline the genetic basis of strokes in general, and highlight key examples of familial forms of stroke.

24.2 Genetics and Genomics of 'Sporadic' Stroke

The majority of strokes are apparently 'sporadic', but considerable evidence demonstrates that genetic risk factors, likely interacting with environmental risk factors, are important even in these cases. Evidence from animals models [4], and also from studies in man of twins and affected sibling-pairs [5, 6], and epidemiological data of familial history of stroke [7] suggest that stroke is heritable. More recently this has been supported by complex trait analysis studies from genome-wide association study (GWAS) data [8]. Heritability is higher for younger onset cases [9].

GWAS in ischaemic stroke have identified a number of risk variants [9–13]. A sticking finding has been the subtype specificity of most loci reported to date, demonstrating that different subtypes of ischaemic stroke have different genetic architecture. GWAS studies have also identified loci for intracerebral haemorrhage [14].

24.3 Genetics of Familial Stroke

Stroke less commonly presents as a key feature of monogenic syndromes. Most monogenic forms of stroke also cause a specific stroke subtype (see Table 24.1 for ischaemic stroke and Table 24.2 for intracerebral haemorrhage, ICH).

The most common monogenic form of stroke is Cerebral Autosomal Dominant Arteriopathy with Subcortical Infarcts and Leukoencephalopathy (CADASIL), which results from mutations in the NOTCH3 gene, and most frequently presents with migraine with aura and/or lacunar strokes, and can progress to dementia. Recently a number of other monogenic forms of small vessel disease have been

Table 24.1 Monogenic or single gene disorders causing ischaemic stroke, classified according to the stroke subtype they result in

Stroke subtype	Monogenic disorders
Small vessel disease	• CADASIL • CARASIL/HTRA1-related autosomal dominant SVD • Retinal Vasculopathy with Cerebral Leukodystrophy (RVCL) • COL4A1/A2 –related small vessel arteriopathy with haemorrhage and intracerebral aneurysms
Large artery atherosclerosis and other arteriopathies	• Familial hyperlipidaemias • Moya-moya disease • Pseudoxanthoma elasticum • Neurofibromatosis type I
Large artery disease—dissection	• Ehlers Danlos Syndrome Type IV • Marfan syndrome • Fibromuscular dysplasia • Arterial Tortuosity Syndrome
Disorders affecting both small and large arteries	• Fabry disease • Homocystinuria • Sickle cell disease
Cardioembolism	• Familial cardiomyopathies • Familial arrhythmias • Hereditary Haemorrhagic Telangiectasia
Prothrombotic disorders	• Factor V Leiden • Prothrombin (F2), Protein S (PROS1), Protein C (PROC), Antithrombin III (AT3) deficiencies
Mitochondrial disorders	• Mitochondrial myopathy, Encephalopathy, Lactic Acidosis and Stroke (MELAS)

The list is not inclusive but includes examples of the major stroke subtypes

Table 24.2 Familial forms of haemorrhagic strokes. Key clinical features are provided for more common syndromes

Stroke subtype	Monogenic disorders
Small vessel disease	• COL4A1/A2* (subcortical haemorrhages) • Hereditary cerebral amyloid angiopathy (lobar haemorrhages)
Large artery disease—rupture of cerebrovascular malformations	Cerebral aneurysms • Familial intracranial aneurysm • Autosomal dominant polycystic kidney disease • COL4A1/A2 Arteriovenous malformation • Hereditary haemorrhagic telangiectasia • Capillary malformation—arteriovenous malformation Venous malformations • Familial cerebral cavernous malformation

*Syndromes marked with an asterix predominantly cause haemorrhagic strokes, but may also cause ischaemic strokes

reported which result in one of more of lacunar stroke, migraine, cognitive impairment, and cerebral microbleeds and ICH [15] (Table 24.3). These are not only important for the individual patient, but are also providing important insights into the pathophysiological mechanisms underlying not only monogenic SVD [16] but also sporadic SVD [17].

Table 24.3 Familial forms of ischaemic strokes

Stroke subtype	Disease	Gene	Pattern of inheritance	Other key clinical features	References
Small vessel disease	CADASIL	NOTCH3	Autosomal dominant	• Migraine with aura • Psychiatric problems e.g. depression • Subcortical cognitive impairment leading to dementia • Seizures • Encephalopathic episodes • White matter hyperintensities often involve anterior temporal poles and external capsules	[18]
	CARASIL/ HTRA1- associated SVD	HTRA1	Autosomal recessive or autosomal dominant	• Subcortical cognitive impairment leading to dementia • Early-onset diffuse alopecia (CARASIL) • Degenerative disc disease (CARASIL)	[19–21]
	Cathepsin A related Arteriopathy with Strokes and Leukoencephalopathy (CARASAL)*	CTSA	Autosomal dominant	• Migraines • Slow and late cognitive impairment • Gait problems • Therapy-resistant hypertension • Dry mouth, dry eyes, muscle cramps	[22]
	RVCL*	TREX1	Autosomal dominant	• Migraines • Visual loss • Subcortical cognitive impairment leading to dementia • Systemic involvement in some patients (Hereditary Systemic Angiopathy) • Subcortical contrast-enhancing mass lesions with surrounding oedema (pseudotumours)	[23]
	FOXC1-related SVD	FOXC1	Autosomal dominant, de novo	• Axenfeld Rieger Syndrome—retinal arteriolar tortuosity, cataracts, glaucoma, ocular anterior segment dysgenesis • Hearing impairment • Hydrocephalus, periventricular heterotopia, cerebellar malformations	[24]
	DAD2 (Deficiency of ADA2)	CECR1	Autosomal recessive	• Intermittent fevers • Subcortical lacunar infarcts before age of 5 • Livedo racemosa • Hepatosplenomegaly • Systemic vasculopathy • Hypogammaglobulinaemia lymphopenia, low IgM	[25]
	Cerebral microangiopathy, leukoencephalopathy with calcifications and cysts	SNORD118	Autosomal recessive	• Leukoencephalopathy, intracranial calcifications and cysts • Age at onset infancy to 50s • Progressive cerebral degeneration • Angiomatous-like blood vessels • Gliosis • Rosenthal fibre deposition	[26]

Stroke subtype	Disease	Gene	Pattern of inheritance	Other key clinical features	References
Small and large vessel disease	Fabry disease*	GLA	X-linked	• Small fibre peripheral neuropathy with acute pain crises • Progressive renal failure • Angiokeratomas • Tortuous retinal vessels, whorl keropathy on slit-lamp exam • Cardiomyopathy and hypertension	[27]
	Pseudoxanthoma elasticum	ABCC6	Autosomal dominant/ recessive	• Hypertension, angina, intermittent claudication, restrictive cardiomyopathy, mitral valve prolapse, gastrointestinal bleeding • Yellow papules on skin • Visual impairment, peau d'orange ocular signs, angioid streaks on retina, neovascularization, retinal haemorrhages	[28]
	Neurofibromatosis 1	NF1	Autosomal dominant	• Neurofibromas, café-au-lait spots, freckling • Lisch nodules in eyes • Neurofibromas, Schwannomas • Dural ectasia • Scoliosis, skeletal dysplasia • Phaeochromocytoma	[29]
	Homocystinuria	CBS (most common)	Autosomal recessive	• Developmental delay and intellectual disability • Arterial and venous thrombotic disease affecting small and large vessels • Dislocation of optic lenses, severe myopia • Skeletal abnormalities, osteoporosis	[30]

*Key clinical features are provided for more common syndromes. Syndromes marked with an asterix primarily cause ischaemic strokes, but may also cause haemorrhagic strokes.

24.4 Diagnosing a Monogenic Cause of Stroke

Monogenic forms of stroke can either be part of a systemic disease, which presents with clinical features affecting multiple organs, or can present primarily with stroke. When stroke is part of a systemic disease, examples of which include Fabry disease and sickle cell disease, the diagnosis is often already known. In contrast, for diseases which present with stroke as the main manifestation, diagnosis and identification of an underlying single gene disorder can be challenging.

Most familial causes of stroke present in young or middle age and the diagnosis should be considered in a patient presenting with stroke at under 60 years, particularly when they have a family history of stroke. However, the majority of young onset strokes will not have an underlying single gene disorder, while increasing numbers of cases of stroke presenting at an older age (for example in the seventh decade for CADASIL) are being reported. Results of specific investigations may also highlight a likely monogenic cause. For example, involvement of the anterior temporal pole on MRI in CADASIL has been shown to be a useful marker of the disease [38].

In all cases it is important that investigations are performed to accurately subtype the stroke. This includes brain imaging with CT or MRI to differentiate an ischemic stroke from a haemorrhagic stroke. Ischemic strokes then require further investigation with imaging of the extra- and intra- cerebral arteries (with CT or MR angiography or ultrasound), investigation of the heart with ECG and echocardiography, and blood tests for lipids and other circulating disease markers. Small lacunar infarcts caused by SVD are frequently not visible on CT brain imaging, and in these cases MRI is important not only to confirm the infarct but also to look for other manifestations of SVD such as white matter hyperintensities and cerebral microbleeds.

If the initial images show an ICH, rather than an infarct, a different series of investigations are required. These can include repeat brain imaging when the blood has resolved to look for an underlying lesion (such as an arteriovenous malformation or a neoplasm), angiography to look for an underlying aneurysm or arterial malformation, and MRI with gradient echo sequences to look for cerebral microbleeds. Cerebral microbleeds characteristically occur in the cortex and grey-white matter junction in amyloid angiopathy, and in the basal ganglia and subcortical structures in hypertensive haemorrhage due to SVD.

If a monogenic cause is suspected, and once the underlying stroke subtype has been determined, appropriate tests can be performed to diagnose monogenic conditions causing that particular stroke subtype. In some cases, this may include a haematological or biochemical test as in sickle cell disease and Fabry disease respectively, while in other cases, and particularly for SVD, genotyping is required. Traditionally this has been performed on a gene-by-gene basis using Sanger sequencing or similar techniques. However, with the increasing availability of next generation sequencing techniques this is increasingly being performed using sequencing arrays which screen multiple genes at the same time. This is particularly useful, for example, for SVD where multiple genes can cause a similar phenotype.

In the remainder of the chapter we present a number of examples of monogenic forms of stroke. We particularly focus on SVD for a number of reasons. Firstly, this includes CADASIL, which is the most common monogenic form of stroke. Secondly because of the recent advances in this area and the identification of multiple non-CADASIL forms of familial SVD. Thirdly because monogenic forms of SVD represent the majority of cases of suspected familial stroke without other systemic disease, and fourthly because they illustrate a number of important features of monogenic stroke including gene-environment interactions and challenges in diagnosis. However, we have also covered sickle cell disease as a non-SVD example of monogenic stroke both because it represents a major problem in some parts of the world, and because identification of the disease and appropriate treatment can reduce the risk of stroke.

24.5 Sickle Cell Disease

Sickle cell disease (SCD) is an autosomal recessive haemoglobinopathy caused by a homozygous glutamic acid-valine substitution in the 6th position of the β-globin chain of haemoglobin. In the resulting haemoglobin (HbS), there are two normal α chains and two mutant β chains. As glutamic acid is a polar amino acid, while valine is non-polar and insoluble, the potential bonds formed by the globin chains are altered, resulting in impaired solubility of the resulting haemoglobin. HbS polymerizes to form fibres known as tactoids, which lead to the distortion of the red cell, which is rigid and dehydrated, and carries a sickle-shaped appearance. The sickled cells are also more adherent to vascular endothelium, thus promoting vessel occlusion [39].

SCD is prevalent in individuals of Sub-Saharan Africans and African Caribbean ancestry, and is also present in the Mediterranean, Middle East and India. Its distribution matches that of the endemic plasmodium falciparum malaria, which exerts a selection pressure, with the sickle gene in heterozygous form conferring protection from malaria [40].

SCD is clinically complex with a high degree of phenotypic heterogeneity, with patients experiencing a range of systemic effects from infancy. One of the key features is vaso-occlusion, which accounts for many systemic complications. Distorted red cells occlude blood vessels and lead to infarction, presenting as painful crises in the bones or joints of hands and feet, acute chest syndrome, pulmonary hypertension, renal papillae damage and stroke [41].

24.5.1 Stroke in SCD

Strokes are a common cause of morbidity and mortality in SCD, affecting up to 3.75% of patients [42]. In affected regions SCD is one of the most common cause of paediatric strokes between the ages of 2–9 years, although they can occur at any age [43]. Strokes in SCD may be ischaemic or haemorrhagic, with ischaemic strokes having a bimodal distribution, peaking around the first and third decade [44], and haemorrhagic strokes being less common, arising at a later age, after the second decade of life [42].

24.5.2 Ischaemic Strokes in SCD

Many strokes in SCD to arise due to narrowing of the major cerebral vessels, primarily the internal carotid artery (ICA) and proximal section of the middle cerebral artery (MCA), resulting in impaired perfusion of territories distal to the stenosis. Sickling of erythrocytes and anaemia results in hyperplasia of the intima of large vessels, a feature seen in 80% of SCD patients with stroke [45].

Beyond an arteriopathy, other mechanisms contribute to strokes in SCD. SCD patients are often in a hypercoagulable state at baseline, with raised levels of markers of coagulation and fibrinolysis, and reduced Protein C and S concentrations [46, 47]. During pain crises, there is also activation of platelets, and sickled erythrocytes may express phosphatidylserine which promotes the activation of prothrombin [48]. Chronic haemolysis of sickled cells depletes circulating nitric oxide, which is essential for maintaining vasomotor tone and preventing platelet aggregation, contributing to ischaemia via vasoconstriction [49]. Chronic hypoxia may also create a state of chronic inflammation, with high circulating proinflammatory cytokines promoting the interaction of sickled cells with the endothelium [50].

Less common causes of stroke are in SCD are underlying cardioembolism and cardiopathies, systolic dysfunction and atrial fibrillation. These are estimated to account for 24% of strokes in adult SCD patients [46]. Adults with SCD also have a high prevalence of posterior circulation aneurysms, and cerebral venous sinus thrombosis is a common event in adults with SCD—both of which may predispose the patient to strokes [51].

24.5.3 Haemorrhagic Strokes in SCD

Large intracerebral artery occlusion may also result in the formation of compensatory collateral subcortical vessels, giving a 'puff of smoke' appearance described as Moya-moya syndrome [52]. These can rupture, leading to ICH and this is often occurs young adulthood rather than childhood [53]. Aneurysms and arteriovenous malformations are common in SCD, and may also predispose individuals to haemorrhagic strokes [54, 55].

24.5.4 Clinically Silent Strokes in SCD

Clinically silent infarcts, and white matter hyperintensities on MRI, are more common than clinically overt strokes in SCD, occurring in more than 22% of patients

[56]. These lesions are associated with cognitive impairment, and are also a recognised risk factor for overt strokes [57].

24.5.5 Risk Factors for Stroke in SCD

A number of clinical biomarkers can serve to predict an individual's risk of developing silent, ischaemic or haemorrhagic strokes in SCD. (Table 24.3 and 24.4) One important tool is the use of transcranial Doppler ultrasonography (TCD) in predicting the risk of stroke in paediatric SCD patients—currently the most accurate prognostic tool available. Raised ICA or MCA flow velocities on TCD serve as a marker of focal stenosis, and can identify those at highest risk of first stroke [58] .

24.5.6 Genetic Risk Factors for Stroke in SCD

As with other clinical phenomena in SCD, the occurrence and severity of stroke between patients can vary widely, and this is likely due to a combination of genetic and environmental risk factors interacting with the sickle cell genotype. Early studies have demonstrated a familial predisposition to cerebral vasculopathy in families with more than one child with SCD, showing that siblings of children with stroke or increased TCD blood flow velocities have an increased risk of stroke [59, 60].

The α-thalassaemia polymorphism, and concentration of foetal haemoglobin (HbF) are well-established modulators of stroke in SCD [61]. HbF decreases the stroke risk by inhibiting HbS polymerization, and genes such as BCL11A, HBS1L-MYB, β-globin genes and quantitative trait loci which affect HbF levels may contribute to this effect [62].

A number of studies have suggested other genes may influence the phenotype. A study of 80 candidate genes involved in vasoregulation, coagulation and other disease-associated processes utilised a Bayesian network approach to identify associations between genes and stroke in 1398 patients with SCD (92 with stroke) [63]. This study identified 31 SNPs in 12 genes as being associated with ischaemic stroke, with interaction between these genes and HbF as a possible mediating mechanism. Several of these genes were involved in the transforming growth factor-beta (TGFβ) pathway, a finding which was partially replicated in a subsequent candidate SNP study [61].

The use of MRI to phenotype stroke subtypes in SCD has also contributed to the discovery of genetic risk factors. In a study of 230 MRI-phenotyped SCA children, 104 SNPs were studied in 65 candidate vascular genes, and demonstrated that SNPs in IL4R, TNFα, and ADRB2 genes were associated with increased risk of large vessel strokes, while VCAM1 and LDLR genes were associated with increased (VCAM1) or decreased (LDLR) small vessel stroke risk [64]. Another variant in VCAM1 was previously also identified as protective against high TCD flow velocity and thus stroke risk in SCD [65].

Table 24.4 Familial forms of haemorrhagic strokes

Stroke subtype	Disease	Gene	Pattern of inheritance	Other key clinical features	References
Small vessel disease	COL4A1/A2* (subcortical haemorrhages)	COL4A1/A2	Autosomal dominant	• Porencephaly, hydroencephaly • Infantile hemiparesis • Visual loss • Developmental delay, cognitive impairment and dementia • Seizures • Nephropathy, myopathy, cardiac involvement • Intracranial aneurysms • Periventricular cysts involving subcortical structures • Retinal vessel abnormalities • HANAC syndrome in some patients: Hereditary Angiopathy, Nephropathy, Aneurysms and Cramps	[31]
	Hereditary CAA (lobar haemorrhages)	APP CST3 ITM2B TTR Gelsolin PPRN	Autosomal dominant	• Dementia • Seizures • Parenchymal plaques • Personality changes	[32, 33]

Large vessel Disease—rupture of vascular malformations	Hereditary Haemorrhagic Telangiectasia (Arteriovenous malformations)	ENG (HHT1) ACRVL1 (HHT2) SMAD4 (Juvenile Polyposis—HHT) GDF2	Autosomal dominant	• Sudden onset, recurrent epistaxis • Mucocutaneous telangiectasia • Visceral organ arteriovenous malformations (lungs, liver, gastrointestinal tract, brain, spinal cord)	[34]
	Autosomal dominant polycystic kidney disease (Intracranial aneurysms)	PKD1 PKD2	Autosomal dominant	• Polycystic kidneys leading to chronic renal failure and hypertension	[35]
	Familial Cerebral Cavernous Malformations (Cavernomas)	KRIT (CCM1) MGC4607 (CCM2) PDCD10 (CCM3)	Autosomal dominant	• CCM1: Hyperkeratotic cutaneous capillary venous malformation, café-au-lait spots, hepatic angiomas • CCM3: scoliosis, cognitive impairment, meningiomas	[36]
	Capillary Malformation—Arteriovenous Malformation	RASA1	Autosomal dominant	• Multiple skin capillary malformations (vascular stains) • Arteriovenous fistulas and malformations • Parkes Weber syndrome (cutaneous capillary malformations associated with underlying micro-AVFs, soft tissue and skeletal hypertrophy) • Infantile haemangiomas	[37]

*Key clinical features are provided for more common syndromes. Syndromes marked with an asterix predominantly cause haemorrhagic strokes, but may also cause ischaemic strokes

Other studies have suggested a potential role for the immune system in the development of stroke in patients with SCD with HLA DPB1 being associated with stroke risk [66].

Genome-wide approaches have been limited in the study of stroke in SCD, and to date have not validated findings in candidate gene or SNP studies [67]. The reader is also directed to a recent comprehensive review of the genetics of SCA-associated cardiovascular disease [68].

24.5.7 Management of Strokes in SCD

Although studies in the acute management of stroke in SCD are limited, there is no clear evidence against the use of thrombolysis in adults with SCD [46]. Supplemental oxygen in the acute setting can also help to maintain blood oxygen saturation at ≥95%, preventing further sickling and blood hyperviscosity [69]. Beyond standard stroke care, exchange blood transfusions are recognised as the standard of care for the primary and secondary prevention of strokes (excluding silent infarcts) [70].

Children with SCD who are at risk of stroke, as identified by high cerebral blood flow velocity on TCD, may have their absolute risk of first stroke being reduced by 9%, and relative risk lowered by 92%, by lowering the proportion of HbS to <30% with exchange transfusion [71]. Cessation of transfusion therapy may result in patients reverting to previous risk status [72]. In SCD children with a previous stroke, the risk of recurrent stroke is as high as 90%, and can be lowered to below 10% by regular exchange blood transfusion [70].

Reducing the proportion of HbS to can improve oxygen saturation through normal red blood cells, reducing further vaso-occlusion, improving tissue perfusion and preventing further ischaemic damage caused by the stroke [46]. A long-term exchange transfusion programme to reduce the proportion of HbS to <20% is thus recommended for children with either prior silent cerebral infarcts or raised TCD velocities [70]. Top-up blood transfusions are not recommended for the acute treatment of stroke as an increased blood viscosity may worsen stroke or painful crises [70].

24.6 Monogenic Forms of Small Vessel Disease

24.6.1 CADASIL

Cerebral Autosomal Dominant Arteriopathy with Subcortical Infarcts and Leukoencephalopathy (CADASIL) is the most common monogenic cause of SVD. CADASIL is caused by cysteine-changing mutations in exons 2–24 of the NOTCH3 gene, which encode the extracellular portion of the Notch 3 protein, a transmembrane receptor [18]. CADASIL is estimated to affect 2–4 per 100,000 population in the UK [73, 74]. Disease-causing NOTCH3 mutations were found in 0.5% of 1000 apparently sporadic young-onset (≤70 years) MRI-defined SVD stroke patients, with this figure rising to 1.5% when considering only patients with confluent white matter hyperintensities on MRI [75].

The clinical features of CADASIL are exclusively neurological. Migraine, usually with aura, is most commonly the earliest feature of disease, with onset usually in the 1920s or 1930s. Subcortical ischaemic lacunar strokes may occur, with an average age of onset of 47 years, and progressive subcortical cognitive impairment can occur in middle age leading to vascular dementia [76]. Depression is common and may precede other symptoms. Less common presentations of CADASIL include an acute reversible encephalopathy or 'coma' episode, which is often misdiagnosed as an acute encephalitis [77].

24.6.1.1 Phenotypic Variation and the Importance of Gene-Gene and Gene-Environment Interactions

Disease severity can vary widely between individuals, both between and within families. Almost all of CADASIL mutations result in the loss or gain of a cysteine amino acid in one of the epidermal growth factor (EGF) repeats in the extra-cellular portion of the Notch 3 protein [78]. Studies have shown no relationship between phenotype and mutation sites [79]. Why the phenotype varies so much between individuals is not well understood but it is thought that both gene-gene and gene-environment interactions are important. Family studies have shown a significant heritability for MRI determined white matter legion volume suggesting additional genes are important in determining phenotypic severity [80]. Conventional cardiovascular risk factors also seem to influence phenotypes. For example, CADASIL carriers who smoke on average develop stroke 10 years earlier [79]. Hypertension also seems to be important with the rate of progression of brain atrophy on MRI related to the level of blood pressure [81], and hypertension related to risk of stroke [77].

24.6.1.2 Diagnosis of CADASIL

CADASIL should be considered in all younger onset cases of lacunar stroke where there are white matter changes such as white matter hyperintensities on the MRI scan. There may be additional clues in the history including migraine with an aura which can be prolonged and confusional. There is usually a family history of clinical features of CADASIL but this is not always immediately clear. Vascular dementia in a relative can frequently be diagnosed as Alzheimer's disease, while particularly in the past CADASIL has been misdiagnosed as multiple sclerosis, so one should always be aware of this diagnosis in the family history. Furthermore, because CADASIL can present in middle age there may be no family history if the parents died relatively young.

As with diagnosis of many forms of SVD, careful assessment of the MRI is crucial. In the case of CADASIL this can reveal features which are almost diagnostic. For example, involvement of the anterior temporal pole has shown to be 90% sensitive and 90% specific [38]. Other features on MRI include confluent involvement of the external capsule, and involvement of the corpus callosum (a structure which is not usually involved in the sporadic small vessel disease although it is frequently involved in multiple sclerosis) [82].

The next step is genetic testing to confirm the diagnosis. Mutations tend to cluster in certain exons particularly exon 4 [78] and this initially led to limited screening to reduce cost and exclude the majority of cases. However, this approach will miss a significant number of cases and many labs now screen all of exons 2–24 in which mutations can occur. Although CADASIL only produces clinical features in the brain, arteries throughout the body are affected by the pathological process. This has led to the use of skin biopsy to detect the characteristic granular osmiophilic material (GOM) which can be seen on Electron Microscopy. However, with the wider availability of genetic testing this is less frequently performed.

Appropriate genetic counselling should be given before genetic testing and we use the Huntingdon's disease protocol. It's important to remember that in an individual with a family history with CADASIL an MRI is essentially a genetic test. If it shows characteristic changes it indicates the individual is a carrier of the mutation.

24.6.1.3 Management of CADASIL

While there is no specific treatment available for CADASIL, aggressive control of conventional cardiovascular risk factors is essential. A study of 200 patients with CADASIL showed that those with poorly controlled hypertension, or those who had a history of smoking, had an increased risk of stroke [77]. We advise our patients not to smoke, to maintain optimal weight and to exercise regularly. We would recommend avoiding the combined oral contraceptive pill, certainly from age 30 upwards. If cholesterol is elevated we often treat with statin therapy although there is no evidence supporting this approach in CADASIL itself, as opposed to more generally in sporadic stroke prevention. We give aspirin or clopidogrel to patients who have suffered ischaemic stroke, and to carriers over the age of 40, but avoid dual antiplatelet therapy and anticoagulants due to a generally increased risk of ICH with these treatments in SVD [83].

Migraines in CADASIL tend to be more complicated than those seen in the general population. Patients with CADASIL are more likely to have atypical migraine auras such as dysphasia and confusion, and can have more prolonged auras [76, 77]. There have been few studies on the management of migraine specifically in CADASIL although drugs used for management of migraine in the general population appear to be similarly effective in CADASIL [84–87]. Although triptans carry a theoretical risk of exacerbating ischaemia in patients with vasculopathy [88], retrospective data from a group of 300 patients with CADASIL suggests that triptans are safe to use and helpful in treating migraines in CADASIL [76].

Depression is frequent in CADASIL, as it is in other forms of SVD. Contributing factors include the stress of a monogenic disease diagnosis, as well as of complications such as stroke. However, there is also a biological reason with white matter lesions thought to disrupt cortical-subcortical pathways involved in mood regulation. It is important to be aware of the diagnosis and treat it with cognitive therapy/counselling and anti-depressants as this can be associated with a markedly improved quality of life.

24.6.1.4 Clinical Case 1

A 54-year-old right-handed female presented with sudden onset of double vision and vomiting, and abnormal eye movements.

She had a history of migraine with aura from the age of 15, experiencing visual changes and numbness in her arm. She did not have any past medical history of depression, seizures, or encephalopathy. She was not hypertensive, and had only smoked briefly as a teenager.

She had an MRI scan which showed an acute infarct in the midbrain with high signal on diffusion-weighted imaging (Fig. 24.1, 1-4), as well as extensive

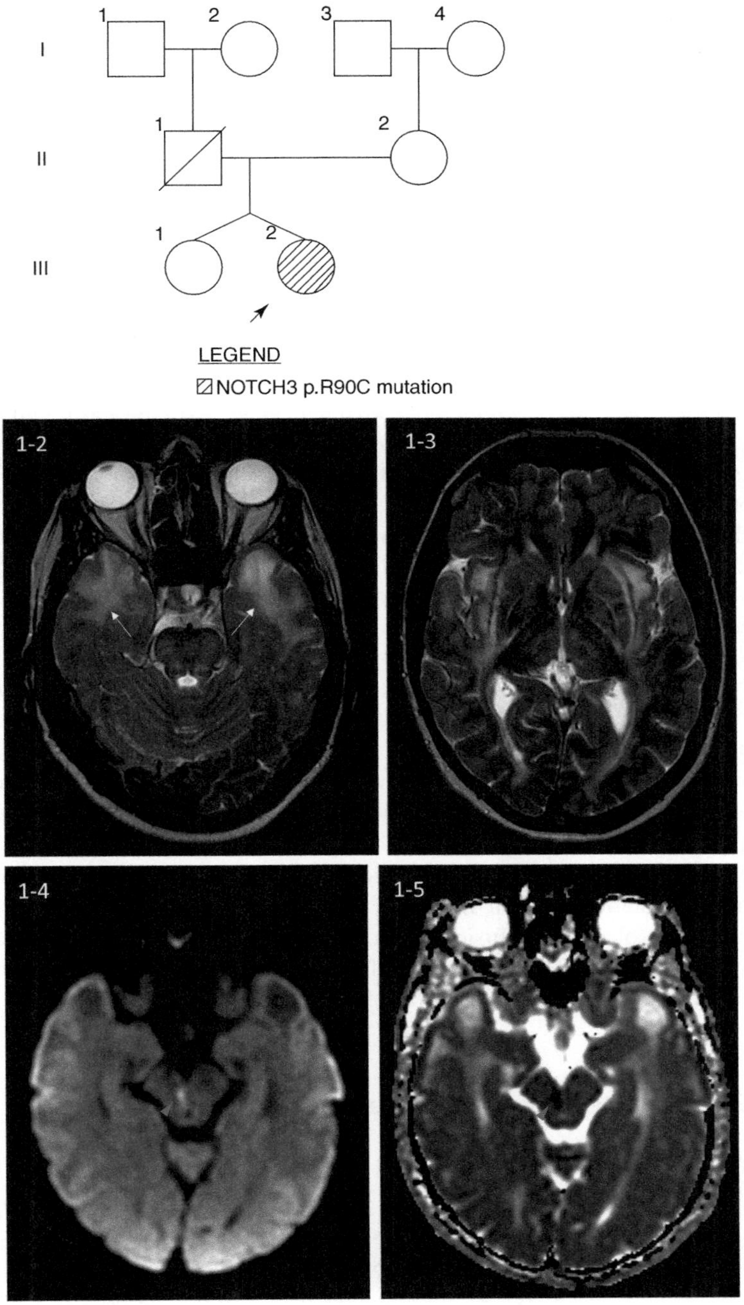

Fig. 24.1 (*inset 1-1*). Pedigree of clinical case 1. Although II.1, II.2 and III.1 had neurological symptoms, there was no clear history of stroke or dementia in the family. (1-2) MR T2-weighted imaging showing white matter intensities involving the anterior temporal poles (arrowed) and (1-3) external capsules. (1-4) Midbrain lesion shown on MR diffusion-weighted imaging, and (1-5) apparent diffusion coefficient imaging (arrowheads). (Copyright Hugh Markus)

white matter changes with prominent involvement of the anterior temporal poles. (Fig. 24.1, 1-2, 1-3).

Her mother was alive at age 83, with a history of migraines and bipolar disease. Her father died at age 72, having had possible complex partial seizures. Her identical twin sister had a history of migraine with aura. Despite the absence of a clear family history of stroke or dementia, the classical involvement of the anterior temporal poles and possible family history led to suspicion of CADASIL (Fig. 24.1). Genetic testing confirmed a p.Arg90Cys mutation on exon 3 of the NOTCH3 gene.

24.6.1.5 Clinical Case 2

A 58-year-old female teacher presented with a confusional episode typical of CADASIL encephalopathy. While teaching she experienced the beginning of what she thought was a migraine with visual disturbance. She was aware of a colleague saying something but could not remember what happened next. She was found to be conscious but poorly responsive to commands.

She was taken to hospital where she suffered four generalised seizures and was treated for encephalitis with acyclovir and antibiotics, as well as anti-epileptics. She continued to experience fluctuating confusion associated with visual hallucinations for the next eight days before regaining full consciousness. She had a past medical history of migraine with visual and sensory aura from the age of 28.

Although there were no known strokes in the family, she had a family history of dementia, with her father being diagnosed of 'Alzheimer's disease' at age 55 and dying at age 63. Her father's identical twin had no strokes or dementia but had not had an MRI scan prior to death also at age 55, and his sister had a diagnosis of 'probable dementia' (Fig. 24.2).

MR imaging of her brain showed confluent T2 hyperintensities in the white matter involving the anterior temporal poles and external capsules. (Fig. 24.2, 2-2, 2-3) A lumbar puncture performed at the time of her first admission was normal and negative for oligoclonal bands. Genetic screening for NOTCH3 mutations revealed a p.Arg151Cys mutation in Exon 4.

This patient's prolonged confusion episode is classical of a CADASIL 'coma' or encephalopathic episode. This is a feature of CADASIL that often follows a typical migraine aura, and can last up to 14 days before resolving completely [89].

24.7 Recently Described Monogenic Forms of SVD Stroke

24.7.1 CARASIL and HTRA1-Related Autosomal Dominant SVD

Cerebral Autosomal Recessive Arteriopathy with Subcortical Infarcts and Leukoencephalopathy (CARASIL) is caused by homozygous mutations in the HTRA1 gene [19]. CARASIL was initially described in a few families in consanguineous Japanese and Chinese populations [19, 90], and subsequently in a consanguineous European family, and a patient with compound heterozygous HTRA1 mutations [91].

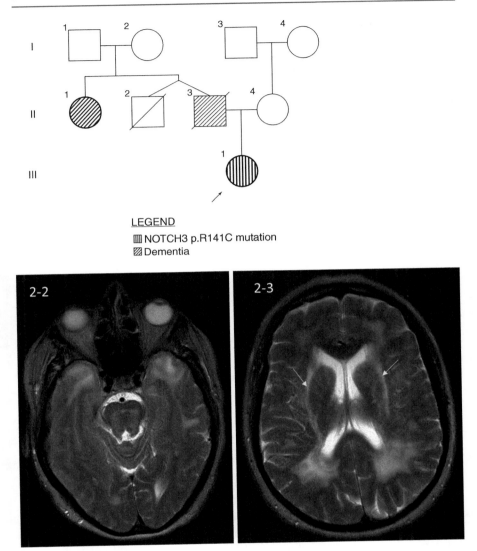

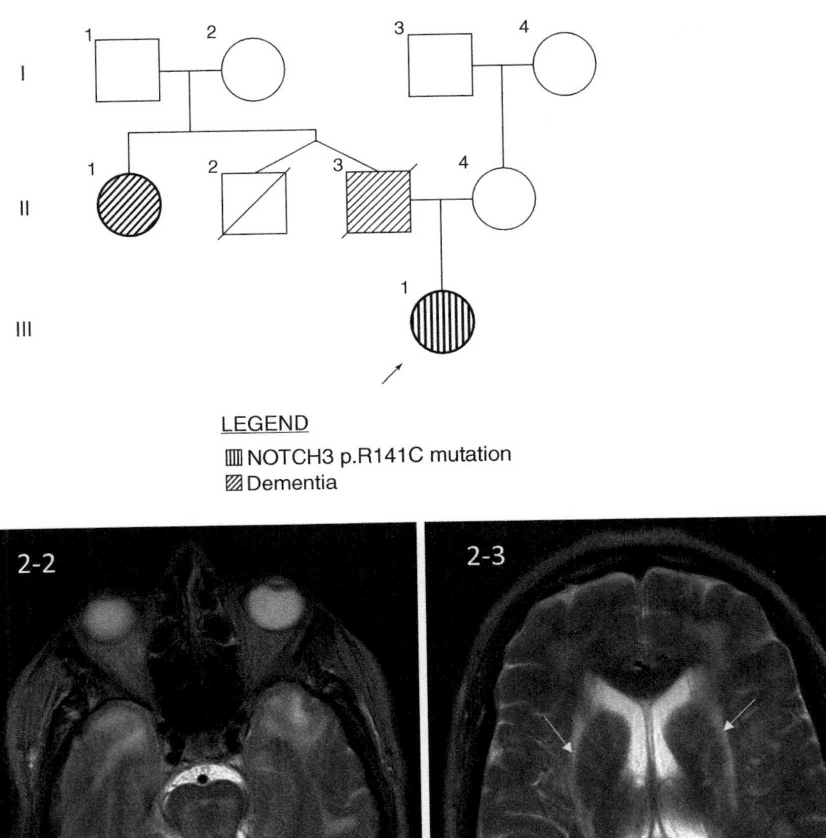

Fig. 24.2 (*inset 2-1*). Pedigree of clinical case 2 showing a family history of dementia (II.3) or suspected dementia (II.1) (2-2) MR T2-weighted imaging showing white matter intensities involving the anterior temporal poles and (2-3) external capsules (arrowed). (Copyright Hugh Markus)

Patients with CARASIL have been described as having a more rapid progression of the neurological features seen in CADASIL. A distinguishing feature of CARASIL is the presence of non-neurological features such as young-onset alopecia and degenerative spinal disc disease. On imaging, these patients may have characteristic arc-shaped hyperintensities extending from the pons to the middle cerebellar peduncles [92]. CARASIL patients have not been found to have the classical imaging feature of anterior temporal pole involvement seen in CADASIL [93].

More recently, whole exome sequencing in 201 Caucasian patients with suspected familial SVD and no NOTCH3 mutations identified heterozygous missense HTRA1 mutations in 10 cases, and segregation of the mutation with disease was also demonstrated in one pedigree. These patients had a later age at onset of disease, and did not report any extra-neurological features seen in CARASIL [20]. A similar study in 113 suspected familial SVD patients with no known genetic cause in Japan also identified four heterozygous missense HTRA1 mutations in six cases [21]. An example of a patient of HTRA1-associated autosomal dominant SVD is described in clinical case 3.

The HTRA1 gene encodes for high temperature requirement serine protease A1 (HtrA1), a homotrimeric serine protease which switches off the TGFβ pathway. This role of this pathway in blood vessel formation and vasoreactivity, as well as vessel and organ fibrosis in disease has been well described [94]. The impact of disease-causing HTRA1 mutations are, however, poorly understood. While most mutations impair protease activity [20], others do not cause a loss-of-function but have been predicted to impact trimer formation and activation [21].

24.7.2 Clinical Case 3

A 45-year-old female presented with a one-year history of migrainous aura without headache. These were stereotyped episodes of left-sided sensory symptoms, characterised by a sensation of flowing water down the left side of her body. She felt that her left hand was clumsy, although she was still able to mobilise with some clumsiness. She denied any speech disturbance or associated headache. These symptoms would last a week, after which she recovered completely.

She had a past history of depression.

She underwent neuropsychological assessment and was found to have impaired attention, information processing skills and some executive function difficulties—features commonly seen in small vessel disease-related cognitive impairment. An MRI of her brain showed widespread hyperintensities in the periventricular white matter and central pons. (Fig. 24.3, 3-2, 3-3).

She had a strong family history of strokes. Her father suffered recurrent strokes from 58, and was also found to have cognitive impairment. Her paternal aunt and uncle both died of strokes in their early 1960s. (Fig. 24.3, 3-1) A screen of exons 2, 3, 4, 5, 6, 8, 11, 18, 19 and 22 of the NOTCH3 gene was performed and no cysteine-changing mutations were found. Whole genome sequencing was performed, and a screen of the HTRA1 gene showed a heterozygous c.854C>T (p.P285L) mutation. This mutation had previously been identified in patients with both autosomal dominant [21] and autosomal recessive (CARASIL) [95] forms of familial SVD. Decreased protease activity was also demonstrated in cellular assays of this mutation [21].

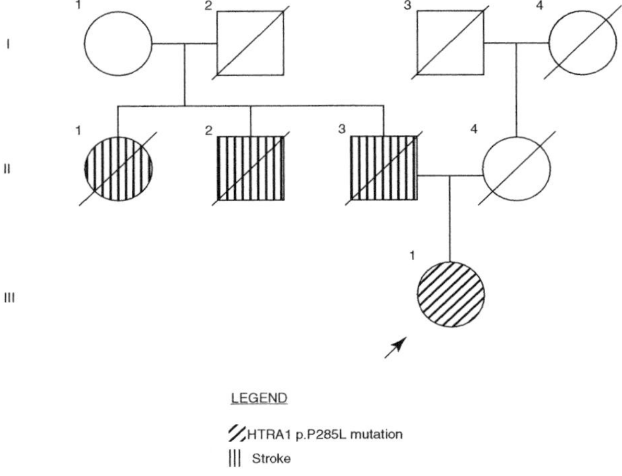

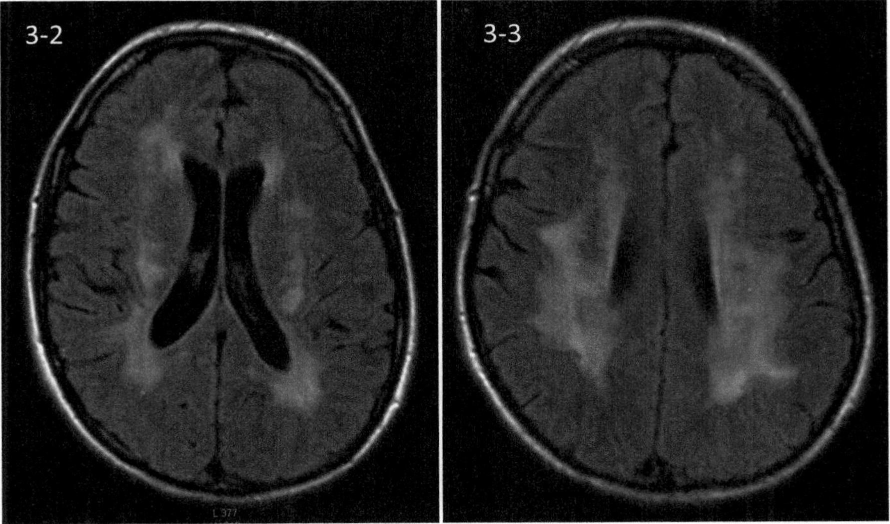

Fig. 24.3 (*inset 3-1*) Pedigree of clinical case 3, showing a clear family history of early-onset strokes in II.1, II.2 and II.3. *Insets 3-2* and *3-3* MR T2-weighted imaging showing confluent white matter hyperintensities not dissimilar to those seen in sporadic cerebral small vessel disease, or CADASIL. (Copyright Hugh Markus)

24.8 Haemorrhagic Strokes

24.8.1 COL4A1/A2-Related SVD: Subcortical Haemorrhages, Infarcts and Aneurysms

Mutations in the COL4A1/2 genes have been recently recognised a cause of lacunar stroke as well as subcortical ICH; i.e. they can cause both ischaemic and haemorrhagic stroke even within the same family. The COL4A1/A2 genes encode Type IV collagen α1 or α2 chains, which are the most abundant type of collagen in humans. COL4A1/A2-related SVD encompasses a broad spectrum of symptoms ranging from porencephaly in infants to adult-onset subcortical ischaemic and haemorrhagic strokes. These were previously described as specific paediatric syndromes, but have now been recognised as being attributable to mutations in the same genes [96, 97].

Patients with COL4A1/A2-related SVD can develop subcortical ICH, ischaemic lacunar infarcts, seizures, cognitive impairment and dementia. They may also have systemic involvement in the form of renal agenesis, nephropathy, visual loss and muscle cramps [98].

Type IV collagen is an integral component of basement membranes. As the most abundant form of collagen in the extracellular matrix, it lends tensile strength, helps to maintain vascular tone and also contributes to endothelial cell function.

The majority of pathogenic mutations in COL4A1 or COL4A2 are missense mutations which substitute a highly conserved glycine residue in the Gly-X-Y repeat region which aid the formation of tropocollagen. The resulting altered three dimensional confirmation of collagen impairs its ability to form heterotrimers in the vascular basement membrane, contributing to vessel wall fragility [99]. There may be some element of genotype-phenotype correlation, as mutations in the CB3[IV] fragment of COL4A1 have been found to be associated with Hereditary Angiopathy with Nephropathy, Aneurysms and muscle Cramps (HANAC) syndrome [100].

Recently common variants in the COL4A2 have been found to be risk factors for sporadic SVD [101].

24.8.2 Clinical Case 4

A 14-year-old boy presented with a subcortical ICH He was tested for and diagnosed with a p.Gly755Arg mutation in exon 30 of the COL4A1 gene. Following this diagnosis, other family members were tested and his 46-year-old mother was found to have same mutation.

Despite the proband's early onset of disease, his mother was relatively asymptomatic and had not had any strokes. She had a history of migraines with aura (visual and/or sensory) from the age of 39. She had no history of depression.

On MR imaging of the brain, she was found to have marked white matter hyperintensities and lacunar infarcts, (Fig. 24.4, 4-2, 4-3) and an aneurysm of the left internal carotid artery in the region of the carotid ophthalmic artery. There was also evidence of microbleeds on gradient echo MRI. (Fig. 24.4, 4-4, 4-5).

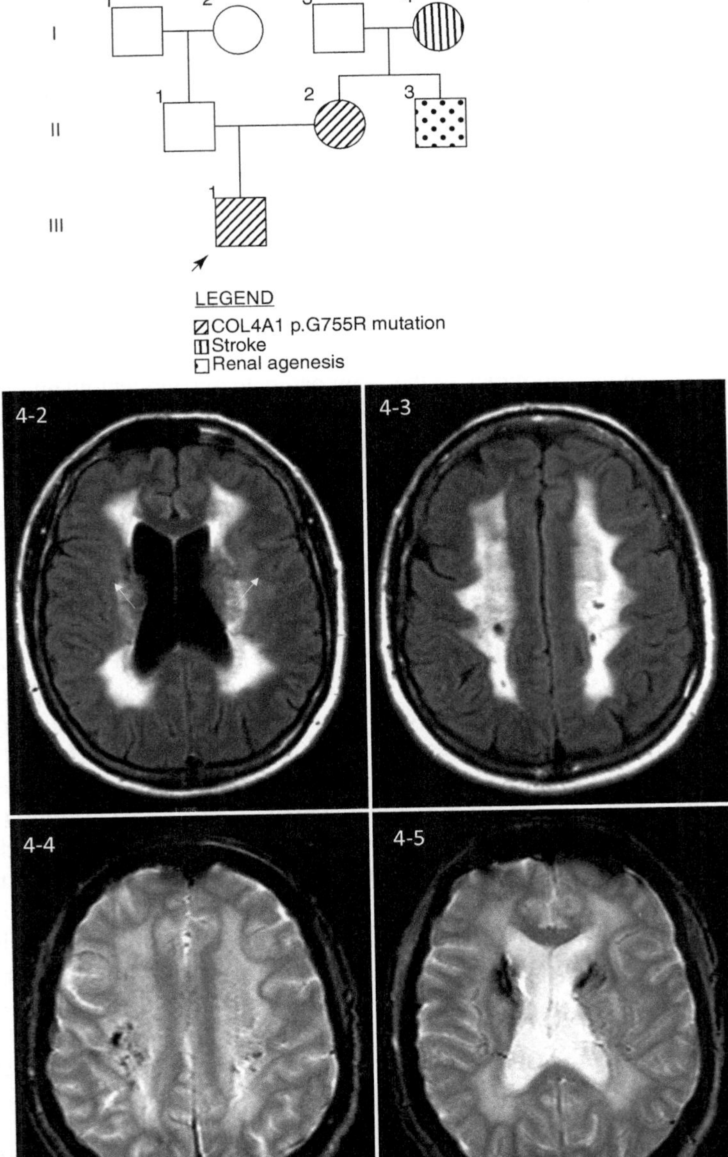

Fig. 24.4 (*inset 4-1*). Pedigree of Clinical Case 4 illustrating a wide variability of phenotypes among mutation carriers. While the proband had a paediatric onset of strokes, II.2 had MRI features of SVD in the fourth decade of life, but no strokes, and II.3 was born without a kidney—a feature previously reported in COL4A1-associated SVD cases. (4-2, 4-3) T2-weighted FLAIR MR images of II.2 showing confluent white matter hyperintensities and silent lacunar infarcts. *Insets 4-4* and *4-5*: Gradient-echo MR images of II.2 showing haemosiderin deposits and microbleeds. (Copyright Hugh Markus)

Her mother died at the age of 73, having had 'facial palsy' at the age of 47, and an episode of self-resolving hemiparesis in her teenage years. Brain imaging showed that she had had a number of strokes and a diagnosis of multiple sclerosis was considered at one point. Her father was 74 and had only a history of cataracts. She had a brother who was born with only one kidney. (Fig. 24.4, 4-1).

24.9 Hereditary Cerebral Amyloid Angiopathy: Lobar or Cortical Haemorrhages

Cerebral amyloid angiopathy (CAA) refers to a small artery vasculopathy which involves the deposition of amyloid fibrils in the small and medium blood vessel walls, and also in the capillaries of the brain parenchyma and leptomeninges [32]. These depositions are altered proteins which have adopted a β-pleated sheet conformation. CAA is most classically characterised by large lobar haemorrhages, but can also cause transient behavioural changes, seizures and cognitive impairment. CAA is definitively diagnosed by brain biopsy or post-mortem histopathological analysis, but the likelihood of CAA can also be determined based on the clinical syndrome and imaging, as described by the modified Boston criteria [102].

CAA most often occurs sporadically in the elderly population, with the deposition of amyloid beta (Aβ) protein in the walls of blood vessels, in association with parenchymal Aβ plaques in Alzheimer's disease [103]. In addition to lobar haemorrhages, CAA patients often have a distinctive distribution of classical SVD features, such as white matter hyperintensities with a predominant posterior distribution, and cerebral microbleeds in the lobar regions as visualised on gradient-echo MR imaging [104]. They may also have cortical superficial siderosis, which is a marker used for radiologically diagnosing CAA according to the modified Boston criteria [102].

CAA may also occur as a familial disease. Several large families worldwide have been identified as having a hereditary form of CAA, and affected individuals tend to have an earlier onset of symptoms than in sporadic CAA. The gene most commonly affected is the amyloid precursor protein (APP), which encodes the amyloid beta protein, and thus CAA arising due to APP mutations may also co-occur with familial Alzheimer's disease.

24.10 Summary and Conclusions

Stroke represents a collection of different aetiologies which lead to a similar clinical syndrome. Most strokes are multifactorial, most commonly occurring in the elderly, although considerable evidence has shown these have a genetic predisposition and GWAS studies are unravelling the specific genetic risk factors.

Stroke less commonly presents as a monogenic disease, where a single gene mutation results in a syndrome which includes early-onset stroke as a key clinical feature. The most common of these is CADASIL, a familial form of SVD which shares many features with sporadic SVD. In recent years, other causative genes have also been identified, such as COL4A1/A2 and HTRA1 which may have a higher prevalence than previously thought.

References

1. Sacco RL, Kasner SE, Broderick JP, et al. An updated definition of stroke for the twenty-first century: a statement for healthcare professionals from the American Heart Association/American Stroke Association. Stroke. 2013;44:2064–89. https://doi.org/10.1161/STR.0b013e318296aeca.
2. Flossmann E, Schulz U, Rothwell P. Systematic review of methods and results of studies of the genetic epidemiology of ischemic stroke. Stroke. 2004;35:212–27. https://doi.org/10.1161/01.STR.0000107187.84390.AA.
3. Meschia JF. Ischaemic stroke: one or several complex genetic disorders? Lancet Neurol. 2003;2:459.
4. Rubattu S, Volpe M, Kreutz R, et al. Chromosomal mapping of quantitative trait loci contributing to stroke in a rat model of complex human disease. Nat Genet. 1996;13:429–34. https://doi.org/10.1038/ng0896-429.
5. Bak S, Gaist D, Sindrup SH, et al. Genetic liability in stroke: a long-term follow-up study of Danish twins. Stroke. 2002;33:769–74.
6. Brass LM, Isaacsohn JL, Merikangas KR, Robinette CD. A study of twins and stroke. Stroke. 1992;23:221–3.
7. Kiely DK, P A W, L A C, et al. Familial aggregation of stroke. The Framingham Study. Stroke. 1993;24:1366–71. https://doi.org/10.1161/01.STR.24.9.1366.
8. Bevan S, Traylor M, Adib-Samii P, et al. Genetic heritability of ischemic stroke and the contribution of previously reported candidate gene and genomewide associations. Stroke. 2012;43:3161–7. https://doi.org/10.1161/STROKEAHA.112.665760.
9. Traylor M, Malik R, Nalls MA, et al. Genetic variation at 16q24.2 is associated with small vessel stroke. Ann Neurol. 2016;81(3):383–94. https://doi.org/10.1002/ana.24840.
10. Bellenguez C, Bevan S, Gschwendtner A, et al. Genome-wide association study identifies a variant in HDAC9 associated with large vessel ischemic stroke. Nat Genet. 2012;44:328–33. https://doi.org/10.1038/ng.1081.
11. Traylor M, Farrall M, Holliday EG, et al. Genetic risk factors for ischaemic stroke and its subtypes (the METASTROKE collaboration): a meta-analysis of genome-wide association studies. Lancet Neurol. 2012;11:951–62. https://doi.org/10.1016/S1474-4422(12)70234-X.
12. Neurology Working Group of the Cohorts for Heart and Aging Research in Genomic Epidemiology (CHARGE) Consortium, Stroke Genetics Network (SiGN), International Stroke Genetics Consortium (ISGC). Identification of additional risk loci for stroke and small vessel disease: a meta-analysis of genome-wide association studies. Lancet Neurol. 2016;15:695–707. https://doi.org/10.1016/S1474-4422(16)00102-2.
13. Traylor M, Mäkelä K-M, Kilarski LL, et al. A novel MMP12 locus is associated with large artery atherosclerotic stroke using a genome-wide age-at-onset informed approach. PLoS Genet. 2014;10:e1004469. https://doi.org/10.1371/journal.pgen.1004469.
14. Woo D, Falcone GJ, Devan WJ, et al. Meta-analysis of genome-wide association studies identifies 1q22 as a susceptibility locus for intracerebral hemorrhage. Am J Hum Genet. 2014;94:511–21. https://doi.org/10.1016/j.ajhg.2014.02.012.
15. Tan RYY, Markus HS. Monogenic causes of stroke: now and the future. J Neurol. 2015;262(12):2601–16. https://doi.org/10.1007/s00415-015-7794-4.
16. Joutel A, Haddad I, Ratelade J, Nelson MT. Perturbations of the cerebrovascular matrisome: a convergent mechanism in small vessel disease of the brain? J Cereb Blood Flow Metab. 2016;36:143–57. https://doi.org/10.1038/jcbfm.2015.62.

17. Tan RYY, Traylor M, Rutten-Jacobs L, Markus HS. New insights into mechanisms of small vessel disease stroke from genetics. Clin Sci. 2017;131(7):515–31.
18. Joutel A, Corpechot C, Ducros A, et al. Notch3 mutations in CADASIL, a hereditary adult-onset condition causing stroke and dementia. Nature. 1996;383:707–10. https://doi.org/10.1038/383707a0.
19. Fukutake T. Cerebral autosomal recessive arteriopathy with subcortical infarcts and leukoencephalopathy (CARASIL): from discovery to gene identification. J Stroke Cerebrovasc Dis. 2011;20:85–93. https://doi.org/10.1016/j.jstrokecerebrovasdis.2010.11.008.
20. Verdura E, Hervé D, Scharrer E, et al. Heterozygous HTRA1 mutations are associated with autosomal dominant cerebral small vessel disease. Brain. 2015;138(Pt 8):2347–58. https://doi.org/10.1093/brain/awv155.
21. Nozaki H, Kato T, Nihonmatsu M, et al. Distinct molecular mechanisms of HTRA1 mutants in manifesting heterozygotes with CARASIL. Neurology. 2016;86:1964–74. https://doi.org/10.1212/WNL.0000000000002694.
22. Bugiani M, Kevelam SH, Bakels HS, et al. Cathepsin A-related arteriopathy with strokes and leukoencephalopathy (CARASAL). Neurology. 2016;87(17):1777–86. https://doi.org/10.1212/WNL.0000000000003251.
23. DiFrancesco JC, Novara F, Zuffardi O, et al. TREX1 C-terminal frameshift mutations in the systemic variant of retinal vasculopathy with cerebral leukodystrophy. Neurol Sci. 2014;36(2):323–30. https://doi.org/10.1007/s10072-014-1944-9.
24. French CR, Seshadri S, Destefano AL, et al. Mutation of FOXC1 and PITX2 induces cerebral small-vessel disease. J Clin Invest. 2014;124:4877–81. https://doi.org/10.1172/JCI75109.
25. Zhou Q, Yang D, Ombrello AK, et al. Early-onset stroke and vasculopathy associated with mutations in ADA2. N Engl J Med. 2014;370:911–20. https://doi.org/10.1056/NEJMoa1307361.
26. Jenkinson EM, Rodero MP, Kasher PR, et al. Mutations in SNORD118 cause the cerebral microangiopathy leukoencephalopathy with calcifications and cysts. Nat Genet. 2016;48(10):1185–92. https://doi.org/10.1038/ng.3661.
27. Mitsias P, Levine SR. Cerebrovascular complications of Fabry's disease. Ann Neurol. 1996;40:8–17. https://doi.org/10.1002/ana.410400105.
28. Chassaing N, Martin L, Calvas P, et al. Pseudoxanthoma elasticum: a clinical, pathophysiological and genetic update including 11 novel ABCC6 mutations. J Med Genet. 2005;42:881–92. https://doi.org/10.1136/jmg.2004.030171.
29. Gutmann DH, Ferner RE, Listernick RH, et al. Neurofibromatosis type 1. Nat Rev. Dis Prim. 2017;3:17004. https://doi.org/10.1038/nrdp.2017.4.
30. Buoni S, Molinelli M, Mariottini A, et al. Homocystinuria with transverse sinus thrombosis. J Child Neurol. 2001;16:688–90. https://doi.org/10.1177/088307380101600913.
31. Renard D, Miné M, Pipiras E, et al. Cerebral small-vessel disease associated with COL4A1 and COL4A2 gene duplications. Neurology. 2014;83:1029–31. https://doi.org/10.1212/WNL.0000000000000769.
32. Revesz T, Holton JL, Lashley T, et al. Genetics and molecular pathogenesis of sporadic and hereditary cerebral amyloid angiopathies. Acta Neuropathol. 2009;118:115–30. https://doi.org/10.1007/s00401-009-0501-8.
33. Vidal R, Frangione B, Rostagno A, et al. A stop-codon mutation in the BRI gene associated with familial British dementia. Nature. 1999;399:776–81. https://doi.org/10.1038/21637.
34. Govani FS, Shovlin CL. Hereditary haemorrhagic telangiectasia: a clinical and scientific review. Eur J Hum Genet. 2009;17:860–71. https://doi.org/10.1038/ejhg.2009.35.
35. Perrone RD, Malek AM, Watnick T. Vascular complications in autosomal dominant polycystic kidney disease. Nat Rev. Nephrol. 2015;11:589–98. https://doi.org/10.1038/nrneph.2015.128.
36. Fischer A, Zalvide J, Faurobert E, et al. Cerebral cavernous malformations: from CCM genes to endothelial cell homeostasis. Trends Mol Med. 2013;19:302–8. https://doi.org/10.1016/j.molmed.2013.02.004.
37. Weitz NA, Lauren CT, Behr GG, et al. Clinical spectrum of capillary malformation-arteriovenous malformation syndrome presenting to a pediatric dermatology practice: a retrospective study. Pediatr Dermatol. 2015;32:76–84. https://doi.org/10.1111/pde.12384.

38. O'Sullivan M, Jarosz JM, Martin RJ, et al. MRI hyperintensities of the temporal lobe and external capsule in patients with CADASIL. Neurology. 2001;56:628–34.
39. Bellingham AJ. The sickling process in relation to clinical manifestations. J Clin Pathol. 1974;8:23–5.
40. Allison AC. Protection afforded by sickle-cell trait against subtertian malarial infection. BMJ. 1954;1:290–4.
41. Bender M, Douthitt Seibel G. Sickle cell disease. 1993. https://www.ncbi.nlm.nih.gov/books/NBK1377/.
42. Ohene-Frempong K, Weiner SJ, Sleeper LA, et al. Cerebrovascular accidents in sickle cell disease: rates and risk factors. Blood. 1998;91:288–94.
43. Gemmete JJ, Davagnanam I, Toma AK, et al. Arterial ischemic stroke in children. Neuroimaging Clin N Am. 2013;23:781–98. https://doi.org/10.1016/j.nic.2013.03.019.
44. Strouse JJ, Jordan LC, Lanzkron S, Casella JF. The excess burden of stroke in hospitalized adults with sickle cell disease. Am J Hematol. 2009;84:548–52. https://doi.org/10.1002/ajh.21476.
45. Kirkham FJ. Therapy Insight: stroke risk and its management in patients with sickle cell disease. Nat Clin Pract Neurol. 2007;3:264–78. https://doi.org/10.1038/ncpneuro0495.
46. Lawrence C, Webb J. Sickle cell disease and stroke: diagnosis and management. Curr Neurol Neurosci Rep. 2016;16:27. https://doi.org/10.1007/s11910-016-0622-0.
47. Schnog JB, Mac Gillavry MR, van Zanten AP, et al. Protein C and S and inflammation in sickle cell disease. Am J Hematol. 2004;76:26–32. https://doi.org/10.1002/ajh.20052.
48. Yasin Z, Witting S, Palascak MB, et al. Phosphatidylserine externalization in sickle red blood cells: associations with cell age, density, and hemoglobin F. Blood. 2003;102:365–70. https://doi.org/10.1182/blood-2002-11-3416.
49. Switzer JA, Hess DC, Nichols FT, Adams RJ. Pathophysiology and treatment of stroke in sickle-cell disease: present and future. Lancet Neurol. 2006;5:501–12. https://doi.org/10.1016/S1474-4422(06)70469-0.
50. Francis RB, Haywood LJ. Elevated immunoreactive tumor necrosis factor and interleukin-1 in sickle cell disease. J Natl Med Assoc. 1992;84:611–5.
51. Hines PC, McKnight TP, Seto W, et al. Central nervous system events in children with sickle cell disease presenting acutely with headache. J Pediatr. 2011;159:472–8. https://doi.org/10.1016/j.jpeds.2011.02.009.
52. Seeler RA, Royal JE, Powe L, Goldberg HR. Moyamoya in children with sickle cell anemia and cerebrovascular occlusion. J Pediatr. 1978;93:808–10.
53. Powars D, Adams RJ, Nichols FT, et al. Delayed intracranial hemorrhage following cerebral infarction in sickle cell anemia. J Assoc Acad Minor Phys. 1990;1:79–82.
54. Powars D, Wilson B, Imbus C, et al. The natural history of stroke in sickle cell disease. Am J Med. 1978;65:461–71.
55. Oyesiku NM, Barrow DL, Eckman JR, et al. Intracranial aneurysms in sickle-cell anemia: clinical features and pathogenesis. J Neurosurg. 1991;75:356–63. https://doi.org/10.3171/jns.1991.75.3.0356.
56. Armstrong FD, Thompson RJ, Wang W, et al. Cognitive functioning and brain magnetic resonance imaging in children with sickle Cell disease. Neuropsychology Committee of the Cooperative Study of Sickle Cell Disease. Pediatrics. 1996;97:864–70.
57. Miller ST, Macklin EA, Pegelow CH, et al. Silent infarction as a risk factor for overt stroke in children with sickle cell anemia: a report from the cooperative study of sickle cell disease. J Pediatr. 2001;139:385–90. https://doi.org/10.1067/mpd.2001.117580.
58. Adams R, McKie V, Nichols F, et al. The use of transcranial ultrasonography to predict stroke in sickle cell disease. N Engl J Med. 1992;326:605–10. https://doi.org/10.1056/NEJM199202273260905.
59. Driscoll MC, Hurlet A, Styles L, et al. Stroke risk in siblings with sickle cell anemia. Blood. 2003;101:2401–4.
60. Sampaio Silva G, Vicari P, Figueiredo MS, et al. Transcranial doppler in adult patients with sickle cell disease. Cerebrovasc Dis. 2006;21:38–41. https://doi.org/10.1159/000089592.

61. Flanagan JM, Frohlich DM, Howard TA, et al. Genetic predictors for stroke in children with sickle cell anemia. Blood. 2011;117:6681–4. https://doi.org/10.1182/blood-2011-01-332205.
62. Lettre G, Sankaran VG, Bezerra MAC, et al. DNA polymorphisms at the BCL11A, HBS1L-MYB, and -globin loci associate with fetal hemoglobin levels and pain crises in sickle cell disease. Proc Natl Acad Sci. 2008;105:11869–74. https://doi.org/10.1073/pnas.0804799105.
63. Hoppe C, Klitz W, Cheng S, et al. Gene interactions and stroke risk in children with sickle cell anemia. Blood. 2004;103:2391–6. https://doi.org/10.1182/blood-2003-09-3015.
64. Sebastiani P, Ramoni MF, Nolan V, et al. Genetic dissection and prognostic modeling of overt stroke in sickle cell anemia. Nat Genet. 2005;37:435–40. https://doi.org/10.1038/ng1533.
65. JGT VI, Tang DC, Savage SA, et al. Variants in the VCAM1 gene and risk for symptomatic stroke in sickle cell disease. Blood. 2002;100:4303–9. https://doi.org/10.1182/blood-2001-12-0306.
66. Hoppe C, Klitz W, Noble J, et al. Distinct HLA associations by stroke subtype in children with sickle cell anemia. Blood. 2003;101:2865–9. https://doi.org/10.1182/blood-2002-09-2791.
67. Flanagan JM, Sheehan V, Linder H, et al. Genetic mapping and exome sequencing identify 2 mutations associated with stroke protection in pediatric patients with sickle cell anemia. Blood. 2013;121:3237–45. https://doi.org/10.1182/blood-2012-10-464156.
68. Geard A, Pule GD, Chelo D, et al. Genetics of sickle cell-associated cardiovascular disease: an expert review with lessons learned in Africa. Omi A J Integr Biol. 2016;20:581–92. https://doi.org/10.1089/omi.2016.0125.
69. Johnson CS. Arterial blood pressure and hyperviscosity in sickle cell disease. Hematol Oncol Clin North Am. 2005;19:827–37. https://doi.org/10.1016/j.hoc.2005.08.006.
70. Estcourt LJ, Fortin PM, Hopewell S, et al. Blood transfusion for preventing primary and secondary stroke in people with sickle cell disease. Cochrane Database Syst Rev. 2017;11:CD003146.
71. Adams RJ, McKie VC, Hsu L, et al. Prevention of a first stroke by transfusions in children with sickle cell anemia and abnormal results on transcranial doppler ultrasonography. N Engl J Med. 1998;339:5–11. https://doi.org/10.1056/NEJM199807023390102.
72. Investigators TOPSP in SCA (STOP 2) T. Discontinuing prophylactic transfusions used to prevent stroke in sickle cell disease. N Engl J Med. 2005;353:2769–78. https://doi.org/10.1056/NEJMoa050460.
73. Razvi SSM, Davidson R, Bone I, Muir KW. The prevalence of cerebral autosomal dominant arteriopathy with subcortical infarcts and leucoencephalopathy (CADASIL) in the west of Scotland. J Neurol Neurosurg Psychiatry. 2005;76:739–41. https://doi.org/10.1136/jnnp.2004.051847.
74. Narayan SK, Gorman G, Kalaria RN, et al. The minimum prevalence of CADASIL in northeast England. Neurology. 2012;78:1025–7. https://doi.org/10.1212/WNL.0b013e31824d586c.
75. Kilarski LL, Rutten-Jacobs LCA, Bevan S, et al. Prevalence of CADASIL and Fabry disease in a Cohort of MRI defined younger onset lacunar stroke. PLoS One. 2015;10:e0136352. https://doi.org/10.1371/journal.pone.0136352.
76. Tan RYY, Markus HS. CADASIL: Migraine, Encephalopathy, Stroke and Their Inter-Relationships. PLoS One. 2016;11:e0157613. https://doi.org/10.1371/journal.pone.0157613.
77. Adib-Samii P, Brice G, Martin RJ, Markus HS. Clinical spectrum of CADASIL and the effect of cardiovascular risk factors on phenotype: study in 200 consecutively recruited individuals. Stroke. 2010;41(4):630. https://doi.org/10.1161/STROKEAHA.109.568402.
78. Joutel A, Vahedi K, Corpechot C, et al. Strong clustering and stereotyped nature of Notch3 mutations in CADASIL patients. Lancet. 1997;350:1511–5. https://doi.org/10.1016/S0140-6736(97)08083-5.
79. Singhal S, Bevan S, Barrick T, et al. The influence of genetic and cardiovascular risk factors on the CADASIL phenotype. Brain. 2004;127:2031–8. https://doi.org/10.1093/brain/awh223.
80. Opherk C, Peters N, Holtmannspötter M, et al. Heritability of MRI lesion volume in CADASIL: evidence for genetic modifiers. Stroke. 2006;37:2684–9. https://doi.org/10.1161/01.STR.0000245084.35575.66.
81. Peters N, Holtmannspotter M, Opherk C, et al. Brain volume changes in CADASIL: a serial MRI study in pure subcortical ischemic vascular disease. Neurology. 2006;66:1517–22. https://doi.org/10.1212/01.wnl.0000216271.96364.50.

82. Singhal S, Rich P, Markus HS. The spatial distribution of MR imaging abnormalities in cerebral autosomal dominant arteriopathy with subcortical infarcts and leukoencephalopathy and their relationship to age and clinical features. AJNR Am J Neuroradiol. 2005;26:2481–7.
83. Investigators TS. Effects of clopidogrel added to aspirin in patients with recent lacunar stroke. N Engl J Med. 2012;367:817–25. https://doi.org/10.1056/NEJMoa1204133.
84. Donnini I, Nannucci S, Valenti R, et al. Acetazolamide for the prophylaxis of migraine in CADASIL: a preliminary experience. J Headache Pain. 2012;13:299–302. https://doi.org/10.1007/s10194-012-0426-9.
85. Forteza AM, Brozman B, Rabinstein AA, et al. Acetazolamide for the treatment of migraine with aura in CADASIL. Neurology. 2001;57:2144–5. https://doi.org/10.1212/WNL.57.11.2144.
86. Weller M, Dichgans J, Klockgether T. Acetazolamide-responsive migraine in CADASIL. Neurology. 1998;50:1505. https://doi.org/10.1212/WNL.50.5.1505.
87. Martikainen MH, Roine S. Rapid improvement of a complex migrainous episode with sodium valproate in a patient with CADASIL. J Headache Pain. 2012;13:95–7. https://doi.org/10.1007/s10194-011-0400-y.
88. MHRA. Imigran 100 mg tablets (sumatriptan succinate) patient information leaflet. In: Medical information and production details. 2013. http://www.medicines.org.uk/emc/medicine/749. Accessed 27 Sept 2015.
89. Schon F, Martin RJ, Prevett M, et al. "CADASIL coma": an underdiagnosed acute encephalopathy. J Neurol Neurosurg Psychiatry. 2003;74:249–52. https://doi.org/10.1136/jnnp.74.2.249.
90. Zheng DM, FF X, Gao Y, et al. A Chinese pedigree of cerebral autosomal recessive arteriopathy with subcortical infarcts and leukoencephalopathy (CARASIL): clinical and radiological features. J Clin Neurosci. 2009;16:847–9. https://doi.org/10.1016/j.jocn.2008.08.031.
91. Mendioroz M, Fernández-Cadenas I, Del Río-Espinola A, et al. A missense HTRA1 mutation expands CARASIL syndrome to the Caucasian population. Neurology. 2010;75:2033–5. https://doi.org/10.1212/WNL.0b013e3181ff96ac.
92. Nozaki H, Sekine Y, Fukutake T, et al. Characteristic features and progression of abnormalities on MRI for CARASIL. Neurology. 2015;85:459–63. https://doi.org/10.1212/WNL.0000000000001803.
93. Yanagawa S, Ito N, Arima K, Ikeda S -i S. Cerebral autosomal recessive arteriopathy with subcortical infarcts and leukoencephalopathy. Neurology. 2002;58:817–20. https://doi.org/10.1212/WNL.58.5.817.
94. Oka C, Tsujimoto R, Kajikawa M, et al. HtrA1 serine protease inhibits signaling mediated by Tgfbeta family proteins. Development. 2004;131:1041–53. https://doi.org/10.1242/dev.00999.
95. Chen Y, He Z, Meng S, et al. A novel mutation of the high-temperature requirement A serine peptidase 1 (*HTRA1*) gene in a Chinese family with cerebral autosomal recessive arteriopathy with subcortical infarcts and leukoencephalopathy (CARASIL). J Int Med Res. 2013;41:1445–55. https://doi.org/10.1177/0300060513480926.
96. Gunda B, Mine M, Kovács T, et al. COL4A2 mutation causing adult onset recurrent intracerebral hemorrhage and leukoencephalopathy. J Neurol. 2014;261(3):500. https://doi.org/10.1007/s00415-013-7224-4.
97. Breedveld G, de Coo IF, Lequin MH, et al. Novel mutations in three families confirm a major role of COL4A1 in hereditary porencephaly. J Med Genet. 2006;43:490–5. https://doi.org/10.1136/jmg.2005.035584.
98. Alamowitch S, Plaisier E, Favrole P, et al. Cerebrovascular disease related to COL4A1 mutations in HANAC syndrome. Neurology. 2009;73:1873–82. https://doi.org/10.1212/WNL.0b013e3181c3fd12.
99. Jeanne M, Labelle-Dumais C, Jorgensen J, et al. COL4A2 mutations impair COL4A1 and COL4A2 secretion and cause hemorrhagic stroke. Am J Hum Genet. 2012;90:91–101. https://doi.org/10.1016/j.ajhg.2011.11.022.
100. Plaisier E, Gribouval O, Alamowitch S, et al. COL4A1 mutations and hereditary angiopathy, nephropathy, aneurysms, and muscle cramps. N Engl J Med. 2007;357:2687–95. https://doi.org/10.1056/NEJMoa071906.

101. Rannikmäe K, Davies G, Thomson PA, et al. Common variation in COL4A1/COL4A2 is associated with sporadic cerebral small vessel disease. Neurology. 2015;84(9):918–26. https://doi.org/10.1212/WNL.0000000000001309.
102. Linn J, Halpin A, Demaerel P, et al. Prevalence of superficial siderosis in patients with cerebral amyloid angiopathy. Neurology. 2010;74:1346–50. https://doi.org/10.1212/WNL.0b013e3181dad605.
103. Vinters HV. Cerebral amyloid angiopathy. A critical review. Stroke. 1987;18:311–24.
104. Thanprasertsuk S, Martinez-Ramirez S, Pontes-Neto OM, et al. Posterior white matter disease distribution as a predictor of amyloid angiopathy. Neurology. 2014;83:794–800. https://doi.org/10.1212/WNL.0000000000000732.

Genetics and Genomics of Systemic Hypertension

25

Patricia B. Munroe, Syeda N.S. Jahangir, and Mark J. Caulfield

Abstract

Since 2007 there has been substantial progress in mapping blood pressure genes, and large-scale genome-wide association studies now indicate over 400 genomic regions. The identity and biological function of genes causing monogenic forms of hypertension have also increased over this time. In this chapter, we describe the main findings from genome-wide association studies across different ancestries utilising different study designs, and discuss new candidate genes and biological pathways. The clinical utility of blood pressure-associated genetic variants are discussed in a genetic risk score framework, and the early results from epigenetic analyses of hypertension are reviewed.

Keywords

Hypertension • Blood pressure • Heritability • Genome-wide association study Genetic risk score • Epigenetics

25.1 Introduction

Hypertension is highly prevalent in the adult population. It is estimated to affect 29% of all adults globally in 2025, and over 50% over the age of 60 years in several regions across the world [1]. It is a major public health concern as it is associated with an increased risk of cardiovascular disease, stroke, renal disease and peripheral artery disease [2–4]. The World Health Organisation estimates that one third of total deaths from cardiovascular disease is related to hypertension, and that

P.B. Munroe (✉) • S.N.S Jahangir • M.J. Caulfield
Department of Clinical Pharmacology, Barts and the London, William Harvey Research Institute, Queen Mary University of London, London, UK
e-mail: p.b.munroe@qmul.ac.uk; ha13489@qmul.ac.uk; m.j.caulfield@qmul.ac.uk

D. Kumar, P. Elliott (eds.), *Cardiovascular Genetics and Genomics*, https://doi.org/10.1007/978-3-319-66114-8_25

complications arising from hypertension accounts for 9.4 million total deaths per year across the globe as well as 45% of mortality due to heart disease, and 51% of mortality due to stroke, with these figures expected to rise [5].

Essential hypertension, also referred to as primary hypertension, is defined as high blood pressure (BP) for which there is no clearly defined aetiology. Most guidelines define hypertension clinically as a systolic BP >140 mmHg, and/or a diastolic BP >90 mmHg [3]. The risk of stroke and ischaemic heart disease mortality doubles for every 20/10 mmHg increase in BP, and therefore from a clinician's perspective, hypertension is best defined as the level of BP, at which treatment to lower BP will result in significant clinical benefit [2]. The latest statistics published by Public Health England, estimate that diseases related to elevated BP cost the NHS over £2.1 billion per year. The estimated prevalence of hypertension in adults over the age of 16 in the UK is 31% in men, and 26% in women, a total of around 12.5 million people in 2015 [4].

Systemic hypertension—high BP in the systemic arteries has been associated with several identifiable risk factors, including age, sex, demographic, environmental, genetic and vascular factors. The most important modifiable risk factors include excess intake of dietary sodium, poor intake of dietary potassium, overweight/obesity (body mass index >25), sedentary lifestyle/lack of physical exercise, increased alcohol intake (> 14 units per week) and physiological stress [3–5].

25.2 Heritability of Hypertension

The first evidence for the genetic basis of hypertension was found in family and twin BP studies. These studies estimated the heritability of BP to be between 48–60% for systolic BP, and 34–67% for diastolic BP, with an overall approximate heritability between 40–50% for both systolic and diastolic BP [6–8]. Heritability studies however, do not permit identification of which genetic differences are most significant, or the mechanism by which they exert their effect on BP.

In the general population, BP readings follow a normal distribution, therefore patients with essential hypertension, will be those that have inherited a collection of genes, and have been exposed to environmental factors favouring hypertension, placing them in the higher end of the normal population distribution of BP [9].

Modern genetic studies are important as they hold the key to examining the biochemical and molecular processes that control BP, which in turn, allow discovery of the interactive physiological regulators that malfunction in patients with hypertension. Findings from genetic studies may allow the development of a new classification of disease based on molecular mechanisms, rather than on the phenotype of the patient [10]. A better understanding of the pathogenesis of the disease will facilitate rational drug development, and allow for targeted pharmacological treatment with a focus on disease subtypes that are more likely to respond to treatment. Genetic screening may also give rise to avoidance of adverse drug effects, using genetic risk factor analysis to facilitate modification, screening, and therapeutic management of people before development of symptoms [10].

25.3 Gene Discovery for Mendelian Forms of Human Hypertension

There are several rare Mendelian forms of hypertension with distinctive co-phenotypes, such as, hypertension and hypokalaemia as observed in Liddle's syndrome and Glucocorticoid Suppressible Hyperaldosteronism. The elucidation of the genetic basis of these Mendelian forms of hypertension has offered some insights into hypertension genomics, and indicate that the mechanisms for some of these rare disorders influence sodium homeostasis. In Table 25.1 we summarise the main clinical features of hypertension syndromes indicating the causal genes for each, the aetiologic mutations in each of these genes typically exhibit large effects on BP [11].

Next generation sequencing (NGS) has facilitated the identification of causative genes for these syndromes, and in 2015, mutations were identified in phosphodiesterase 3A (*PDE3A*) in a Turkish kindred with early onset hypertension with brachydactyly type E (HTNB) [12]. Frederick Luft and colleagues had spent over 10 years tracking down the disease gene for this condition. The Turkish study involved whole genome sequencing of family members, to identify a heterozygous missense mutation in *PDE3A*, which encodes a cyclic GMP (cGMP) and AMP (cAMP) phosphodiesterase with a prominent role in the heart, vascular smooth muscle cells (VSMC), oocytes and platelets. Re-sequencing of 48 affected individuals in 6 unrelated families identified 6 independently clustered heterozygous mutations in exon 4 of *PDE3A*, which exhibit a gain-of-function effect on cAMP hydrolysis, and cause enhanced cell proliferation. Evidence was found for mechanisms mediating VSMC hyperplasia and increased peripheral vascular resistance. The authors suggested that VSMC-expressed PDE3A as a possible therapeutic target for the treatment of hypertension.

Alongside the discovery of genes causing Mendelian forms of hypertension—analyses have been undertaken to assess association of variants in the monogenic genes with BP phenotypes in the general population. The existence of rare genetic variants may provide an explanation to the significant degree of inter-individual blood pressure variance. The rare independent variant hypothesis was initially tested by Ji and colleagues, in 2008 [13]. This study involved sequencing of candidate genes that encode the Na-K-2Cl cotransporter (*SLC12A1*), the inward rectifier K+ channel (*KCNJ1*), and the Na-CL cotransporter (*SLC12A3*) in 3125 individuals registered in the Framingham Heart Study. Homozygous mutations in these genes causes Bartter's (*SLC12A1*, *KCNJ1*) or Gitelman's (*SLC12A3*) disease, salt-wasting hypotensive disorders. It was hypothesized that rare, heterozygous mutations in these candidate genes may predispose individuals to salt wasting in the kidneys, leading to a subsequent lowering of BP. It was discovered that patients with rare, independent variants within the three candidate genes had clinically significant lower BP, and were less likely to develop hypertension. The average systolic BP of rare mutation carriers was 5.7 mmHg lower at age 40, and 9 mmHg lower at age 60. The mutations were rare, as only 1% of the study population possessed a relevant mutation. Consequently, mutations within such genes is unlikely to provide a

Table 25.1 Mendelian disorders with systemic hypertension

Disorder	OMIM#	Inheritance	Phenotype	Chr	Gene
Pseudohypoaldosteronism type 2; Familial Hyperkalaemic Hypertension; Gordons syndrome	603136	AD	Hypertension and ↑K+, metabolic acidosis	2q36	Cullin-3 (*Cul3*)
	605775	AD & AR		5q31	Kelch-like protein 3 (*KLHL3*)
	605232	AR		12p13	Protein kinase, lysine deficient 1 (*WNK 1*)
	601884	AR		17q21	Protein kinase, lysine deficient 4 (*WNK 4*)
Hypertension associated with *PPARγ* mutations	601487	AD	Hypertension & Insulin resistance, type 2 diabetes	3p25	Peroxisome proliferator-activated receptor gamma (*PPARγ*)
Hypertension exacerbated by pregnancy	605115	AD	Early hypertension, exacerbated by pregnancy	4q31.23	Mineralocorticoid receptor (*NR3C2*)
Glucocorticoid remediable aldosteronism	103900	AD	Hypertension with other variable features	8q24.3	11 β-hydroxylase/aldosterone synthase (*CYP11B1/CYP11B2*) chimera
Congenital Adrenal Hyperplasia with 11β-hydroxylase deficiency	202010	AR	Hypertension with other variable features	8q	11 β-hydroxylase (*CYP11B1*)
Congenital Adrenal Hyperplasia with 17α-hydroxylase deficiency	202110	AR	Hypertension	10q24.32	17 α-hydroxylase (*CYP17A1*)
Hypertension & brachydactyly	112410	AD	Hypertension & brachydactyly	12p	Phosphodiesterase 3A (*PDE3A*)
Apparent mineralocorticoid excess	207765	AR	Hypertension & ↓K+, metabolic alkalosis, ↓renin, ↓↓ aldosterone	16q	11 β-hydroxysteroid dehydrogenase (*HSD11B2*)
Liddle's syndrome	600228	AD	Hypertension & ↓K+, metabolic alkalosis, ↓renin, ↓ aldosterone	12p13.31	Sodium channel non-voltage-gated 1, α subunit (*SCNN1A*)
	600670	AD		16p12.2	β subunit (*SCNN1B*)
	600761	AD		16p12.2	γ subunit (*SCNN1G*)

OMIM online Mendelian inheritance in man (https://www.omim.org), *AD* autosomal dominant, *AR* autosomal recessive, *K* potassium, *Chr* chromosome

definitive reason for BP variance in large populations, and it is likely that there is a role for rare mutation in other BP related genes.

More recently international BP consortia using much larger sample sizes have investigated this hypothesis using data from genotyping arrays with low frequency and rare variants [14]. No significant enrichment of BP variants has been observed in monogenic BP genes [14]. However, large genome-wide association studies (GWAS) have discovered both common and rare genetic variants (minor allele frequency, MAF <1%) in three genes causing monogenic hypertension (*CYP17A1*, *DBH*, and *PDE3A*) [14–17]. These analyses indicate genetic variation in monogenic genes does occur, however variants in these genes do not explain the cause of the disease in the majority of patients with clinical hypertension.

25.4 Genome Wide Association Studies

Contemporary genomic tools permit the genotyping of millions of single nucleotide polymorphisms (SNPs) on a single microarray in a reliable, efficient, and most significantly, cost-effective manner. The GWAS approach uses dense maps of SNPs located throughout the human genome to investigate associations without bias between genetic variants and the phenotype, with no preconception of the identity of the genes involved. This approach can be considered one of the first direct applications of the Human Genome Project and the HapMap project, and allows new information to be discovered concerning previously unidentified loci. International collaborative projects between researchers have facilitated the use of extremely large sample sizes for BP gene discovery and replication. GWAS have identified many genetic factors contributing to the control of BP, and have reported a multitude of loci associated with BP or hypertension, owing to the reproducibility of GWAS and replication of results across different ethnic backgrounds. Some of these findings from these studies may become potential targets for drug therapy, for both prevention and management of hypertension [18].

A model for the genetics of complex traits has been the 'common disease-common variant hypothesis', which suggests that common disease is due to allelic variants with a MAF greater than 5% in the population, and a small individual effect size [19]. GWAS addresses this precise spectrum of genetic variation, which is useful when the disease under investigation is caused by a few common variants that associate specifically with the disease [19]. However, in the case of several different loci contributing small amounts to the disease phenotype being studied, GWAS is less successful and the genetic signal is lost within the background noise of the multiple genetic loci [20].

In 2007, two major GWAS investigating for hypertension were published, by Levy et al., and the Welcome Trust Case Control Consortium (WTCCC) respectively published two major hypertension GWAS [21, 22]. The work of Levy et al., was conducted on individuals participating in the Framingham Heart Study, and was a study of BP at two different time points and long term average BP using more than 100,000 polymorphic genetic markers [21]. The WTCCC study included hypertensive subjects from the British Genetics of Hypertension (BRIGHT) study, and used over 500,00 polymorphic genetic markers, to compare their genotype with control subjects from the general population [22]. Neither study managed to identify robust signals associated with hypertension on a genome wide level as the power to detect the small contribution of multiple genetic loci on BP was too small. Following on from these studies, the approach was to increase the sample size for subsequent GWAS.

25.5 Large-Scale Meta-Analysis of GWAS

The first robust signals from GWAS investigating hypertension originated from two large consortia, the Global Blood Pressure Genetics (Global BPgen) consortium and the Cohorts for Heart and Aging Research in Genomic Epidemiology (CHARGE) consortium which tested approximately 2.5 million genotyped or imputed SNPs for association with BP in 34,333 and 29,136 subjects of European ancestry, respectively [23, 24]. Meta-analysis on a large scale involves combining the data of several studies together to detect SNPs with smaller effect sizes. The Global BPgen study identified 8 loci with genome-wide significance. The variants were near the *CYP17A1*, *CYP1A2*, *FGF5*, *SH2B3*, *MTHFR*, *ZNF652*, and *PLCD3* genes and chromosome 10 open reading frame 107 (*c10orf107*) [23]. The CHARGE study identified significant associations with systolic BP for 13 SNPs, with diastolic BP for 20 SNPs, and with hypertension for 10 SNPs, and reported 8 independent BP loci [24]. Three of these loci were common to both studies. Of the genomic regions identified by these meta-analyses, two of the 13 regions contained genes that were previously indicated to contribute to susceptibility of hypertension. These include the atrial natriuretic peptide A and B-type natriuretic peptide genes (*NPPA* and *NPPB*) on chromosome 1p32, and the *CYP17A1* gene on chromosome 10q24, which causes a rare Mendelian form of mineralocorticoid hypertension [25].

Following these studies, the International Consortium for Blood Pressure (ICBP) used a multi-stage design in ~200,000 participants of European ancestry to identify 29 SNPs from 28 loci with statistically robust associations for BP, including 16 novel loci, and 6 loci that contained genes suspected or known to contribute to BP control; *GUCY1A3–GUCY1B3*, *NPR3–C5orf23*, *ADM*, *FURIN–FES*, *GOSR2*, *GNAS–EDN3* [15]. A genetic risk score (GRS) based on the cumulative effect of all 29 BP-associated variants was found to be associated with risk of stroke, coronary artery disease and left ventricular hypertrophy. No associations were observed with kidney disease or function. The described variants increased further to over 100 using bespoke genotyping arrays including the ITMAT-Broad-CARE (IBC) array comprising 50,000 candidate genes SNPs [26–28], and Cardio-Metabochip [16], though the effect size for each SNP was small, on average 1 mmHg for systolic BP, and 0.5 mmHg for diastolic BP, typical of most genetic variants identified for disease, which tend to be common, and possess a small effect size [29].

The most recent GWAS have taken advantage of access to Biobank samples and longitudinal electronic health records (EHR) to discover new loci. A study by Hoffman et al., used records on 99,785 Genetic Epidemiology Research on Adult Health and Aging (GERA) cohort individuals to provide over 1.3 million BP measurements for a GWAS on long-term average pulse pressure and systolic and diastolic BP [30]. Among 75 significant loci, 39 new loci were identified and replicated in the combined ICBP and UK Biobank study. Merging data from GERA and ICBP produced 36 additional new loci, most of which were replicated in UK Biobank, and merging all three cohorts identified 241 additional significant loci, although no replication dataset was available. The BP associated SNPs were found to be enhanced in the aorta and tibial artery. The benefit of using clinical readings from EHR includes access to large sample sizes of data, and data that shows a long-term average of several independent clinical measurements from a variety of clinical visits, which simulation and experimental studies show can reduce phenotype variability, thus increasing the statistical power of a study [30, 31].

Another study by Warren et al., reported association of BP among approximately 140,000 UK Biobank participants of European ancestry, taken from a prospective cohort of 500,00 individuals aged 40–69 (using data from baseline BP measurements), with independent replication in large international cohorts [31]. Robust validation was reported for 107 independent loci (not previously reported at the time of analysis), including new independent variants at 11 previously reported BP loci.

25.6 Limited Contribution of Rare Genetic Variants to BP in the General Population

The majority of genetic variants associated with BP are common with relatively small effects (~1 mmHg SBP and ~0.5 mmHg per allele). Until recently, targeted experiments to address the contribution of low and rare frequency variants to BP traits were largely unexplored. In September 2016, the results from two large meta-analyses of Exome chip genotypes were reported [14, 17]. The Exome chip is comprised of mostly rare (MAF ≤ 0.01) and low frequency (0.01 < MAF < 0.05) non-synonymous coding variants. These large analyses reported three rare variant associations (MAF < 0.1%) at *COL21A1*, *RBM47*, *RRAS* and three low frequency variant associations at *SVEP1*, *PTPMT1*, *NPR1*. The effect size per allele of the rare variants was ~2.0 mmHg per allele. Gene-based analyses including coding variants with MAF < 1% in the Exome chip studies discovered further associations at two new genes (*A2ML1* and *NPR1*).

The more recently fabricated GWAS arrays also contain bespoke Exome content, similar to the Exome chip. The recent reports by Hoffman and Warren did not find any rare variant lead associations [30, 31]. However, conditional analysis of known loci identified a rare variant was at the *CDH17*; rs138582164 locus, this is an exonic stop gain mutation in the *GEM* gene [31]. This is a finding that will require validation.

25.7 GWAS in Individuals of Non-European Ancestry

GWASs have also been carried out in large cohorts of subjects of non-European ancestry. In 2010, a large GWAS meta-analyses identified a genetic variant near *CASZ1* in subjects with Japanese ancestry [32]. The following year, the Asian

Genetic Epidemiology Network Blood Pressure (AGEN-BP) consortium identified 6 significant associations with BP from a meta-analysis of GWAS including 19,608 subjects of East Asian ancestry, only a few of these associations corresponded with findings from the ICBP meta-analyses that included only subjects of European ancestry [33]. The prevalence of hypertension is greater in African Americans, and the manifestations of cardiovascular disease are more severe compared to any other ethnic group in the USA. One of the largest meta-analyses of GWAS in African Americans was published in 2013 by Franceschini et al., which included 29,378 individuals from 19 cohorts and replication in additional samples of individuals with African American, European and East Asian ancestry [34]. Three novel BP loci (*RSPO3*, *PLEKHG1* and *EVX1-HOXA*) were identified from the combined trans-ethnic meta-analyses. In 2017, a study by Liang et al. in individuals of African ancestry identified three further BP loci (*TARID/TCF21*, *LLPH/TMBIM4* and *FRMD3*), this study analysed 21 cohorts comprising of 31,968 individuals of African ancestry, and performed validation in 54,396 individuals from multi-ethnic samples. The BP-associated SNPs at *TARID/TCF21*, *LLPH/TMBIM4* and *FRMD3* and *GRP20/CDH1* were specific to individuals of African ancestry [35]. Functional annotation showed enrichment for genes expressed in immune and kidney cells, as well as in heart and vascular tissue cells.

In 2012, Kato et al., noted that approximately one quarter of BP associated loci (8/34) reported in four meta-analyses of GWAS are common across three ethnic groups—Europeans, East Asians and South Asians [36]. Trans-ancestry meta-analyses are useful for discovering novel BP associated loci, but they also enable fine mapping of common casual variants. Kato et al., went on to follow up these findings in 2015 by reporting a large trans-ancestry GWAS, and replication study of BP phenotypes (systolic and diastolic BP, mean arterial pressure and hypertension) among 320,251 individuals of East Asian, European and South Asian ancestry [37]. Genetic variants at 12 novel loci were associated with BP, and 19 novel SNPs were identified with little heterogeneity between the different ethnic groups. These SNP associations indicated candidate genes involved in vascular smooth muscle (*IGFBP3, KCNK3, PDE3A* and *PRDM6*) and renal function (*ARHGAP24*, *OSR1*, *SLC22A7* and *TBX2*).

In Table 25.2 we provide a summary of the results from large GWAS studies that have been undertaken thus far in non-European individuals, there have been limited studies undertaken solely in individuals of African descent (both discovery and replication). These early results indicate there is only a handful of variants that have ethnic-specific associations with BP traits [33, 35]. A comparison of BP-associated variants between individuals of Asian descent and Europeans indicate some are shared, however there is less sharing of BP-associated variants between Africans and East Asians, and between Africans and European individuals. The lack of cross validation of BP-associated variants in African individuals could in part be related to issues with power as smaller sample sizes have been investigated to date. It is notable however, that BP variants discovered in Europeans are combined into GRS, the GRS is significantly associated with BP traits in both Asian and African ancestries indicating a shared aetiology of BP and hypertension [15, 16].

Table 25.2 BP loci discovery in individuals of non-European ancestry

SNP	Chr	Position, Hg38	Genotype	RA	RAF				Effect size			Gene	Trait	PMID
					AFR	AMR	ASN	EUR	EUR	ASN	AFR			
East Asian ancestry														
rs880315	1	10736809	C/T	C	0.17	0.47	0.65	0.34	*	0.72		*CASZ1*	DBP	20479155
rs17030613	1	112648185	C/A	C	0.08	0.24	0.48	0.24	^	0.34		*ST7L*	DBP	21572416
rs16849225	2	164050310	C/T	T	0.08	0.19	0.44	0.22	^	–0.2		*FIGN*	SBP	21572416
rs6825911	4	110460482	C/T	C	0.45	0.75	0.51	0.77	^	0.36		*ENPEP*	DBP	21572416
rs1173766	5	32804422	C/T	T	0.64	0.53	0.64	0.56	^	–0.25		*NPR3*	SBP	21572416
rs11066280	12	112379979	T/A	A	0	0	0.24	0		–1.34		*ALDH2*	DBP	21572416
rs35444	12	115114632	A/G	G	0.44	0.35	0.26	0.41	^	–0.46		*TBX3*	DBP	21572416
rs16998073	4	80263187	T/A	T	0.12	0.26	0.33	0.29	*	1.43	*	*FGF5*	SBP	21572416
rs1004467	10	102834750	A/G	T	0.79	0.82	0.66	0.91	*	1.47		*CYP17A1*	SBP	21572416
rs17249754	12	89666809	G/A	A	0.17	0.12	0.36	0.14	*	–0.94		*ATP2B1*	SBP	21572416
rs1275988	2	26691496	T/C	C	0.15	0.68	0.23	0.58	^	0.37		*KCNK3*	MAP	26390057
rs1344653	2	19531084	A/G	A	0.36	0.46	0.17	0.4	*	–0.27		*OSR1*	PP	26390057
rs2014912	4	85794517	T/C	T	0.81	0.8	0.79	0.86	^	0.62		*ARHGAP24*	SBP	26390057
rs13359291	5	123140763	A/G	G	0.16	0.2	0.59	0.18	^	–0.53		*PRDM6*	SBP	26390057
rs9687065	5	149011577	A/G	A	0.08	0.16	0.23	0.2	^	0.26		*ABLIM3*	DBP	26390057
rs1563788	6	43340625	T/C	C	0.72	0.38	0.35	0.34	^	–0.51		*ZNF318*	SBP	26390057
rs10260816	7	45970501	C/G	C	0.38	0.36	0.75	0.45	^	0.32		*IGFBP3*	PP	26390057
rs2107595	7	19009765	A/G	G	0.22	0.22	0.36	0.18	^	0.31		*HDAC9*	PP	26390057
rs751984	11	61510774	T/C	T	0.18	0.25	0.47	0.13	^	0.33		*SYT7*	MAP	26390057
rs12579720	12	20020830	C/G	C	0.31	0.66	0.45	0.74	^	–0.32		*PDE3A*	DBP	26390057
rs740406	19	2232222	A/G	A	0.31	0.15	0.26	0.07		–0.55		*AMH*	PP	26390057
rs2240736	17	61408032	T/C	C	0.63	0.51	0.44	0.73	^	–0.35		*TBX2*	MAP	26390057

(continued)

Table 25.2 (continued)

SNP	Chr	Position, Hg38	Genotype	RA	RAF				Effect size			Gene	Trait	PMID
					AFR	AMR	ASN	EUR	EUR	ASN	AFR			
African ancestry														
rs1717027	3	41946428	T/C	T	0.3	0.81	0.84	0.8	^		0.49	*ULK4*	DBP	23972371
rs13209747	6	126794309	T/C	C	0.13	0.4	0.48	0.46	^		−0.56	*RSPO3*	SBP	23972371
rs17080102	6	150683634	C/G	G	0.12	0.17	0.05	0.07	^		0.74	*PLEKHG1*	DBP	23972371
rs17428471	7	27298248	T/G	T	0.17	0.09	0.05	0.07	^		1.2	*EVX1-HOXA*	SBP	23972371
rs1401454	11	16228637	T/C	C	0.46	0.54	0.54	0.42	^		−0.45	*SOX6*	DBP	23972371
rs76987554	6	133759717	C/T	T	0.09	0.01	0	0			−1.85	*TARID*	SBP	28498854
rs115795127	9	83378986	T/C	T	0.14	0	0	0			N/A	*FRMD3*	CPASSOC	28498854
rs7006531	8	94098516	G/A	A	0.19	0.02	0	0			1.16	*CDH17*	PP	28498854
rs78192203	8	141364973	T/A	T	0.22	0.02	0	0			0.77	*GPR20*	CPASSOC	28498854
rs113866309	12	66123168	C/T	C	0.02	0.01	0	0			3.28	*LLPH*	PP	28498854

SNP single nucleotide polymorphism, *Chr* chromosome, Position Hg38 refers to position of the SNP in the human genome reference panel, *RA* reference allele taken from HaploRegV1.4 (http://archive.broadinstitute.org/mammals/haploreg/haploreg.php), *RAF* reference allele frequency taken from HaploRegV1.4, *gene* refers to the nearest gene to the associated SNP, *AFR* African, *AMR* American, *ASN* Asian, *EUR* European, *trait* the trait which the effect size relates to, *SBP* systolic blood pressure, *DBP* diastolic blood pressure, *PP* pulse pressure, *MAP* mean arterial pressure, The effect size is taken from the replication sample (if available) from the referenced paper (PMID) for that ancestry. The * indicates if the exact SNP is genome-wide significant in this ancestry for a BP trait, and ^ indicates $P < 0.05$, these results are taken from PhenoScanner (http://www.phenoscanner.medschl.cam.ac.uk/phenoscanner). *CPASSOC* is the single or multi-trait statistic

25.8 Blood Pressure Genetic Risk Score and Prediction of Cardiovascular Risk

Each BP-associated variant discovered in a GWAS individually only has a small effect size thus has no predictive value. However, the overall predictive information can be increased by combining the effects of multiple genetic variants together into a GRS. Blood pressure GRSs are commonly used to assess association with hypertension and cardiovascular outcomes, and strong associations have been reported across several cardiovascular traits (for example: coronary artery disease, stroke, carotid intima thickness) [15, 16, 31]. A GRS constructed from BP-associated variants is highly significant for association with hypertension as the binary clinical outcome. This was originally illustrated by ICBP in 2011 using a GRS of 29 SNPs ($P = 3.1 \times 10^{-33}$) [38].

Using data from 5639 individuals from the 1958 Birth Cohort, a GRS based on all currently published BP variants (N = 332 were available in this dataset from N = 348) increases the percentage trait variance explained by over 2-fold, with much higher statistical significance levels, compared to the GRS based on only the original 29 identified SNPs [15]: from 0.81% ($P = 7.31 \times 10^{-12}$) to 2.02% ($P = 5.06 \times 10^{-27}$) for association with SBP residuals after adjustment for sex and BMI; from 0.81% ($P = 7.07 \times 10^{-12}$) to 1.85% ($P = 7.33 \times 10^{-25}$) for association with DBP; and from 0.27% ($P = 5.54 \times 10^{-5}$) to 0.55% ($P = 1.34 \times 10^{-8}$) for association with hypertension (Fig. 25.1). Furthermore, the odds of hypertension for those at highest genetic risk in the top 20% of the GRS compared to those at lowest genetic risk in the bottom 20% of the GRS increases from 1.50 (95% CI: 1.22–1.85, $P = 1.01 \times 10^{-4}$) for the 29-SNP GRS to 1.78 (95% CI: 1.45–2.18, $P = 2.64 \times 10^{-8}$) for the full GRS, showing a better capacity for risk stratification as the number of variants added to the GRS increases. If other variants with larger effect sizes are identified risk stratification may increase further in the future.

The clinical utility of a BP-GRS as this time however is limited, even with the addition of 300 more signals. However, it may be useful for either screening subgroups of high-risk individuals, or for use in GRS models for stratified risk prediction to identify patients at high risk of hypertension earlier in life, that may enable lifestyle intervention strategies. Recently, Warren et al. created a GRS including 107 novel loci and 163 previously reported and LD filtered to $r^2 > 0.2$ and tested the impact on BP levels and hypertension risk. A comparison of individuals in the highest quintile of the distribution of the GRS in individuals age >50 years to the lowest quintile indicated a two-fold higher risk of hypertension (OR = 2.32, 95% CI = 1.76 to 3.06, $P = 2.8 \times 10^{-9}$) and the authors suggested that a BP-GRS may have some potential clinical and public health implications [31].

25.9 Missing Heritability

Despite the discovery of a multitude of validated SNPs for BP, the associated variants have a small effect, and the cumulative proportion of heritability accounts for approximately 3.5% of phenotypic variance in BP studies, a large difference from

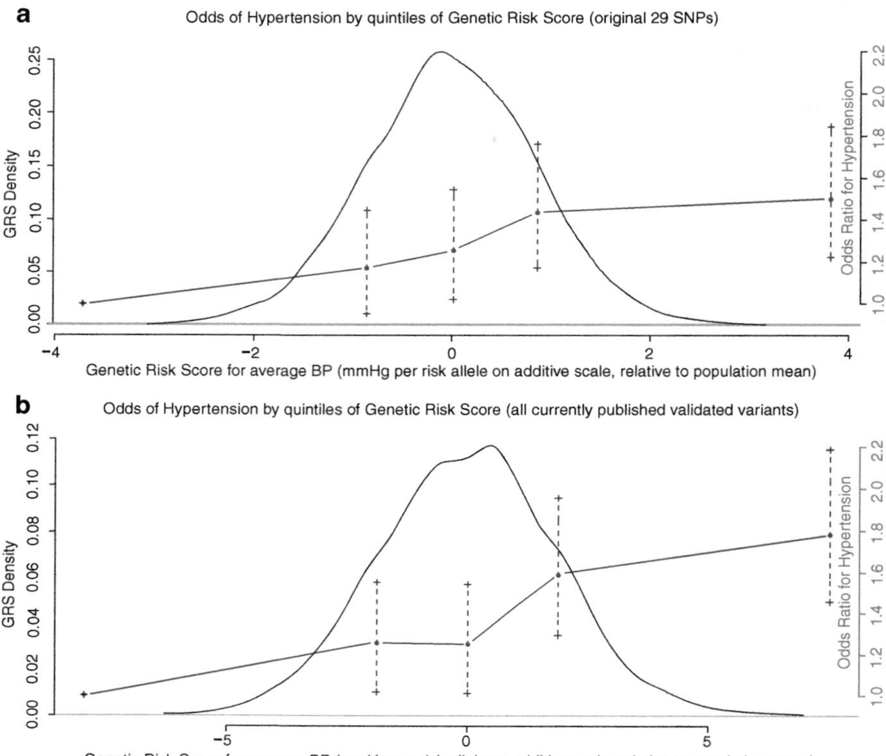

Fig. 25.1 Genetic risk score and the Odds of Hypertension. The density plots show the distribution (left-hand y-axis) of the blood pressure (BP) genetic risk score (GRS) within N = 5639 individuals from the 1958 Birth Cohort. In plot (**a**) the GRS is based on the 29 BP-associated SNPs from the ICBP study [15]. In Plot (**b**) the GRS is based on all the currently published and validated BP-associated variants: after filtering by LD ($r^2 < 0.2$), 348 independent BP genetic signals remain, of which 332 were available from 1958 Birth Cohort 1000 Genomes imputed data. For each model, two GRS, for SBP and DBP, were constructed according to trait-increasing alleles and weighted by effect size estimates. The average of these scores was used as the average BP-GRS, which was centered at mean zero (x-axis). At each quintile of the GRS, the Odds Ratio for Hypertension (right-hand y-axis), comparing each of the upper four GRS quintiles against the lowest reference quintile, is indicated together with standard error bars, in order to show the increase in hypertension risk as genetic risk increases

the heritability estimates of 30–50% from twin and family studies. This is presumed to be a consequence of many of the causal loci not yet being identified, a phenomenon referred to as 'missing heritability'. Heritability reflects the degree of phenotypic resemblance between relatives and depend on both shared genetic factors contributing to the trait and environmental factors and interactions within the genome [7]. Whereas GWAS have concentrated on identifying genetics factors by modelling the main effects of common SNPs, a focus on modelling gene-environment (G × E) and gene-gene (G × G) interactions may help to uncover additional causal factors in human disease [6]. Hypertension is well known to be modulated by various lifestyle factors. In GWAS for hypertension related phenotypes, significant G × E interactions have been identified with alcohol consumption, BMI, smoking, education levels and sodium intake, all of which are modifiable risk factors through a change in lifestyle. Findings from these studies warrant further research into the G × E interaction to help discover causal genetic loci that are contributing to missing heritability [6]. No large-scale studies on G × G have been reported.

However, missing heritability does not automatically correspond to missing variants, and may be a consequence of over-estimation of heritability. The proportion of heritability explained by a set of variants is the ratio of heritability caused by these variants (estimated directly from their observed effects), to the total heritability estimated indirectly from population data [39]. The estimation of heritability can increase or decrease, with no changes in genetics, when there is a change in environmental variation. Current heritability estimates represent a specific population under a specific environment. However environmental conditions differ between populations and across generations. Therefore, the observed heritability of BP is not a reflection of the true degree of genetic effect, rather it reflects the degree of variation in environmental effects [7]. Heritability estimates may also be influenced by errors in measurement, in previous studies it has been shown that minimising measurement errors using ambulatory BP reading, or long-term average BP leads to higher estimates of heritability [7]. Missing heritability may also been a consequence of the undetected causal variation at known GWAS loci, that are unable to be quantified by GWAS markers, as well as the presence of additional unidentified variants with small effect sizes that have been not been detected with strong significance [40].

25.10 Epigenetics

Epigenetics is the study of potentially heritable changes in gene expression that does not involve changes to the underlying DNA sequence, a change in phenotype without a change in genotype [41]. This can occur by way of DNA methylation, histone modification, nucleosome positioning, transcription control with DNA-binding proteins and non-coding RNAs and translation control with microRNAs and RNA binding proteins [42]. Epigenetic mechanisms have been proposed as a potential cause for the missing heritability of essential hypertension and the most studied has been DNA methylation [43]. Methylation occurs when a methyl group becomes bound to position 5 of the cytosine ring, forming 5-methyl-cytosine, at specific dinucleotide sites called CpGs. These CpGs are short sequences of DNA with high linear frequency 5′-CpG-3′ sequences and are frequently located in gene promoter regions. Functionally, DNA methylation suppresses gene transcription resulting in silencing of a gene [41, 43].

The advent of high-throughput technologies has allowed epigenetic features to be comprehensively and quantitatively profiled across the genome. Different degrees of DNA methylation have been associated with variable onset, timing, and severity of essential hypertension. Global genomic DNA methylation can be quantified be measuring the level of 5-methyl-cytosine in a DNA sample [49]. Smolarek et al. found a correlation between decreased levels of 5-methyl-cytosine with increased hypertension severity in samples of peripheral blood [44]. Friso et al. found that *HSD11B2* gene promoter methylation was associated with essential hypertension onset via disruption to body tetrahydrocortisol-tetrahydrocortisone ratio [45]. Wang et al. found that the *PRCP* gene was hypomethylated in hypertensive individuals, resulting in interfered cleavage of angiotensin II and III [46].

The most robust data for the involvement of DNA methylation in BP regulation comes from a study by Kato et al. [37]. An investigation of the relationship between the sentinel BP SNPs with local DNA methylation in 1904 South Asians revealed a two-fold enrichment between sequence variation and DNA methylation. The authors demonstrated that SNPs influencing BP are associated with methylation at multiple CpG sites, and that the observed effect of SNPs on BP is related to the effect predicted through association with methylation. Further epigenetic studies may help to explain some of the BP variance mediated by changes in gene expression.

25.11 Novel Hypertension Pathways

One of the most important outcomes from GWAS is the identification of new BP loci, and new biological mechanisms. There is a time-lag however in translating GWAS findings to physiology. Evidence has recently emerged of a novel pathway, mediated by the uromodulin gene (*UMOD*) in sodium homeostasis and BP regulation. Uromodulin is a protein exclusively expressed by epithelial cells in the thick ascending limb of the loop of Henle in the kidney [47]. Interest in uromodulin was first indicated by an early GWAS showing an association between common SNPs in the upstream region of the *UMOD* gene with renal function and hypertension. A GWAS of BP extremes showed that the minor G allele of a *UMOD* promoter SNP, rs13333226, was associated with reduced urinary *UMOD* excretion, and a reduced risk of hypertension [48]. Confirmation of the essential role of uromodulin in sodium homeostasis and BP was subsequently demonstrated in a set of complementary experiments in mouse models [49, 50]. Graham et al. reported *umod* knockout mice had significantly lower systolic BP than wild-type mice, and were resistant to salt-induced changes of BP [49]. In contrast, Trudu et al. found that overexpression of *UMOD* caused a dose-dependent increase in *UMOD* expression and excretion, which was associated with increased BP [50]. These studies also showed that treatment with furosemide (loop diuretic that inhibits sodium, chloride and potassium reabsorption in the thick ascending limb of the loop of Henle) increased urinary sodium excretion and decreased BP in both transgenic mice, and in hypertensive individuals homozygous for the uromodulin increasing allele. These findings suggested that hypertensive patients in possession of the UMOD increasing allele may benefit from loop diuretic treatment, rather that thiazide diuretics, particularly those patients with resistant hypertension burdened with the problem of fluid volume overload [49, 50].

25.12 Future Directions

There are now over 400 different genetic variants associated with BP that have been identified and validated by GWAS meta-analyses. Many of the SNPs discovered are common, and have a relatively small effect size, in contrast to rare variants, which exert a larger effect on BP [11]. Analyses of rare SNPs associated with BP has been inadequate so far, as only a small proportion of rare coding SNPs have been interrogated. Next-generation sequencing technology permits the detection of rare variants through deep sequencing of the entire genome at a reduced cost. Genetic sequencing studies of BP are still in the preliminary stages, and early studies have shown that it is crucial these studies possess large sample sizes [18]. The establishment of national biobanks is likely to facilitate these studies, as they permit large well-powered studies for the analysis of rare variants, and interactions. For example, in the USA the National Institutes of Health will grant $142 million to the Mayo Clinic over 5 years, to establish the world's largest research-cohort biobank for the Precision Medicine Initiative Program, a longitudinal research study aiming to enroll over a million or more American participants [51, 52]. In the UK, the 100,000 Genomes Project aims to sequence 100,000 whole genomes from approximately 75,000 NHS patients with rare diseases, cancer, or their families [53]. This project may aid in the discovery of further candidate genes that showed no previous association with BP.

Gene × Environment (G × E) interactions, relevant to the underlying pathophysiology of hypertension, present a promising opportunity for the discovery of novel BP loci. G × E studies may help to account for non-additive genetic variance, which is typically ignored when genome-wide markers are used to research complex traits such as hypertension [18]. Non-additive genetic variance describes the genetic variation due to interactions between genes, and may have a significant impact on total genetic variation of complex traits [55]. A Gene-Lifestyle Interactions Working Group has recently been funded by the National Institute of Health to facilitate the first large, concerted, multi-ancestry study to systematically evaluate gene-lifestyle interactions [56]. The National Heart, Lung and Blood Institute (NHLBI) have also assembled a working group of multidisciplinary experts to explore the relationship between epigenetic modifications of genomic DNA and etiology, progression and prevention of hypertension [55]. Many epigenetic studies are limited by the nature of their sample, given blood is studied rather than effector tissues. Further research will be required in both human and animal models to reveal the specific mechanisms involved and apply this knowledge for therapeutic purposes [57].

Despite the last decade witnessing a continued expansion of our understanding of the genetics of hypertension, the picture remains complex, and much of the heritability of blood pressure continues to be unexplained. The enhanced understanding of genetic factors, will allow us to predict an individual's susceptibility to hypertension, and provide an appropriately tailored management plan, to both prevent and manage hypertension in clinical settings. Improvement in these areas will have major consequences for public health, and reduce the burden of chronic disease caused by hypertension, especially cardiovascular disease, on a worldwide scale.

Acknowledgements We wish to acknowledge the support of the NIHR Cardiovascular Biomedical Research Centre at Barts and The London, Queen Mary University of London, UK and would like to thank Dr. Helen Warren for assistance in preparation of Fig. 25.1, and analysis of BP traits in the 1958 Birth Cohort dataset.

References

1. Kearney PM, Whelton M, Reynolds K, Muntner P, Whelton PK, He J. Global burden of hypertension: analysis of worldwide data. Lancet. 2005;365(9455):217–23.
2. World Health Organisation. Global Health Observatory (GHO) Data-Mean Systolic Blood Pressure (SBP). 2017. Available from: http://www.who.int/gho/ncd/risk_factors/blood_pressure_prevalence_text/en/.
3. Carretero OA, Oparil S. Essential hypertension. Part I: definition and etiology. Circulation. 2000;101(3):329–35.
4. Public Health England. Health matters: combating high blood pressure [Internet]. 2017.
5. World Health Organisation. A global brief on hypertention [Internet]. 2013.
6. Waken RJ, de Las Fuentes L, Rao DCA. Review of the genetics of hypertension with a focus on gene-environment interactions. Curr Hypertens Rep. 2017;19(3):23.
7. Padmanabhan S, Caulfield M, Dominiczak AF. Genetic and molecular aspects of hypertension. Circ Res. 2015;116(6):937–59.
8. Salfati E, Morrison AC, Boerwinkle E, Chakravarti A. Direct estimates of the genomic contributions to blood pressure heritability within a population-based cohort (ARIC). PLoS One. 2015;10(7):e0133031.
9. Butler MG. Genetics of hypertension. Current status. J Med Liban. 2010;58(3):175–8.
10. Delles C, Padmanabhan S. Genetics and hypertension: is it time to change my practice? Can J Cardiol. 2012;28(3):296–304.
11. Munroe PB, Barnes MR, Caulfield MJ. Advances in blood pressure genomics. Circ Res. 2013;112(10):1365–79.
12. Maass PG, Aydin A, Luft FC, Schachterle C, Weise A, Stricker S, et al. PDE3A mutations cause autosomal dominant hypertension with brachydactyly. Nat Genet. 2015;47(6):647–53.
13. Ji W, Foo JN, O'Roak BJ, Zhao H, Larson MG, Simon DB, et al. Rare independent mutations in renal salt handling genes contribute to blood pressure variation. Nat Genet. 2008;40(5):592–9.
14. Surendran P, Drenos F, Young R, Warren H, Cook JP, Manning AK, et al. Trans-ancestry meta-analyses identify rare and common variants associated with blood pressure and hypertension. Nat Genet. 2016;48(10):1151–61.
15. International Consortium for Blood Pressure Genome-Wide Association Studies, Ehret GB, Munroe PB, Rice KM, Bochud M, Johnson AD, et al. Genetic variants in novel pathways influence blood pressure and cardiovascular disease risk. Nature. 2011;478(7367):103–9.
16. Ehret GB, Ferreira T, Chasman DI, Jackson AU, Schmidt EM, Johnson T, et al. The genetics of blood pressure regulation and its target organs from association studies in 342,415 individuals. Nat Genet. 2016;48(10):1171–84.
17. Liu C, Kraja AT, Smith JA, Brody JA, Franceschini N, Bis JC, et al. Meta-analysis identifies common and rare variants influencing blood pressure and overlapping with metabolic trait loci. Nat Genet. 2016;48(10):1162–70.

18. Zheng J, Rao DC, Shi G. An update on genome-wide association studies of hypertension. Appl Bioinforma. 2015;2:10.
19. Ehret GB. Genome-wide association studies: contribution of genomics to understanding blood pressure and essential hypertension. Curr Hypertens Rep. 2010;12(1):17–25.
20. Geller DS. New developments in the genetics of hypertension: what should clinicians know? Curr Cardiol Rep. 2015;17(12):122.
21. Levy D, Larson MG, Benjamin EJ, Newton-Cheh C, Wang TJ, Hwang SJ, et al. Framingham Heart Study 100K Project: genome-wide associations for blood pressure and arterial stiffness. BMC Med Genet. 2007;8(Suppl 1):S3.
22. Wellcome Trust Case Control Consortium. Genome-wide association study of 14,000 cases of seven common diseases and 3,000 shared controls. Nature. 2007;447(7145):661–78.
23. Newton-Cheh C, Johnson T, Gateva V, Tobin MD, Bochud M, Coin L, et al. Genome-wide association study identifies eight loci associated with blood pressure. Nat Genet. 2009;41(6):666–76.
24. Levy D, Ehret GB, Rice K, Verwoert GC, Launer LJ, Dehghan A, et al. Genome-wide association study of blood pressure and hypertension. Nat Genet. 2009;41(6):677–87.
25. Dominiczak AF, Munroe PB. Genome-wide association studies will unlock the genetic basis of hypertension: pro side of the argument. Hypertension. 2010;56(6):1017–20. Discussion 25.
26. Johnson T, Gaunt TR, Newhouse SJ, Padmanabhan S, Tomaszewski M, Kumari M, et al. Blood pressure loci identified with a gene-centric array. Am J Hum Genet. 2011;89(6):688–700.
27. Ganesh SK, Tragante V, Guo W, Guo Y, Lanktree MB, Smith EN, et al. Loci influencing blood pressure identified using a cardiovascular gene-centric array. Hum Mol Genet. 2013;22(8): 1663–78.
28. Tragante V, Barnes MR, Ganesh SK, Lanktree MB, Guo W, Franceschini N, et al. Gene-centric meta-analysis in 87,736 individuals of European ancestry identifies multiple blood-pressure-related loci. Am J Hum Genet. 2014;94(3):349–60.
29. Burrello J, Monticone S, Buffolo F, Tetti M, Veglio F, Williams TA, et al. Is there a role for genomics in the management of hypertension? Int J Mol Sci. 2017;18(6)
30. Hoffmann TJ, Ehret GB, Nandakumar P, Ranatunga D, Schaefer C, Kwok PY, et al. Genome-wide association analyses using electronic health records identify new loci influencing blood pressure variation. Nat Genet. 2017;49(1):54–64.
31. Warren HR, Evangelou E, Cabrera CP, Gao H, Ren M, Mifsud B, et al. Genome-wide association analysis identifies novel blood pressure loci and offers biological insights into cardiovascular risk. Nat Genet. 2017;49(3):403–15.
32. Takeuchi F, Isono M, Katsuya T, Yamamoto K, Yokota M, Sugiyama T, et al. Blood pressure and hypertension are associated with 7 loci in the Japanese population. Circulation. 2010;121(21):2302–9.
33. Kato N, Takeuchi F, Tabara Y, Kelly TN, Go MJ, Sim X, et al. Meta-analysis of genome-wide association studies identifies common variants associated with blood pressure variation in east Asians. Nat Genet. 2011;43(6):531–8.
34. Franceschini N, Fox E, Zhang Z, Edwards TL, Nalls MA, Sung YJ, et al. Genome-wide association analysis of blood-pressure traits in African-ancestry individuals reveals common associated genes in African and non-African populations. Am J Hum Genet. 2013;93(3):545–54.
35. Liang J, Le TH, Edwards DRV, Tayo BO, Gaulton KJ, Smith JA, et al. Single-trait and multi-trait genome-wide association analyses identify novel loci for blood pressure in African-ancestry populations. PLoS Genet. 2017;13(5):e1006728.
36. Kato N. Ethnic differences in genetic predisposition to hypertension. Hypertens Res. 2012;35(6):574–81.
37. Kato N, Loh M, Takeuchi F, Verweij N, Wang X, Zhang W, et al. Trans-ancestry genome-wide association study identifies 12 genetic loci influencing blood pressure and implicates a role for DNA methylation. Nat Genet. 2015;47(11):1282–93.
38. Ehret GB, Munroe PB, Rice KM, Bochud M, Johnson AD, Chasman DI, et al. Genetic variants in novel pathways influence blood pressure and cardiovascular disease risk. Nature. 2011;478(7367):103–9.

39. Zuk O, Hechter E, Sunyaev SR, Lander ES. The mystery of missing heritability: genetic interactions create phantom heritability. Proc Natl Acad Sci U S A. 2012;109(4):1193–8.
40. Visscher PM, Brown MA, McCarthy MI, Yang J. Five years of GWAS discovery. Am J Hum Genet. 2012;90(1):7–24.
41. Raftopoulos L, Katsi V, Makris T, Tousoulis D, Stefanadis C, Kallikazaros I. Epigenetics, the missing link in hypertension. Life Sci. 2015;129:22–6.
42. Zhao Q, Kelly TN, Li C, He J. Progress and future aspects in genetics of human hypertension. Curr Hypertens Rep. 2013;15(6):676–86.
43. Wise IA, Charchar FJ. Epigenetic modifications in essential hypertension. Int J Mol Sci. 2016; 17(4):451.
44. Smolarek I, Wyszko E, Barciszewska AM, Nowak S, Gawronska I, Jablecka A, et al. Global DNA methylation changes in blood of patients with essential hypertension. Med Sci Monit. 2010;16(3):CR149–55.
45. Friso S, Pizzolo F, Choi SW, Guarini P, Castagna A, Ravagnani V, et al. Epigenetic control of 11 beta-hydroxysteroid dehydrogenase 2 gene promoter is related to human hypertension. Atherosclerosis. 2008;199(2):323–7.
46. Wang X, Falkner B, Zhu H, Shi H, Su S, Xu X, et al. A genome-wide methylation study on essential hypertension in young African American males. PLoS One. 2013;8(1):e53938.
47. Rindler MJ, Naik SS, Li N, Hoops TC, Peraldi MN. Uromodulin (Tamm-Horsfall glycoprotein/uromucoid) is a phosphatidylinositol-linked membrane protein. J Biol Chem. 1990;265(34):20784–9.
48. Padmanabhan S, Melander O, Johnson T, Di Blasio AM, Lee WK, Gentilini D, et al. Genome-wide association study of blood pressure extremes identifies variant near UMOD associated with hypertension. PLoS Genet. 2010;6(10):e1001177.
49. Graham LA, Padmanabhan S, Fraser NJ, Kumar S, Bates JM, Raffi HS, et al. Validation of uromodulin as a candidate gene for human essential hypertension. Hypertension. 2014;63(3):551–8.
50. Trudu M, Janas S, Lanzani C, Debaix H, Schaeffer C, Ikehata M, et al. Common noncoding UMOD gene variants induce salt-sensitive hypertension and kidney damage by increasing uromodulin expression. Nat Med. 2013;19(12):1655–60.
51. Collins FS, Varmus H. A new initiative on precision medicine. N Engl J Med. 2015;372(9):793–5.
52. Frellick M. Mayo clinic gets $142 million for precision medicine biobank. 2016. Available from: http://www.medscape.com/viewarticle/864089.
53. England G. The 100,000 genomes project. 2017. Available from: https://www.genomicsengland.co.uk/.
55. Su G, Christensen OF, Ostersen T, Henryon M, Lund MS. Estimating additive and non-additive genetic variances and predicting genetic merits using genome-wide dense single nucleotide polymorphism markers. PLoS One. 2012;7(9):e45293.
56. Rao DC, Sung YJ, Winkler TW, Schwander K, Borecki I, Cupples LA, et al. Multiancestry study of gene-lifestyle interactions for cardiovascular traits in 610 475 individuals from 124 cohorts: design and rationale. Circ Cardiovasc Genet. 2017;10(3)
57. Cowley AW Jr, Nadeau JH, Baccarelli A, Berecek K, Fornage M, Gibbons GH, et al. Report of the National Heart, Lung, and Blood Institute Working Group on epigenetics and hypertension. Hypertension. 2012;59(5):899–905.

Inherited Pulmonary Arterial Hypertension

26

Sophie Herbert and Robert M.R. Tulloh

Abstract

Pulmonary hypertension is now a well recognised disease and is no longer regarded as rare. As new therapies come on line, the disease comes into recognition by cardiologists, respirologists, rheumatologists and paediatricians.

The genetic basis is also becoming clearer, not only in the idiopathic form, but also in the forms secondary to chromosomal abnormalities, micro-deletions and systemic disease.

The present chapter aims to introduce the reader to the genetic and molecular abnormalities in pulmonary hypertension, predominantly pulmonary arterial hypertension (PAH). However it must be realised that the field is now very large, with over 4500 gene mutations recognised to be implicated in pulmonary hypertension. This chapter covers some of the interesting areas in this field, including the genetic changes in idiopathic PAH and the changes seen in association with congenital heart disease. The molecular changes that accompany this gives an insight to the cellular abnormalities in such disease.

Keywords

Pulmonary hypertension • Inherited pulmonary arterial hypertension • Idiopathic pulmonary arterial hypertension

S. Herbert • R.M.R. Tulloh (✉)
Department of Congenital Heart Disease, Bristol Heart Institute, Bristol, UK
e-mail: Robert.Tulloh@bristol.ac.uk

D. Kumar, P. Elliott (eds.), *Cardiovascular Genetics and Genomics*,
https://doi.org/10.1007/978-3-319-66114-8_26

26.1 Introduction

Pulmonary Hypertension (PH) is a chronic condition affecting significantly both respiratory and cardiac function. PH has a high associated mortality due to the cardio-respiratory functional compromise. It is recognised more and more commonly—affecting 1% of the population [1].

Pulmonary arterial hypertension (PAH) is one of five types of PH and is identified as Group 1 of the World Health Organisation (WHO) classification (Table 26.1). It derives from increased pulmonary vascular resistance secondary to vasculature proliferation, hypertrophy and impaired endothelial growth [3, 4]. The increased resistance causes increased pressure on the right heart leading to strain and damage, resulting in symptoms including, hypoxaemia, dyspnoea, fatigue, syncope, and eventually fluid retention with peripheral oedema [5].

PAH is formally defined as a mean pulmonary arterial pressure >25 mmHg on right heart catheterisation with a raised pulmonary vascular resistance of more than 3 Wu.m^2 and no evidence of left heart disease, with a mean left atrial or capillary wedge pressure

Table 26.1 Classification of pulmonary hypertension (PH) [2]

Category
1. Pulmonary arterial hypertension (PAH) 1. Idiopathic PAH (IPAH) 2. Heritable PAH (HPAH) includes: BMPR2, ALK1, endoglin (with or without hereditary haemorrhagic telangiectasia) 3. Drugs and toxin induced 4. Associated with 1. Connective tissue disease 2. HIV 3. Portal hypertension 4. Congenital heart disease 5. Schistosomiasis 6. Chronic haemolytic anaemia 5. Persistent pulmonary hypertension of the newborn 1. Pulmonary veno-occlusive disease and/or Pulmonary haemangiomatosis
2. PH related to left heart disease 1. Systolic dysfunction 2. Diastolic dysfunction 3. Valvular disease
3. PH related to chronic lung disease and/or hypoxia 1. Chronic obstructive pulmonary disease 2. Interstitial lung disease 3. Other pulmonary diseases 4. Sleep-disorder breathing 5. Alveolar hypoventilation disorders 6. Chronic high altitude 7. Developmental
4. PH related to chronic thromboembolic disease (CTEPH)
5. PH with unclear multifactorial mechanisms a. Haematological disorders b. Systemic disorders c. Metabolic disorders d. Others

of <15 mmHg [2]. In practice, echocardiography is used for screening with evidence of a dilated right heart, a high peak velocity of tricuspid regurgitation of more than 2.7 m/s [6]. Within the WHO PAH classification, there are multiple causes including idiopathic disease, heritable causes, congenital heart disease, toxin related, PAH associated with connective tissue disease and persistent PAH of the new born [2].

In this chapter, we are mostly concerned with PAH, in terms of inherited causes of pulmonary arterial hypertension. We shall now discuss some cases to highlight important features. All cases are anonymised, with changed ages and characteristics to maintain patient anonymity.

26.2 Case 1

A 12 year old boy is seen in the general paediatric clinic because of tiredness and lethargy. He was previously well, but has been unable to play a game of football for the last 6 months. He had two episodes of breathlessness while running to school and fainted on one occasion while playing in the garden. All his family is well, with an older sister, two healthy parents and no sudden unexplained deaths.

When seen in the clinic, he was tall, had hypertelorism, normal character pulses, blood pressure and oxygen saturations. On palpation of his precordium, he has a right ventricular heave, loud pulmonary second heart sound and a soft diastolic murmur. Chest radiograph shows cardiomegaly and dark lung fields.

His ECG showed right atrial hypertrophy, right axis deviation and right ventricular hypertrophy.

His echocardiogram (Fig. 26.1) shows dilated right heart with reduced function. The tricuspid regurgitation peak jet velocity is 4 m/s, indicating that his right

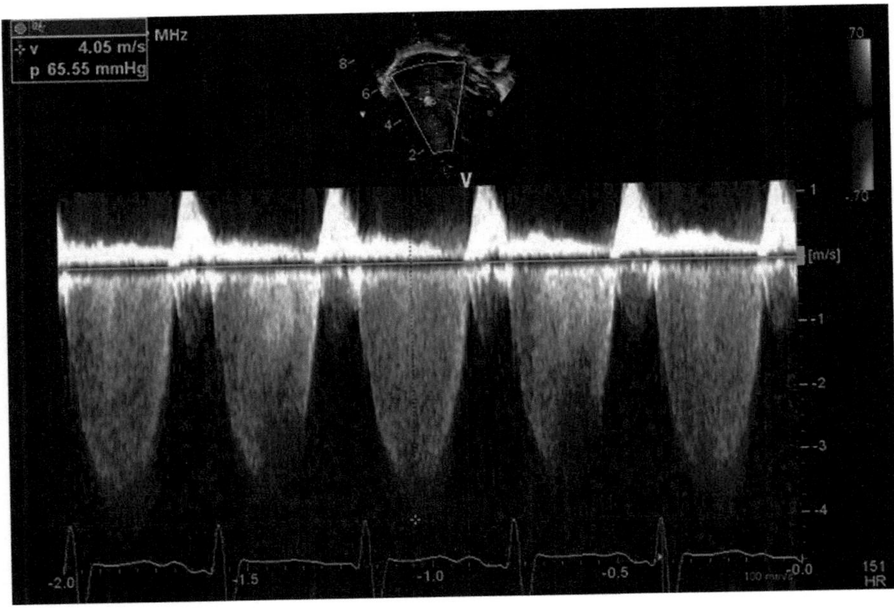

Fig. 26.1 Patient echocardiogram

ventricular and hence pulmonary artery systolic pressure is around 70 mmHg (normal <36 mmHg).

He has the full pulmonary hypertension investigations performed following the protocol. CT scan of his lungs shows patchy mosaic appearance, but no evidence of pulmonary emboli. The other results are shown in the table. Of note, he has a low 6 minute walk distance with a fall in peripheral oxygen saturation and also a degree of liver dysfunction, and was found to have a mutation in the BMPR2 gene.

He was treated with intravenous Epoprostenol via a centrally placed indwelling line, with medicine supplies sent to his home after 1 week in hospital for training. His right heart pressures fell substantially, confirmed on repeat cardiac catheterisation and he was able to return to school, living a fairly normal existence, even going swimming, with a waterproof container for the line.

He stayed remarkably stable for 7 years, but was noticed to have rising pulmonary pressures on his routine echocardiogram and a worsening 6 min walk test. Additional therapy was introduced as Tadalafil and Ambrisentan. This held him stable for 18 months but he continued to deteriorate. He had already been referred for lung transplantation, which was now urgent and fortunately he received one before too long.

Sadly, whilst in recovery from transplantation, his 39-year-old mother was noted to be more breathless on walking the dog. She was referred to cardiology and was recognised to have pulmonary hypertension too. Rapid assessment in the PH clinic that week, revealed her to also have BMPR2 mutation and so also had heritable PAH. She responded well to oral medication, and both members of the family go home together, wondering what their futures hold.

26.2.1 Learning Points

This case highlights a typical presentation with respiratory symptoms, often described as 'non-wheezing asthma' [7]. The boy is the index case and demonstrates all the features of idiopathic pulmonary arterial hypertension. Although most often seen in young ladies, this disease can affect any age. The mother presents at a later age, showing genetic anticipation so often seen, with earlier age of presentation with each successive generation.

The usual survival with no therapy is 2.8 years, but the advent of oral and intravenous therapy has altered this substantially [8]. Now, we have children and adults with IPAH who may survive a decade or more. New therapies are being added every year, giving hope to the patients.

26.3 Case 2

A 4 month old baby was seen in the cardiology clinic because it is known to have Trisomy 21 (Down's syndrome) and complete atrio-ventricular septal defect. It would be expected that he would be breathless and in heart failure. However, he was feeding well and was gaining weight normally.

When seen in the cardiac clinic, he was found to have signs of increased pulmonary vascular resistance, with peripheral oxygen saturations of 88%, no breathlessness, but a right ventricular heave with loud pulmonary second sound. His Echocardiogram showed that there was no volume loading of the left heart, but the right ventricle was dilated with evidence of right to left shunt across the septum.

Time is given for the pulmonary vascular resistance to fall further, but at 9 months of age, cardiac catheterisation was performed, which demonstrated a raised pulmonary vascular resistance of 9 Wu.m^2. He was therefore not deemed to be suitable for cardiac surgery and was followed up in clinic.

Many years later, at age 20 years old he was seen in the Adult congenital heart disease pulmonary hypertension clinic, as part of the National Pulmonary Hypertension service. His exercise tolerance had fallen over the last few months, he was in WHO class III and so he was commenced on tadalafil and then macitentan in addition, both as oral therapy. His WHO class improved to II and his quality of life score (emPHasis 10) was better. He was stable and followed in the clinic for many years longer, with life expectancy being into the fifth or sixth decade.

26.3.1 Learning Points

Chromosomal anomalies, such as Trisomy 21 and Trisomy 18 are commonly associated with poor development of the alveolae [9–11]. This leads to an increased pulmonary vascular resistance and can mean inoperability. In addition such people may have bronchomalacia or gastro-oesophageal reflux that makes the lung disease significantly worse. It is worth considering somatic syndromes as a cause when pulmonary vascular disease is diagnosed and conversely, consider there might be an underlying chromosomal anomaly or gene deletion that might be associated with a newly discovered PAH.

The first randomised controlled trial for therapy in pulmonary hypertension was BREATHE-5, which used a dual endothelin receptor antagonist—Bosentan, to demonstrate improvement in clinical markers in patients with Eisenmenger syndrome (PAH due to congenital heart disease) as compared with placebo [12]. This spawned a whole leash of new therapies and to management guidelines for PAH [13]. A variety of therapies are now available for such patients.

26.4 Molecular Changes

Multiple genetic diseases have been documented to contribute to PAH disease burden directly and indirectly. Genes directly contributing to PAH include numerous heritable causes that can be split into Familial PAH (2 or more family members affected) or simple PAH (spontaneous mutation). The diagnosis of heritable PAH is with right heart catheterisation, exclusion of other causes of PH and positive genetic testing. 6% of PAH patients have a positive family history and a median age of diagnosis at 36 years but the range includes the extremes of age [14]. The most important genetic defect is in the BMPR2 gene (Bone morphogenetic protein receptor type II) which accounts for 75% of heritable PAH [15, 16].

The BMPR2 gene is found on chromosome 2q33 and encodes a serine-threonine kinase BMP receptor where Tissue Growth Factor (TGF-β) binds [17, 18]. The majority of the BMPR2 abnormalities lead to frameshift and nonsense mutations [19]. Limited functional analysis of this gene dysfunction has been documented, but the data suggests replacement of important cysteine molecules affects receptor migration to the surface. Failure of BMP receptor production increases the TGF-β in the pulmonary vasculature leading to a pro-fibrotic state [20]. Interestingly, it is thought, 20% of idiopathic PAH have a similar BMPR2 genetic abnormality [21]. BMPR2 gene defects can be both familial and in simplex PAH. The penetrance of the defect is 20% with a higher female to male ratio at 2.5 [22, 23]. In addition, it has been shown that there is an increased incidence of BMPR2 mutations in PAH associated with congenital heart disease but the significance of this is as yet uncertain [24].

Other mutations in genes can directly increase PAH susceptibility including Vasoactive Intestinal Polypeptide (VIP) on chromosome 10, which is involved in smooth muscle relaxation [25]. Activin Receptor Like Type 1 (ACVR1) on chromosome 12 acts similarly to BMPR2 gene by increasing TGF-β and ALK-1 in hereditary haemorrhagic telangiectasia [26, 27]. Caveolin 1 (CAV 1) on chromosome 7 is involved in regulating cell growth and division therefore mutations contribute to disordered proliferation [28].

The penetrance of these conditions is increased in the female sex but also exposure to environmental triggers including RSV infection, premature delivery, congenital heart disease, 22q11.2 deletion, gastro-oesophageal reflux, and drug and toxin exposure can further increase susceptibility of phenotypic presentation (Fig. 26.2) [29, 30].

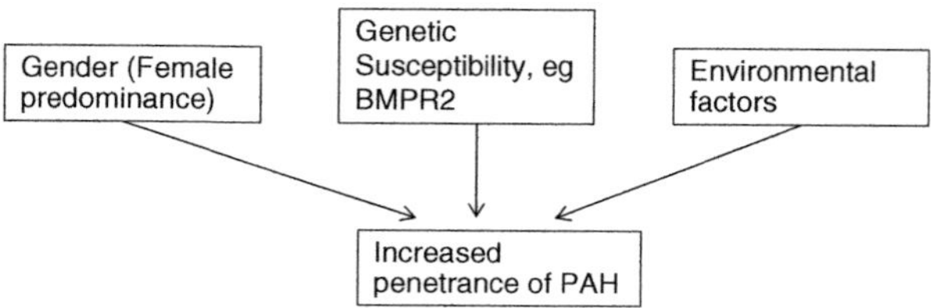

Fig. 26.2 Contributing factors to increased penetrance of PAH

Within the WHO group 1 category of PAH there are also a group of diseases that PAH is indirectly associated with, that can be attributed to genetic abnormalities. Congenital heart disease (CHD) is a significant contributor to PAH. CHD, particularly with a left to right shunt, increases the pulmonary circulating volume damaging the vasculature. Over time, the pressure inside the lungs can exceed that of the left heart due to hypertrophy and proliferation of the vasculature. This leads to a reversal of the shunt, which is a phenomenon, called Eisenmenger's syndrome (ES). ES is the most severe form of CHD associated PAH, and is associated with challenging cyanosis and hypoxaemia and has a poor prognosis [31].

The most common genetic abnormality worldwide associated with CHD is Trisomy 21, Down's Syndrome (DS) [32]. Around 50% of patients with DS have CHD, however there are multiple factors in this patient group contribute to PH, including gastro-oesophageal reflux disease, obstructive airways, abnormal lung development, and obesity [9, 33, 34]. The most common cardiac abnormality is atrio-ventricular septal defect—AVSD [3].

The majority of patients with DS have not inherited their condition; the most common way to acquire the genetic defect is with a meiosis problem in the maternal gamete. A small proportion of patients with DS have non-disjunction where there is translocation from both the maternal and paternal genes [35].

Diagnosis of DS can be made prenatally by chorionic villus sampling or amniocentesis or postnatally with genetic karyotyping if diagnosis is suspected based on dysmorphic features. It is important that once diagnosis is made that echocardiography is performed to rule out CHD, as irreversible pulmonary vasculature changes can develop within 6 months [3].

Other genetic causes for CHD and therefore potentially PAH includes Trisomy 13 (80% prevalence of CHD) and 18 (nearly 100%) which are typically associated with a poor outcome, and X Chromosome abnormalities Turner's (XO, 45) (30%) and Klinefelter's syndrome (XXY, 47) (50%) [36].

Within group 1 of the WHO PH classifications also is PAH associated with connective tissue disease (CTD). CTD includes vascular injury, autoimmunity, tissue inflammation and organ dysfunction, hence their association with PAH [37]. CTD include Systemic Lupus Erythematosus (SLE), systemic sclerosis, and less frequently rheumatoid arthritis, dermatomyositis and Sjogren's Syndrome and the prevalence of PAH in CTD is 13% (range 2.8–32%). CTD genes are inherited but they are not always associated with disease onset, it is a complex combination of genetics and environmental factors that pre-dispose to PAH.

Cantú syndrome is a condition associated with both congenital heart disease and inflammatory disease. The abnormal ABCC9 gene on chromosome 12 leads to frameshift and missense mutations when encoding an ATP sensitive potassium channel [38]. It is unknown how excessive opening in the channel leads to hypertrichosis, congenital heart disease, macrocephaly and typical facies appearance. These patients are at increased risk of developing PAH.

Chronic haemolytic anaemia (CHA) is a pathological disease process where red blood cells are broken down. CHA is a cause of PAH and there are multiple genetic and acquired causes for this disease. Genetic diseases include, hereditary spherocytosis, thalassaemia, sickle cell disease, and glucose-6-phosphate dehydrogenase (g6pd) deficiency.

All chronic haemolytic anaemias have different genetic causes but contribute to pulmonary arterial hypertension by interfering with the nitric oxide (NO) pathway, which is responsible for vasodilation. Increased haemolysis results in increased circulating haemoglobin which reacts with and destroys NO leading to a lack of vasoconstriction in the pulmonary vasculature [39].

Disorders of haemoglobin production include the thalassaemias and sickle cell disease. Thalassaemias are abnormalities within either the alpha or beta chain of haemoglobin and have a spectrum of clinical presentations from incompatibility of life with alpha-thalassaemia major to mild chronic anaemia with the beta-thalassaemias [40]. The most common affecting haemolysis are the beta-thalassaemia intermedia and major [41]. The HBB gene defect in beta-thalassaemia is located on chromosome 11 [42] and Beta-thalassaemia major is diagnosed in early life and requires life long transfusion therapy for survival whilst beta-thalassaemia intermedia is associated with a better prognosis including survival without regular transfusions [41]. 60% to 75% of patients with a beta-thalassaemia will have an incidental finding of PAH [43, 44].

Sickle cell disease is an autosomal recessive condition that is also associated with an abnormality of the HBB gene called HbS on chromosome 11 [42]. Non-functional beta haemoglobin is formed leading to a change in the shape of the red blood cell from characteristic biconcave disk to crescent shape, 10% of patients will develop PAH [45].

Less common causes of CHA associated PAH include G6PD deficiency, which is a defect in red cell metabolism that leads to haemolysis. It has X-linked recessive inheritance and therefore affects males predominantly [46]. Defects in red blood cell membrane production include hereditary spherocytosis resulting in abnormally shaped spherical red blood cells. These causes of CHA are relevant to PAH when other clinical factors are present including, chronic splenectomy, coagulation abnormalities, oxidative stress, and iron overload [47, 48].These factors potentiate the effects of all CHA associated PAH.

People with PAH have a high mortality in pregnancy, particularly post-partum with only around a 60% survival and pregnancy should be advised against in this population [49]. However, pre-pregnancy counselling in the patients who do not possess PAH is of paramount importance if the patient or family members are at an increased genetic risk. This is particularly important for patients possessing high-risk gene defects for example BMRP2.

26.5 Molecular Aspects of BMPR2 and Other Mutations in the Pathway

Genetic studies have demonstrated that 70% or more of patients with hereditary PAH [50] and 10%–20% of patients with sporadic IPAH, are heterozygous for a mutation in bone morphogenetic protein (BMP) receptor type 2 (BMPR2). BMPR2

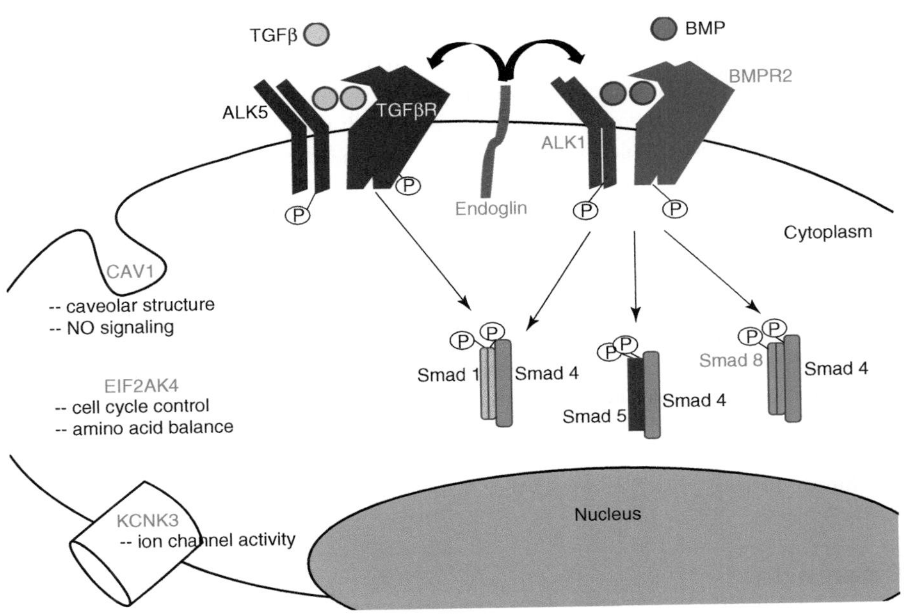

Fig. 26.3 Simplified schematic of the proteins encoded by the genes with mutations known to associate with pulmonary arterial hypertension (PAH), with a focus on the BMP signaling pathway but addition of recently described mutations. Genes with mutations known to associate with PAH include BMPR2, ALK1, Endoglin, Smad 9 (encodes SMAD 8), CAV1, KCNK3, and EIF2AK4. Possible resultant signaling or effects of protein actions are briefly listed. Of note, Smad-independent effects of BMP signaling abnormalities are not shown but may contribute to PAH pathogenesis, such as alterations in cytoskeletal dynamics, cell survival, and mitochondrial metabolism. BMPR2 indicates bone morphogenic protein receptor type 2; and TGF-β, transforming growth factor-β. From [51]; with permission

is a member of the TGF-β superfamily of growth factor receptors (Fig. 26.3). Different functions of BMPR2 are affected by different mutations including the ligand-binding domain and the signalling mechanism. Penetrance of heritable PAH is low, 80% of family members with BMPR2 mutation, never develop PAH [52]. Interestingly, 8% of patients with congenital heart disease and left to right shunts, leading to PAH also have mutations in BMPR2 [24]. More recent studies have made better links with Smad activation and microRNAs (especially miRNA 21) [53]. Loss of BMPR2 causes proliferation of pulmonary artery smooth muscle cells in response to TGF-β1 and BMP2.

26.6 Treatment and Summary

Treatment of PAH requires a multi-disciplinary team approach lead by a PH specialist, firstly by correcting any underlying disease, for example CHD and completing genetic testing and screening family members. A full description of the treatment available for PAH is beyond the scope of this chapter. In summary, oral monotherapy includes phosphodiesterase-5 inhibitors (sildenafil), second line therapy (usually dual therapy) with endothelin receptor agonists (bosentan, macitentan, ambrisentan). Finally severe disease is treated with the prostanoids (Epoprostenol infusion or Iloprost inhalation) or sometimes with lung transplantation [2]. New therapies recently introduced include direct stimulation of soluble guanylate cyclase by Riociguat [54] especially for chronic thromboembolic PH not amenable to surgical therapy and also Selexipag [55] a new IP3 stimulator—with the intention of providing an oral alternative to the parenteral therapies of the prostanoids.

PAH is a chronic condition associated with a poor prognosis due to irreversible effects on the pulmonary and cardiac function. There are multiple genes associated with PAH including gene defects directly resulting in PAH, eg. BMPR2, or other diseases that have side effects of PAH, eg. CHD and CHA. Efforts need to be taken to diagnose PAH as early as possible to prevent long-term morbidity. Clinical suspicion should be kept high for a genetic cause contributing to PAH particularly if there is a family history.

References

1. Hoeper MM, Humbert M, Souza R, Idrees M, Kawut SM, Sliwa-Hahnle K, Jing ZC, Gibbs JS. A global view of pulmonary hypertension. Lancet Respir Med. 2016;4:306–22.
2. Galie N, Hoeper MM, Humbert M, Torbicki A, Vachiery JL, Barbera JA, Beghetti M, Corris P, Gaine S, Gibbs JS, Gomez-Sanchez MA, Jondeau G, Klepetko W, Opitz C, Peacock A, Rubin L, Zellweger M, Simonneau G, Guidelines ESCCFP. Guidelines for the diagnosis and treatment of pulmonary hypertension: the Task Force for the Diagnosis and Treatment of Pulmonary Hypertension of the European Society of Cardiology (ESC) and the European Respiratory Society (ERS), endorsed by the International Society of Heart and Lung Transplantation (ISHLT). Eur Heart J. 2009;30:2493–537.
3. King P, Tulloh R. Management of pulmonary hypertension and Down syndrome. Int J Clin Pract Suppl. 2011;174:8–13.
4. Rabinovitch M. Pathobiology of pulmonary hypertension. Annu Rev Pathol. 2007;2:369–99.
5. Iacobazzi D, Suleiman MS, Ghorbel M, George SJ, Caputo M, Tulloh RM. Cellular and molecular basis of RV hypertrophy in congenital heart disease. Heart. 2016;102:12–7.
6. Hoeper MM. The new definition of pulmonary hypertension. Eur Respir J. 2009;34:790–1.
7. Tulloh R. Etiology, diagnosis, and pharmacologic treatment of pediatric pulmonary hypertension. Paediatr Drugs. 2009;11:115–28.
8. Lopez Reyes R, Nauffal Manzur D, Garcia Ortega A, Menendez Salinas MA, Ansotegui Barrera E, Balerdi Perez B. Clinical characteristics and survival of patients with pulmonary hypertension: a 40-month mean follow-up. Clin Respir J. 2017;11:103–12.
9. Espinola-Zavaleta N, Soto ME, Romero-Gonzalez A, Gomez-Puente Ldel C, Munoz-Castellanos L, Gopal AS, Keirns C, Lupi-Herrera E. Prevalence of congenital heart disease and pulmonary hypertension in Down's syndrome: an echocardiographic study. J Cardiovasc Ultrasound. 2015;23:72–7.
10. Hawkins A, Langton-Hewer S, Henderson J, Tulloh RM. Management of pulmonary hypertension in Down syndrome. Eur J Pediatr. 2011;170:915–21.
11. Saji T. Clinical characteristics of pulmonary arterial hypertension associated with Down syndrome. Pediatr Int. 2014;56:297–303.
12. Berger RM, Beghetti M, Galie N, Gatzoulis MA, Granton J, Lauer A, Chiossi E, Landzberg M. Atrial septal defects versus ventricular septal defects in BREATHE-5, a placebo-controlled

study of pulmonary arterial hypertension related to Eisenmenger's syndrome: a subgroup analysis. Int J Cardiol. 2010;144:373–8.
13. Humbert M, Galie N. What's new in the European Society of Cardiology/European Respiratory Society Pulmonary Hypertension Guidelines? Eur Heart J. 2016;37:4–5.
14. Austin ED, Loyd JE. Heritable forms of pulmonary arterial hypertension. Semin Respir Crit Care Med. 2013;34:568–80.
15. Cogan J, Austin E, Hedges L, Womack B, West J, Loyd J, Hamid R. Role of BMPR2 alternative splicing in heritable pulmonary arterial hypertension penetrance. Circulation. 2012;126:1907–16.
16. Cogan JD, Vnencak-Jones CL, Phillips JA 3rd, Lane KB, Wheeler LA, Robbins IM, Garrison G, Hedges LK, Loyd JE. Gross BMPR2 gene rearrangements constitute a new cause for primary pulmonary hypertension. Genet Med. 2005;7:169–74.
17. Li G, Tang L, Jia P, Zhao J, Liu D, Liu B. Elevated plasma connective tissue growth factor levels in children with pulmonary arterial hypertension associated with congenital heart disease. Pediatr Cardiol. 2016;37:714–21.
18. West J, Cogan J, Geraci M, Robinson L, Newman J, Phillips JA, Lane K, Meyrick B, Loyd J. Gene expression in BMPR2 mutation carriers with and without evidence of pulmonary arterial hypertension suggests pathways relevant to disease penetrance. BMC Med Genet. 2008;1:45.
19. Hamid R, Hedges LK, Austin E, Phillips JA 3rd, Loyd JE, Cogan JD. Transcripts from a novel BMPR2 termination mutation escape nonsense mediated decay by downstream translation re-initiation: implications for treating pulmonary hypertension. Clin Genet. 2010;77:280–6.
20. Daniels CE, Wilkes MC, Edens M, Kottom TJ, Murphy SJ, Limper AH, Leof EB. Imatinib mesylate inhibits the profibrogenic activity of TGF-beta and prevents bleomycin-mediated lung fibrosis. J Clin Invest. 2004;114:1308–16.
21. Thomson J, Machado R, Pauciulo M, et al. Sporadic primary pulmonary hypertension is associated with germline mutations of the gene encoding BMPR-2, a receptor member of the TGF-Beta family. J Med Genet. 2000;37:741–5.
22. Austin ED, Cogan JD, West JD, Hedges LK, Hamid R, Dawson EP, Wheeler LA, Parl FF, Loyd JE, Phillips JA 3rd. Alterations in oestrogen metabolism: implications for higher penetrance of familial pulmonary arterial hypertension in females. Eur Respir J. 2009;34:1093–9.
23. Newman JH, Wheeler L, Lane KB, Loyd E, Gaddipati R, Phillips JA 3rd, Loyd JE. Mutation in the gene for bone morphogenetic protein receptor II as a cause of primary pulmonary hypertension in a large kindred. N Engl J Med. 2001;345:319–24.
24. Harrison RE, Berger R, Haworth SG, Tulloh R, Mache CJ, Morrell NW, Aldred MA, Trembath RC. Transforming growth factor-beta receptor mutations and pulmonary arterial hypertension in childhood. Circulation. 2005;111:435–41.
25. Haberl I, Frei K, Ramsebner R, Doberer D, Petkov V, Albinni S, Lang I, Lucas T, Mosgoeller W. Vasoactive intestinal peptide gene alterations in patients with idiopathic pulmonary arterial hypertension. Eur J Hum Genet. 2007;15:18–22.
26. Harrison RE, Flanagan JA, Sankelo M, Abdalla SA, Rowell J, Machado RD, Elliott CG, Robbins IM, Olschewski H, Mclaughlin V, Gruenig E, Kermeen F, Halme M, Raisanen-Sokolowski A, Laitinen T, Morrell NW, Trembath RC. Molecular and functional analysis identifies ALK-1 as the predominant cause of pulmonary hypertension related to hereditary haemorrhagic telangiectasia. J Med Genet. 2003;40:865–71.
27. Thomas M, Docx C, Holmes AM, Beach S, Duggan N, England K, Leblanc C, Lebret C, Schindler F, Raza F, Walker C, Crosby A, Davies RJ, Morrell NW, Budd DC. Activin-like kinase 5 (ALK5) mediates abnormal proliferation of vascular smooth muscle cells from patients with familial pulmonary arterial hypertension and is involved in the progression of experimental pulmonary arterial hypertension induced by monocrotaline. Am J Pathol. 2009;174:380–9.
28. Mathew R. Pulmonary hypertension and metabolic syndrome: possible connection, PPARgamma and Caveolin-1. World J Cardiol. 2014;6:692–705.

29. Rose JA, Cleveland JM, Rao Y, Minai OA, Tonelli AR. Effect of age on phenotype and outcomes in pulmonary arterial hypertension trials. Chest. 2016;149:1234–44.
30. Wardle AJ, Tulloh RM. Evolving management of pediatric pulmonary arterial hypertension: impact of phosphodiesterase inhibitors. Pediatr Cardiol. 2013;34:213–9.
31. Bradford R, Tulloh R. Diagnosis and Management of Pulmonary hypertension in adult congenital heart disease. Br J Cardiac Nurs. 2008;3:138–45.
32. Freeman SB, Taft LF, Dooley KJ, Allran K, Sherman SL, Hassold TJ, Khoury MJ, Saker DM. Population-based study of congenital heart defects in Down syndrome. Am J Med Genet. 1998;80:213–7.
33. Tulloh RM. Congenital heart disease in relation to pulmonary hypertension in paediatric practice. Paediatr Respir Rev. 2005;6:174–80.
34. Yu S, Yi H, Wang Z, Dong J. Screening key genes associated with congenital heart defects in Down syndrome based on differential expression network. Int J Clin Exp Pathol. 2015;8:8385–93.
35. Antonarakis SE, Lyle R, Dermitzakis ET, Reymond A, Deutsch S. Chromosome 21 and down syndrome: from genomics to pathophysiology. Nat Rev Genet. 2004;5:725–38.
36. Richards AA, Garg V. Genetics of congenital heart disease. Curr Cardiol Rev. 2010;6:91–7.
37. Yang X, Mardekian J, Sanders KN, Mychaskiw MA, Thomas J 3rd. Prevalence of pulmonary arterial hypertension in patients with connective tissue diseases: a systematic review of the literature. Clin Rheumatol. 2013;32:1519–31.
38. Bienengraeber M, Olson TM, Selivanov VA, Kathmann EC, O'Cochlain F, Gao F, Karger AB, Ballew JD, Hodgson DM, Zingman LV, Pang YP, Alekseev AE, Terzic A. ABCC9 mutations identified in human dilated cardiomyopathy disrupt catalytic KATP channel gating. Nat Genet. 2004;36:382–7.
39. Reiter CD, Wang X, Tanus-Santos JE, Hogg N, Cannon RO 3rd, Schechter AN, Gladwin MT. Cell-free hemoglobin limits nitric oxide bioavailability in sickle-cell disease. Nat Med. 2002;8:1383–9.
40. Olivieri NF. The beta-thalassemias. N Engl J Med. 1999;341:99–109.
41. Giardina PJ, Hilgartner MW. Update on thalassemia. Pediatr Rev. 1992;13:55–62.
42. Panigrahi I, Agarwal S. Genetic determinants of phenotype in beta-thalassemia. Hematology. 2008;13:247–52.
43. Du ZD, Roguin N, Milgram E, Saab K, Koren A. Pulmonary hypertension in patients with thalassemia major. Am Heart J. 1997;134:532–7.
44. Farmakis D, Aessopos A. Pulmonary hypertension associated with hemoglobinopathies: prevalent but overlooked. Circulation. 2011;123:1227–32.
45. Potoka KP, Gladwin MT. Vasculopathy and pulmonary hypertension in sickle cell disease. Am J Physiol Lung Cell Mol Physiol. 2015;308:L314–24.
46. Verrelli BC, Mcdonald JH, Argyropoulos G, Destro-Bisol G, Froment A, Drousiotou A, Lefranc G, Helal AN, Loiselet J, Tishkoff SA. Evidence for balancing selection from nucleotide sequence analyses of human G6PD. Am J Hum Genet. 2002;71:1112–28.
47. Phrommintikul A, Sukonthasarn A, Kanjanavanit R, Nawarawong W. Splenectomy: a strong risk factor for pulmonary hypertension in patients with thalassaemia. Heart. 2006;92:1467–72.
48. Walter PB, Fung EB, Killilea DW, Jiang Q, Hudes M, Madden J, Porter J, Evans P, Vichinsky E, Harmatz P. Oxidative stress and inflammation in iron-overloaded patients with beta-thalassaemia or sickle cell disease. Br J Haematol. 2006;135:254–63.
49. Regitz-Zagrosek V, Seeland U, Geibel-Zehender A, Gohlke-Barwolf C, Kruck I, Schaefer C. Cardiovascular diseases in pregnancy. Dtsch Arztebl Int. 2011;108:267–73.
50. International PPH Consortium, Lane KB, Machado RD, Pauciulo MW, Thomson JR, Phillips JA 3rd, Loyd JE, Nichols WC, Trembath RC. Heterozygous germline mutations in BMPR2, encoding a TGF-beta receptor, cause familial primary pulmonary hypertension. Nat Genet. 2000;26:81–4.
51. Austin ED, Loyd JE. The genetics of pulmonary arterial hypertension. Circ Res. 2014;115: 189–202.

52. Hamid R, Cogan JD, Hedges LK, Austin E, Phillips JA 3rd, Newman JH, Loyd JE. Penetrance of pulmonary arterial hypertension is modulated by the expression of normal BMPR2 allele. Hum Mutat. 2009;30:649–54.
53. Li Q, Zhang D, Wang Y, Sun P, Hou X, Larner J, Xiong W, Mi J. MiR-21/Smad 7 signaling determines TGF-beta1-induced CAF formation. Sci Rep. 2013;3:2038.
54. Ghofrani HA, D'Armini AM, Grimminger F, Hoeper MM, Jansa P, Kim NH, Mayer E, Simonneau G, Wilkins MR, Fritsch A, Neuser D, Weimann G, Wang C, Group C-S. Riociguat for the treatment of chronic thromboembolic pulmonary hypertension. N Engl J Med. 2013;369:319–29.
55. Simonneau G, Torbicki A, Hoeper MM, Delcroix M, Karlocai K, Galie N, Degano B, Bonderman D, Kurzyna M, Efficace M, Giorgino R, Lang IM. Selexipag: an oral, selective prostacyclin receptor agonist for the treatment of pulmonary arterial hypertension. Eur Respir J. 2012;40:874–80.

Genetics and Genomics of Sudden Unexplained Cardiac Death

27

Efstathios Papatheodorou, Mary N. Sheppard, and Elijah R. Behr

Abstract

The aetiology of sudden cardiac death (SCD) and sudden arrhythmic death syndrome (SADS) is not fully explored. Expert cardiac pathology and detailed familial clinical evaluation can identify an inherited cardiac disease in up to 50% of the cases and subsequently guide the genetic investigation in the living family members. Post-mortem genetic testing, known as the "molecular autopsy", has been increasingly used in the last 15 years as a complementary diagnostic tool. Advances in next-generation sequencing technologies, allowing the use of whole exome sequencing of expanding panels of genes, provide further insight into the pathogenesis of SCD and SADS. However, identification of numerous variants of unknown significance, emphasises the importance of cautious genetic interpretation. In this review, we present the diagnostic process followed in characteristic young SCD and SADS cases. We describe current evidence regarding cardiac pathology, appropriate familial clinical evaluation, and genetic analysis performed in relatives or in the proband's DNA.

E. Papatheodorou (✉)
Cardiovascular and Cell Sciences Research Institute, St George's University Hospital, Tooting, London, UK
e-mail: spapathe@sgul.ac.uk

M.N. Sheppard
CRY Cardiovascular Pathology Unit, Institute of Cardiovascular and Cell Sciences, St. George's University Hospital, Tooting, London, UK
e-mail: m.sheppard@sgul.ac.uk

E.R. Behr
Reader in Cardiovascular Medicine, Cardiovascular and Cell Sciences Research Institute, Tooting, London, UK
e-mail: ebehr@sgul.ac.uk

D. Kumar, P. Elliott (eds.), *Cardiovascular Genetics and Genomics*,
https://doi.org/10.1007/978-3-319-66114-8_27

Keywords
Sudden cardiac death • Sudden arrhythmic death syndrome • Molecular autopsy • Autopsy findings • Ion channelopathies • Cardiac pathology • Cardiomyopathy

27.1 Introduction

Sudden cardiac death (SCD) is defined as an acute change in cardiovascular status with the time to death being up to 1 h. In unwitnessed cases, the definition also includes victims last seen alive and functioning normally less than 24 h before being found dead [1]. The annual incidence of SCD in the general population, ranges from 40 per 100,000 in Asia [2] to 100 per 100,000 in the USA [1]. There are an estimated 70,000 SCDs in the UK and 300,000–400,000 SCD in the USA per annum [3]. The vast majority of these deaths can be attributed to coronary artery disease and heart failure. The incidence of SCD increases with age in both men and women, because the prevalence of ischemic heart disease increases with age. SCD has a much higher incidence in men than women, reflecting sex differences in the incidence of coronary heart disease [4]. The epidemiology of SCD in the young (≤35 years), however, is not established adequately. Estimates of its annual incidence range from 0.7 to 6.2 per 100,000 (Table 27.1), depending upon the age ranges included, the definitions used, the presence of an expert autopsy, the use of autopsy reports and/or death certificates and differences in populations investigated such as athletes or military recruits [17, 19, 21]. The proportion of sudden deaths that remains unexplained after post-mortem cardiac investigation and toxicological analysis is termed the Sudden Arrhythmic Death Syndrome (SADS) [29]. "Sudden infant death syndrome" (SIDS) or "sudden unexpected death in infancy" (SUDI) are also used in cases under 1 year of age when the cause of death remains unexplained despite detailed autopsy and forensic investigation [29].

Whereas coronary artery disease is identified as the major cause of death in older individuals, in the younger age group inherited cardiac disease and/or SADS predominate [30]. Non-inherited cardiac disease such as Wolff-Parkinson-White (WPW) syndrome, coronary artery spasm, coronary anatomy anomalies, concussion of the heart from non-penetrating blunt trauma to the anterior chest in athletes (Commotio Cordis), malignant mitral valve prolapse or myocarditis are also recognised as occasional causes of SCD [18, 31]. In the athletic population, hypertrophic cardiomyopathy (HCM) [32, 33], arrhythmogenic right ventricular cardiomyopathy (ARVC) [11] or SADS [26] have all been reported as the dominant cause of death in different series. Subsequent clinical and genetic diagnostic workup identifies a genetic cause responsible for the death in up to 50% of the SADS victims and their families [34–37]. In this review, we present characteristic young SCD and SADS cases and the concomitant diagnostic process including the autopsy, familial clinical evaluation and the genetic analysis performed in relatives or in the proband's DNA.

Table 27.1 Main studies of sudden cardiac death in the young

Study	Population studied	Age	SADS yield N (%)	Annual incidence of SADS[a]	Annual incidence of SCD[a]
Molander [5]	Sweden, 1974–1979	1–20	4/31 (13%)	0.14	1.1
Neuspiel and Kuller [6]	USA, 1972–1980	1–21	29/207 (14%)	0.64	4.6
Anderson et al. [7]	USA, New Mexico 1977–1988	5–39	39/650 (6%)	0.39	6.6
Shen et al. [8]	USA, 1960–1989	20–40	7/54 (13%) <35 47.8%	0.80	6.2
Maron et al. [9]	USA, Minnesota, 1985–1997	Athletes 13–19			0.20
Chugh et al. [10]	USA, Minneapolis 1984–1996	>20	14/270 (5%)		
Corrado et al. [11]	Italy, Veneto 1979–1998	1–35	16/273 (6%)		
Wisten et al. [12]	Sweden, 1992–1999	15–35	38/181 (21%)	0.19	0.9
Morentin et al. [13]	Spain, Bizkaia 1991–1998	1–35	19/107 (18%)	0.43	2.4
Corrado et al. [14]	Italy, Veneto 1979–1999	12–35	18/300 (6%)	0.06	1 2.1 athletes
Eckart et al. [15]	USA, 1977–2001, military recruits	>18	44/126 (35%)		
Doolan et al. [16]	Sydney, Australia 1994–2002	≤35	60/193 (31%)		
Puranik et al. [17]	Australia, 1995–2004	5–35	124/427 29%		
Fabre and Sheppard [18]	UK, 1994–2003	15–35	144/223 (64.5%)		
Papadakis et al. [19]	UK, England Wales	1–34	226/1677 (14%)	0.24	1.8
Chugh et al. [20]	USA, Oregon 2002–2005	<18	23/25 (92%) SIDS		1.7 0.8 SIDS
Winkel et al. [21]	Denmark 2000–2006	1–35	136/314 (33%)	0.8	2.4
Eckart et al. [22]	USA, 1998–2008	>18	39/187 (21%) 41% in <35 11% >35	1.2 < 35 2.0 > 35	6.7 males, 1.4 females
Margey et al. [23]	Ireland, 2005–2007	14–35	31/116 (26.7%)	0.76	2.8
Pilmer et al. [24]	Ontario, Canada, 2008	2–40	48/174 28%		0.7 (2–18) 2.4 (19–29) 5.3 (30–40)

(continued)

Table 27.1 (continued)

Study	Population studied	Age	SADS yield N (%)	Annual incidence of SADS[a]	Annual incidence of SCD[a]
Harmon et al. [25]	USA 2004–2008	Athletes	11/36 (31%)		
Finocchiaro et al. [26]	UK 1994–2014	Athletes	149/357 (41%)		
Anastasakis et al. [27]	Greece, Attica 2002–2010	1–35	63/349 (18%)	0.5	1.8
Bagnall et al. [28]	Australia, New Zealand 2010–2012	1–35	198/490 (40%)	0.5	1.3

[a]Annual incidence when available in population-based studies is reported per 100,000 persons

27.2 Clinical Examples

27.2.1 Case 1

A 3 years-old young girl collapsed having just arrived at her aunt's home. She had experienced no prior cardiac events and had no prior medical history of note. An autopsy performed by a specialist cardiac pathologist did not reveal any cardiac pathology. There was a subtle lymphocytic infiltrate seen in the heart insufficient to make a diagnosis of acute myocarditis (Fig. 27.1a). DNA was extracted from the spleen at post-mortem and was stored in the molecular genetics laboratory. A diagnosis of SADS was advocated and the victim's family was invited to an Inherited Cardiac Diseases Clinic for cardiac evaluation.

The family had also suffered the sudden death of her father due to subarachnoid haemorrhage few months after the birth of his daughter. At his autopsy there was evidence of significant coronary atherosclerosis. There was a strong history of coronary artery disease in the father's side but no history of premature sudden cardiac death. The proband's older brother and mother were investigated with a comprehensive cardiac protocol which included a resting ECG, an exercise treadmill test, 24-h ambulatory ECG monitoring and a 2D echocardiogram. These investigations were within normal limits (Fig. 27.1b). Her mother also underwent ajmaline provocation testing and an epinephrine challenge. The ajmaline test did not induce any evidence of the type 1 Brugada ECG pattern and the epinephrine challenge did not induce any sustained or significant QT prolongation or any significant ventricular arrhythmia.

Genetic results from a next generation sequencing (NGS) of a 77 panel analysis of the proband's DNA however revealed a likely pathogenic variant in the ryanodine receptor gene (*RYR2*, c.12013G>A). Cascade genetic analysis of the deceased's mother and brother and DNA extracted from a block retained from the father's autopsy did not identify the variant indicating a likely de novo variant and permitting reassurance of the mother and her son and discharge from clinical care.

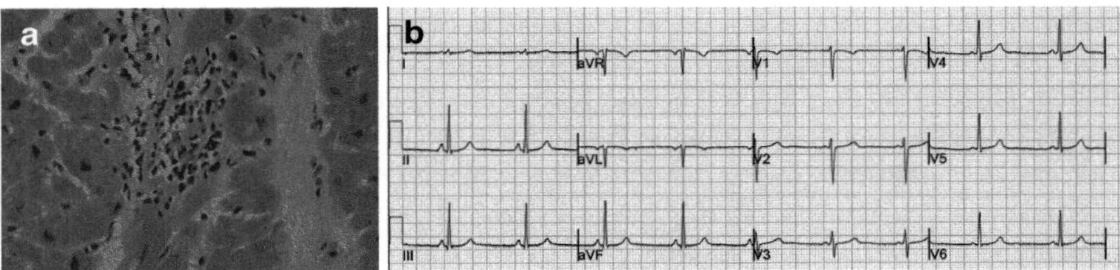

Fig. 27.1 (**a**) Single lymphocytic focus in the microscopic evaluation of the proband's heart. (**b**) Normal resting ECG of the proband's mother

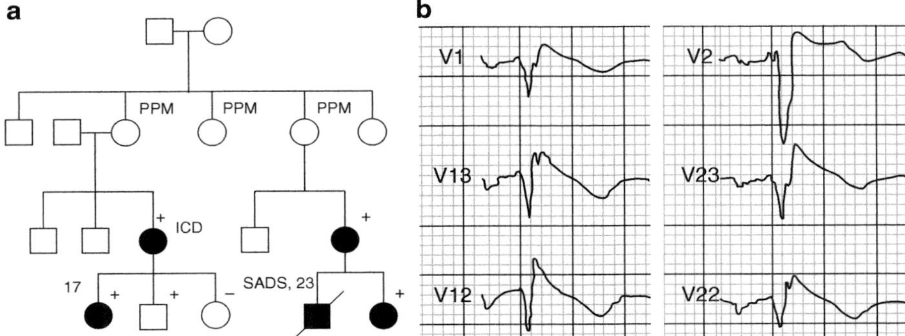

Fig. 27.2 (**a**) 3 generation family pedigree. Circles indicate female; squares indicate male; symbols with a slash indicate deceased subjects and coloured black symbols indicate clinically diseased persons. Symbols with a positive sign indicate mutation carriers whereas a minus sign indicates mutation-free subjects. The age reported in subjects with SD indicates the age at the event. (**b**) Right precordial leads placed on the 4th (V1, V2), 2nd (V12, V22) and 3rd (V13, V23) intercostal space recorded at the 6th minute of an ajmaline provocation testing in the proband's second cousin. An unequivocal type 1 Brugada pattern is recorded with J point elevation >2 mm, coved ST segment appearance and symmetric negative T wave (in all leads except V2)

27.2.2 Case 2

A 23 year-old Caucasian male was found deceased during his sleep. He had been fit and healthy and never complained of any cardiac symptoms prior to his death. A specialist cardiac autopsy did not reveal any cardiac pathology. Cardiac investigations in the family revealed a spontaneous type 1 Brugada ECG pattern in the victim's mother and a definite Brugada type 1 during an ajmaline provocation testing in his sister (Fig. 27.2). Targeted genetic analysis in the proband's mother and sister, revealed a pathogenic *SCN5A* mutation (c.4385T>A, p.Leu1462Gln). Due to low quality DNA, genetic screening in the DNA of the deceased was not possible. From the family history, there were 3 more unexplained deaths in distant relatives and several relatives had received a pacemaker. Insights from the extended family showed that a maternal 1st cousin has been diagnosed with sick sinus syndrome and had a pacemaker implanted several years ago. Due to symptomatic episodes of ventricular tachycardia the device was upgraded to an implantable cardiovertor defibrillator (ICD). She was treated with flecainide but she had several inappropriate and appropriate shocks. Following the death of her distant nephew and the information that BrS was found in the family, she was tested for *SCN5A* mutations and was found to bear the same mutation as her 1st cousin. Cascade genetic analysis revealed that her two children were also *SCN5A* carriers. Her 17 years-old daughter exhibited a type 2 Brugada pattern on her ECG.

27.2.3 Case 3

A 39 year-old Caucasian male died suddenly and unexpectedly during light jogging. He had been fit and healthy and never complained of any cardiac symptoms prior to his death. A specialist cardiac autopsy was performed and revealed fibrosis of the intraventricular septum (Fig. 27.3a). Subsequently, DNA was extracted from the spleen at post-mortem and was stored in the molecular genetics laboratory. There was an additional premature sudden death in the proband's maternal uncle who died at the age of 17. The post-mortem-report from 1966 stated 'vagal inhibition' as the cause of death. Given the pathological diagnosis of idiopathic fibrosis and the family history of two sudden deaths, the family was invited to the Inherited Cardiac Diseases Clinic for cardiac evaluation. The proband's younger sister and his parents were investigated with a comprehensive cardiac protocol which included a resting ECG, an exercise treadmill test, 24-h ambulatory ECG monitoring and a 2D echocardiogram as baseline investigations.

A mild phenotype of dilated cardiomyopathy (DCM) with left ventricular (LV) enlargement and moderately impaired systolic function was identified in the proband's sister. A cardiac MRI revealed mid-wall fibrosis with late gadolinium enhancement in the left apical and mid septal walls and LV hypo-perfusion (Fig. 27.3b, c). Her 24-h tape revealed over 4000 polymorphic ventricular ectopics with several runs of non-sustained ventricular tachycardia. Borderline left ventricular dimensions with low normal systolic function and a high burden of ventricular and supraventricular arrhythmias were also identified in the proband's mother. Both patients received optimised heart failure medication and an ICD for primary prevention. Additionally, the proband's mother was started on full anticoagulation therapy. Predictive genetic testing for commonest genes implicated in arrhythmogenic dilated cardiomyopathy (*LMNA*, *TTN*, *MYH7*, *TNNT2*) and left-dominant ARVC (*DSG2*, *PKP2*, *DSP*) was performed. Two variants of unknown significance in *LMNA* and *TTN* genes were identified in the proband's mother. A 77-panel NGS analysis in the proband's DNA confirmed the presence of the *TTN* stop gain variant (c.65935A>T p.(Arg21979) which was then classified as likely pathogenic using the American College of Medical Genetics consensus statement guidelines [38].

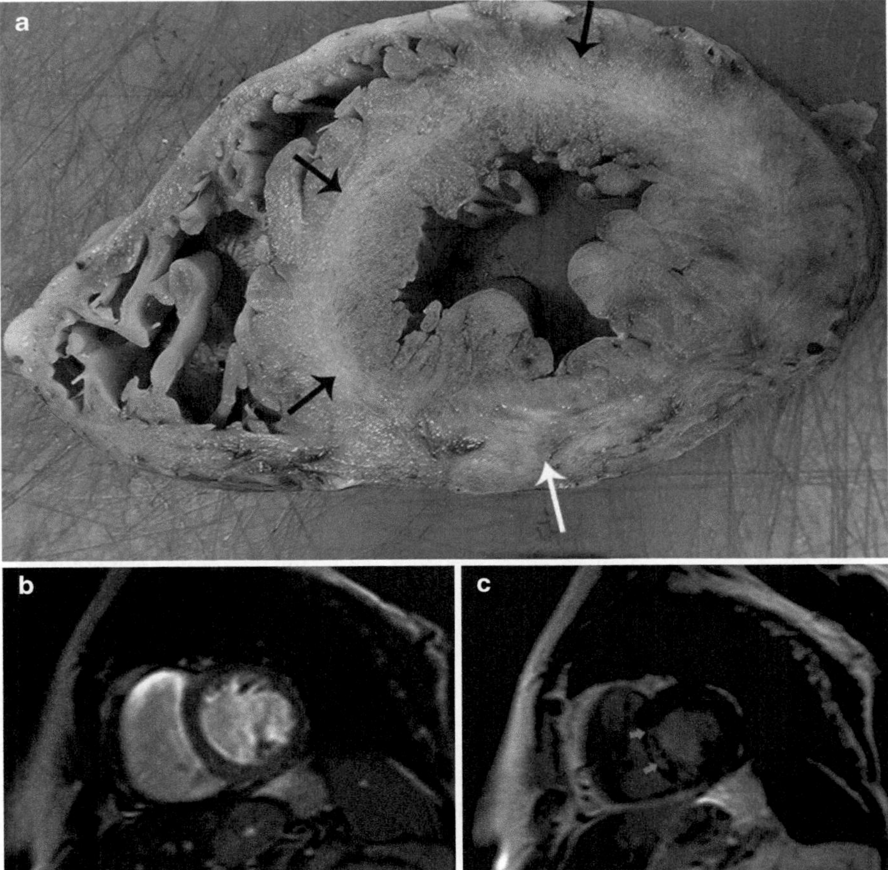

Fig. 27.3 *Upper panel* (**a**) Macroscopic findings in the proband with sudden cardiac death. Note the pale appearance of the left ventricular myocardium (black arrows) indicating circumferential mid wall fibrosis. The myocardium appears brighter in the inferior wall with almost transmural extension of the fibrosis (white arrow). *Lower panel*: Cardiac MRI images in the proband's mother. (**b**) Short axis cine still showing normal biventricular size and function (**c**) Midventricular short-axis late gadolinium enhancement indicating mid wall circumferential fibrosis (red arrows)

27.3 Discussion

27.3.1 The Role of Cardiac Pathology

An accurate post-mortem diagnosis is the first step in the assessment of SCD and allows optimal clinical and genetic evaluation of families in cases with a suspected genetic cause. Lack of resources, time constraints and limited preservation of

Table 27.2 Equivocal findings during autopsy

Autopsy finding	Normal finding in	Pathological change in
Right ventricular fatty infiltration	Females, obese, elderly	ARVC
Idiopathic LVH	Athletes	HCM
MV ballooning	Female gender, elderly	MV prolapse
Left ventricular myocyte disarray	Left ventricular anteroseptal and posteroseptal walls	Subclinical HCM
Inflammatory foci with or without fibrosis		Focal myocarditis
Idiopathic Fibrosis		DCM, ARVC, HCM

ARVC arrhythmogenic right ventricular cardiomyopathy, *HCM* hypertrophic cardiomyopathy, *LVH* left ventricular hypertrophy, *MV* mitral valve, *DCM* dilated cardiomyopathy

autopsy tissue represent the main factors for absence or deficiency of histopathological examination. This leads to reduced quality autopsies and erroneous diagnoses. Even when an autopsy with adequate histopathological analysis is performed, normal macroscopic and microscopic variation can be misinterpreted as pathological, impeding the correct clinical evaluation in the family and misdirecting the genetic process. Expert cardiac pathology can detect subtle findings of unknown significance that cannot be categorised diagnostically (Table 27.2; Fig. 27.4). Accurate interpretation of these cases is crucial, especially when idiopathic fibrosis or left ventricular hypertrophy (LVH) are detected, since familial evaluation and/or post-mortem genetic testing (the 'molecular autopsy') identify a similar yield of primary arrhythmia syndromes and cardiomyopathies compared to series of SADS cases [39, 40]. On the other hand, cardiac pathology may be missed by general autopsy, mislabelling cases as SADS and leading families into an unnecessary, time-consuming expensive and distressing process. Moreover, a detailed autopsy study of the conduction system is extremely consuming and unsatisfactory in the investigation of most sudden deaths [41].

The proportion of morphologically normal hearts at autopsy vary widely, ranging from 5% to 65%. Data from population-based studies estimate annual incidences of SADS from 0.19 to 2.0 per 100,000. Discrepancies in the identification of SADS are commonly recognised in series from expert cardiac pathology centres when compared to general pathology. Although a referral bias to specialist centres is a major limitation in defining the true aetiology of SCD, this disparity mainly reflects the low sensitivity and specificity of cardiac autopsy performed by general pathologists [18]. De Norohna et al. directly analysed the interpretation of autopsies in young sudden death victims given by general pathologists and specialist cardiac pathologists and showed an incongruence of almost 59% in diagnoses. General pathologists tended to diagnose pathology rather than designate the heart as structurally normal with 37% of normal hearts being described as pathologically abnormal. ARVC and myocarditis were the most commonly over-reported misdiagnoses given in normal hearts. Fatty infiltration of the right ventricle and normal myocyte

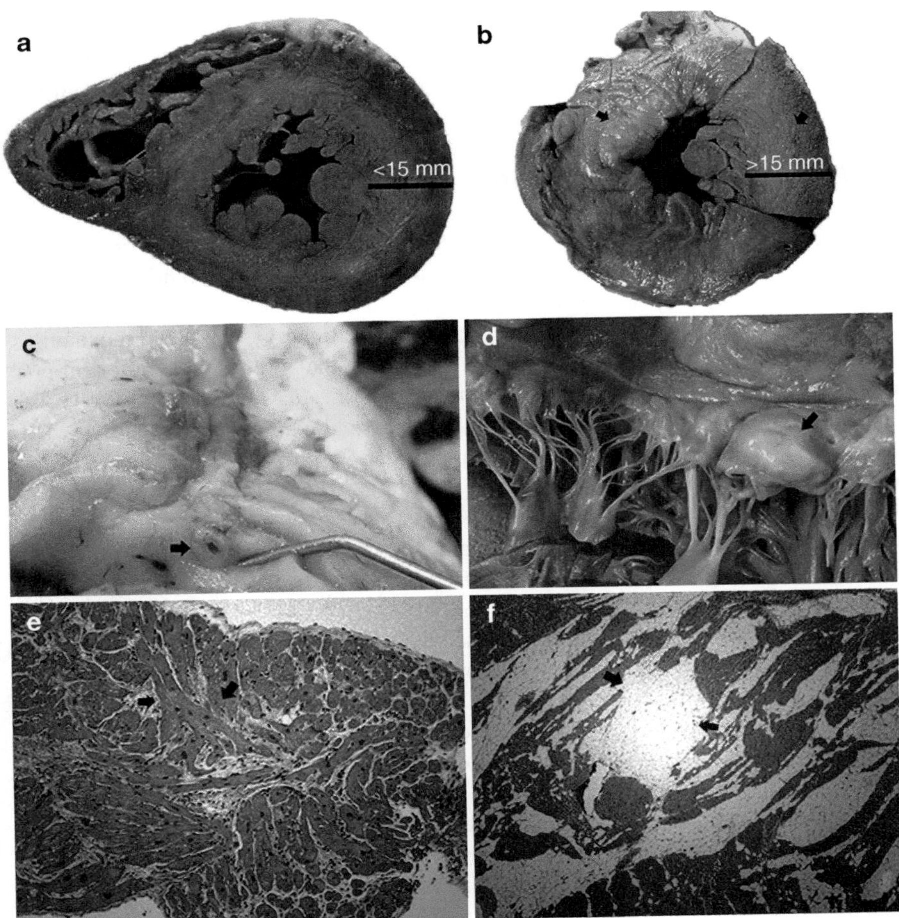

Fig. 27.4 Findings of unknown significance during autopsy (**a**) Macroscopically normal heart (**b**) Isolated RV fatty infiltration (**c**) MV ballooning (**d**) Isolated left ventricular disarray (**e**) Isolated left ventricular hypertrophy (**f**) Non-significant coronary artery disease

disarray in the anteroseptal and posteroseptal LV walls were the main misinterpreted findings; mislabelling autopsies as ARVC and HCM respectively. In contrast, a number of hearts which general pathologists labelled as normal did actually have pathology [42].

These data indicate that the true incidence of structurally normal hearts is underestimated and underdiagnosed by general pathologists whereas cardiomyopathies and coronary artery disease are over-diagnosed. The significance of expert cardiac autopsy has been emphasized and is recognized as a class I indication by a consensus statement from the Heart Rhythm Society (HRS), European Heart Rhythm Association (EHRA), and the Asia Pacific HRS [29]. Best practice guidelines set by the Royal College of Pathologists and the Association for European Cardiovascular

Pathology also recommend referral of whole hearts to specialist centres with high volume and recognized expertise [43]. There is still however significant variance in the use of expert autopsy amongst different countries and within the same country.

27.3.2 Circumstances of Death

A careful anamnesis of the specific circumstances of death and of any prior symptoms in the victim is helpful in designing the consequent genetic and clinical process since it may imply a distinct pathophysiological mechanism liable for the death. Deaths during sleep or at rest suggest a non-adrenergic mediated mechanism in contrast to deaths during exertion or stress where the adrenergic component predominates [30]. Exertion as an inciting event implies HCM, ARVC, Wolff-Parkinson-White syndrome or an underlying channelopathy, such as subtype 1 of long QT syndrome (LQTS) or catecholaminergic polymorphic ventricular tachycardia (CPVT) as potential causes of death. On the other hand, the incidence of ventricular arrhythmias in Early Repolarisation Syndrome (ERS), coronary artery spasm and Brugada syndrome (BrS) exhibits marked circadian variations with significant peaks of cardiac arrest and appropriate shocks observed during sleep or increased vagal activity [44–46].

Analysis of gender and trigger-specific data reveal that deaths during sleep or at rest are more common than deaths during exercise or with emotional stress [47]. Our group analysed approximately 1000 SADS cases with 82% of the deaths occurring during rest or at sleep [48]. Male sex and age <18 years were independently associated with exercise/stress related deaths. Prior syncope (4.1%), documented arrhythmia (3.4%), and family history of sudden death (4.2%) were relatively uncommon. Data from autopsy series in the athletic population have shown that the higher risk of SCD in athletes is strongly related to congenital coronary artery anomaly, ARVC and premature coronary artery disease [14]. In a recent analysis of 357 athletes, ARVC and left ventricular fibrosis most strongly predicted SCD during exertion [26]. Additional circumstantial, age and gender-specific characteristics have been associated with different cardiac causes for SCD and SADS as illustrated in Table 27.3.

27.3.3 Pathophysiology of SCD/SADS

The pathophysiology of SCD is complex and varies between different pathologies. The most common electrophysiological mechanism in ischaemic SCD is ventricular tachycardia degenerating primarily to ventricular fibrillation and later to asystole. Bradyarrhythmia or electromechanical dissociation are also implicated particularly in patients with advanced heart disease [4], or conditions affecting the cardiac conduction system such as desminopathies, laminopathies or premature cardiac conduction disease (PCCD).

Table 27.3 Age, gender and triggers specific correlations of conditions causing SCD and SADS

	Gender	Age	Triggers
ARVC			Exercise, athletic activity
HCM		Late adolescence-early adulthood	Exercise
LQTS1	Male children female adults	Younger age	Exercise, swimming, pharmacological
LQTS2	Post-partum in females		Auditory stimuli, stress, pharmacological
LQTS3			Sleep, pharmacological
BrS	Male	Young middle age adults	Fever, sleep, post-prandial, pharmacological
SQTS		Late adolescence-early adulthood	
Coronary Spasm			Rest, morning
CPVT	Male	Childhood - early adolescence	Exercise, Stress
WPW syndrome			Exercise, Athletic activity

ARVC arrhythmogenic right ventricular cardiomyopathy, *HCM* hypertrophic cardiomyopathy, *LQTS* long QT syndrome, *BrS* Brugada syndrome, *SQTS* short QT syndrome, *CPVT* catecholaminergic polymorphic ventricular tachycardia, *WPW* Wolff-Parkinson-White

In patients with a morphologically normal heart at post-mortem, various genetic or acquired cardiac abnormalities are the main contributors to the initiation of life-threatening arrhythmias such as polymorphic ventricular tachycardia and torsade de pointes. In arrhythmia syndromes, primary genetic defects lead to dysfunctional cardiac ion channel subunits or interacting proteins and subsequently to impaired electrical properties of the heart. This consists of an underlying substrate susceptible to ventricular arrhythmias especially when interacting with a transient event such as emotional stress or exercise (CPVT, LQTS), fever (BrS), pharmacological challenge (BrS, LQTS) or increased vagal tone (BrS, LQTS), causing syncope or cardiac arrest [30]. In patients with the WPW syndrome, pre-excited and rapidly conducted atrial fibrillation may lead to high ventricular rates and cardiac arrest [49]. Commotio cordis, can lead to fatal cardiac arrest, due to either myocardial trauma or the mechano-electrical triggering of a ventricular tachyarrhythmia during the vulnerable period of the T wave [50].

27.3.4 Clinical Evaluation of SADS Victims

Familial cardiological evaluation can identify an inherited cardiac disease and guide the genetic investigation in the family [29]. Various extensive or more limited clinical protocols have been used in the clinical assessment of SADS victims (Fig. 27.5), including personal and family history, physical examination, resting 12-lead ECG

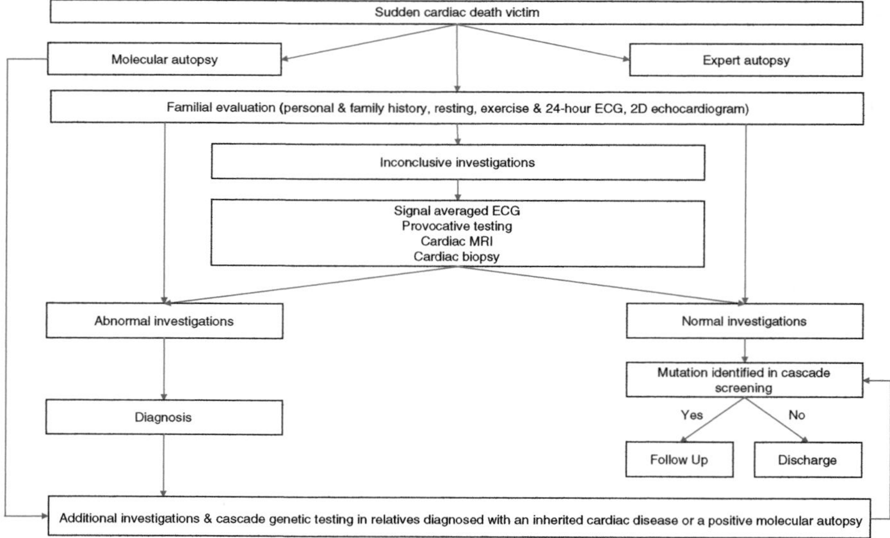

Fig. 27.5 Flow diagram of the standard clinical protocol in families of sudden cardiac death victims

(including high right ventricular leads), echocardiography, exercise, and ambulatory ECGs [34, 51–55]. Further investigations are usually guided by the initial results. A detailed analysis of the victim's prior symptoms or contingent clinical encounters (including any previous ECGs) as well as the circumstances of death and pathology reports is pertinent and the first step in the familial evaluation. A systematic assessment of the family tree in search of any additional sudden deaths or deaths associated with drowning, car accidents or SIDS, a specific pattern of inheritance (X-linked) and relevant clinical phenotypes such as syncopal episodes or relatives with pacemakers or ICDs can provide precious hints regarding the presence of an inherited cardiac disease [56].

The mean yield of studies of familial evaluation in SADS is 32% with a range of 18%–53% (Fig. 27.6). This variability is very much dependent on the population, the availability of autopsy and expert autopsy, and the rigor of the investigative protocol used. Arrhythmia syndromes predominate with average yields for LQTS, BrS and CPVT of 13% (5–18%), 6% (2.3%–39%) and 4% (0–12%) respectively. Despite a normal expert cardiac autopsy, some families manifest cardiomyopathy with an estimated mean yield of 6% (0–16%). Variable expressivity and incomplete penetrance are hallmarks in inherited cardiac diseases and should be expected in the familial evaluation of SADS victims [57].

After comprehensive evaluation, if no abnormalities are detected in first-degree relatives, the risk of future cardiac events related to inherited cardiac disease is generally low [30]. Affected family members are given appropriate treatment and/or interventions such as beta-blockers, pacemakers or ICDs. Usually any potential genetic testing is guided by the clinical phenotype found in the family or the cardiac

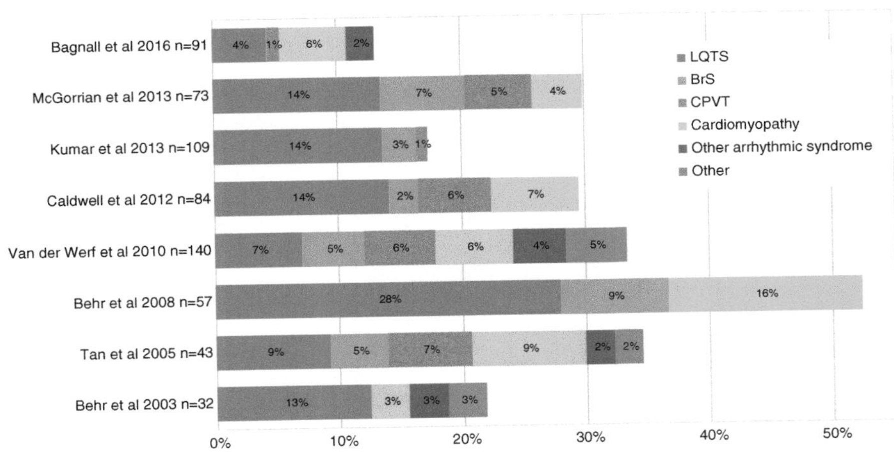

Fig. 27.6 Clinical yield of studies assessing SADS

condition suspected. Cascade genetic analysis can then identify several asymptomatic mutation carriers who will require regular clinical follow up. Once a diagnosis is made the actual proportion of molecular diagnoses in those with a clinical phenotype ranges from 23%–47% overall in all reported series [30]. The identification of the specific mutation or mutations in the DNA of the victim can confirm the suspected cause of SCD and provide the sufficient segregation analysis to clarify the causal relationship and pathogenicity of a specific genetic variant.

27.4 Molecular Autopsy in SADS: Initial Experience

27.4.1 The Evidence

The alternative approach of post-mortem genetic testing in SADS victims, known as the molecular autopsy [58], has been increasingly explored in the last 15 years (Table 27.4). Preliminary case reports indicated an additive value of targeted testing of ion channel genes in the assessment of SADS victims (5, 6). Subsequent small case series, investigating less than 20 SADS victims and using Sanger sequencing technologies, corroborated initial results reporting a molecular autopsy yield for the major LQTS and CPVT genes of up to 35%.

Initial studies often utilised formalin-fixed paraffin embedded (FFPE) tissue as a source of DNA that has severe limitations when used for comprehensive mutational analysis as it can be degraded by the process and over time. When validating different DNA extraction procedures, DNA from FFPE is considered error-prone and unreliable in comprehensive evaluation of SADS associated genes [76]. Given these shortcomings, the guidelines of the Association for European Cardiovascular Pathology recommend 10 ml of EDTA blood and 5 g of heart and spleen or liver tissues to be either frozen and stored at −80 °C, or alternatively preserved in a tissue

Table 27.4 Main studies assessing genetic testing in the assessment of SADS

Study	Genes tested	Source of DNA	Number of cases	Age of population studied (y)	Overall Yield (%)	CPVT1 LQT1–3 Yield (%)	Minor arrhythmia genes yield (%)	Cardiomyopathy genes yield (%)
Di Paolo et al. [59]	LQTS panel	FFPE	10	13–29	20	20	0	–
Chugh et al. [60]	LQTS panel	FFPE	12	22–51	17	17	0	–
Creighton et al. [61]	*RYR2* (22 exons)	Frozen tissues	14	1–43	21	21	–	–
Doolan et al. [62]	*KCNQ1*, *SCN5A*	FFPE	59	1–35	0	0	–	–
Nishio et al. [63]	*RYR2* (24 exons)	Autopsy blood samples	18	2–42	11	11	–	–
Gladding et al. [64]	LQTS panel	Guthrie cards	19	1–34	21	21	0	–
Skinner et al. [65][a]	LQTS panel	Autopsy frozen blood or tissue	33	1–40	15	12	3	–
Tester et al. [37]	LQTS panel, *KCNJ2*, *ANK1* *CACNA1C*:TS1, *RYR2* (18 exons)	Autopsy frozen blood or tissue	173	1–69	26	25	1	–
Winkel et al. [66][a]	*KCNQ1 KCNH2 SCN5A*	Dried blood spot samples or autopsy blood	44	1–35	11	11	–	–
Larsen et al. [67]	*RYR2* (29 exons)	Autopsy frozen blood	36	0–40	11	11	–	–

(continued)

Bagnall et al. [68]	31 genes panel - WES	Autopsy frozen blood	29	1–40	31	10	7	14
Nunn et al. [69]	135 genes panel - targeted exome sequencing	Autopsy frozen blood or tissue	59	1–51	29	8	17	14
Anderson et al. [70]	100 gene panel WES	Whole blood, blood spot card or frozen tissue	21	2–19	14	–	9	5
Hertz et al. [71]	100 genes NGS	Frozen blood/ tissues	52	<50	28	6	8	15
Narula et al. [72]	117 genes WES	Frozen blood	14	12–29	14	0	7	7
Zhang et al. [73]	PKP2	Autopsy frozen tissue	25	24 ± 3	12	–	–	12
Huang et al. [74]	PKP2	Blood samples	119	>18	1	–	–	1
Bagnall et al. [28][a]	69–101 genes panel, exome sequencing	Whole blood samples	113	1–35	27	9	5	17
Lahrouchi et al. [75]	77 genes NGS	Autopsy frozen blood or tissue	302	17–33	13	10.5	0.7	2

FFPE formalin-fixed paraffin embedded tissue, *LQTS panel KCNQ1*, *KCNH2*, *SCN5A*, *KCNE1*, *KCNE2* genes, *MA* major arrhythmia genes (LQT1–3 and *RYR2* genes), *mA* minor arrhythmia genes, *CM* cardiomyopathy genes

[a]Population-based studies, *WES* whole exome sequencing, *NGS* next generation sequencing

storage solution capable of protecting cellular RNA (“RNA later”) at 4 °C for up to 2 weeks as part of the standard autopsy for SADS [43]. Collection of blood and/or suitable tissue for molecular autopsy is a class I recommendation in the HRS and EHRA recommendations for genetic testing in inherited arrhythmias [29, 77].

A large series of 173 consecutive cases tested for the main LQTS and CPVT1 genes finding a yield of 26% [37]. Overall, 45 putative pathogenic mutations, absent in up to 700 controls were identified in 45 cases. This study also provided interesting gender, personal and family history and trigger specific associations with genotype. Female gender, family history of premature SCD, personal history of cardiac symptoms and exercise-related death were associated with a higher genetic yield. Almost half of SADS cases with a family history of premature SCD were identified with a putative pathogenic mutation. Cases aged 1 to 10 years with an exertion-induced death had a yield that was significantly higher than that of 11- to 20-year-olds with exertion-induced death. In contrast, for those individuals who died during sleep, the 11- to 20-year-olds had a higher yield than the 1- to 10-year-olds. These results are in accordance with known susceptibility of *KCNQ1* and *RYR2* mutations to exertional arrhythmias [30].

Due to the circumstances of sudden death and family history, these earlier series may have reflected a referral bias, leading to an overestimation of the expected yield of ion channel genes. Further studies (see Table 27.4) conducted population-based studies leading to distinctly lower yields of around 15% [62, 66]. However, these studies predominantly assessed a limited range of ion channels genes and a restricted number of exons in the *RYR2* gene due to the limitations of Sanger sequencing.

27.4.2 Molecular Autopsy in the Whole Exome Sequencing (WES) Era

Advances in next-generation sequencing technologies have led to cost-efficient and rapid genetic analysis from comparatively small amounts of DNA. Most recent studies (Table 27.4) benefited from the use of whole exome sequencing, investigating expanding panels of genes, including all major disease-associated arrhythmia syndrome and cardiomyopathy genes, as well as less frequently involved genes. Evidence arising from these comparatively small studies still emphasised the dominant role of the main LQTS genes in the aetiology of SADS. The presence of pathogenic *RYR2* variants was however significantly lower in these exome studies [68, 69]. This may be due to smaller numbers or a stricter frequency cut-off for variant calling comparing to the initial Sanger sequencing molecular autopsy series.

Since cardiomyopathies are expected to be picked up at autopsy, systematic testing of genes associated with structural cardiac disease had not been performed in the initial era of molecular autopsy. The use of exome sequencing also enabled the analysis of cardiomyopathy-related genes, the role of which remains largely unexplored in SADS cases. Loporcaro et al. first reported results from a whole exome sequencing specific analysis of 90 genes in a single case of a 16-years-old female SADS victim. Unexpectedly a pathogenic variant in MYH7 was identified, a gene that has been associated previously with hypertrophic cardiomyopathy (HCM) [78]. Subsequently, pathogenic variants in genes associated with ARVC (*DSP*, *DSC2*, *PKP2*), HCM (*MYH7*, *MYH6*) and DCM (*TTN*, *LMNA*) have been identified in studies of WES molecular autopsy [68, 69, 72]. In one of the highest cardiomyopathy yields reported so far, Zhang et al. reported a 12% of *PKP2* possibly pathogenic variants in SADS victims [73].

Most recently a population based study conducted in New Zealand and Australia [28] performed genetic analysis of at least 59 cardiac arrhythmia and cardiomyopathy genes in 113 SADS cases. The investigators found 36 clinically relevant cardiac gene mutations in 31 of 113 SADS cases (27%) with only 10 variants (9%) in the four 'usual' molecular autopsy genes (*RYR2*, *KCNQ1*, *KCNH2*, and *SCN5A*). Interestingly, 20 rare variants were found when the major, minor, and rare cardiomyopathy genes were analysed. The one major caution however is the increased background genetic noise evident in these genes and the challenge of interpretation of rare variants which are often of uncertain significance (VUSs). This may lead to a relative over estimation of the true impact of these genes on the risk of SADS. Indeed, in the largest to date study, including 302 SADS victims, an NGS panel of 77 candidate genes and more stringent criteria in the variant classification, as indicated by the ACMG guidelines were used [75]. The authors identified a pathogenic or likely pathogenic variant in 13% of cases and the majority of variants were found in the major ion channelopathy genes. Although a small number of variants in the cardiomyopathy genes was also identified, the ratio of rare VUS to pathogenic or likely pathogenic cardiomyopathic variants was extremely unfavorable in this cohort.

Nonetheless these data tend to confirm the small proportion of inherited cardiomyopathy that is systematically reported in major series of familial clinical evaluation [79]. They also support the inclusion of genes associated with structural cardiac diseases when investigating SADS albeit with cautious interpretation of results.

How can this phenomenon be explained? Subtle structural and histological changes can be missed during autopsy, even in an expert setting, or may not have developed in the hearts of children. There is however mounting evidence from experimental and clinical studies of arrhythmogenesis in preclinical cases of cardiomyopathies without an overt phenotype of cardiac dilatation, hypertrophy or dysfunction. Diminished *PKP2* expression has been associated with reduced connexin 43 content and significant redistribution to the intracellular space [80], altered sodium current properties and impaired action potential propagation velocity [81]. These mechanisms are implicated in the structural instability of the cardiomyocyte junction and arrhythmogenic potential and may precede fibro-fatty replacement in ARVC. Connexin mislocalization resulting in significant alterations in conduction-repolarization kinetics before any overt structural changes, have also been reported due to mutations in desmoplakin [82]. The authors provided a hypothesis for sudden deaths in pre-clinical ARVC as associated with adrenergic drive, contending that different mechanisms are implicated in different disease phases. Additionally, a preclinical phase without cardiac expression but predominant arrhythmogenic features (ventricular or supra-ventricular arrhythmia or conduction defects) is now well recognised in the early phase of genetic diseases which eventually manifest with a dilated cardiomyopathy phenotype, such as lamin A/C and neuromuscular disorders [83].

27.4.3 Molecular Autopsy in Non-Diagnostic Structural Autopsy Positive SADS Cases

Hertz et al. [71] performed next generation sequencing in 52 cases of SCD victims in whom the autopsy revealed non-diagnostic findings of structural disease such as isolated LVH, increased heart weight, mild dilation of one or more chambers, moderate to severe fibrosis and fatty replacements or scattered inflammatory foci in the myocardium. In total, 28 (54%) individuals had hypertrophy, either isolated or with fibrosis and/or fatty infiltration. They compared the findings with 20 cases of SCD in which the autopsy was diagnostic for ARVC and HCM. Potentially pathogenic mutations were equally distributed in cardiomyopathy (47%) and channelopathy (53%) associated genes. Variants in ion channel genes with likely functional effects were found in 8 cases with idiopathic fibrosis, fibro-fatty infiltration and/or hypertrophy. These findings are in agreement with a previous clinical study by Papadakis et al. that compared clinical yields from familial evaluation between 163 SADS victims and 41 victims with post-mortem structural findings of uncertain significance and reported similar percentages of inherited cardiac disease in the two groups. Ion channel disease such as LQTS and BrS were detected in these cases. Remarkably, an arrhythmia syndrome was identified in almost 50% of families of the 19 SCD cases where idiopathic LVH or myocardial fibrosis was reported at postmortem [40].

Although it is plausible to hypothesise that non-specific structural change could represent an innocent bystander not implicated in the pathogenesis of SCD, these data highlight the complexity and diversity in the phenotypic spectrum of inherited cardiac disease. Current evidence suggests that a small proportion of channelopathies can also exhibit structural changes; albeit predominantly subtle and easily missed during autopsy. Specific *RYR2* variants have been reported in patients with isolated fatty infiltration of the right ventricular apex [63] and even in individuals exhibiting an ARVC phenotype [84]. Detailed morphometric analysis for post-mortem myocardial collagen identified epicardial surface and interstitial fibrosis in the right ventricular outflow tract of male SADS victims in families with BrS [85]. A DCM phenotype with cardiac dilatation and dysfunction is well recognized in the spectrum of *SCN5A* mutations [86], further enhancing the hypothesis that ion channels genes can be implicated in cardiomyopathies.

Moreover, structural cardiac disorders have been associated with higher risk of SCD in patients with channelopathies. Coronary artery disease is recognized as an independent risk factor in LQTS patients [87], whereas case studies in Japanese patients [88] have reported a possible contribution of myocardial ischemia in the pathogenesis of the characteristic Brugada electrocardiographic changes.

27.4.4 Mode of Death and Yield of the Molecular Autopsy

Molecular autopsy in cases of SCD related to specific triggers has been reported to associate with a higher frequency of positive molecular autopsy findings. Tester et al. [89] found cardiac ion channel mutations (*KCNH2*, *RYR2*) in nearly 30% of victims with a swimming-related drowning. Anderson et al. reported a pathogenic mutation detection rate of 44% in victims with an exercise-related sudden death, using direct DNA sequencing (*KCNQ1*, *KCNH2*, and *SCN5A*) initially, followed by a 100-gene panel extracted by whole exome sequencing [70]. The overall yield was significantly higher among 1–10 year olds than those 11–19 years of age. Remarkably, only 5 of the 100 interrogated sudden death genes hosted a pathogenic mutation in their cohort. Comprehensive personal and family history with documentation of the circumstances of death may therefore guide the following post-mortem genetic testing and may improve the yields of causative gene defects.

27.4.5 Genetic and Genomic Pitfalls

WES studies have led to the identification of increasing numbers of VUS, whose role in the pathogenesis of SADS remains to be understood. In silico tools and amino acid conservation measures are unreliable as sole evidence of pathogenicity of a variant [30]. Clinical phenotype in surviving genetically affected family members, demonstration of a de novo event by analysis of unaffected parents and/or evidence of a significant functional effect in a model system could provide more solid evidence in favour of pathogenicity. Indeed, these parameters are included in current guidelines for variant interpretation by the American College of Medical Genetics [38]. Given the absence of any phenotype in the proband victims, small family sizes and the variable penetrance of inherited arrhythmias and cardiomyopathies, family co-segregation studies and phenotype-genotype correlations are usually hard to determine. Furthermore, functional studies are costly and not always feasible to be performed in the clinical setting. Additionally, evidence of functional significance of genetic variant in model systems may not translate directly into clinically relevant phenotypes and thus may not be of clinical importance.

For example, rare variants have been identified in one of the three major LQTS-susceptibility genes (*KCNQ1*, *KCNH2*, or *SCN5A*) in 4% of healthy white and 6–8% of healthy black individuals [90]. Moreover, Refsgaard et al. recently demonstrated that a large proportion of 33 variants previously associated with LQTS are very unlikely to be monogenic causes of LQTS and of them, four variants (*KCNH2* P347S; *SCN5A*: S216L, V1951L; and *CAV3* T78M) were identified in 3% of a control population [91]. Another Danish study [92] also reported a higher than anticipated frequency of cardiomyopathy associated variants in the general population.

Genetic studies are also expected to provide further insights into the role of common variants that have been associated with arrhythmic risk and SCD [93–95]. These may be prevalent variably in different ethnic groups and may modulate the clinical phenotype manifested by patients with inherited arrhythmia syndromes

[96]. Over-presentation or under-presentation of these polymorphisms in SADS cohorts could imply increased susceptibility to sudden death. Doolan et al. [62] identified the *SCN5A* S1103Y polymorphism, with an expected heterozygote frequency of 13% among healthy black controls and functional effects, in 33% of black and in 17% of Hispanic SADS victims. The drug-induced LQTS associated D85N-*KCNE1* polymorphism was identified in 5 of 154 (3.2%, all male) white unexplained sudden death patients compared with the expected prevalence of 1.0% in the general white population. Tester et al. [37] reported a significant association of sleep-related deaths in otherwise pathogenic mutation–negative SADS victims with functional polymorphisms in *SCN5A* (S216L, S1103Y, R1193Q, V1951L, F2004L, and P2006A). Huang et al. reported a significantly higher frequency of two polymorphisms in the nitric oxide synthase gene (NOS1AP) in a Chinese population of SADS victims [97].

It is justifiable therefore to hypothesise that a spectrum of genomic variation ranging from common genetic modifiers and potentially pathogenic mutations impacts upon SADS risk. These variants need to be interpreted with caution given the dramatic consequences of potential "false-positive results". Further analysis of intronic and untranslated regions of genes associated with SADS, currently largely unexplored, should provide information on other potential genetic interactions.

27.4.6 The role of the Molecular Autopsy: Expanding and Evolving

Current international consensus statements [29, 77] recommend a comprehensive or targeted (*RYR2*, *KCNQ1*, *KCNH2*, and *SCN5A*) ion channel genetic testing especially in the presence of highly specific indicators of a clinical diagnosis of LQTS or CPVT such as emotional stress, acoustic trigger or drowning in the circumstances of death (class IIA recommendation). In total, molecular autopsy has been reported in over 800 SADS cases so far, with a reported yield of 0–29% (Table 27.4). Mutations in the main ion channel genes implicated in LQTS and CPVT have been identified in up to 25% of the SADS victims although the actual yields seem lower in population based studies and stringency of variant calling. Although yields of rare variants are higher when including other genes, clear pathogenic variants are relatively rare.

Thus the molecular autopsy, especially in the WES era, has become a potent tool for investigating the genetic basis of SADS. In the future it may identify novel loci and genes involved in arrhythmogenesis and thus provide critical insights in the pathogenesis of SCD. Large-scale prospective population studies involving genotype–phenotype correlation and analysing genomic data are necessary to improve understanding of the complex and diverse aetiology of sudden arrhythmic death and the role of common and rare variation in cardiomyopathy and other 'minor' channelopathy genes. A multidisciplinary approach, involving expert cardiac pathology, thorough and extend cardiac evaluation of SADS relatives in specialist centres and molecular autopsy with close cooperation of forensic pathologists, clinical genetics, and cardiologists is indispensable in the appropriate clinical evaluation and counselling of those left behind.

Learning and Key Points

- A cardiac autopsy should be performed in every victim of unexpected sudden death. Blood and/or suitable tissues should be stored during the autopsy for subsequent genetic analysis when a cause of death is not identified or suspected to be heritable.
- Expert cardiac pathology is indispensable in the assessment of SADS and can differentiate pathological from normal findings.
- Autopsy findings of uncertain significance such as idiopathic fibrosis or idiopathic left ventricular hypertrophy should be interpreted accurately and treated as SADS.
- Systematic and comprehensive cardiological evaluation for surviving first-degree relatives is imperative in determining the cause of death, in guiding the genetic investigation in the family and in providing co-segregation information for appropriate genotype-phenotype correlations.
- Molecular autopsy is a complementary diagnostic tool providing useful genetic information regarding the pathogenesis of SADS. Cautious interpretation of genetic variants of unknown significance is critical.

References

1. Myerburg RJ. Sudden cardiac death: exploring the limits of our knowledge. J Cardiovasc Electrophysiol. 2001;12(3):369–81.
2. Murakoshi N, Aonuma K. Epidemiology of arrhythmias and sudden cardiac death in Asia. Circ J. 2013;77:2419–31.
3. Chugh SS, Jui J, et al. Current burden of sudden cardiac death: multiple source surveillance versus retrospective death certificate-based review in a large U.S. community. J Am Coll Cardiol. 2004a;44(6):1268–75.
4. Zipes DP, Wellens HJ. Sudden cardiac death. Circulation. 1998;98(21):2334–51.
5. Molander N. Sudden natural death in later childhood and adolescence. Arch Dis Child. 1982;57(8):572–6.
6. Neuspiel DR, Kuller LH. Sudden and unexpected natural death in childhood and adolescence. JAMA. 1985;254(10):1321–5.
7. Anderson RE, et al. A population-based autopsy study of sudden, unexpected deaths from natural causes among persons 5 to 39 years old during a 12-year period. Hum Pathol. 1994;25(12):1332–40.
8. Shen WK, et al. Sudden unexpected nontraumatic death in 54 young adults: a 30-year population-based study. Am J Cardiol. 1995;76(3):148–52.
9. Maron BJ, Gohman TE, Aeppli D. Prevalence of sudden cardiac death during competitive sports activities in Minnesota High School athletes. J Am Coll Cardiol. 1998;32(7):1881–4.
10. Chugh SS, Kelly KL, Titus JL. Sudden cardiac death with apparently normal heart. Circulation. 2000;102(6):649–54.
11. Corrado D, Basso C, Thiene G. Sudden cardiac death in young people with apparently normal heart. Cardiovasc Res. 2001;50(2):399–408.

12. Wisten A, et al. Sudden cardiac death in 15-35-year olds in Sweden during 1992-99. J Intern Med. 2002;252(6):529–36.
13. Morentin B, Suárez-Mier MP, Aguilera B. Sudden unexplained death among persons 1–35 years old. Forensic Sci Int. 2003;135(3):213–7.
14. Corrado D, et al. Does sports activity enhance the risk of sudden death in adolescents and young adults? J Am Coll Cardiol. 2003;42(11):1959–63.
15. Eckart RE, et al. Sudden death in young adults: a 25-year review of autopsies in military recruits. Ann Intern Med. 2004;141(11):829–34.
16. Doolan A, Langlois N, Semsarian C. Causes of sudden cardiac death in young Australians. Med J Aust. 2004;180(3):110–2.
17. Puranik R, et al. Sudden death in the young. Heart Rhythm. 2005;2(12):1277–82.
18. Fabre A, Sheppard MN. Sudden adult death syndrome and other non-ischaemic causes of sudden cardiac death. Heart. 2006;92(3):316–20.
19. Papadakis M, et al. The magnitude of sudden cardiac death in the young: a death certificate-based review in England and Wales. Europace. 2009;11(10):1353–8.
20. Chugh SS, et al. Population-based analysis of sudden death in children: the Oregon Sudden Unexpected Death Study. Heart Rhythm. 2009;6(11):1618–22.
21. Winkel BG, et al. Nationwide study of sudden cardiac death in persons aged 1–35 years. Eur Heart J. 2011;32(8):983–90.
22. Eckart RE, et al. Sudden death in young adults: an autopsy-based series of a population undergoing active surveillance. J Am Coll Cardiol. 2011;58(12):1254–61.
23. Margey R, et al. Sudden cardiac death in 14- to 35-year olds in Ireland from 2005 to 2007: a retrospective registry. Europace. 2011;13(10):1411–8.
24. Pilmer CM, et al. Scope and nature of sudden cardiac death before age 40 in Ontario: a report from the Cardiac Death Advisory Committee of the Office of the Chief Coroner. Heart Rhythm. 2013;10(4):517–23.
25. Harmon KG, et al. Pathogeneses of sudden cardiac death in national collegiate athletic association athletes. Circ Arrhythm Electrophysiol. 2014;7(2):198–204.
26. Finocchiaro G, et al. Etiology of sudden death in sports: insights from a United Kingdom regional registry. J Am Coll Cardiol. 2016;67(18):2108–15.
27. Anastasakis A, et al. Sudden unexplained death in the young: epidemiology, aetiology and value of the clinically guided genetic screening. Europace. 2017. https://doi.org/10.1093/europace/euw362. [Epub ahead of print].
28. Bagnall RD, et al. A prospective study of sudden cardiac death among children and young adults. N Engl J Med. 2016;374(25):2441–52.
29. Priori SG, et al. HRS/EHRA/APHRS expert consensus statement on the diagnosis and management of patients with inherited primary arrhythmia syndromes. Heart Rhythm. 2013;10(12):1932–63.
30. Miles CJ, Behr ER. The role of genetic testing in unexplained sudden death. Trans Res. 2015;168:59–73.
31. Sheppard MN, Steriotis AK, Sharma S. Letter by Sheppard et al regarding article, "Arrhythmic mitral valve prolapse and sudden cardiac death". Circulation. 2016;133(13):e458.
32. Maron BJ, et al. Demographics and epidemiology of sudden deaths in young competitive athletes: from the United States National Registry. Am J Med. 2016;129(11):1170–7.
33. Pelliccia A, Zipes DP, Maron BJ. Bethesda Conference #36 and the European Society of Cardiology Consensus Recommendations revisited a comparison of U.S. and European criteria for eligibility and disqualification of competitive athletes with cardiovascular abnormalities. J Am Coll Cardiol. 2008;52(24):1990–6.
34. Behr E, et al. Cardiological assessment of first-degree relatives in sudden arrhythmic death syndrome. Lancet (London, England). 2003;362(9394):1457–9.
35. Behr ER, et al. Sudden arrhythmic death syndrome: a national survey of sudden unexplained cardiac death. Heart. 2007;93(5):601–5.
36. Tan HL, et al. Sudden unexplained death: heritability and diagnostic yield of cardiological and genetic examination in surviving relatives. Circulation. 2005;112(2):207–13.

37. Tester DJ, et al. Cardiac channel molecular autopsy: insights from 173 consecutive cases of autopsy-negative sudden unexplained death referred for postmortem genetic testing. Mayo Clin Proc. 2012;87(6):524–39.
38. Richards S, et al. Standards and guidelines for the interpretation of sequence variants: a joint consensus recommendation of the American College of Medical Genetics and Genomics and the Association for Molecular Pathology. Genet Med. 2015;17(5):405–24.
39. Hertz CL, et al. Next-generation sequencing of 34 genes in sudden unexplained death victims in forensics and in patients with channelopathic cardiac diseases. Int J Legal Med. 2015;129(4):793–800.
40. Papadakis M, et al. Sudden cardiac death with autopsy findings of uncertain significance: potential for erroneous interpretation. Circ Arrhythm Electrophysiol. 2013;6(3):588–96.
41. Sheppard MN. Aetiology of sudden cardiac death in sport: a histopathologist's perspective. Br J Sports Med. 2012;46(Suppl 1):i15–21.
42. de Noronha SV, et al. The importance of specialist cardiac histopathological examination in the investigation of young sudden cardiac deaths. Europace. 2014;16(6):899–907.
43. Basso C, et al. Guidelines for autopsy investigation of sudden cardiac death. Virchows Arch. 2008;452(1):11–8.
44. Kim S-H, et al. Circadian and seasonal variations of ventricular tachyarrhythmias in patients with early repolarization syndrome and Brugada syndrome: analysis of patients with implantable cardioverter defibrillator. J Cardiovasc Electrophysiol. 2012;23(7):757–63.
45. Takigawa M, et al. Seasonal and circadian distributions of ventricular fibrillation in patients with Brugada syndrome. Heart Rhythm. 2008;5(11):1523–7.
46. Yasue H, et al. Circadian variation of exercise capacity in patients with Prinzmetal's variant angina: role of exercise-induced coronary arterial spasm. Circulation. 1979;59(5):938–48.
47. Reddy PR, et al. Physical activity as a trigger of sudden cardiac arrest: the Oregon Sudden Unexpected Death Study. Int J Cardiol. 2009;131(3):345–9.
48. Mellor G, et al. Clinical characteristics and circumstances of death in the sudden arrhythmic death syndrome. Circ Arrhythm Electrophysiol. 2014;7(6):1078–83.
49. Pappone C, et al. Risk of malignant arrhythmias in initially symptomatic patients with Wolff-Parkinson-White syndrome: results of a prospective long-term electrophysiological follow-up study. Circulation. 2012;125(5):661–8.
50. Sharma S, Papadakis M. Improved survival rates from commotio cordis: a case for automatic external defibrillator provision during high-risk sports. Heart Rhythm. 2013;10(2):224–5.
51. Behr ER, et al. Sudden arrhythmic death syndrome: familial evaluation identifies inheritable heart disease in the majority of families. Eur Heart J. 2008;29(13):1670–80.
52. Caldwell J, et al. The clinical management of relatives of young sudden unexplained death victims; implantable defibrillators are rarely indicated. Heart. 2012;98(8):631–6.
53. Kumar S, et al. Familial cardiological and targeted genetic evaluation: low yield in sudden unexplained death and high yield in unexplained cardiac arrest syndromes. Heart Rhythm. 2013;10(11):1653–60.
54. Mcgorrian C, et al. Family-based cardiac screening in relatives of victims of sudden arrhythmic death syndrome. Europace. 2013;15(7):1050–8.
55. Van Der Werf C, et al. Diagnostic yield in sudden unexplained death and aborted cardiac arrest in the young: the experience of a tertiary referral center in The Netherlands. Heart Rhythm. 2010;7(10):1383–9.
56. Rapezzi C, et al. Diagnostic work-up in cardiomyopathies: bridging the gap between clinical phenotypes and final diagnosis. A position statement from the ESC Working Group on Myocardial and Pericardial Diseases. Eur Heart J. 2013;34(19):1448–58.
57. Charron P, et al. Genetic counselling and testing in cardiomyopathies: a position statement of the European Society of Cardiology Working Group on Myocardial and Pericardial Diseases. Eur Heart J. 2010;31(22):2715–28.
58. Ackerman MJ, et al. Molecular diagnosis of the inherited long-QT syndrome in a woman who died after near-drowning. N Engl J Med. 1999;341(15):1121–5.
59. Di Paolo M, et al. Postmortem molecular analysis in victims of sudden unexplained death. Am J Forensic Med Pathol. 2004;25(2):182–4.

60. Chugh SS, Senashova O, et al. Postmortem molecular screening in unexplained sudden death. J Am Coll Cardiol. 2004b;43(9):1625–9.
61. Creighton W, et al. Identification of novel missense mutations of cardiac ryanodine receptor gene in exercise-induced sudden death at autopsy. J Mol Diagn. 2006;8(1):62–7.
62. Doolan A, et al. Postmortem molecular analysis of KCNQ1 and SCN5A genes in sudden unexplained death in young Australians. Int J Cardiol. 2008;127(1):138–41.
63. Nishio H, Iwata M, Suzuki K. Postmortem molecular screening for cardiac ryanodine receptor type 2 mutations in sudden unexplained death: R420W mutated case with characteristics of status thymico-lymphatics. Circ J. 2006;70(11):1402–6.
64. Gladding PAA, et al. Posthumous diagnosis of long QT syndrome from neonatal screening cards. Heart Rhythm. 2010;7(4):481–6.
65. Skinner JR, et al. Prospective, population-based long QT molecular autopsy study of postmortem negative sudden death in 1 to 40 year olds. Heart Rhythm. 2011;8(3):412–9.
66. Winkel BG, et al. The prevalence of mutations in KCNQ1, KCNH2, and SCN5A in an unselected national cohort of young sudden unexplained death cases. J Cardiovasc Electrophysiol. 2012;23(10):1092–8.
67. Larsen MK, et al. Postmortem genetic testing of the ryanodine receptor 2 (RYR2) gene in a cohort of sudden unexplained death cases. Int J Legal Med. 2013;127(1):139–44.
68. Bagnall RD, et al. Exome analysis–based molecular autopsy in cases of sudden unexplained death in the young. Heart Rhythm. 2014;11(4):655–62.
69. Nunn LML, et al. Diagnostic yield of molecular autopsy in patients with sudden arrhythmic death syndrome using targeted exome sequencing. Europace. 2015;93(7422):655–62.
70. Anderson JH, et al. Whole exome molecular autopsy following exertion-related sudden unexplained death in the young. Circ Cardiovasc Genet. 2016;9(3):259–65.
71. Hertz CL, et al. Next-generation sequencing of 100 candidate genes in young victims of suspected sudden cardiac death with structural abnormalities of the heart. Int J Legal Med. 2016;130(1):91–102.
72. Narula N, et al. Post-mortem whole exome sequencing with gene-specific analysis for autopsy-negative sudden unexplained death in the young: a case series. Pediatr Cardiol. 2015;36(4):768–78.
73. Zhang M, et al. PKP2 mutations in sudden death from arrhythmogenic right ventricular cardiomyopathy (ARVC) and sudden unexpected death with negative autopsy (SUDNA). Circ J. 2012;76(1):189–94.
74. Huang L, et al. Molecular autopsy of desmosomal protein plakophilin-2 in sudden unexplained nocturnal death syndrome. J Forensic Sci. 2016;61(3):687–91.
75. Lahrouchi N, et al. Utility of post-mortem genetic testing in cases of sudden arrhythmic death syndrome. J Am Coll Cardiol. 2017;69(17):2134–45.
76. Carturan E, et al. Postmortem genetic testing for conventional autopsy-negative sudden unexplained death: An evaluation of different DNA extraction protocols and the feasibility of mutational analysis from archival paraffin-embedded heart tissue. Am J Clin Pathol. 2008;129(3):391–7.
77. Ackerman MJ, et al. HRS/EHRA expert consensus statement on the state of genetic testing for the channelopathies and cardiomyopathies: this document was developed as a partnership between the Heart Rhythm Society (HRS) and the European Heart Rhythm Association (EHRA). Europace. 2011;13(8):1077–109.
78. Loporcaro CG, et al. Confirmation of cause and manner of death via a comprehensive cardiac autopsy including whole exome next-generation sequencing. Arch Pathol Lab Med. 2014;138(8):1083–9.
79. Raju H, Behr ER. Unexplained sudden death, focussing on genetics and family phenotyping. Curr Opin Cardiol. 2013;28(1):19–25.
80. Oxford EM, et al. Connexin43 remodeling caused by inhibition of plakophilin-2 expression in cardiac cells. Circ Res. 2007;101(7):703–11.
81. Sato PY, et al. Loss of plakophilin-2 expression leads to decreased sodium current and slower conduction velocity in cultured cardiac myocytes. Circ Res. 2009;105(6):523–6.

82. Gomes J, et al. Electrophysiological abnormalities precede overt structural changes in arrhythmogenic right ventricular cardiomyopathy due to mutations in desmoplakin-A combined murine and human study. Eur Heart J. 2012;33(15):1942–53.
83. Pinto YM, et al. Proposal for a revised definition of dilated cardiomyopathy, hypokinetic non-dilated cardiomyopathy, and its implications for clinical practice: a position statement of the ESC working group on myocardial and pericardial diseases. Eur Heart J. 2016;37(23):1850–8.
84. Tiso N. Identification of mutations in the cardiac ryanodine receptor gene in families affected with arrhythmogenic right ventricular cardiomyopathy type 2 (ARVD2). Hum Mol Genet. 2001;10(3):189–94.
85. Nademanee K, et al. Fibrosis, connexin-43, and conduction abnormalities in the brugada syndrome. J Am Coll Cardiol. 2015;66(18):1976–86.
86. McNair WP, et al. SCN5A mutations associate with arrhythmic dilated cardiomyopathy and commonly localize to the voltage-sensing mechanism. J Am Coll Cardiol. 2011;57(21):2160–8.
87. Sze E, et al. Long QT syndrome in patients over 40 years of age: increased risk for LQTS-related cardiac events in patients with coronary disease. Ann Noninvasive Electrocardiol. 2008;13(4):327–31.
88. Yamaki M, et al. Possible contribution of ischemia of the conus branch to induction or augmentation of Brugada type electrocardiographic changes in patients with coronary artery disease. Int Heart J. 2010;51(1):68–71.
89. Tester DJ, et al. Unexplained drownings and the cardiac channelopathies: a molecular autopsy series. Mayo Clin Proc. 2011;86(10):941–7.
90. Kapa S, et al. Genetic testing for long-qt syndrome: distinguishing pathogenic mutations from benign variants. Circulation. 2009;120(18):1752–60.
91. Refsgaard L, et al. High prevalence of genetic variants previously associated with LQT syndrome in new exome data. Eur J Hum Genet. 2012;20(8):905–8.
92. Andreasen C, et al. New population-based exome data are questioning the pathogenicity of previously cardiomyopathy-associated genetic variants. Eur J Hum Genet. 2013;21(9):918–28.
93. Ackerman MJ, et al. Spectrum and prevalence of cardiac sodium channel variants among black, white, Asian, and Hispanic individuals: implications for arrhythmogenic susceptibility and Brugada/long QT syndrome genetic testing. Heart Rhythm. 2004;1(5):600–7.
94. Bezzina CR, et al. Common sodium channel promoter haplotype in asian subjects underlies variability in cardiac conduction. Circulation. 2006;113(3):338–44.
95. Splawski I, et al. Variant of SCN5A sodium channel implicated in risk of cardiac arrhythmia. Science (New York, NY). 2002;297(5585):1333–6.
96. Priori SG, Napolitano C. Molecular underpinning of 'good luck'. Circulation. 2006;114(5):360–2.
97. Huang J, et al. Genetic variants in KCNE1, KCNQ1, and NOS1AP in sudden unexplained death during daily activities in Chinese Han population. J Forensic Sci. 2015;60(2):351–6.

Specific Issues in Clinical Genetics and Genetic Counselling Practices Related to Inherited Cardiovascular Conditions

28

Angus Clarke and Siv Fokstuen

Abstract

The genetically determined cardiomyopathies and arrhythmias are usually inherited as autosomal dominant traits with a wide range of inter- and intra-familial clinical variability concerning age at onset, penetrance, degree of symptoms and risk of cardiac death. In addition they are all characterized by extensive genetic and allelic heterogeneity. It has become obvious that molecular testing in clinical practice has an important impact on the management of patients and their families. With the introduction of high throughput sequencing (HTS) platforms, which allow simultaneous screening of a large number of genes, the time and the cost of DNA sequencing has been greatly reduced. Molecular testing of inherited cardiac disorders is now performed routinely in diagnostic genetics laboratories.

Keywords

Cardiomyopathy • Long QT • Uncertainty • Incidental findings • Variant(s) of uncertain significance (VUS or VOUS) • Communication • Ethics • Counselling

A. Clarke (✉)
All Wales Medical Genetics Service, University Hospital of Wales, Cardiff, Wales, UK

Cardiff University School of Medicine, Institute of Medical Genetics, Cardiff, Wales, UK
e-mail: clarkeaj@cf.ac.uk

S. Fokstuen
Department of Genetic Medicine and Laboratories, University Hospitals of Geneva, Geneva, Switzerland
e-mail: Siv.Fokstuen@unige.ch

D. Kumar, P. Elliott (eds.), *Cardiovascular Genetics and Genomics*,
https://doi.org/10.1007/978-3-319-66114-8_28

28.1 Introduction

The genetically determined cardiomyopathies and arrhythmias are usually inherited as autosomal dominant traits with a wide range of inter- and intra-familial clinical variability concerning age at onset, penetrance, degree of symptoms and risk of cardiac death. In addition they are all characterized by extensive genetic and allelic heterogeneity. It has become obvious that molecular testing in clinical practice has an important impact on the management of patients and their families. With the introduction of high throughput sequencing (HTS) platforms, which allow simultaneous screening of a large number of genes, the time and the cost of DNA sequencing has been greatly reduced. Molecular testing of inherited cardiac disorders is now performed routinely in diagnostic genetics laboratories.

HTS technology can be used in different ways. Many diagnostic laboratories offer "targeted gene panels", in which there is a focus on a set of genes known to be associated with specific cardiac disorders. Others provide whole exome sequencing (WES) which covers almost all protein-coding sequences or even whole genome sequencing (WGS) that includes nearly all non-coding sequences as well. Targeted gene panels have been shown to generate results identical to Sanger sequencing and have the advantage of being faster and cheaper with a better coverage and sensitivity than WES and WGS [1, 2]. Although WES and WGS make it possible to perform an unbiased search for mutations in all human genes, this approach may be less appropriate for routine diagnostic purposes as not every part of the coding sequence is sufficiently covered, which may lead to false negative results. In addition, issues related to management of the huge amount of data generated by WES and especially by WGS remain to be solved before these approaches are suitable for routine use in a clinical setting [3]. In this context, special attention also has to be paid to incidental findings, which are results that are not related to the indication for ordering the investigation but that may nonetheless be of medical value or utility to the ordering physician and the patient.

Given both the complexity of the genetics of the inherited cardiac disorders and the new challenges of HTS technologies, highly sensitive and competent genetic counselling, including the provision of information and support for decision making to enable consent, are essential components of the genetic testing process [4–6]. In this chapter we will highlight some of the challenges encountered in clinical practice.

28.2 Clinical Cardiac Genetics

Clinical cardiac genetics has established itself as the joint activity of two subspecialties, i.e., of cardiologists focusing on inherited cardiac disorders, and clinical geneticists and genetic counsellors working with families affected by cardiac conditions. The joint working of these two groups can be to the great benefit of patients and families, especially where they coordinate their activities and come together to discuss cases. Occasionally, when an MDT clinic has been established, they may see patients jointly.

Two features of inherited cardiac disorders create the "perfect storm" for difficult clinical and family scenarios. First, some of these disorders can result in sudden cardiac death at a young age, so that the distress—the sadness caused by these deaths, and the fear that more deaths may occur—can be especially marked. The risk of further deaths can hang over an entire extended family. Secondly, while genetic testing for variants in genes that contribute to inherited cardiac disorders is available, the interpretation of test results can be especially difficult and the reinterpretation of previously reported results has proven necessary rather too often for complacency about the process and worth of testing. More will be said about both these aspects of clinical cardiac genetics.

In this chapter, we examine some of the social and ethical difficulties that arise in relation to inherited cardiac disorders from a perspective informed by what has been learned assessing patients and managing families with these conditions and other genetic disorders.

28.3 The Inevitability of Uncertainty

One of the most difficult challenges in clinical cardiac genetics is how to manage the disclosure and follow-up of a variant of uncertain significance (VUS), especially in families with a history of sudden cardiac death (SCD). As most laboratories tend to screen for many genes, the probability of identifying a VUS is quite high [7]. Although there are no published European guidelines, many laboratories report the VUS, especially if they are found in genes well-established as causing disease. Depending upon the details of the consent provided in advance of testing by the patient, the clinical geneticist or cardiologist may or may not disclose the VUS. A problem may arise, if the doctor who ordered the molecular test did not inform the patient properly before testing about the range of different possible results. In these situations, the patient may feel disappointed or even disturbed. If the patient was correctly informed beforehand, he/she will usually not be so surprised but may still be disappointed. As some patients consent to molecular testing specifically to enable their relatives and especially their children to have predictive testing, they may be quite disappointed, as there is a general consensus that a VUS should not be used for predictive testing.

In families with several affected persons, cosegregation analysis may provide strong evidence for causation. However, in case of a de novo VUS in a sporadic case, the uncertainty remains. Even in the case of an inherited VUS carried by a clinically unaffected parent, the uncertainty remains, as most inherited cardiac disorders and especially the cardiomyopathies show incomplete penetrance and/or a late age of onset of symptoms. Thus, the identification of a VUS changes nothing in the clinical follow-up of the affected patient and of his/her relatives, as they have to continue the regular cardiac monitoring. It is however important to report the VUS to clinical databases like ClinVar in order to advance genetic knowledge. It is also important to interrogate the databases regularly, in case the VUS can be reassigned as more definitely pathgenic or benign. There are no guidlines about how often this should be done and the laboratories are not "obligated" to do so; however, if the interpretation of a variant has changed it is recommended to issue a new report to the referring physician, who should then inform the patient. The most efficient way to follow the development of knowledge of a VUS is probably to reevaluate the variants at the regular clinical follow-ups of the patient.

Even more challenging is the identification of a VUS in a gene which so far has not been associated with the cardiac phenotype of the patient, for instance a VUS in the *MYBPC3* gene in a young patient with clear long QT syndrome and normal echocardiography. Further discoveries about the variant may reveal that it finally represents a benign variant, or a definitely or likely pathogenic variant associated with cardiomyopathy, or finally that the spectrum of phenotypes associated with *MYBPC3* variants has enlarged and also includes long QT syndrome. As long as the situation has not been clarified, the patient will be monitored for his long QT syndrome and probably also by regular echocardiography for an eventual cardiomyopathy.

As the detection rate for a pathogenic or likely pathogenic variant varies a lot between the different inherited cardiomyopathies and arrhythmias, and as it does not exceed in the best scenario the rate of $\approx$80% (example reflecting the situation of long QT syndrome), the question of reviewing those families with a negative molecular test result has to be addressed. Although these situations are quite common, there are so far no guidelines on how to best manage them. The same approach may be valuable for the re-evaluation of the pathogenicity of other variants. Most laboratories transmit the responsibility to recontact the laboratory in 2–3 years time to the referring physician, and this advice may or may not be followed. In cardiogenetic expert centers where the cardiologist, clinical geneticist and molecular biologist work closely together, negative molecular results as well as previously reported variants are usually reviewed at the regular multidisciplinary clinical follow-up, which may be once a year. These families are therefore automatically "updated" concerning recent progress in knowledge of variant interpretation and/or concerning new genes which it may be useful to analyse. It is well known that severely affected patients, especially patients with severe hypertrophic cardiomyopathy, may carry more than one pathogenic variant. It is therefore important to address the question of screening in the extended families of those who have already had a clear result with "only" a single pathogenic variant identified. This option should especially be discussed when the molecular analysis has been performed a long time ago and with a restricted molecular testing approach (often a rather small gene panel). Therefore, for optimal counselling and clinical management of patients and their families, it is essential to work as a team, ideally in expert centers. This facilitates multidisciplinary case discussion and the constant review of the indication for genetic testing, counselling strategies and interpretation of sequencing results.

The simultaneous molecular analysis of all known genes responsible for the different subtypes of inherited cardiomyopathies and/or arrhythmias raises the possibility of identifying a class 4 or 5 variant in a gene which is not thought to be a good match for the clinical phenotype of the patient. This is illustrated by the following situation:

A young man, of 22 years, who had been diagnosed at the age of 16 years with left ventricular dilated cardiomyopathy, underwent molecular analysis for 65 genes responsible for all subtypes of inherited cardiomyopathies. His family history was unremarkable for cardiac problems. Both parents (the father 52 years old, the mother 51 years) and his younger sister had cardiac monitoring with normal echocardiography. We found a novel nonsense class 4 variant in the Desmoplakin gene (DSP), which has been thought usually to cause ARVD. However, some reports have shown that desmosomal genes may also be associated with DCM [8, 9]. This molecular result illustrates the well known heterogeneity and clinical overlap of cardiomyopathies which may surprise the cardiologist as well as the patient and his family. It is therefore very important to mention this phenomenon before molecular testing of large panels of cardiomyopathy and/or arrythmia genes. Usually, the cardiac phenotype is then re-evaluated and the diagnosis may need to be reconsidered, especially in young patients where the full cardiac phenotype may not yet be visible. Interestingly, *DSP* variants seem to be associated with left ventricular involvement in ARVD [10]. The patient did not wish that his parents, who both had normal cardiac monitoring, be tested for the same variant as he did not want them to feel guilty for his cardiac disease. After some time for reflection, the parents finally underwent predictive testing as they wished to know whether it would be important for them to inform other family members. The results showed that the father carried the same variant. Penetrance of mutations in *DSP* is generally no higher than 50%. Thus, it is not surprising that cardiac monitoring of the 52 year old father was normal and, fortunately, it is rather unusual to develop ARVD after 50 years of age. It is nervertheless not easy to cope with such a result. The healthy younger sister (20 years) now had a 50% risk of carrying the same variant. She quite quickly wished to know her *DSP* genotype which, again fortunately, was normal.

28.4 Family History and the Family Dimension

The understanding of "heart disease" in most families with an inherited cardiac disorder starts from the same point as in the rest of the population, with an awareness that heart disease is potentially fatal and that it can "run in families." In the more usual and familiar types of heart disease, especially coronary artery disease, there is often a recognition that individuals' own behaviors contribute to their health or their pattern of disease. Fieldwork in South Wales during the late 1980s revealed the widespread currency of ideas about the type of person who would be at risk of heart disease—the "coronary candidate"—existing alongside the contrary notions of luck, fate, destiny, and chaos [11, 12], which were reinforced by the observation of counter-examples of individuals whose state of health or disease contradicted the messages of health promotion campaigns. Such simultaneously held but essentially incompatible perspectives can become impregnable systems of belief, allowing adherents to account satisfactorily for any observed pattern of events without their beliefs about heart disease being challenged by cases of, for example, obese smokers living to a ripe old age, succumbing neither to coronary artery disease (CAD) nor to lung cancer. Subsequent work in Scotland has emphasized the extent to which gender has also long been seen within popular culture as relevant to the risk of heart disease, with men understood to be at higher risk [13].

Health professionals wish to make use of family history information to identify those at increased risk of serious health problems. If the genome sequence of the whole population were known from birth, and if this sequence information could be interpreted with confidence, then there might be little reason to gather family history information. However, in our present, imperfect state of knowledge, a significant family history of serious disease will often indicate those who are at increased risk of the same or a related disorder. In the field of cancer genetics, a family history of specific cancer types can provide a very useful way of identifying those most likely to benefit from surveillance for early signs of disease or, in some cases, primary disease prevention. It can indicate those at increased risk of disease, who are most likely to benefit from more detailed clincal assessment and genetic investigation. This can be understood as sifting out the individuals at high, essentially Mendelian, risk of disease from all the rest—those who have been affected through a combination of weaker contributing factors, including Gene-x-Environment interactions, whose relatives may be at slightly above average risk but not at high risk.

The family history information of relevance to cardiac disease includes not only information about relatives who suffered from easily recognised cardiac symptoms (e.g., angina, "heart attacks," or sudden cardiac death), but also those with stroke or with loss of consciousness (including a label of epileptic seizures) or primarily respiratory symptoms such as shortness of breath on exercise or at night. Research into the popular understanding of family history has shown that many lay (non-health professional) individuals think very differently from informed health professionals about "having a family history of heart disease." A family history may not be attributed any significance by the individual unless several close relatives have been affected, and the relevance may be discounted if the individual sees himself or herself as being different from the affected person/s in some crucial respect/s [14]. Most cardiac risk factors, such as obesity, hypercholesterolemia, or hypertension, may not lead to symptoms until a serious or fatal event occurs. The asymptomatic individuals may therefore regard themselves, comfortingly, as *not* being at increased risk, when professionals might prefer not to give such reassurance. Similar factors operate even for many with cardiac symptoms, who delay seeking medical attention or deny that the symptoms are cardiac. Inadequate access to services is another factor that can lead to a failure to access services in the context of unmet health needs, which can excerbate social inequities in health [15].

Enquiries into the family history of heart disease in primary health care can be awkward, with professionals not always feeling sufficiently confident to integrate the family history into the context of other risk factors [16]. Professionals in U.K. primary health care are more familiar with collecting and interpreting family history information concerning breast and bowel cancer, for which they have been referring patients appropriately for specialist genetic assessment for two decades [17]. Their confidence may improve in relation to heart disease as the cardiac family history comes to be recorded more frequently and as referral guidelines are developed and promulgated.

An additional practical problem that may arise within some jurisdictions is that of legal restrictions placed upon the collection and storage of information from individuals about their relatives, or at least the self-fulfilling assumption (on the part of health professionals) that such restrictions exist. Such data protection legislation has usually been motivated by a desire to allow individuals effective control over the information held about them by commercial or other organizations but may be unhelpful if applied too rigidly within the context of health care. If I believe that my Aunt Mabel is affected by a condition X or Y, and I pass that "information" to my physician, is that information mine (I am reporting my belief) or does it belong to my aunt (as the person about whom the belief is held)? Does the physician have an obligation to check the accuracy of the information? If the information is kept in my medical records and not linked to Mabel's, does that make a difference? There are clearly some tangled issues here that may require unscrambling [18]; these issues will become very much more complex as the feasibility of linking the electronic patient records of family members becomes greater [19]. Family histories of cancer can be checked quite readily within the United Kingdom (UK), without the need to obtain consent from multiple members of each family, because of the established system of cancer registries. Should similar systems be put in place for other disorders, including cardiac disease? Within countries where health care is organised through private systems, or multiple provider insurance-based systems, how readily is information pooled to the best advantage of all concerned?

There is another approach to these issues, which has the virtue of treating family situations equitably, whether or not the condition is one where specific information about the mutation in that family would be required for genetic testing to be most effective or at least most efficient. This is to distinguish between the fact of the genetic disease being present in the family and the precise nature of that family's mutation. Simply knowing that person X has disease Y is sufficient to make genetic testing available to all who want it in some contexts, but in other contexts it is necessary (or at least very helpful) to know the precise mutation. Knowing that one person has Huntington's disease (HD) or a chromosome translocation would usually be sufficient for family members to have testing, while knowing that a relative has Duchenne muscular dystrophy, cystic fibrosis, or a susceptibility to breast cancer may not be enough. The major Mendelian cardiac disorders are more complex than those other conditions, being genetically heterogeneous at the level both of the locus and of the mutation; it is therefore important in these diseases to identify the mutation in an affected individual before carrying out predictive testing on an unaffected relative. By treating as fully confidential the diagnosis in the affected individual, family members will only become aware of this if the patient chooses to release that information to them: it is the diagnosis that is confidential. Once that information is known in the family, it may be helpful to regard the mutational basis of the condition as information that is not an essentially personal item but rather belongs to the laboratory or the health care system, or perhaps to the family, but not solely to the single patient. On this understanding, knowledge of the gene locus and the precise mutation should be available for use by the laboratory to test other family members without specific consent from their affected relative [20].

In addition to these questions of information, there may be practical and/or legal restrictions upon access to DNA or tissue stored from deceased family members. The Human Tissue Act in England and Wales introduced systems for regulating access to banked DNA samples for genetic testing and to stored tissue that might be required for pathological analysis of any sort. This has placed a regulatory burden that is sometimes seen as unduly onerous, an obstacle to both research and clinical practice. The situation in other countries varies widely, even within Europe.

28.5 Molecular Genetic Diagnostics of Inherited Cardiac Disorders

Before considering some of the major inherited cardiac disorders individually, we will address some of the difficulties of interpretation of genetic variants found using Next Generation Sequencing (also known as High Throughput or Massively Parallel Sequencing). There are five principal categories of disease encountered in the cardiac genetics clinic:

1. The inherited cardiomyopathies (CMPs), especially hypertrophic cardiomyopathy (HCM) but also including dilated CMP (DCM), restricive CMPathy (RCM), left ventricular non-compaction cardiomyopathy (LVNC) and arrhythmogenic right ventricular dysplasia (ARVD).
2. The inherited dysrhythmias, including mainly the long QT syndromes, Brugada syndrome and more rarely catecholaminergic polymorphic ventricular tachycardia (CPVT) [164].
3. Congenital heart disease, as an isolated phenomenon or as part of a chromosomal or syndromic disorder. This sometimes requires life-long medical supervision. In most centres, specific consultations for the cardiac follow-up and assessment of adults with congenital heart malformations have been established. The adult cardiac phenotypes of some congenital disorders and the risk of recurrence in the children of affected individuals are both becoming clearer as survival into adult life improves. The cognitive limitations of some affected adults mean that both compliance with medical advice and consenting to procedures and interventions can generate problems in clinical practice.
4. The inherited connective tissue disorders, especially Marfan syndrome and other rare disorders of the thoracic aorta that lead to aneurysm, like Loeys–Dietz syndrome or the vascular type of Ehlers–Danlos syndrome, remain an important element in cardiovascular genetics. Continuing developments in drug therapy, imaging, and surgery require that affected individuals should have access to specialist cardiac assessment; local factors will determine whether this is best arranged through the cardiac genetics clinic or a separate, specialist cardiac service but the multiple medical, surgical, and psychological needs of those with Marfan syndrome mean that a purely cardiac clinic is not sufficient to meet their needs.
5. Coronary artery disease (CAD) and the familial forms of hypercholesterolaemia, which predispose to CAD [163, 165].

The disease contexts that cause most distress for families, anxiety for professionals and uncertainty for all concerned, are the inherited cardiac conditions that can lead to sudden cardiac death in young adults or even children. The large majority of sudden cardiac deaths in adults are caused by coronary artery disease (CAD) and in only about 4% of sudden unexplained cardiac deaths in the community is the heart structurally normal [21, 22]. Experience from a major referral centre in the United Kingdom [23] showed that almost 60% of the 453 hearts examined postmortem of individuals aged >15 years without atherosclerosis were structurally normal but that 23% showed features of cardiomyopathy or right ventricular dysplasia and >15% showed other definite pathologies. These studies highlight both the need for and the scarcity of the specialist cardiac pathology services, including histopathology, that are required for health services to deal appropriately with the surviving family members of young adults who have died suddenly and whose relatives may be at high risk of a similar fate.

Such accounts written by pathologists make poignant reading for clinicians who meet with the families of the deceased. A typical scenario would be the grieving young mother, whose husband has recently died without any warning—perhaps on the sports field—and who has two young children, both potentially at risk of serious cardiac pathology that could cause problems at any stage of life. She may find it difficult to communicate with her deceased husband's family, who are themselves also in shock, but whose cooperation may be necessary for the adequate assessment of any risk to the children. Without a firm diagnosis in the deceased, it is difficult for the cardiologist or clinical geneticist to deal satisfactorily with the family. A normal cardiac examination and ECG give little reassurance to the clinician in these circumstances even if it temporarily satisfies the family. The legal system in many countries is only interested to determine whether a death was natural or otherwise, and pursuing the investigation beyond that point can be expensive so the coroner may be unwilling to authorise additional expenditure. At least in England and Wales, the coroner is now able to arrange for the taking of tissue samples that can be stored and made available, perhaps years later, if the family chooses to look further into the cause of death.

It has become clear from several series of "molecular autopsies" that simple genetic investigations will identify the likely cause in about one third of cases of a sudden cardiac death in a child or young adult [24–26], or even of an infant [27]. This means that a likely or definitely pathogenic variant will be found in at least one gene in which mutations are already known to be implicated in sudden cardiac deaths.

While variants in many gene loci have been identified as pathogenic—causing a cardiomyopathy or a dysrhythmia, for example—there remains much uncertainty in the interpretation of sequence variants in these genes [4]. Many variants once thought to be definitely pathogenic have subsequently been found at levels in the population too high for them to be credible as causes, in isolation, of a transmissible, Mendelian cardiac disorder. This has especially been shown for long QT syndrome. Indeed, it is easy to over-interpret any departure from the 'standard' gene sequence. One consequence of this complexity, that makes it difficult to interpret the pathogenicity of a gene variant without very careful study, is to make clinicians cautious in the interpretation of exome analyes (or, *a fortiori*, whole genome sequencing) because they will uncover variants in "relevant" genes whose significance may be very difficult to determine.

If the proband in a family survives a near-fatal cardiac event, or presents with cardiac symptoms such as syncope, dyspnea, angina, or palpitations, the chance of attaining a clear diagnosis is much greater and the level of family distress will often be much less. It is then possible to approach the investigations more calmly and more efficiently. However, the former, more difficult circumstances, following a sudden cardiac death in a young adult, provide the most difficult cases both diagnostically and interactionally. It is these cases that set the ethos of the developing subspecialty.

28.6 Patient Experiences

In this and the following sections, we include some comments made by patients and families about their experiences of the cardiac genetics service.

A 41-year-old lady who had heart transplantation at the age of 32 years because of early onset (2 years) severe familial HCM (her father died from heart failure at the age of 43 years) said:

> "My mother did her best but it was very difficult and at the time nobody offered psychological support for the family, which really should have been seen as necessary. I remember it was so hard to see my mum suffering that I forbade her to come to the hospital, which of course was a catastrophe for her but for me it was survival. This was really bad… you know how crucially important the emotional side is with the heart and the problem is different for the patient, the mother, and the healthy brothers and sisters. I think that something has to be done here."

Preparing an individual to think through decisions about testing and perhaps having to confront an adverse result can be demanding on staff—on their time and their emotional energy—as can be the provision of intensive emotional support after a result [28]. Cardiologists are necessarily involved very closely in these clinics but do not usually have the time or the full set of knowledge and skills to conduct these clinics without genetics support [29]. They are also less familiar with managing those at risk but without symptoms, who are entirely "well".

A mother who lost her 17-year-old son from sudden cardiac death caused by ARVD said:

> "It is true that a team with a cardiologist, a geneticist, and a psychiatrist is ideal. When we asked questions of our cardiologist about genetics he could not answer. When he then had your [clinical genetics] letter he was very grateful and said that then he knew something. So it is true that a multidisciplinary approach is essential.
>
> I think the most important thing is to take time. You took the time. We did not have the impression of being here for only half an hour; what can you say in half an hour? You took the time to discuss with us, to listen to us, it's true that sometimes it was very long but it is

really very important. It was especially important when the question arose of predictive testing in our son. It was not only to do the blood sampling but he had to ask himself, 'What am I going to do with this, what does it mean, what will be the consequences?' and then he has the choice."

It is also possible for cardiac-trained nurses to participate in these clinics alongside and complementing the genetic counsellors [30].

Another issue to be considered is insurance, especially the potential consequences for obtaining life and health insurance. The possibility of adverse consequences for obtaining insurance is likely to be at least as difficult a problem in cardiac genetics as it has become in relation to HD and familial cancers [31, 32].

28.7 Specific Clinical Considerations

In this section specific issues in major clinical groups of inherited cardiac diseases are examined.

28.7.1 Inherited Cardiomyopathies

The European Society of Cardiology adopted a clinically oriented classification of cardiomyopathies (CMs) into specific morphological and functional phenotypes with a subclassification into familial and nonfamilial forms (Fig. 28.1; [33]). The most common CM in clinical practice is HCM with a prevalence of 1 in 500, a prevalence similar to familial hypercholesterolemia (FH). Dilated cardiomyopathies (DCM) are important but less frequent and less frequently inherited. Some 25–50% of DCM patients in Western populations have evidence for familial disease with predominantly autosomal dominant inheritance [34] and the counselling issues

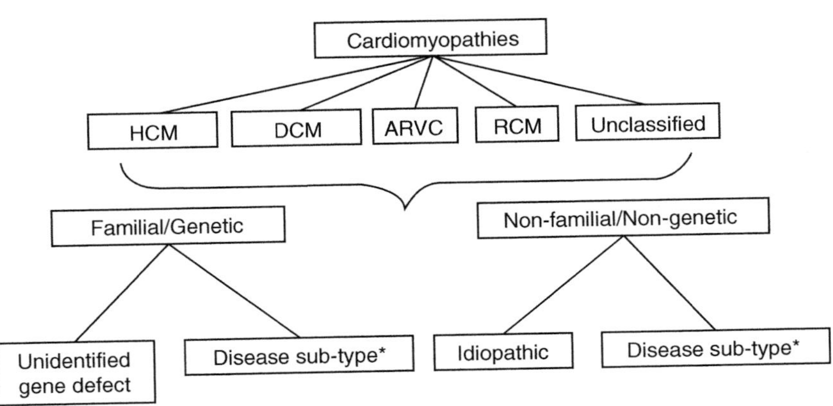

Fig. 28.1 Reprinted from Elliott et al. Classification of the cardiomyopathies: a position statement from the European Society of Cardiology Working Group on Myocardial and Pericardial Diseases. *Eur Heart J.* 2008;29(2):270–276, with permission

are complex [35]. The exact prevalence of restrictive cardiomyopathy (RCM) and of left ventricular non-compaction cardiomyopathy are unknown but these are probably the least common types of CM. RCM may be idiopathic, familial, or result from various systemic disorders, in particular amyloidosis, sarcoidosis, carcinoid heart disease, or scleroderma and has always been difficult to define [33]. Finally, arrhythmogenic right ventricular dysplasia (ARVD), is rather uncommon (1:5000) but a frequent cause of sudden cardiac death in young people.

In this section we will focus on HCM, not only because of its frequency but also because so far it is the best studied cardiomyopathy from a genetic and molecular point of view and it represents the major cause of sudden death in the young and in athletes [36].

The proportion of those who develop cardiac problems (either symptoms or sudden unexpected death) before 70–75 years is substantial but uncertain and lower than has been reported from highly selected clinic populations [37, 38], as is true for other inherited disorders subject to ascertainment bias (e.g., *BRCA1* and *BRCA2* mutation carriers). The prevalence of those with overt disease is of course lower still. The diagnosis and management of HCM is evolving [39] but the prognosis given to patients and families in clinic may sometimes be more pessimistic than is warranted because of this bias in publications toward the reporting of subgroups with a higher rate of sudden death and other serious complications; the extent of incomplete penetrance is still being evaluated but seems to be greater for disease-associated mutations at some loci than others.

As our awareness of the clinical uncertainties increases, our interpretation of molecular genetic variation has had to become more sophisticated. The mutation detection strategies employed to screen patients for disease-associated mutations are improving as high-throughput DNA sequencing methods are introduced into clinical practice [40]. The yield (sensitivity) of mutation screening is therefore improving but the interpretation of some identified variants remains difficult; when can a novel variant safely be assigned the blame for causing the disease in a family? Clarifying such results can require further intensive family studies or technically challenging and time-consuming molecular functional studies. When mutation screening is discussed with families, they need to be aware that the results of a family study may give sufficient confidence that predictive testing becomes feasible but, equally, they may fail to do this: they may disprove pathogenicity of the suspect variant or they may simply not generate enough new information to be decisive. Once a pathogenic or likely pathogenic variant has been identified in a kindred, the offer of testing family members for the known variant is usually less likely to cause confusion but can still present asymptomatic individuals at risk with complex challenges.

The need for caution in the interpretation of the significance of molecular results has been reinforced with several recent publications. Das et al. [41] showed that the reassessment of results previously reported to patients was necessary as the interpretation of several HCM-related genetic variants had changed over a few years, with some likely pathogenic results being reinterpreted as benign and vice versa. The scale of this need for reassessment is substantial, as emphasised in a major study from Walsh et al. [42], who drew on exome data from the ExAc Consortium to show that there were many false claims of variant pathogenicity and some instances of overly cautious under-interpretation of pathogenic variants as being of uncertain significance. There are several systematic difficulties in this area including the under-representation of ethnic minorities in available population exome databanks, leading to the over-interpretation of low frequency benign alleles in some population groups as pathogenic because the greater allele frequency in the minority population had not been appreciated [43].

Furthermore, the scope for intersection between variants at different loci is only now becoming clear. In the past, when Sanger sequencing was used, the search for variants in candidate genes would often cease once a plausible pathogenic variant had been found. Now, with large gene panels and exome analyses being used, it is becoming clear that variants in two or more relevant genes may be found, with perhaps one major variant "causing" the disease and another variant acting as disease modifier [44]. There is much more to be learned about these processes and mechanisms of disease. In our present state of understanding, however, it can be helpful to limit the information with which we are presented by the diagnostic laboratory. Thus, the use of focused panels of HCM-related genes may be more helpful than the use of large "cardiac gene panels" (whether "genuine" panels, when sequence is only generated from genes on the panel, or "virtual," when exome sequencing is performed but only genes known to be relevant to the phenotype are included in the sequence analysis) or a full exome [45].

The difficulty of giving an accurate prognosis in this clinically and genetically very heterogeneous condition, and the overestimation in published series of the risk of cardiac disease because of ascertainment bias, need to be discussed openly with those who may be at increased risk. Exaggerated risk estimates could lead some to reject genetic testing who might otherwise benefit from it either medically or psychologically. The questions posed by families seem, however, in the limited published experience, to focus more on predictive testing and reproductive risks than on the information volunteered by professionals, especially the details of diagnosis and prognosis [46].

In one study of families with a known pathogenic mutation, the uptake of predictive testing among at-risk relatives who attended for genetic counselling was very high while the proportion of at-risk first-degree relatives who attended the genetics clinic within 12 months of a mutation being identified in the family (making a predictive test available) was less than 40% [47]. The authors concluded that efforts must be made to increase the uptake of genetic counselling. Care must be taken, however, not to achieve a higher rate of clinic attendance through offering better treatment or greater certainty in the interpretation of molecular test results than can be justified on the evidence. Rather than the problem being one of family ignorance, it may be that ambivalence about the treatments on offer, including implantable defibrillators, may contribute to this shortfall. Another reason may be that only relatives already actively seeking a predictive test attend the genetic counselling clinic and those who prefer not to know have no interest in coming.

It would clearly be very important that the relatives at risk are well informed about the aims of the genetic counselling clinic. They should know that the genetics consultation would aim to provide a session of information put into a realistic context that can support their making the decision whether or not to proceed with a genetic test, and that there is no obligation to accept testing when they attend the clinic. It is clear that further research is required in several domains: to develop improved treatments, to describe the experiences of patients and families from their own perspectives and so to make these descriptions more accessible to professionals, and to explore with families the factors affecting the acceptability of those genetic tests and those treatments that are available.

28.7.2 Long QT Disorders and Brugada Syndrome

The genetic dissection of the long QT disorders, and their relationship to the epilepsies and other channelopathies, has been a fascinating story of scientific progress over the two decades from 1995. This progress and its clinical applications were carefully set out in a consensus report from the U.S. National Heart Lung and Blood Institute, moving on from a focus on the ion channels themselves to the macromolecular signaling complex of which it is a part and whose disruption leads to a dysrhthmogenic cardiomyopathy [48]. The clinical application of this genetic knowledge has shown that the factors likely to trigger a dysrrhythmia (loud noise, swimming, other strenuous exercise, sleep/rest) differ as between the different gene loci involved [49]. It has also been shown that ethnic background and variation at other loci can influence the frequency and severity of symptoms caused by the same disease-associated mutation within one gene—the A341V mutation in the *KCNQ1* locus [50] and other mutations are known to cause different phenotypic effects even in different members of the same family. Attempts have been made to relate variation in a particular gene to survival; how this interacts with gender and the duration of the QT interval have been studied. The authors proposed a scheme for risk stratification among patients with LQTS based on the gene mutated (*LQT1*, *LQT2*, or *LQT3*), QT measurement and sex. The risk categories were high (>50%), intermediate (30%–49%), and low (<30%). A first cardiac arrest or SCD was highest among female patients with a mutation in the *LQT2* gene and male patients with a mutation in the *LQT3* gene. As in HCM-related genetic variation, the cosegregation of two disease-associated mutations within a family can also occur, sometimes in different genes, causing unusually severe disease in those family members who inherit both mutations [51].

Brugada syndrome is said to be responsible for up to 12% of all sudden deaths and approximately 20% of deaths occurring in patients with structurally normal hearts. The mean age of SCD is approximately 40 years. Clinical presentations may also include the sudden infant death syndrome (SIDS) [52] and the sudden unexpected nocturnal death syndrome, a typical presentation in young individuals from Southeast Asia [53]. An implantable cardioverter-defibrillator (ICD) is essentially the only recommended form of therapy as drugs are mostly ineffective.

Brugada syndrome and LQTS can both be caused by defects in the *SCN5A* gene. In general, those *SCN5A* mutations implicated in LQT3 cause gain of function of the ion channel, whereas the ones implicated in the Brugada syndrome cause a loss of channel function [54]. However, mutations that are associated with both diseases have been described in the same family, supporting the concept that these two disorders are part of a spectrum of “sodium channelopathies” [55].

Substantial progress has been made in understanding the basic science of these conditions—the molecular genetics and the electrophysiology—and on the management of cardiac risk in family members. However, the interpretation of variants in relevant genes has had to undergo very substantial reassessment over the past few years. A detailed report has been published of the experience of one kindred, in which a variant in KCNQ1 had been misinterpreted as pathogenic. Many family members were thought to be at high risk of sudden cardiac death, with one even having a defibrillator implanted that, in hindsight, was unnecessary. Intensive molecular sleuthing showed that the cause of cardiac death in a family member had been a pathogenic variant in a different gene, and the KCNQ1 variant was shown to be benign [56]. This salutary tale has served as lesson to many practitioners, and is reinforced by the difficulty demonstrated recently of interpreting the pathogenicity of variants in *SCN5A* and *KCNH2* (in particular), when they have been found incidentally in pharmacogenetic studies, not in association with a cardiac phenotype [57]. This need for caution is echoed in the the paper of Riuro et al. [58], where bioinformatic analyses of sequences from single individuals were shown to be prone to misinterpretation, and that family segregation studies could be most helpful in confirming (or refuting) the otherwise tentative conclusions of an analysis. However, by virtue of the sudden death phenotype itself, such studies can be especially difficult as there may not be enough family members to achieve sufficient evidence of linkage.

28.8 The Cardiac Genetics Clinic

The application of recently acquired genetics knowledge to the management of families must be performed with great care, as emphasised by the review of molecular diagnostic misinterpretations indicated above. The role of the cardiac genetic clinic, the required clinical approach, and the benefits for patients who attend have been well described [59, 60]. When a definitely pathogenic mutation is found in the case of a sudden cardiac death or a near-miss event, then standard cardiac management can be followed. When there is no family or personal history, however, and when the variant identified is not known to be associated with disease in the patient's ethnic group, more caution is needed. The consensus advice on the prevention of sudden cardiac death from the American College of Cardiology and the American Heart Association Task Force on Performance Measures has been commendably cautious, placing the emphasis very much on cardiac functional and physiological testing and de-emphasising the role of genetic tests, while allowing that these will have a role in specific circumstances [61]. This is consistent with the previous recommendations on cardiac genetic testing from 2012 [62].

One issue that requires attention is how families experience and cope with being told that several of them could die at any moment. This must differ greatly from the experience of an individual being told that she has, perhaps, 4–6 months to live. To be told (for example) that your death may be triggered by loud noise, by swimming in cold water or by strenuous exertion is likely to have immense but individually different consequences for the way such individuals and families live their lives. Very frightening is of course the fact that you could die during sleep. Adults known to be affected by LQT syndrome, and so known to be at risk of sudden cardiac death, experience worry and limitations in their lives. They appreciate advice from an expert regional clinic as it avoids confusion and the misinformation that may come from less well informed professionals, and they focus much of their concern on their children and grandchildren [63]. Similarly, families who have faced the sudden cardiac death of a young relative and have experience of a cardiac genetics evaluation, report finding this very helpful, and recommend that professionals should advise those in this position that referral for expert evaluation is recommended [64].

The decision whether to be tested for a plausibly causal genetic factor that may put you at risk of your family's cardiac disorder is not simple. The process of making this decision has now been reported in several studies, although the picture is still incomplete. Ormondroyd et al. [65] have shown, in the context of HCM and LQT, that several aspects of the patient's understanding of their situation need to be explored thoroughly, such as their appreciation of risk in the absence of obvious symptoms and in the recognition that the result may not yield a dichotomous "Yes/No" but rather a point on a spectrum. Indeed, it is important they appreciate that genetic testing in their family may be uninformative [66]. Manuel and Brunger [67] studied families at risk of ARVC and identified six factors whose impact on the testing decision can usefully be considered (the availability of a valid test; deaths in the family; signs and symptoms of disease; gender; family relationships and sense of obligation; availability of family support).

The impact of cardiac genetic testing has been assessed using cardiac-specific 'quality of life' (QoL) measures before and after testing, indicating that some individuals at risk find this stressful and that a positive (adverse) genetic test result can—understandably—add to this stress at follow-up 12 months after testing [68, 69]. As in comparable cancer genetics settings, very little effect of testing is seen when very general QoL measures are used, instead of indicators of cardiac-specific anxiety [70]. The sensitivity of such measures is poor.

Another important topic to mention here, albeit briefly, is the assessment of cardiac risk in athletes. There are numerous reports of the sudden death of apparently healthy young men during competitive sports and a post-mortem diagnosis of HCM, LQT or Brugada syndrome will sometimes be made, especially after a "molecular autopsy" and family studies. The best approach to screening athletes for cardiac risk is still open to debate. Multiple difficulties arise in the clinical assessment of athletes, including that of "athlete's heart" (cardiac training) [71]. A proportionate and balanced view is adopted in the report of Al-Khatib et al. [61] although some jurisdictions, such as Italy, recommend more intensive assessments.

28.9 Genetic Testing of Children

Testing children can raise particular difficulties. To be given cardiac risk information about one's child may result in not only immediate but also sustained distress [72] and one may ask the question whether one would do more harm than good discussing these topics or, at least, generating genetic test results about risk to children. The crumb of comfort is that children identified as carrying such a mutation do not seem to suffer from it in the way their parents do [73], although that was a preliminary finding.

Many parents of a child with serious developmental problems are initially desperate to find out why their child has these problems, and some use their knowledge of the diagnosis to exert influence over the actions of the health care and education professionals involved with their child [74]; the "need" for a diagnosis may lessen with time as it becomes clear that no cure will be forthcoming, whatever the diagnosis. Similarly, and very understandably, many parents of a child at risk of a later-onset genetic disorder wish to find out whether their child has inherited the family's genetic disorder and is at risk of serious problems. This parental concern relates to the question of how positively professionals present the benefits and hazards of different approaches to cardiac management and genetic testing—what *evaluation* do they convey in addition to the mere facts? Testing even young children for disease manifestations, including the use of ECG and cardiac echo, will clearly be entirely appropriate, when there is an established medical intervention available to treat, defer, or prevent complications of the condition, as is especially true for LQT disorders and sometimes for cardiomyopathies.

There will always be difficult areas of professional judgment as to the border between research and service, and how to manage a complex case that is not being included within a research study. Predictive genetic testing of healthy children could be viewed as rather different from testing adults because, in the absence of cardiac symptoms, physical signs, ECG, or echocardiographic evidence of current pathology, there will usually be no implications for medical management in the event of a positive genetic test result. On the other hand, not carrying out a genetic test that is available would impose continuing practical and emotional burdens on the child's family and would incur the continued costs of cardiac surveillance. Therefore, when it is available, it will usually be reasonable to discuss the offer of genetic testing with the parents of children at risk of an inherited cardiac disorder that could develop during childhood, especially for children who are very active in sports.

In practice, the focus of decision making by a child's parents will often depend upon the contextual air of optimism or caution within which the physician wraps his/her assessment of the medical interventions that could be offered if the child does carry the relevant mutation. This, in turn, depends upon how the physician sees the border between research and standard clinical practice. It would be possible for a clinical researcher to subject at-risk children to the potentially hazardous pharmacological provocation of electrophysiological anomalies, for example, out of both a wish to find out more about the disease (this could be termed "intellectual curiosity") and a wish to clarify the situation for this particular child; the balance between these motivations is crucial and the professional has to restrain her "curiosity" (and the legitimate wish to expand our knowledge of these diseases) when it would entail subjecting the child to additional discomfort, pain, or hazard that has not been discussed with the parents and, where appropriate, approved in advance by an ethics review process. The cardiologist is likely to possess a greater understanding of both what is at stake and of the risks for the child than any other party involved: this is a great responsibility that calls for a very finely developed sense of professionalism. Monitoring this borderland is tremendously difficult and institutional attempts to prevent all misjudgment are likely to prevent all progress.

In the absence of medical interventions established as useful and applicable in childhood, or when the inherited disorder is unlikely to develop until adult life, then the case for predictive genetic testing in a child is much weaker [75, 76]. A special situation may arise when a child wishes to participate in competitive sports. The consequence of a positive test result would be the exclusion from this possibility that may be very difficult to accept. Thus, careful preparation and discussion of alternative options are mandatory before testing in such situations.

Adults who wished to have molecular testing, when it is available, would be able to access this through a clinical genetics unit and with the support of pre- and post-test genetic counselling. The question will then arise as to whether professionals should accede to requests for testing made by adolescents of less than 18 years. In the United Kingdom, such requests are usually discussed carefully with the teenager and testung may go ahead if the professional assesses the teenager as possessing sufficient maturity. The extent of "counselling" in advance of the test will vary with the minor's maturity and the extent to which a test result can usefully inform medical decisions or shape the teenager's approach to life decisions. There will be more tendency to defer testing if there is no clinical benefit. The legal context and professional guidance in other European jurisdictions varies, as it does internationally. A natural next question is how professionals should respond to a healthy but at-risk young adult who requests predictive genetic testing but who, upon assessment, appears to be of questionable maturity [77, 78]. If there were no medical indication for testing at that time, it would be defensible in those circumstances to defer testing while maintaining contact and encouraging further reflection. In relation to inherited cardiac disease, however, these issues are usually of little relevance as the core question is whether, or to what extent, medical surveillance and intervention, or lifestyle advice grounded in good evidence, would be available.

An adolescent or young adult who is told that sudden loud noise or exercise or cold water or even sleep could kill them may respond in a very different fashion from their parents—or parent, if one parent has already died in just such circumstances. The stage is set for distress and conflict. We need to know more about what parents say to their at-risk children and what different patterns of coping are employed; some of the research required may be observational but some must surely entail listening to the accounts of survivors and the bereaved who are living through these difficulties.

Some accounts of the genetic testing of adolescents have been reported, especially in some HCM families in the Netherlands which (unusually, and most usefully) incorporate a longitudinal dimension. However, the family situations and responses to risk and to testing differ and it is difficult to envisage a single, simple approach that will 'usually' be appropriate [79, 80]. These studies have shown that testing minors can lead to regrets, sometimes because of fears about problems with insurance and sometimes because of the medical advice that is given if a minor is found to be at risk, such as exercise restrictions. While these findings are the most thoughtful and thorough such reports available, they merely "scratch the surface": there is so much more to be learned and understood. Similarly complex issues arise in families at risk of LQT syndrome, where the question of disclosure of information or privacy within the family can also be prominent [81].

28.10 Family Communication

One of the areas that has proved most difficult in clinical genetics practice is that of difficulties with the communication of genetic information within families [82, 83]. For the full medical, as well as personal and social, benefits of the diagnosis of a genetic disorder to accrue, those diagnosed within a family must transmit the relevant information to their relatives. Problems with this transmission of information about the risk of disease and the health benefits of early intervention take different forms depending upon whether the information is to be passed "vertically" to a child or parent, or "horizontally" to a sibling, cousin, or other relative and depending upon the availability of preventive and/or therapeutic strategies.

The difficulties felt by parents in transmitting such information to a child have long been clear in the context of polycystic kidney disease, where there is great potential for denial of the problem to lead subsequently both to psychological distress and to serious clinical consequences [84, 85]. Similar problems have been documented in relation to other autosomal dominant disorders for which the children of an affected adult will be at risk—most notably Huntington's Disese (HD) [86] and the Mendelian familial cancer disorders. Some difficulties have also been apparent in relation to the transmission of information about genetic carrier status, especially in relation to sex-linked disorders and balanced chromosome translocations [87, 88]. A focus group study of the impact of genetic conditions on families has shown that families (but not professionals) have raised the difficulties parents have in communicating with their children as one of their major problems [89, 90]. Parents want to discuss such topics with their children but often find it very difficult; they may require active support from professionals if they are to share information in the most helpful fashion. Parents and doctors may often think to protect their child in not telling the truth and failing to explain the reasons for their medical visits, but for the child's well-being and trust it seems essential for them to understand, in an age-appropriate way, why she or he needs regular cardiac follow-up and what kind of investigations have to be done. As was said by the 41-year-old lady with an early onset severe familial HCM (already mentioned above):

"I got no explanation as to why I regularly had to go to the cardiac clinic, it was a family secret. I did not understand why I had to go and my sister did not. I just heard a few things but it was not an open discussion and that was very frightening for me. I don't recommend people to do that.

Later I heard different things like, "because of that disorder she will not have children"; but it was never an open discussion. The doctors never told me clearly what is going on and that was terrible. Finally I understood that I had the same disorder as my father and I saw how his situation got steadily worse. It got to the point where he couldn't do anything anymore, not even kneeling. I saw that it was terrible and that created a climate of fear in the family."

Passing information horizontally to other members of the family involves additional considerations. There are many reasons why the flow of information through family networks can be problematic, including the reluctance of individuals to pass on disturbing information to unaware relatives [91], the question of who counts as family [92], and the preexisting pattern of relationships within each family [93]. There may be specific individuals within a family system, who feel a duty of care toward specific others, to whom they would then be bound to disclose information that becomes available; furthermore, the disclosure may be the duty *of these particular individuals* so that it would be an abrogation of their role for others to perform this task [82]. There are the related but distinct issues that arise from generating such information that would then need to be passed to others; for example, some women affected by hereditary breast and ovarian cancer feel a sense of obligation to have a test performed, even if they might personally prefer not to do so, so that the family's mutation can be found. Only then does predictive testing become feasible for their female relatives [94, 95]. An interesting feature in some families is the emergence of a key family organizer who facilitates communication within the family and may organize family gatherings to ensure that all have access to the information or are able to participate [92, 96].

We have more comments from the same mother already mentioned above, who had lost one of her two sons from sudden cardiac death due to ARVD. She developed the disorder herself after cascade screening of the family, and genetic testing in her revealed a pathogenic mutation in one of the genes associated with ARVD. She said:

> "There was no problem when I announced to my family that I have the same cardiac problem as (our son had) and that all my brothers and sisters need to do a cardiac evaluation, but when the mutation was identified and I informed one of my sisters about the possibility of predictive testing she said: "Fine, so we go and do the blood sampling". I said, "No, no, this is not the way it should be done. It is essential to do this through a geneticist and discuss all the issues and possible consequences". So, I told them that they *have to* go to a geneticist, that they have to give me the address of the geneticist, and that I am going to send him or her the information. This is because you just can't simply do the blood sampling. What are you going to do afterward? If you have the mutation what are you going to do?"

Most patients and family members agree, when asked, that information about the heart disease or cardiac genetic tests of one person should be passed to others in the family, for whom it may also be important [97]. However, such opinions are often gathered when they are hypothetical; patients or relatives may feel differently when faced with concrete situations. Professionals can then experience difficulty when important information is not passed through a family in the way they think it should be. Under what circumstances would it be permissible, or perhaps obligatory, for them to break their usual obligation to maintain confidentiality because of a greater duty to prevent harm to others? This raises larger questions of the obligations of a physician; do we have duties solely to the individual(s) in front of us, or also to their absent kin, or to society at large and "the general good?" The usual response of professionals in such circumstances, where there may be a conflict between the duties to protect confidentiality and at the same time to disclose personal information, is not to force disclosure but to work with the family over time to help them achieve the disclosure in an emotionally safe but effective manner [98]. There have, however, been calls to define the circumstances in which professionals may or should disclose a patient's personal information to others without consent [99]. These have arisen largely within the anglophone world of utilitarian ethics where the difficulties of reducing incommensurable qualities to a single scalar dimension often seem not to be fully appreciated; even a sophisticated account of this view reduces essentially to the attempt to compare the outcomes likely to result from the available courses of action and then selecting the one assessed as leading to fewer harms [100]. This effectively writes out of the account any prior Hippocratic commitment of the physician or health care professional and assumes that all manner of consequences can be reduced to a single dimension. This position is less highly regarded in continental Europe.

Efforts made by professionals to support their clients' disclosure of information to their relatives recognizes the vulnerability of those given unwelcome information and the time it can take for them to process the information and acknowledge their obligations [101] rather than trying to insist that they should act immediately, as if they were able instantly to weigh up these issues calmly, with objectivity and detachment. It also recognizes the complexity of relationships within a family, in which forceful medical intervention could do real harm [102]. This gentle approach has been shown often to be effective [103] and in some circumstances can be helped through a group approach [104, 105]. The need for such professionally supported communication is clear in the context of FH [106].

There have been helpful reviews of family communication of genetic information [107–109]. Such work is useful in allowing us to anticipate some of the difficulties that may arise in families confronting sudden death resulting from an inherited cardiac disorder.

28.11 Risks and Certainties

One component of genetic counseling in cardiac genetics is conveying information about risks: risks to the patient or client, risks to their relatives, and ways of modifying these risks. At one level this can entail a narrowly informational process, the impersonal transfer of cold facts; at another level, it can entail a personal contact between counsellor and client when both engage with the personal meaning and significance of the information.

To focus on the narrowly factual, one can assess the effectiveness of techniques—contrasting verbal or numerical (probabilistic) or visual descriptions of risk—but this has to be just a start (e.g., [110]). The tendency for genetic counselling clients to convert a probability statement into the resolution of a dichotomy—converting a *maybe* into a *yes* or a *no*—has been recognized for decades [111, 112], so that a genetic counsellor must engage with the personal context [113] and the significance of the possible outcome events. This approach is necessary to help the client appreciate the genuine uncertainties involved. This dialogical approach to risk communication has been well described in nongenetic [114] and genetic contexts [115] although the ways in which genetic counseling clients use their understandings of risk in making decisions is yet another matter.

Decisions about genetic testing will be influenced by the professional, who has framed the choice (to have the test or not), by the client's understanding of their biological situation [116], and by the client's judgments about their own personal emotional responses and their assessment of the likely responses of others in their family. When the decision is not to go ahead with testing, however, or when no test is available or when the risk information simply hangs there, without one single specific decision to be made, the influence or impact of the professional will be felt in a different way. The clients will go away and live their lives but they will take with them the manner in which the information was provided; this applies not only but especially to "bad news." If these long-lasting memories of us professionals are not to be entirely negative, then we need to know our clients as individuals—as far as possible within the proper constraints of professional conduct.

It is our personal relationship with clients, arising from empathy but without sentimentality, which gives us the opportunity to help them face these decisions. We need to explain the facts and risks to enable them to make a realistically grounded decision but we also have to help them (those who want the help) to think through the consequences of the different possible courses of action open to them. That requires a respectful relationship that can develop over time. The centrality of the ongoing relationship between genetics services and their clients has been recognized as crucial in family-based research [117] and in a professional consensus of leading genetic counselors in the United States [28].

The influence of risk perception on decision making has been studied in the context of predictive genetic testing for HD and the familial cancers. It will be important to explore the same processes in relation to familial cardiac disorders. Although this process has begun, and has been referred to above, there is much more to do. We suspect that professionals would like their clients to be making cool, rational judgments about genetic testing and practical aspects of risk management while many clients will be making decisions on quite different grounds. Whereas cardiologists, even more than genetics professionals, are likely to perceive the LQT disorders and HCMs as amenable to useful medical interventions, so that decisions about genetic testing could be made on the basis of a rational decision process, many at-risk individuals will feel differently and will perhaps stay away from both genetics and cardiology clinics. They are likely to make decisions more comparable to those made by people at risk of HD than would apply in the context of an effectively preventable cancer predisposition (such as familial polyposis coli or one of the multiple endocrine neoplasia syndromes). Substantial numbers will persist in preferring not to be tested until the family experiences of treatment confirm that the outcomes are substantially better than they have yet seen. This is particularly true for young and asymptomatic at-risk relatives. The medical benefits of predictive testing in this situation often appear to be uncertain. This arises firstly because only limited data may so far be available about the natural history of healthy carriers. Secondly, the expression of the disease may be highly variable even within a family and the clinician can predict neither the age at onset of the disease nor its severity, although phenotype-genotype correlations, especially for LQTS and HCM, may be of some help. Thirdly, it may be that no medical treatment is effective in preventing or in lowering the occurrence of the disease. Restriction of physical activity might be recommended but its ability to counter sudden death in healthy (so far unaffected) carriers of their family's mutation will often be uncertain.

The only treatment that might prevent sudden death from dysrhythmia is an implantable defibrillator. This is not currently the general recommendation for healthy mutation carriers, although this option may be discussed in the context of a family with sudden death, especially in the young. For these reasons it is actually not possible to make a firm recommendation in favour of predictive genetic testing for inherited cardiac disorders because the balance of (dis)advantages will depend on so many factors, including the dangers of a particular mutation or set of variants, the likely response of this set of variants to the available treatments, and very individual and personal choices made by patients about how they would like to live their lives. If a predictive test is positive, then strict medical follow-up is required that will allow the early diagnosis of symptoms and lead to improved therapeutic management. This strategy, however, can also be followed without genetic testing of the healthy at-risk relative. Interestingly, one study showed that only 76% of mutation carriers after predictive testing for HCM received regular cardiac follow-up which seems to indicate a need for better patient and/or physician education [118]. If the test is negative, the individual will be reassured and the result will probably improve his or her well-being, although there might be adverse psycho-emotional reactions as has been shown for HD, deriving from issues of family dynamics [119]. So far the main reasons why an individual would ask for predictive cardiac genetic testing would be the psychological burden related to uncertainty and/or the wish to know the risk of transmission of the disease to their offspring [46] and/or the situation of a young sportive adolescent who wish to continue his/her intense physical activities. The psychological burden of uncertainty could, however, be replaced after an unfavorable test result by a new psychological burden of the knowledge of an increased risk of a (possibly fatal) cardiac event but with major uncertainties about the level of risk under any particular circumstances and the likely response to interventions. Not everybody wants to know for sure about this if no demonstrably effective prevention and/or therapies have been developed.

Knowledge that one carries a gene predisposing to a cardiac disorder also has implications for reproductive decisions—it raises for discussion the eventual possibility of a prenatal diagnosis if the mutation in the family is known. It has been possible to perfrom prenatal diagnosis for inherited cardiac disorders for many years [120] and this raises complex medical, psychological, and ethical issues. From the medical point of view, the termination of an affected pregnancy may be regarded as indicated in families with malignant forms of the disease (i.e., with several cardiac deaths in the young or deaths associated with heart failure). However, the variable expression even within a given family, and the difficulty of predicting the potential phenotype, counterbalance the value of prenatal diagnosis. As for many other inherited, mostly adult-onset disorders with wide clinical heterogeneity, no general rules can be given and decisions should be made after case-by-case discussion and according to a consensus between the parents and the medical team.

28.12 Professional Optimism and Family Scepticism

Underlying these differences in perspective there may be, on the one hand, a degree of professional optimism about the worth of one's craft and, on the other hand, the at-risk client may manifest either some measure of denial as a psychological defense, some anxiety as to what shape treatment might take or some scepticism of the professional's claims—or some combination of these. A very real issue for professionals is how to present information in a "balanced" way when what is being made available is both highly variable between centres and rapidly developing over time, so that a specialist's practice is likely to be somewhat ahead of what is justified by the published evidence. The influence of the professional on the client (who is the cardiologist's *potential* patient) will be exerted not so much by what is said but rather through the way in which the information is given; this involves both the degree of professional optimism and enthusiasm, the professional's convincing display of competence and the achievement of a sense of personal contact between client and professional. It will be immensely important for professionals in this field to develop their self-awareness skills, to work whenever possible with a colleague from a different discipline within the same multidisciplinary team, and to seek awareness-enhancing psychological supervision. Those wishing to borrow insights from studies of HD may like to look at the findings of in-depth interviews with genetic counselling clients from HD families (such as [121–123]).

28.13 Family Cascade Testing, the Paradigm of Familial Hypercholesterolaemia (FH)

28.13.1 Familial Hypercholesterolemia (FH)

FH was the first genetic condition to be recognized as an important cause of heart disease, specifically of coronary artery disease (CAD), and biochemical testing has long been available to confirm the diagnosis and assist in dietary and pharmacological management. The primary diagnosis in a family used to be made largely by testing those with early-onset CAD or physical signs of hypercholesterolaemia for raised cholesterol. Increasingly, however, the recognition of FH has been achieved through the opportunistic screening of adults with or without symptoms of CAD, often in primary care or preventive health checks, or direct-to-consumer, including over-the-counter. For an interesting variation on this approach, see below [124].

The emergence of services for FH through this biochemical approach has led to its usually being managed as a metabolic disorder by medical biochemists, in contrast to other inherited cardiac conditions that are increasingly managed jointly by cardiologists and genetics professionals. The later arrival of molecular genetic testing in the management of FH, as well as the limited utility of genetic testing as a primary diagnostic tool in FH, has led to a highly focused role for genetic testing in the cascade testing of the relatives of established cases for whom a pathogenic mutation in *LDLR* or another relevant gene has been found. Molecular testing of the *APOB* and *PCSK9* genes as well as *LDLR* may be required to find rhe family's mutation(s) and, still, a pathogenic mutation will often not be found. There have been periodic reassessments of whether it would be feasible to offer individualized risk assessments on the basis of single nucleotide polymorphism (SNP) typing but the consensus has long been that such applications would not be warranted [125–127]. Such information adds little to more conventional methods of assessing risk of cardiovascular disease [128], especially as measures of the apolipoproteins have been shown to give more accurate risk assessments than any of the cholesterol ratios [129]. We know that susceptibility screening can also cause confusion and has the potential to reinforce inequities in health [130]. The identification of those with a "predisease" state generates feelings of uncertainty and places additional demands on the health care system [131, 132]. Recent re-evaluation of the polygenic influence on serum cholesterol shows an accumulation of polygenic variants of individually small effect that are likely to be contributing to the high cholesterol levels [133]. Given that the interventions to be recommended on the basis of serum lipid measurements would not be modified by such genetic data, SNP-based population screening is not recommended; the situation has not changed over some 20 years [134, 135].

Family cascade testing must therefore persevere with biochemical testing in those many familes without a pathogenic FH mutation, although molecular genetic cascade testing is preferred where possible because biochemical tests are not always definitive in family members who do not yet have overt disease [136]: this is especially true in the young [137, 138]. This approach has increased the absolute numbers of those diagnosed with the condition in the Netherlands, with a major, beneficial impact on the proportion of known affected persons under appropriate medical management [139], and this approach to cascade screening is also being adopted in the UK.

Before the advent of safe and effective cholesterol-lowering drugs, one consequence of finding a raised serum cholesterol (not specifically FH) was that some individuals responded paradoxically with unhelpful behaviors—feeling either fatalistically doomed to develop CAD or completely invulnerable (reviewed in [134, 140]). The introduction of the statin drugs changed this: since then, patients with FH have generally regarded this as treatable and have recognized the need to alter behavior [141], although those with FH in whom a causative mutation has been found appear more likely to trust medication than dietary intervention [142]. This may be an instance of a more general phenomenon, with those at increased risk of disease through an established genetic factor placing more trust in rationally designed pharmacological interventions than in "merely" behavioural or lifestyle changes [143]. There are few grounds for the optimistic belief that genetic testing for susceptibility to disease has a sustained, beneficial impact on lifestyle, such as smoking cessation and compliance with recommendations on diet and exercise [144–146]. This, in turn, carries lessons for the circumstances under which it may be appropriate to introduce population screening tests for disease susceptibility, especially the strength of the evidence that the interpretation of a test result should be not only valid but also of established clinical utility [134]. The therapeutic effectiveness of statins for treating FH, however, is not in doubt [147, 148], and they are effective in reducing the risk of stroke as well as myocardial infarction [149].

Where there are clear practical benefits from early diagnosis, as with FH, the question arises as to how health services can best be structured with the goal of maximizing the numbers of at-risk people who are identified before they have developed disease complications. They can then decide whether they wish to be investigated, or not, and take appropriate precautions, or not. The strategic choice lies between a population screening approach and a family-based system of offering testing to the first- and second-degree relatives of identified patients, "cascading" out or "snowballing" through the family. The fact that mutation-based genetic testing is much more sensitive and specific than a cholesterol-based population screening test indicates that the family-based approach may be superior, at least for those families in which a definitely pathogenic mutation has been found. The family-based approach has been shown to be more cost-effective [150] as well as clinically rational; a population-based screening program for FH using an assay for serum cholesterol does not meet the U.K.'s public health criteria for a screening program [151, 152].

Cascade testing gives families an opportunity to escape from the pattern of disease that has affected previous generations, not only for FH but for other inherited, single gene (Mendelian) cardiac disorders for which pathogenic mutations have been identified. How should such services operate? How should the family cascading be implemented?

We know from studies in Netherlands that most of those contacted, but not all, welcome this [153]. The practical details of screening programmes can be crucial [154]. Even small differences in the operational procedures of a genetic screening program may have a major impact on how it is perceived and the ethical issues it raises (in the context of newborn screening, see [155]). The FH programme relies on contact details for relatives being provided by the index case patients, who may or may not prepare their relatives for being contacted [156–158]. The clear potential for major health benefits generally outweighs the sense of intrusion that could otherwise result from such unsolicited contact [159]. This will not necessarily be the case where the benefits from genetic testing are not so clear and would therefore not be transferable to some other cardiac disease contexts; it may also not apply in countries with different health care systems—where the cost of testing and treatment would have to be met by the individual or where the cost of health insurance may deny health care to the poor and to those with inherited predispositions to disease ("pre-existing conditions").

The particular needs of healthy but mutation-carrying (likely-to-become-affected) children also require consideration. It has been suggested that population screening for serum cholesterol could be applied to children between the ages of

1 and 9 years, as discrimination on the basis of cholesterol levels between those with FH and those without (i.e., distinguishing between the two groups) is best in childhood [160]. There are powerful reasons for caution with this approach, however, on clinical and cost-effectiveness grounds as well as from a consideration of the psychological and social consequences of such an approach [152, 161, 162]. However, an interesting approach to this—offering opportunistic cholesterol screening to >10,000 infants at a clinic visit for immunisation—has been assessed favourably in a pilot study, with the immediate benefit being the detection and treatment of FH in affected but previously undiagnosed parents [42]. However, this project was clearly driven by enthusiasts and may not warrant adoption for the population without further and more critical evaluation.

Conclusions

Clinical genetics and genetic counselling have been shaped by their experiences of working both with families and with colleagues from other disciplines. Clinical genetics at first emerged from pediatrics and neurology and then its pattern of working changed when developments in cancer genetics led to many referrals for such concerns. This led to a greater focus on adult patients and to the coordination of medical management on behalf of so far unaffected family members—for example, the surveillance for tumors. Genetics professionals work alongside oncologists and other specialists, retaining their role of working with families rather than individual patients and especially with the healthy but at-risk relatives. Genetics professionals (both medically qualified clinical geneticists and genetic counsellors or genetic nurses) now work alongside specialists from several other medical subspecialties including cardiology. What role will they have 10–20 years into the future?

Most cardiac disease is of "complex" etiology, which may to some extent be clarified by large genetic epidemiological studies but for which population screening approaches are unlikely to have a high predictive value. Genetic tests may be useful in guiding treatment for those with overt disease or in the cascade, "follow-up" arms of population screening programs to identify those affected by FH, but those activities will not usually be carried out by genetic specialists: genetic testing for therapeutic guidance (i.e., pharmacogenetics) will be performed by generalists and population screening for FH and similar predispositions to cardiac disease will be an activity conducted within primary health care.

The central, core role of genetics professionals will remain with the uncommon, Mendelian genetic disorders and genetic counselling will continue to focus on predictive testing, especially where tests are not clearly necessary for good medical management, and on reproductive issues where individuals need to make very personal decisions after careful consideration. However, an increasing proportion of our work may be dealing with the impact on families of incidental or additional findings from genomic investigations initiated by other, mainstream specialists who may be unwilling to apply such findimgs to the overall healyh care of their patients and their patients' extended families.

In the Mendelian cardiac disorders, the difficult issues will remain of (i) promoting family communication while respecting individuals' right to confidentiality, (ii) making "well" (i.e., "wisely") those difficult decisions about genetic testing and medical surveillance on behalf of young children and in the context of reproduction, (iii) managing those situations of uncertainty where variants are found in genes that are implicated in the inherited cardiac disorders, but when the variant found is not already known to cause the disorder (i.e., is of uncertain significance), and (iv) addressing the non-cardiac genetic findings of cardiac patients having genomic investigations (i.e., incidental or additional findings). Category (iii) will include many patients being investigated by other (non-cardiac) specialists, who are then found to carry a variant of (possible) significance for their risk of cardiac disease, just as category (iv) will comprise patients who begin as "cardiac patients" but are then drawn into a wider web of health concerns.

The disease-related context of sudden death ensures that these decisions are going to remain difficult and loaded with a high emotional charge, whatever scientific progress brings in terms of improved understanding, until a real cure becomes available (not just an ICD). We can offer a supportive relationship with a self-aware professional not only to the affected patients seen in clinic but also to their family members. We can also offer the best available interpretation of the significance of novel genetic variants and review these interpretations as new evidence accumulates, including the possibilities of gene editing and other rational and gene-based (if not always genetic) treatments.

These contributions will complement the therapeutic skills of our colleagues in cardiology and will indeed help to ensure that as many at-risk family members as possible will benefit from those skills.

References

1. Pua CJ, Bhalshankar J, Miao K, et al. Development of a comprehensive sequencing assay for inherited cardiac condition genes. J Cardiovasc Trans Res. 2016;9:3–11.
2. Sikkema-Raddatz B, Johansson LF, de Boer EN, et al. Targeted next-generation sequencing can replace Sanger sequencing in clinical diagnostics. Hum Mutat. 2013;34(7):1035–42.
3. Biesecker LG, Green RC. Diagnostic clinical genome and exome sequencing. N Engl J Med. 2014;370(25):2418–25.
4. Andreasen C, Nielsen JB, Refsgaard L, et al. New population-based exome data are questioning the pathogenicity of previously cardiomyopathy-associated genetic variants. Eur J Hum Genet. 2013;21:918–28.
5. Green RC, Berg JS, Grody WW, et al. ACMG recommendations for reporting of incidental findings in clinical exome and genome sequencing. Genet Med. 2013;15(7):565–74.
6. Lopes LR, Zekavati A, Syrris P, et al. Genetic complexity in hypertrophic cardiomyopathy revealed by high-throughput sequencing. J Med Genet. 2013;50(4):228–39.
7. Rehm HL, Berg JS, Brooks LD, Bustamante CD,Evans JP, Landrum MJ, Ledbetter DH, Maglott DR, Martin CL, Nussbaum RL, Plon SE, Ramos EM, Sherry ST, and Watson MS. ClinGen — The Clinical Genome Resource. N Engl J Med. 2015;372:2235–42. https://doi.org/10.1056/NEJMsr1406261
8. Elliott P, O'Mahony C, Syrris P, et al. Prevalence of desmosomal protein gene mutations in patients with dilated cardiomyopathy. Circ Cardiovasc Genet. 2010;3:314–22.

9. Garcia-Pavia P, Syrris P, Salas C, et al. Desmosomal protein gene mutations in patients with idiopathic dilated cardiomyopathy undergoing cardiac transplantation: a clinicopathological study. Heart. 2011;97:1744–52.
10. Cox MGPJ, van der Zwaag PA, van der Werf C, et al. Arrhythmogenic right ventricular dysplasia/cardiomyopathy pathogenic desmosome mutations in index-patients predict outcome of family screening: Dutch arrhythmogenic right ventricular dysplasia/cardiomyopathy genotype-phenotype follow-up study. Circulation. 2011;123:2690–700.
11. Davison C, Frankel S, Smith GD. The limits of lifestyle: re-assessing "fatalism" in the popular culture of illness prevention. Soc Sci Med. 1992;34(6):675–85.
12. Davison C, Smith GD, Frankel S. Lay epidemiology and the prevention paradox: the implications of coronary candidacy for health education. Sociol Health Illn. 1991;13:1–19.
13. Emslie C, Hunt K, Watt G. Invisible women? The importance of gender in lay beliefs about heart problems. Sociol Health Illn. 2001;23:203–33.
14. Hunt K, Emslie C, Watt G. Lay constructions of a family history of heart disease: potential for misunderstandings in the clinical encounter? Lancet. 2001;357:1168–71.
15. Tod AM, Read C, Lacey A, Abbott J. Barriers to uptake of services for coronary heart disease: qualitative study. BMJ. 2001;323:214–7.
16. Hall R, Saukko PM, Evans PH, Qureshi N, Humphries SE. Assessing family history of heart disease in primary care consultations: a qualitative study. Fam Pract. 2007;24:435–42.
17. Emery J, Lucassen A, Murphy M. Common hereditary cancers and implications for primary care. Lancet. 2001;358:56–63.
18. Lucassen A, Parker M, Wheeler R. Implications of data protection legislation for family history. BMJ. 2006;332:299–301.
19. Temple IK, Westwood G. Do once and share: clinical genetics. Department of Health—Connecting for Health. 2006.
20. Clarke A. Should families own genetic information? No. BMJ. 2007;335:23.
21. Bowker TJ, Wood DA, Davies MJ, et al. Sudden, unexpected cardiac or unexplained death in England: a national survey. QJM. 2003;96(4):269–79.
22. Roberts R, Brugada R. Genetics and arrhythmia. Annu Rev Med. 2003;54:257–67.
23. Fabre A, Sheppard MN. Sudden adult death syndrome and other nonischaemic causes of sudden cardiac death. Heart. 2006;92:316–20.
24. Cann F, Corbett M, O'Sullivan D, et al. Phenotype-driven molecular autopsy for sudden cardiac death. Clin Genet. 2017;91:22–9.
25. Christiansen SL, Hertz CL, Ferrero-Miliani L, et al. Genetic investigation of 100 heart genes in sudden unexplained death victims in a forensic setting. Eur J Hum Genet. 2016;24:1797–802.
26. Semsarian C, Ingles J, Wilde AAM. Sudden cardiac death in the young: the molecular autopsy and a practical approach to surviving relatives. Eur Heart J. 2015;36:1290–6.
27. Hertz CL, Christiansen SL, Larsen MK, et al. Genetic investigations of sudden unexpected deaths in infancy using next-generation sequencing of 100 genes associated with cardiac diseases. Eur J Hum Genet. 2016;24:817–22.
28. McCarthy Veach P, Bartels D, LeRoy BS. Coming full circle: a reciprocal engagement model of genetic counseling practice. J Genet Couns. 2007;16(6):713–28.
29. van Langen IM, Birnie E, Leschot NJ, et al. Genetic knowledge and counselling skills of Dutch cardiologists: sufficient for the genomics era? Eur Heart J. 2003;24:560–6.
30. Royse SD. Implications of genetic testing for sudden cardiac death syndrome. Br J Nurs. 2006;15:1104–7.
31. Bombard Y, Penziner E, Suchowersky O, et al. Engagement with genetic discrimination: concerns and experiences in the context of Hunrtington disease. Eur J Hum Genet. 2008;16:279–89.
32. Treloar TS, Barlow-Stewart K, Stranger M, Otlowski M. Investigating genetic discrimination in Australia: a large scale survey of clinical genetics clients. Clin Genet. 2008;74:20–30.
33. Elliott P, Andersson B, Arbustini E, et al. Classification of the cardiomyopathies: a position statement from the European Society of Cardiology Working Group on Myocardial and Pericardial Diseases. Eur Heart J. 2008;29(2):270–6.

34. Burkett EL, Hershberger RE. Clinical and genetic issues in familial dilated cardiomyopathy. J Am Coll Cardiol. 2005;45(7):969–81.
35. Hanson EL, Hershberger RE. Genetic counselling and screening issues in familial dilated cardiomyopathy. J Genet Couns. 2001;10:397–415.
36. Maron BJ, Shirani J, Poliac LC, et al. Sudden death in young competitive athletes. Clinical, demographic, and pathological profiles. JAMA. 1996;276(3):199–204.
37. ACC/ESC (American College of Cardiology/European Society of Cardiology). Clinical expert consensus document on hypertrophic cardiomyopathy. J Am Coll Cardiol. 2003;42:1687–713.
38. Yu B, French JA, Jeremy RW, et al. Counselling issues in familial hypertrophic cardiomyopathy. J Med Genet. 1998;35:183–8.
39. Semsarian C, Members of the CSANZ Cardiovascular Genetics Working Group. Guidelines for the diagnosis and management of hypertrophic cardiomyopathy. Heart Lung Circ. 2007;16:16–8.
40. Fokstuen S, Lyle R, Munoz A, et al. A DNA resequencing array for pathogenic mutation detection in hypertrophic cardiomyopathy. Hum Mutat. 2008;29(6):879–85.
41. Das KJ, Ingles J, Bagnall RD, Semsarian C. Determining pathogenicity of genetic variants in hypertrophic cardiomyopathy: importance of periodic reassessment. Genet Med. 2014;16(4):286–93.
42. Walsh R, Thomson KL, Ware JS, Exome Aggregation Consortium, et al. Reassessment of Mendelian gene pathogenicity using cardiomyopathy cases and 60,706 reference samples. Genet Med. 2017;19(2):192–203.
43. Manrai AK, Funke BH, Rehm HL, et al. Genetic misdiagnoses and the potential for health disparities. N Engl J Med. 2016;375:655–65.
44. Mouton JM, van der Merwe L, Goosen A, et al. MYBPH acts as modifier of cardiac hypertrophy in hypertrophic cardiomyopathy (HCM) patients. Hum Genet. 2016;135(5):477–83.
45. Ouellette AC, Jacob Mathew J, Manickaraj AK, et al. Clinical genetic testing in pediatric cardiomyopathy: is bigger better? Clin Genet. 2017. https://doi.org/10.1111/cge.13024.
46. Charron P, Héron D, Gargiulo M, et al. Genetic testing and genetic counselling in hypertrophic cardiomyopathy: the French experience. J Med Genet. 2002;39:741–6.
47. Christiaans I, Birnie E, Bonsel GJ, Wilde AAM, van Langen IM. Uptake of genetic counselling and predictive DNA testing in hypertrophic cardiomyopathy. Eur J Hum Genet. 2008;16(10):1201–7.
48. Lehnart SE, Ackerman MJ, Benson DW, et al. A National Heart Lung and Blood Institute and Office of Rare Diseases Workshop Consensus Report about the diagnosis, phenotyping, molecular mechanisms and therapeutic approaches for primary cardiomyopathies of gene mutations affecting ion channel function. Circulation. 2007;116:2325–45.
49. Schwartz PJ, Priori SG, Spazzolini C, et al. Genortype-phenotype correlation in the long-QT syndrome. Gene-specific triggers for life-thereatening arrhythmias. Circulation. 2001;103:89–95.
50. Crotti L, Spazzolini C, Schwartz PJ, et al. The common long-QT syndrome mutation KCNQ1/A341V causes unusually severe clinical manifestations in patients with different ethnic backgrounds. Towards a mutation-specific risk stratification. Circulation. 2007;116:2366–75.
51. Beckmann BM, Wilde AAM, Kääb S. Dual inheritance of sudden death from cardiovascular causes. N Engl J Med. 2008;358:2077–8.
52. Priori SG, Napolitano C, Giordano U, et al. Brugada syndrome and sudden cardiac death in children. Lancet. 2000;355(9206):808–9.
53. Roberts R. Genomics and cardiac arrhythmias. J Am Coll Cardiol. 2006;47(1):9–21.
54. Veldkamp MW, Viswanathan PC, Bezzina C, et al. Two distinct congenital arrhythmias evoked by a multidysfunctional Na(+) channel. Circ Res. 2000;86(9):E91–7.
55. Grant AO, Carboni MP, Neplioueva V, et al. Long QT syndrome, Brugada syndrome, and conduction system disease are linked to a single sodium channel mutation. J Clin Invest. 2002;110(8):1201–9.

56. Ackerman BA, Bartos DC, Kapplinger JD, et al. The promise and peril of precision medicine: phenotyping still matters most. Mayo Clin Proc. 2016;91(11):1606–16.
57. van Driest SL, Wells QS, Stallings S, et al. Association of arrhythmia-related genetic variants with phenotypes documented in electronic medical records. JAMA. 2016;315(1):47–57.
58. Riuro H, Campuzano O, Berne P, et al. Genetic analysis, in silico prediction, and family segregation in long QT syndrome. Eur J Hum Genet. 2015;23:79–85.
59. Ingles J, Lind J, Phongsavan P, Semsarian C. Psychosocial impact of specialized cardiac genetic clinics for hypertrophic cardiomyopathy. Genet Med. 2008;10:117–20.
60. Ingles J, Semsarian C. Sudden cardiac death in the young: a clinical genetic approach. Int Med J. 2007;37:32–7.
61. Al-Khatib SM, Yancy CW, Solis P, et al. AHA/ACC clinical performance and quality measures for prevention of sudden cardiac death: a report of the American College of Cardiology/American Heart Association Task Force on Performance Measures. J Am Coll Cardiol. 2017;69(6):712–44.
62. Ashley EA, Hershberger RE, Caleshu C, et al. Genetics and cardiovascular disease: a policy statement from the American Heart Association. Circulation. 2012;126:142–57.
63. Andersen J, Øyen N, Bjorvatn C, Gjengedal E. Living with long QT syndrome: a qualitative study of coping with increased risk of sudden cardiac death. J Genet Couns. 2008;17:489–98.
64. van der Werf C, Onderwater AT, van Langen IM, Smets EMA. Experiences, considerations and emotions relating to cardiogenetic evaluation in relatives of young sudden cardiac death victims. Eur J Hum Genet. 2014;22(2):192–6.
65. Ormondroyd E, Oates S, Parker M, et al. Pre-symptomatic genetic testing for inherited cardiac conditions: a qualitative exploration of psychosocial and ethical implications. Eur J Hum Genet. 2014;22:88–93.
66. Predham S, Hathaway J, Hulait G, et al. Patient recall, interpretation, and perspective of an inconclusive long QT syndrome genetic test result. J Genet Couns. 2017;26:150–8.
67. Manuel A, Brunger F. Making the decision to participate in predictive genetic testing for arrythmogenic right ventricular cardiomyopathy. J Genet Couns. 2014;23:1045–55.
68. Hamang A, Eide GE, Rokne B, et al. General anxiety, depression, and physical health in relation to symptoms of heart-focused anxietya cross sectional study among patients living with the risk of serious arrhythmias and sudden cardiac death. Health Qual Life Outcomes. 2011;9:100.
69. Hamang A, Eide GE, Rokne B, et al. Predictors of heart-focused anxiety in patients undergoing genetic investigation and counseling of long QT syndrome or hypertrophic cardiomyopathy: a one year follow-up. J Genet Couns. 2012;21:72–84.
70. Ingles J, Yeates L, O'Brien L, et al. Genetic testing for inherited heart diseases: longitudinal impact on health-related quality of life. Genet Med. 2012;14(8):749–52.
71. Maron BJ. Sudden death in young athletes. N Eng J Med. 2003;349:1064–75.
72. Hendricks KSWH, Grosfeld FJM, van Tintelen JP, et al. Can parents adjust to the idea that their child is at risk of sudden death?: psychological impact of risk for long QT syndrome. Am J Med Genet. 2005;138A:107–12.
73. Smets EMA, Stam MMH, Meulenkamp TM, et al. Health-related quality of life of children with a positive carrier status for inherited cardiovascular diseases. Am J Med Genet. 2008;146A:700–7.
74. Starke M, Möller A. Parents' needs for knowledge concerning the medical diagnosis of their children. J Child Health Care. 2002;6:245–57.
75. Clinical Genetics Society. The genetic testing of children. Report of a Working Party of the Clinical Genetics Society (UK) (chair, Clarke A). J Med Genet. 1994;31:785–97.
76. European Society of Human Genetics. Genetic testing in asymptomatic minors: recommendations of the European Society of Human Genetics. Eur J Hum Genet. 2009;17:720–1.
77. Gaff C, Lynch E, Spencer L. Predictive testing of eighteen year olds: counseling challenges. J Genet Couns. 2006;15:245–51.

78. Richards FH. Maturity of judgement in decision making for predictive testing for nontreatable adult-onset neurogenetic conditions: a case against predictive testing of minors. Clin Genet. 2006;70:396–401.
79. Geelen E, van Hoyweghen I, Doevendans PA, Marcelis CLM, Horstman K. Constructing 'Best Interests': genetic testing of children in families with hypertrophic cardiomyopathy. Am J Med Genet A. 2011a;155A(8):1930–8.
80. Geelen E, van Hoyweghen I, Horstman K. Making genetics not so important: family work in dealing with familial hypertrophic cardiomyopathy. Soc Sci Med. 2011b;72(2011):1752–9.
81. Cohen LL, Stoleman M, Walsh C, et al. Challenges of genetic testing in adolescents with cardiac arrythmia syndromes. J Med Ethics. 2012;38:163–7.
82. Keenan KF, Simpson SA, Wlson BJ, et al. 'It's their blood not mine': who's responsible for (not) telling relatives about genetic risk? Health Risk Soc. 2005;7:209–26.
83. Kenen R, Ardern-Jones A, Eeles R. We are talking but are they listening? Communication patterns in families with a history of breast/ovarian cancer (HBOC). Psycho-Oncology. 2004;13:335–45.
84. Clarke A, Sarangi S, Verrier Jones K. Voicing the lifeworld: parental accounts of responsibility in genetic consultations for Polycystic Kidney Disease. Soc Sci Med. 2011;72:1743–51.
85. Manjoney DM, McKegney FP. Individual and family coping with polycystic kidney disease: the harvest of denial. Int J Psychiatry Med. 1978;9:19–31.
86. Etchegary H. Discovering the family history of Huntington disease (HD). J Genet Couns. 2006;15:105–17.
87. Järvinen O, Aalto A-M, Lehesjoki A-E, et al. Carrier testing of children for two X linked diseases in a family based settzing: a retrospective long term psychosocial evaluation. J Med Genet. 1999;36:615–20.
88. Jolly A, Parsons E, Clarke A. Identifying carriers of balanced chromosomal translocations: interviews with family members. In: Clarke A, editor. The genetic testing of children. Oxford, Washington DC: Bios Scientific Publishers; 1998. p. 61–90.
89. McAllister M, Payne K, Nicholls S, et al. Improving service evaluation in clinical genetics: identifying effects of genetic diseases on individuals and families. J Genet Couns. 2007;16(1):71–83.
90. Metcalfe A, Coad J, Plumridge GM. Family communication between children and their parents about inherited genetic conditions: a meta-synthesis of the research. Eur J Hum Genet. 2008;16(10):1193–200.
91. Adelsward V, Sachs L. The messenger's dilemmas—giving and getting information in genealogical mapping for hereditary cancer. Health Risk Soc. 2005;5:125–38.
92. Featherstone K, Bharadwaj A, Clarke A, Atkinson P. Risky relations: family and kinship in the era of new genetics. Oxford: Berg Publishers; 2006.
93. Peterson SK, Watts BG, Koehly LM, et al. How families communicate about HNPCC genetic testing: findings from a qualitative study. Am J Med Genet. 2003;119C:78–86.
94. Foster C, Eeles R, Ardern-Jones A, et al. Juggling roles and expectations: dilemmas faced by women talking to relatives about cancer and genetic testing. Psychol Health. 2004;19:439–55.
95. Hallowell N, Foster C, Eeles R, et al. Balancing autonomy and responsibility: the ethics of generating and disclosing genetic information. J Med Ethics. 2003;29:74–9.
96. Dudok de Wit AC, Tibben A, Frets PG, et al. BRCA1 in the family: a case description of the psychological implications. Am J Med Genet. 1997;71:63–71.
97. Vavolizza RD, Kalia I, Aaron KE, et al. Disclosing genetic information to family members about inherited cardiac arrhythmias: an obligation or a choice? J Genet Couns. 2015;24:608–15.
98. Clarke A, Richards MPM, Kerzin-Storrar L, et al. Genetic professionals' reports of nondisclosure of genetic risk information within families. Eur J Hum Genet. 2005;13:556–62.
99. Clarke A. Challenges to genetic privacy. The control of personal genetic information. In: Harper PS, Clarke A, editors. Genetics, society and clinical practice. Oxford: Bios Scientific Publishers; 1997b. p. 149–64.
100. American Society of Human Genetics Statement. Professional disclosure of familial genetic information. Am J Hum Genet. 1998;62:474–83.

101. Forrest LE, Curnow L, Delatycki MB, et al. Health first, genetics second: exploring families' experiences of communicating genetic information. Eur J Hum Genet. 2008a;16(11):1329–3.
102. Gilbar R. Communicating genetic information in the family: the familial relationship as the forgotten factor. J Med Ethics. 2007;33:390–3.
103. Forrest LE, Burke J, Bacic S, Amor DJ. Increased genetic counselling support improves communication of genetic information in families. Genet Med. 2008b;10:167–72.
104. McKinnon W, Naud S, Ashikaga T, et al. Results of an intervention for individuals and families with BRCA mutations: a model for providing medical updates and psychosocial support following genetic testing. J Genet Couns. 2007;16:433–56.
105. Speice J, McDaniel SH, Rowley PT, Loader S. Family issues in a psychoeducational group for women with a BRCA mutation. Clin Genet. 2002;62:121–7.
106. van den Nieuwenhoff HWP, Mesters I, Gielen C, de Vries NK. Family communication regarding inherited high cholesterol: why and how do patients disclose genetic risk? Soc Sci Med. 2007;65:1025–37.
107. Gaff C, Clarke AJ, Atkinson PA, et al. Process and outcome in communication of genetic information within families: a systematic review. Eur J Hum Genet. 2007;15:999–1011.
108. Nycum G, Avard D, Knoppers BM. Factors influencing intrafamilial communication of hereditary breast and ovarian cancer genetic information. Eur J Hum Genet. 2009;17(7):872–80.
109. Wilson BJ, Forrest K, van Teijlingen ER, et al. Family communication about genetic risk: the little that is known. Community Genet. 2004;7:15–24.
110. Lipkus IM, Hollands JG. The visual communication of risk. J Natl Cancer Inst Monogr. 1997;25:149.
111. Lippman-Hand A, Fraser FC. Genetic counselling: provision and reception of information. Am J Med Genet. 1979a;3:113–27.
112. Lippman-Hand A, Fraser F. Genetic counselling: the post-counselling period: I. Patients' perceptions of uncertainty. Am J Med Genet. 1979b;4:51–71.
113. Julian-Reynier C, Welkenhuysen M, Hagoel L, et al. Risk communication strategies: state of the art and effectiveness in the context of cancer genetic services. Eur J Hum Genet. 2003;11:725–36.
114. Edwards A, Elwyn G, Mulley AI. Explaining risks: turning numerical data into meaningful pictures. BMJ. 2002;324:827–30.
115. O'Doherty K, Suthers GK. Risky communication: pitfalls in counselling about risk, and how to avoid them. J Genet Couns. 2007;16:409–17.
116. Krynski TR, Tenenbaum JB. The role of causality in judgement under uncertainty. J Exp Psychol Gen. 2007;136:430–50.
117. Skirton H. The client's perspective of genetic counseling. A grounded theory study. J Genet Couns. 2001;10:311–29.
118. Christiaans I, van Lange IM, Birnie E, et al. Genetic counseling and cardiac care in predictively tested hypertrophic cardiomyopathy mutation carriers: the patients' perspective. Am J Med Genet A. 2009;149A:1444–51.
119. Gargiulo M, Lejeune S, Tanguy ML, et al. Long-term outcome of presymptomatic testing in Huntington disease. Eur J Hum Genet. 2009;17(2):165–71.
120. Charron P, Héron D, Gargiulo M, et al. Prenatal molecular diagnosis in hypertrophic cardiomyopathy: report of the first case. Prenat Diagn. 2004;24(9):701–3.
121. Dudok de Wit AC, Tibben A, Duivenvoorden HJ, et al. Distress in individuals facing predictive DNA testing for autosomal dominant late-onset disorders: comparing questionnaire results with in-depth interviews. Am J Med Genet. 1998;75:62–74.
122. Smith JA, Michie S, Stephenson M, Quarrel O. Risk perception and decision-making processes in candidates for genetic testing for Huntington's disease: an interpretative phenomenological analysis. J Health Psychol. 2002;7:131–44.
123. Taylor SD. Predictive genetic test decisions for Huntington's disease: context, appraisal and new moral imperatives. Soc Sci Med. 2004;58:137–49.

124. Wald DS, Bestwick JP, Morris JK, et al. Child–parent familial hypercholesterolemia screening in primary care. N Engl J Med. 2016;375:1628–37.
125. Humphries SE, Ridker PM, Talmud PJ. Genetic testing for cardiovascular disease susceptibility: a useful clinical management tool or possible misinformation? Arterioscler Thromb Vasc Biol. 2004;24:628–36.
126. Janssens ACJW, Gwinn M, Bradley LA, et al. A crtitical appraisal of the scientific basis of commercial genomic profiles used to assess health risks and personalize health interventions. Am J Hum Genet. 2008;82:593–9.
127. Muntwyler J, Lüscher TF. Assessment of cardiovascular risk: time to apply genetic risk factors? Eur Heart J. 2000;21:611–3.
128. Hippisley-Cox J, Coupland C, Vinogradova Y, et al. Predicting cardiovascular risk in England and Wales: prospective derivation and validation of QRISK2. BMJ. 2008;336:1475–82.
129. McQueen MJ, Hawken S, Wang X, et al. Lipids, lipoproteins, and apolipoproteins as risk markers of myocardial infarction in 52 countries (the INTERHEART study): a case-control study. Lancet. 2008;372:224–33.
130. Saukko PM, Ellard S, Richards SH. Patients' understanding of genetic susceptibility testing in mainstream medicine: qualitative study on thrombophilia. BMC Health Serv Res. 2007;7:82.
131. Timmermans S, Buchbinder M. Patients-in-waiting: living between sickness and health in the genomics era. J Health Soc Behav. 2010;51(4):408–23.
132. Troughton J, Jarvis J, Skinner C, et al. Waiting for diabetes: perceptions of people with pre-diabetes: a qualitative study. Patient Educ Couns. 2008;72:88–93.
133. Talmud PJ, Shah S, Whittall R, et al. Use of low-density lipoprotein cholesterol gene score to distinguish patients with polygenic and monogenic familial hypercholesterolaemia: a case-control study. Lancet. 2013;381(9874):1293–301.
134. Clarke A. The genetic dissection of multifactorial disease. The implications of screening for susceptibility to disease. In: Harper PS, Clarke A, editors. Genetics, society and clinical practice. Oxford: Bios Scientific Publishers; 1997a. p. 93–106.
135. Chaufan C. How much can a large population study on genes, environments, their interactions and common diseases contribute to the health of the American people? Soc Sci Med. 2007;65:1730–41.
136. Humphries SE, Cranston T, Allen M, et al. Mutational analysis in UK patients with a clinical diagnosis of familial hypercholesterolaemia: relationship with plasma lipid traits, heart disease risk and utility in relative tracing. J Mol Med. 2006;84:203–14.
137. Heath KE, Humphries SE, Middleton-Price H, Boxer M. A molecular genetic service for diagnosing individuals with familial hypercholesterolaemia (FH) in the United Kingdom. Eur J Hum Genet. 2001;9:244–52.
138. Humphries SE, Galton D, Nicholls P. Genetic testing for familial hypercholesterolaemia. QJM. 1997;90:169–81.
139. Umans-Eckenhausen MAW, Defesche JC, Sijbrands EJG, et al. Review of first 5 years of screening for familial hypercholesterolaemia in the Netherlands. Lancet. 2001;357:165–8.
140. Clarke A. Population screening for genetic susceptibility to disease. BMJ. 1995;311:35–8.
141. Senior V, Smith JA, Michie S, Marteau TM. Making sense of risk: an interpretive phenomenological analysis of vulnerability to heart disease. J Health Psychol. 2002;7:157–68.
142. Marteau T, Senior V, Humphries SE, et al. Psychological impact of genetic testing for familial hypercholesterolemia within a previously aware population: a randomized controlled trial. Am J Med Genet A. 2004;128A:285–93.
143. Senior V, Marteau TM. Causal attributions for raised cholesterol and perceptions of effective risk-reduction: self-regulation strategies for an increased risk of cotronary heart disease. Psychol Health. 2007;22:699–717.
144. Joyner MJ. Seven questions for personalized medicine. JAMA. 2015;314(10):999–1000.
145. Marteau TM, French DP, Griffin SJ, et al. Effects of communicating DNA-based disease risk estimates on risk-reducing behaviours (review). Cochrane Libr. 2010;10:1–74.

146. McBride CM, Koehly LM, Sanderson SC, Kaphingst KA. The behavioural response to personalised genetic risk information: will genetic risk profiles motivate individuals and families to choose more healthful behaviours? Annu Rev Public Health. 2010;31:89–103.
147. Scientific Steering Committee on behalf of the Simon Broome Register Group. Mortality in treated heterozygotes for familial hypercholesterolaemia: implications for clinical management. Atherosclerosis. 1999;142:105–12.
148. Smilde TJ, van Wissen S, Wollersheim H, et al. Effect of aggressive versus conventional lipid lowering on atherosclerosis progression in familial hypercholesterolaemia (ASAP): a prospective randomised, double-blind trial. Lancet. 2001;357:577–81.
149. Sever PS, Poulter NR, Dahlof B, Wedel H, Beevers G, Caulfield M, Collins R, Kjeldsen SE, Kristinsson A, McInnes G, Mehlsen J, Nieminen MS, O'Brien ET, Ostergren J, ASCOT Investigators. The Anglo-Scandinavian Cardiac Outcomes Trial lipid lowering arm: extended observations 2 years after trial closure. Eur Heart J. 2008;29(4):499–508.
150. Marks D, Wonderling D, Thorogood M, et al. Cost effectiveness analysis of different approaches of screening for familial hypercholesterolaemia. BMJ. 2002;324:1303.
151. UK National Screening Committee. Criteria for appraising the viability, effectiveness and appropriateness of a screening programme. London: Department of Health; 2009.
152. UK National Screening Committee. Screening for familial hypercholesterolaemia in children. London: Department of Health; 2016.
153. Horstman K, Smand C. Detecting familial hypercholesterolaemia: escaping the family history? In: de Vries G, Horstman K, editors. Genetics from laboratory to society. societal learning as an alternative to regulation. Basingstoke: Palgrave Macmillan; 2008. p. 90–117.
154. Newson A, Humphries SE. Cascade testing in familial hypercholesterolaemia: how should family members be contacted? Eur J Hum Genet. 2005;13:401–8.
155. Parsons EP, Clarke AJ, Hood K, et al. Feasibility of a change in service delivery: the case of optional newborn screening for Duchenne muscular dystrophy. Community Genet. 2000;3(1):17–23.
156. London IDEAS Genetics Knowledge Park. Department of health familial hypercholesterolaemia cascade testing audit project. Recommendations to the Department of Health. 2007.
157. van Maarle MC, Stouthard MEA, van den Mheen PJM, et al. How disturbing is it to be approached for a genetic cascade screening programme for familial hypercholesterolaemia? Community Genet. 2001;4:244–52.
158. van den Nieuwenhoff HWP, Mesters I, Nellissen JJTM, et al. The importance of written information packages in support of case-finding within families at risk for inherited high cholesterol. J Genet Couns. 2006;15:29–40.
159. Suthers GK, Armstrong J, McCormack J, Trott D. Letting the family know: balancing ethics and effectiveness when notifying relatives about genetic testing for a familial disorder. J Med Genet. 2006;43:665–70.
160. Wald DS, Bestwick JP, Wald NJ. Child-parent screening for familial hypercholesterolaemia: screening strategy based on a meta-analysis. Br Med J. 2007;335:599–603.
161. Hopcroft KA. Child-parent screening may have adverse psychological effects. BMJ. 2007;335:683.
162. Senior V, Marteau TM, Peters TJ. Will genetic fatalism for predisposition for disease result in fatalism? A qualitative study of parents' responses to neonatal screening for familial hypercholesterolaemia. Soc Sci Med. 1999;48:1857–60.
163. Chow CK, Dominiczak AF, Pell JP, et al. Families of patients with premature coronary heaert disease: an obvious but neglected target for primary prevention. BMJ. 2007;335:481–5.
164. Priori SG, Schwartz PJ, Napolitano C, et al. Risk stratification in the long-QT syndrome. N Engl J Med. 2003;348(19):1866–74.
165. Samani NJ, Erdmann J, Hall AS, et al. Genomewide association analysis of coronary artery disease. N Engl J Med. 2007;357:443–53.

Multi-Disciplinary Management of Inherited Cardiovascular Conditions

29

Gerry Carr-White and Robert Leema

Abstract

The complex and chronic nature of inherited cardiovascular conditions (ICCs) require a multi-disciplinary approach to provide holistic care. This ensures appropriate diagnosis, risk assessment, management, cascade screening and/or genetic testing; and psychological support for patients and their families. In this chapter, we describe the rationale and ideal setting for a multi-disciplinary team approach and the unique contribution of various professionals and groups within the team.

Case studies are used to illustrate the multiple needs of families affected by ICCs and the pivotal role of the multi-disciplinary team in delivering and coordinating their care. This includes the comprehensive services required by the family of a child with sudden arrhythmic death syndrome where decisions were being made for individual care as well as reproductive choices in a highly emotional situation; and that of a patient with multiple symptoms requiring a unifying diagnosis.

Keywords

Inherited cardiovascular conditions • Cardiovascular genetics • Multi-disciplinary clinic

G. Carr-White (✉) • R. Leema
Guys and St Thomas' NHS Foundation Trust, South East Thames Regional Genetics Centre, Guys Hospital, London, UK
e-mail: Gerry.Carr-White@gstt.nhs.uk; Leema.Robert@gstt.nhs.uk

D. Kumar, P. Elliott (eds.), *Cardiovascular Genetics and Genomics*, https://doi.org/10.1007/978-3-319-66114-8_29

29.1 Introduction

In many countries multi-disciplinary approach has become widely accepted in management of patients with long term conditions. In the UK, this approach has been endorsed by the Department of Health as a core model for managing chronic diseases [1]. The need for multi-disciplinary work has emerged as a result of increase in complex, specialized medical knowledge and promotion of the patient's role in their own care.

Multidisciplinary teams (MDT) bring together professionals from different disciplines with specialist knowledge, skills and expertise, aiming to provide high quality care for patients. Team members are involved in the assessment, diagnosis, treatment and care of individual patients. Main activities of an MDT are regular meetings (weekly, fortnightly, monthly) and/or multi-disciplinary clinics (i.e. a number of consultations with different team members during a single patient's visit). The clinical decision making process results in MDT recommendations which are evidence based, in line with standard treatment protocols (where possible), and patient-centered.

There is great variability in effectiveness of multi-disciplinary teams across disciplines and within disciplines across different geographical regions [2]. Data have demonstrated that multidisciplinary decisions or interventions improve clinical outcomes for individual patients [heart failure MDTs [3], cancer MDTs [4], stroke rehabilitation MDTs [5] etc.]. Despite all identified benefits, there is still limited evidence on overall cost-effectiveness of multi-disciplinary approach in clinical practice [6].

In this chapter we discuss the specifics of multidisciplinary team work within Inherited Cardiovascular Conditions (ICC) service.

29.2 Complex Nature of Inherited Cardiovascular Conditions

Inherited cardiovascular conditions (ICC) are rare, complex and very variable group of disorders. Four main categories of ICC are:

- *Inherited arrhythmias*, caused by mutations in genes encoding proteins that are involved in action potential (Long QT syndrome, Short QT syndrome, Brugada syndrome, Catecholaminergic Polymorphic Ventricular Tachycardia CPVT)
- *Cardiomyopathies*, caused by mutations in genes encoding proteins of the contractile system of cardiomyocytes (Hypertrophic Cardiomyopathy, Dilated Cardiomyopathy, Restrictive Cardiomyopathy, Left ventricular non-compaction, Arrhythmogenic Right Ventricular Dysplasia)
- *Inherited aortopathies*, manifesting as catastrophic blood vessel rupture, caused by mutations in genes encoding for connective tissue proteins (Marfan syndrome, Loeys-Dietz syndrome, Elher Danlos Syndrome)
- *Muscular dystrophies*, a systemic genetic conditions that cause skeletal muscle weakness and sometimes affect heart's conduction system or heart muscle, causing

arrhythmias and/or cardiomyopathies (Emery-Dreifuss muscular dystrophy, Myotonic dystrophy, Duchene muscular dystrophy, Becker's muscular dystrophy, Limb-girdle muscular dystrophy)

29.2.1 Epidemiology of ICC

Epidemiological data on prevalence of ICCs are incomplete. This is because of the rarity of conditions in general population, genetic heterogeneity, incomplete penetrance, and difficulty in distinguishing ICCs from common multi-factorial conditions with similar symptoms. NHS Commissioning board [7] have estimated that total prevalence of ICCs is 340,000 cases in the UK (including 120,000 individuals affected by familial hypercholesterolemia). Collectively ICCs potentially represent significant burden of disease in the UK population.

29.2.2 Genetics of ICC

These are largely monogenic disorders with variable penetrance (not all individuals with a disease causing mutation will show clinical symptoms, or these are latent in the absence of triggering factors). Most ICCs show a great deal of genetic heterogeneity-one condition can be caused by numerous mutations in many different genes. In the last decade, the complexity of ICCs has been magnified with advances in technology that enabled better understanding of their underlying genetic basis. With next generation sequencing, simultaneous testing of multiple genes is available in shorter period of time and at significantly lower cost. However, with the use of available technology, genetic test results may reveal sequence changes that are not easy to interpret. Therefore, both clinical and genetic findings need to be carefully considered when *establishing a diagnosis* in the index case.

29.2.3 Clinical Management of Individuals with ICC

Individuals with suspected ICC require specialist assessment. Patient's pathway within an established ICC service involves investigations to establish the diagnosis (including genetic testing), surveillance and clinical management of the condition, family screening, establishing the risk for future offspring and reproductive options if applicable.

Establishing the diagnosis includes analyzing: personal and family history, electrocardiogram (including exercise ECG, ambulatory ECG, or signal-averaged ECG), echocardiography, routine and specialized blood tests (including metabolic investigations), specialized cardiovascular imaging (CMR, cardiac CT), electrophysiology investigations (Ajmalin test, electrophysiology studies), and if appropriate genetic testing.

Once a diagnosis is established, management of ICC involves advice on avoidance of triggering factors (exercise or certain medications), treatment with medications and/or device implantation, if appropriate, interventional treatment (alcohol septal ablation, septal myectomy in management of obstructive HCM; aortic root replacement and Aortic Valve Replacement in aortopathies), and where necessary surveillance and preventative measures. A minority of individuals affected by ICC is at risk of sudden cardiac death, and therefore significant part in management of ICC is recognizing those at risk (*risk stratification*).

If genetic basis of the diagnosis is established, cascade predictive testing is offered to all first degree relatives. If applicable, Geneticist estimates the risk of future offspring being affected by the condition and discusses various reproductive options that may provide avoidance of the condition in subsequent generations.

29.2.4 Looking After Families of Individuals with ICC

The nature of ICCs includes the need to extend investigations to the families of affected individuals. All of their first degree relatives are eligible for 'cascade' testing. This can involve clinical assessment for the possibility of shared phenotypes, or genetic testing if a disease causing mutation was identified in the index case. Cascade genetic testing has been shown for some ICCs to be cost-effective [8, 9]. Family members who have not inherited familial mutation can be reassured and also spared regular clinical testing. With advances in genetic testing, looking after families with ICC includes discussing the options for avoiding presence of ICC in future offspring (prenatal diagnostic options and pre-implantation genetics).

29.3 Multidisciplinary Management for Inherited Cardiovascular Conditions

Care for the individuals with ICC and their families is provided in centers with specialists who have expertise in managing a full range of inherited cardiovascular conditions. ICC services are usually based in major tertiary centers, where regional genetic service is also available. The complex and varied nature of ICCs, implications for other family members, and increase in specialized medical knowledge created a clear need for ICCs to be managed by multi-disciplinary teams. Multidisciplinary work within ICC services is shaped by unique and complex characteristics of inherited cardiovascular conditions. The aim is to provide holistic care for the patients and their families.

Review of ICC service showed that there is a great variability in service provision across the UK, both in terms of quality and quantity [10]. Some services provide 'one stop' multidisciplinary clinics where patient has the opportunity to be seen by different specialists during one visit only. Particularly complex cases are discussed in multidisciplinary setting during regular MDT meetings. Another model for ensuring provision of service for the whole population of a region is 'hub and spoke' model. More specialized elements of care are delivered within tertiary centers whilst less specialized aspects of care are provided by district cardiology services. For remote areas service is provided through 'satellite' (outreach) clinics.

Team members and their roles may differ in different centers, but here we describe the main roles of the ICC multidisciplinary team. The *core* team members are Cardiologist, Geneticist and Cardiogenetic nurse. Holistic care is provided in liaison of core MDT members with other specialist services.

29.3.1 Consultant Cardiologist

The role of cardiologist is to make a clinical diagnosis, assess the risk of sudden cardiac death, and be involved in ongoing clinical management of the patients. For a successful role, it is necessary to have expertise in interpretation of cardiological investigations and this involves experience in echocardiography, specialized cardiac imaging, and electrophysiology. Regular specialist follow-up and advice on cardiac management requires expertise in heart failure and management of arrhythmias. Cardiologist with specialist interest in ICC also has a good understanding of the value of genetic testing in diagnosis and management of patients with ICC.

Inherited cardiovascular conditions MDT includes Cardiologists from different sub-specialties: Electrophysiologists, Cardiac Imaging Consultants, Heart failure specialists with interest in Inherited Cardiovascular Conditions, specialists in Adult Congenital Heart Conditions, and for assessment of feasibility of septal myectomy in HCM patients, expertise of Interventional Cardiologists.

Some inherited cardiac conditions present in childhood, and therefore the role of Pediatric cardiologist is equally important. The necessary expertise involves knowledge of age-specific clinical management and insight into psychological, social, and ethical issues in management of conditions with genetic basis in children. There is also a significant role in transition of care of adolescents to adult services that is led by Pediatric Cardiologist.

29.3.2 Consultant Clinical Geneticist

The role of geneticists is primarily in the diagnosis of ICC, and requires expert knowledge of both phenotype and genotype of ICC. This involves clinical expertise in recognizing dysmorphic features associated with rare genetic syndromes, and knowledge of rare metabolic and neuromuscular conditions associated with cardiac involvement. Based on clinical assessment geneticist may make recommendations on diagnostic genetic testing strategies in individual cases. Geneticist is also involved in interpretation of genetic test results including uncertain findings, and provides advice on utility of genetic testing within the family. Part of managing families with ICC involves not only cascade genetic testing but also providing counseling on the recurrence risk for future offspring, and options for prenatal and pre-implantation diagnosis. In some couples other reproductive options may be suitable (egg/sperm donor, surrogacy etc.) and geneticists coordinates the referral to Reproductive Medicine specialists.

ICC Multidisciplinary team usually involves Cardiac geneticist and when required Consultant Geneticist with specialist interest in Pre-Implantation Genetic Diagnosis.

29.3.3 Specialist Cardiac Genetic Nurse

The role of cardiac genetic nurses is in coordinating the care for patient with ICC and their families. This entails arranging specialized investigations, clinical appointments, and links with other specialized services depending on individual needs. They also provide emotional and psychological support to affected individuals and their families. Part of this role is to provide clear and easy to understand information on the condition and its symptoms. Within many multi-disciplinary teams specialist cardiac genetic nurses are the first point of contact for patients' queries.

29.3.4 Genetic Counselor

Genetic counselor has multiple roles within ICC multidisciplinary team, and this varies across the services. They are involved in taking family history and drawing up detailed family tree, as well as developing and keeping genetic registers and other records. Counselors also have a role in eliciting patient's expectations and concerns and based on that provide appropriate psychological support. They are involved in counseling family members who are undergoing predictive genetic testing. This requires knowledge of natural history of ICCs as well as understanding of support networks that provide education and support to patients. They are also involved in counseling on the recurrence risk and options for prenatal diagnosis.

29.3.5 Cardiac Physiologist

Cardiac physiologists involved in care of patients with ICC have expertise in echocardiography, electrophysiology, or cardiopulmonary exercise testing. They work closely with cardiologist in interpreting abnormalities specific to ICCs.

29.3.6 Cardiac Pathologist

The role of pathologist is in establishing the cause of death where underlying ICC is suspected. This sometimes involves referral to cardiac pathologists who specialize in sudden cardiac death. Their role is also in guiding further investigations including genetic testing, and with appropriate permission, retention of tissues for further testing in future.

29.3.7 Clinical Scientist

Clinical scientists have a major role in provision of laboratory genetic test results from accredited genetic laboratories. They are involved in planning the most appropriate testing strategies for individual referrals. They are responsible for interpretation of genetic test results, and for recommendations on further investigations and testing of other family members.

29.3.8 Other Specialist Services

Some ICCs are systemic disorders and their management requires involvement of other specialists. Patients with Marfan syndrome require follow-up by ophthalmologist, and rheumatologist. Heart is affected in different rare inherited metabolic disorders and these patients require follow-up by specialists in Metabolic medicine. Similarly, neuromuscular conditions with cardiac involvement require significant input from Neurology services. The role of ICC multidisciplinary service is to ensure good links with other related specialties.

29.3.9 Support Groups and Voluntary Organizations

Support groups and voluntary organizations provide valuable practical and psychological support for patients. Support groups often organize patient information sessions with updates on the new developments in the field. It is sometimes that within ICC service patients find out about the support groups in the first instance. Here we provide a (non-exhaustive) list of support groups in the UK.

Cardiomyopathy UK www.cardiomyopathy.org
CRY-Cardiac Risk in the Young www.c-r-y.org.uk
SADS UK- Sudden Arrhythmic Death Syndrome www.sads.org.uk
Arrhythmia alliance www.heartrhythmcharity.org.uk
Marfan Association UK www.marfan-association.org.uk

On the following pages we discuss clinical cases where the role of multidisciplinary work of ICC service has been vital in providing integrated holistic care for patients and their families.

29.4 Clinical Cases

29.4.1 Case 1

29.4.1.1 Case History

Following tragic sudden death of an 18 months old girl, her parents were referred for genetic counseling to their Regional Genetics Service. At the time of the appointment molecular test results were available.

She was the first child to healthy, unrelated Caucasian parents. *Detailed history* revealed that she was born at 38 weeks of gestation via normal delivery. The labour was induced, as her mother suffered from preeclampsia, but there were no complications. The baby had a tongue tie and a torticolis. Her physical and mental development were normal, and she was a healthy child. In retrospect, her parents described two unusual episodes that they witnessed long before the tragic death of their daughter. On one occasion, she was in a car seat when her eyes suddenly appeared hooded, and her head was leaning backward. She did not appear to be asleep at the time. When her father lifted her head, she started crying. On another occasion she was in a car seat when she appeared to have a blank expression on her face for about 10 min. Soon thereafter she started crying. She was well in herself prior to both episodes and there was no history of seizure activity. The consultant Clinical Geneticist reviewed her photographs at the time of genetics appointment, but no unusual facial features were observed.

On the day when she passed away, the family were visiting friends who were based in the neighboring county. She was well in herself and for a few hours she was playing in the park. In the course of the day, she had an episode of a loose stool, but no diarrhea. Before going to bed, she had a warm meal and her body felt warm. She had some milk to settle down, but soon thereafter she became limp, her eyes rolled backwards and she became unresponsive. Her parents started CPR and ambulance arrived within 10 min of the event.

After the girl's sudden death, a *post mortem examination* was performed on coroner's request. It revealed that there were no anatomical cardiovascular abnormalities. There were no anatomical abnormalities in other internal organs. Microbiology, virology and toxicology testing was unremarkable. There was no evidence of metabolic disease (Oil-Red-O stain was used as a screening test for metabolic disorders). Neuropathology examination showed acute global cerebral hypoxia which was consistent with clinical presentation. Karyotype was normal female 46 (XX).

By the time of genetic appointment the results of parental studies were available. Genetic testing in the mother revealed that she had the genetic change in the KCNQ1 gene and both genetic changes in SCN5A gene were detected in the father. During focused history taking, the father reported occasional episodes of palpitations and lightheadedness when getting up from a sitting position, but there were no syncopal episodes. He has been fit and well. He had regularly run several miles twice a week and in the past he completed a marathon. The mother had two near-fainting episodes, first one a few years earlier as she was anticipating a bad news from her doctor (stress fracture of the hip), and one during the labour. She has otherwise been fit and well, and engaged in moderate intensity exercise.

Based on the above findings the next steps in understanding the clinical importance of the variants were *segregation studies* in wider family, and establishing any *genotype-phenotype correlation* in individual family members.

Three generation *family history* was also obtained during the appointment. Details of this are in Fig. 29.1. On the maternal side of the family there was history of sudden death in infancy, in maternal great uncle. The cause of death on death certificate was documented as suffocation secondary to suppurative bronchitis.

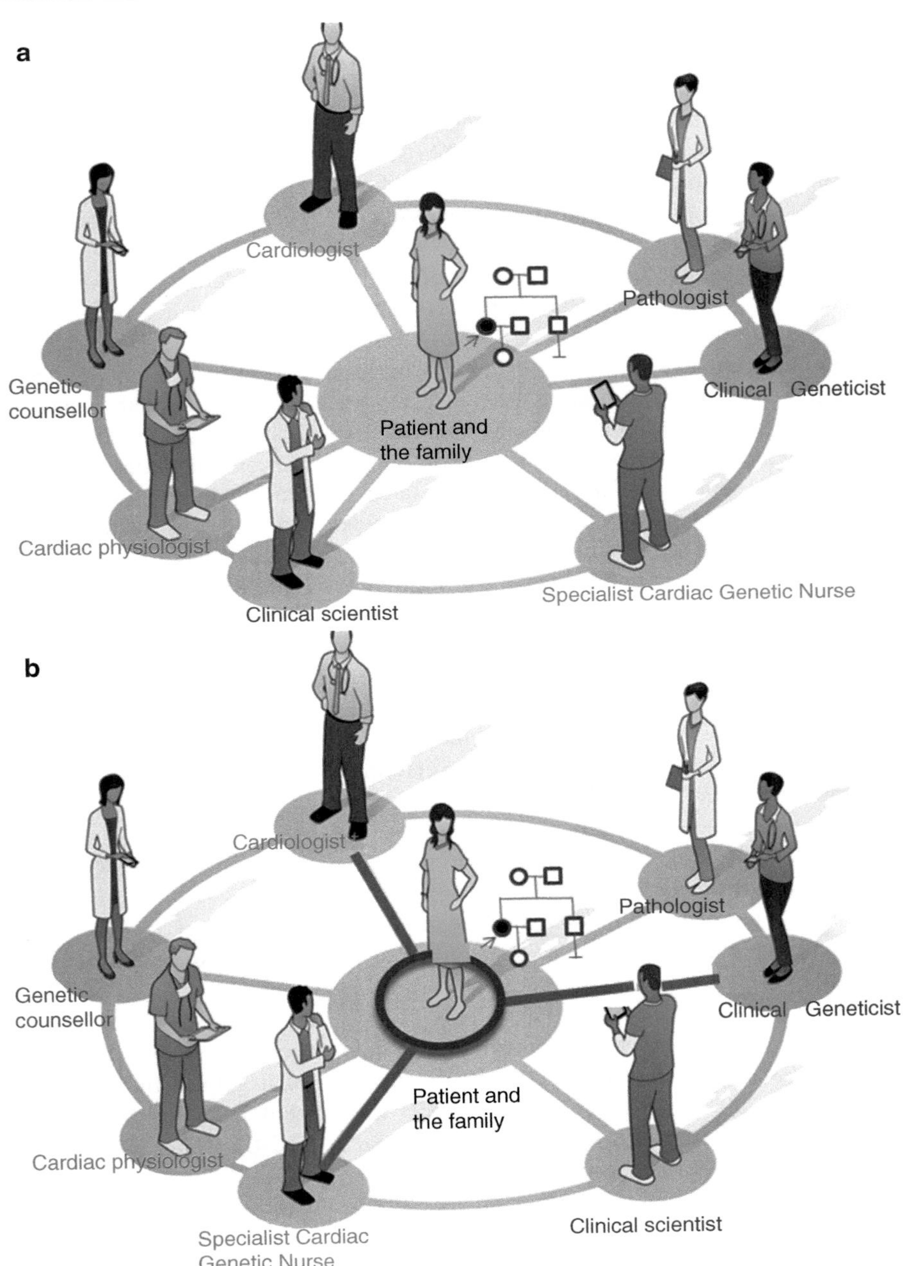

Fig. 29.1 (**a**) Patient-centred care within ICC service. (**b**) Patient-centred care within ICC service. Core ICC MDT members highlighted in blue

Other than that, there has been no other history of sudden cardiac death and deceased members of the family on maternal side lived up to 60 years or even older. On paternal side of the family there was no history of sudden cardiac death, and deceased members of the family lived well beyond 60 years of age. Based on family tree, there was no clear presence of a condition associated with sudden cardiac death or other cardiac symptoms that was being passed down through generations. As a matter of fact, sudden cardiac death in 18 months old girl appeared to be almost entirely an isolated event.

Based on genetic test results in parents, clinical screening for genotype-phenotype correlation was indicated. They both have undergone ECG, echocardiography, imaging with cardiac MRI, exercise test, 24 h Holter monitoring, and Ajmaline test. All tests were entirely normal in mother, who was found to carry a variant of uncertain significance in KCNQ1 gene, previously reported in association with Long QT syndrome, but overall of uncertain significance. The conclusion was that there was no phenotypical evidence of Long QT syndrome in her. Except for cardiac MRI the results of the same tests were normal in the father. He was thought to be in risk of developing symptoms associated with Brugada syndrome, as he was found to be a carrier of a pathogenic mutation in SCN5A gene and in the same copy of the gene a carrier of another variant of unknown significance. His MRI revealed mildly impaired left ventricular function (52%), and mildly dilated right ventricle with normal function. It was agreed that these findings would be were reevaluated after he stopped exercising for 3 months. Reassessment did not show any changes in his left ventricular function. This has remained stable, 2 years since initial diagnosis. As the father is a carrier of a pathogenic mutation in SCN5A gene responsible for Brugada syndrome, the advice given to him in terms of managing his risk of arrhythmia has been:

- to be cautious with medications known to be contraindicated in Long QT syndrome and Brugada syndrome;
- to have aggressive treatment in the case of infection or high fever;
- to engage in moderate intensity exercise and avoid professional resistance training.

His clinical management in terms of monitoring has been thoroughly discussed at the ICC MDT meeting, with particular emphasis on management from electrophysiology point of view. The multidisciplinary team recommendation was that he would not need repeat of Ajmaline test, but annual ECG, 24 h Holter monitoring, and echocardiogram were recommended.

For better understanding of pathogenicity of variants, further segregation studies in wider family were performed. This showed that KCNQ1 variant was maternally inherited in the mother. Deceased girl's maternal grand-mother had undergone clinical investigations (ECG, echocardiogram, 24 h Holter monitoring) and there was no clinical evidence of Long QT or Brugada syndrome.

On the father's side variant of unknown significance (VUS) in SCN5A gene was paternally inherited, whilst likely pathogenic variant appears to have arisen de novo in the father. Deceased girl's paternal grandfather was found to have left bundle branch block (LBBB) and moderately impaired left ventricular function (with prominent trabeculations in the left ventricle). He has been known to have a long-standing hypertension, and he complained of left sided non-specific chest pains and exertional shortness of breath. There was no history of pre-syncopal or syncopal episodes. With increase in the dose of antihypertensives some of his symptoms have improved. He has undergone further investigations and 24 h Holter monitor did not reveal any arrhythmia. Previously his coronary angiogram showed normal coronaries. He was due to have a stress MRI, which is reported normal.

Along with detailed investigations within the family, for better understanding of the genetic findings, the couple (parents of the deceased girl) was also keen to expand family, and to have children. This was another reason why understanding the genetic basis of sudden death in their first child was important. With all investigations into the cause of sudden death in their daughter, it was difficult to say whether pathogenic variant of SCN5A gene was solely responsible for her risk of sudden death. It may well have been that a combination of all three variants has increased her own risk (our knowledge does not extend to this realm as yet). If we assumed that this was due to presence of all three variants the risk for this couple to have another child with similar risk of sudden cardiac death would be 1 in 4 (25%). However, if we take that SCN5A variant was definitely pathogenic, and arose de novo in the father, there was 50% risk of this variant to be passed on to the offspring. The difficulty would be to estimate the risk of sudden cardiac death associated solely with pathogenic SCN5A variant. With this in mind the couple were keen to explore options for avoiding the condition in the offspring.

P*renatal diagnostic testing* was discussed with them in the first instance. It is performed either through choriovillious sampling (CVS) after 11 weeks of pregnancy, or amniocentesis after 16 weeks of pregnancy. Based on the results, in the couple's future pregnancies prenatal diagnosis could have been offered for pathogenic variant in SCN5A only, but not for the other two variants of unknown significance. Risk of miscarriage with prenatal diagnostic testing is 1–2%, and it is generally accepted if a couple would consider termination of pregnancy (if the fetus was affected). After discussing pros and cons of prenatal diagnostic testing the couple decided that this was not something they wanted to make a use of.

They were keen to explore the option of *pre-implantation genetic diagnosis* (PGD). Therefore they were referred to Consultant Genetic Counsellor for PGD within Regional Genetics Service. Even though the principles of this technique have been known for a few decades, it is still relatively new in clinical practice. It involves identifying genetic defects in embryos created through in vitro fertilization (IVF). Following this, only unaffected embryos are transferred to the uterus for implantation. This is a complex and lengthy process (Pre-implantation Genetic diagnosis (PGD), [11]) and at the time, SCN5A mutations, as a cause of Brugada syndrome, were not licensed by the Human Fertilisation Embriology Authority (HFEA) for use in PGD. Setting up PGD for a new condition involves several different stages and in total takes up approximately 18 months. Details of the process are outlined in Fig. 29.2.

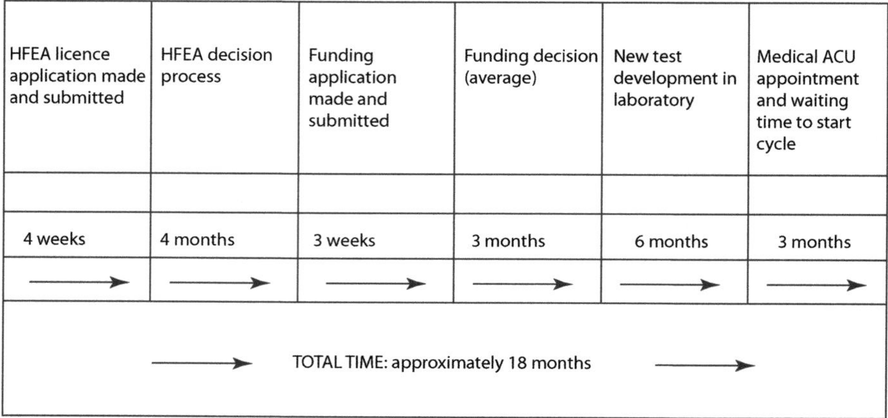

HFEA licence application made and submitted	HFEA decision process	Funding application made and submitted	Funding decision (average)	New test development in laboratory	Medical ACU appointment and waiting time to start cycle
4 weeks	4 months	3 weeks	3 months	6 months	3 months
⟶	⟶	⟶	⟶	⟶	⟶
⟶ TOTAL TIME: approximately 18 months ⟶					

Fig. 29.2 Standard timeline for setting up PGD for a new condition

After detailed counseling on what the process would involve the couple decided to go for alternative reproductive option—using a sperm donor (and thus avoid possibility of SCN5A pathogenic variant being passed on). This required involvement of Fertility Medicine team and they were referred appropriately. Process was successful, and the couple now has a daughter.

Their second daughter has 50% chance of having inherited variant of unknown significance in KCNQ1 gene from her mother. However, there is no benefit of genetic testing in her for a VUS. She was clinically reviewed by Pediatric Cardiology team and was found to have a normal electrocardiogram and echocardiogram. There was no phenotypical evidence of Long QT syndrome in her. She will remain under regular Cardiology follow up.

29.4.1.2 Discussion

This complex case illustrates the need for multi-disciplinary team coordinated care for the family following a tragic death of an 18 month olds girl. Management of all aspects of Sudden Arrhythmic Death Syndrome would not be possible, by any one individual service only. Chapter 8 of the National Service Framework in the UK requires NHS to provide dedicated clinic to assess families with appropriately trained staff [12].

The care for the family was primarily coordinated by Cardiac Genetic Nurse, who was the first point of contact for any queries. Answering questions to all family members individually often involved having good access to a number of specialist services. It also involved psychological support in managing anxiety in different family members. Communication was via emails and telephone conversations, but also as part of clinic appointments with multidisciplinary ICC service. Cardiac Genetic Nurse was also involved in obtaining post mortem report, genetic test results, family physician's reports, local general cardiac investigation reports, etc. Detailed history from the parents, as well as three generation family tree was obtained by Cardiac Genetic Nurse.

Based on genetic test results clinical screening of different family members required involvement of: Consultant Electrophysiologist, Heart failure consultant with specialist interest in ICCs, and Pediatric Cardiologist who assessed the couple's second daughter. For assessment of members of a wider family local Cardiology services were also involved.

Interpretation of genetic test results of individual members of the family required input from Consultant Cardiac Geneticist and Clinical Scientist. Performing of segregation studies was also carried out with involvement of Cardiac Geneticist. Their role was also in counseling the couple on recurrence risk in future offspring, and offering the options for prenatal diagnosis, and pre-implantation genetics. The couple explored different strategies in minimizing the risk of sudden cardiac death in offspring, before deciding to proceed with the option of a sperm donor. Advice and management plan has been highly individualized in this particular case, and required further input from Consultant in Pre-Implantation Genetics, and input from Reproductive Medicine team.

In conclusion, management of families with the history of SADS is complex and lengthy process that involves comprehensive multidisciplinary team approach.

29.4.1.3 Summary and Learning Points

In deceased 18 months old girl, based on clinical history and post mortem examination diagnosis of *Sudden Arrhythmic Death Syndrome (SADS)* was suspected and therefore *molecular autopsy* was performed (see Tables 29.1, 29.2, 29.3, 29.4, 29.5 Her DNA was tested in 2012 for the mutations in the following genes: KCNQ1, KCNH2, KCNE1, KCNE2, and SCN5A. It revealed three genetic variants that in given clinical context may be of significance.

Table 29.1 Learning points [13]

For *diagnosis* of sudden arrhythmic death syndrome (SADS) the following points need to be fulfilled
• Sudden death in patients between the ages 1–40 without previous cardiac history
• Patients were seen well and alive 12 h prior to death
• Coroner's post mortem confirmed structurally normal heart
• Toxicology screen was normal
Underlying *causes* of SADS
• Long QT syndrome
• Brugada syndrome
• Catecholaminergic polymorphic ventricular tachycardia
Focused *history* taking
• Important to find out if there have been any previous syncope, seizures, pre-syncope
• Important to elicit any major triggers relevant for inherited arrhythmia syndrome: exercise, emotional stimuli sleep and rest

Table 29.2 Learning points

Delete row
Delete
Molecular autopsy refers to extracting DNA during postmortem examination from blood or other organ tissues (heart spleen, liver) for molecular analysis; in this case it involved genetic testing for mutations in the genes known to be associated with SADS

Table 29.3 Certified diagnostic molecular laboratories consider a number of lines of evidence when *evaluating sequence variant pathogenicity* [14]

These involve
1. Variant databases including Locum Specific Databases
2. Presence or absence on Single Nucleotide Polymorphism (SNP) databases
3. Testing matched controls
4. Co-occurrence (in trans) with known deleterious variants
5. Co-seggregation with the disease in the family
6. Occurrence of a new variant concurrent with the (sporadic) incidence of the disease
7. Species conservation
8. In silico prediction of pathogenic effect
9. In silico splice site prediction
10. RNA studies
11. Functional studies
12. Loss of heterozygosity
13. An integrated evaluation of sequence variants

Table 29.4 Following in depth analysis of available lines of evidence, variants are classified by the certified laboratories in five classes

Class 1 clearly not pathogenic
Class 2 unlikely pathogenic
Class 3 unknown significance (VUS)
Class 4 likely to be pathogenic
Class 5 clearly pathogenic

Table 29.5 Learning points—screening of SADS families

• Counseling is integral part of screening of families with SADS
• Implications of genetic testing and clinical screening need to be well understood by family members
• Possible outcomes of screening need to be clearly explained before the screening

In *SCN5A gene* she was found to have two variants-

1. Heterozygous for c.1066G>A (p.Asp356Asn)

Analysis of pathogenicity of this variant revealed that:

- It has previously been reported in the literature in association with Brugada syndrome and Brugada-like syndrome in infancy [15, 16].
- It has not previously been detected in apparently normal control samples.
- p.Asp356 amino acid residue is highly conserved across species and lies within a functionally important region of the protein.
- p.Asp356Asn represents substitution of a negatively charged amnio acid to uncharged amino acid.
- In vitro functional studies have demonstrated that this variant affects protein function [16].

Based on laboratory analysis of the variant and literature search the overall conclusion was that this variant is highly likely to be pathogenic and this was consistent with the diagnosis of Cardiac Sodium Channelopathy.

2. Heterozygous for c.5260A>T (p.Thr1754Ser)

Investigations into pathogenicity of this variant revealed that:

- This variant has not previously been reported in the literature.
- p.Thr1754 is highly conserved across species.
- p.Thr1754 is located in the functionally important region of the protein and pathogenic missense variants have been reported in this domain with both Long QT syndrome and Brugada syndrome.
- p.Thr1754Ser is exchange of two small, uncharged, polar amino acids.

Overall laboratory concluded that the pathogenicity of this variant was uncertain and further analysis including parental studies were recommended.

In *KCNQ1 gene* she was found to be heterozygous for c.458C>T (p.Thr153Met). Analysis of the pathogenicity of this variant revealed that:

- This variant has been reported in the literature in association with Long QT syndrome. The variant has been detected with a frequency of 1 in 1000 in NHLBI Exome Sequencing Project (ESP) cohort [17].
- p.Thr153Met is conserved across vertebrates and lies within a functionally important domain of the protein
- p.Thr153Met is an uncharged polar to non polar amino acid exchange

Overall, laboratory concluded that this is a variant of uncertain pathogenicity and further analysis was recommended including parental studies.

29.4.2 Clinical Case 2

29.4.2.1 Case History

A 54 years old man was referred by his GP to one stop ICC clinic based on his personal and family history.

He had been a fit and well man, who at the age of 18 noticed decrease in strength of his legs. The weakness was initially progressive, but remained restricted to distal lower limbs. Clinically there was symmetrical muscle wasting in the calves and shins, and there were reduced ankle reflexes. Based on clinical findings he was diagnosed with Charcot-Marie-Tooth disease. His symptoms remained static for nearly 14 years and his diagnosis on a further neurology review was made to be that of a distal spinal muscular atrophy (DSMA). As his symptoms were stable, he did not require Neurology input for nearly 9 years.

In the meantime, at the age of 49 he presented with an episode of lightheadedness and was found to be in atrial flutter. His treatment included medical management, DC cardioversion, and flutter ablation. He also required dual chamber permanent pacemaker insertion for AV block. He remained under Cardiology follow-up as he occasionally experienced palpitations (awareness of fast irregular heart beat) and was found to be in paroxysmal atrial fibrillation (AF burden on pacing check <1%).

At the age of 52, he was seen by Neurology service on his own request, following a road traffic accident (patient was a driver of a car involved in the accident). He was worried about the RTA impact on his underlying neurological condition. Clinically, it was thought that his neurological condition had not deteriorated. He went on to have an MRI spine which did not reveal any significant abnormalities. He also had nerve conduction studies which were somewhat equivocal showing both neuropathic and myopathic features. Findings in this gentleman, from neurological perspective, were most consistent with distal motor neuropathy and mutation analysis of *BSCL2*gene was performed. No mutations were identified in this patient in *BSCL2* gene.

His family history was reviewed during his appointment with ICC team. It revealed that his father died suddenly at the age of 78 with a pacemaker in situ. Post-mortem examination was performed and it showed that the cause of death was myocardial ischaemia. Patient's father had four brothers and one sister, all of whom had pacemakers at some stages of their lives. Two paternal uncles died of heart related complications. One of the cousins on the paternal side died suddenly (no prior symptoms reported) at the age of 44, but post-mortem examination was not performed. Except for our patient no other family member had any muscular involvement. Patient himself has three children and he was concerned if his condition had any implications for their health. Family pedigree is on Fig. 29.3.

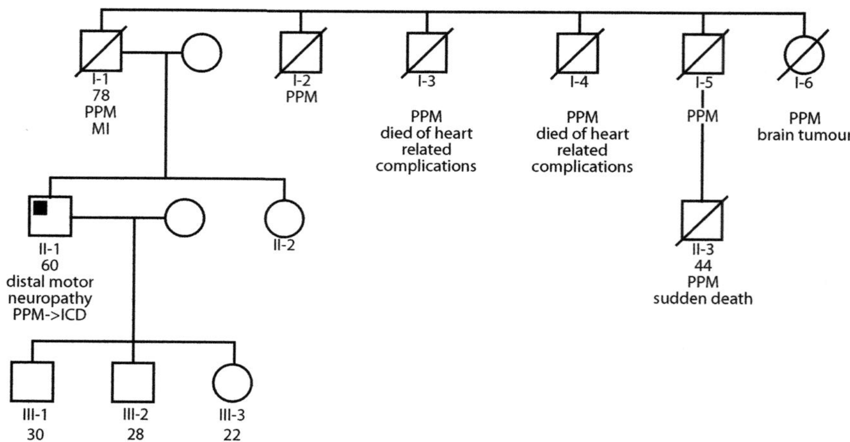

Fig. 29.3 Family pedigree for clinical case 2

Table 29.6 Lamin A/C phenotypes [18]

• The laminopathies are a diverse group of conditions caused by mutations in the LMNA gene (MIM*150330)
• LMNA encodes the nuclear envelope proteins lamin A and lamin C by utilization of an alternative splice site in exon 10
• More than 10 distinct phenotypes have been associated with lamin A/C mutations (Table 29.7)

Initial review of patient's personal and family history did not give clear clues towards unifying diagnosis of an inherited condition. There was a suggestion that muscle biopsy may be a way forward in revealing the underlying cause of his presentation. Diagnosis of laminopathy Table 29.6 or possible channelopathy was also considered (during clinical review with Consultant Clinical geneticist), but there were no sufficient phenotypical features to support investigations in these directions. Therefore, the case was discussed at ICC MDT meeting and recommendation was made to clinically screen patient's first degree relatives for any cardiac abnormalities.

As family clinical screening was underway, patient had further review in Neurogenetics clinicby one of the experts in the field. This was initiated by the team to consider genetic testing by an NCG service service. His symptoms have deteriorated somewhat over time, but were still restricted to the distal legs. Dropped foot gait was clinically prominent. Patient remained physically active, attending the gym 3 times a week where he did both cardio and weight exercises, with the aim of keeping fit and healthy. His phenotype was considered in the context of possible inherited condition and phenotypically his presentation was in keeping with Charcot-Marie-Tooth. As there has been personal and family history of a conduction disease, testing for mutations in *Lamin A/C* was requested. Various *Lamin A/C* phenotypes are in learning points Table 29.7.

Prior to mutation analysis in _*Lamin A/C* gene patient had genetic counseling. The session involved understanding of the possible outcomes of genetic testing:

1. If a mutation in *Lamin A/C* gene was found, that would be the explanation of his symptoms and this might have impact on further management of his condition. Predictive testing for the same mutation in that case can be offered to all his first degree relatives.
2. If a variant of unknown clinical significance was found in the *Lamin A/C gene* this might not provide the explanation for patient's symptoms and there will be uncertainty if the variant had disease causing properties. Predictive genetic testing could not be offered to his first degree relatives, but family studies might be recommended.
3. If no mutation was found in *Lamin A/C gene*, no further insight would be gained into genetic basis of his condition, but it might mean that other explanations for his presentation may need to be considered.

Table 29.7 Clinical phenotypes associated with lamin A/C mutations

Syndromes associated with LMNA mutations	Clinical features	Inheritance
Emery-Dreiffus muscular dystrophy (MD)	Muscle weakness, contractures, cardiac involvement (DCM and arrythmia)	AD/AR
Isolated heart disorders	Conduction disease	AD
	Dilated cardiomyopathy	
	Malignant ventricular arrhythmia	
Limb-girdle MD	Hip and shoulder girdle muscle weakness; DCM; AV block and sudden cardiac death;	AD
Severe congenital form of MD	Severe hypotonia, delayed motor development, failure to thrive, respiratory insufficiency	AD
Charcot Marie tooth axonal neuropathy	Pes cavus	AR
	Feet deformities	
	Distal muscle weakness	
	Areflexia/Hyporeflexia	
Familial partial Lipodystrophy of Dunnigan type, FPLD	Abnormal fat distribution (loss of fat in limbs, trunk and gluteal region); insulin-resistant diabetes	AD
Hutchinson-Gilford progeria	Premature ageing (median life expectancy 13.4 years); absence of subcutaneous fat tissue; osteoporosis	AD/AR
Restrictive dermopathy, lethal	Tight, rigid skin, with skin fissures and erosions, dysmorphic facial features, multiple internal organ involvement leading to premature birth, stillbirth or in, liveborns often die within the first week.	AR
Mandibulo acral dysplasia	Craniofacial and skeletal abnormalities, abnormal fat distribution	AR
Heart-hand syndrome, Slovenian type	Brachydactyly more in feet, proximal muscle weakness, AV block, DCM, malignant ventricular arrythmia	AD

Mutation analysis of *Lamin A/C gene* revealed that the patient was heterozygous for a mutation c.949G>A (p.Glu317Lys) in exon 6. This mutation has been previously reported as pathogenic in Leiden Muscular Dystrophy database (http://www.dmd.nl/). Molecular analysis also included testing for any insertions or deletions within the gene (MLPA), but no abnormality was found. Based on the clinical findings the sequence mutation was the explanation of patient's personal and family history. Further to genetic test result, the next step in clinical management of the patient was to determine his risk of sudden cardiac death.

Results of studies looking at the risk of sudden cardiac death in *Lamin A/C* mutation carriers were available at the time (Tables 29.8 and 29.9). They demonstrated that *Lamin A/C* mutation carriers are at risk of sudden cardiac death because of malignant ventricular arrhythmias [20]. Implantation of an ICD in this group of patients based on the results of the studies seemed justifiable, although studies did not directly look at efficacy of ICD implantation or it effect on survival. Therefore

Table 29.8 Independent risk factors for malignant ventricular arrhythmias in lamin A/C mutation carriers ([19])

• Non-sustained ventricular tachycardia
• Left ventricular ejection fraction <45% at the first clinical contact
• Male sex
• Non-missense mutations (ins/del/truncating mutations)
Malignant ventricular arrhythmias occur typically in individuals with at least 2 of these factors.

Table 29.9 Independent risk factors for malignant ventricular arrhythmias in lamin AC mutation carriers [19]

• Non-sustained ventricular tachycardia
• Left ventricular ejection fraction <45% at the first clinical contact
• Male sex
• Non-missense mutations (ins/del/truncating mutations)
Malignant ventricular arrhythmias occur typically in individuals with at least 2 of these factors

Table 29.10 Summary of results of clinical and genetic testing within family presented in clinical case 2

Individual	Genetic test results	Cardiac or neurological symptoms	ECG	Holter	Echo	ETT	Amalin test	CMR
II-2	???	Asymptomatic	Normal	Normal	Normal	?	?	?
III-1	Not a mutation carrier	Palpitations	Normal	1 dropped beat; nocturnal Wenchenbach	Normal	?	?	?
III-2	Mutation carrier	Muscle twitches that last for weeks	Normal	Normal	?	Normal	Negative	Normal
III-3	Mutation carrier	Asymptomatic	Normal	Normal	Normal	?	??	

following further ICC MDT discussion the patient had ICD implanted. He remains under follow up by Cardiology and Neurology team.

His first degree family members underwent both clinical screening and predictive genetic testing. Combined outcome of clinical and genetic testing is in the Table 29.10.

29.4.2.2 Discussion

This interesting case illustrates complexity of inherited cardiovascular conditions, and difficulties in making clinical and genetic diagnosis. Patient's history of neurological problem spans period of nearly 40 years, starting in the era when there was no knowledge of *Lamin A/C* mutations. Reaching the diagnosis required input from various specialists over prolonged period of time. The recommendation for *Lamin*

A/C gene testing was instigated by Neurologist in this particular case. Neurology clinical findings were most consistent with Charcot-Marie-Tooth (autosomal recessive form of peripheral nerve laminopathy). This highlights the need for involvement of multiple professionals in care of patients with ICC.

Even when diagnosis was reached and confirmed by genetic testing, clinical management of the patient remained a challenge. This is primarily due to scarce evidence for benefit of any interventions in this relatively small group of patients. In situations like this review of literature may be a starting point, but overall clinical decision is best reached in multidisciplinary setting, taking into account patient's wishes and their individual circumstances [21].

29.4.2.3 Summary and Learning Points

Establishing the diagnosis in patients with laminopathies is rarely a straightforward, particularly taking into account the number of different phenotypes patients present with. Furthermore, identifying those at risk of sudden cardiac death represents clinical challenge and decisions on management of individual patients are best reached in multidisciplinary setting.

Charcot-Marie-Tooth syndrome

- Charcot–Marie–Tooth (CMT) disease or hereditary motor and sensory neuropathy is traditionally classified according to clinical, electrophysiological, morphological and genetic criteria.
- CMT disorders are divided into two groups on the basis of nerve conduction studies. Type 1—demyelinating type and Type 2—axonal type
- Dominant, Recessive and X-linked types of inheritance have been described.
- Autosomal recessive axonal CMT (AR CMT2) is associated with mutations in lamin A/C.
- Weakness and amyotrophy of the upper limbs and involvement of the proximal muscles of the lower limbs are frequent in Lamin A/C associated AR CMT2.

Lamin A/C phenotypes: [18]

- The laminopathies are a diverse group of conditions caused by mutations in the LMNA gene (MIM*150330).
- LMNA encodes the nuclear envelope proteins lamin A and lamin C by utilization of an alternative splice site in exon 10.
- More than 10 distinct phenotypes have been associated with lamin A/C mutations (Table 29.1)
- DCM with conduction system disorders is one of the well recognised phenotypes of laminopathy

In this family,

- The proband had consistent clinical features of CMT2 and had long standing clinical diagnosis

- Although there have been several reports of conduction abnormalities, dilated cardiomyopathy has not been associated with CMT2.
- The presence of a significant FH of pacemaker insertions and heart failure on assessment in the ICC service raised the possibility of two distinct pathologies in our proband.
- Laminopathy as a possible explanation for early onset cardiomyopathy with conduction abnormalities was explored
- Multidisciplinary involvement with cardiology, neurology and genetic teams lead to the diagnosis of laminopathy in this family.
- Genetic testing is still ongoing in the proband for CMT2.

Independent risk factors for malignant ventricular arrhythmias in lamin A/C mutation carriers: [19]

- Non-sustained ventricular tachycardia
- Left ventricular ejection fraction <45% at the first clinical contact
- Male sex
- Non-missense mutations (ins/del/truncating mutations)

Malignant ventricular arrhythmias occur typically in individuals with at least two of these factors.

- (MNCV): (1) demyelinating types (CMT1) with (MNCV) with MNCV 438

Acknowledgments Special acknowledgements are made to both Tootie Bueser and Jelena Blagojevic, both of whom have contributed to the writing of this chapter.

References

1. Raine R, et al. Improving the effectiveness of multidisciplinary team meetings for patients with chronic diseases: a prospective observational study. Health Serv Deliv Res. 2014;2(37):1–72.
2. Taylor C, et al. Measuring the quality of MDT working: an observational approach. BMC Cancer. 2012;12:202.
3. Holland R, et al. Systematic review of multidisciplinary interventions in heart failure. Heart. 2005;91:899–906. https://doi.org/10.1136/hrt.2004.048389.
4. Keesson EM, et al. Effects of multidisciplinary team working on breast cancer survival: retrospective, comparative, interventional cohort study of 13,722 women. BMJ. 2012;344:e2718.
5. Clarke DJ. The role of multidisciplinary team care in stroke rehabilitation. Prog Neurol Psychiatry. 2013;17(4):5–8.
6. Ke KM, et al. Are multidisciplinary teams in secondary care cost-effective? A systematic review of the literature. Cost Eff Res Alloc. 2013;11:7.
7. England NH 14 NHS standard contract for cardiology: inherited cardiac conditions (all ages). NHS England; 2013.
8. Ingles J, et al. A cost-effectivness model of genetic testing for the evaluation of families with hypertrophic cardiomyopathy. Heart. 2012;98(8):625–30.
9. Wodsworth S, et al. DNA testing for hypertrophic cardiomyopathy: a cost-effectivness model. Eur Heart J. 2010;31(8):926–35.

10. Burton H, Alberg C, Stewart A. Heart to heart: inherited cardiovascular conditions services A needs assessment and service review. Cambridge: PHG Foundation; 2009. www.phgfoundation.org
11. Guy's and St Thomas NHS Foundation Trust, 2008 Centre for Preimplantation Genetic Diagnosis. http://www.guysandstthomas.nhs.uk/resources/our-services/acu/pgd-booklet.pdf
12. Department of Health. National service framework for coronary heart disease. Chapter Eight: arrhythmias and sudden cardiac death. 2005. http://www.dh.gov.uk/prod_consum_dh/groups/dh_digitalassets/@dh/@en/documents/digitalasset/dh_4105 280.pdf. Accessed 5 Feb 2013.
13. Vyas V, Lambiase PD. The investigation of sudden arrhythmic death syndrome (SADS)-the current approach to family screening and the future role of genomics and stem cell technology. Front Physiol. 2013;4:199.
14. Walleis Y et al. Practice guidelines for the evaluation of pathogenicity and the reporting of sequence variants in clinical molecular genetics. Assoc Clin Genet Sci. 2013. http://www.acgs.uk.com/media/774853/evaluation_and_reporting_of_sequence_variants_bpgs_june_2013_-_finalpdf.pdf.
15. Kapplinger JD, et al. An international compendium of mutations in the SCN5Aencoded cardiac sodium channel in patients referred for Brugada syndrome genetic testing. Heart Rhythm. 2010;7(1):33–46.
16. Makiyama T, et al. High risk for bradyarrhythmic complications in patients with Brugada syndrome caused by SCN5A gene mutations. J Am Coll Cardiol. 2005;46(11):2100–6.
17. Kapplinger JD, et al. Spectrum and prevalence of mutations from the first 2,500 consecutive unrelated patients referred for the FAMILION® long QT syndrome genetic test. Heart Rhythm. 2009;6(9):1297–303.
18. Rankin J, Ellard S. The laminopathies: a clinical review. Clin Genet. 2006;70(4):261–74.
19. van Rijsingen IA, et al. Risk factors for malignant ventricular arrhythmias in lamin A/C mutation carriers. J Am Coll Cardiol. 2012;59(5):493–500.
20. Meune C, et al. Primary prevention of sudden death in patients with lamin A/C gene mutations. N Engl J Med. 2006;354(2):209–10.
21. National Cancer Action Team The characteristics of an effective multidisciplinary team (MDT). 2010.

Interventions and Implantable Devices for Inherited Cardiac Conditions

30

Zaheer Yousef and Mark Drury-Smith

Abstract
Inherited cardiac conditions comprise many different structural and cardiac rhythm abnormalities. Many are asymptomatic and can be detected as an incidental finding or during routine medical screening and require pedigree evaluation, risk stratification, and ongoing long-term surveillance. Structural inherited cardiac conditions (ICC) can cause heart failure with primary heart muscle defects, impaired ventricular function, pump failure or sudden cardiac death. The arrhythmic ICC can present with a range of arrhythmias as a result of different channalopathies and notably brady and tachy arrhythmias and sudden cardiac death (SCD).

Keywords
Inherited cardiac conditions (ICC) • Cardiac devices • Cardiac resynchronization therapy • Sudden cardiac death (SCD)

30.1 Introduction

Inherited cardiac conditions comprise many different structural and cardiac rhythm abnormalities. Many are asymptomatic and can be detected as an incidental finding or during routine medical screening and require pedigree evaluation, risk stratification, and ongoing long-term surveillance. Structural inherited cardiac conditions (ICC) can cause heart failure with primary heart muscle defects, impaired ventricular function, pump failure or sudden cardiac death. The arrhythmic ICC can present with a range of arrhythmias as a result of different channalopathies and notably brady and tachy arrhythmias and sudden cardiac death (SCD) (Fig. 30.1).

Z. Yousef (✉) • M. Drury-Smith
Department of Cardiology, University Hospital of Wales, Cardiff, UK
e-mail: zaheer.yousef@wales.nhs.uk; mark.drury-smith@wales.nhs.uk

D. Kumar, P. Elliott (eds.), *Cardiovascular Genetics and Genomics*,
https://doi.org/10.1007/978-3-319-66114-8_30

30.2 Cardiac Devices

Cardiac devices in ICC primarily include permanent pacemakers (PPM) and implantable cardiac defibrillators (ICDs). These devices can be either the sole treatment for patients or as part of the treatment strategy for patients with ICC.

Transvenous permanent pacing and defibrillator systems consist of a generator which is connected to the cardiac endocardium or epicardial surface by one or more leads (Figs. 30.2 and 30.3).

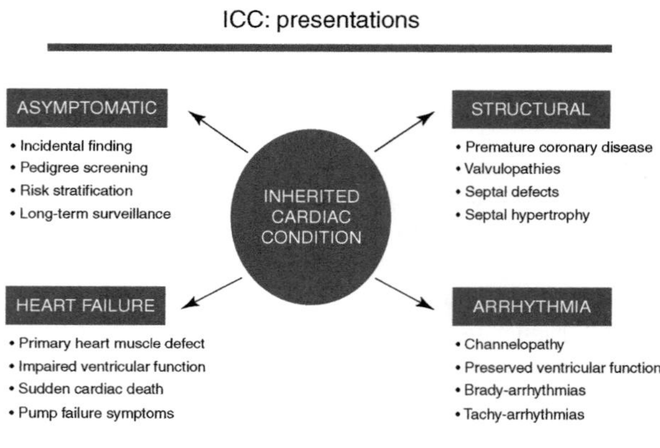

Fig. 30.1 A summary outlining the wide range of presentations for inherited cardiac conditions

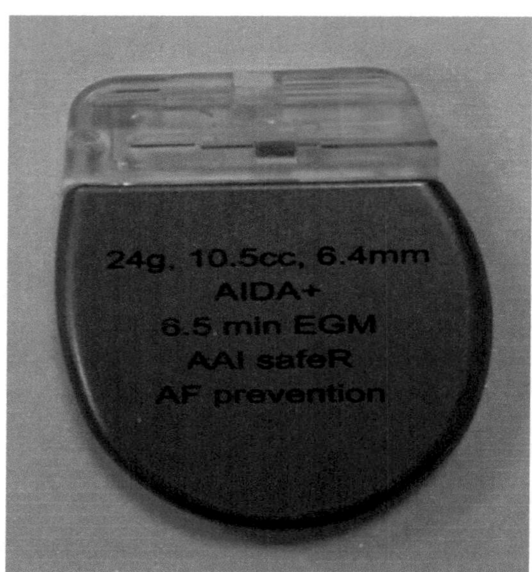

Fig. 30.2 Pacemaker pulse generator

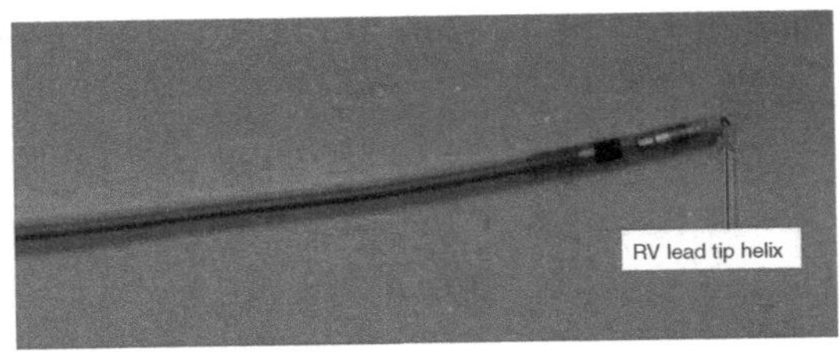

Fig. 30.3 Permanent pacemaker leads

30.2.1 Implantation

Device implantation is a procedure performed by cardiologists in either an operating room or catheterization laboratory designed with appropriate standards of ventilation and temperature control for sterile procedures. The procedure is performed under strict aseptic technique and in sterile conditions with thorough attention required to reduce the risk of device related infections.

The procedure is more commonly performed under local anaesthetic, with the occasional use of intravenous sedation and analgesia. This is to improve patient comfort during the procedure. However, rarely devices are implanted under general anaesthetic. The most common reason for this option would be patients suffering with severe anxiety whom would otherwise be unable to tolerate the procedure under local anaesthetic.

The main reasons for implantation under local anaesthetic include firstly, avoidance of the need for an anaesthetist. Secondly, the use of local anaesthetic avoids the potential pitfalls which maybe encountered in patients with a range of medical problems and co morbidities undergoing a general anaesthetic.

Cardiac devices are most commonly implanted in the region 2–3 cm inferior to the left clavicle and medial to the deltopectoral groove. The second most common site is the same region but on the right side.

The left side is most commonly used due to the fact that most patients are right hand dominant. This is important because following pacemaker implantation, a period of reduced range of arm movement in the operated side is advised to reduce the likelihood of pacemaker lead displacement. Another reason for implantation on the left side is that there is often a less acute angle between the subclavian vein and innominate vein compared to the right side. This makes manipulation of the leads easier. However, one disadvantage of a left sided approach is the small incidence of a persistent left sided superior vena cava which drains into the coronary sinus rather than into the right heart directly [1].

Prior to the surgical incision, the site is cleaned thoroughly with an aseptic solution and the surrounding area covered with sterile drapes to create a sterile operating area. During the procedure, the patient is continuously monitored with a combination of blood pressure, electrocardiograms (ECGs), and pulse oximetry.

Under local anaesthetic, a surgical skin incision is made either as a horizontal line parallel to the clavicle or vertically in the deltopectoral groove. The choice of incision is sometimes operator dependent depending on their preferred means of vascular access (Fig. 30.4).

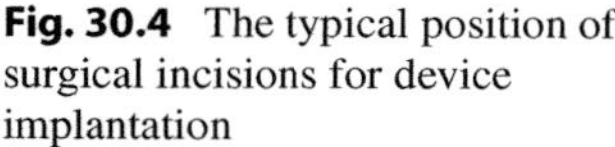

Fig. 30.4 The typical position of surgical incisions for device implantation

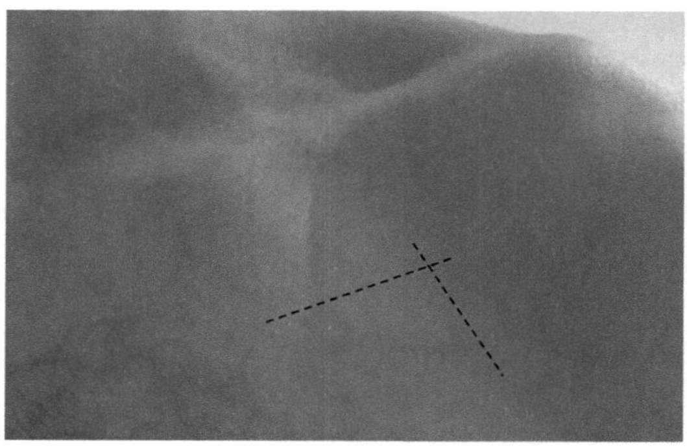

In transvenous cardiac devices, venous access is typically achieved through one of three potential different access points. The veins used are either the subclavian, axillary or cephalic veins.

The seldinger technique is used to gain venous access to the subclavian and axillary veins. The cephalic vein is located in the deltopectoral groove and often requires surgical dissection to locate it and under direct vision, a venotomy to gain venous access for implantation of the leads. The main advantage of the cephalic vein approach is with regards safety as it avoids the potential complication of a pneumothorax or haemothorax [1].

Once venous access is achieved, a guide wire is passed and 'peel' away sheaths are used to allow for insertion of the leads into the right heart chambers.

There are atrial and ventricular pacing leads which are fixed in the right atrium and ventricle respectively. ICD leads are positioned into the right ventricle. In the case of biventricular devices, left ventricular leads are placed in cardiac veins through the coronary sinus. Implantation of the leads is performed using fluoroscopy to correctly position the leads. There are principally two types of pacing leads, and this refers to how the leads are fixed to the endocardium. Active fixation leads have a helix mechanism which is 'screwed' into the endocardial surface. Passive fixation leads have tiny 'prongs' that anchor into the right ventricular trabeculations. There are potential advantages and disadvantages for both types of leads.

Active fixation leads have the advantage that they can be placed in a variety of different positions including in the right ventricular septum and lateral atrial wall. This option is important in patients whom may have for example, scar tissue and hence different pacing positions can be tried to ensure the best possible parameters. Passive atrial and ventricular leads are invariably limited to either the right atrial appendage or ventricular apex respectively. In addition, active fixation leads tend to be preferred in younger patients because of their easier removal of chronic implants in the case of system extraction for device related infection [1].

Once the leads have been correctly positioned, the leads are secured with internal sutures and then connected to the pulse generator or 'box'. The generator is buried in a 'pocket' which is in the infraclavicular region close to the area of venous access. The pocket is located either just above prepectoral fascia layer or placed subpectorally. A subpectoral pocket is typically employed in patients with very little subcutaneous tissue, large generators and the concern of future erosion.

30.2.2 Post Procedure Management

Following implantation of cardiac devices, post procedure management includes ordering of a posteroanterior and lateral chest radiographs. This is to ensure satisfactory lead positioning and to exclude a pneumothorax in patients whom have had their device implanted using the subclavian or axillary approach. In addition, the wound should be checked to ensure adequate haemostasis and the absence of a haematoma. The device should be interrogated to ensure satisfactory functioning prior to discharge from hospital (Fig. 30.5).

The patient should be offered analgesia and general advice with regards to limiting the movement of ipsilateral arm particularly overstretching movements to minimise the risk of lead displacements for the first few weeks. The wound should be kept dry for a week.

In addition, the patient should be made aware of potential driving restrictions imposed following device implantation. The current Driver and Vehicle Licensing Agency (DVLA) guidelines [2] are shown in Table 30.1.

30.2.3 Complications

Patients whom undergo implantation of cardiac devices are unfortunately potentially at risk of device related complications. These complications can be classified

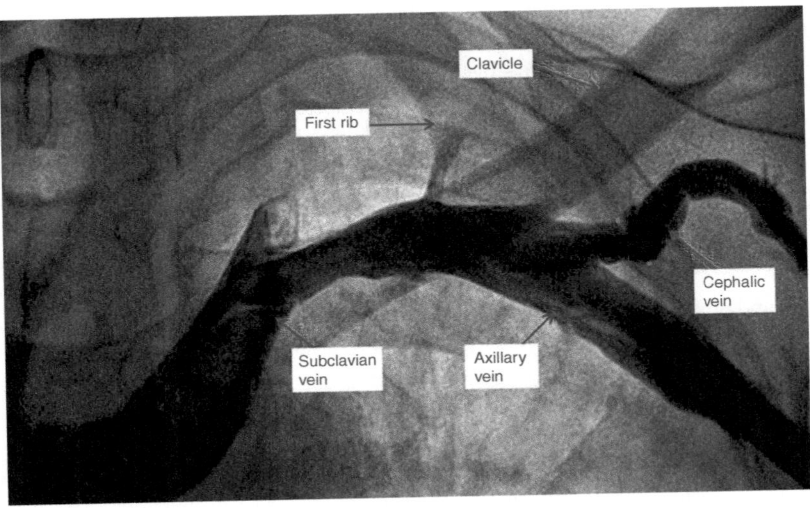

Fig. 30.5 Venogram demonstrating the venous system of the upper limb

Table 30.1 Driver and Vehicle Lincesing Agency (DVLA) guidelines for cardiac devices

Device	Group 1—car and motorcycle drivers	Group 2—bus and lorry drivers
PPM	Driving may resume after 1 week	Driving may resume after 6 weeks
ICD—for sustained ventricular arrhythmia associated with incapacity	Driving must stop for 6 months following ICD implant	Driving must stop permanently
ICD—with any shock therapy and/or pacing for symptomatic tachycardia	Driving must stop for 6 months	Driving must stop permanently
ICD—with any revision of electrodes or alteration of drug treatment	Driving may resume 1 month after electrode revision or drug alteration	Driving must stop permanently
ICD—with defibrillator box change	Driving may resume 1 week after box change	Driving must stop permanently
ICD—if shock therapy delivery was due to an inappropriate cause such as atrial fibrillation	Driving may resume 1 month after complete control of any cause	Driving must stop permanently
Prophylactic ICD—asymptomatic individuals	Driving may resume 1 month after implant	Driving must stop permanently

Table adapted from the DVLA guidelines [2]

as acute or delayed depending when they occur in relationship to the timing of the device implant. Acute complications are considered to occur during or soon after the procedure. Delayed complications can occur from days to weeks and even years following the procedure. The potential complications can be further subdivided into a complication relating to either to the vascular access, the lead, the generator, the wound or the patient. A meta-analysis of over 4000 patients, demonstrated an early complication occurs in 5.1% of patients greater than 75 years of age compared to 3.4% of patients aged less than 75 years [3].

In one series [4], the most frequent acute ppm complication lead displacement, followed by pneumothorax and then cardiac perforations. A meta-analysis [5] demonstrated lead displacement rates are higher in CRT devices (5.7%) compared with ICD devices (1.8%). This is predominately due to the additional left ventricular (LV) lead. The long-term complications of CRT devices in particular infections occurred at a rate of 1.0% per year. Device-related events are more frequent in CRT-D than in single- or dual-chamber ICDs [6].

Intrinsic device programming can also result in complications including pacemaker syndrome, and inappropriate shocks. Extrinsic factors, such as electromagnetic interference and physically manipulating the device, can also result in problems (Table 30.2).

30.3 Permanent Pacemakers (PPM)

Permanent pacemakers are indicated in patients with bradyarrhythmias. Many of the indications for pacing have evolved over the last few decades. These have been based on experience without the benefit of randomized clinical trials. This is because of the absence of alternative options to treat bradycardias. There are

Table 30.2 Complications of implantable cardiac devices

Complication	Acute
Vascular related	Pneumothorax hemothorax
	Blood vessel damage including arterial or venous structures
	Nerve damage
	Air embolism
	Foreign body embolism
Lead related	Lead displacement
	Cardiac perforation with tamponade
	Arrhythmias—either brady or tachy
	Lead damage
	Damage to the tricuspid valve
Generator related	Haematoma
	Pain
	Lead and generator connection issues
Complication	Delayed
Lead related	Lead displacement
	Lead related endocarditis
	Upper limb thrombosis
	Lead damage/fracture
	Lead failure
	Inappropriate shocks
Generator related	Haematoma
	Infection
	Pain at site of device
	Erosion of device
	Scar
	Pacemaker syndrome

Table adapted from Cardiac Pacing and ICDs by Ellenbogen K.A., Wood M.A. [1]

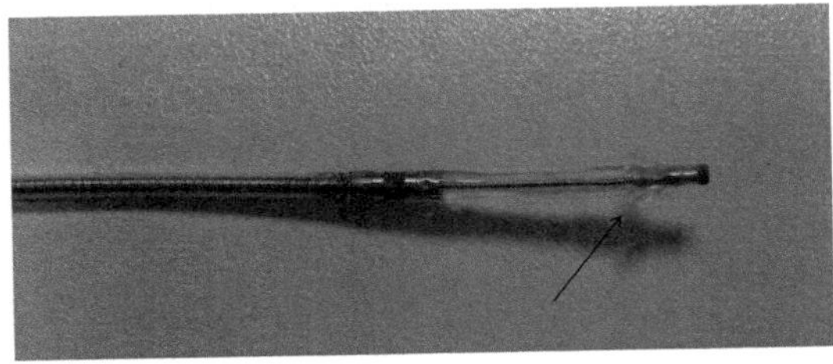

Fig. 30.6 Photograph demonstrating the 'prongs' of a passive pacemaker lead

however, a few special circumstances pacemakers are implanted for alternative reasons. Bradyarrhythmia's which require cardiac pacing can be caused by a variety of different aetiologies [7]. However, the indication for pacing is determined mainly by the severity and the patient's clinical presentation rather than the potential cause of bradycardia. It is however important to exclude potentially reversible causes prior to PPM implantation (Fig. 30.6) [7].

Table 30.3 Pacemaker indications

Class 1	Class 3
– Symptomatic sinus node disease	– PPM implantation not indicated in asymptomatic sinus node disease
– 3rd degree and 2nd degree AV block	– PPM implantation not indicated in patients with AV block due to reversible causes
– Alternating bundle-branch block	– PPM implantation not indicated for asymptomatic type I 2nd degree AV block at the supra-his level
– Recurrent unpredictable syncope due to dominant cardioinhibitory carotid sinus syndrome	– PPM implantation not indicated for asymptomatic patients with bundle-branch block
	– PPM implantation not indicated in asymptomatic patients with the absence of a documented cardioinhibitory reflex

Adapted from the current European [8] and American [9] guidelines

Table 30.4 Conditions and preferred pacemaker modes

Condition	Preferred pacemaker modes
– Sinus node disease	Dual-chamber PPM
– AV block with sinus rhythm	Dual-chamber PPM preferred to single chamber ppm
– AV block with AF	Single chamber PPM
– Intermittent documented bradycardia	Dual-chamber PPM
– Reflex asystolic documented bradycardia	Dual-chamber PPM
– Carotid sinus syncope	Dual-chamber PPM

Adapted from the current European [8] and American [9] guidelines

The current European [8] and American [9] guidelines for cardiac pacing differentiate between sinus node disease and atrioventricular (AV) heart block. The current class 1 indications are symptomatic sinus node disease and either third or second-degree type 2 AV heart block irrespective of symptoms [7] Table 30.3.

Permanent pacing can either be dual or single-chamber (ventricular and atrial). There are different pacing modes and these have been compared in a variety of large multi-centre, randomized trials and meta-analyses. These have demonstrated, particularly in patients with sinus node disease, that dual-chamber pacing reduces the incidence of atrial fibrillation (AF) and PPM syndrome [10]. This has the effect of resulting in an improved quality of life [11] (Table 30.4) (Fig. 30.7).

30.3.1 Clinical Case: 1

A 20-year-old man with Myotonic dystrophy, was admitted to hospital following recurrent episodes of transient loss of consciousness. On admission, this man's examination was normal with no abnormalities of his blood pressure. His 12-lead ECG showed first degree heart block and LBBB.

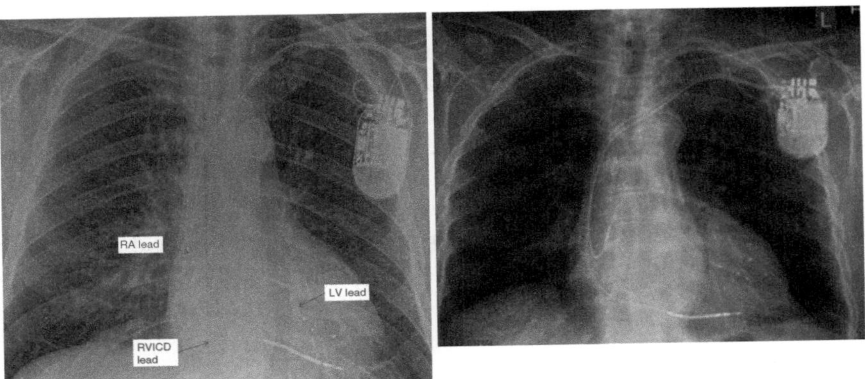

Fig. 30.7 Chest radiograph demonstrating the typical positions of the pulse generator, right atrial (RA) and right ventricular (RV) leads following device implantation. Chest radiograph demonstrating the typical lead positions of the left ventricular (LV), right ventricular (RV) and right atrial (RA) leads

An TTE demonstrated a structurally normal heart. His other investigations, including bloods were within normal limits.

A diagnosis of likely intermittent complete heart block as a cause of his transient loss of consciousness was made.

He subsequently underwent implantation of a dual chamber permanent pacemaker without complication. At follow up, over the following year, he remained well with no further episodes of loss of consciousness.

30.4 Cardiac Resynchronization Therapy (CRT)

In addition to single and dual chamber pacing devices, cardiac resynchronization therapy (CRT) is used, i.e. biventricular pacing modes. The class 1 indications for CRT are patients with chronic heart failure with a left bundle branch block (LBBB) electrocardiogram (ECG) appearance with a QRS duration greater than >130 ms in patients with severe left ventricular ejection fraction (LVEF), less than 35% and symptomatic heart failure despite optimal medical management [12]. In addition, patients with impaired left ventricular (LV) function whom require right ventricular (RV) pacing due to high grade AV heart block [12].

CRT has been shown to restore atrioventricular, inter and intra-ventricular synchrony. In addition, it improves LV function, reduces functional mitral regurgitation and helps induce LV reverse remodelling. This results in improved LV filling time and function, and a reduction in LV end-diastolic- and end-systolic volumes, mitral regurgitation and septal dyskinesis [13]. This has the effect of improving cardiac symptoms and reducing morbidity and mortality [14, 15].

The CARE-HF [16] and COMPANION [17] trials demonstrated HF hospitalizations and all-cause mortality with CRT-P compared to medical therapy improved symptoms and reduced all-cause mortality by 22% and HF hospitalizations by 35% respectively.

The patients most likely to respond and benefit from CRT are women with a non-ischaemic cardiomyopathy. This has been suggested to be due to the lack of scar tissue. The presence of a wide QRS duration and in particular the presence of a LBBB morphology. These factors have been shown to predict patients whom will have a beneficial response to CRT. The reasons patients are either 'responders' or 'nonresponders' has been suggested to relate to the degree of reverse or favourable LV remodelling [18] (Tables 30.5, 30.6, and 30.7).

The majority of these trials enrolled patients with LV impairment of less than 35% and a wide QRS morphology greater than 130 ms (Fig. 30.8).

30.4.1 Clinical Case: 2

40-year-old man presented to the hospital with a 6 month history progressively worsening shortness of breath and reduced exercise tolerance. On admission, the patient's examination revealed peripheral pitting oedema extending to his thighs bilaterally. In addition, on admission, the patient had mildly impaired renal function but normal full blood count. An ECG on admission showed sinus rhythm and the presence of LBBB, (QRS 150 ms).

During this man's admission in hospital, he underwent several investigations including, a coronary angiogram which demonstrated smooth coronary arteries. An transthoracic echocardiogram (TTE) which showed a dilated LV with severe LV systolic function. A urine and blood cardiomyopathy screen was within normal limits.

The patient was treated with diuretics and commenced on medical therapy including an ACE inhibitor, beta blocker and mineralocorticoid receptor antagonist. The patient was subsequently discharged with the plan for ongoing up titration of his optimal medical therapy.

Table 30.5 Cardiac resynchronization therapy

Class 1 indication
– Patients with heart failure, sinus rhythm, left bundle branch block with a QRS duration greater than 130 ms with severe LV ejection fraction less than 35% despite optimal medical therapy
– Patients with reduced LV ejection fraction whom required RV pacing with high grade AV heart block

Adapted from the current European [12] and American [9] guidelines

Table 30.6 Cardiac resynchronization therapy—favourable characteristics predicting response

– Women
– Non-ischaemic aetiology
– LBBB morphology
– Wider QRS duration

Adapted from the current European guidelines [12]

Table 30.7 A selection of the major CRT-P/D trial including the designs and outcome results

Major CRT-P/D trials	Design	Outcome
MUSTIC-SR	Single-blinded, crossover, randomized trial. CRT versus optimal medical therapy	Improvement in 6 min walk test, NYHA class, quality of life and VO2, reduction in LV volumes and MR and reduced hospitalizations
PATH-CHF	Single-blinded, crossover, randomized trial	Improvement in NYHA class, quality of life and 6 min walk test and reduced hospitalizations
MIRACLE	Double-blinded, randomized trial. CRT versus optimal medical therapy	Improvement in NYHA class, LVEF quality of life and 6 min walk test and reduction in LV volume and mitral regurgitation
CARE-HF	Double-blinded randomized trial. Optimal medical therapy versus CRT-P	Reduction in all-cause mortality and hospitalization Improvement in NYHA class and quality of life
COMPANION	Double-blinded randomized trial. Optimal medical therapy versus CRT-P/or versus CRT-D	Reduction in all-cause all-cause mortality or hospitalization
MADIT-CRT	Single-blinded, randomized trial. CRT-D versus. ICD,	Reduction in heart failure hospitalizations and all-cause mortality and LV volumes
RAFT	Double-blinded randomized trial. CRT-D versus. ICD	Reduction in all-cause mortality heart failure hospitalizations.
MIRACLE-ICD	Double-blinded, randomized trial. CRT-D versus ICD,	Improvement in NYHA class, quality of life, peak VO2

Adapted from ESC guidelines [2]

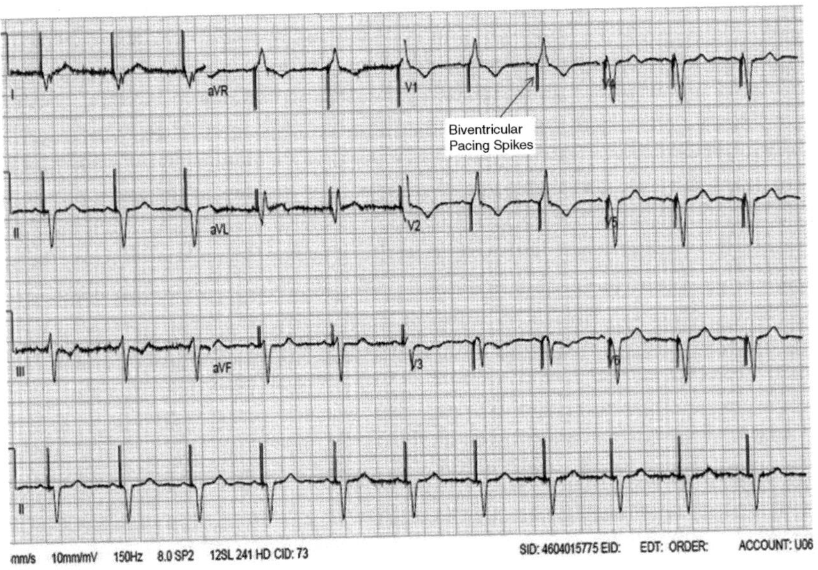

Fig. 30.8 An ECG demonstrating the biventricular pacing

Following 3 months of optimal medical therapy, a repeat TTE continued to show the persistence of severe LV systolic function. Therefore, the patient subsequently underwent implantation of a CRT device with the aim to improve the patient's symptoms and to improve his cardiac function.

30.5 Sudden Cardiac Death in Inherited Cardiac Conditions

30.5.1 Definition

Sudden Cardiac Death (SCD) is defined as a diagnosis of exclusion with a variety of potential conditions being the cause. A sudden death occurring in an individual older than 1 year of age is known as sudden unexplained death syndrome (SUDS) [19]. Sudden arrhythmic death syndrome (SADS) is a term used to describe SCD in the absence of an identifiable cause and in the presence of a structurally normal heart on autopsy [20].

30.5.2 Epidemiology and Etiology

It has been shown that the mortality rate for SCD is higher in men (6.7) than in women (1.4) per 100,000 person-years [21]. Approximately 80% of patients with SCD have been shown to be due to a structural cardiac condition. In individuals aged less than 35 years of age, the leading cause of death has been shown to be SUD, whilst in individuals over the age of 35, the leading cause is coronary artery disease (CAD). For SUD the incidence below 35 and above 35 years of age is 1.2 and 2 per 100,000 person-years, respectively [15]. Whilst CAD as a cause of SCD below 35 and above years has been shown to be 0.7 and 13.7 per 100,000 person-years respectively [21].

The table below demonstrates cardiac conditions which cause SCD. These can vary and can be classified depending on an individual's age (Table 30.8).

Cardiac arrest occurs most commonly in individuals with underlying structural heart abnormalities. It has been shown that in people over the age of 40 years pre-existing CAD is the most common cause. In this group, many individuals will have unknown CAD [22]. In younger individuals, HCM and LQTs have been shown to be the most prevalent cause [22]. LV ejection fraction, notably severe LV systolic dysfunction, has been shown to be the most reliable indicator to prognosticate and predict an increased risk of sudden death in individuals with CAD [23]. In contrast to risk stratification in patients with other causes is more variable and specific to the condition.

Table 30.8 Cardiac conditions that cause sudden cardiac death

Younger individuals	Older individuals
Hypertrophic cardiomyopathy	Coronary artery disease
Anomalous coronary artery	Valvular heart disease
Channelopathies	Hypertensive cardiomyopathy
Myocarditis	Ischaemic cardiomyopathy
Idiopathic dilated cardiomyopathy	

30.5.3 Pharmacological Therapy

There are no antiarrhythmic drugs, other than beta-blockers, to have been shown in randomized clinical trials (RCTs) to be effective in the primary management of patients in the prevention of SCD [24].

Overall, beta-blockers are first-line therapy in the management of patients with VT and the prevention of SCD [24]. Beta-blockers effectively block a patient's sympathetic drive, suppress ventricular ectopic beats, slow the sinus rate and inhibit excessive calcium release [24]. These are factors important in arrhythmia formation.

Amiodarone is another commonly used medication in the prevention of SCD. Its mechanism of action is on sodium and potassium channels. However, as per the Sudden Cardiac Death in Heart Failure Trial (SCD-HeFT) trial, amiodarone has been shown to have no favourable effect on survival when compared to placebo, in RCTs [25]. In addition, amiodarone is associated with a variety of drug interactions and side effects which limits its patient tolerability (www.evidence.nhs.uk/formulary/bnf/current/a1/amiodarone).

Other pharmacological therapy may involve discontinuation of medications which may be pro-arrhythmic [24].

In patients with LV dysfunction and heart failure the drugs including, ACEi or angiotenson receptor blockers, beta-blockers and MRA have been shown to reduce rates of SCD. This is likely due to their ability to inhibit or delaying adverse cardiac remodeling [26, 27].

30.6 Implantable Cardiac Defibrillators (ICD)

ICDs are recommended in two clinical settings, as primary prevention of SCD and as secondary prevention for those individuals who have survived a life threatening event.

The benefit of an ICD has been demonstrated for primary prevention in both ischaemic and non-ischaemic cardiomyopathies. The SCD-HeFT trial demonstrated a 23% decreased risk of death with an ICD [25]. Whilst the DEFINITE trial demonstrated that implantation of an ICD significantly reduced the risk of sudden death from an arrhythmia [28]. A meta-analysis of five primary prevention ICD trials enrolling 1854 patients with a non-ischaemic cardiomyopathy, demonstrated that the use of an ICD was associated with a significant 31% reduction in total mortality (Figs. 30.9 and 30.10) [29].

In view of the above trials, the current ESC guidelines [24] recommend ICD implantation to reduce SCD in patients with LV dysfunction. This is defined as an ejection fraction of less than 35%. This can be as a result of either an ischaemic or non-ischaemic cause. The patient should also have been on optimal medical therapy for at least 3 months. Individuals require a life expectancy of greater than 1 year with a good functional status to be considered for an ICD [24].

An ICD is recommended as secondary prevention for patients who have survived a cardiac arrest from VF or have had haemodynamically significant VT in the absence of reversible causes. These patients should have been receiving optimal medical

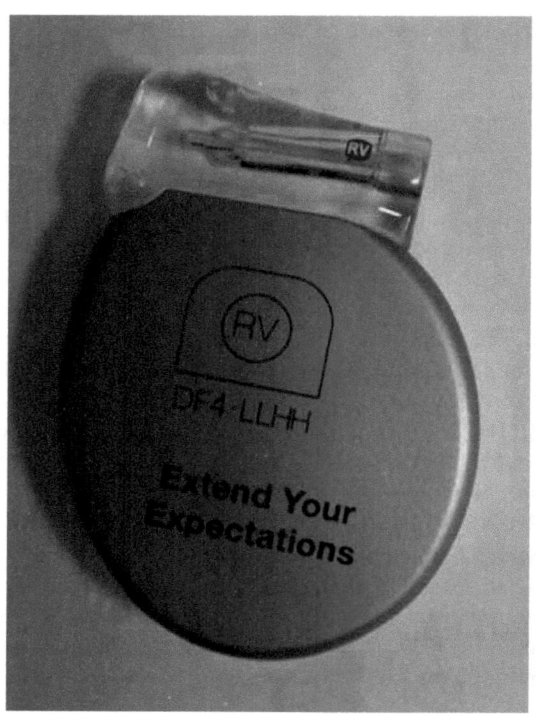

Fig. 30.9 A transvenous single chamber ICD

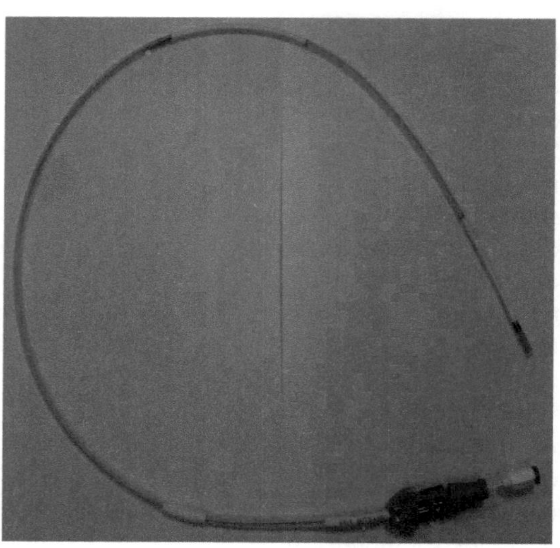

Fig. 30.10 An right ventricular ICD lead

therapy with a predicted functional status in excess of 1 year [24]. These recommendations are as a result of a meta-analysis of three ICD secondary prevention trials. These were, Antiarrhythmic drugs Versus Implantable Defibrillator (AVID), Canadian Implantable Defibrillator Study (CIDS) and Cardiac Arrest Study Hamburg (CASH). This meta-analysis demonstrated that ICD therapy was associated with a 50% reduction in arrhythmic mortality and a 28% reduction in total mortality [30].

As previously discussed, there are clear benefits of ICD implantation in the setting of both primary and secondary prevention of SCD. However, transvenous ICD implantation is associated potential complications. One study, demonstrated an overall complication rate of 11% [31] Whilst in a more recent study over a 12 year period, ICD and CRT-D implantation was associated with a 20% incidence of inappropriate shocks, 6% rate for device-related infection, and an incidence of 17% for lead related complications [32].

In view of the potential lead related complications of transvenous ICDs, the concept of subcutaneous ICDs (S-ICD) has more recently been developed. S-ICDs do not require leads in or on the heart. They provide therapy with a left lateral pulse generator and parasternal electrode configuration that is placed under the skin outside the thoracic cavity [33]. The results of two large prospective studies, IDE and EFFORTLESS S-ICD Registry, have demonstrated appropriate system performance comparable with conventional ICDs [34, 36].

S-ICDs are a potential treatment option for patients whom have difficult venous access and patients at particular risk of bacteraemia and infections [34]. In addition, it has been suggested that they may be appropriate for young patients with inherited cardiac conditions at risk of SCD who would otherwise have the prospect of lifelong device therapy and the potential complications associated with this [36].

S-ICDs are however not appropriate in patients who require pacing for bradycardia, CRT or when antitachycardia pacing is used to treat ventricular arrhythmias [36] Table 30.9.

30.7 Inherited Cardiac Conditions Affecting the Myocardium

30.7.1 Dilated Cardiomyopathy

30.7.1.1 Definition and Epidemiology

Dilated cardiomyopathy (DCM) is defined by the presence of left ventricular dilatation and left ventricular systolic dysfunction in the absence of abnormal loading conditions or coronary artery disease sufficient to cause global systolic impairment [37]. The exact prevalence and incidence of DCM is unknown but it has been suggested to affect 1 in 2500 individuals and have an incidence of approximately 7 per 100,000 per year [38]. In many cases the DCM is inherited and is therefore termed familial DCM (FDC) [37].

Table 30.9 Indications for ICD implantation in inherited cardiac conditions

Primary prevention	Secondary prevention
– Patients with symptomatic heart failure and severe LVSD (less than 35%) after 3 months of optimal medical therapy who are expected to survive for 1 year	– Patients with haemodynamically compromising VT and VF who are expected to survive for 1 year
– Patients with ARVC who have 1 or more risk factors for SCD	– Patients with unexplained syncope, significant LV dysfunction, and nonischemic DCM
– Patients with cardiac sarcoidosis, giant cell myocarditis, or Chagas disease	– Patients with Brugada syndrome who have had syncope. Patients with Brugada syndrome who have documented VT that has not resulted in cardiac arrest
	– Patients with catecholaminergic polymorphic VT who have syncope and/or documented sustained VT while receiving beta blockers
	– Patients with long-QT syndrome who are experiencing syncope and/or VT while receiving beta blockers

Adapted from the current European [24] and American [9] guidelines

30.7.1.2 Management and Device Therapy

The management of patients with DCM involves medical, device therapy and potentially surgical treatment.

Device therapy in DCM is recommended in the guidelines as previously discussed. This can be in the form of PPM, CRT or ICD therapy. This is largely dependent on the individual patient characteristics and condition involved.

30.8 Hypertrophic Cardiomyopathy

30.8.1 Definition and Clinical Presentation

Hypertrophic cardiomyopathy (HCM) is a condition characterised by the presence of increased left ventricular (LV) wall thickness that cannot be explained by abnormal loading conditions [37]. In an adult, LV wall thickness greater than15 mm in one or more LV myocardial segments is required for the definition [37, 39]. There are many conditions causing left ventricular hypertrophy [40, 41]. Many individuals with HCM have few, if any, symptoms. In certain individuals the diagnosis can be incidental or the result of screening. However, patients can experience angina, breathlessness, palpitations, presyncope, syncope and sudden cardiac arrest [42].

30.8.2 Device Therapy and Management

In patients with HCM the management and potential interventions aims to alleviate symptoms, prevent complications and stratify and reduce sudden cardiac death

(SCD). The potential interventions include pharmacological therapy, surgical and procedural treatments and device therapy. These interventions vary depending on the presence or absence of an LVOTO [43].

In many asymptomatic patients no specific treatments are necessary only general advice. This includes advice against participation in competitive sports and for patients to be discouraged from intense physical activity. This is particularly important in patients whom have risk factors for SCD and LVOTO.

30.8.3 Device Therapy

Three randomised controlled trials [44–46] have shown only a modest overall benefit with a reduction in LVOT gradient and symptoms with dual chamber permanent pacing in symptomatic HCM patients whom are refractory to medical therapy. The average LVOT gradient reduction was approximately 40 mm Hg. They have however shown no significant effect on quality of life, exercise capacity, peak oxygen consumption or septal wall thickness. However, in a small group of patients over the age of 65 years, pacing has been shown to improve HCM patient's functional capacity [42]. In addition, the placebo effect of pacing in HCM patients has also been demonstrated with a subjective improvement in symptoms [46].

The optimal AV interval has been shown to be short, around 100 ms. Pacing parameters should be optimized to achieve maximum pre-excitation of the right ventricular apex [47]. Current ESC guidelines [43] recommend permanent pacing should be considered in patients with an LVOT gradient greater than 50 mm Hg, whom are in sinus rhythm and on maximal drug therapy who are not suitable for other invasive treatment.

Permanent pacing has been shown to achieve a symptomatic and haemodymanic improvement in HCM patients with mid-cavity obstruction. This is uncommon but an important subset of patients with obstructive HCM [48].

30.9 Sudden Cardiac Death (SCD) in Hypertrophic Cardiomyopathy

The annual mortality, annual cardiac mortality, and annual mortality due to sudden death in HCM in one study has been shown to be 1.3%, 0.8%, and 0.6%, respectively [49]. There are three distinctive modes of death in HCM. The first is SCD, the second progressive heart failure and thirdly HCM-related stroke associated with atrial fibrillation [50].

In adults, SCD risk stratification is required as part of the management and ongoing interventions. The evidence suggests risk assessment should comprise of clinical and family history, 48-hour ambulatory ECG, TTE, CMR and a symptom-limited exercise test. Clinical features that are associated with an increased SCD risk are shown in the table below. The risk of SCD should be assessed at the first patient clinical assessment and re-evaluated at one to 2 year intervals or whenever there is a change in clinical status (Table 30.10).

Table 30.10 Risk factors for sudden cardiac death in HCM

– Young age
– Non-sustained ventricular tachycardia on ambulatory ECG monitoring
– LV maximum wall thickness of ≥30 mm
– Family history of SCD
– Increased left atrial size
– Left ventricular outflow tract obstruction
– Abnormal exercise blood pressure response (a failure to increase systolic blood pressure by a 20 mm Hg from rest to peak exercise or a fall of >20 mm Hg from peak blood pressure

Table adapted from the ESC guidelines [42]

Table 30.11 Indications for ICD implantation in HCM

– Survivors of cardiac arrest due to VT or VF or spontaneous sustained VT causing syncope or haemodynamic compromise with a life expectancy greater than 1 year
– Patients with an estimated 5-year risk of sudden death ≥6% and a life expectancy of greater than 1 year

The HCM Risk of SCD calculation is as follows [42]

$$\text{ProbabilitySCD at 5 years} = 1 - 0.998 \exp(\text{Prognostic index})$$

This calculation can be used to characterise patients into low, intermediate or high risk for SCD.

An ICD has been shown to be the treatment of choice for primary or secondary prevention in high-risk patients with HCM. Whilst pharmacological treatment with antiarrhythmic medications such as amiodarone, beta-blockers or calcium channel blockers have not be shown to be protective against SCD in HCM [51]. In one study, 10% of patients taking drugs, and specifically 20% of patients taking amiodarone, experienced SCD [51]. The current ESC guidelines [42], recommend an ICD as secondary prevention in patients whom have survived a cardiac arrest due to ventricular tachycardia (VT) or ventricular fibrillation (VF), or who have spontaneous sustained VT causing syncope or haemodynamic compromise, and have a life expectancy of greater than 1 year. In addition, ICDs should be considered in high risk HCM patients of SCD [42] Table 30.11.

It has been shown that in high-risk HCM patients, ICD interventions for life-threatening ventricular tachyarrhythmias are frequent and highly effective. In one series [52], ICD interventions appropriately terminated VT/VF in 20% of cases. Intervention rates were approximately 10% per year for secondary prevention after cardiac arrest. It has been shown that, 35% of ICD discharges occurred in primary prevention patients who had undergone implantation for only a single risk factor [52]. Therefore it has been suggested, a single marker of high risk for sudden death may be sufficient to justify consideration for prophylactic defibrillator implantation in selected patients with HCM. This however needs to be balanced against the risk of device related complications [52].

30.9.1 Clinical Case: 3

A 73-year-old lady with a history of HCM, whilst attending the cardiology outpatient clinic, complained of deteriorating symptoms notably, shortness of breath on exertion with a resultant reduction in exercise tolerance and frequent palpitations. This lady's past medical history included a history of permanent atrial fibrillation (AF) for which she was on warfarin and small dose of a beta blocker.

In view of this patient's deterioration, a repeat TTE and 48 hour holter monitor were requested. The TTE showed the presence of preserved LV systolic function but a mid-cavity obstruction. Her 48 hour holter monitor demonstrated periods of fast AF with rates of up to 140 bpm and asymptomatic pauses.

This patient's risk for SCD was calculated to be low and in view of her TTE findings and holter monitor underwent implantation of a single chamber permanent pacemaker in an attempt to improve the mid cavity obstruction and allow for more aggressive rate control of her fast AF.

Following implantation of her permanent pacemaker, her symptoms were significantly improved. This case highlights the use of pacing in small group of elderly patients with HCM.

30.10 Rarer Inherited Cardiac Conditions Predominantly Affecting Myocardium

In addition to DCM and HCM, a number of other inherited syndromes cause defects that are responsible for systemic as well as cardiac manifestations, most notably affecting skeletal muscle. A selection of these disorders are summarised in Table 30.12.

These rare inherited disorders can cause conduction tissue disease either brady or tachyarrhythmias. However, there is little evidence to support disease specific treatments. Therefore, the current recommendations for device therapy in these groups of patients should in general be based upon conventional indications as previously discussed [8].

30.11 Inherited Primary Arrhythmia Conditions

There are several different conditions which can be classified into the group of inherited cardiac problems. These conditions can predispose patients to a variety of potential problems but in particular and probably most importantly predispose individuals to a high risk of sudden cardiac death. Table 30.13 demonstrates a selection of different arrhythmia related inherited conditions.

30.11.1 Clinical Case: 4

A 36-year-old man was admitted to hospital feeling generally unwell with a high fever of 38° C. On admission, he complained of a productive cough with green sputum.

Table 30.12 Rarer cardiac conditions predominantly affecting myocardium

Condition	Gene defect	Symptoms/Signs	Investigation/ findings	Management
Duchenne muscular dystrophy (DMD)	Defective gene on X chromosome responsible for dystrophin	Teenage years. Proximal limb muscle weakness. Miral regurgitation and heart failure	Elevated creatine kinase conduction abnormalities involving AV node and arrhythmias particularly supraventricular. DCM	ACE inhibitors and beta blockers for LV dysfunction PPM for conduction disturbances
Becker muscular dystrophy	Defective gene on X chromosome responsible for dystrophin	Later age of onset compared to DMD. Proximal limb muscle weakness. Heart failure	Elevated creatine kinase conduction abnormalities of the AV node with can progress to complete heart block	Conventional heart failure medication and device implantation for LV dysfunction and brady/ tachy arrhythmias
Emery-Dreifuss muscular dystrophy (EDMD)	X-linked recessive, autosomal dominant, or autosomal recessive involving the emerin or lamin A/C genes	First or second decade. Slowly progressive muscle weakness and wasting in humeroperoneal distribution	Elevated creatine kinase AV conduction abnormalities, AF, DCM	Conventional heart failure medication and device implantation for LV dysfunction and brady/ tachy arrhythmias
Facioscapulohumeral dystrophy (FSHD)	Autosomal dominant inheritance chromosome 4q35	Slowly progressive muscle weakness involving the facial, scapular, upper arm, lower leg, and hip girdle muscles	Conduction defects, arrhythmias, and cardiomyopathy	Conventional heart failure medication and device implantation for LV dysfunction and brady/ tachy arrhythmias

(continued)

Table 30.12 (continued)

Condition	Gene defect	Symptoms/Signs	Investigation/ findings	Management
Myotonic dystrophy	Autosomal dominant inheritance and variable penetrance and clinical anticipation	Myotonia, weakness and wasting affecting facial muscles and distal limb muscles, frontal balding in males, cataracts, multiple endocrinopathies, and low intelligence or dementia. Heart failure, syncope, SCD	Conduction defects, ventricular arrhythmias, AF, DCM	Conventional heart failure medication and device implantation for LV dysfunction and brady/ tachy arrhythmias
Friedreich ataxia	Autosomal recessive inheritance Frataxin gene mutations	Progressive ataxia of limbs, heart failure	Arrhythmias, cardiomyopathy	Conventional heart failure medication and device implantation for LV dysfunction and brady/ tachy arrhythmias
Hereditary hemochromatosis	Autosomal recessive inheritance. HFE gene mutations	Diabetes mellitus, bronze skin changes, heart failure	Conduction disturbances, DCM	Phlebotomy. Iron chelation agents

Table adapted from, The ESC Textbook of Cardiovascular Medicine, ESC and American guideline documents [8, 24, 41, 51, 53]

His blood tests revealed high inflammatory markers and a chest x-ray showed consolidation. This man was seen by the medical team and commenced on appropriate antibiotics. His ECG is shown below.

Whilst in the accident and emergency department, this man collapsed and suffered a cardiac arrest. He was successfully treated for ventricular fibrillation (VF) with one direct current shock. He was subsequently transferred to the coronary care unit. A diagnosis of Brugada syndrome was made and after appropriate treatment underwent implantation of a ICD. In addition, he was advised to avoid provoking drugs and ensure prompt treatment of any pyrexial illness.

ECG 2: An ECG demonstrating ST-segment elevation greater than 2 mm in a patient with Brugada syndrome.

Table 30.13 Various arrhythmia-related inherited conditions

Condition	Epidemiology	Gene defect	Symptoms/Signs	Investigation findings	Risk stratification for SCD	Treatments
Long QT syndrome (LQTS)	1:2000 most likely in males before 12 years and after this age in females	Three main genes include, KCNQ1 (LQT1), KCNH2 (LQT2), and SCN5A (LQT3)	Asymptomatic, recurrent syncope, sudden death	Corrected QT interval of greater than 480 ms	Corrected QT interval, LQT2 genotype, previous cardiac events	Avoidance of QT-prolonging drugs and specific triggers
						Beta-blockers for symptomatic patients
						ICDs in conjunction with beta-blockers for cardiac arrest survivors
						Left cardiac sympathetic denervation for recurrent syncope despite beta-blockade, in patients with arrhythmia
						Storms with an ICD or when an ICD is contraindicated
Timothy syndrome (TS)	Rare	Autosomal dominant	Structural heart defects, dysmorphic facial features, syndactyly, seizures, developmental delay and autism	Prolonged QT interval on ECG		ICDs in conjunction with beta-blockers for cardiac arrest survivors

Andersen–Tawil syndrome (ATS)	Rare	Autosomal dominant hereditary multisystem disorder with variable expression	Ventricular arrhythmias, periodic paralysis, dysmorphic features	Prolonged QT interval, prominent U wave, polymorphic or bidirectional VT		ICDs in conjunction with beta-blockers for cardiac arrest survivors
Brugada syndrome (BrS)	1 in 5000 to 10,000 in Western countries and more prevalent in South Asia. Most common in males particularly in the third to fourth decade	Autosomal dominance with incomplete penetrance. Genes predominantly involved SCN5A and CACN1Ac	Asymptomatic, sudden cardiac death precipitation include Na channel blockers, pyrexia, vagotonic agents, excessive alcohol, large meals	ST elevation and incomplete RBBB on ECG.	High-risk patients include spontaneous ECG, history of syncope, aborted cardiac arrest and spontaneous sustained ventricular arrhythmias. Lowest risk patients have a negative phenotype and diagnostic ECG after provocation	ICD for high risk group. Avoid provoking drugs. Avoid excessive alcohol and large meals. Prompt treatment of any pyrexial illness

(continued)

Table 30.13 (continued)

Condition	Epidemiology	Gene defect	Symptoms/Signs	Investigation findings	Risk stratification for SCD	Treatments
Catecholaminergic Polymorphic VT (CPVT)	1 in 10,000 most common in the first decade of life	Autosomal dominant RyR2 gene. Autosomal recessive CASQ2 gene	Asymptomatic, recurrent syncope, sudden death prompted by physical activity or emotional stress	Normal ECG and echocardiogram abnormal exercise stress test with bidirectional or polymorphic VT		Beta-blockers for documented spontaneous or stress-induced ventricular arrhythmias. ICD for a cardiac arrest, recurrent syncope or documented VT. Therapy-refractory cardiac events avoidance of competitive sports, strenuous exercise and stressful environments
Short QT syndrome (SQTS)	Occurs in all age groups, including children in their first months of life, and tends to occur at the age of 40 years is	Five genes involved including KCNH2, KCNQ1, KCNJ2, CACNA1C and CACNB2b	Asymptomatic, syncope, sudden death	Corrected QT interval of less than 340 ms	Risk factors for cardiac arrest not clear	ICD for survivors of an aborted cardiac arrest, and/or documented spontaneous sustained VT
Idiopathic ventricular fibrillation	Rare, more often young male patients	Unknown cause	Syncope, sudden death	Normal ECG structurally normal heart	Spontaneous arrhythmias triggered by narrow-complex ventricular ectopics	ICD for survivors of cardiac arrest

Table adapted from, The ESC Textbook of Cardiovascular Medicine, ESC and American guideline documents [8, 24, 41, 51, 53]

Table 30.14 Key points about cardiac devices in inherited cardiac conditions

Condition	Device
– Symptomatic bradycardia	– Permanent pacemaker either single or dual chamber
– Severe LV systolic dysfunction and wide QRS complex (LBBB)	– Biventricular device either with pacemaker or ICD
– Survivor of cardiac arrest	– Secondary prevention ICD
– High risk of SCD	– Primary prevention ICD

30.11.2 Clinical Case: 5

A 32-year-old man, whilst having a pre-assessment for orthopaedic surgery was found to have the ECG below. He was subsequently referred to the cardiology out-patient clinic for further investigations and treatment.

After further assessment, he denied any symptoms such as palpitations or black-outs. He had no family history of sudden cardiac death. He subsequently underwent an TTE which was normal demonstrating a structurally normal heart.

In view of this patient being asymptomatic and having no significant family history and the ECG findings being incidental, his risk of sudden cardiac death was considered to be low. Therefore, the patient was advised to avoid QT-prolonging drugs. In addition, he was offered a trial of unselective beta-blockers.

Conclusion

There are many inherited cardiac conditions which have a varied morbidity and mortality. These conditions require a range of different investigations and cardiac interventions. These interventions can take the form of general lifestyle advice, avoidance of particular high risk activities, a range of medical treatments, procedural interventions including device implantation. Key points about this chapter are outlined in Table 30.14.

References

1. Marine JE, Brinker JA Techniques o pacemaker implantation and removal. In: Ellenbogen KA, Wood MA Cardiac pacing and ICDs. 2008 Blackwell Hoboken 204-281
2. Assessing fitness to drive: a guide for medical professionals. Updated 10 August 2016. https://www.gov.uk/government/uploads/system/uploads/attachment_data/file/526635/assessing-fitness-to-drive-a-guide-for-medical-professionals.pdf.
3. Armaganijan LV, Toff WD, Nielsen JC, Andersen HR, Connolly SJ, Ellenbogen KA, Healey JS. Are elderly patients at increased risk of complications following pacemaker implantation? a meta-analysis of randomized trials. Pacing Clin Electrophysiol. 2012;35(2):131–4. https://doi.org/10.1111/j.1540-8159.2011.03240x. Epub 2011 Oct 31
4. Link MS, Estes NA, Griffin JJ, Wang PJ, Maloney JD, Kirchhoffer JB, Mitchell GF, Orav J, Goldman L, Lamas GA. Complications of dual chamber pacemaker implantation in the

elderly. Pacemaker selection in the elderly (PASE) investigators. J Interv Card Electrophysiol. 1998;2(2):175–9.
5. van Rees JB, de Bie MK, Thijssen J, Borleffs CJ, Schalij MJ, van Erven L. Implantation-related complications of implantable cardioverter-defibrillators and cardiac resynchronization therapy devices: a systematic review of randomized clinical trials. J Am Coll Cardiol. 2011;58(10):995–1000.
6. Landolina M, Gasparini M, Lunati M, Iacopino S, Boriani G, Bonanno C, Vado A, Proclemer A, Capucci A, Zucchiatti C, Valsecchi S, Ricci RP, Santini M. Cardiovascular centers participating in the clinical service project. Long-term complications related to biventricular defibrillator implantation. Rate of surgical revisions and impact on survival: insights from the Italian clinical service database. Circulation. 2011;123:2526–35.
7. Mond HG, Irwin M, Morillo C, Ector H. The world survey of cardiac pacing and cardioverter defibrillators: calendar year 2001. Pacing Clin Electrophysiol. 2004;27:955–64.
8. Brignole M, Auricchio A, Baron-Esquivias G, Bordachar P, Boriani G, Breithardt O, Cleland J, Deharo J, Delgado V, Elliott PM, Gorenek B, Israel CW, Leclercq C, Linde C, Mont L, Padeletti L, Sutton R, Vardas PE. ESC guidelines on cardiac pacing and cardiac resynchronization therapy the Task Force on cardiac pacing and resynchronization therapy of the European Society of Cardiology (ESC). Developed in collaboration with the European Heart Rhythm Association (EHRA). Eur Heart J. 2013;34:2281–329.
9. Epstein AE, DiMarco JP, Ellenbogen KA, Estes NA, Freedman RA, Gettes LS, Gillinov AM, Gregoratos G, Hammill SC, Hayes DL, Hlatky MA, Newby LK, Page RL, Schoenfeld MH, Silka MJ, Stevenson LW, Sweeney MO, Tracy CM, Epstein AE, Darbar D, DiMarco JP, Dunbar SB, Estes NA, Ferguson TB Jr, Hammill SC, Karasik PE, Link MS, Marine JE, Schoenfeld MH, Shanker AJ, Silka MJ, Stevenson LW, Stevenson WG, Varosy PD. 2012 ACCF/AHA/HRS focused update incorporated into the ACCF/AHA/HRS 2008 guidelines for device-based therapy of cardiac rhythm abnormalities: a report of the American College of Cardiology Foundation/American Heart Association Task Force on Practice Guidelines and the Heart Rhythm Society. American College of Cardiology Foundation; American Heart Association Task Force on Practice Guidelines; Heart Rhythm Society. J Am Coll Cardiol. 2013;61(3):e6–75. https://doi.org/10.1016/j.jacc.2012.11.007. Epub 2012 Dec 19
10. Connolly SJ, Kerr CR, Gent M, Roberts RS, Yusuf S, Gillis AM, Sami MH, Talajic M, Tang AS, Klein GJ, Lau C, Newman DM. Effects of physiologic pacing versus ventricular pacing on the risk of stroke and death due to cardiovascular causes. Canadian trial of physiologic pacing investigators. N Engl J Med. 2000;342:1385–91.
11. Lamas GA, Orav EJ, Stambler BS, Ellenbogen KA, Sgarbossa EB, Huang SK, Marinchak RA, Estes NA, Mitchell GF, Lieberman EH, Mangione CM, Goldman L. Quality of life and clinical outcomes in elderly patients treated with ventricular pacing as compared with dual-chamber pacing. Pacemaker selection in the elderly investigators. N Engl J Med. 1998;338:1097–104.
12. Ponikowski P, Voors AA, Anker SD, Bueno H, Cleland JG, Coats AJ, Falk V, González-Juanatey JR, Harjola VP, Jankowska EA, Jessup M, Linde C, Nihoyannopoulos P, Parissis JT, Pieske B, Riley JP, Rosano GM, Ruilope LM, Ruschitzka F, Rutten FH, van der Meer P, Authors/Task Force Members. 2016 ESC guidelines for the diagnosis and treatment of acute and chronic heart failure: The Task Force for the diagnosis and treatment of acute and chronic heart failure of the European Society of Cardiology (ESC). Developed with the special contribution of the Heart Failure Association (HFA) of the ESC. Eur J Heart Fail. 2016;18(8):891–975. https://doi.org/10.1002/ejhf.592. Epub 2016 May 20.
13. Cha YM. Cardiac resynchronization therapy. In: Ellenbogen KA, Kaszala K, editors. Cardiac pacing and ICDs. Hoboken: Wiley, Blackwell; 2014.
14. Abraham WT, Fisher WG, Smith AL, Delurgio DB, Leon AR, Loh E, Kocovic DZ, Packer M, Clavell AL, Hayes DL, Ellestad M, Trupp RJ, Underwood J, Pickering F, Truex C, McAtee P, Messenger J. Cardiac resynchronization in chronic heart failure. MIRACLE Study Group. Multicenter InSync randomized clinical evaluation. N Engl J Med. 2002;346(24):1845–53.

15. DJ B, Bradley EA, Baughman KL, Berger RD, Calkins H, Goodman SN, Kass DA, Powe NR. Cardiac resynchronization and death from progressive heart failure: a meta-analysis of randomized controlled trials. JAMA. 2003;289(6):730–40.
16. Cleland JGF, Daubert J-C, Erdmann E, Freemantle N, Gras D, Kappenberger L, Tavazzi L. Longer-term effects of cardiac resynchronization therapy on mortality in heart failure [the CArdiac REsynchronization-Heart Failure (CARE-HF) trial extension phase]. Eur Heart J. 2006;27:1928–32.
17. Bristow MR, Saxon LA, Boehmer J, Krueger S, Kass DA, De Marco T, Carson P, DiCarlo L, DeMets D, White BG, DeVries DW, Feldman AM. Comparison of Medical Therapy, Pacing, and Defibrillation in Heart Failure (COMPANION) Investigators. Cardiac-resynchronization therapy with or without an implantable defibrillator in advanced chronic heart failure. N Engl J Med. 2004;350(21):2140–50.
18. Sohaib SMMA, Finegold JA, Nijjer SS, Hossain R, Linde C, Levy WC, Sutton R, Kanagaratnam P, Francis DP, Whinnett ZI. Opportunity to increase life span in narrow QRS cardiac resynchronization therapy recipients by deactivating ventricular pacing: evidence from randomized controlled trials. JACC Heart Fail. 2015;3:327–36.
19. Fowler S, Priori S. Clinical spectrum of patients with a Brugada ECG. Curr Opin Cardiol. 2009;24:74–81.
20. Priori S, Wilde A, Horie M, Cho Y, Behr ER, Berul C, Blom N, Brugada J, Chiang CE, Huikuri H, Kannankeril P, Krahn A, Leenhardt A, Moss A, Schwartz PJ, Shimizu W, Tomaselli G, Tracy C. Executive summary: HRS/EHRA/APHRS expert consensus statement on the diagnosis and management of patients with inherited primary arrhythmia syndromes. Europace. 2013;15:1389–406.
21. Eckart R, Shry E, Burke A, McNear J, Appel D, Castillo-Rojas L, Avedissian L, Pearse L, Potter R, Tremaine L, Gentlesk P, Huffer L, Reich S, Stevenson W. Department of defense cardiovascular death registry group. Sudden death in young adults: an autopsy-based series of a population undergoing active surveillance. J Am Coll Cardiol. 2011;58(12):1254–61.
22. van der Werf C, Hofman N, Tan HL, van Dessel P, Alders M, van der Wal AC, van Langen IM, Wilde AA. Diagnostic yield in sudden unexplained death and aborted cardiac arrest in the young: the experience of a tertiary referral center in The Netherlands. Heart Rhythm. 2010;7:1383–9.
23. Moss AJ, Zareba W, Hall WJ, Klein H, Wilber DJ, Cannom DS, Daubert JP, Higgins SL, Brown MW, Andrews ML. Prophylactic implantation of a defibrillator in patients with myocardial infarction and reduced ejection fraction. N Engl J Med. 2002;346:877–83.
24. Priori SG, Blomstrom-Lundqvist C, Mazzanti A, Blom N, Borggrefe M, Camm J, Elliott PM, Fitzsimons D, Hatala R, Hindricks G, Kirchhof P, Kjeldsen K, Kuck K, Hernandez-Madrid A, Nikolaou N, Norekva TM, Spaulding C, Van Veldhuisen DJ. 2015 ESC guidelines for the Management of Patients with ventricular arrhythmias and the prevention of sudden cardiac death. The Task Force for the management of patients with ventricular arrhythmias and the prevention of sudden cardiac death of the European Society of Cardiology (ESC). Eur Heart J. 2015;36:2793–867.
25. Bardy GH, Lee KL, Mark DB, Poole JE, Packer DL, Boineau R, Domanski M, Troutman C, Anderson J, Johnson G, McNulty SE, Clapp-Channing N, Davidson-Ray LD, Fraulo ES, Fishbein DP, Luceri RM, Ip JH. Sudden Cardiac Death in Heart Failure Trial (SCD-HeFT) Investigators. Amiodarone or an implantable cardioverter-defibrillator for congestive heart failure. N Engl J Med. 2005;352(3):225–37.
26. Alberte C, Zipes DP. Use of nonantiarrhythmic drugs for prevention of sudden cardiac death. J Cardiovasc Electrophysiol. 2003;14:S87–95.
27. Pitt B, Remme W, Zannad F, Neaton J, Martinez F, Roniker B, Bittman R, Hurley S, Kleiman J, Gatlin M. Eplerenone post-acute myocardial infarction heart failure efficacy and survival study investigators. Eplerenone, a selective aldosterone blocker, in patients with left ventricular dysfunction after myocardial infarction. N Engl J Med. 2003;348(14):1309–21. Epub 2003 Mar 31

28. Kadish A, Dyer A, Daubert JP, Quigg R, Estes NA, Anderson KP, Calkins H, Hoch D, Goldberger J, Shalaby A, Sanders WE, Schaechter A, Levine JH. Defibrillators in Non-Ischemic Cardiomyopathy Treatment Evaluation (DEFINITE) Investigators. Prophylactic defibrillator implantation in patients with nonischemic dilated cardiomyopathy. N Engl J Med. 2004;350(21):2151–8.
29. Desai AS, Fang JC, Maisel WH, Baughman KL. Implantable defibrillators for the prevention of mortality in patients with nonischemic cardiomyopathy. A meta-analysis of randomized controlled trials. JAMA. 2004;292(23):2874–9.
30. Connolly SJ, Hallstrom AP, Cappato R, Schron EB, Kuck KH, Zipes DP, Greene HL, Boczor S, Domanski M, Follmann D, Gent M, Roberts RS. Meta-analysis of the implantable cardioverter defibrillator secondary prevention trials. AVID, CASH and CIDS studies. Antiarrhythmics vs implantable defibrillator study. Cardiac arrest study Hamburg. Canadian implantable defibrillator study. Eur Heart J. 2000;21:2071–8.
31. Reynolds MR, Cohen DJ, Kugelmass AD, Brown PP, Becker ER, Culler SD, Simon AW. The frequency and incremental cost of major complications among medicare beneficiaries receiving implantable cardioverter-defibrillators. J Am Coll Cardiol. 2006;47:2493–7.
32. van der Heijden AC, Borleffs CJ, Buiten MS, Thijssen J, van Rees JB, Cannegieter SC, Schalij MJ, van Erven L. The clinical course of patients with implantable cardioverter-defibrillators: extended experience on clinical outcome, device replacements, and device-related complications. Heart Rhythm. 2015;12(6):1169–76. https://doi.org/10.1016/j.hrthm.2015.02.035. Epub 2015 Mar 4
33. Bardy GH, Smith WM, Hood MA, Crozier IG, Melton IC, Jordaens L, Theuns D, Park RE, Wright DJ, Connelly DT, Fynn SP, Murgatroyd FD, Sperzel J, Neuzner J, Spitzer SG, Ardashev AV, Oduro A, Boersma L, Maass AH, Van Gelder IC, Wilde AA, van Dessel PF, Knops RE, Barr CS, Lupo P, Cappato R, Grace AA. An entirely subcutaneous implantable cardioverter-defibrillator. N Engl J Med. 2010;363:36–44.
34. Lambiase PD, Barr C, Theuns DA, Knops R, Neuzil P, Johansen JB, Hood M, Pedersen S, Kaab S, Murgatroyd F, Reeve HL, Carter N, Boersma L. Worldwide experience with a totally subcutaneous implantable defibrillator: early results from the EFFORTLESS S-ICD registry. Eur Heart J. 2014;35:1657–65.
35. Burke MC, Gold MR, Knight BP, Barr CS, Theuns DAMJ, Boersma LVA, Knops RE, Weiss R, Leon AR, Herre JM, Husby M, Stein KM, Lambiase PD. Safety and efficacy of the totally subcutaneous implantable defibrillator: 2-year results from a pooled analysis of the IDE study and EFFORTLESS registry. J Am Coll Cardiol. 2015;65:1605–15.
36. Jarman JW, Lascelles K, Wong T, Markides V, Clague JR, Till J. Clinical experience of entirely subcutaneous implantable cardioverter-defibrillators in children and adults: cause for caution. Eur Heart J. 2012;33:1351–9.
37. Elliott P, Andersson B, Arbustini E, Bilinska Z, Cecchi F, Charron P, Dubourg O, Kuhl U, Maisch B, McKenna WJ, Monserrat L, Pankuweit S, Rapezzi C, Seferovic P, Tavazzi L, Keren A. Classification of the cardiomyopathies: a position statement from the European Society of Cardiology working group on myocardial and pericardial diseases. Eur Heart J. 2008;29:270–6.
38. Taylor MR, Carniel E, Mestroni L. Cardiomyopathy, familial dilated. Orphanet J Rare Dis. 2006;1:27.
39. Charron P, Forissier JF, Amara ME, Dubourg O, Desnos M, Bouhour JB, Isnard R, Hagege A, Benaiche A, Richard P, Schwartz K, Komajda M. Accuracy of European diagnostic criteria for familial hypertrophic cardiomyopathy in a genotyped population. Int J Cardiol. 2003;90:33–8.
40. Yousef Z, Elliott PM, Cecchi F, Escoubet B, Linhart A, Monserrat L, Namdar M, Weidemann F. Left ventricular hypertrophy in Fabry disease: a practical approach to diagnosis. Eur Heart J. 2013;34(11):802–8. https://doi.org/10.1093/eurheartj/ehs166. Epub 2012 Jun 26
41. Maron BJ, Towbin JA, Thiene G, Antzelevitch C, Corrado D, Arnett D, Moss AJ, Seidman CE, Young JB. Contemporary definitions and classification of the cardiomyopathies: an American Heart Association Scientific Statement from the Council on Clinical Cardiology, Heart Failure and Transplantation Committee; Quality of Care and Outcomes Research and Functional

Genomics and Translational Biology Interdisciplinary Working Groups; and Council on Epidemiology and Prevention. Circulation. 2006;113:1807–16.

42. Elliott PM, Anastasakis A, Borger MA, Borggrefe M, Cecchi F, Charron P, Hagege AA, Lafont A, Limongelli G, Mahrholdt H, McKenna WJ, Mogensen J, Nihoyannopoulos P, Nistri S, Pieper PG, Pieske B, Rapezzi C, Rutten FH, Tillmanns C, Watkins H. 2014 ESC guidelines on diagnosis and management of hypertrophic cardiomyopathy: the Task Force for the diagnosis and management of hypertrophic cardiomyopathy of the European Society of Cardiology (ESC). Eur Heart J. 2014;35(39):2733–79. https://doi.org/10.1093/eurheartj/ehu284. Epub 2014 Aug 29
43. Sorajja P, Ommen SR, Holmes DR Jr, Dearani JA, Rihal CS, Gersh BJ, Lennon RJ, Nishimura RA. Survival after alcohol septal ablation for obstructive hypertrophic cardiomyopathy. Circulation. 2012;126:2374–80.
44. Nishimura RA, Trusty JM, Hayes DL, Ilstrup DM, Larson DR, Hayes SN, Tajik AJ ATG. Dual-chamber pacing for hypertrophic cardiomyopathy: a randomized, double-blind, crossover trial. J Am Coll Cardiol. 1997;29:435–41.
45. Kappenberger L, Linde C, Daubert C, McKenna W, Meisel E, Sadoul N, Chojnowska L, Guize L, Gras D, Jeanrenaud X, Ryden L. Pacing in hypertrophic obstructive cardiomyopathy. A randomized crossover study. PIC study group. Eur Heart J. 1997;18:1249–56.
46. Maron BJ, Nishimura RA, McKenna WJ, Rakowski H, Josephson ME, Kieval RS. Assessment of permanent dual-chamber pacing as a treatment for drug-refractory symptomatic patients with obstructive hypertrophic cardiomyopathy. A randomized, double-blind, crossover study (M-PATHY). Circulation. 1999;99:2927–33.
47. Topilski I, Sherez J, Keren G, Copperman I. Long-term effects of dual-chamber pacing with periodic echocardiographic evaluation of optimal atrioventricular delay in patients with hypertrophic cardiomyopathy. 50 years of age. Am J Cardiol. 2006;97:1769–75.
48. Begley D, Mohiddin S, Fananapazir L. Dual chamber pacemaker therapy for mid-cavity obstructive hypertrophic cardiomyopathy. Pacing Clin Electrophysiol. 2001;24(11):1639–44.
49. Kofflard MJ, Ten Cate FJ, van der Lee C, van Domburg RT. Hypertrophic cardiomyopathy in a large community-based population: clinical outcome and identification of risk factors for sudden cardiac death and clinical deterioration. J Am Coll Cardiol. 2003;41:987–93.
50. Maron BJ, Olivotto I, Spirito P, et al. Epidemiology of hypertrophic cardiomyopathy-related death:revisited in a large non-referral-based patient population. Circulation. 2000;102:858–64.
51. Melacini P, Maron BJ, Bobbo F, Basso C, Tokajuk B, Zucchetto M, Thiene G, Iliceto S. Evidence that pharmacological strategies lack efficacy for the prevention of sudden death in hypertrophic cardiomyopathy. Heart. 2007;93:708–10.
52. Maron BJ, Spirito P, Shen WK, Haas TS, Formisano F, Link MS, Epstein AE, Almquist AK, Daubert JP, Lawrenz T, Boriani G, Estes NA, Favale S, Piccininno M, Winters SL, Santini M, Betocchi S, Arribas F, Sherrid MV, Buja G, Semsarian C, Bruzzi P. Implantable cardioverter-defibrillators and prevention of sudden cardiac death in hypertrophic cardiomyopathy. JAMA. 2007;298(4):405–12.
53. Eckardt L, Brugada P, Morgan J, Breithardt G. Ventricular tachycardia. In: Camm AJ, Lüscher TF, Serruys PW, editors. The ESC textbook of cardiovascular medicine. 2nd ed. Oxford: Blackwell Publishing.

Inherited Cardiovascular Conditions: Phenotype-Genotype Data Mining and Sharing, and Databases

31

J. Peter van Tintelen and Paul A. van der Zwaag

Abstract

With the advances of genetics in cardiovascular disease, increasingly more information on genetics and its associated phenotypes is becoming available, often online. The physician dealing with cardiovascular genetic disorders has to be able to interpret genetic test results and implement this in patient care including genetic counseling, risk assessment and, possibly personalized, treatment.

To be able to navigate through the online resources available, we summarized some databases and online tools on the interpretation of genetic variants; i.e. databases that assess the pathogenicity using in silico computional models, databases with data on the presence of variants in control populations and disease or gene specific databases that summarize variants and its associated phenotypes.

In addition to these variant-interpretation databases, databases to aid the clinician in making a diagnosis, predicting a positive genetic test or risk assessment are summarized. Finally websites that facilitate data-sharing are mentioned.

Even though these tools are very useful, one has to be aware that online data are not always up-to-date and the interpretation of data that are used, especially in patient care, always need a critical review. This should be considered a multidisciplinary teams effort that involve amongst others cardiologists, clinical and molecular geneticists, and genetic counselors.

Keywords

Genetics • Mutation • Pathogenicity • Database • Data-sharing • On-line tools

---

J.P. van Tintelen (✉)
Department of Clinical Genetics, Academic Medical Center, Amsterdam, The Netherlands
e-mail: p.vantintelen@amc.nl

P.A. van der Zwaag
Department of Genetics, University Medical Center Groningen, Groningen, The Netherlands
e-mail: p.a.van.der.zwaag@umcg.nl

D. Kumar, P. Elliott (eds.), *Cardiovascular Genetics and Genomics*,
https://doi.org/10.1007/978-3-319-66114-8_31

31.1 Introduction

With the advances in human genetics including the implementation of Next Generation Sequencing techniques to study large numbers of genes in large patients cohorts, large amounts of data overwhelm the clinician working in the field of cardiovascular genetics. A clinician nowadays has to be able to deal with this data, in addition to being able to diagnose, treat and follow-up patients with some times rare diagnoses. Reasons to have the skills to be able to "navigate" in the genetics field, is that a specific variant or multiple variants may have been identified in a patient with a specific cardiovascular genetic condition like hypertrophic cardiomyopathy (HCM) or long QT syndrome (LQTS); or because a specific variant is found in an individual patient that has been genetically evaluated for another reason, yet genetic analyses reveal a variant in a gene that is labeled as an actionable gene according to the American College of Medical Genetics and Genomics (ACMG) [1]. Following the rapid technological advances in the field of molecular genetics, the identification of variants itself is no longer a bottleneck. It is the assessment and classification of variants that is challenging and requires multidisciplinary teams at least consisting of cardiologists, clinical geneticists/genetic counselors, molecular geneticists and bioinformaticians [2].

The main goal is to correctly interpret a variant as resulting in an abnormal protein with an effect on cardiovascular function or not. If leading to an abnormal protein and consequently an effect on the phenotype, it is important to know the associated clinical phenotype including information on penetrance and clinical variability. This information is not only crucial for the clinician following up this patient, but also for clinical geneticists and others counseling these patients and their family members [3].

To facilitate the process of evaluating variants, collecting information on clinical phenotypes associated with specific gene mutations, and risk-assessment, an overview of potential useful online resources is provided in this chapter.

31.2 Interpretation of Variants

31.2.1 Resources Used to Assess Pathogenicity of Variants

Whether a specific variant leads to an abnormal protein and thereby is potentially disease-causing is based upon several factors, such as the gross effect of a mutation (leading to a truncated protein based upon a nonsense mutation, an insertion or deletion out side the reading frame or a mutation affecting splicing e.g.), or the effect of the variant at nucleotide and therefore amino acid level in case of missense mutations. The standards and guidelines for this interpretation are summarized in a guideline by the ACMG [4] The impact of a missense change depends on criteria such as the evolutionary conservation of an amino acid or nucleotide, the location and context within the protein sequence, the biochemical consequence of the amino acid substitution, its predicted effect on protein function and the presence or absence of the variant in control populations. Several online resources are available that are used to evaluate these aspects and some of these integrate several of these "factors". Multiple software packages are available to aid in the interpretation of identified variants. The use of these resources may help to correctly classify these variants in one of the main categories of pathogenicity; (class 5) pathogenic, (4) likely pathogenic, (3) uncertain significance, (2) likely benign, or (1) benign.

31.2.2 A Computational Predictive Programs (In Silico Analyses)

Several in silico tools can aid in the interpretation of sequence variants. The algorithms underlying these tools determine the effect of a sequence variant at the nucleotide and amino acid level, including the effect of a variant on the primary and alternative gene transcripts, and compute a potential impact of the variant on the protein. The most widely used tools can be categorized in those predicting the effect of missense mutations and those predicting whether a mutation affects splicing. The most commonly used in silico tools for missense variant interpretation are PolyPhen2 [5], SIFT [6] and MutationTaster [7]. A more extensive list of these tools and those used for splice site variant interpretation can be found in Table 31.1. With the increasing use of whole genome sequencing, more extensive tools also evaluate the effect of noncoding sequences [8].

The use of multiple software programs for sequence variant interpretation is recommended because the different programs each have their own strengths and weaknesses, depending on the algorithm; the combined predictions are however considered a single piece of evidence in interpretation of variants.

31.2.3 Databases with Control Populations

Population databases (Table 31.2) can be helpful to get an impression of the frequencies of specific variants or variability within a gene in large populations. One has to keep in mind however that specific information on disease status is often lacking from these control individuals, so these data are not specifically from individuals with confirmed absence of cardiovascular genetic disease, especially considering the age-dependent and incomplete penetrance of many cardiovascular genetic diseases. In addition, detailed information on pathogenic effects of variants is often limited. One also has to keep in mind that in specific cohorts, multiple members from a single family may be included.

One of the most commonly used population database is the ExAC (Exome Aggregation Consortium) database (www.exac.broadinstitute.org) [9]. It consists of genome data of over 60,000 unrelated individuals from diverse disease-genetic and population genetic studies. To illustrate that one needs to interpret the presence of variants in these control databases very cautiously; for example the single most prevalent HCM causing mutation in two large cohorts from the UK and the US, *MYBPC3* c.1504C>T (p.Arg502Trp), was identified three times in the ExAC database [10]. This is not surprising, given the high prevalence of HCM (1:500) and highlights the importance of careful utilization of these databases.

Table 31.1 Commonly used in silico predictive tools/software used for sequence variant interpretation (from [4])

Category	Name	Website	Basis
Missense prediction	MutationAssessor	http://mutationassessor.org	Evolutionary conservation
	SIFT	http://sift.jcvi.org	Evolutionary conservation
	MutationTaster	http://www.mutationtaster.org	Protein structure/function and evolutionary conservation
	PolyPhen-2	http://genetics.bwh.harvard.edu/pph2	Protein structure/function and evolutionary conservation
	CADD	http://cadd.gs.washington.edu	Contrasts annotations of fixed/nearly fixed derived alleles in humans with simulated variants
Splice site prediction	GeneSplicer	http://www.cbcb.umd.edu/software/GeneSplicer/gene_spl.shtml	Markov models
	Human Splicing Finder	http://www.umd.be/HSF/	Position-dependent logic
	MaxEntScan	http://genes.mit.edu/burgelab/maxent/Xmaxentscan_scoreseq.html	Maximum entropy principle
	NetGene2	http://www.cbs.dtu.dk/services/NetGene2	Neural networks
	NNSplice	http://www.fruitfly.org/seq_tools/splice.html	Neural networks
	FSPLICE	http://www.softberry.com/berry.phtml?topic=fsplice&group=programs&subgroup=gfind	Species-specific predictor for splice sites based on weight matrices model

Table 31.2 Examples of population databases [4]

Population databases	Website	
Exome Aggregation Consortium	http://exac.broadinstitute.org/	Exome sequencing results of >60,000 individuals from various projects (disease-specific/population based)
Exome Variant Server	http://evs.gs.washington.edu/EVS	Exome sequencing results of large cohorts; collection of different studies
1000 Genomes Project	http://browser.1000genomes.org	Variant database from 26 populations
dbSNP	http://www.ncbi.nlm.nih.gov/snp	Short genetic variations from different databases
dbVar	http://www.ncbi.nlm.nih.gov/dbvar	Structural variations from different sources

Table 31.3 Disease-specific mutation databases

Database	Online Resource (URL)	Specific utility
Clinvar	www.ncbi.nlm.nih.gov/clinvar	
OMIM	www.omim.org	
Human Gene Mutation Database	www.hgmd.org	
Atlas of cardiac genetic variation (HCM, DCM and ARVC)	https://cardiodb.org	
ARVC	www.arvcdatabase.info	
Marfan syndrome (FBN1)	www.umd.be/FBN1	
Familial hypercholesterolemia	www.jojogenetics.nl	
Leiden Open Variation Database	http://www.lovd.nl	
IF databases	www.interfil.org	Contains genes encoding intermediate filament proteins like DES, LMNA
TTN	https://cardiodb.org/titin/	
Factor IX Variant Database	www.factorix.org/	

It is to be expected that the size of this and other databases will continue to grow, because several disease related and population related genome sequencing initiatives are going on such as the large scale Precision Medicine Initiative of the NIH in the USA (https://www.nih.gov/precision-medicine-initiative-cohort-program) and the 100 K Genomes Project in the UK (www.genomicsengland.co.uk). But also smaller projects, with more national genetic data can be useful such as the genome of the Netherlands with data of 250 trios (www.nlgenome.nl) [11].

31.2.4 Disease and Gene Specific Databases

Disease and gene specific (Table 31.3) databases primarily contain variants found in patients with a specific disease or lists variants in genes including an assessment of the variants' pathogenicity. One has to be aware that these disease and gene-specific databases often contain variants that are incorrectly classified, including incorrect claims published in peer-reviewed literature. The reason for this is that many databases do not perform a primary review of evidence. In addition, the level of evidence may change over time; i.e. a mutation initially considered pathogenic, may turn out to be an innocent variant after additional studies. Some examples are the *PKP2* c.419C>T; p. (Ser140Phe) and *DSC2* c.2686_2687dupGA; p.A897KfsX4 variations in arrhythmogenic right ventricular cardiomyopathy (ARVC) [12, 13]. Also for *FBN1* mutations in Marfan Syndrome, discrepancies in databases have been described [14].

Notably, based on the reported classification in the Human Genome Mutation Database (HGMD), 11.7, 19.6, and 20.1% of individuals in the ExAC database have reported HCM, dilated cardiomyopathy (DCM), and ARVC variants, respectively

[10]. Given the prevalence of these diseases, these numbers are far too high and should alert the user that the HGMD classification could be an overestimate of the variant pathogenicity.

In addition, one has to keep in mind that many databases are often not completely up to date, because these databases are maintained by professionals who update the databases next to their professional activities, which is a challenging task like we encounter for the ARVC related mutation database [15, 16].

With these limitations in mind, these databases can however be very helpful in getting a quick overview of a specific variant, including relevant references to literature which can greatly facilitate interpretation of a variant.

31.3 Online Tools for Clinicians

31.3.1 Diagnostic Aids

Clinical criteria to diagnose specific cardiovascular genetic disorders can be very extensive such as the clinical criteria for ARVC where depolarization/repolarization abnormalities on ECG, arrhythmias, the results of imaging and family history, have to be scored to make a diagnosis [17]. These criteria can be filled out online to calculate at https://ocrr.ca/pdg/public.php.

Making a diagnosis might even get more complicated, if a cardiovascular genetic disorder has multisystem manifestations such as Marfan syndrome where skeletal, ophthalmologic and cardiac features can be present [18]. To easily access normograms for aortic size related to body service and to facilitate interpretation and scoring of features in Marfan syndrome, online diagnostic tools/calculators are available (see http://www.marfan.org/dx/home).

31.3.2 Calculators to Predict a Positive Genotype

The yield of genetic testing in cardiovascular genetic disease is generally dependent on several factors such as age of diagnosis, specific cardiac features and a positive family history for disease. Because resources for genetic testing are sometimes limited or genetic testing is not reimbursed, it may be helpful to predict which patients have a high pretest chance to have a mutation. For HCM, one of the most common genetic cardiac diseases, these calculators are available and based upon: age of diagnosis, gender, maximal LV wall thickness, morphology of septal hypertrophy, a family history of SCD or HCM and a history of hypertension [19, 20].

31.3.3 Risk Calculators

Cardiovascular genetic diseases are often associated with premature death, for example due to end-stage heart failure or ventricular arrhythmias. Therapeutic options, like placing an ICD, may prevent such dismal outcome. However, not infrequently the placement of an ICD is associated with serious complications and inappropriate ICD therapy as has also been described in inherited cardiac disease [21]. Therefore the implantation of an ICD has to be precisely timed to prevent sudden death; not too early because of the complications and not too late so that a patient does not benefit from it [22].

For HCM a calculator is available to predict the 5-years risk of SCD and based upon this prediction the indication for an ICD implantation is discussed. This tool makes use of seven variables that can be filled out online (http://www.doc2do.com/hcm/webHCM.html) [23].

31.3.4 Datasharing

Sharing data on variants and phenotypes is important to better understand the role of variants in specific disorders and its pathogenicity, but also to study potential genotype-phenotype relationships. These are helpful for genetic counseling, but also for treatment; for example, non-missense mutations in the *LMNA* gene are considered a risk factor in the presence of a second risk factor. This conclusion might justify the implantation of an ICD given the high risk for malignant ventricular arrhythmias [24]. These data were collected from a large European cohort underscoring the importance for collaboration and sharing data in improving therapies and risk stratification for rare genetic disorders. Making data available to other researchers will enable researchers worldwide to work with much larger and richer data and material sets of higher quality compared to what is locally available. An efficient and transparent research portal may help enable researchers worldwide to work with a much larger and richer data and material set of higher quality compared to what is currently possible. An on-line catalogue may aid to this goal. For some cardiovascular genetic diseases such a catalogue to create an overview of the available clinical data, bio-samples, and imaging archive from the existing and on-going registries has been built (http://www.durrercenter.nl/catalogue/). By using the FAIR Data principle (Findable, Accessible, Interoperable and Re-useable) this task should boost the exploitation and re-use of expensively gathered patient data. For example, the aggregate data from a number of studies is made available by the German Centre for Heart and Circulation Research (DZHK) (https://dzhk.de/en/resources/data-catalogue/), which is considered an essential step towards the controlled provision of data and biomaterials, leading to increased value of these collections to the scientific community.

Conclusion

Several online tools are available that are useful in determining the pathogenicity of variants identified in genetic diagnostics, making a diagnosis, predicting a positive test result and risk assessment. One has to be aware that some online databases are outdated. In the near future, sharing data will become increasingly common, in particular in rare genetic diseases. Different groups around the globe have launched a number of online catalogues that facilitate data sharing.

References

1. Green RC, Berg JS, Grody WW, et al. American college of medical genetics and genomics ACMG recommendations for reporting of incidental findings in clinical exome and genome sequencing. Genet Med. 2013;15:565–74.
2. Mogensen J, van Tintelen JP, Fokstuen S, et al. The current role of next-generation DNA sequencing in routine care of patients with hereditary cardiovascular conditions: a viewpoint paper of the European Society of Cardiology working group on myocardial and pericardial diseases and members of the European Society of Human Genetics. Eur Heart J. 2015;36:1367–70. https://doi.org/10.1093/eurheartj/ehv122.
3. Choi Y, Sims GE, Murphy S, et al. Predicting the functional effect of amino acid substitutions and indels. PLoS One. 2012;7:e46688.
4. Richards S, Aziz N, Bale S, et al. ACMG laboratory quality assurance committee. Standards and guidelines for the interpretation of sequence variants: a joint consensus recommendation of the American College of Medical Genetics and Genomics and the Association for Molecular Pathology. Genet Med. 2015;17:405–24.
5. Adzhubei IA, Schmidt S, Peshkin L, et al. A method and server for predicting damaging missense mutations. Nat Methods. 2010;7:248–9.
6. Kumar P, Henikoff S, Ng PC. Predicting the effects of coding non-synonymous variants on protein function using the SIFT algorithm. Nat Protoc. 2009;4:1073–81.
7. Schwarz JM, Rödelsperger C, Schuelke M, Seelow D. MutationTaster evaluates disease-causing potential of sequence alterations. Nature Methods. 2010;7:575–576. https://doi.org/10.1038/nmeth0810-575.
8. Kircher M, Witten DM, Jain P, et al. A general framework for estimating the relative pathogenicity of human genetic variants. Nat Genet. 2014;46:310–5. https://doi.org/10.1038/ng.2892.
9. Monkol Lek M, Karczewski KJ, Minikel EV, et al. Analysis of protein-coding genetic variation in 60,706 humans. Nature. 2016;536:285–91. https://doi.org/10.1038/nature19057.
10. Walsh R, Thomson KL, Ware JS, et al. Reassessment of Mendelian gene pathogenicity using 7,855 cardiomyopathy cases and 60,706 reference samples. Genet Med. 2016;19(2):192–203. https://doi.org/10.1038/gim.2016.90. [Epub ahead of print]
11. Genome of the Netherlands Consortium. Whole-genome sequence variation, population structure and demographic history of the Dutch population. Nat Genet. 2014;46:818–25. https://doi.org/10.1038/ng.3021.
12. Christensen AH, Kamstrup PR, Gandjbakhch E, et al. Plakophilin-2 c.419C>T and risk of heart failure and arrhythmias in the general population. Eur J Hum Genet. 2016;24:732–8. https://doi.org/10.1038/ejhg.2015.171.
13. De Bortoli M, Beffagna G, Bauce B, et al. The p.A897KfsX4 frameshift variation in desmocollin-2 is not a causative mutation in arrhythmogenic right ventricular cardiomyopathy. Eur J Hum Genet. 2010;18:776–82. https://doi.org/10.1038/ejhg.2010.19.
14. Groth KA, Gaustadnes M, Thorsen K, et al. Difficulties in diagnosing Marfan syndrome using current FBN1 databases. Genet Med. 2016;18:98–102. https://doi.org/10.1038/gim.2015.32.
15. Lazzarini E, Jongbloed JD, Pilichou K, et al. The ARVD/C genetic variants database: 2014 update. Hum Mutat. 2015;36:403–10.
16. van der Zwaag PA, Jongbloed JD, van den Berg MP, et al. A genetic variants database for arrhythmogenic right ventricular dysplasia/cardiomyopathy. Hum Mutat. 2009;30:1278–83.
17. Marcus FI, McKenna WJ, Sherrill D, et al. Diagnosis of arrhythmogenic right ventricular cardiomyopathy/dysplasia: proposed modification of the task force criteria. Circulation. 2010;121:1533–41. https://doi.org/10.1161/CIRCULATIONAHA.108.840827.
18. Loeys BL, Dietz HC, Braverman AC, et al. The revised Ghent nosology for the Marfan syndrome. J Med Genet. 2010;47:476–85. https://doi.org/10.1136/jmg.2009.072785.
19. Bos JM, Will ML, Gersh BJ, et al. Characterization of a phenotype-based genetic test prediction score for unrelated patients with hypertrophic cardiomyopathy. Mayo Clin Proc. 2014;89:727–37. https://doi.org/10.1016/j.mayocp.2014.01.025.

20. Gruner C, Ivanov J, Care M, et al. Toronto hypertrophic cardiomyopathy genotype score for prediction of a positive genotype in hypertrophic cardiomyopathy. Circ Cardiovasc Genet. 2013;6:19–26. https://doi.org/10.1161/CIRCGENETICS.112.963363.
21. Olde Nordkamp LR, Postema PG, et al. Implantable cardioverter-defibrillator harm in young patients withinherited arrhythmia syndromes: a systematic review and meta-analysis of inappropriate shocks and complications. Heart Rhythm. 2016;13:443–54. https://doi.org/10.1016/j.hrthm.2015.09.010.
22. Olde Nordkamp LR, Wilde AA, Tijssen JG, et al. The ICD for primary prevention in patients with inherited cardiac diseases: indications, use, and outcome: a comparison with secondary prevention. Circ Arrhythm Electrophysiol. 2013;6:91–100. https://doi.org/10.1161/CIRCEP.112.975268.
23. O'Mahony C, Jichi F, Pavlou M, et al. A novel clinical risk prediction model for sudden cardiac death in hypertrophic cardiomyopathy (HCM risk-SCD). Eur Heart J. 2014;35:2010–20. https://doi.org/10.1093/eurheartj/eht439.
24. van Rijsingen IA, Arbustini E, Elliott PM, et al. Risk factors for malignant ventricular arrhythmias in lamin a/c mutation carriers a European cohort study. J Am Coll Cardiol. 2012;59:493–500. https://doi.org/10.1016/j.jacc.2011.08.078.

Glossary: Commonly Used Terms and Phrases in Cardiovascular Genetics and Genomics[1]

Abbreviations

AA	Antiarrhythmic
AF	Atrial fibrillation
ARVC	Arrhythmogenic right ventricular cardiomyopathy
ATP	Antitachycardia pacing
BRS	Brugada syndrome
CABG	Coronary artery bypass graft
CAD	Coronary artery disease
CASH	Cardiac arrest study Hamburg
CHD	Coronary heart disease
CHF	Congestive heart failure
CIDS	Canadian implantable defibrillator study
CNV	Copy number variation
DCM	Dilated cardiomyopathy
DFT	Defibrillation threshold
DNA	Deoxyribose nucleic acid
ECG	Electrocardiography
EF	Ejection fraction
EPS	Electrophysiologic study
ESC	European society of cardiology
HCM	Hypertrophic cardiomyopathy
IBD	Identity by descent
ICD	Implantable cardioverter defibrillator
ICD	Implantable cardioverter device
iLVNC	Isolated left ventricular noncompaction
iNVM	Isolated noncompaction of the ventricular myocardium
LOS	Length of stay
LQTS	Long Q-T syndrome

[1] Disclaimer: The glossary is compiled from author's personal collection, suggestions from other professionals and on-line resources. All terms, abbreviations and phrases are commonly used in both clinical and scientific practices. There should not be any copyright or ownership infringement.

D. Kumar, P. Elliott (eds.), *Cardiovascular Genetics and Genomics*,
https://doi.org/10.1007/978-3-319-66114-8

LV	Left ventricle
LVNC	Left ventricular noncompaction
MRI	Magnetic resonance imaging
mtDNA	Mitochondrial DNA
NGS	Next generation genome sequencing
NVM	Noncompaction of the ventricular myocardium
OMIM	On-line Mendelian inheritance in man
ORF	Open reading frame
PCR	Polymerase chain reaction
PGD	Pre-implantation genetic diagnosis
PVC	Premature ventricular contraction
RCM	Restrictive cardiomyopathy
RNA	Ribose nucleic acid
RT-PCR	Reverse transcriptase polymerase chain reaction
RV	Right ventricle
SADS	Sudden arrhythmic death syndrome
SCD	Sudden cardiac death
SUD	Sudden unexplained death
SVT	Supraventricular tachycardia
VF	Ventricular fibrillation
VT	Ventricular tachycardia
WGS	Whole genome sequencing
WES	Whole exome sequencing

Terms and Phrases

Ablation The removal, isolation or destruction of cardiac tissue or conduction pathways involved in arrhythmias.

Acrocentric A chromosome having the centromere close to one end.

Algorithm A step-by-step method for solving a computational problem or a set of precise rules or procedures programmed into a pacemaker or defibrillator that are designed to solve a specific clinical problem.

Allele An alternative form of a gene at the same chromosomal locus.

Allelic Heterogeneity Different alleles for one gene.

Alternative Splicing A regulatory mechanism by which variations in the incorporation of coding regions (see exon) of the gene into messenger RNA (mRNA) lead to the production of more than one related protein, or isoform.

Amino Acid A chemical subunit of a protein. Amino acids polymerize to form linear chains linked by peptide bonds called polypeptides. All proteins are made from twenty naturally occurring amino acids.

Amplification Refractory Mutation System (ARMS) An allele-specific PCR amplification reaction.

Annealing The association of complementary DNA (or RNA) strand to form the double-stranded structure.

Anonymous DNA DNA not known to have a coding function.

Annotation The descriptive text that accompanies a sequence in a database method.

Antibody A protein produced by the immune system in response to an antigen (see antigen). Antibodies bind to their target antigen to help the immune system destroy the foreign entity.

Anticipation A phenomenon in which the age of onset of a disorder is reduced and/or severity of the phenotype is increased in successive generations.

Anticodon The three bases of a tRNA molecule that form a complementary match to an mRNA codon and thus allow the tRNA to perform the key translation step in the process of information transfer from nucleic acid to protein.

Antigen A molecule that is perceived by the immune system to be foreign.

AntiTachycardia Pacing (ATP) Short, rapid, carefully controlled sequences of pacing pulses delivered by an ICD and used to terminate a tachycardia in the atria or ventricles.

Apoptosis Programmed cell death

Arrest (Cardiac) Cessation of the heart's normal rhythmic electrical and/or mechanical activity which causes immediate haemodynamic compromise.

Arrhythmogenic Right Ventricular Cardiomyopathy/Dysplasia A new term of arrhythmogenic cardiomyopathy (AC) is preferred due to biventricular involvement in most cases of ARVC/ARVD

Arrhythmia Any heart rhythm that falls outside the accepted norms with respect to rate, regularity, or sequence of depolarisation. (Any abnormal or absent heart rhythm.)

ATP Antitachycardia pacing

Atrial Fibrillation (AF) Very fast, disorganised heart rhythm that starts in the atria.

Atrial Flutter (AFL) Fast, organised atrial rhythm.

Atrial Tachycardia (AT) A rapid heart rate that starts in the atria (includes AF, and AFL).

Atrioventricular (AV) Node A section of specialised neuromuscular cells that are part of the normal conduction pathway between the atria and the ventricles. (A junction that conducts electrical impulses from the atria to the ventricles of the heart.)

Atrioventricular (AV) Synchrony The normal activation sequence of the heart in which the atria contract and then, after a brief delay, the ventricles contract. The loss of AV synchrony can have significant haemodynamic effects. Dual chamber pacemakers are designed to attempt to maintain AV synchrony.

Atrium The heart is divided into four chambers. Each of the two upper chambers is called an atrium. (Atria is the plural form of atrium.) Either of the two upper chambers of the heart, above the ventricles that receive blood from the veins and communicate with the ventricles through the tricuspid (right) or mitral (left) valve.

Autosome Any chromosome other than a sex chromosome (X or Y) and the mitochondrial chromosome.

Autozygosity In an inbred person, homozygosity for alleles identical by descent.

Autozygosity Mapping A form of genetic mapping for autosomal recessive disorders in which affected individuals are expected to have two identical disease alleles by descent.

Bacterial Artificial Chromosome (BAC) DNA vectors into which large DNA fragments can be inserted and cloned in a bacterial host.

Bioinformatics An applied computational system which includes development and utilization of facilities to store, analyse and interpret biological data.

Biotechnology The industrial application of biological processes, particularly recombinant DNA technology and genetic engineering.

Basic Local Alignment Search Tool (BLAST) A fast database similarity search tool used by the NCBI that allows the world to search query sequences against the GeneBank database over the web.

Blastocyst The mammalian embryo at the stage at which it is implanted into the wall of the uterus.

Bradycardia/Bradyarrhythmia) A heart rate that is abnormally slow; commonly defined as under 60 beats per minute or a rate that is too slow to physiologically support a person and their activities.

Candidate Gene Any gene which by virtue of a known property (function, expression pattern, chromosomal location, structural motif, etc.) is considered as a possible locus for a given disease.

Cardiac Arrest Failure of the heart to pump blood through the body. If left untreated, it is dangerous and life-threatening.

Cardioversion Termination of an atrial or ventricular tachyarrhythmia (other than ventricular fibrillation) by a delivery of a direct low energy electrical current which is synchronised to a specific instant during the heart beat (during to the ventricular depolarisation). Synchronisation of the shock prevents shocking during periods which could cause ventricular fibrillation.

Carrier A person who carries an allele for a recessive disease (see heterozygote) without the disease phenotype but can pass it on to the next generation.

Carrier Testing Carried out to determine whether an individual carries one copy of an altered gene for a particular recessive disease.

Cell Cycle Series of tightly regulated steps that a cell goes through from its creation to division to form two daughter cells.

"Central Dogma" A term proposed by Francis Crick in 1957- 'DNA is transcribed into RNA which is translated into protein'.

Complementary DNA (cDNA) A piece of DNA copied in vitro from mRNA by a reverse transcription enzyme.

CentiMorgan (cM) A unit of genetic distance equivalent to 1% probability of recombination during meiosis. One centiMorgan is equivalent, on average, to a physical distance of approximately 1 megabase in the human genome.

Centromere The constricted region near the center of a chromosome that has critical role in cell division.

Chimera A hybrid, particularly a synthetic DNA molecule that is the result of ligation of DNA fragments that come from different organisms or an organism derived from more than one zygote.

Chromosome Subcellular structures which contain and convey the genetic material of an organism.

Chromosome Painting Fluorescent labelling of whole chromosomes by a FISH procedure in which labelled probes each consist of complex mixture of different DNA sequences from a single chromosome.

Chronic Lead A pacemaker or ICD lead which has been implanted in the past.

Chronotropic Incompetence The inability of the heart to increase its rate appropriately in response to increased activity or metabolic need, e.g., exercise, illness, etc.

Class I Antiarrhythmic Drugs Drugs which act selectively to depress fast sodium channels, slowing conduction in all parts of the heart (e.g. Quinidine, Procainamide, Flecainide, Encainide, Propafenone)

Class II Antiarrhythmic Drugs Drugs which act as beta-adrenergic blocking agents (e.g. Propanolol, Metoprolol, Atenolol)

Class III Antiarrhythmic Drugs Drugs which act directly on cardiac cell membrane, prolong repolarisation and refractory periods, increase VF threshold, and act on peripheral smooth muscle to decrease peripheral resistance (e.g. amiodarone, sotalol)

Clinical Sensitivity The proportion of persons with a disease phenotype who test positive

Clinical Specificity The proportion of persons without a disease phenotype who test negative.

Clone A line of cells derived from a single cell and therefore carrying identical genetic material.

Cloning Vector A DNA construct such as a plasmid, modified viral genome (bacteriophage or phage), or artificial chromosome that can be used to carry a gene or fragment of DNA for purposes of cloning (for example, a bacterial, yeast or mammalian cell).

Coagulation Factors Various components of the blood coagulation system. The following factors have been identified: (Synonyms which are or have been in use are included). · Factor I (fibrinogen); · Factor II (prothrombin); · Factor III (thromboplastin, tissue factor); · Factor IV (calcium); · Factor V (labile factor); · Factor VII (stable factor); · Factor VIII (antihemophilic globulin [AHF], antihemophilic globulin [AHG], antihemophilic factor A Factor VIII: C); · Factor IX (plasma thromboplastin component [PTC], Christmas factor, antihemophilic factor B); Factor X (Stuart factor, Prower factor, Stuart-Prower factor); · Factor XI (plasma thromboplastin antecedent [PTA], antihemophilic factor C); · Factor XII (Hageman factor, surface factor, contact factor); · Factor XIII (fibrin stabilizing factor [FSF], fibrin stabilizing enzyme, fibri-nase); Other factors: (prekallikrein [Fletcher factor], and high molecular weight kininogen [Fizgerald]).

Coding DNA (Sequence) The portion of a gene that is transcribed into mRNA.

Codon A three-base sequence of DNA or RNA that specifies a single amino acid.

Comparative Genomics The comparison of genome structure and functional across different species in order to further understanding of biological mechanisms and evolutionary processes.

Comparative Genome Hybridization (CGH) Use of competitive fluorescence in situ hybridization to detect chromosomal regions that are amplified or deleted, especially in tumours.

Complementary DNA (cDNA) DNA generated from an expressed messenger RNA through a process known as reverse transcription.

Complex Diseases Diseases characterized by risk to relatives of an affected individual which is greater than the incidence of the disorder in the population

Complex Trait One which is not strictly Mendelian (dominant, recessive, or sex linked) and may involve the interaction of two or more genes to produce a phenotype, or may involve gene-environment interactions.

Computational Therapeutics An emerging biomedical field concerned with the development of techniques for using software to collect, manipulate and link biological and medical data from diverse sources. It also includes the use of such information in simulation models to make predictions or therapeutically relevant discoveries or advances.

Computer Aided Diagnosis [CAD] A general term used for a variety of artificial intelligence techniques applied to medical images. CAD methods are being rapidly developed at several academic and industry sites, particularly for large-scale breast, lung, and colon cancer screening studies. X-ray imaging for breast, lung and colon cancer screening are good physical and clinical models for the development of CAD methods, related image database resources, and the development of common metrics and methods for evaluation. [Large-scale screening applications include (a) improving the sensitivity of cancer detection, (b) reducing observer variation in image interpretation, (c) increasing the efficiency of reading large image arrays, (d) improving efficiency of screening by identifying suspect lesions or identifying normal images, and (e) facilitating remote reading by experts (e.g., telemammography).]

Congenital Any trait, condition or disorder that exists from birth.

Consanguinity Marriage between two individuals having common ancestral parents, commonly between first cousins; an approved practice in some communities who share social, cultural and religious beliefs. In genetic terms two such individuals could be heterozygous by descent for an allele expressed as 'coefficient of relationship', and any offspring could be therefore homozygous by descent for the same allele expressed as 'coefficient of inbreeding'.

Conserved Sequence A base sequence in a DNA molecule (or an amino acid sequence in a protein) that has remained essentially unchanged throughout evolution.

Constitutional Mutation A mutation which is inherited and therefore present in all cells containing the relevant nucleic acid (same as germ line mutation)

Contig A consensus sequence generated from a set of overlapping sequence fragments that represent a large piece of DNA, usually a genomic region from a particular chromosome.

Copy Number The number of different copies of a particular DNA sequence in a genome.

Copy Number Variation (CNV) Variation in copy number sequences, likely to be of pathogenic importance for certain complex disease traits.

CpG Island Short stretch of DNA, often less than 1 kb, containing CpG dinucleotides which are unmethylated and present at the expected frequency. CpG islands often occur at transcriptionally active DNA.

Cytoplasm The internal matrix of a cell. The cytoplasm is the area between the outer periphery of a cell (the cell membrane) and the nucleus (in a eukaryotic cell).

Defibrillation Termination of an erratic, life-threatening arrhythmia of the ventricles by a high energy, direct current delivered asynchronously to the cardiac tissue. The defibrillation discharge will often restore the heart's normal rhythm.

Denaturation Dissociation of complementary strands to give single-stranded DNA and/or RNA.

Demographic Transition The change in the society from extreme poverty to a stronger economy, often associated by a transition in the pattern of diseases from malnutrition and infection to the intractable conditions of middle and old age, for example cardiovascular disease, diabetes, and cancer.

Diagnostics Data gathered by an ICD or pacemaker to evaluate patient rhythm status, verify system operation, or assure appropriate delivery of therapy options.

Diploid A genome (the total DNA content contained in each cell) that consists of two homologous copies of each chromosome.

Disease A fluid concept influenced by societal and cultural attitudes that change with time and in response to new scientific and medical discoveries. The human genome sequence will dramatically alter how we define, prevent, and treat disease. Similar collection of symptoms and signs (phenotype) may have very different underlying genetic constitution (genotype). As genetic capabilities increase, additional tools will become available to subdivide disease designations that are clinically identical (see taxonomy of disease).

Disease Etiology Any factor or series of related events directly or indirectly causing a disease. For example, the genomics revolution has improved our understanding of disease determinants and provided a deeper understanding of molecular mechanisms and biological processes (see 'Systems Biology').

Disease Expression When a pathogenic genotype is manifested in the phenotype.

Disease Management A continuous, coordinated health care process that seeks to manage and improve the health status of a patient over the entire course of a disease. The term may also apply to a patient population. Disease management services include disease prevention efforts and as well as patient management.

Disease Phenotype Includes disease related changes in tissues as judged by gross anatomical, histological and molecular pathological changes. Gene and protein expression analysis and interpretation studies, particularly at the whole genome level are able to distinguish apparently similar phenotypes.

Diversity, Genomic The number of base differences between two genomes divided by the genome size.

DNA (Deoxyribonucleic Acid) The chemical that comprises the genetic material of all cellular organisms.

DNA Cloning Replication of DNA sequences ligated into a suitable vector in an appropriate host organism (see Cloning vector).

DNA Fingerprinting Use of hypervariable minisatellite probe (usually those developed by Alec Jeffreys) on a Southern blot to produce an individual-specific series of bands for identification of individuals or relationships.

DNA Library A collection of cell clones containing different recombinant DNA clones.

DNA Sequencing Technologies through which the order of base pairs in a DNA molecule can be determined.

Domain A discrete portion of a protein with its own function. The combination of domains in a single protein determines its overall function.

Dominant An allele (or the trait encoded by that allele) which produces its characteristic phenotype when present in the heterozygous form.

Dominant Negative Mutation A mutation which results in a mutant gene product which can inhibit the function of the wild-type gene product in heterozygotes.

Dosage Effect The number of copies of a gene; variation in the number of copies can result in aberrant gene expression or associated with disease phenotype.

Drug Design Development of new classes of medicines based on a reasoned approach using gene sequence and protein structure function information rather than the traditional trial- and- error method.

Drug Interactions Refer to adverse drug interaction, drug–drug interaction, drug–laboratory interaction, drug–food interaction, etc. It is defined as an action of a drug on the effectiveness or toxicity of another drug.

Dual-Chamber Pacemaker A pacemaker with two leads (one in the atrium and one in the ventricle) to allow pacing and/or sensing in both chambers of the heart to artificially restore the natural contraction sequence of the heart. (Also called physiologic pacing.)

Electronic Health Record [EHR] A real-time patient health record with access to evidence-based decision support tools that can be used to aid clinicians in decision-making, automating and streamlining clinician's workflow, ensuring that all clinical information is communicated. It can also support the collection of data for uses other than clinical care, such as billing, quality management, outcome reporting, and public health disease surveillance and reporting.

Ejection Fraction A measure of the output of the heart with each heartbeat (stroke volume divided by end-diastolic volume)

Electrocardiogram (ECG) A printout from an electrocardiography machine used to measure and record the electrical activity of the heart.

Electromagnetic Interference (EMI) Equipment and appliances that use magnets and electricity have electromagnetic fields around them. If these fields are strong, they may interfere with the operation of the ICD.

Electrophysiology (EP) Study The use of programmed stimulation protocols to assess the electrical activity of the heart in order to diagnose arrhythmias.

Embryonic Stem Cells (ES cells) A cell line derived from undifferentiated, pluripotent cells from the embryo.

Enhancer A regulatory DNA sequence that increases transcription of a gene. An enhancer can function in either orientation and it may be located up to several thousand base pairs upstream or down stream from the gene it regulates.

ENTREZ An online search and retrieval system that integrates information from databases at NCBI. These databases include nucleotide sequences, protein sequences, macromolecular structures, whole genomes, OMIM, and MEDLINE, through PubMed.

Environmental Factors May include chemical, dietary factors, infectious agents, physical and social factors.

Enzyme A protein which acts as a biological catalyst that controls the rate of a biochemical reaction within a cell.

Epigenetic A term describing non-mutational phenomenon, such as methylation and histone modification that modify the expression of a gene.

Euchromatin The fraction of the nuclear genome which contains transcriptionally active DNA and which, unlike heterochromatin, adopts a relatively extended conformation.

Eukaryote An organism whose cells show internal compartmentalization in the form of membrane-bounded organelles (includes animals, plants, fungi and algae).

Exon The sections of a gene that code for all of its functional product. Eukaryotic genes may contain many exons interspersed with non-coding introns. An exon is represented in the mature mRNA product-the portions of an mRNA molecule that is left after all introns are spliced out, which serves as a template for protein synthesis.

Expression Sequences Tag (EST) Partial or full complement DNA sequences which can serve as markers for regions of the genome which encode expressed products.

Family History An essential tool in clinical genetics. Interpreting the family history can be complicated by many factors, including small families, incomplete or erroneous family histories, consanguinity, variable penetrance, and the current lack of real understanding of the multiple genes involved in polygenic (complex) diseases

Fibrillation A chaotic and unsynchronised quivering of the myocardium during which no effective pumping occurs. Fibrillation may occur in the atria or the ventricles.

Fluorescence In Situ Hybridization (FISH) A form of chromosome in situ hybridization in which nucleic acid probe is labelled by incorporation of a flurophore, a chemical group that fluoresces when exposed to UV irradiation.

Founder Effect Changes in allelic frequencies that occur when a small group is separated from a large population and establishes in a new location.

Founder Mutation Specific mutation in a particular gene present in an ethnic migrant population that is prevalent in the indigenous population.

Frame-Shift Mutation The addition or deletion of a number of DNA bases that is not a multiple of three, thus causing a shift in the reading frame of the gene. This shift leads to a change in the reading frame of all parts of a gene that are downstream from the mutation leading to a premature stop codon, and thus to a truncated protein product.

Functional Genomics The development and implementation of technologies to characterize the mechanisms through which genes and their products function and interact with each other and with the environment.

Gain-of-Function Mutation A mutation that produces a protein that takes on a new or enhanced function.

Gene The fundamental unit of heredity; in molecular terms, a gene comprises a length of DNA that encodes a functional product, which may be a polypeptide (a whole or constituent part of a protein or an enzyme) or a ribonucleic acid. It includes regions that precede and follow the coding region as well as introns and exons. The exact boundaries of a gene are often ill-defined since many promoter and enhancer regions dispersed over many kilobases may influence transcription.

Gene-Based Therapy Refers to all treatment regimens that employ or target genetic material. This includes (1) transfection (introducing cells whose genetic make-up is modified) (2) antisense therapy, and (3) naked DNA vaccination.

Gene Expression The process through which a gene is activated at a particular time and place so that its functional product is produced-i.e transcription into mRNA followed by translation into protein.

Gene Expression Profile The pattern of changes in the expression of a specific set of genes that is relevant to a disease or treatment. The detection of this pattern depends upon the use of specific gene expression measurement technique.

Gene Family A group of closely related genes that make similar protein products.

Gene Knockouts A commonly used technique to demonstrate the phenotypic effects and/or variation related to a particular gene in a model organism, for example in mouse (see Knock-out); absence of many genes may have no apparent effect upon phenotypes (though stress situations may reveal specific susceptibilities). Other single knockouts may have a catastrophic effect upon the organism, or be lethal so that the organism cannot develop at all.

Gene Regulatory Network A functional map of the relationships between a number of different genes and gene products (proteins), regulatory molecules, etc. that define the regulatory response of a cell with respect to a particular physiological function.

Gene Therapy A therapeutic medical procedure that involves either replacing/manipulating or supplementing non-functional genes with healthy genes. Gene therapy can be targeted to somatic (body) or germ (egg and sperm) cells. In somatic gene therapy the recipient's genome is changed, but the change is not passed along to the next generation. In germ-line gene therapy, the parent's egg or sperm cells are changed with the goal of passing on the changes to their offspring.

Genetics Refers to the study of heredity, gene and genetic material. In contrast to genomics, the genetics is traditionally related to lower-throughput, smaller-scale emphasis on single genes, rather than on studying structure, organisation and function of many genes.

Genetic Architecture Refers to the full range of genetic effects on a trait. Genetic architecture is a moving target that changes according to gene and genotype frequencies, distributions of environmental factors, and such biological properties as age and sex.

Genetic Code The relationship between the order of nucleotide bases in the coding region of a gene and the order of amino acids in the polypeptide product. It is universal, triplet, non-overlapping code such that each set of three bases (termed a codon) specifies which of the 20 amino acids is present in the polypeptide chain product of a particular position.

Genetic Counseling An important process for individuals and families who have a genetic disease or who are at risk for such a disease. Genetic counseling provides patients and other family members information about their condition and helps them make informed decisions.

Genetic Determinism The unsubstantiated theory that genetic factors determine a person's health, behaviour, intelligence, or other complex attributes.

Genetic Engineering The use of molecular biology techniques such as restriction enzymes, ligation, and cloning to transfer genes among organisms (also known as recombinant DNA cloning).

Genetic Epidemiology A field of research in which correlations are sought between phenotypic trends and genetic variation across population groups.

Genetic Map A map showing the positions of genetic markers along the length of a chromosome relative to each other (genetic map) or in absolute distances from each other.

Genetic Susceptibility Predisposition to a particular disease due to the presence of a specific allele or combination of alleles in an individual's genome.

Genome The complete set of chromosomal and extra-chromosomal DNA/RNA of an organism, a cell, an organelle or a virus.

Genome Annotation The process through which landmarks in a genomic sequence are characterized using computational and other means; for example, genes are identified, predictions made as to the function of their products, their regulatory regions defined and intergenic regions characterized (see Annotation).

Genome Project The research and technology development effort aimed at mapping and sequencing the entire genome of human beings and other organisms.

Genomics The study of the genome and its action. The term is commonly used to refer large-scale, high-throughput molecular analyses of multiple genes, gene products, or regions of genetic material (DNA and RNA). The term also includes the comparative aspect of genomes of various species, their evolution, and how they relate to each other (see comparative genomics).

Genotype The genetic constitution of an organism; commonly used in reference to a specific disease or trait.

Genetic Discrimination Unfavourable discrimination of an individual, a family, community, or an ethnic group on the basis of genetic information. Discrimination may include societal segregation, political persecution, opportunities for education and training, lack or restricted employment prospects, and adequate personal financial planning, for example life insurance and mortgage.

Genomic Drugs Drugs based on molecular targets; genomic knowledge of the genes involved in diseases, disease pathways, and drug-response

Genomic Instability An increased tendency of the GENOME to acquire MUTATIONS when various processes involved in maintaining and replicating the genome are dysfunctional

Genomic Profiling Complete genomic sequence of an individual including the expression profile. This would be targeted to specific requirements, for example most common complex diseases (diabetes, hypertension and coronary heart disease).

Genetic Screening Testing a population group to identify a subset of individuals at high risk for having or transmitting a specific genetic disorder

Genetic Test An analysis performed on human DNA, RNA, genes and/or chromosomes to detect heritable or acquired genotypes. A genetic test also is the analysis of human proteins and certain metabolites, which are predominantly used to detect heritable or acquired genotypes, mutations or phenotypes.

Genetic Testing Strictly refers to testing for a specific chromosomal abnormality or a DNA (nuclear or mitochondrial) mutation already known to exist in a family member. This includes diagnostic testing (post-natal or pre-natal), pre-symptomatic or predictive genetic testing or for establishing the carrier status. The individual concerned should have been offered full information on all aspects of the genetic test through the process of 'non-judgemental and non-directive' genetic counselling. Most laboratories require a formal fully informed signed consent before carrying out the test. Genetic testing commonly involves DNA/RNA-based tests for single gene variants, complex genotypes, acquired mutations and measures of gene expression. Epidemiologic studies are needed to establish clinical validity of each method to establish sensitivity, specificity, and predictive value.

Germ-Line Cells A cell with a haploid chromosome content (also referred to as a gamete); in animals, sperm or egg and in plants, pollen or ovum.

Germ-Line Mosaic (Germinal mosaic, gonadal mosaic, gonosomal mosaic): an individual who has a subset of germline celles carrying a mutation which is not found in other germline cells.

Germ-Line Mutation A gene change in the body's reproductive cells (egg or sperm) that becomes incorporated into the DNA of every cell in the body of offspring; germline mutations are passed on from parents to offspring, also called hereditary mutation.

Haploid Describing a cell (typically a gamete) which has only a single copy of each chromosome (i.e. 23 in man).

Haplotype A series of closely linked loci on a particular chromosome which tend to be inherited together as a block.

Heart Block A condition in which electrical impulses are not conducted in the normal fashion from the atria to the ventricles. May be caused by damage or disease processes within the cardiac conduction system.

Hemodynamics The forces involved in circulating blood through the cardiovascular system. The heart adapts its haemodynamic performance to the needs of the body, increasing its output of blood when muscles are working and decreasing output when the body is at rest.

Heterozygote Refers to a particular allele of a gene at a defined chromosome locus. A heterozygote has a different allelic form of the gene at each of the two homologous chromosomes.

Heterozygosity The presence of different alleles of a gene in one individual or in a population—a measure of genetic diversity.

Holter Monitoring A technique for the continuous recording of electrocardiographic (ECG) signals, usually over 24 h, to detect and diagnose ECG changes. (Also called ambulatory monitoring.)

Homology Similarity between two sequences due to their evolution from a common ancestor, often referred to as homologs.

Homozygote Refers to same allelic form of a gene on each of the two homologous chromosomes.

Human Genome Project A programme to determine the sequence of the entire three billion bases of the human genome.

Human Gene Transfer The process of transferring genetic material (DNA or RNA) into a person; an experimental therapeutic procedure to treat certain health problems by compensating for defective genes, producing a potentially therapeutic substance, or triggering the immune system to fight disease. This may help improve genetic disorders, particularly those conditions that result from inborn errors in a single gene (for example, sickle cell anemia, hemophilia, and cystic fibrosis), and as well as with complex disorders, like cancer, heart disease, and certain infectious diseases, such as HIV/AIDS.

Implantable Cardioverter Defibrillator (ICD) An ICD is an implanted device used to treat abnormal, fast heart rhythms. Several types of therapies are used by the ICD, including cardioversion, defibrillation, and antitachycardia pacing.

Identity by Descent (IBD) Alleles in an individual or in two people that are identical because they have been inherited from the same common ancestor, as opposed to identity by state (IBS), which is coincidental possession of similar alleles in unrelated individuals. (see Consanguinity).

Immunogenomics Refers to the study of organisation, function and evolution of vertebrate defense genes, particularly those encoded by the Major Histocompatibility Complex (MHC) and the Leukocyte Receptor Complex (LRC). Both complexes form integral parts of the immune system. The MHC is the most important genetic region in relation to infection and common disease such as autoimmunity. Driven by pathogen variability, immune genes have become the most polymorphic loci known, with some genes having over 500 alleles. The main function of these genes is to provide protection against pathogens and they achieve this through complex pathways for antigen processing and presentation.

Informatics The study of the application of computer and statistical techniques to the management of information. In genome projects, informatics includes the development of methods to search databases quickly, to analyze DNA sequence information, and to predict protein sequence and structure from DNA sequence data.

Intron A non-coding sequence within eukaryotic genes which separates the exons (coding regions). Introns are spliced out of the messenger RNA molecule created from a gene after transcription, prior to protein translation (protein synthesis).

Ischemia Insufficient blood flow to tissue due to blockage in the blood flow through the arteries.

Isoforms/Isozymes Alternative forms of protein/enzyme.

In Situ Hybdridization Hybridization of a labelled nucleic acid to a target nucleic acid which is typically immobilized on a microscopic slide, such as DNA of denatured metaphase chromosomes (as in fluorescent in situ hybdridization [FISH]) or the RNA in a section of tissue (as in tissue in situ hybridization [TISH]).

In Vitro (Latin) literally "in glass", meaning outside of the organism in the laboratory, for example a tissue culture.

In Vivo (Latin) literally "in life", meaning within a living organism.

Knock-out A technique used primarily in mouse genetics to inactivate a particular gene in order to define its function.

Lead In an ICD system, the wire or catheter which conducts energy from the ICD to the heart, and from the heart to the ICD.

Left Ventricular Dysfunction A heart condition in which the heart is unable maintain normal cardiac output due to a deficiency in the left ventricle.

Library A collection of genomic or complementary DNA sequences from a particular organism that have been cloned in a vector and grown in an appropriate host organism (e.g. bacteria or yeast).

Ligase An enzyme which can use ATP to create phosphate bonds between the ends of two DNA fragments, effectively joining two DNA molecules into one.

Linkage The phenomenon whereby pairs of genes which are located in close proximity on the same chromosome tend to be co-inherited.

Linkage Analysis A process of locating genes on the chromosome by measuring recombination rates between phenotypic and genetic markers (see Lod score)

Linkage Disequilibrium The non-random association in a population of alleles at nearby loci.

Locus The specific site on a chromosome at which a particular gene or other DNA landmark is located.

Lod Score A measure of likelihood of genetic linkage between loci; a lod score greater than +3 is often taken as evidence of linkage; one that is less than −2 often taken as evidence against linkage.

Loss-of-Function Mutation A mutation that decreases the production or function (or both) of the gene product.

Loss of Heteorozygosity (LOH) Loss of alleles on one chromosome detected by assaying for markers for which an individual is constitutionally heterozygous.

Lyonization The process of random X chromosome inactivation in mammals.

Marker A specific feature at an identified physical location on a chromosome, whose inheritance can be followed. The position of a gene implicated in a particular phenotypic effect can be defined through its linkage to such markers.

Meiosis Reductive cell division occurring exclusively in testis and ovary and resulting in the production of haploid cells, including sperm cells and egg cells.

Mendelian Genetics Classical genetics, focuses on *monogenic* genes with high *penetrance*. The Mendelian genetics is a true *paradigm* and is used in discussing the mode of inheritance (see Monogenic disease).

Messenger RNA (mRNA) RNA molecules that are synthesized from a DNA template in the nucleus (a gene) and transported to ribosomes in the cytoplasm where they serve as a template for the synthesis of protein (translation).

Microarrays-Diagnostics A rapidly developing tool increasingly used in pharmaceutical and genomics research and has the potential for applications in high-throughput diagnostic devices. Microarrays can be made of DNA sequences with known gene mutations, polymorphisms, and as well as selected protein molecules.

Microsatellite DNA Small array (often less than 0.1 kb) of short tandemly repeated DNA sequences.

Minisatellite DNA An intermediate size array (often 0.1 to 20 kb long) of short tandemly repeated DNA sequences. Hypervaiable minisatellite DNA is the basis of DNA finderprinting and many VNTR markers.

Missense Mutation Substitution of a single DNA base that results in a codon that specifies an alternative amino acid.

Mitochondria Cellular organelles present in eukaryotic organisms which enable aerobic respiration and generate the energy to drive cellular processes. Each mitochondria contains a small amount of circular DNA encoding a small number of genes (approximately 50).

Mitosis Cell division in somatic cells.

Model Organism An experimental organism in which a particular physiological process or disease has similar characteristics to the corresponding process in humans, permitting the investigation of the common underlying mechanisms.

Modifier Gene A gene whose expression can influence a phenotype resulting from mutation at another locus.

Molecular Genetic Screening Screening a section of the population known to be at a higher risk to be heterozygous for one of the mutations in the gene for a common autosomal recessive disease, for example, screening for cystic fibrosis in the North-European populations and beta-thalassaemia in the Mediterranean and Middle-East population groups.

Molecular Genetic Testing Molecular genetic testing for use in patient diagnosis, management, and genetic counselling; this is increasingly used in presymptomatic (predictive) genetic testing of 'at-risk' family members using a previously known disease-causing mutation in the family.

Mosaic A genetic mosaic is an individual who has two or more genetically different cell lines derived from a single zygote.

Motif A DNA-sequence pattern within a gene that, because of its similarity to sequences in other known genes, suggests a possible function of the gene, its protein products, or both.

Multifactorial Disease Any disease or disorder caused by interaction of multiple genetic (polygenic) and environmental factors.

Multigene Family A set of evolutionary related loci within a genome, at least one of which can encode a functional product.

Mutation A heritable alteration in the DNA sequence.

Myocardial Infarction Death of a portion of the heart muscle tissue due to a blockage or interruption in the supply of blood to the heart muscle.

Myocardium The middle and the thickest layer of the heart wall, composed of cardiac muscle.

Natural Selection The process whereby some of the inherited genetic variation within a population will affect the ability of individuals to survive to reproduce (fitness).

Neutral Mutation A change or alteration in DNA sequence which has no phenotypic effect (or has no effect on fitness).

New-Born Screening Performed in newborns in state public health programs to detect certain genetic diseases for which early diagnosis and treatment are available.

Non-Coding Sequence A region of DNA that is not translated into protein. Some non-coding sequences are regulatory portions of genes, others may serve structural purposes (telomoeres, centromeres), while others may not have any function.

Nonconservative Mutation A change in the DNA or RNA sequence that leads to the replacement of one amino acid with a very dissimilar one.

Nonsense Mutation Substitution of a single DNA base that leads in a stop codon, thus leading to the truncation of a protein.

Northern Blot Hybridization A form of molecular hybridization in which target consists of RNA molecules that have been size fractioned by gel electrophoresis and subsequently transferred to a membrane.

Nucleotide A subunit of the DNA or RNA molecule. A nucleotide is a base molecule (adenine, cytosine, guanine and thymine in the case of DNA), linked to a sugar molecule (deoxyribose or ribose) and phosphate groups.

Nullizygous Lacking any copy of a gene or DNA sequence normally found in chromosomal DNA usually resulting from homozygous deletion in an autosome or from a single deletion in sex chromosomes in male.

Oncogene An acquired mutant form of a gene which acts to transform a normal cell into a cancerous one.

On-line Mendelian Inheritance in Man (OMIM) Victor McKusick's regularly updated electronic catalog of inherited human disorders and phenotypic traits accessible on NCBI network. Each entry is designated by a number (MIM number).

Open Reading Frame (ORF) A significantly long sequence of DNA in which there are no termination codons. Each DNA duplex can have six reading frames, three for each single strand.

Ortholog One of set of homologous genes or proteins that perform similar functions in different species, i.e. identical genes from different species, for example SRY in humans and Sry in mice.

Paralog Similar genes (members of a gene family) or proteins (homologous) in a single species or different species that perform different functions.

Penetrance The likelihood that a person carrying a particular mutant gene will have an altered phenotype (see Phenotype).

Pulse Field Gel Eletrophoresis (PFGE) A form of gel electrophoresis which permits size fractionation of large DNA molecules.

Pharmacogenomics The identification of the genes which influence individual variation in the efficacy or toxicity of therapeutic agents, and the application of this information in clinical practice.

Phenotype The clinical and/or any other manifestation or expression, such as a biochemical immunological alteration, of a specific gene or genes, environmental factors, or both.

Physical (Gene) Map A map showing the absolute distances between genes.

Point Mutation The substitution of a single DNA base in the normal DNA sequence.

Polygenic Trait or Character A character or trait determined by the combined action of a number of loci, each with a small effect.

Polymerase Chain Reaction (PCR) A molecular biology technique developed in the mid-1980s through which specific DNA segments may be amplified selectively.

Polymorphism The stable existence of two or more variant allelic forms of a gene within a particular population, or among different populations.

Positional Cloning The technique through which candidate genes are located in the genome through their co-inheritance with linked markers. It allows genes to be identified that lack information regarding the biochemical actions of their functional product.

Post-transcriptional Modification A series of steps through which protein molecules are biochemically modified within a cell following synthesis by translation of messenger RNA. A protein may undergo a complex series of modifications in different cellular compartments before its final functional form is produced.

Predictive Testing Determines the probability that a healthy individual with or without a family history of a certain disease might develop that disease.

Predisposition, Genetic Increased susceptibility to a particular disease due to the presence of one or more gene mutations, and/or a combination of alleles (haplotype), not necessarily abnormal, that is associated with an increased risk for the disease, and/or a family history that indicates an increased risk for the disease.

Predisposition Test A test for a genetic predisposition (incompletely penetrant conditions). Not all people with a positive test result will manifest the disease during their lifetimes

Pre-implantation Genetic Diagnosis (PIGD) Used following in vitro fertilization to diagnose a genetic disease or condition in a pre-implantation embryo.

Premature Atrial Contraction (PAC) A contraction in the atrium which is initiated by an ectopic focus and occurs earlier than the next expected normal sinus beat.

Premature Ventricular Contraction (PVC or VPD) A contraction in the ventricle which is initiated by an ectopic focus and occurs earlier than the next expected normal sinus or escape rhythm beat.

Prenatal Diagnosis Used to diagnose a genetic disease or condition in a developing fetus.

Presymptomatic Test Predictive testing of individuals with a family history. Historically, the term has been used when testing for diseases or conditions such as Huntington's disease where the likelihood of developing the condition (known as *penetrance*) is very high in people with a positive test result.

Primer A short nucleic acid sequence, often a synthetic oligonucleotide, which binds specifically to a single strand of a target nucleic acid sequence and initiates synthesis, using a suitable polymerase, of a complementary strand.

Probe A DNA or RNA fragment which has been labelled in some way, and used in a molecular hybridization assay to identify closely related DNA or RNA sequences.

Prokaryote An organism or cell lacking a nucleus and other membrane bounded organelles. Bacteria are prokaryotic organisms.

Promoter A combination of short sequence elements to which RNA polymerase binds in order to initiate transcription of a gene.

Protein A protein is the biological effector molecule encoded by sequences of a gene. A protein molecule consists of one or more polypeptide chains of amino-acid subunits. The functional action of a protein depends on its three-dimensional structure, which is determined by its aminoacid composition.

Proteome All of the proteins present in a cell or organism.

Proteomics The development and application of techniques to investigate the protein products of the genome and how they interact to determine biological functions.

Proto-Oncogene A cellular gene which when mutated is inappropriately expressed and becomes an oncogene.

Pseudoautosomal Region (PAR) A region on the tips of mammalian X chromosomes which is involved in recombination during male meiosis.

Pesudogene A DNA sequence which shows a high degree of sequence homology to a nonallelic functional gene but which is itself nonfunctional.

Recessive An allele that has no phenotypic effect in the heterozygous state.

Recombinant DNA Technology The use of molecular biology techniques such as restriction enzymes, ligation, and cloning to transfer genes among organisms (see genetic engineering).

Regulatory Mutation A mutation in a region of the genome that does not encode a protein but affects the expression of a gene.

Regulatory Sequence A DNA sequence to which specific proteins bind to activate or repress the expression of a gene.

Repeat Sequences A stretch of DNA bases that occurs in the genome in multiple identical or closely related copies.

Replication A process by which a new DNA strand is synthesized by copying an existing strand, using it as a template for the addition of a complementary bases, catalyzed by a DNA polymerase enzyme.

Reproductive Cloning Techniques aimed at the generation of an organism with an identical genome to an existing organism.

Restriction Enzymes A family of enzymes derived from bacterial that cut DNA at specific sequences of bases.

Restriction Fragment Length Polymorphism (RFLP) A polymorphism due to difference in size of allelic restriction fragments as a result of restriction site polymorphism.

Ribonucleic Acid (RNA) A single stranded nucleic acid molecule comprising a linear chain made up from four nucleotide subunits (A, C, G and U). There are three types of RNA messenger, transfer and ribosomal.

Risk Communication An important aspect of genetic counselling which involves pedigree analysis, interpretation of the inheritance pattern, genetic risk assessment, and explanation to the family member (or the family).

Reverse Transcriptase-PCR (RT-PCR) A PCR reaction in which the target DNA is a cDNA copied by reverse transcriptase from an mRNA source.

Screening Carrying out of a test or tests, examination(s) or procedure(s) in order to expose undetected abnormalities, unrecognized (incipient) diseases, or defects: examples are early diagnosis of cancer using mass X-ray mammography for breast cancer and cervical smears for cancer of the cervix.

Segregation The separation of chromosomes (and the alleles they carry) during meiosis; alleles on different chromosomes segregate randomly among the gametes (and the progeny).

Sensitivity (of a Screening Test) Extent (usually expressed as a percentage) to which a method gives results that are free from false negatives; the fewer the false negatives, the greater the sensitivity. Quantitatively, sensitivity is the proportion of truly diseased persons in the screened population who are identified as diseased by the screening test.

Sex Chromosome The pair of chromosomes that determines the sex (gender) of an organism. In man one X and one Y chromosomes constitute a male compared to two X chromosomes in a female.

Sex Selection Preferential selection of the unborn child on the basis of the gender for social and cultural purposes. However, this may be acceptable for medical reasons, for example to prevent the birth of a male assessed to be at risk for an x-linked recessive disease. For further information visit: http://www.bioethics.gov/topics/sex_index.html

Shotgun Sequencing A cloning method in which total genomic DNA is randomly sheared and the fragments ligated into a cloning vector, also referred to as 'shotgun' cloning.

Signal Transduction The molecular pathways through which a cell senses changes in its external environment and changes its gene expression patterns in response.

Silent Mutation Substitution of a single DNA base that produces no change in the aminoacid sequence of the encoded protein.

Single-Nucleotide Polymorphism (SNP) A common variant in the genome sequence; the human genome contains about ten million SNPs.

Sinoatrial (SA) Node The heart's natural pacemaker located in the right atrium. Electrical impulses originate here and travel through the heart, causing it to beat.

Somatic All of the cells in the body which are not gametes (germ-line).

Southern Blot Hybridization A form of molecular hybridization in which the target nucleic acid consists of DNA molecules that have been size fractioned by gel electrophoresis and subsequently transferred to a nitrocellulose or nylon membrane.

Splicing A process by which introns are removed from a messenger RNA prior to translation and the exons adjoined.

Stem Cell A cell which has the potential to differentiate into a variety of different cell types depending on the environmental stimuli it receives.

Stop Codon A codon that leads to the termination of a protein rather than to the addition of a amnioacid. The three stop codons are TGA, TAA, and TAG.

Sudden Cardiac Death (SCD) Death due to cardiac causes within 1 h of the onset of symptoms, with no prior warning, usually caused by ventricular fibrillation.

Supraventricular Tachycardia (SVT) A tachycardia originating from above the ventricles.

Syncope Fainting, loss of consciousness, or dizziness which may be due to a transient disturbance of cardiac rhythm (arrhythmia) or other causes.

Synteny A large group of genes that appear in the same order on the chromosomes of two different species.

Systems Biology Refers to simultaneous measurement of thousands of molecular components (such as transcripts, proteins, and metabolites) and integrate these disparate data sets with clinical end points, in a biologically relevant manner; this model can be applied in understanding the etiology of disease.

Tachycardia (Tachyarrhythmia) Rapid beating of either or both chambers of the heart, usually defined as a rate over 100 beats per minute.

Telomere The natural end of the chromosome.

Therapeutic Cloning The generation and manipulation of stem cells with the objective of deriving cells of a particular organ or tissue to treat a disease.

Transcription The process through which a gene is expressed to generate a complementary RNA molecule on a DNA template using RNA polymerase.

Transcription Factor A protein which binds DNA at specific sequences and regulates the transcription of specific genes.

Transcriptome The total messenger RNA expressed in a cell or tissue at a given point in time.

Transfection A process by which new DNA is inserted in a eukaryotic cell allowing stable integration into the cell's genome.

Transformation Introduction of foreign DNA into a cell and expression of genes from the introduced DNA; this does not necessarily include integration into host cell genome.

Transgene A gene from one source that has been incorporated into the genome of another organism.

Transgenic Animal/Plant A fertile animal or plant that carries an introduced gene(s) in its germ-line.

Translation A process through which a polypeptide chain of amino acid molecules is generated as directed by the sequence of a particular messenger RNA sequence.

Tumour Suppressor Gene A gene which serves to protect cells from entering a cancerous state; according to Knudson's "two-hit" hypothesis, both alleles of a particular tumour suppressor gene must acquire a mutation before the cell will enter a transformed cancerous state.

Unequal Crossing Over Recombination between nonallelic sequences on nonsister chromatids of homologous chromosomes.

Ventricle One of the two lower chambers of the heart. (See Atrium)

Ventricular Fibrillation (VF) Very fast, chaotic, quivering heart contractions that start in the ventricles. During VF, the heart does not beat properly. This often results in fainting. If left untreated, it may result in cardiac arrest. Blood is not pumped from the heart to the rest of the body. Death will occur if defibrillation is not initiated within 6 min from the onset of VF.

Ventricular Tachycardia (VT) A rapid heart rate that starts in the ventricles. During VT, the heart does not have time to fill with enough blood between heart beats to supply the entire body with sufficient blood. It may cause dizziness and light-headedness.

Western Blotting A process in which proteins are size-fractioned in a polyacrylamide gel prior to transfer to a nitrocellulose membrane for probing with an antibody.

X-Chromosome Inactivation Random inactivation of one of the two X chromosomes in mammals by a specialized form of genetic imprinting (see Lyonization).

Yeast Artificial Chromosome (YAC) An artificial chromosome produced by combining large fragments of foreign DNA with small sequence elements necessary for chromosome function in yeast cells.

Yeast Two-Hybrid System A genetic method for analysing the interactions of proteins.

Zinc Finger A polypeptide motif which is stabilized by binding a zinc atom and confers on proteins an ability to bind specifically to DNA sequences; commonly found in transcription factors.

Zoo Blot A Southern blot containing DNA samples from different species.

Index

D. Kumar, P. Elliott (eds.), *Cardiovascular Genetics and Genomics*,
https://doi.org/10.1007/978-3-319-66114-8

B

C

E

L

N

O

P

R